MEDICAL HERBALISM
The Science and Practice
of Herbal Medicine

David Hoffmann, FNIMH, AHG

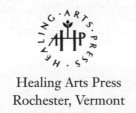

Healing Arts Press
Rochester, Vermont

Healing Arts Press
One Park Street
Rochester, Vermont 05767
www.InnerTraditions.com

Healing Arts Press is a division of Inner Traditions International

Note to the reader: This book is intended as an informational guide. The remedies, approaches, and techniques described herein are meant to supplement, and not to be a substitute for, professional medical care or treatment. They should not be used to treat a serious ailment without prior consultation with a qualified health care professional.

Library of Congress Cataloging-in-Publication Data
Hoffmann, David, 1951–
  Medical herbalism : the science and practice of herbal medicine / David Hoffmann.
      p. ; cm.
Includes bibliographical references and index.
  ISBN-978-089281749-8 (hardcover)
 1. Herbs—Therapeutic use. 2. Medicinal plants.
  [DNLM: 1. Phytotherapy—methods. 2. Holistic Health. 3. Plants,
Medicinal. WB 925 H711m 2003] I. Title.
  RM666.H33H6444 2003
  615'.321—dc22

                        2003017536

Printed and bound in China by Shenzhen Reliance Printing

20 19

Text design and layout by Priscilla Baker
This book was typeset in Janson, with Agenda and Trajan as display typefaces

DEDICATION

For Lois Stopple,
What can I say, after 600 odd pages (odd pages indeed), I'm tongue tied! You have healed me heart and soul, with the celebration of life and joy that you are. This book may have been written by me, but it was midwifed by you.

> *Sweet blossom come on under the willow*
> *We can have high times if you'll abide*
> *We can discover the wonders of nature*
> *Rolling in the rushes down by the riverside*
>
> *She's got everything delightful*
> *She's got everything I need*
> *A breeze in the pines in the summer night moonlight*
> *Crazy in the sunlight, yes, indeed*
>
> —THE GRATEFUL DEAD (WHO ELSE . . .)

ACKNOWLEDGMENTS

My deepest appreciation to Cheri Quincy, DO, for the continuing encouragement and support. Thank you for your confidence in me, even when I couldn't even spell the word!

It is with love and gratitude that I acknowledge my friends and colleagues in the North American community of herbalists for making this escapee from Thatchers' Britain so welcome. The ideas in this book have been gestating over the years in discussions with many, many herbalists. The U.S. herb world is blessed with an atmosphere of openness and mutual support that is unique and deeply nurturing. We can thank Rosemary Gladstar for so very much . . .

There is so much I could say to each of you, so I'm copping out and simply "naming names." No special order, I love you all: Cascade Anderson-Geller, Paul Bergner, Jane Bothwell, Mark Blumenthal, Don Brown, Ryan Drum, Rosemary Gladstar, Mindy Green, Christopher Hobbs, Tori Hudson, Feather Jones, Gail Julian, Kathi Keville, Tierona Low Dog, David LaLucerne, Rob McCaleb (and everyone at the Herb Research Foundation), Anne McIntyre, Terence McKenna, Bill Mitchel, Pam Montgomery, Rob Montgomery, Michael Moore, 7 Song, Ric Scalzo, Ed Smith, Sara Smith, Paul Stamets, Jill Stansbury, Autumn Summers, Jonathan Treasure, Gail Ulhrich, Roy Upton, Marty Wall, David Winston, Linda Wolf, Tom Wolf, Matthew Wood, Dusty Yeo.

This book is much better than it deserves to be because of the superlative guidance of herbalist/editor extroadinaire Evelyn Leigh. Thank you for being so knowledgeable, insightful, literate, and understanding of this aging deadhead. You made the process pleasant, rewarding (or is that rewording?), and even entertaining.

To Jeanie Levitan, the first editor to give me her toothbrush! All authors should hope to be blessed with guidance from someone with your erudition and warmth. To Jamaica Burns for editorial help above and beyond the call of duty. Sorry about the obscure Chinese citations.

I want to thank the many groups of students I have had the honor of working with over the years. You all know who you are. In case you've forgotten, you went to one (or more!) of the following institutions: the California School of Herbal Studies, the Rocky Mountain Center of Botanical Studies, Bastyr University, National College of Naturopathic Medicine, California Institute of Integral Studies, and the National College of Phytotherapy.

Sonoma County reference librarians have been a great help during the writing of this book. What would we do without libraries?

To Sasha Shulgin, Grant Morrison, Hakim Bey, Jerry Garcia, and Ozric Tentacles for the help with sanity maintenance (and furtherance . . .).

CONTENTS

Part Two

TREATMENT APPROACHES BY BODY SYSTEM

APPENDICES

INTRODUCTION

This is an exciting and very challenging time to be involved in herbal medicine. There is a growing openness to the insights of clinical herbalism from practitioners of other health care modalities, and a plethora of peer-reviewed work on herbs being published by the research community. Many new insights have been put forth, and many traditional ideas are being reassessed and either rejected or embraced anew.

Above all, this is a time of change for Western medicine, both holistic and orthodox. While herbs have a unique and valuable contribution to make, no clear context has yet been defined for Western holistic medicine. In such a rapidly evolving clinical and research milieu, a book of this sort can at best serve as a building block, a step on the road toward a more cohesive vision for the future of Western holistic healing.

With this book I have endeavored to lay a foundation for the skilled use of herbal medicine within a holistic practice by bringing together the modern scientific movement with traditional herbal practice. The book is intended for practitioners and students of medical herbalism, as well as practitioners of other modalities who are interested in the principles and practice of Western herbal medicine.

A cursory look at the contents reveals two distinct sections of the book.

Part 1 surveys the scientific underpinnings of medical herbalism, the chemistry and pharmacology that may help clarify the mechanisms of herbal activity and clinical efficacy. While this information may be unfamiliar and challenging for many herbalists, I feel it is important for traditional practitioners to have at least a rudimentary grasp of this subject as we move into the 21st century.

Part 2 deals with the practical therapeutics of the major body systems and the pathologies that affect them. It is based on my own 25 years of clinical experience, the experience and knowledge accrued by the Eclectic and Physiomedical physicians of the United States, and the practices developed by the National Institute of Medical Herbalists in the United Kingdom.

Despite the seeming dichotomy of these two major sections of the book, I have attempted throughout to marry biomedical theory with the clinical experience of the medical herbalist. As a clinician who began his own herbal practice in 1978, I have seen that Western herbal medicine is based upon a body of knowledge and experience that has as much clinical value as any other field of medicine. Thus the guidelines for protocol development given throughout the book are based firmly on this bedrock of Western herbalism. I have not rejected the clinical approaches of medical herbalism in favor of peer-reviewed research. Even acknowledging the wealth of research occurring, there is not yet enough clinically relevant material to justify changing tried-and-true approaches, an issue that is explored throughout the book.

The focus of the medicinal plant research community, however, is rarely on the protocols used in herbal medicine, but instead on the plants themselves as sources of novel (and thus patentable) chemical structures. A disquieting trend in North American herbalism is the tendency to be influenced by the marketplace and herbal fashion. I have made a point of avoiding such hype in the treatment section of the book. The following statement, made by the 19th-century Eclectic physician John King in writing about *Grindelia squarrosa*, is as relevant today as it was 100 years ago:

> The fact is, that many physicians have a great proneness to run after new remedies, especially when introduced under some pretentious name, and to place a marvelous credulity in the statements of interested parties, who are incapable of determining accurate conclusions as to the value of a remedy.[1]

Herbalism is a fundamentally conservative activity, although I must say it is the only aspect of my life where any trace of conservative tendencies will be found!

OVERVIEW OF THE BOOK
PART 1

Chapter 1

Places Western herbalism in a philosophical, therapeutic, ecological, and multicultural context. This chapter introduces the relationship between science and herbal medicine, looking at the scientific method and the language of research. A discussion of pharmacognosy is followed by a review of large-scale screening programs to assess the therapeutic potential of the world's flora. The importance of the conservation of medicinal plants and the work of organizations such as United Plant Savers is discussed.

Chapter 2
Explores the diversity of medicinal plants through taxonomy and the insights of the Linnaean system of nomenclature—actually much more interesting than is often appreciated!

Chapters 3–8
Plant chemistry is the basis of the therapeutic uses of herbs. In these chapters, I discuss the nature of primary and secondary plant metabolites as a foundation for a review of the main categories of constituents considered to be of therapeutic importance. Each chapter includes an overview of structure, botanical distribution, and generalizations about pharmacology, followed by a discussion of representative molecules described in the herbal literature. Important groups, such as sesquiterpene lactones, saponins, and flavonoids, are covered in depth.

Chapter 9
An introduction to the principles of pharmacology relevant to herbal medicine, covering the broad principles of pharmacokinetics and pharmacodynamics. Using herbal examples wherever possible, the chapter explores a range of pharmacological actions.

Chapter 10
An introduction to the basics of toxicology as they relate to issues concerning the safety and toxicity of medicinal plants. A discussion of contraindications and drug–herb interactions is followed by a review of toxic plant constituents.

Chapter 11
Explores the formulation and preparation of herbal medicines. The various pharmaceutical forms are discussed, with examples from official pharmacopoeias as well as folk medicine.

PART 2
Chapter 12
Presents a model of holistic herbal medicine that is applied throughout the rest of the book, and describes the process of developing a protocol that addresses specific pathologies while supporting the unique individual involved. The criteria for establishing dosage and formulation specifics are given, along with an outline of the structure of the subsequent treatment chapters.

Chapters 13–24
The therapeutic approach to each body system is explored in turn, focusing on prevention and wellness but also addressing a range of conditions that may be approached herbally. Phytotherapeutic approaches to the health needs of the young and the elderly are also discussed. The holistic context is always emphasized. Where lists or tables are given, the sequence of herbs reflects my opinion of relative importance.

I must emphasize that the suggested prescriptions are NOT to be considered "herbal formulae." The importance of their inclusion lies in the process of developing a treatment program that takes advantage of the strengths of herbalism in addressing individual needs, not simply pathologies. I have emphasized the application of the model and identification of any resulting patterns of relationship between plant and pathology in an attempt to empower the reader as he or she faces clinical realities.

In practice, however, theory is often secondary to reality. The suggested prescriptions come from personal observation of many herbally treated cases. Any conclusions or ideas presented come from an interpretation of such observations and of the healing process in the people who have honored me by allowing me to work with them. In instances where I have no solid foundation in practice, I have referred to colleagues who do.

Chapter 25
A review of the main herbal actions with an exploration of the mechanisms underlying their activity (where known). The primary herbal examples are given, along with a discussion of the other actions of these plants.

Chapter 26
An herbal materia medica, in the traditional sense, covering 150 of the plants most commonly used in European and North American phytotherapy. A description of the structure used throughout these entries is presented at the beginning of the chapter. The traditional uses of the plant are covered, along with relevant research data.

Appendices
- Glossary of herbal, medical, and phytochemical terms.
- Meanings of some Latin binomials. Here translations can be found into English of the meanings of the Latin or Greek words used in botanical binomials.

- Translation lists of the common names of herbs to their Latin binomial and, similarly, the Latin binomial to the common name.
- Pharmacy terms. A listing of Latin pharmacy terms and their shorthand descriptors, which are often encountered when reading older books on herbal medicine.
- Weight and measure conversion tables.
- Taxonomic classification of medicinal plants.
- Information sources and useful URLs. A brief guide to finding herbal information using modern bibliographic databases, emphasizing the relevance of Medline and MeSH terms. (The World Wide Web addresses given were current as of July 2003.)
- Bibliography. This select bibliography focuses on works

relevant to the practice of Western herbalism. I have emphasized the writings of herbal clinicians who not only present relevant information, but also place it within the context of real clinical experience. References are given for phytochemistry, pharmacology, and toxicology. The suggested readings at the end of each chapter are not meant to be a comprehensive list of resources. Rather, they reflect my opinion of what is most relevant to the clinical experience.

References

1. Felter and Lloyd, *King's American Dispensatory*, vol. 1 and 2, 1892. Reprint. Sandy, OR: Eclectic Medical Publications, 1983.

Part One

❧

INTRODUCTION TO PRINCIPLES
AND PRACTICES

1

HERBS, HOLISM, AND SCIENCE

Phytotherapy is a thriving medical modality that uses whole plants to treat whole people, facilitating the healing process within the framework of holistic medicine. It is both an art and a science. With its roots in the past, it is still relevant and meaningful in the present, offering great potential contributions to modern medicine.

Herbalism has a scope of use as wide as any form of medicine, as herbs may be used for any condition that is medically treatable. This statement is not meant to imply that herbs are a panacea for the ills of humanity! However, the ecological integration of plant activity with human physiology offers the potential for facilitating the healing process at any time in any situation.

A new understanding of health is dawning. This new understanding reflects changes in both attitude and approach, and is often referred to as *holistic medicine*. This is a small part of a profound transformation now taking place in the way our culture views itself and the issues that affect it. This has been called a *paradigm shift:* a change in the patterns of belief and perception that our culture holds about itself. Such shifts have happened many times before. From a historical point of view, the transformation of society from the medieval worldview to what we now call the Renaissance is strikingly clear. However, to the people of the time, the process of change was either imperceptible or totally confusing, except to those with the vision of, for example, a Leonardo da Vinci.

The current development of new patterns of expectation and explanation is, of course, affecting the field of medicine. Questions are being raised about every aspect of medicine, from the nature of health and disease to appropriate therapeutic techniques.

How, then, do we define health in the context of this new paradigm? The World Health Organization (WHO) provides the clearest definition. Its simplicity only serves to highlight its profound relevance:

> Health is a state of complete physical, emotional, mental and social well being and not merely the absence of disease or infirmity.

This is a wonderfully precise encapsulation of the point of view of holistic medicine. The holistic approach to medicine begins with the assumption that health is a positive and active state, that it is an inherent characteristic of whole and integrated human beings. From a holistic standpoint, a person is not a patient with a disease syndrome, but a whole being. Acknowledgment of this wholeness means that the therapist must appreciate the mental, emotional, spiritual, social, and environmental aspects of his or her patients' lives—not just the physical. A holistic practitioner of any particular therapy has a deep respect for the individual's inherent capacity for self-healing. This facilitates a relationship of active partnership in the healing process, as opposed to an unequal dynamic between expert healer and passive recipient.

The concept of relating to the whole person is, of course, not new. It is an inherent part of the healer's heritage. Beginning with Hippocrates, teachers through the ages have guided every student doctor, herbalist, and nurse toward a deeply caring support of the patient. Today's emphasis on holistic medicine is an attempt to correct the tendency in modern medicine to equate "health care" with the treatment of disease entities.

Holism is not limited to any medical technique or theory. Rather, it provides a context in which the whole person is considered—his or her physical as well as mental and emotional health, including quality of life and relationships. A medical doctor may be a holistic practitioner, as can a medical herbalist or an osteopath. A framework that embraces a whole range of therapeutic modalities—whether labeled orthodox or alternative—becomes apparent. These modalities may all be used in a relevant and coherent way in the treatment of the whole of a person, not just symptoms or syndromes.

Bearing in mind that this is a time of flux, we can articulate some provisional ideas about holistic medicine. Holistic medicine emphasizes the uniqueness of the individual coming to the healer for care. The importance of tailoring treatment to meet the broad needs of each individual is fundamental, as is the need to understand and treat people in the contexts of their families, communities, and culture.

Because holistic medicine views health as a positive state of well-being, not simply the absence of disease, it emphasizes the promotion of health and the prevention of disease. It employs therapeutic modalities that mobilize the individual's innate capacity for self-healing. Holistic practitioners emphasize the role of the individual in their own healing process, and much responsibility is handed back to the patient. While swift and authoritative medical or surgical intervention may still be necessary on occasion, holism focuses on helping people understand health in order to help themselves, stressing education and self-care over treatment and the resulting dependency. Holistic practitioners also recognize the social and economic conditions that perpetuate ill health, and a commitment to change these factors is as much a part of holistic medicine as is the emphasis on individual responsibility.

A unique and important characteristic of any holistic approach is the practice of viewing illness as an opportunity for self-discovery. This has many significant implications for the caring professions, perhaps best exemplified by the hospice movement. The holistic approach includes a concern for the quality of life in each of its stages and a commitment to improving this quality of life.

The therapeutic importance of the setting within which health care takes place is also fundamental to holistic practice. Part of the problem with medical care is the alienation and dehumanization that tends to accompany institutional and laboratory settings. When the healing process becomes too far removed from the humanity of the people involved, nothing is left but chemistry and surgery. There must be a meeting of the hearts of doctor and patient, not just skill and symptoms.

Taken together, all of this clearly shows why holistic medicine transforms its practitioners as well as its patients. What, then, is the contribution of medical herbalism within this healing framework and the emerging holistic paradigm? As a healing technique, medical herbalism is inherently in tune with nature. Because herbalism works within the context of humanity's shared ecological and evolutionary heritage with the plant kingdom, it has been described as *ecological healing*.

Another of the enduring strengths of herbalism is that it has solid foundations in traditional healing, but is at the same time a part of modern science and medicine. Paradoxically, herbalism is both a wonderfully simple and a staggeringly complex therapy. It is as simple as picking cleavers from the hedgerow or chewing on chickweed stems, and as complex as the multitude of biochemical interactions that occur among all of a plant's chemical constituents and the various aspects of human metabolism and physiology. The degree and depth of interaction is breathtaking.

Practitioners of phytotherapy have the unique opportunity to introduce their patients to their medicine! A bridge can be built between person and herb, empowering the patient to be present and responsible in the healing process. A gift to a patient of a packet of herb seeds encourages a direct experience of the life of the plant. This experience of herbal vitality can turn an impersonal medicine into a living entity with which the individual can develop a deeper rapport. The patient will receive not only the medicinal benefit of the herb, but also the enlivening, empowering experience of growing and preparing his or her own healing medicine.

DEFINING HERBS AND HERBALISM

The word *herb* implies different things to different people, and definitions varying according to area of interest and personal bias. What, then, is herbalism? Simply defining *herbalism* as "the study of herbs" begs the question. This lack of clarity reflects the changing fortunes of herbalism in English-speaking cultures over the centuries.

At one time, herbalism was an honorable profession that laid the foundations of modern medicine, botany, pharmacy, perfumery, and chemistry. As these areas of study developed and the cultural infatuation with technology took hold, herbalism was relegated to history books or the realm of pleasantly quaint country craft. This left us with a word that has a variety of uses but no cultural core. As herbalism develops anew, in what has been called the "herbal renaissance," it is time for us to reclaim this little word.

Each usage of the word *herb* is relevant to a particular area of study, but this limits the applicability of the word to herbalism in general. *The Complete Oxford Dictionary* contains almost four pages (in very small print) of words derived from *herb* and *herbalist*. The primary definition of *herb* reads:

> A plant of which the stem does not become woody or persistent (as in a shrub or tree), but remains more or less soft and succulent, and dies down to the ground (or entirely) after flowering.

The second definition indicates that the term *herb* is

> . . . applied to plants of which the leaves or stem and leaves are used for food or medicine, or in some way for their scent or flavor.

The Merriam-Webster Collegiate Dictionary provides the following entry:

herb (ûrb, hûrb) *n.* 1. A plant whose stem does not produce woody, persistent tissue and generally dies back at the end of each growing season. 2. Any of various often aromatic plants used especially in medicine or as seasoning. 3. *Slang.* Marijuana.

Botanists view herbs as nonwoody plants—that is, plants that do not contain woody lignin fibers. *Dorling's Medical Dictionary* similarly defines an herb as "a plant whose stems are soft and perishable, and which are supported chiefly by turgor pressure." Of course, this then implies that trees like witch hazel (*Hamamelis virginiana*), ginkgo (*Ginkgo biloba*), and hawthorn (*Crataegus laevigata*) are not herbs. And what about mushrooms?

The science of *ecology*, or the study of interrelationships among plants, animals, and the environment, uses the word *herb* in a very specific way. In descriptions of complex communities such as forests, herbs are plants that are less than 12 inches high that complete their life cycles in the "herb layer." Again, this suggests that trees and shrubs like sarsaparilla (*Smilax* spp.) and cramp bark (*Viburnum opulus*) are not herbs.

The culinary arts have explored the use of plants in many delicious ways, but the understanding of what constitutes an herb is restricted in this field to plants that smell and taste wonderful. These are plants that are usually rich in pleasantly aromatic volatile oils, such as basil, peppermint, and oregano. No chef would think of creating culinary delights with stinking iris (*Iris foetidissima*), skunk cabbage (*Symplocarpus foetida*), or goldenseal (*Hydrastis canadensis*). This does not mean these plants are not herbs, but simply that they are not appropriate for cooking because they do not taste good.

In the various branches of medicine, the word *herb* usually implies a plant that is a healing remedy, either in its crude form or as a source of pharmacologically active chemicals. This useful but limited interpretation leads to a situation in which only pharmacologically potent plants are recognized as herbs and gentle tonic remedies are ignored.

One general definition often given states that an herb is "any useful plant." However, in return, an environmentalist might ask, What plant is *not* useful? Indeed, it could be argued that the Pacific poison oak (*Toxicodendron diversilobum*), for example, is exceptionally useful. In California, it is one of the first plants to establish itself on disturbed ground after disruption due to human activity. In a way, we might view this plant as a type of vulnerary

(wound-healing) covering, as it tends to keep humans off the land on which it grows! Because the wholeness of the environment is vital for individual human health, all plants in our environment have a medicinal role to play in planetary terms.

From the perspective of phytotherapy, an herb is any plant that may be used in the field of health and wholeness. Plants may be herbs in the strictly botanical sense, such as remedies like white horehound (*Marrubium vulgare*). However, they may also be a part of a plant of any kind, as with the flowers of marigold (*Calendula officinalis*), the heartwood of the lignum vitae tree (*Guaiacum officinale*), the seeds of chasteberry (*Vitex agnus-castus*), or the roots of coneflower (*Echinacea angustifolia*).

As a subject, *herbalism* was once the descriptor for what is now called botany, again pointing to the important past role of herbalism. *The Collins Dictionary of the English Language* defines an herbalist as a person who grows, sells, collects, or specializes in the use of herbs, especially medicinal herbs. "Herbalist" was once the term used to describe botanists, although modern botanists would likely be offended!

Webster's Revised Unabridged Dictionary defines *herbalism* as the "knowledge of herbs" and an herbalist as "one who grows, collects, or specializes in the use of herbs, especially medicinal herbs." A secondary definition refers to the herb doctor: "One who practices healing with herbs. Also called herbalist."

From a very broad perspective, I define an herb as a plant in relationship with humanity. Thus, herbalism becomes the study and exploration of the interactions between humanity and the plant *kindom* (see box on page 9). Such a point of view highlights the range and depth of human dependence on plants. This relationship is at the core of agriculture, forestry, carpentry, construction, clothing manufacture, medicine, and so on. In fact, as coal is geologically processed wood, this broad view includes the petrochemical industry as a subset of modern herbalism!

THERAPEUTIC ECOLOGY

A common idea among holistically orientated practitioners of all modalities is that a human being is a self-healing individual, and, at best, all a medical practitioner can do is facilitate this profound inner process. Addressing pathology is relatively straightforward, but, as emphasized in the WHO's definition, health is much more an active state of well-being than the absence of disease. Such vitalistic insights do not negate the importance of medicine and the healing arts, but rather provide a context within which to view them.

A self-healing individual is enmeshed in a therapeutic *ecology*, so called because the various components exist in relationship to each other and the wider world. The individual is the core of this therapeutic ecology, embraced by four groups or branches of therapies: medicine, bodywork, psychology, and spiritual techniques.

The term *medicine* is used here to mean anything that is ingested for healing purposes. Medicinal approaches include medical herbalism, homeopathy, naturopathy, and drug-based orthodox medicine. All have in common the use of some form of medicine that is taken into the body to achieve the therapeutic goal. While the specifics vary, all such medicines can be seen as fruits of the earth. Whether herbs or synthetic drugs, they share a common origin in the physical world.

Bodywork includes all approaches that do something with or to the physical body. It focuses on structural factors as either causative of or contributing to illness. This category includes the manipulative therapies, such as osteopathy, chiropractic, and the various forms of massage, as well as surgery. Personal lifestyle ideally will also contribute exercise, dance, or some other expression of bodily vitality.

Therapies that work with the psyche embrace a whole array of psychological techniques essential for identifying and treating the emotional and mental factors that contribute to health and disease. All the branches of psychotherapy are involved here, but especially the more holistically oriented approaches of humanistic and transpersonal psychology. A conscious and free-flowing emotional life is fundamental to achieving inner harmony. This does not mean that everyone must undergo in-depth psychotherapy, but that some attention should be given in a form appropriate for each individual's emotional needs. Mental factors are critical, as we are what we think.

Spiritual factors in human healing are increasingly recognized by Western medicine. Meditative and prayer-based techniques help the individual align their being with higher spirit. Others involve interaction with a practitioner who works with the energy body of the patient. Some openness to spirituality is vital in healing. This might take the form of appreciating an uplifting sunset, feeling touched by poetry or art, believing in an established religion, or simply experiencing a dogma-free joy in being alive.

Holism tells us to focus on an individual's unique situation, not simply to treat a diagnosed disease syndrome. In the context of therapeutic ecology, one person diagnosed with colitis might recuperate best when treated with dietary advice, herbs, and osteopathic manipulation, while another might respond better to drugs, psychoanalysis, and surgery. Practitioners have firmly held opinions about the pros and cons of one approach or another, but the patient is always more important than the doctor's belief system.

Such therapeutic relationships point to the possibilities for mutual support. Such support may come in the

---

The Plant Kindom

My use here of *kindom,* rather than *kingdom,* is deliberate. On a political level, I see the use of the word *kingdom*—as in "plant kingdom"—as yet another example of the dominant culture's linguistic straitjacket. As I still hold a British passport, I know what a kingdom is like, and I can assure you that the plants have no imperialist aspirations! If we must use such terms, then why not plant *queendom,* or, better yet, plant *kindom*?

I feel strongly that the practice of holistic medicine is a culturally transformative act. One of the names for an herbalist in ancient Greece was *rhizotomoi,* because herbalists collected rhizomes. I've been suggesting to all my herbal friends that we should be called *radicles,* after the growing tip of a plant's root. A plant radicle is one of the strongest things in nature. Just think of little shepherd's purse *(Capsella bursa-pastoris)* cracking through sidewalks!

The depth of this relationship goes far beyond social and economic issues to the actual life-sustaining mechanisms of planetary ecology. The health and well-being of the biosphere is governed by the green mantle of the Earth. Humanity's rapacious exploitation and destruction of the forests and seas strike at the very core of the planet's life-support mechanisms. It is becoming evident that in order to survive the multifaceted crisis at hand, humanity must learn some environmental humility, including how to cooperate with nature. Herbalism is a unique and important expression of this cooperation.

form of compensation for the weaknesses inherent in a particular therapy; for example, homeopathic remedies cannot put a splint on a fractured arm. From a more positive perspective, cooperation can lead to the development of a synergistic support system in which the whole of any treatment program becomes more than the sum of its parts. Cooperation among practitioners of different therapeutic modalities can create a geodesic relationship of extraordinary potential and strength. In such a scenario, differences lead to a celebration of the richness of therapeutic diversity and are no longer a cause for acrimonious debate and conflict.

A key insight for practitioners is to understand the limits of both their therapies and themselves. We can take for granted that well-qualified practitioners will be skilled in their chosen healing art, but true holistic healers will think beyond their training to focus on the overall needs of the sick person. This raises some questions about educational standards that cannot be meaningfully explored here. However, the point must be made that a medical doctor who completes a short training in acupuncture does not suddenly become an acupuncturist, just as a chiropractor who attends a brief workshop on herbs is not transformed into a medical herbalist overnight.

COMPLEMENTARY, ALTERNATIVE, OR ORTHODOX?

The terms *alternative* and *orthodox* are often applied in attempts to differentiate among various therapeutic modalities. However, given the rapidly changing cultural climate affecting the healing professions, it is a mistake to talk of phytotherapy as a form of "alternative" medicine. Is it an alternative to acupuncture, osteopathy, or psychiatry? Of course not. These different therapeutic modalities complement one another, creating a complex of relationships in which the whole is much more than the sum of the parts. In light of the unique strengths and weaknesses offered by each approach, mutual support and cooperation is the way toward truly holistic health service. Within the context of the patient's needs, all medical modalities are *complementary*.

Shared medical endeavors are often frustrated by communication blocks, some of which stem from differences in the language used by practitioners of various modalities. Apparent disparities in vocabulary and jargon may mask fundamental agreement in ideas and approach. On the other hand, lack of clarity can obscure important differences in both guiding principles and techniques. All too often, dogmatic attachments to words and specific formulations of belief, opinion, and theory exist. If the "correct" words or phrases are not used, then the speaker must be wrong!

Entrenched disagreement between dedicated orthodox and holistic practitioners becomes irrelevant when seen in the context of therapeutic ecology. Characteristics of open-mindedness and tolerance should be common to all involved in health care, whether practitioners, researchers, or patients. Medical modalities with foundations outside of the biomedical model should not be ignored or discounted simply because they exemplify a different belief system. They should be respected because they represent an enrichment of possibilities, not scorned as a challenge to the status quo.

Such mutually supportive endeavors in health care bear many kinds of fruit, and everyone involved will benefit. Health service administrators will appreciate the economic savings gleaned from a reduced dependence upon costly medical technology. A proportion of procedures and treatments that currently utilize expensive drugs or surgery may be replaced by more appropriate techniques from other healing modalities. For example, run-of-the-mill gallbladder removal might be avoided through the skilled use of appropriate herbs.

TYPES OF HERBALISM

Herbalism is common to all peoples and cultures of the world. The shared experience of alleviating suffering through the use of plant medicines bridges cultural divides, religious differences, and racial conflicts. A relationship exists between each culture and its plant environment, in which the herbalist plays a pivotal role. Herbalism is more than knowledge about healing plants—it encompasses all of the experience and wisdom born of this relationship between humanity and plants.

As a number of modalities use plants in their healing work, confusion exists as to their differences. Plant treatments are at the core of many of the diverse medical systems of the world, including Indian ayurveda, traditional Chinese medicine, and Islamic unani medicine. Among Western therapies, homeopathy, aromatherapy, and the Bach flower remedies also make extensive use of herbs. Many drugs currently used in orthodox medicine were either derived from plant constituents or are actual plant products.

As affirmed by the WHO, all medicine is modern as long as it is directed toward the goal of providing health care. The essential differences among these various systems of medicine are related to their cultural contexts, rather than their goals, techniques, or effects. The WHO recognizes that all traditions have value and that any particular worldview is limited, as it operates only within the belief system of one tradition. Thus, the view of reality from the cloisters of a Western medical school is as limited and limiting as that from a shaman's hut in West Africa. All perspectives have value in any worldwide approach to enhancing health for all.

HERBALISM AND HOMEOPATHY

Homeopathy is an important system of medicine that utilizes plants in the treatment of disease, though in a way fundamentally different from that of medical herbalism. There is a common misconception that these two healing modalities are the same, because they both employ plants. Indeed, herbs are used in both approaches, but in radically divergent ways that reflect differences in philosophy and therapeutic technique. A holistic perspective can help establish a complementary relationship between the two, but only when the strengths and weaknesses of each are acknowledged and understood. There is not sufficient space here to give homeopathy the attention it deserves. Instead, we will simply compare the use of herbs in these two different approaches.

As with other approaches to holistic medicine, homeopathy looks at the patient's total picture, body and mind, within the social setting of his or her life. The system originated in Germany around 1800 with the work of Samuel Hahnemann. He treated disease with very low doses of drugs that at higher doses produce symptoms similar to those of the disease itself. This is the basis of the homeopathic principle that "like treats like."

About 60% of homeopathic remedies are botanical in nature; the rest are minerals, animal products, or *nosodes* (highly diluted extracts of diseased tissue). The medicines are administered in extremely diluted form and are thought to work by influencing the vital force within the human body. The more the dose of the remedy is reduced, the more its potency is enhanced. This is why the homeopathic process of dilution is known as *potentiation*. The dilation of 1 part of the active remedy in 10 parts of the solvent (usually water) is known as a potency of 1X. A 1 in 100 dilution is 2X, and so on, up to a dilution of 200X. A homeopathic mother tincture is similar to an ordinary herbal tincture.

A problem that impedes mutual understanding between the two therapies is the application of the "like treats like" concept. Many of the herbs in the homeopathic materia medica are prescribed in dilution to treat symptom pictures that would supposedly be caused by a full dose of the herb. This is easy to understand with very strong or poisonous herbs, such as belladonna and gelsemium.

However, the medical herbalist has more trouble with the homeopath's ideas about many of the remedies shared by both systems. An example is the homeopathic remedy pulsatilla, known as pasqueflower (*Pulsatilla vulgaris*) to the herbalist. A comparison of the physical symptom picture given for the homeopathic remedy is very similar to the herbal indications for the plant. The fact that the herb is used to treat similar conditions in both approaches would appear to contradict the core idea behind homeopathy.

The value of homeopathy in health care is not in question here, but its use of plants is in no way "herbal." A selection of one or the other therapeutic modality should be based upon attraction to the philosophical context, recognizing that there is little or no real sharing of the principles of botanical medicine.

An interesting piece of lexicography becomes relevant here. The word *allopathic* is increasingly applied to orthodox medicine, even though the word is not found in the textbooks used in medical schools. In fact, it is a word coined by Hahnemann, partially to describe herbalism! *Webster's Revised Unabridged Dictionary* defines *homeopathy* and *allopathy* thus:

homeopathy \ho-me-o-p'a-thy\, n. [Gr. likeness of condition or feeling; like (fr. same; cf. Same) + to suffer: cf. F. hom['e]opathie.] The art of curing, founded on resemblances; the theory and its practice that disease is cured (tuto, cito, et jucunde) by remedies which produce on a healthy person effects similar to the symptoms of the complaint under which the patient suffers, the remedies being usually administered in minute doses. This system was founded by Dr. Samuel Hahnemann, and is opposed to allopathy, or heteropathy.

---

allopathy \al-lo-p'a-thy\, n. [Gr. other + suffering, to suffer: cf. G. allopathie, F. allopathie. See Pathos.] That system of medical practice which aims to combat disease by the use of remedies which produce effects different from those produced by the special disease treated; a term invented by Dr. Samuel Hahnemann to designate the ordinary practice, as opposed to homeopathy.

A brief note on the history of this fascinating profession: Herbalism has thrived in all cultures of the world and in all historical periods, even, until the very recent past, in the industrialized West. The rich and colorful history of herbalism is the history of humanity itself. As a constant and vital thread in human life, it is alive and well. As a branch of medicine, it has occasionally found itself on the wrong side of the establishment, but this ebb and flow of acceptance is just an artifact of changing fashions and opinions. No attempt will be made to explore the fascinating history of herbalism here, as others have done it extremely well. The interested reader should consult the excellent *Green Pharmacy*, by Barbara Griggs, the best and most comprehensive history of Western herbalism yet written.

QUESTIONING AUTHORITY IN HERBALISM

Herbalism is an aspect of human culture that takes many forms. While this rich diversity is a gift deserving of celebration, it can also be a cause of much misunderstanding. There appears to be an inherent antagonism between those who see herbalism as an expression of a green flowering in human consciousness and those who view it as a vehicle for the pharmacology of secondary plant products. Differing worldviews obviously lead to divergent goals, assumptions, and visions, but, more important, unless there is a recognition and acknowledgment of the differences among frames of reference, meaningful dialogue becomes problematic.

For example, consider table 1.1, taken from the November 15, 1998, edition of the American Medical Association (AMA) journal *Family Practice News*, which is sent regularly to general practitioners. In the journal's Clinical Rounds section, this table was presented under the headline "Herbal Products Being Evaluated Under an IND Investigation." (IND stands for Investigational New Drug Application, a request for authorization from the Food and Drug Administration to administer an investigational drug or biological product to humans.)

If the AMA considers sharks (an animal), zinc (a metal), and arginine (an amino acid) to be herbs, there is a profound educational discrepancy at work here.

It is time for herbalists to lose what might be described as our ghetto mentality, a sense of inferiority developed through years of cultural disdain for and active suppression of our therapeutic modality. However, this will also entail abandoning our negative, knee-jerk reaction to the "system," which often takes the reprehensible form of an arrogant condemnation of medical doctors and a delusion of standing on higher moral ground. On the other hand, those working within the established scientific, medical, and legislative communities must acknowl-

Table 1.1. Herbal Products Being Evaluated Under an IND Application [November 1998]

HERB	INDICATIONS
Antineoplastons	Cancer
Arginine	Cancer
Chinese herbal	HIV-associated chronic synovitis Plantar warts Postmenopausal hot flashes
Ginkgo biloba	Cognitive impairment
Green tea extract	Cancer
Melatonin	Chronobiology, reproduction
Ozone therapy	Transfusion-related diseases
Saw palmetto	Benign prostatic hypertrophy
Shark cartilage	Cancer
St. John's wort	Depression
Vitamin D	Cancer
Zinc	Head and neck cancer

edge the need to apply scientific objectivity in assessing the existing evidence about herbs. If phytotherapy is illuminated with the light of critical evaluation, much of value will be found.

WHERE IS THE EVIDENCE?

Today, practitioners and consumers alike are being bombarded by claims and counterclaims, information and misinformation about herbs. The confusion is compounded by different, often hidden, agendas. Explanations for the actions of herbs range from mechanistic science to channeled guidance, and creative advertising copy further obscures the facts behind the rhetoric. Where is the road map when we need it?

The only relevant question is whether any new therapy actually works. What outcome will the patient observe? Is there evidence of any kind that real people will experience real improvement? My intention here is not to imply that herbs don't work or to deny traditional experience. Rather, we must attempt to assess the validity of claims, especially new claims emanating from marketers, in order to facilitate the healing work that is central to herbalism. It is time to apply some critical herbal thinking to the process of questioning authority—bearing in mind that questioning is not the same thing as rejecting.

Among those who question almost anything they hear from medical doctors, the pharmaceutical industry, or the FDA, some appear willing to unquestioningly embrace any new idea or product that magazines advertise. The existence of this kind of gullibility is lamentable. Critical thinking and some degree of discrimination are needed to keep herbalism from drowning in the sea of misrepresentation, spurious theorizing, and fraudulent claims that characterize today's herbal marketplace. Natural medicine is not simply anything that does not require a prescription.

Particularly worrisome is the tendency among some practitioners to embrace marketing trends and fashionable theories by rushing to try new protocols. I suggest this is tantamount to experimenting with patients by using them to perform field trials of new, unproven, and nontraditional methods.

Let me make clear that in the material that follows, I am not attempting to make judgments about right or wrong or to promote my personal belief system. I am simply encouraging phytotherapists to inquire about the evidence behind new therapies and protocols, so that we can make informed decisions based on something more substantial than marketing claims. One must always bear in mind the basic principles of pharmacology when considering research relevant to plants. The complex interactions among the numerous constituents in a medicinal herb must be taken seriously on pharmacokinetic grounds.

Australian phytotherapist Kerry Bone, FNIMH, has suggested some important guidelines.

> Phytotherapists must avoid pseudoscience. If we intend to incorporate scientific knowledge into our therapies, let it be good science. Be on your guard for:
>
> - Hypotheses presented as undisputed facts
> - Hypotheses which can neither be proved nor disproved, that is, circular arguments
> - Conclusions based on insufficient evidence
> - Extrapolating from a narrow context of results, e.g., from *in vitro* data to the clinic, without consideration of factors such as dose, metabolism, absorption and distribution
> - Claiming scientific persecution (this does occur, of course, but is usually an excuse)
> - Developing theories which bear no relationship to experimental findings[1]

Proanthocyanidins and Pycnogenol

Pycnogenol is a legal trademark that refers to a patented process for extracting flavonoids and other substances from pine bark. The product consists of 50% to 65% proanthocyanidins. Although the proanthocyanidins present in Pycnogenol likely have health benefits, not much published research exists to support their use in specific conditions. The evidence cited in the marketing of Pycnogenol is largely extrapolated from more general research on flavonoids and proanthocyanidins.

Is this appropriate? One can expect a wide range of biological effects from the more than 4,000 individual flavonoids and 250 proanthocyanidins that have been identified. The plethora of literature on Pycnogenol cites a number of medical studies that used this specific source of proanthocyanidins. However, most of the claims made for the product itself are extrapolations from research on the general benefits of proanthocyanidins and flavonoids. To some extent, the rationale for such extrapolation is sound, as flavonoids do function as antioxidants. However, individual flavonoids often display striking differences in activity.

For example, pine bark has been called a "super antioxidant" 50 times more powerful than vitamin E. The basis for this claim is a study that compared the antioxidant properties of various proanthocyanidins. However, these did not come from pine bark, but from green tea leaves and persimmons.[2] While the marketers claim that pine bark contains a unique mix of proanthocyanidins, so do green tea and persimmons. Of the six proanthocyanidins analyzed in the study, only one was actually 50 times more effective than vitamin E, and only in quenching one type of free radical. Furthermore, proanthocyanidins are water-soluble and vitamin E is oil-soluble, which invalidates the comparison from another angle. The body needs both water- and fat-soluble antioxidants for effective antioxidant protection. Also, a diverse intake of antioxidants is far better than intake of only one or two isolated antioxidants.[3]

An overemphasis on proanthocyanidins increases the risk that other flavonoids and polyphenols will be underemphasized. As discussed in chapters 7 and 9, the isoflavones genistein and daidzein appear to reduce the risk of prostate and breast cancers. Ellagic acid, related more closely to gallates than to proanthocyanidins, is also a potent antioxidant and cancer inhibitor. The citrus flavonoids, hesperidin, quercetin, rutin, and tangeretin, are abundant and effective. Consider some recent research findings:

- Hesperidin raises blood levels of high-density lipoprotein (HDL) and lowers levels of low-density lipoprotein (LDL) and triglycerides. It also possesses significant anti-inflammatory and analgesic properties.[4]
- Quercetin reduces inflammation associated with allergies, can inhibit the growth of head and neck cancers, and inhibits the activity of reverse transcriptase.[5,6,7]
- Tangeretin induces apoptosis (programmed cell death) in leukemia cells, but does not harm normal cells.[8]

In one Pycnogenol study, described as an investigation of the effects of the product on human immunodeficiency virus (HIV), mice were infected with a retrovirus known to cause leukemia.[9] Pycnogenol improved immune function in mice with depressed immune function. Pycnogenol also increased the activity of natural killer cells, which attack both cancer cells and virus-infected cells.

However, in this study, the researchers did not use HIV, but a mouse retrovirus identified as LP-BM5. A study involving mice and a leukemia virus cannot be accepted as a model for an HIV study. The commonly accepted animal subject for HIV experiments is the monkey, and the commonly accepted viral agent is simian immunodeficiency virus. The antioxidant activity of Pycnogenol and other types of proanthocyanidins may well have some value in the treatment of AIDS. However, the insights garnered from research to date are not specific to Pycnogenol, but rather demonstrate that free radicals fuel replication of HIV and antioxidants slow it.[10]

Horsetail and Silica

Horsetail (*Equisetum arvense*) has been used to maintain the health and vitality of skin, nails, and hair for many generations in a number of world herbal traditions. The explanation often given for the effectiveness of this application is that the plant contains silica.

This raises a number of questions that I have seen addressed in very little objective material. There are two primary issues: bioavailabilty of silica and evidence for a role played by silicon in the body. I emphasize evidence here, rather than opinion or theory. I have found numerous statements about a role in joint capsule physiology, but no references directing me to research to back up this claim. A review of the MedLine database and the standard reference books on human physiology produced no literature identifying a role for silicon in human metabolism.

Even if there is a role for silicon, where is the evidence that horsetail is a source? Silica itself is silicon dioxide, one form of which is quartz. Quartz, for all intents and purposes, is insoluble in water or alcohol—after all, if it were soluble in water, there would be no sand on the beaches. Thus, it is appropriate to ask whether there is any silica in horsetail tea or extract. A further twist in the convolution of confusion is the way in which horsetail formulations are sometimes sold as "vegetable silica," implying that the need for silica is an established fact and that the traditional use of horsetail is as a source of silica. Again I ask, Where is the evidence?

This all becomes rather surreal with the invocation of a singular process termed "biotransmutation," whereby the silicon is supposedly transmuted into calcium in the body. We are moving into the realm of alchemy here, but I would have no problem with this if some evidence existed to support this claim. It strikes me as rather convenient that silicon is the only substance for which I have ever seen this aspect of human physiology invoked. If our bodies can biotransform one element into another, why limit the application of this process to silicon? Why, then, are there are deficiency problems at all?

Let me reiterate here that I am questioning not the efficacy of the herb but the explanation of mechanism given to explain its actions. I have come across a purely circular argument that comes to the conclusion that because horsetail works, it must be because it contains silica. This is based on a simple lack of knowledge of phytochemistry, as a much simpler hypothesis would invoke flavonoid effects. Such attachment to hypotheses leads to a dogmatic adherence to belief systems that is detrimental for all involved.

Why get enmeshed in bizarre intellectual convolutions to attempt justifications for an outdated hypothesis? It might be worth invoking Occam's razor here. The axiom states that

> . . . entities should not be multiplied needlessly, giving precedence to simplicity, so that of two competing theories, the simplest explanation is to be preferred.

This is interpreted to mean that the simplest of two or more theories is preferable, and that any explanation should first be attempted in terms of what is already known. In other words, after all possibilities have been considered, in all likelihood the correct answer to a problem is the simplest explanation.

Essiac, Safety, and Oxalic Acid

An herbal combination called Essiac has become well known in the United States. It has gained a reputation as a risk-free herbal approach to the treatment of cancer and other chronic conditions. My intention here is not to disparage its potential contribution to the treatment of cancer, but to highlight some of the challenges faced in modern herbal therapeutics by examining a largely overlooked safety consideration.

There is an important contraindication to the use of Essiac that is rarely mentioned, even by well-trained herbalists who should be able to see it. Essiac consists of a combination of four herbs, burdock root (*Arctium lappa*), slippery elm bark (*Ulmus rubra*), sheep sorrel (*Rumex acetosella*), and turkey rhubarb (*Rheum palmatum*). One of these components, sheep sorrel, is a rich source of oxalic acid. Intake of oxalic acid or its salts increases the risk of developing kidney stones. In all of the propaganda surrounding Essiac, I have seen no mention of this problem.

HERBS AND PHYTOTHERAPY

A distinction must be made between two separate but overlapping issues: that herbs are relevant medicinal substances and that phytotherapy is a valid therapeutic modality whose practitioners have unique skills and clinical experience. The clinical issues faced by a practitioner are not the same as the quality-control problems that confront product manufacturers and marketers. Different concerns pertinent to each of these two issues will lead to different but equally relevant insights.

The quality of attention now being given to medicinal plants by science and government must be expanded to include an assessment of the insights and protocols of the phytotherapist. A personal example may help clarify this point. At the height of the media frenzy over the "discovery" that St. John's wort can help alleviate mild depression, I was asked to present a paper on the topic of "Herbal Alternatives to Prozac." This quest to identify an herbal alternative to Prozac is a perfect example of how the real gifts of herbalism can be deflected by underlying assumptions. By phrasing the topic in this way, we are forced to respond to the issue in terms of the efficacy and pharmacological mechanism of Prozac, rather than by highlighting the potential contribution of phytotherapy to the treatment of depression.

It would, in fact, be more appropriate to consider holistic alternatives to the current vogue for psychopharmaceutical solutions. The fact that Prozac (fluoxetine) is an effective serotonin reuptake inhibitor has led to its use as a pharmacological antidepressant, but its efficacy begs the fundamental question about the cause of depression.

No herbal serotonin reuptake inhibitors of any consequence have been identified, leading me to conclude that there are no herbal alternatives to Prozac. However, this does not mean there are no herbal approaches to treating depression. My point here is that a competent herbal practitioner, trained to consider approaches to maintaining wellness in addition to treating specific pathologies, will be able to help an individual with depression in a variety of ways. Articulating herbal approaches to depression in terms of alternatives to specific drugs allows the drug companies to set the herbal agenda.

HERBAL IMPERIALISM

Attempts to bridge and integrate the various herbal traditions of the world can be problematic, and always require a high level of critical thinking. Here are a couple of examples of what might be termed *intellectual imperialism*, an assumption in the Western mind-set that we can spontaneously understand the concepts and visions of another culture.

There is a wealth of knowledge and experience in the traditional Chinese medicine (TCM) community, but not all herbalists who use these insights have the necessary training in the principles of TCM. For example, consider the widely held idea in North American herbalism that, according to TCM, *dang gui (Angelica sinensis)* is a woman's herb and ginseng (*Panax ginseng*) is a man's herb. This is nonsense! The assumption is a gross simplification of the TCM concept that *dang gui* is one of the most yielding yin tonics and ginseng is the strongest yang tonic. Yin and yang *do not* translate simply as "woman and man."

In a similar vein, Western herbalists may try to interpret the TCM concept of organs in terms of their understanding of anatomical organs, or according to the Western biomedical model. However, the TCM concept of organs is energetic and an expression of the TCM five-element theory. To take a diagnosis of "insufficient liver chi" to mean that dandelion root (*Taraxacum officinale*) and milk thistle (*Silybum marianum*) are indicated misses the point entirely.

HERBAL MARKETPLACE VERSUS HERBAL MEDICINE

Another discomforting modern dynamic is that the herbal tradition suddenly finds itself in an environment apparently created and maintained for the benefit of the "marketplace." The importance of critical thinking in the evaluation of information about herbs—particularly information generated by marketers—has never been greater. How else can practitioners and consumers make decisions about protocol development or even which products to buy?

I would argue that market forces and healing are mutually exclusive. The rapidly growing industry addressing the material needs of complementary medicine is a manifestation of market forces—it is not a healing modality or a "holistic" anything. It is merely an expression of the same rapacious economic forces that treat nature as a resource to control and profit from, and will only serve to obliterate cultural, biological, and herbal diversity.

Embracing economics as the driving force in herbalism leads directly to standardization, not only in product development, but also in the development of treatment protocols. Regulators and manufacturers who want to centralize control and standardize methods ignore individual uniqueness, except as a complicating factor. Practitioner knowledge and wisdom is rarely acknowledged, so regulations, product lines, and research are predicated on abstract theories and piecemeal information. Thus, reductionist, product-based medicine relies on controlling the patient's healing process. Surely holistic medicine would reject such an approach as a matter of principle.

SAFETY, RISK, AND TOXICITY

Safety and all it entails are major concerns for anyone involved in health care. Any meaningful discussion of safety, risk, and toxicity must take into account pharmacology, epidemiology, and statistics, as well as perceptual issues. Chapter 10 addresses these issues in terms of the herbs themselves, but here we will focus on the need for critical thinking in assessing the safety of herbs.

Statements made by "experts" are often unquestioningly accepted as insightful, considered opinion. But who are the experts in these situations? As an example, consider hawthorn (*Crataegus laevigata*), an invaluable herb discussed in chapter 14 of this book. The German Commission E Monograph cites no warnings, contraindications, side effects, or drug interactions for hawthorn.[11] Varro Tyler, Ph.D., Professor Emeritus of Pharmacognosy at Purdue University, provides an excellent review of the published studies on hawthorn in his best-selling book, *The Honest Herbal*. However, at the end of his review, he comes to a somewhat tangential conclusion.

> Its toxicity is low as well, becoming evident only in large doses. Until additional research has been carried out, prospective users of hawthorn for heart and circulation problems should consider all the consequences. Users of self-selected medicines almost always do so as a result of self-diagnosis. This is a very dangerous practice when such vital systems of the human body as the heart and blood vessels are involved. For this reason, self-treatment with hawthorn is neither advocated nor condoned.[12]

Surely this conclusion concerns self-medication, not any risk posed by hawthorn.

As another example, Dr. Ryan Huxtable, an expert on the pharmacology of plant toxins, makes a very illuminating statement in a paper on neurotoxins in herbs.

> The modern flora has evolved in the face of continual assault from mammals, which are ultimately dependent on the plant kingdom.[13]

This comment highlights one of the fundamental differences among the conceptual frameworks in which these discussions take place. Some see the natural world as a Darwinian battleground where natural selection enforces the concept of survival of the fittest. This, in turn, leads to an emphasis on defense as the driving force behind the diversity of secondary metabolites, as in ". . . plants and those using them coexist in an uneasy balance of chemical power."[14] This is the antithesis of the vitalist worldview held by most herbalists and naturopaths, who would rather see the relationship between "plants and those using them" characterized as *coevolutionary mutualism*.

THE HEALING POWER OF NATURE

In light of the issues just discussed, let us look at some of the principles of naturopathic medicine. The *healing power of nature* is the inherent self-organizing and healing process, present in all living systems, that establishes, maintains, and restores health. The naturopathic physician's role is to facilitate and augment this process by identifying and removing obstacles to health and recovery and by supporting the creation of a healthy internal and external environment.

Identify and Treat the Causes

Illness does not occur without cause.

Underlying causes of illness and disease must be identified and removed before complete recovery can occur. Symptoms may be caused by disease, but can also serve as expressions of the body's attempt to defend itself, to adapt and recover, or to heal itself. The naturopathic physician seeks to treat the causes of disease, rather than merely to eliminate or suppress symptoms.

Treat the Whole Person

Health and disease result from a complex of physical, mental, emotional, genetic, environmental, social, and other factors.

Naturopathic medicine recognizes that the harmonious functioning of all aspects of the individual is essential to health.

The multifactorial nature of health and disease requires a personalized and comprehensive approach to diagnosis and treatment.

Such principles must be applied in practice and used as a touchstone for interpreting the plethora of data and theories we wade through. As powerful and enticing as pharmacological reductionism is, it might also be seen as "immunosuppressive" to the vitalist perspective!

A PLEA FOR HERBAL TRADITIONS

The perspectives of holism and wellness now entering the practice of medicine must be taken seriously, not simply used as marketing ploys. One of the implications of this idea is that the holistic treatment of illness must encompass a positive vision of wellness, at the same time acknowledging that wellness is a process, not an endpoint. A constellation of components contribute to wellness:

Social	Physiological/metabolic
Work	Genetic
Cultural	Intellectual
Environmental	Emotional
Behavioral	Spiritual
Nutritional	

As discussed earlier, each of these components has an impact on the whole individual, and holistic medicine endeavors to address each within a therapeutic ecology. This leads to some immediate implications for the herbalist. Holism is a context, not a belief system or a specific physical form, and as such, herbal products are not and cannot be holistic in their own right.

The mere use of herbal medicines does not make a treatment holistic. In fact, using an herbal tincture as a natural alternative to a prescription medication relegates the herb to the status of an organic drug delivery system! What makes herbs part of holistic treatment is the context within which the herbs are prescribed and used.

There is at least one clear conclusion that can be drawn from the concept that holistic medicine treats the whole person and not the disease. The use of commercial formulas cannot be holistic, as these formulations do not recognize the uniqueness of the individuals who will be taking them. A formula may well be effective in addressing symptoms or even facilitating a cure, but that is not the issue. This point is further reinforced by the belief that holistic medicine doesn't merely treat symptoms, but addresses the underlying cause of disease. However, when herbs are used as an adjunct to another therapeutic modality, formulas may be appropriately used as supportive agents to treatment protocols that have been developed from a holistic perspective.

This all leads me to some specific conclusions about the challenging interface that exists between traditional herbalism and the plethora of research findings now available. There is inherent value in traditional herbalism, and we must not abandon traditional protocols and remedies because of a lack of modern research. However, as herbalists, we must familiarize ourselves with the language and processes of research so that we can establish a meaningfully dialogue with the scientific community. This dialogue must take the form of a two-way exchange, encompassing not only what we have to share, but also what we need to learn.

SCIENCE AND PHYTOTHERAPY

Any conceptual framework for phytotherapy must be broad enough to embrace the whole spectrum of human knowledge. This is simply an acknowledgment of the fact that any holistic approach to human health care must be as expansive as humanity itself. However, for a moment, let us limit our perspective to examine some of the ways in which science can add to the practitioner's understanding of how herbs work.

Almost all branches of the biological sciences are relevant to the phytotherapist, as is much of chemistry, and the application of science to herbs is as relevant as it is to any other Western healing modality.

The Scientific Method

Science is any system of knowledge concerned with the physical world and its phenomena that entails unbiased observation and systematic experimentation. In general, a science involves a pursuit of knowledge about general truths or the operation of fundamental laws. The scientific method, then, is part of the endeavor to construct an accurate, reliable, consistent, and nonarbitrary representation of the world. It attempts to minimize the influence of the bias or prejudice of the experimenter when a hypothesis or theory is tested.

Hypotheses and Theories

In science, the words *hypothesis* and *theory* relate to the stage of acceptance or knowledge about physical phenomena. A hypothesis is an idea to work from. It forms the basis of a preliminary explanation or line of reasoning, and is a limited statement about cause and effect in specific situations. The word *theory* refers to an idea that is widely accepted as a correct explanation. When a hypothesis explains many observations and leads to predictions that are continually supported by experiments, it may then be called a scientific theory.

A scientific theory represents a hypothesis (or a group of related hypotheses) that has been confirmed through repeated experiments. The steps of the scientific method may be described as follows.

1. Observation
2. Defining the problem or question
3. Formulating a hypothesis
4. Testing the hypothesis with a controlled experiment
5. Observing and recording results
6. Forming conclusions by confirming or modifying the hypothesis
7. Reporting results

Experimental tests may lead either to the confirmation or the ruling out of the hypothesis. The scientific method requires that a hypothesis be ruled out or modified if its predictions are clearly and repeatedly incompatible with the results of experimental tests. Because experimentation is a necessary part of the scientific method, a theory must be testable. If a theory cannot be tested because, for example, it has no observable ramifications, it does not qualify as a scientific theory.

The Language of Research

In the language of research, otherwise familiar words may take on entirely different and very specific meanings. For example, the use of the words *validity* and *reliability* in science can cause confusion if misunderstood. In everyday language, *validity* implies legitimacy and *reliability* suggests stability and dependability. In the language of research, these terms have a precise meaning. A study has validity if it measures what it claims to measure. The reliability of a study is a reflection of the likelihood that subsequent experiments will yield the same results.

A research sample is a small group of people (or animals, or objects) who are the subject of observation during the process of research. Thus, each individual in the study is called a research subject. The term *sample* means exactly what it seems to mean: It is a group taken as a sample of some larger group. This larger group is called the research population. Researchers cannot study whole populations, only samples. To this end, they target a population to study, but select a smaller sample from this target population to serve as the actual research subjects.

Sampling is the process of selecting a research sample. The results of a study cannot be generalized beyond the boundaries of the sample. If women are studied, the results of the research apply only to women. If men 40 to 60 years of age are studied, the results apply only to men 40 to 60 years of age. For this reason, it is important to know the makeup of research samples in order to interpret claims based on studies.

In scientific research, a variable is a condition in the experiment that changes, or varies, while other conditions remain constant. A dependent variable is usually the focus in a research study that investigates how variables change in response to one other.

The herbalist may come across a number of different types of research studies.

Controlled study. The responses of one group (the experimental group) are compared with a second, untreated group (the control group).

Placebo-controlled study. Here, an experimental treatment is compared with a placebo, an inert substance that appears to be identical to the treatment. This represents an attempt to distinguish between the *placebo effect*—the tendency of people to experience symptomatic improvement even when nothing but a sugar pill is taken—and the actual effects of treatment. If a treatment works, the effects it produces should be more pronounced than those seen in subjects receiving a placebo.

Blinded studies. If subjects are "blind" to the nature of a study and do not know whether or not they are receiving the active medication, the outcome is less likely to be influenced by their expectations. This is a way to work around research bias.

Double-blind studies. This means that neither patients nor researchers know which treatment patients are receiving. This type of study also helps researchers avoid special treatment of subjects based on whether they are receiving the active or the placebo substance, as the researchers do not know which subjects are which. Thus, there is less chance that the results of these studies will be influenced in an undesirable manner.

Randomized, double-blind, placebo-controlled, multi-center trial. This is a clinical study that takes into account a number of potential bias factors. *Randomized* means that the patients are randomly assigned to receive either the study drug or a placebo. Because the study is double blind, neither subjects nor researchers know who is receiving what treatment. *Multicenter* means the study was conducted at several different research centers.

PUBLISHED PHYTOTHERAPEUTIC RESEARCH

The usual avenue for communicating experimental results is through publication in a peer-reviewed journal. Peer-reviewed journals publish studies only after a thorough review of those studies by a group of the researcher's peers, fellow researchers who are able to evaluate the merits of the research. However, publication does not guarantee the quality of a study, and a published study is not necessarily more reliable or valid than an unpublished one.

A number of different kinds of articles may be found in peer-reviewed journals. Journal articles are based on a single investigation and published as a contribution to the progress of science. Review articles and meta-analyses are based upon analysis of existing literature on a given topic and evaluate the research performed to date.

PHARMACOGNOSY AND WAYS TO ASSESS HERB QUALITY

A number of options are available for the assessment of herb quality. These range from the plethora of scientific techniques used in pharmacognosy to the traditional skills employed by the herbalist.

The term *pharmacognosy* is derived from two Greek words, *pharmakon* (drug) and *gnosis* (knowledge). The scope of this field encompasses the study of the physical, chemical, biochemical, and biological properties of drugs, drug substances, and potential drug substances of natural origin, as well as the search for new drugs from natural sources. At one time, it was necessary for pharmacists to have extensive knowledge in this area, because many medicinal products were obtained from plants. However,

---

Basic Structure of a Peer-Reviewed Journal Article

Summary or abstract: This includes a concise statement of the goal or hypothesis of the study, explains how the endeavor was undertaken, highlights results of the study, and provides a concluding thought that puts it all into perspective. Because they must be concise, abstracts select highlights only.

Introduction: The introduction provides background information on the topic as well as the rationale for undertaking the study. The introduction may also offer an extended review of existing literature on the topic.

Methodology: This section details study design and the data-collection techniques that the researchers employed, and also describes in detail the analytical and evaluative procedures used to derive results.

Results: This is where findings are presented, along with some analysis and interpretation of the data.

Discussion, comments, or conclusion: Here, the study authors provide a further analysis of the results, and may compare and contrast their results with the conclusions of other studies in order to place their results in perspective. This is usually the most speculative part of the paper.

References: The list of references gives an indication of how far the authors went in reviewing published research. An extensive, well-done bibliography that provides access to other articles is invaluable.

as the culturally dominant medical modality in the United States moved away from natural products, most pharmacy schools dropped their courses in pharmacognosy.

Methods Currently Utilized to Evaluate Herbs and Extracts

A number of approaches to the evaluation of herb quality are available, ranging from the use of human senses to the application of advanced technology.

Organoleptic

Organoleptic analysis represents the simplest and the most human form of evaluation. *Organoleptic* means "impression of the organs." Organoleptic analysis of plant material involves the use of the senses, including sight, smell, taste, touch, and occasionally even hearing, to identify the plant and evaluate its quality. The appearance of a plant or extract can be so specific that it practically identifies itself, but identification may be difficult in other cases—for example, if the herb is in powdered form. If visual analysis is not enough, perhaps the plant or extract has a characteristic odor or taste that can assist in identification or help the herbalist assess freshness or quality.

Microscopic

Microscopic evaluation is valuable in the initial identification of herbs. It is also an indispensable technique for identifying the plant by characteristic tissue features, recognizing small fragments of crude or powdered herbs, or detecting adulterants or contaminants, such as insects, animal feces, mold, and fungi. Every plant possesses a characteristic tissue structure, which can be demonstrated through the study of tissue arrangement, cell walls, and configuration when samples are properly mounted in stains, reagents, and media.

Physical

In crude plant evaluation, physical methods are often used to determine solubility, specific gravity, melting point, water content, degree of fiber elasticity, and other physical characteristics.

Chemical

Various chemical analysis methods are used to determine percentages of active principles, alkaloids, flavonoids, enzymes, vitamins, essential oils, fats, carbohydrates, protein, ash, acid-insoluble ash, or crude fiber present. The final analytical process relies on more precise assays for determining quality. Sophisticated techniques, such as gas chromatography (GC), thin layer chromatography (TLC), and high-pressure liquid chromatography (HPLC), are often used to separate out molecules to provide a chemical "fingerprint" or profile of the constituents contained in the plant or extract. These techniques are useful in identifying herbs, but also invaluable in standardizing extracts to chosen active ingredients or marker compounds.

Biological

The plant or extract may be evaluated by various biological methods, mostly animal tests, to assess pharmacological activity, potency, and toxicity.

Official Standards

Official standards usually serve as the reference by which the authenticity and quality of an herb is established. These standards can be found in pharmacopoeias and other official publications. Examples include *The United States Pharmacopoeia* (USP), *The National Formulary* (NF), *The European Pharmacopoeia* (EP), *The British Pharmacopoeia* (BP), and *The British Pharmacopoeial Codex* (BPC).

The USP, which is published every five years by the U.S. Pharmacopoeial Convention, describes and defines approved therapeutic agents and sets standards for purity and assays. Agents are included in the USP on the basis of their therapeutic value. The NF, formerly published by the American Pharmaceutical Association, contained standards of purity and methods of assay for some drugs, as well as formulae and methods of manufacture for a variety of pharmaceutical preparations. Drugs were included in the NF on the basis of demand as well as therapeutic value. The U.S. Food and Drug Administration recognizes the NF and the USP as official standards, and the two are now published as a single volume.

The pharmacognosy literature contains precise descriptions of dried plant material that follow an all-purpose scheme for describing plant parts. The particulars of these descriptions sometimes differ from purely biological descriptions, because in pharmacognosy, one is frequently concerned with dried structures that may have been subjected to manipulation during preparation for the market. In addition, certain points important in pharmacognosy are of little value in descriptions of systematic biology.

SCREENING PROGRAMS

The pharmaceutical industry and academic institutions both conduct screening programs to identify plants that might be worthy of further study. The interdisciplinary approach taken to obtain an exploitable pure plant con-

Official Standards in Practice

Official standards provide qualitative and quantitative measures that must be met in order for the quality of a medicinal plant or extract to be considered good enough for use.

Sampling. Official standards often specify the best technique for taking a representative sample of an herb from a large consignment.

Preliminary examination. This involves the use of human senses to assess characteristics such as general appearance, presence of appropriate plant parts, odor, and taste.

Foreign matter. Because the natural world is not clean and tidy (thankfully!), official standards state what percentage of foreign matter is allowed in each sample. For example, the hairy leaves of mullein are allowed to contain more foreign matter than the smooth, shiny leaves of bearberry.

Microbial contamination. For some herbs, official standards specify the allowable content of microbes, such as *Escherichia coli*.

Toxic residues. Residues commonly found in herbs include pesticides and fumigants. In our all-too-polluted world, it is next to impossible to obtain completely toxin-free herb or food materials, so standards have been set for "acceptable" levels of such residues.

Moisture content. Measuring the water content of dried herbs gives some indication of the likelihood of spoilage. This consideration also has economic importance, as it affects the weight of herbs in commerce. A whole array of methods have been developed to assess moisture content. The most often cited is *loss on drying*, which measures the amount of weight lost through water evaporation. More precise techniques involve the separation and measurement of moisture, as well as chemical, spectroscopic, and electronic methods for measuring moisture content.

Ash values. This is given as a percentage representing the amount of inorganic ash that should remain after a sample of dried herb is incinerated.

Volatile oil content. This standard states the minimum acceptable standard for the percentage of volatile oil that should be present in a sample of a given dried herb.

Swelling index. This is the volume in milliliters occupied by 1 gram of herb after it has soaked in water for four hours.

R_F *value.* This is a measurement of the rate of flow that a compound has in specific chromatographic analysis techniques.

Refractive index and optical rotation. These are measurements of the optical properties of compounds and liquids.

Quantitative chemical tests. These are analytical methods for measuring specific compounds or groups of compounds.

stituent involves botany, pharmacognosy, pharmacology, chemistry, and toxicology, as illustrated in the steps outlined here.

1. Selection, collection, botanical identification
2. Preparation of plant material
3. Extraction with suitable solvents
4. Preliminary separations
5. Biological and pharmacological screening of crude extracts
6. Chromatographic separation of pure bioactive constituents, guided by bioassay

7. Structure determination
8. Analysis and pharmacological profiling of pure compounds
9. Toxicological testing
10. Partial or total synthesis
11. Preparation of derivatives for the study of structure-activity relationships

Selection of Plant Material

The basis upon which plants are selected for study is often pivotal to the success of screening efforts. Random collection is one possible method, but better results have been achieved when selection is based on certain criteria.

* Plants used in traditional medicine are more likely to yield pharmacologically active compounds.
* Chemotaxonomic insights are often valuable. For example, if researchers are looking for xanthones, they might best start by investigating families known to contain this class of phenolics, such as Gentianaceae, Polygalaceae, and Clusiaceae.
* Field observations are important. If a bush or a tree shows no signs of attack by pests or microorganisms, there is a good chance that insecticidal or antimicrobial metabolites are present. Foaming in aqueous plant extracts may indicate the presence of saponins.

Separation and Identification

To identify constituents, it is necessary to separate fractions of the extract to find out where the biological activity lies. A range of chromatographic techniques are used to facilitate this process.[15] Chromatography separates chemicals by taking advantage of the fact that mixtures of substances in a moving stream of gas or liquid travel at different rates through a stationary substance. This stationary substance is usually a finely divided solid, a sheet of filter material, or a thin film of a liquid on the surface of a solid. Very complex mixtures can be separated by this method, making chromatography ideal for the separation of chemicals found in herbs. It is impossible to achieve complete separation with any single method, so a multistep process is often used.

Thin Layer Chromatography

In thin layer chromatography (TLC), an extract made with an appropriate solvent is dropped onto a strip of filter paper. After drying, the paper is hung inside an airtight chamber with a liquid solvent at the bottom. The bottom of the strip is in the solvent, and as the solvent moves up the paper, the different constituents move at different rates because of differences in their molecular weight and shape. Compounds moving with the solvent front have characteristic retention times (R_F values) that facilitate identification of compounds. If the constituents separated on the paper are colorless, the paper is removed, dried, and treated to make specific chemicals visible. The main application of TLC is in separating out samples for further analysis.

Column Chromatography

Column chromatography can improve separation of individual components. The technique uses a glass column packed with a resin that serves as the *stationary phase*, through which a solvent, or the *mobile phase*, passes. Solutes in the solvent move through the column at different rates, thus separating the compounds. If the stationary phase is a solid, the system is called *adsorption chromatography*, and if the stationary phase is a liquid, the system is called *partition chromatography*.

High-Performance Liquid Chromatography

High-performance liquid chromatography (HPLC) operates on a principle similar to that of column chromatography, but has advantages of high speed, resolution, sensitivity, and ease of sample recovery. An HPLC detector is used to monitor the concentration of solutes in the mobile phase after separation. Detectors may measure refractive index, dielectric constant, molecular and atomic spectroscopy, electrochemistry, and electrolytic conductivity.

Gas Chromatography

Gas chromatography (GC) is a powerful analytical tool for separating and identifying constituents in relatively pure mixtures. The herbal extract is vaporized by heating and then moved through the column in a stream of gas—for example, helium, hydrogen, nitrogen, or argon. The vapors move at different rates, separating into clear zones as they move through the column and emerging via some detector.

Gas Chromatography-Mass Spectrometry

Final identification of a constituent usually depends upon gas chromatography-mass spectrometry (GC-MS). GC-MS is a selective and sensitive method of analyzing compounds. However, the compounds to be analyzed must first be thoroughly purified.

Mass spectrometry itself is a powerful analytical tool that yields structural information about unknown molecules. GC-MS instruments combine the ability to separate chemical mixtures (the GC component) with a very sensitive detector of the molecules' mass spectrum (the MS component). The mass spectrum obtained is compared with those of thousands of compounds in a database. The ultimate goal is accurate identification of a compound.

Bioassays

The availability of suitable *bioassays*, or biological test methods, is central to any scientific investigation of plants with biological activities. The majority of pharmaceuticals have a known chemical composition that can be assayed via quantitative analyses. However, herbs cannot be assayed satisfactorily in this way, and so are tested by biological methods. These bioassays help investigators determine potency by observing the reactions of living organisms or tissues.

Investigators employ broad-based screening (screens that cover a wide area of biological activity) to find out if the plant has any pharmacological potential. Specialized screening utilizes one or two sufficiently accurate bioassays to detect a particular property, such as anti-inflammatory activity. In some cases, adequate information may be obtained through in vitro studies, but additional tests may be undertaken in animals.

Primary Screening Bioassays

Brine Shrimp Lethality Test

The brine shrimp (*Artemia salina*) lethality bioassay is sensitive to a broad spectrum of bioactivity, providing an initial screen that can be backed up with more specific bioassays.

Crown-Gall Tumor Bioassay

This test assesses inhibition of crown-gall tumor on potato disks, and is fairly accurate in predicting *in vivo* antileukemic activity in mice.

Starfish or Sea Urchin Assay

The eggs of the starfish, *Asterina pectinifera*, have permeable cell membranes, so exposure of fertilized eggs to chemicals will lead to different outcomes. This assay can help determine which substances should be investigated as antineoplastic agents.

Bioassays for Antibiotic Activity

A range of simple tests have been developed to screen for antibiotic activity. These will determine the strength or activity of an herb or constituent in killing bacteria grown in a laboratory.

Plant Growth Regulator Activity

Tests for effects on the regulation of growth in plants can provide insights into immunosuppressant and antifungal activities of plants and extracts.

Specialized Screening Bioassays

Testing for Hepatoprotective Properties

Two approaches have been developed to screen for activity relevant to the treatment of liver disease. In the first approach, investigators induce liver damage in experimental animals and then estimate the beneficial effects of plant extracts with liver function tests that measure factors such as enzyme levels and hexobarbital sleeping times. The other approach involves removing part of the liver by biopsy and measuring the rate of regeneration after treatment with a test substance. This test takes advantage of the regenerative powers of the liver, as the liver has the ability to recover completely even after surgical resection of as much as 90% of the organ.

Because liver disease is often induced by drugs, toxins, viral infections, or reactions to immunogenic agents, appropriate test methods should mimic natural causes.

Chemical: Acetaminophen- or carbon tetrachloride–induced damage

Immunological: Complement-mediated cytotoxicity induced by immunization with specific antigens

Consider milk thistle (*Silybum marianum*) and its complex of flavolignans known as silymarin. This herb is used to treat many types of liver disease, including severe toxicity related to ingestion of the death cap mushroom (*Amanita phalloides*), which has a fatality rate higher than 50%. Treatment with silymarin (or its principal component, silibinin) within 48 hours of mushroom ingestion usually guarantees a satisfactory outcome.[16] Milk thistle and many other plants have demonstrated activity in screening tests using mice with carbon tetrachloride-induced hepatotoxicity.

Rapid Screening for Hepatoprotective Effects

For rapid screening, investigators employ an in vitro method using cultured hepatocytes, a type of liver cell. First, they isolate liver cells using collagenase, add a hepatotoxin, and culture the sample. They then assess liver function by measuring transaminase activity in the hepatocytes. After this initial screening, animals can be treated or pretreated with plant extracts, and the results determined either by assessing liver function (for example, by measuring enzyme levels) or by evaluating a parameter that is affected by liver function.

Hexobarbital Sleeping Time

Hexobarbital induces a consistent pattern of sleep in the unfortunate experimental animals, so any change in sleep time suggests a disturbance in metabolism of the sedative. An increase in sleeping time implies a reduction in the liver's ability to metabolize hexobarbital. Carbon tetrachloride produces such a change, and is known to cause dose-dependent acute hepatotoxicity. This hepatotoxicity occurs because cytochrome P_{450} enzymes transform carbon tetrachloride into free radicals, inducing lipid peroxidation and eventual death of the hepatocytes.

Regardless of the hepatoxin employed, this basic test method may be applied to assess hepatoprotection.[17] When milk thistle is added, the increase in sleeping time normally produced by carbon tetrachloride is reduced by up to 60%, suggesting that the herb defends the liver against the toxin.

Assessment of Liver Enzyme Levels

Blood levels of the enzymes aminotransferase, aspartate aminotransferase (AST), and alanine aminotransferase (ALT) are useful indicators of liver disease. AST is present in the liver, heart, muscle, kidney, and brain, and catalyzes the conversion of aspartate to oxaloacetate and glutamate. Necrosis or membrane damage releases the enzyme into circulation, so it can be measured without the need to resort to taking liver samples. Increases in AST are seen in any condition involving necrosis of hepatocytes, myocardial cells, or skeletal muscle cells. High levels indicate liver damage, including that due to viral hepatitis and toxicity, as well as cardiac infarction and muscle injury.

ALT catalyzes the conversion of alanine to pyruvate and glutamate and is released in a similar manner, but is more specific to liver function. As with AST, increases in serum levels of ALT are seen in conditions involving necrosis of hepatocytes, myocardial cells, erythrocytes, or skeletal muscle cells. High levels of ALT usually indicate acute hepatitis or other liver damage.

THE U.S. NATIONAL CANCER INSTITUTE

Since 1955, the U.S. National Cancer Institute (NCI) has carried out a search for potential cancer drugs, with a goal of screening all the flowering plants of the world to identify antitumor activity! So far, NCI has screened 176,000 extracts from 41,000 plant samples collected from 25 countries. The University of Illinois obtains samples from Southeast Asia, the Missouri Botanical Garden collects in

Africa, and the New York Botanical Garden gathers plants from Central and South America. Each center collects 1,200 samples per year, and different plant parts constitute discrete samples.

Collectors submit detailed documentation for each sample, including taxonomic details, plant part, date, site of collection, habitat, and, if possible, medicinal uses and methods of preparation employed by indigenous peoples. Researchers determine the structures of extracts that show significant activity and analyze them for active chemicals. Chemicals showing sufficient anticancer activity are advanced to preclinical development.

Currently used test systems are classified as either cytotoxicity-based bioassays or mechanism-based bioassays. Cytotoxicity-based assays may indicate activity in cancers that proliferate rapidly, such as leukemia, lymphoma, and a few rare tumors, but are inadequate indicators of activity in slow-growing solid tumors of humans. New in vitro screening strategies generally test 80 to 100 human cell lines of major tumors.[18]

Mechanism-based assays are designed by analogy with specific types of molecular responses mediated by clinically effective antitumor agents. Bioassays have been developed to recognize compounds that inhibit carcinogenesis by preventing the formation of carcinogens, blocking binding of the carcinogen to its target, or preventing tumor development. For example, one assay for blocking agents examines the effect of compounds on the detoxifying enzyme glutathione-S-transferase. Another is a mutation assay known as the Ames test, which assesses mutagenicity by assessing the effects of substances on the mutation rate of the bacterium *Salmonella typhimurium*.

Positive results in mechanism-based assays suggest potential biological activity, but cannot determine whether a substance will actually generate a clinical response. Thus, final identification of anticancer agents requires subsequent evaluation with advanced testing systems, followed by clinical trials.

Although many antitumor compounds have been isolated through these screening procedures, few have been found to be clinically effective against slow-growing solid tumors. This is a consequence of using rapidly dividing tumors in the primary screens. The development of chemotherapy agents that destroy only fast-growing cells grew directly out of the use of mouse tumor cell lines in drug-screening assays. Fast-growing mouse tumor lines provide quick turnaround times and minimize animal handling costs. The agents most effective against these cell lines are also most effective against fast-growing human tumors. However, most solid cancers in humans

Taxonomic Distribution of Higher Plants Containing Anticancer Compounds[19]

Gymnosperm Families

Cephalotaxaceae, Podocarpaceae, and Taxaceae

Angiosperm Orders and Families

Magnoliales: Annonaceae
Ranunculales: Menispermaceae
Myrtales: Thymelaeaceae
Celastrales: Celestraceae
Euphorbiales: Euphorbiaceae
Sapindales: Rutaceae, Simaroubaceae
Gentianales: Apocynaceae
Liliales: Liliaceae

grow relatively slowly, and therefore do not respond well to these agents.

Antitumor activity is a complex process, and it is well known that isolated constituents may not elicit the same clinical response as a preparation of the whole plant. The total therapeutic activity is often greater than or at least different from the activities of the individual chemicals. It is common for a fraction from a plant extract with significant biological activity to contain no single constituent that demonstrates the activity observed with the whole plant.

Few compounds reach clinical trials. A low therapeutic index, a poor ratio of maximum tolerated dose to minimum effective dose, undesirable side effects, or high toxicity may outweigh beneficial antitumor activity. Of 25,000 screens of both synthetic and natural materials conducted annually by the NCI, only 8 to 12 compounds will be selected for preclinical testing, and only 6 to 8 of these will actually enter clinical trials.[20]

THE WORLD HEALTH ORGANIZATION AND HERBAL MEDICINE

The World Health Organization (WHO) recognizes that herbalism is common to all cultures of the world and actively promotes the development of what it calls traditional medicine. The Traditional Medicine Program was established by the WHO in 1977. The WHO Resolution EB63.R4 of that year expressed the following idea:

> . . . the need for the governments of the countries interested in the use of traditional medical practice to give adequate support to engaging traditional medical practitioners in primary health care teams as and when appropriate, to the utilization of appropriate technology in these traditional medical practices and to undertake adequate measures for effective regulation and control of traditional medical practices.[21]

This resolution led to a worldwide effort by the WHO to enhance traditional medicine. To the WHO, traditional medicine implies all of the knowledge and practices used in the prevention, diagnosis, and elimination of physical, mental, or social imbalance. This knowledge is based on the experience and observation of generations. It includes highly developed, complex systems such as ayurveda and traditional Chinese medicine as well as collections of simple, local home remedies.

Traditional medicine fits perfectly into the WHO's wonderfully holistic definition of health as a state of complete physical, emotional, mental, and social well-being, not merely the absence of disease or infirmity. From this perspective, one can begin to appreciate the potential for open dialogue and integration between current scientific approaches to health and the older traditional techniques. All perspectives have value in any worldwide approach to health for all. The WHO's role is not to endorse any and all forms of traditional medicine, but instead to ensure that traditional medicine is examined critically and with an open mind.

In 1994, Resolution WHA47.27 called on the WHO director general to

> . . . consider the contribution WHO might make to promoting respect for, and maintenance of, indigenous knowledge, traditions and remedies, in particular, their pharmacopoeia.

The WHO Rationale for Promoting Traditional Medicine

- Traditional medicine has intrinsic value, and in recognition of this fact, it should be promoted and its potential developed for the wider use and benefit of mankind.
- Traditional medicine has certain advantages over imported systems of medicine, because as an integral part of the people's culture, it is particularly effective in solving certain cultural health problems.

- Traditional medicine contributes greatly to scientific medicine, thus justifying its development from the Western biomedical perspective.

A number of countries are cooperating with WHO through programs that integrate traditional approaches with the scientific techniques of modern medicine. One report from a WHO committee proposes some interesting prerequisites for integration.

- Valid factual data must be provided to overcome the current lack of information. This data may then be used to help convince decision makers, health care professionals, and the general population of the value of integration.
- There must be legal recognition of traditional therapies and practitioners to ensure sociopolitical acceptability and access to resources.
- Dialogue among practitioners of different systems should be established early in any integrative effort. This should eliminate prejudice and hopefully encourage the adoption of more acceptable attitudes.

THE CONSERVATION OF MEDICINAL PLANTS

The WHO is among a number of international bodies concerned with the protection of medicinal plants. In March 1988, the WHO, the International Union for Conservation of Nature and Natural Resources (IUCN), and the World Wildlife Fund (WWF) convened a conference on medicinal plant conservation, which was held in Chiang Mai, Thailand.[22]

The stimulus for this conference was the unprecedented loss of plant species observed by scientists worldwide. Between 1600 and 1900, about 75 species of plants and animals became extinct because of human activity. During the first 70 years of this century, about the same number of species became extinct. These numbers, however, are small when compared to the number of extinctions that were projected to occur during the final 20 years of the last century. Earth is on the verge of experiencing an extinction of species unparalleled in human experience. The IUCN estimated that if present trends continue, 60,000 higher plant species could become extinct or near extinct by the middle of the twenty-first century. The 60,000 figure accounts for approximately one in four of all higher plants.

The core Chiang Mai Declaration is extremely significant, especially if we remember that this came from scientists and international bureaucrats.

The 2002 IUCN Red List of Threatened Species

Biodiversity loss is one of the world's most pressing crises, and there is growing global concern about the status of the biological resources on which so much of human life depends. It has been estimated that the current species extinction rate is between 1,000 and 10,000 times higher than it would naturally be. Many species are declining to critical population levels; important habitats are being destroyed, fragmented, and degraded; and ecosystems are being destabilized through climate change, pollution, invasive species, and direct human impact. The IUCN Red List is the world's most comprehensive inventory of the global conservation status of plants and animals.

The updated 2002 IUCN Red List of Threatened Species is available as a searchable database at www.redlist.org. Users can search for species by common or scientific name to find out about status, distribution, habitats, threats, and other information that supports the listing.

There are nine categories of threat in the IUCN Red List system: extinct, extinct in the wild, critically endangered, endangered, vulnerable, near threatened, least concern, data deficient, and not evaluated. A species is listed as threatened if it falls in the critically endangered, endangered, or vulnerable category. Classification is accomplished through a set of five quantitative criteria that form the heart of the system. These criteria are based on biological factors related to extinction risk and include rate of decline, population size, area of geographic distribution, and degree of population and distribution fragmentation.

The categories are defined as follows:

- A taxon is "extinct" when there is no reasonable doubt that the last individual has died.
- A taxon is "extinct in the wild" when it is known to survive only under cultivation, in captivity, or as a naturalized population (or populations) well outside its past range.
- A taxon is "critically endangered" when the best available evidence indicates that it meets any of the criteria for critically endangered, and is therefore considered to be facing an extremely high risk of extinction in the wild.
- A taxon is "endangered" when the best available evidence indicates that it meets any of the criteria for endangered, and is therefore considered to be facing a very high risk of extinction in the wild.
- A taxon is "vulnerable" when the best available evidence indicates that it meets any of the criteria for vul-

Saving Lives by Saving Plants

We, the health professionals and the plant conservation specialists who have come together for the first time at the WHO/IUCN/WWF International Consultation on Conservation of Medicinal Plants, held in Chiang Mai, 21–26 March 1988, do hereby reaffirm our commitment to the collective goal of "Health for All by the Year 2000" through the primary health care approach and to the principles of conservation and sustainable development outlined in the World Conservation Strategy. We:

- Recognize that medicinal plants are essential in primary health care, both in self-medication and in national health services
- Are alarmed at the consequences of loss of plant diversity around the world
- View with grave concern the fact that many of the plants that provide traditional and modern drugs are threatened
- Draw the attention of the United Nations, its agencies and Member States, other international agencies and their members and nongovernmental organizations to:
  — The vital importance of medicinal plants in health care
  — The increasing and unacceptable loss of these medicinal plants due to habitat destruction and unsustainable harvesting practices
  — The fact that plant resources in one country are often of critical importance to other countries
  — The significant economic value of the medicinal plants used today and the great potential of the plant kingdom to provide new drugs
  — The continuing disruption and loss of indigenous cultures, which often hold the key to finding new medicinal plants that may benefit the global community
  — The urgent need for international cooperation and coordination to establish programs for conservation of medicinal plants to ensure that adequate quantities are available for future generations

We, the members of the Chiang Mai International Consultation, hereby call on all people to commit themselves to Save the Plants That Save Lives.

nerable, and is therefore considered to be facing a high risk of extinction in the wild.

- A taxon is "near threatened" when it has been evaluated against the criteria but does not qualify for critically endangered, endangered, or vulnerable now, but is close to qualifying or is likely to qualify for threatened status in the near future.
- A taxon is categorized as "least concern" when it has been evaluated against the criteria and does not qualify for critically endangered, endangered, vulnerable, or near threatened. Widespread and abundant taxa are included in this category.
- A taxon is "data deficient" when there is inadequate information to make a direct or indirect assessment of its risk of extinction based on its distribution or population status.

The 1997 IUCN Red List of Threatened Plants was the first such comprehensive listing ever undertaken for plants on a global scale. Analyses of the data in the 1997 Red List revealed the following unsettling information.

- Of the estimated 270,000 known species of vascular plants, 33,798 species were considered at risk of extinction. These plants are found in 369 plant families scattered throughout 200 countries.
- Of these plants, 91% can be considered to be found only in a single country (a statistical generalization). A limited geographic distribution can make a species much more vulnerable and may reduce options for its protection.
- A great number of species known to have medicinal value are at risk. For example, 75% of species from the

yew family, a source of important cancer-fighting compounds, are threatened. In the willow family, from which aspirin is derived, 12% of species are threatened.[23]

Many herbalists are profoundly concerned about any potential impact of their activities on natural communities. The term "wildcrafting" has been used to describe a harvest of wild plants that takes into account ecological balance so that it does not threaten the survival of the plant species. Keeping in mind ecological principles, a wildcrafter ideally harvests wild plants in a sustainable manner, or with the goal of increasing their number and health.

United Plant Savers

In the United States, a nonprofit organization called United Plant Savers (UpS) is working to help protect American medicinal plants.

The organization was formed in a spirit of hope, by herbalists committed to protecting and replanting threatened species and to raising public awareness of the plight of wild medicinal plants. Its membership reflects the diversity of American herbalism and includes wildcrafters, seed collectors, manufacturers, growers, botanists, practitioners, medicine-makers, educators, and plant lovers from all walks of life.

For further information contact United Plant Savers, PO Box 77, Guysville, OH 45735, (740) 662-0041, www.unitedplantsavers.org.

United Plant Savers publishes a list of herbs used in commerce that, because of overharvesting or loss of habitat, or by nature of their innate rareness or sensitivity, are at risk of a significant decline in numbers within their current range. As of December 1998, this list included:

American ginseng (*Panax quinquefolius*)
Beth root (*Trillium* spp.)
Black cohosh (*Cimifuga racemosa*)
Bloodroot (*Sanguinaria canadensis*)
Blue cohosh (*Caulophyllum thalictroides*)
Echinacea (*Echinacea* spp.)
Goldenseal (*Hydrastis canadensis*)
Helonias root (*Chamaelirium luteum*)
Kava kava (*Piper methysticum*)
Lady's slipper (*Cypripedium* spp.)
Lomatium (*Lomatium dissectum*)
Osha (*Ligusticum porterii*)
Partridgeberry (*Mitchella repens*)
Peyote (*Lophophora williamsii*)
Slippery elm (*UImus rubra*)

Sundew (*Drosera* spp.)
True unicorn (*Aletris farinosa*)
Venus's flytrap (*Dionaea muscipula*)
Wild yam (*Dioscorea villosa*)

Another list of wild medicinal plants indicates those in need of attention and further research. United Plant Savers is watching these herbs and collecting information on levels of commercial usage while monitoring the viability of these plants within their current range.

Arnica (*Arnica* spp.)
Butterfly weed (*Asclepias tuberosa*)
Calamus (*Acorus calamus*)
Chaparro (*Casatela emoryi*)
Elephant tree (*Bursera microphylla*)
Eyebright (*Euphrasia* spp.)
Gentian (*Gentiana* spp.)
Goldthread (*Coptis* spp.)
Lobelia (*Lobelia* spp.)
Maidenhair fern (*Adiantum pendatum*)
Mayapple (*Podophyllum peltatum*)
Oregon grape (*Mahonia* spp.)
Pink root (*Spigelia marilaandica*)
Pipsissewa (*Chimaphila umbellata*)
Spikenard (*Aralia racemosa*)
Stone root (*Collinsonia canadensis*)
Stream orchid (*Epipactis gigantea*)
Turkey corn (*Dicentra canadensis*)
Virginia snakeroot (*Aristolochia serpentaria*)
White sage (*Salvia apiana*)
Yerba mansa (*Anemopsis californica*)
Yerba santa (*Eriodictyon californica*)

References

1. Mills S, Bone K. *Principles and Practice of Phytotherapy: Modern Herbal Medicine*. Edinburgh: Churchill Livingstone, 1999.

2. Uchida S, et al. *Medical Science Research* 1987; 15:831–2.

3. Chen H, Tappel AL. *Free Radical Biology & Medicine* 1994; 16:437–44.

4. Monforte MT, et al. *Farmaco* 1995 Sept; 50:595–9.

5. Middleton E Jr. *International Archives of Allergy and Immunology* 1995; 107:435–6.

6. Castillo MH, et al. *American Journal of Surgery* 1989; 158:351–5.

7. Spedding G, et al. *Antiviral Research* 1989; 12:99–110.

8. Hirano T, et al. *British Journal of Cancer* 1995; 72:1380–8.

9. Cheshier JE, et al. *Life Sciences* 1995 Dec 22; 58:87–96.

10. Sappey C, et al. *AIDS Research and Human Retroviruses* 1994; 10:1451–61.

11. Bisset, ed. *Herbal Drugs & Phytopharmaceuticals*. Boca Raton, FL: CRC Press, 1994.

12. Tyler V. *The Honest Herbal*. Binghamton, NY: Haworth Press, 1993.

13. Huxtable R. Neurotoxins in herbs and food plants. In: Isaacson, Jensen, eds. *The Vulnerable Brain and Environmental Risks*. Vol 1. New York: Plenum Press, 1992.

14. Ibid.

15. Li F, Sun S, Wang J, Wang D. Chromatography of medicinal plants and Chinese traditional medicines. *Biomedical Chromatography* 1998 Mar; 12(2):78–85.

16. Vogel G, Temme I. Curative antagonism of liver damage caused by phalloidin with silymarin as a model of anti-hepatotoxin therapy. *Arzneimittel-Forschung* 1969; 19:613–5.

17. Kiso Y, et al. Assay method for antihepatotoxic activity using complement mediated cytotoxicity in primary culture hepatocytes. *Planta Medica* 1987; 52(3):2417.

18. Shoemaker, et al. Development of human tumor cell line panels for use in disease oriented drug screening. In: Hall TC, ed. *Prediction of Response to Cancer Therapy*. New York: Alan R. Liss, 1988.

19. Barclay AS, Perdue RE. Distribution of anticancer activity in higher plants. *Cancer Chemotherapy Reports*. Part 1 1976; 60:1081.

20. Cragg GM, et al. Drug discovery and development at the United States National Cancer Institute: International collaboration in the search for new drugs from natural sources. Proceedings of the Eighth Asian Symposium on Medicinal Plants and Spices and other Natural Products; 1994 Jun 13–16: Melake, Malaysia.

21. *WHO Technical Report*. The promotion and development of traditional medicine 1978; 622.

22. Akerele O, Heywood V, Synge H. *The Conservation of Medicinal Plants*. Cambridge, UK: Cambridge University Press, 1991.

23. Walter KS, Gillett HJ, eds. 1997 IUCN Red List of Threatened Plants. Compiled by the World Conservation Monitoring Centre IUCN. The World Conservation Union, Gland, Switzerland, 1998.

2

&

CLASSIFICATION OF MEDICINAL PLANTS

Medicinal plants can be categorized in a variety of ways, reflecting various interests and fulfilling different purposes. Categorizations may clarify potentially useful therapeutic relationships, suggest avenues of research for the pharmacologist (for example, in the screening of plants for anticancer activity), and even provide the environmentalist with data for the seemingly endless struggle to protect the environment against the ravages of human activities. Here are some of the more common methods by which plants may be classified.

Alphabetical
Plants may be listed alphabetically either by Latin binomial or common name. While this method of classification may facilitate access to information, it offers the practitioner no therapeutic insights.

Taxonomic
Based upon botanical systematics, plants are arranged according to botanists' current opinions as to which class, order, family, genus, or species they belong.

Morphologic
Here, remedies are grouped according to shared anatomical features: leaves, flowers, fruits, seeds, aerial parts, whole plant, rhizomes, bark, or roots. Such remedies are known in pharmacognosy as *organized drugs* because they are morphologically whole, or actual plant parts. *Unorganized drugs*, on the other hand, are plant materials that have no cellular structure, such as extracts, gums, resins, oils, fats, and waxes.

Therapeutic
There are a number of different ways to classify plants according to their pharmacological effects.

Action-based. Because an action-based arrangement provides some indication of the effect of a plant on the human body, this method of classification offers valuable information to the holistic practitioner.

Body system or organ affinity. This approach highlights plants appropriate for different parts of the human body.

Medical system. Herbs have different therapeutic indications depending upon the system within which the practitioner is working, whether ayurveda, the Western biomedical approach, or traditional Chinese medicine.

Biochemical. This type of classification groups plants according to their content of chemical constituents, such as saponins, alkaloids, or flavones. The many limitations of such an approach stem from the tendency of some scientists to perceive plants merely as organic drug sources.

Biogenetic. This approach categorizes plants by genetic taxonomy and evolutionary relationships among plant biochemicals. Other than academic, this categorization is of little value to the phytotherapist.

Geographical. This type of classification is based on ethnobotanical uses, or ways in which plants are used by people in different parts of the world.

PLANT TAXONOMY AND PHYTOTHERAPY

The scientific name of a plant, or Latin binomial, can be a great source of information. Scientific names are all too often overlooked, as many people are intimidated by Latin. However, if one gains a basic understanding of how botanical names are derived and what they can tell us about plants, intimidation can be transformed into empowerment—or at least simple bewilderment!

There is at least one vitally important reason for phytotherapists to be concerned with understanding how plants are named. When using plants in medicine, it is essential to know exactly which herb is being prescribed. Botanical names are exact and internationally recognized, and each Latin binomial refers to one plant and one plant only. Common names, on the other hand, vary from place to place, and much confusion can result when several plants are called by the same common name.

The coining of botanical names occurs in the field of taxonomy. This is the branch of science devoted to the arrangement of living organisms into categories based on natural similarities, such as structure, development, biochemical or physiological function, and evolutionary history. Theoretically, this field of study helps scientists identify relationships among different ancient and modern groups, can indicate the evolutionary pathways along which present-day organisms may have developed, and provides a coherent basis for comparing experimental data about different plants and animals. As many characteristics as possible are incorporated, including the organism's anatomy, biochemistry, embryology, molecular biology, behavior, and distribution.

Traditionally, organisms have been classified into two kingdoms, plant and animal. Now, for a number of practical and theoretical reasons, scientists utilize the five-kingdom system. In this system, organisms are classified according to whether they are prokaryotic (single-celled, like bacteria, with no internal membranes or organelles) or eukaryotic (composed of one or more cells containing membrane-bound nuclei and organelles), and whether they obtain food by photosynthesis, ingestion, or absorption of organic matter from their surroundings.

Carolus Linnaeus, a Swedish botanist, introduced the modern system of classification in 1753. The basic unit in the Linnaean system is the species: a group of organisms that resemble each other more closely than those of any other group and are capable of mating with one another to produce fertile offspring.

Species are arranged into higher groupings that are progressively more inclusive. Species that are closely related are grouped together into a genus. Genera with similar characteristics and origins are grouped into families. Families, in turn, are grouped into orders, orders into classes, and classes into divisions (if plants) or phyla (if animals). Finally, related phyla or divisions are placed together into kingdoms.

Sometimes it is desirable to make a finer distinction between two consecutive ranks. In that case, an additional rank is inserted between the original two, and the prefix sub- or super- added to one of the main ranks. Between an order and a family, for example, there may be several suborders. Each suborder may contain several superfamilies, and each superfamily several families.

The Five Kingdoms

The Monera. This group includes bacteria and blue-green algae, single-celled or colony-forming prokaryotes. If colonial, no specialization or division of labor occurs among the cells. Organisms are classified by the nature of their cell walls, type of motility, and mode of nutrition.

The Protista. These organisms have eukaryotic cell structures, as do all other living things except those in the Monera. Two major subgroups are the algae, which photosynthesize, and protozoans, which live by ingesting or absorbing organic matter.

The Fungi. These multicellular, plantlike organisms live by absorbing nutrients from their surroundings. Classified by body structure and type of reproduction, this group includes yeasts, molds, slime molds, and mushrooms.

The Plantae. These are many-celled organisms that usually live by photosynthesis. They have leaves or leaflike structures adapted for photosynthesis, stems or stemlike structures that hold the leaves, and roots specialized for anchoring the plant in a growth medium and absorbing water. The plants fall into two groups: bryophytes (liverworts and mosses), which have no tissues for transporting water and minerals from roots, and the more numerous vascular plants, a group that includes both ferns and seed-producing plants.

The Animalia. These are the organisms we know as animals, including sponges, coelenterates (such as jellyfish), annelids (earthworms and leeches), mollusks (snails and squid), arthropods (insects, spiders, and lobsters), echinoderms (starfish and sea urchins), and vertebrates (fish, amphibians, reptiles, birds, and mammals).

Refer to appendix 7 for a list highlighting some of the kingdoms, classes, orders, families, and genera in which major phytotherapeutic agents are found, with some examples of important species.

A plant is identified by a Latin *binomial*, or two-part name. The first name identifies the genus, which is a group of species more closely related to one another than to any other group. The second, or specific epithet, identifies a particular species within a genus. Binomials are written in italics. The genus name always begins with a capital letter, while the species epithet always begins with a small or lowercase letter. An example of a generic name is *Eupatorium*, which is used for every species of *Eupatorium*.

Eupatorium cannabinum: hemp agrimony
Eupatorium perfoliatum: boneset
Eupatorium purpureum: gravel root

The specific epithet describes exactly which of all species we are talking about. For example, *Eupatorium cannabinum* is the *Eupatorium* with leaves resembling those of *Cannabis. Eupatorium perfoliatum* is the *Eupatorium* with leaves that appear to be perforated by the stem, and *Eupatorium purpureum* is the *Eupatorium* with purplish flowers. The abbreviations sp. and spp. are used to denote one specie or several species of a particular genus, respectively. For example, "*Eupatorium* spp." indicates that we are talking about a number of species in the *Eupatorium* genus.

Species are sometimes divided into subsets known as subspecies (abbreviated as ssp.), varieties (abbreviated as var.), and forms. For example, the name *Lavandula angustifolia* ssp. *angustifolia* differentiates this subspecies of lavender from *Lavandula angustifolia* ssp. *pyrenaica*. Some plants are hybrids of two other plants of the same genus, which is denoted by an "x" between the genus and species names, as in *Mentha* x *piperita* var. *piperita*. In these two

The Linnaean System of Classification

As an example of how the system is applied, consider *Salvia divinorum,* the divine sage.

Kingdom: Plantae

Division: Magnoliophyta (angiosperms)

Class: Magnoliopsida (dicotyledons). Class names end in *-opsida.*

Subclass: Asteridae. Subclass names end in *-idae.*

Order: Lamiales. Order names usually end in *-ales.*

Family: Lamiaceae. Family names usually end in *-aceae.*

Genus: *Salvia.* The genus name should be capitalized and either italicized or underlined.

Species: *Salvia divinorum* Epling et Játiva. The species name is always preceded by its genus name. Species names begin with a lowercase letter and, like genus names, are italicized or underlined. For complete accuracy, the binomial is followed by the name of the botanical authority who first described the species.

The International Code of Botanical Nomenclature (ICBN) governs the naming of plants. The ICBN, in turn, is regulated by the Nomenclature Section of an International Botanical Congress. The current botanical code is the Tokyo edition, revised in accordance with decisions made by the XV International Botanical Congress, held in Yokohama in 1993 and published in 1994.[1] A similar code has been developed for cultivated plants. The International Code of Nomenclature for Cultivated Plants is regulated by the International Commission for the Nomenclature of Cultivated Plants (ICNCP).[2] Six principles form the basis of the code.

1. Botanical nomenclature is independent of zoological nomenclature.
2. Names of taxonomic groups are determined through the use of nomenclatural types, or specimens.
3. Nomenclature of taxonomic groups is based on priority of publication.
4. Each taxonomic group can have only one correct name, the earliest that is in accordance with the rules, although there are some exceptions.
5. Scientific names are given in Latin.
6. With some exceptions, the rules are retroactive.

examples, the plants are so well known and distinguishable by scent and taste that they are usually written simply as *Lavandula angustifolia* and *Mentha* x *piperita*.

In this book, the full botanical name is usually given in the text, so that if you need to verify botanical details, you will be able to look up the correct plant. Otherwise, please refer to appendix 3 for English common names for Latin binomials and vice versa.

Plant and family names are occasionally changed to reflect new discoveries or clarifications. Thus Roman chamomile, formerly in the genus *Anthemis*, is now a member of the genus *Chamaemelum*. Family names have changed too, and the major groups Compositae, Cruciferae, Labiatae, Leguminosae, and Umbelliferae, among others, have each been renamed after an important genus of the family. Thus, the composite family has become Asteraceae, named after the aster genus, and the cruciferous or mustard family has been renamed Brassicaceae. The two-lipped flowers of the mint family are now in Lamiaceae, the leguminous plants in Fabaceae, and the umbelliferous plants in Apiaceae. Plants may be reclassified into different families, too. For example, *Hypericum* has been moved from Hypericaceae to Clusiaceae.

The botanical authority who named the species is listed after the species name. The authority is usually abbreviated and the correct abbreviation can be found in any flora, although abbreviations are not universally standardized. Parentheses have a special meaning in taxonomy. For example, the name *Vernonia noveboracensis* (L.) Michx. reveals that André Michaux transferred to the genus *Vernonia* a species originally included in another genus *(Serratula)* by Linnaeus. The parentheses indicate a corrected name. Other conventions include "Britt. et Rose" or "Britt. & Rose" for N. L. Britton and J. N. Rose, indicating that they published the name together. "Muhl. ex Willd." indicates that the name is ascribed to G. H. E. Muhlenberg but was published by K. L. Willdenow.

Although some of these taxonomic details may seem trivial, actually they are important. Except in the case of "conserved names" officially designated by the ICBN, the publication date of a botanical name determines its priority and hence which of several possible synonyms is most valid. The ICBN provides rules to govern all possible situations related to nomenclature, but when one is preparing a taxonomic monograph, determining the correct plant name can still require quite extensive historical and botanical research.

DERIVATION OF BOTANICAL NAMES

Botanical Latin is significantly different from classical Latin. William Stearn provides a fascinating study of this subject in his essential text, *Botanical Latin* (see Suggested Reading). Stearn has succeeded in making Latin interesting and engaging to this author—no mean feat!

The Latin names used in taxonomy can be grouped into categories based upon their derivation. A few examples are given here.

Mythological Names

A variety of names are taken from classical mythology.

Nymphaea: the water lily, from the Latin Nympha, goddess of waters, meadows, and forest
Paeonia: from the Greek Paionia, physician of the gods
Achillea: from the Greek Achilles, hero of Homer's *Iliad*, whose bleeding ankle was treated with yarrow

Geographical or Ecological Names

These may refer to the plant's habitat or some other geomorphologic feature.

montana: growing in mountainous places
riparius: growing by rivers and streams
nivalis: from the Latin *nivis*, growing in or near snow
hydrocotyle: living in water

Place Names

These are often self-explanatory.

alabamensis: Alabama
californica: California
sinensis: China

Uses or Properties

As many early botanists were also doctors, some names reflect their knowledge of the therapeutic uses of the plants, or materia medica.

cardiaca: helps the heart
officinalis: once in the official pharmacopoeia
catharticus: a purgative or cathartic

Classical Names

Apparently every name of a plant used in classical Greek has been used in modern nomenclature, and these have been modified until they form a large number of the designations in common use. Consider *Psyllium* from the Greek word *psylla*, or flea. *Psylla* was the Greek name for psyllium, the seeds of which resemble fleas.

Betonica: from Vettonica, the name of a medicinal plant from the region of Spain once called Vectones or Vettones

Anethum: from the Greek *anethon*, meaning anise or dill

Ligusticum: from the Latin name of a plant growing in Liguria, Italy

Names Commemorating People

Botanists have been ingenious in their use of binomials to commemorate people. A botanist might name a plant after the first botanist to describe the species for which a genus is named, a respected teacher, or, it seems, just about anyone else!

Lobelia: named for Matthias de l'Obel, a Flemish botanist (1538–1616)

Eschscholzia: named after the 19th-century German botanist Johann Friedrich von Eschscholtz

Larrea: named for Juan Antonio de la Larrea

Historical Names

These are derived from names of historical figures. For example, *Agrimonia eupatoria* is named for Eupator, also known as Mithradates the Great, King of Pontus, northern Anatolia (120–63 B.C.). Eupatoria was a city on the west coast of the Crimean Peninsula, which legend locates as the place where Jason and the Argonauts retrieved the Golden Fleece.

Asclepias, named for Asklepios, Greek god of medicine and healing

Artemisia, named for the Greek goddess Artemis, the virgin goddess of the hunt

Narcissus, from the character of the same name in Greek mythology, who was renowned for his beauty

Anatomical Names

These names highlight visible plant features, as in *Hypericum perforatum* (St. John's wort), which is characterized by small perforations along the leaf edges. Indications of size are also common. For example, *Plantago major* describes the greater plantain.

millefolium: finely cut, from the Latin *mille* (thousand) and *folium* (leaf)

crispus: from the Latin *crispus,* meaning curled

pendulus: from the Latin *pendulus,* meaning hanging down

Color Names

A rich vocabulary applies here, as is fitting for the wide spectrum of color manifested in flowers and leaves.

Whites

niveus: snow white
galacto, lacteus: milk white
albidus: whitish

Blacks

ater, mela, or *melano:* pure black
niger: black
anthracinus: coal-black

Browns

fuscus, phaeo: brown
porphyreus: red-brown
hepaticus: liver-colored

Yellows

aureus, auratus, chryso: golden yellow
luteus, xantho: yellow
favus, luteolus, lutescens, flavidus, flavescens: pale yellow

Greens

viridis, chloro: green
glaucus, thalassicus, glaucescens: sea green
flavovirens: yellowish green

Blues

cyaneus, cyano: Prussian blue
caeruleus: blue
azureus: sky blue

Reds

ruber, erythro: red
roseus, rhodo: rosy
purpureus: purple

Aroma Names

Some binomials suggest that the plant has a strong odor, either pleasant or unpleasant. It must be remembered in these days of fashionable aromatherapy that not all plants have a sweet bouquet! Disagreeable odors are suggested by such names as *foetidus,* as in *Symplocarpus foetidus* (skunk cabbage).

odorata: from the Latin *odoratus,* meaning sweet-smelling

myroxylon: from the Greek *myron,* meaning sweet-smelling oil, and *xylon,* wood

References

1. Greuter W, Barrie FR, Burdet HM, et al., eds. International code of botanical nomenclature (Tokyo code). *Regnum Vegetabile* No. 131. Koeltz Scientific Books, Konigstein. 1994.

2. Trehane P, Brickell CD, Baum BR, et al., *1995 International Code of Nomenclature for Cultivated Plants*. Wimborne, UK: Quarterjack Publishing, 1995.

Suggested Reading

Stearn WT. *Botanical Latin*. Newton-Abbot, UK: David & Charles, 1992.

Walters DR, Keil DJ. *Vascular Plant Taxonomy*. Dubuque, Iowa: Kendall/Hunt, 1996.

3

᎒᎒

AN INTRODUCTION TO PHYTOCHEMISTRY

> To many people, a "chemical" is something to be avoided, an evil and artificial corruption of nature. However, everything tangible is a chemical. All that is good is chemical, just as all that is bad. All that is natural is chemical, just as all that is artificial.[1]

The fundamental physical nature of herbal medicine is chemical, as is the fundamental physical nature of the human body. In the chapters that follow, I shall discuss the constituents of plants that are often called the "active ingredients." However, as I will contend often throughout this book, the effects of a plant can rarely be attributed to a single constituent. More often, effects are due to the various ways in which a whole plant complex interacts with the human body.

Consider the example of the widely used British herb meadowsweet (*Filipendula ulmaria*). As is discussed in chapter 26, it is used as a mild yet effective anti-inflammatory, astringent, and carminative agent. It is specifically relevant for the treatment of musculoskeletal inflammations, as well as a range of digestive problems, including children's diarrhea. Theory tells us that the "active ingredient" of this herb is a group of compounds called salicylates, found in the aerial parts of the plant. Undoubtedly, salicylates play a vital role in the activity of meadowsweet, but they are also renowned for their unfortunate tendency to cause gastritis (inflammation of the gastric mucosa, or the lining of the stomach).

If we take the concept of active ingredients literally, meadowsweet should be contraindicated for people with gastric inflammation. However, the most common use of the herb is to mitigate arthritis pain, and it is usually taken by people who already have some degree of gastritis related to use of nonsteroidal anti-inflammatory drugs (NSAIDs). Clinical observation and historical tradition both confirm that meadowsweet can be very effective in reducing such gastric inflammation. So what is going on here? In the absence of detailed pharmacological research on the whole plant, we can only surmise that actions other than those of salicylates also contribute to the effects of this herb. Such cases inevitably lead the herbalist to conclude, "The whole is more than the sum of the parts."

The herbal remedies of the world vary in strength from potentially lethal poisons to gentle tonics that might be considered to be foods. This variation in the potency of pharmacological impact is chemically based and has a profound effect on the therapeutic selection of herbs for any individual. Herbs may be loosely categorized into the following broad groups.

Normalizers. These herbs gently nourish the body in ways that support natural processes of growth, health, and renewal. They are primarily tonics and "herbal foods." Nettles (*Urtica dioica*), cleavers (*Galium aparine*), and chickweed (*Stellaria media*) are good examples.

Effectors. Herbs that have an observable impact upon the body are used in the treatment of specific illnesses. Based on their mechanisms of action, the effects of these herbs may in turn be divided into two groups.

- *Whole plant actions* are the result of some complex of interactions between the chemistry of the whole plant and the human body. Examples include echinacea (*Echinacea* spp.) and meadowsweet (*Filipendula ulmaria*).
- *Effects of specific active chemical(s)* are generally strong enough to mask any evidence of whole plant effects. Because of the presence of these intense chemicals, such herbs are potentially poisonous if taken at the wrong dose or in the wrong way. The cardioactive herb foxglove (*Digitalis purpurea*) and the opium poppy (*Papaver somniferum*) are good examples.

As demonstrated in part 2 of this book, the herbalist focuses on the use of mild normalizers and gentle effectors, and uses strong effectors only if absolutely necessary. In fact, potent effectors are hardly used at all in herbalism. They are, however, the foundation of pharmacological medicine.

The activity of most herbs is more complex than a mere representation of the effects of an "active ingredient." Nonetheless, a review of active plant constituents can be illuminating for the phytotherapist. For example, as seen in table 3.1, it is often possible to identify major contributors to the known actions of an herb.

Table 3.1. Herbs and Constituents

CONSTITUENT GROUP	HERB EXAMPLES
Carbohydrates	
Mycopolysaccharides	Shiitake mushroom (Lentinus edodes)
Inulin	Elecampane (Inula helenium)
Mucopolysaccharides	Marshmallow root and leaf (Althaea officinalis)
Glycosides	
Cardiac glycosides	Lily of the valley (Convallaria majalis)
Cyanogenic glycosides	Wild cherry bark (Prunus serotina)
Lipids	
Fatty acids	Evening primrose oil (Oenothera biennis)
Terpenes	
Monoterpenes	Peppermint oil (Mentha piperita)
Iridoid	Gentian (Gentiana lutea)
Sesquiterpenes	Clove (Syzygium aromaticum)
Sesquiterpene lactones	Feverfew (Tanacetum parthenium)
Diterpenes	Horehound (Marrubium vulgare)
Triterpenes	Wild yam (Dioscorea villosa)
Phenolics	
Simple phenolics	Meadowsweet (Filipendula ulmaria)
Phenylpropanoids	Turmeric (Curcuma longa)
Coumarins	Angelica (Angelica archangelica)
Naphthoquinones	Sundew (Drosera rotundifolia)
Anthraquinones	Purging buckthorn (Rhamnus cathartica)
Flavonoids	Hawthorn (Crataegus laevigata)
Isoflavonoids	Red clover (Trifolium pratense)
Lignans	Milk thistle (Silybum marianum)
Tannins	Agrimony (Agrimonia eupatoria)

CONSTITUENT GROUP	HERB EXAMPLES
Alkaloids	
Piperidines	Lobelia (Lobelia inflata)
Tropanes	Henbane (Hyoscyamus niger)
Purines	Guarana (Paullinia cupana)
Isoquinolines	Bloodroot (Sanguinaria canadensis)
Indoles	Ma huang (Ephedra sinica)
Quinolizidines	Scotch broom (Cytisus scoparius)

PRIMARY AND SECONDARY PLANT METABOLITES

The chemical constituents found in plants are often classified as either primary or secondary metabolites. In all living beings, chemical compounds are synthesized and broken down via a series of chemical reactions, each mediated by an enzyme. This complex of processes is known as metabolism, which comprises catabolism (breakdown) and anabolism (synthesis).

All organisms possess similar metabolic pathways for the synthesis and use of certain essential chemicals: sugars, amino acids, common fatty acids, nucleotides, and the polymers derived from them (including polysaccharides, proteins, lipids, RNA, and DNA). This is primary metabolism, and these compounds, which are essential for the survival and well-being of the organism, are primary metabolites. In plants, such compounds are responsible for the primary life processes of respiration, photosynthesis, growth, development, and other essential functions.

Plants also use other metabolic pathways to produce compounds that often have no readily apparent function. These are the secondary metabolites, and their pathways of synthesis and utilization constitute secondary metabolism. Secondary metabolites are derived from primary metabolites but have a more limited distribution in the wonderful diversity of plants, often being restricted to a particular taxonomic group. These secondary compounds appear to play no direct role in a plant's primary metabolism, but apparently have an ecological function. They may attract pollinators, help the plant adapt to environmental stressors, or serve as chemical defenses against microorganisms, insects and other predators, or even other plants.

The dividing line between primary and secondary

metabolism is not absolute. For example, many steroid alcohols (sterols) have an essential structural role in organisms, and must therefore be considered primary metabolites.[2] In addition, these two types of metabolism are profoundly interconnected. Primary metabolism provides the small molecules that are employed as starting materials for all of the important secondary metabolic pathways.

Secondary metabolites can be broadly divided into three groups, according to their route of biosynthesis: terpenes, phenolics, and nitrogen-containing compounds. Terpenes are lipids synthesized from acetyl coenzyme A via the mevalonic acid pathway. Phenolic compounds are aromatic substances formed in various ways via the shikimic or malonic acid pathway. The nitrogen-containing secondary products, such as alkaloids, are biosynthesized primarily from amino acids.

A couple of fascinating unanswered questions arise here. How many secondary plant metabolites are there, and how many can occur in a single plant? New molecules are being isolated and characterized at a rate of about 3,000 per year, and the best estimate of the total number known appears to be 80,000 to 100,000 isolated compounds of determined structure. *The Dictionary of Natural Products*, by far the most comprehensive database of natural products, lists 170,000 compounds, but this covers all natural sources, including marine and microbial.[3] However, the literature is unexpectedly lacking in estimates of total numbers of constituents in a single plant cell.

The classes of plant constituents discussed in the chapters that follow are those most strongly implicated in the activity of medicinal plants. The primary metabolites are, of course, essential for health, as they form the basis of the human diet. However, as already noted, there are times when no clear division exists between primary and secondary metabolites. This is the case with the fundamentally important primary metabolites known as carbohydrates and lipids. These are discussed in this book from the perspective of herbal pharmacological activity, not nutrition.

The discussion of other phytochemicals focuses on the three main groups of secondary metabolites: terpenes, polyphenols, and alkaloids. These are pivotal to any chemistry-based understanding of herb activity. Bear in mind, however, that it is not always possible to identify the chemical mechanisms that explain the actions of herbs. This should not be interpreted to mean that the herbs in question do not work, but rather implies a lack of research. In turn, lack of research on a plant usually implies that no one has received a research grant!

ORGANIC CHEMISTRY

This book is not intended to provide a foundation in chemistry. It is assumed that the basics of chemistry and the conventions of organic chemistry are familiar to the reader. A brief glossary of relevant terms can be found at the end of this chapter. However, a few words must be said about the structures and formulas used in this book.

The molecules discussed in the following pages are organic. That is, they are compounds that contain carbon and hydrogen. Compounds that are not organic are called inorganic. Some very simple carbon compounds, particularly those that do not contain hydrogen (carbon dioxide, chalk, and other carbonates, for example), are considered inorganic compounds. The term *organic* does not mean that the compounds are necessarily made by biological organisms (although that was once thought to be the case), but indicates that the compounds contain carbon and hydrogen.

Carbon plays a special role in the natural world because it has a unique ability to form links with itself. A few other elements can link to themselves, but none as extensively as carbon, and none yields as many stable structures. It may be helpful to think of the organic compounds found in plants as chains or rings of carbon atoms that form a carbon frame to which other groups of atoms are attached. These *functional groups* are often the chemically active parts of organic molecules. Their addition to a carbon frame results in the formation of a new compound with different functions and reactions from that associated with the bare hydrocarbon. Some principal functional groups are illustrated in table 3.2.

A carbon-carbon double bond is normally a chemically sensitive part of a molecule, one that is liable to react. One of the bonds opens, and a group of atoms can attach to each of the carbon atoms originally joined together by the bond. A double bond is also responsible for holding a molecule in a rigid shape. Single bonds act like hinges, enabling molecules to fold into many different shapes, but a double bond is rigid and cannot be twisted. A molecule will probably be more chemically active if it possesses double carbon-carbon bonds, and the absence of multiple bonds is a sign that a molecule is flexible.

The variety of structures that carbon can form is due in part to its ability to form single, double, and triple bonds with other atoms, including carbon atoms. This structural fecundity can give rise to very intricate networks. However, this also makes it difficult to create two-dimensional representations of many bond orientations around carbon atoms. Thus, the structure of secondary metabolites as depicted on paper should always be taken with a grain of salt.

Table 3.2. Representative Functional Groups

GROUP	STRUCTURE
Hydroxyl/alcohol	—OH
Aldehyde	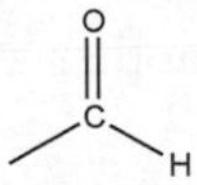
Ketone	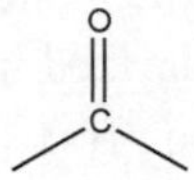
Acid/carboxyl	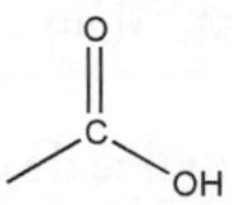
Ester	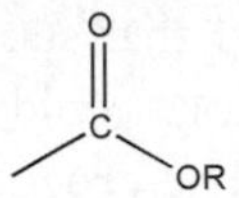
Amide	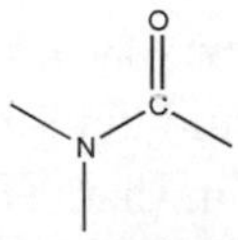
Double bond	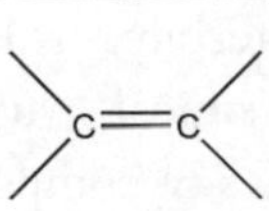
Triple bond	

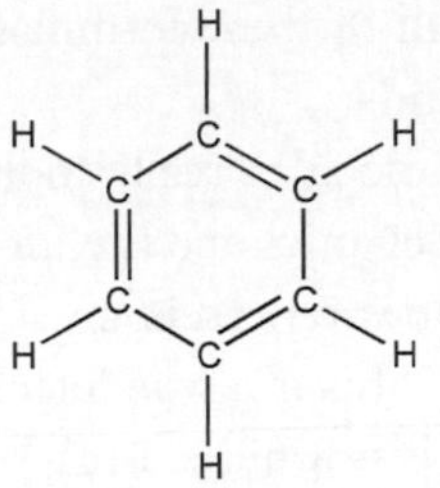

Fig. 3.1. Benzene ring

Fig. 3.2. Carbon-carbon bonds in benzene molecule

In the line formula, the hydrogen atoms are ignored, and only the carbon-carbon bonds are shown.

The related compound toluene is shown as:

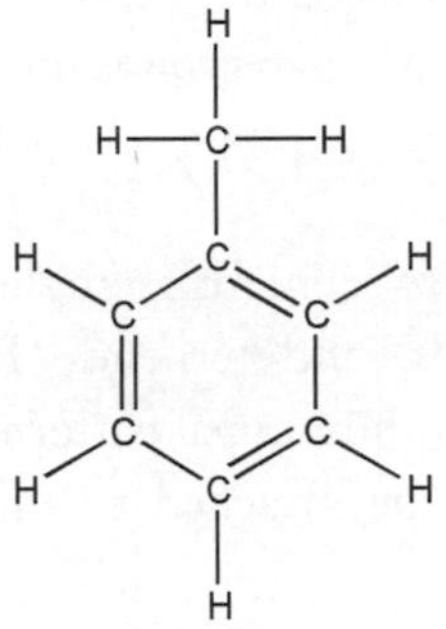

Fig. 3.3. Toluene

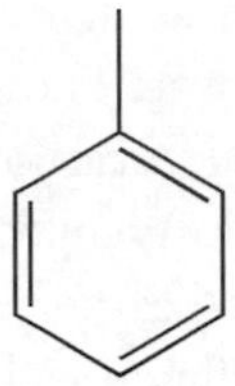

Fig. 3.4. Carbon-carbon bonds of the toluene molecule

with the single spike representing a CH_3 group.

Atoms other than carbon are always shown explicitly, as in allicin.

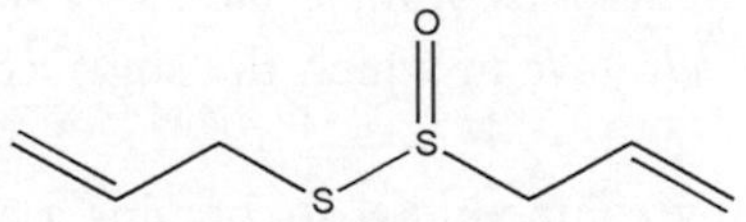

Fig. 3.5. Allicin

The orientation of the bonds around a carbon atom depends upon the number of bonds present. Thus, in a three-dimensional representation, the usual four bonds may be arranged as a tetrahedron, so that all four bonds are equally spaced about the central carbon atom, separated by 109.5-degree angles. This means that strings of hydrocarbons appear to zigzag, regardless of whether or not they contain double bonds.

Chemists often represent a molecular structure by a line formula, which shows only the links and virtually ignores the atoms. As an example, consider benzene. The benzene molecule is a hexagonal arrangement of six carbon atoms and six hydrogen atoms.

This convention greatly simplifies the depiction of organic structures. In the following chapters, I have provided a line formula whenever it seems likely to be useful. It is sometimes helpful to specify the kinds of atoms that make up a molecule and the number of atoms of each type. When such a molecular formula is written, the symbol for each element is followed by a subscript numeral indicating the number of atoms of that element in the molecule. Again using allicin as an example, the formula below shows that the compound consists of six carbon atoms, ten hydrogen atoms, one oxygen atom, and two sulfur atoms.

$$C_6H_{10}OS_2$$

However, one must realize that all of these formulas represent nothing more than shorthand.

No one knows what atoms or molecules really look like. This is the realm of quantum mechanics and the uncertainty principle. The spherical shapes represent an attempt to visualize probability spaces. This is a wonderful level of reality to contemplate, but it is not herbalism!

COMMONLY USED TERMS AND CONCEPTS

Here are some terms and concepts that the reader will encounter frequently in the phytochemical discussions.

aglycone: A molecule that can exist with or without a sugar group attached. Without the sugar group, they are known as *aglycones*. When they contain a sugar group, they are known as *glycosides*.

aromatic ring: A carbon ring structure seen, for example, in phenolic compounds, alkaloids, and terpenes. It consists of 6 carbon atoms in a flat, hexagonal pattern. Different functional groups may be attached to the ring.

conformation: The three-dimensional arrangement of the atoms of a molecule.

compound: A chemical composed of more than one type of atom.

functional group: In organic molecules, these are particular groups of atoms in which characteristic chemical reactions take place. Functional groups can be found in many different kinds of molecules.

glucoside: A *glycoside* in which the sugar constituent is glucose.

glycoside: Any compound that contains a carbohydrate molecule. These can be converted into a sugar and a nonsugar component (an *aglycone*), and are named specifically for the sugar contained, as in glucoside (named for glucose), pentoside (pentose), and fructoside (fructose).

hydrolysis: The splitting of a compound into fragments by the addition of water.

isomers: Two or more compounds with the same molecular composition. The number of possible structural isomers increases with the size of the molecule.

ligand: An ion, a molecule, or a molecular group that binds to another chemical entity to form a larger complex.

optical isomerism: Compounds that have the same molecular formula but differ in the way they rotate the plane of polarized light.

oxidation: The process by which oxygen is added or electrons removed from a molecule.

pH: A measure of acidity or alkalinity. Neutral pH is 7, acidic is less than 7, and alkaline (or basic) is higher than 7.

phenolic: A molecule containing an *aromatic ring* bearing one or more hydroxyl groups.

precipitate: A solid that is separated from a solution.

R: Shorthand that stands for a variable group, meaning that the group could have any of a number of structures.

reduction: The process by which electrons are added or oxygen lost.

stereoisomer: Two molecules that contain the same numbers and kinds of atoms bonded in the same order, but differ in that certain bonds are oriented differently in space.

structure-activity relationship: The relationship between chemical structure and pharmacological activity for a series of compounds.

References

1. Atkins PW. *Molecules*. New York: Scientific American Library, 1987.

2. Mann J. *Secondary Metabolism*. Oxford; New York: Oxford University Press, 1987.

3. Buckingham J. *Dictionary of Natural Products*. London; New York: Chapman & Hall, 1994.

4

CARBOHYDRATES

Carbohydrates are primary metabolites universally present in living beings on our planet. As the first product of photosynthesis, carbohydrates are the starting point for all phytochemicals, and also, by extension, for all animal biochemicals. More carbohydrates occur in nature than any other type of natural compound. The most abundant single organic substance on Earth is cellulose, a polymer of glucose, which is the main structural material of plants.

Functions of Carbohydrates

- Primary nutritional components for all animals
- Nutritional energy sources for metabolism in both plants and animals
- Sources of carbon in metabolic processes
- Forms of energy storage in the body
- Sources of flavor and sweetness in food
- Primary dietary fiber sources
- Important structural elements of cells and tissues (for example, cellulose in plant cell walls)
- Components of cell-to-cell contact and biological recognition processes

The name *carbohydrate* was originally assigned to compounds believed to be hydrates of carbon, of the general formula $C_n(H_2O)_n$. Of course, we now know that many other molecules are also hydrates of carbon, so the word has become an interesting reflection on the early history of biochemistry. The definition of *carbohydrate* has been modified and broadened to include polyhydroxy aldehydes and ketones, alcohols and acids, and simple derivatives of these compounds, as well as the products formed by their condensation into oligosaccharides or polysaccharides. In fact, many compounds of unusual structure that do not conform to the general formula are now included in the expanded group of compounds known as carbohydrates.

The following material focuses upon carbohydrates that play a role in the therapeutic activity of medicinal plants. Carbohydrates are also fundamentally important in human nutrition, but this subject has been adequately covered in many excellent nutrition textbooks.

CLASSIFICATION OF CARBOHYDRATES

In biochemistry, sugars and carbohydrates are now commonly termed *saccharides*. The name is derived from the Latin word *saccharum*, meaning "sugar." Carbohydrates are usually classified according to size and thus solubility. For example, a monosaccharide contains one sugar, a disaccharide contains two, and a polysaccharide contains many sugars. In general, the larger the molecule, the less soluble it is in water. Most carbohydrates in plants are bound as oligosaccharides or polysaccharides or attached to a range of different aglycones as glycosides. Much variation occurs in the way they are linked in plant glycosides, oligosaccharides, or polysaccharides.

Carbohydrates may be classified according to the number and relationships of the monosaccharide groups present.

Monosaccharides have three to nine carbon atoms, although five or six is most common.

Oligosaccharides are molecules formed by the combination of 10 or fewer monosaccharides. The bond between them is called a glycosidal bond. *Disaccharides*, a subcategory of oligosaccharides, are extremely important in nutrition.

Polysaccharides have 10 or more monosaccharide units. This group can be broken into subcategories of *homopolysaccharides* and *heteropolysaccharides*. *Glycosides* are formed via a bond between a sugar (a monosaccharide or oligosaccharide) and a nonsugar molecule (known as the *aglycone* or genin). The numerous glycosides found in plants are of great importance to herbal medicine and are discussed later in this chapter.

Major Categories of Carbohydrates

Monosaccharides

Oligosaccharides
- Prebiotics

Disaccharides
- Lactose
- Maltose
- Sucrose

Polysaccharides (glycans)

Homopolysaccharides
- Glucans
- β-D-glucans
- Starches (amylose and amylopectin)
- Glycogen
- Cellulose
- Dextrans
- Fructans
- Galacturonans
- Inulins

Heteropolysaccharides
- Arabinogalactans
- Glucomannans
- Galactomannans
- Pectins
- Xyloglucans
- Glycosaminoglycans
- Glycoproteins
- Mucopolysaccharides

Polysaccharides from fungi (mycopolysaccharides)

Polysaccharides from algae

Glycosides
- Glucosinolates
- Cyanogenic glycosides
- Flavonoid glycosides
- Anthraquinone glycosides
- Cardiac glycosides
- Saponin glycosides

MONOSACCHARIDES

Monosaccharides are described by the general formula $C_n(H_2O)_n$. Each monosaccharide can exist as more than one optically active isomer. However, only one form is normally encountered. Glucose is usually the D-isomer, rhamnose the L-isomer, and so on. Each sugar can theoretically exist in both a pyrano (6-membered) and furano (5-membered) ring form, although one or the other is usually favored. Glucose normally takes up the pyrano configuration, whereas fructose usually occurs in the furano form.

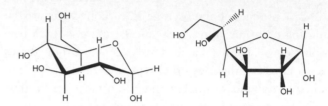

Fig. 4.1. Pyrano (6-membered) and furano (5-membered) ring forms of D-glucose

To fully convey the chemistry and hence the biochemical role of monosaccharides would necessitate an exploration of technicalities that are beyond the scope of this book. Please refer to Suggested Reading at the end of this chapter for further reading on this topic.

Principal Plant Monosaccharides

Tetroses ($C_4H_8O_4$)

These do not occur in free form in plants but play vital roles in the biosynthesis of polyphenols. Threose and erythrose are examples.

Pentoses ($C_5H_{10}O_5$)

Ribose is a pentose monosaccharide that is found universally in nucleic acids. Arabinose and xylose are present in a range of polysaccharides as well as various glycosides.

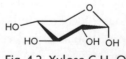

Fig. 4.2. Xylose $C_5H_{10}O_5$

Hexoses ($C_6H_{12}O_6$)

The hexoses glucose and fructose are the free sugars or monosaccharides that are found most often in plants, along with the disaccharide sucrose.

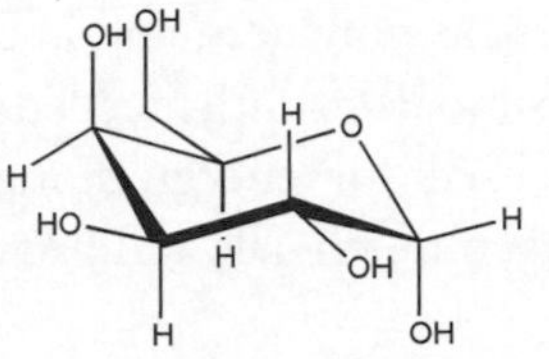

Fig. 4.3. Galactose $C_6H_{12}O_6$

Deoxysugars

In deoxysugars, one or two alcohol groups have been lost via reduction.

2-deoxy-D-ribose ($C_5H_{10}O_4$)

L-rhamnose ($C_6H_{12}O_5$)

Amino Sugars

Amino sugars are constituents of many polysaccharides, glycolipids, and glycoproteins. More than 60 are known. They contain from three to nine carbon atoms. Five-carbon pentoses and 6-carbon hexoses are most abundant.

D-glucosamine ($C_6H_{13}NO_5$)

D-galactosamine ($C_6H_{13}NO_5$)

Five sugars are commonly found as components of glycosides and polysaccharides: two are hexoses (glucose and galactose), two are pentoses (xylose and arabinose), and one is a methylpentose (rhamnose). Fructose is a common component of oligosaccharides, such as sucrose, and of the polysaccharides known as fructans.

OLIGOSACCHARIDES

Oligosaccharides are composed of monosaccharides or their derivatives linked together via glycosidal bonds. The plant world contains a wide variety of oligosaccharides. The term is derived from the Greek word *oligos*, meaning "few"; oligosaccharides contain between two and ten sugar units. Their various names reflect the number of monosaccharides they contain, as in disaccharide (2 saccharides) and trisaccharides (3 saccharides).

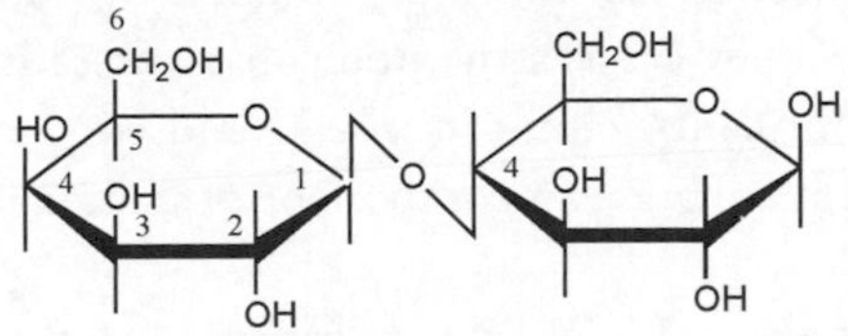

Fig. 4.4. Lactose

Prebiotics

A *prebiotic* is defined as an indigestible food ingredient that selectively stimulates the growth or activity of certain bacteria in the colon. To be effective, prebiotics must escape digestion in the upper gastrointestinal tract and be used by a limited number of the microorganisms that make up the colonic microflora. Prebiotics are principally oligosaccharides that stimulate the growth of *Bifidobacteria*, and are referred to as bifidogenic factors. Prebiotics may have anticarcinogenic, antimicrobial, hypolipidemic, and glucose-modulating activities.

POLYSACCHARIDES

Polysaccharides, also known as *glycans*, are defined as high molecular-weight polymers created through the condensation of a large number of monosaccharide molecules. Like oligosaccharides, polysaccharides are built up of monosaccharide units and their derivatives. They differ from oligosaccharides in that their molecules contain from 10 to as many as several thousand units. The most frequently occurring building block is D-glucose, though D-mannose, D- and L-galactose, D-xylose, L-arabinose, uronic acids (D-glucuronic acid, D-galacturonic acid, and

Table 4.1. Disaccharides and Trisaccharides

TYPE	NAME	MONOSACCHARIDE COMPONENTS	OCCURRENCE
Disaccharide	Sucrose	Glucose, fructose	Sugarcane, sugar beet
	Maltose	Glucose, glucose	Enzymatic breakdown of starch
	Lactose	Glucose, galactose	Milk
Trisaccharide	Gentianose	Glucose, glucose, fructose	*Gentiana* spp.
	Planteose	Glucose, fructose, glucose	*Psyllium* seeds
	Raffinose	Rhamnose, glucose, fructose	Many seeds (e.g., cottonseed)

L-iduronic acid), and amino sugars (D-glucosamine and D-galactosamine) also occur. Unlike oligosaccharides, many polysaccharides are insoluble in water.

Polysaccharides fulfill a number of fundamental functions. They act as structural substances: for example, cellulose in plants, chitin in insects and crustaceans, and chondroitin sulfate as a component of mammalian cartilage tissue.

They also serve as energy reserves, in the forms of starch and inulin in plants and glycogen in animals. The lubricant function of hyaluronic acid and the anticoagulant activity of heparin provide some specific examples.

Polysaccharides can be subdivided according to structure into homopolysaccharides and heteropolysaccharides.

Homopolysaccharides

Homopolysaccharides are composed of building blocks of a single type of monosaccharide. Depending on the type of monosaccharide they contain, homopolysaccharides are given various names, such as glucans, fructans, mannans, and xylans.

Glucans

Although glucose is the most important sugar for energy metabolism in most cells, it is not present to any great extent in the form of a free monosaccharide. Cells store glucose for future use as polymers, and in this form, glucose can be stored compactly until needed. The two major polysaccharides used for energy storage are starch in plants and glycogen in animals and bacteria.

Starch

Starch is a constituent of some algae and all higher plants. It occurs both as amylose, an unbranched molecule, and amylopectin, a branched molecule. Amylose consists chiefly of linear chains of glucose and is water-soluble. Amylopectin, also water-soluble, is a highly branched molecule that is substantially larger than amylose. Starch molecules contain between 100 and 6,000 units of glucose.

Cellulose

Cellulose is the most abundant organic compound in plants and the most abundant single polymer in the biosphere. It is also a *homopolymer* of glucose (a large polymer that consists entirely of a single monomer, in this case glucose). However, the glycosidic linkages in cellulose are in the β-configuration instead of the α-configuration of starch and glycogen. Cellulose is insoluble in water because of the high affinity of the polymer chains for one another. Its individual polymeric chains have molecular weights of 50,000 or greater. Unlike those of amylose, the linear chains are very rigid and lie parallel to each other, stabilized by intra- and intermolecular hydrogen bridges.

Mycopolysaccharides

Mycopolysaccharides and polysaccharide-protein complexes make up the cell walls of various fungi. Their principal bioactive substances are believed to be the β-D-glucans.[4] The properties of the various myco-β-D-glucans depend upon a range of chemical characteristics, such as molecular weight, branching patterns, solubility in water, and tertiary structure.

Edible Fungi Rich in β-glucans

Agaricus blazel (himematsutake)	*Schizophyllum commune* and
Auricularia auricula (wood ear)	*Sclerotina sclerotiorum* (button mushrooms)
Flammulina velutipes (enoki)	*Tremella fuciformis* (tremella)
Grifola frondosa (maitake)	*Ustilago maydis* (huitlacoche)
Lentinus edodes (shiitake)	*Wolfporia cocos* (poria)

Medicinal Fungi Rich in β-glucans

Coriolus versicolor (coriolus mushroom)	*Ganoderma lucidum* (reishi)

The mycopolysaccharides may have anticarcinogenic, immune-modulating, antimicrobial, anti-inflammatory, cardioprotective, hepatoprotective, nephroprotective, hypoglycemic, and anticaries effects.[5] An important example discussed elsewhere is lentinan, from *Lentinus edodes*. Please refer to chapter 9 for more information.

The chains interact in parallel bundles of about 2,000 chains. Each bundle constitutes a single *microfibril*. Many microfibrils arranged in parallel bundles constitute a *macrofibril*, which can be seen under the light microscope. In higher plants, cellulose occurs in association with other polysaccharides, with proteins, and also with lignin.

β-D-*glucans*

β-D-glucans, usually called β-glucans, comprise a class of indigestible polysaccharides located primarily in the cell walls. They are widely distributed in such sources as oats, barley, yeast, bacteria, algae, and mushrooms. Oat β-glucan is a soluble, viscous polysaccharide made up of mixed-linkage units of the sugar D-glucose. The different linkages break up the uniform structure of the β-glucan molecule, increasing its solubility and flexibility.

Oat bran contains more than 5.5% β-glucan, and rolled oats and whole oat flour about 4%. Oat β-glucan has cholesterol-lowering effects.[1] It has demonstrated some immune-enhancing effects and may be helpful for some people with diabetes.[2,3] Please refer to chapter 9 for more information on β-glucans.

Dextrans

Dextrans are extracellular polysaccharides formed from sucrose by certain species of bacteria. They consist of linear chains of D-glucopyranose units with occasional branchings. Dextran-forming bacteria occur primarily in the mouth and are the causative agents of plaque.

Fructans

Fructans are polymers of fructose stored in some plants as reserve material instead of starch. They have a much lower molecular weight than starch and are water-soluble. The branched fructans are found mainly in grasses, while linear fructans (for example, inulin) are particular common in Asteraceae plants.

Inulins

Inulins are composed mainly of fructose units and typically have a terminal glucose. The bond between fructose units in inulins is a β-(2,1) glycosidic linkage. Plant inulins contain 2 to 150 fructose units.

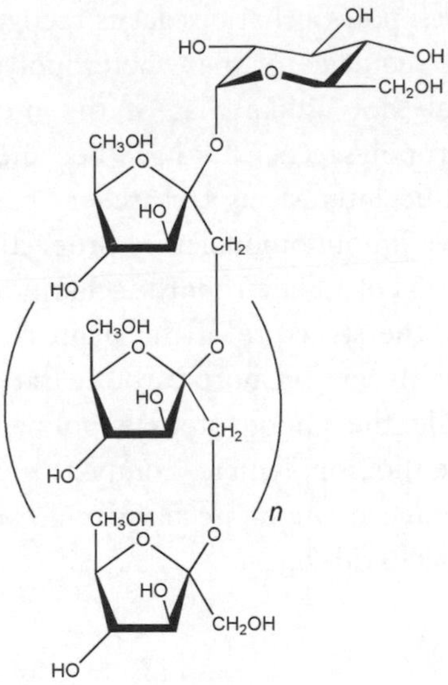

Fig. 4.5. Inulin

Inulins are present in onions, leeks, garlic, bananas, asparagus, and artichokes, among other vegetables and fruits. Because of their sweet taste and texture, inulins are added to various foods in the form of powders produced by the food chemical industry. They are only slightly digested in the small intestine and fermented by a limited number of colonic bacteria. The sources of inulins marketed as nutritional supplements and functional foods are the roots of chicory *(Cichorium intybus)* and Jerusalem artichoke *(Helianthus tuberosus)*.

Inulins may have antitumor, antimicrobial, hypolipidemic, and hypoglycemic properties. They may also have antiosteoporotic activity, as they appear to help improve mineral absorption and balance.[6]

Herbs Containing Inulins

Arctium lappa (burdock)
Cichorium intybus (chicory)
Cynara scolymus (globe artichoke)
Echinacea spp. (echinacea)
Inula helenium (elecampane)
Taraxacum officinale (dandelion root)

Heteropolysaccharides

Heteropolysaccharides are composed of building blocks of two or three different types of monosaccharides. For the most part, heteropolysaccharides are branched-chain molecules linked to a protein framework by covalent bonds.

Branched-chain polysaccharides linked to proteins give the proteins unique molecular signatures that guide them to their final destinations and facilitate specific interactions among free proteins or proteins attached to cells. Cell-wall polysaccharides act as recognition signals, so the sugar sequence of these heteropolysaccharides is informational, not unlike that of the nucleic acids in DNA. Heteropolysaccharides have become the focus of much scientific interest, as researchers have discovered that they have immunomodulatory properties.

The myriad plant heteropolysaccharides are classified according to the structure of the main chain, to which side chains with one or more carbohydrate units are attached. While the energy-storage polysaccharides and cellulose are homopolymers composed exclusively of glucose, a range of monosaccharides are used to build heteropolysaccharides:

D-mannose
D- and L-galactose
D-xylose
L-arabinose
D-glucuronic acid
L-iduronic acid
N-acetyl-D-glucosamine
N-acetyl-D-galactosamine
N-acetylneuraminic acid

Glycosaminoglycans

In terms of structure, the simplest and best known of the heteropolysaccharides are the glycosaminoglycans. These are long, unbranched polysaccharides composed of repeating disaccharide subunits in which one of the two sugars is either N-acetylglucosamine or N-acetylgalactosamine. Glycosaminoglycans are negatively charged. This causes the polymeric chains to adopt a stretched or extended conformation, which increases their spheres of influence and generates a high viscosity in the surrounding region.

Glycosaminoglycans are usually found in extracellular spaces, where they produce a viscous matrix that resists compression. This matrix confers many benefits: It can allow a passageway for cell migration, create lubrication between joints, and provide rigidity to structures such as cartilage and the eyeball.

Hyaluronic acid is a heteropolymer of D-glucuronic acid and N-acetyl-D-glucosamine. It is considerably larger than most glycosaminoglycans, reaching molecular weights greater than one million. Hyaluronic acid is formed by the successive addition of glucuronic acid and N-acetylglucosamine residues to the ends of a growing chain. Hyaluronic acid is usually found in a complex with protein.

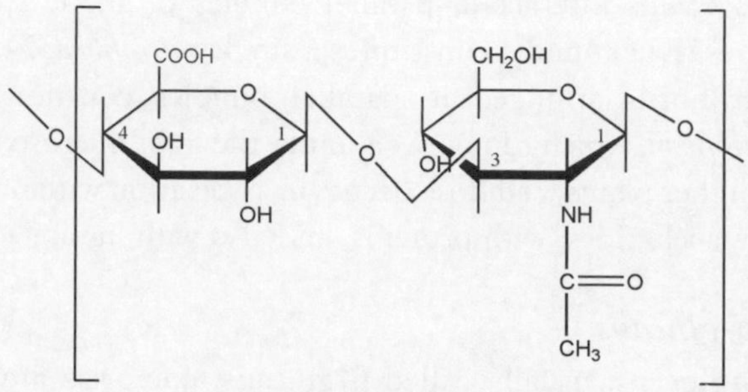

Fig. 4.6. Hyaluronic acid

Hyaluronic acid is a universal component of the extracellular fluid that fills the spaces between the cells of body tissues. Extracellular fluid is packed with proteins (collagen) and glycosaminoglycans. This forms a gel-like matrix in which proteins are embedded and through which water, oxygen, and solutes have to pass to get to the cells. Hyaluronic acid is the main component of this extracellular matrix. Hyaluronic acid solutions have remarkable viscosity and tensile properties. When no pressure is applied to the solution, it is highly viscous and rigid. If pressure is applied, the water is squeezed out and the strands move past one another. Thus, hyaluronic acid solutions behave as biological shock absorbers in connective tissue. Hyaluronic acid plays an important role in tissue hydration, lubrication, and cellular function, and is able to hold more water than any other natural substance.

Arabinogalactans

Arabinogalactans are water-soluble polysaccharides widely found in plants, fungi, and bacteria. They are composed of D-galactose and L-arabinose residues in the form of a β-D-(1-3)-galactan main chain with side chains made up of galactose and arabinose units of various lengths. In plants, arabinogalactans occur as arabinogalactan proteins. These proteins are proteoglycans involved in plant growth and development; they may also be involved in signal transduction in plants.

Dietary arabinogalactans come primarily from carrots, radishes, tomatoes, pears, and wheat, among other plant foods. Gum arabic, a common food additive, is composed of highly branched arabinogalactan. Arabinogalactans are also found in medicinal plants, such as *Echinacea* spp., and in the medicinal mushroom *Ganoderma lucidum*. Arabinogalactans are thought to contribute to the immune-enhancing activities of such herbs.

Larch arabinogalactan is a mixture of several different arabinogalactans mainly derived from the wood of the western larch (*Larix occidentalis*) but also present in other species of larch. Research suggests that larch arabinogalactan may have immune-enhancing activity; in vitro studies revealed that it stimulated the activity of human natural killer cells and enhanced the function of certain other immune-system components. In other laboratory studies, it inhibited the metastasis of tumor cells to the liver.[7,8]

Glucomannans

A glucomannan is a hydrocolloidal polysaccharide composed of D-glucose and D-mannose residues bonded together in β-1,4 linkages. Approximately 60% of the polysaccharide is D-mannose and approximately 40% is D-glucose.

Dietary glucomannan is a soluble fiber derived from konjac flour. Konjac flour itself comes from the tubers of various *Amorphophallus* species, relatives of the philodendron houseplant. When ingested, glucomannan swells and causes an increase in stool bulk, making it useful as a laxative. It may also help control serum glucose and lipid levels.

Pectins

Pectins are linear polysaccharides containing about 300 to 1,000 monosaccharides, principally D-galacturonic acid. The D-galacturonic acid residues are linked together by α-1,4 glycosidic linkages.

Pectins are found in the cell walls of many fruits but are most concentrated in citrus and apples. As fruit ripens, an insoluble precursor is converted to soluble pectin and becomes gelatinous.

Pectin is widely employed in the food industry as a gelling agent. It is also combined with the clay kaolin for use in the management of diarrhea. Research suggests that pectin has cholesterol-lowering and antithrombotic properties and may help protect against colorectal cancer.

GLYCOPROTEINS

A rapidly advancing area in biochemistry is that concerned with the structure and metabolism of saccharides that are covalently attached to proteins (as in glycoproteins) and lipids (as in glycolipids). The carbohydrates in these complexes vary in composition, in the way they are linked, in their branching patterns, and in the type of sugars that terminate each branch.

Glycoproteins are proteins to which carbohydrates are linked by glycosidic bonds. The carbohydrates vary in size, from mono- or disaccharides to polysaccharides, and may be located at various positions on the polypeptide chain. There is good reason to believe that most proteins are, in fact, glycoproteins. In other words, there are more proteins that contain covalently bound carbohydrates than proteins that are devoid of carbohydrates.

The molecular size of glycoproteins ranges from 15,000 to greater than one million. They differ not only in the types and relative proportions of sugars they contain, but also in the number of side chains present. Some glycoproteins are of small molecular size and contain only one carbohydrate chain per molecule. At the other extreme, we have proteins that contain some 800 saccharide chains in each molecule, such as sheep submaxillary mucin. Attachment of sugars to proteins increases the solubility of proteins.

Glycoproteins cover the linings of the respiratory and intestinal tracts, are responsible for the viscosity of saliva and cervical mucus, and lubricate the eyeball in the eye socket.

Mucopolysaccharides (Proteoglycans)

A group of compounds often classified as glycoproteins are the mucopolysaccharides, or proteoglycans, of connective tissue, including the chondroitin sulfates, heparin, and keratan sulfate. To distinguish them from other glycoproteins, they are called *proteoglycans* and their carbohydrate chains *glycosaminoglycans*.

Mucopolysaccharides differ from typical glycoproteins in that they contain long polysaccharide chains made up of about 100 monosaccharide units. Mucopolysaccharides typically consist of a protein core to which many long-chain linear heteropolysaccharides are covalently linked. These are made up largely of repeating disaccharide units. In these disaccharides, one sugar is always an amino sugar, either glucosamine or galactosamine.

Another constituent common to most mucopolysaccharides is sulfate groups, linked by ester bonds to the hydroxyl groups of their monosaccharide constituents, and in some cases also by amide linkages to the amino groups of glucosamine. By virtue of their carboxyl and sulfate groups, mucopolysaccharides are highly charged anions.

Mucopolysaccharides occur in many animal tissues and fluids, including connective tissue, which is a particularly rich source. In skin, bone, cartilage, and ligaments, mucopolysaccharides join with collagen or elastin fibers to form the matrix or "ground substance" in which the connective tissue cells (or fibroblasts) are embedded.

Postulated Functions of Protein-Bound Carbohydrates

1. Physicochemical properties of glycoproteins (viscosity)
   - Activity of cells and tissues

2. Molecule-membrane interactions
   - Secretion
   - Clearance of glycoproteins from plasma
   - Reaction of cell surface with viruses, blood group antisera, and lectins
3. Membrane-membrane interactions
   - Secretion
   - Differentiation and growth
   - Contact inhibition
   - Adhesion and aggregation of cells
   - Segregation of cells within the organism— for example, the homing of lymphocytes
   - Gamete recognition

GLYCOSIDES

The multitude of glycosides found in plants are all compounds that contain a sugar unit attached to a noncarbohydrate molecule, which is called the aglycone.

Sugar + Aglycone = Glycoside

On first consideration, this seems straightforward enough, until one considers the variety of both sugars and aglycones found in nature. From a biochemical perspective, saponins, flavones, and cardiac glycosides might all be grouped together in a single category—a situation guaranteed to confuse the nonspecialist. The important point for the practitioner to remember is that glycosides, because of their sugar component, are more easily absorbable, and thus the aglycone is more readily bioavailable. This increased bioavailability appears to be the reason that so many diverse molecules naturally occur as glycosides.

A number of ways have been developed to categorize glycosides, each of which reflects different interests.

Classification of Glycosides

By sugar unit. A glycoside based on glucose is called a glucoside; rhamnose will produce a rhamnoside, and so on. In nature, most glycosides are formed from 5-carbon pentose sugars or 6-carbon hexose sugars. The sugar may be a mono-, di-, or oligosaccharide.

According to the nature of the aglycone-sugar linkage. Different chemical bondings are possible in the aglycone-sugar linkage, each having potentially different chemical and physiological effects. The most common are the *O*-glycosides, in which an oxygen atom acts as the link. *C*-glycosides, with carbon links, play an important role as anthraquinone laxatives, such as aloin in aloe. Other linkages include sulfur-based

S-glycosides and nitrogen-based *N*-glycosides. As with other carbohydrate-based molecules, the bond might be either an α- or a β-glycoside; β-glycosides are more common.

By specific aglycone. This categorization is often the most useful for the purposes of phytotherapy, as seen in the following examples.

Simple Phenolic Glycosides: Arbutin and Salicin

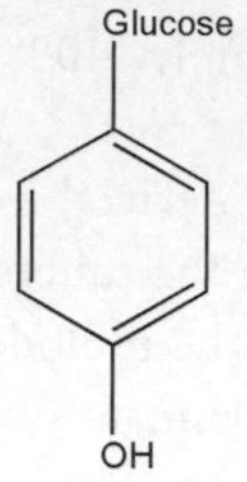

Fig. 4.7. Arbutin

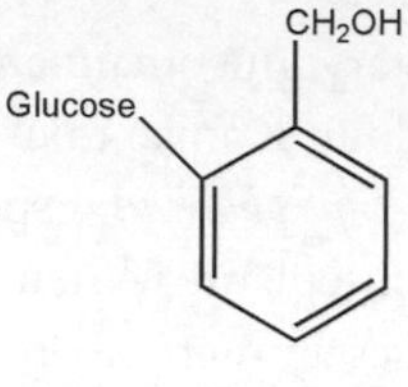

Fig. 4.8. Salicin

Flavonoid Glycoside: Rutin

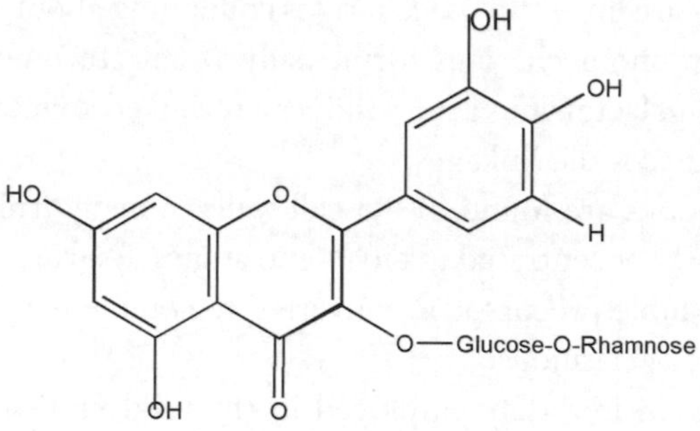

Fig. 4.9. Rutin

Anthraquinone Glycoside: Sennoside A

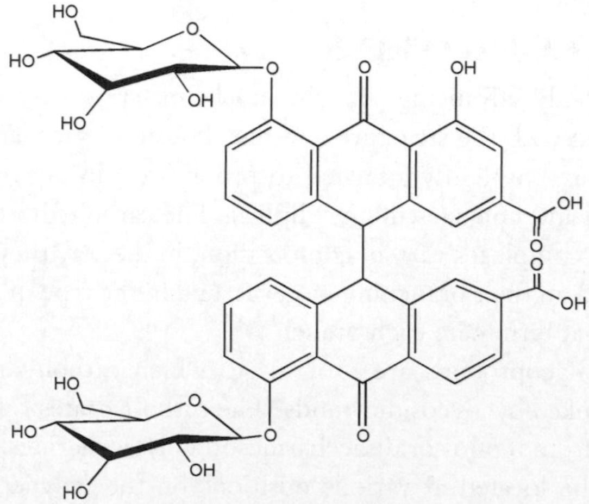

Fig. 4.10. Sennoside A

Steroid and Saponin Glycoside: Ginsenosides

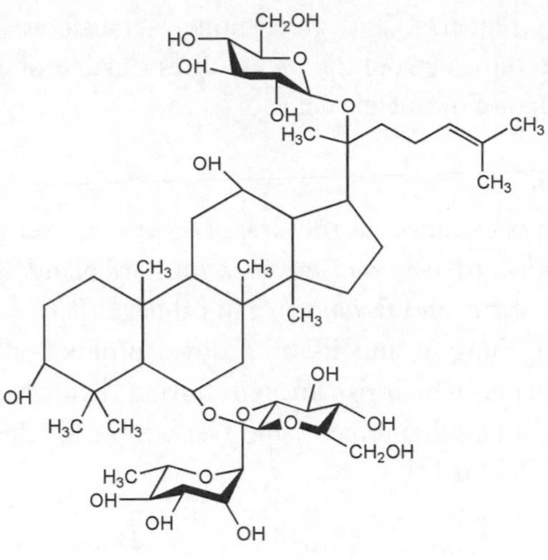

Fig. 4.11. Ginsenoside Re

Many pharmacologically important constituents occur in plants as glycosides. While modification by the sugar component is possible, the effect of a glycoside is mainly determined by the nature of its aglycone. Thus, in this book, we will consider glycosides in the context of their aglycones, not as a separate group. However, I will discuss two unique groups here, namely the cyanogenic and the isothiocyanate glycosides.

Cyanogenic Glycosides

Bitter almonds (*Prunus dulcis* var. *amara*) produce a poison, hydrogen cyanide (HCN), a fact that has been known since antiquity. Cyanide occurs in the intact nut in a bound form as a cyanogenic glycoside. The plant releases its characteristic smell of bitter almonds only when the tissue is damaged, which causes either enzymatic or nonenzymatic hydrolysis of the glycoside. The immediate hydrolytic product is a cyanohydrin, which spontaneously decomposes to HCN and an aldehyde or ketone.

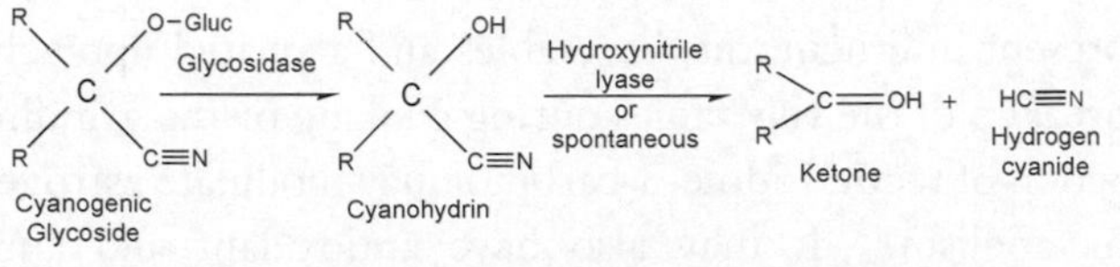

Fig. 4.12. Cyanogenic glycoside hydrolysis

At least 1,000 species representing 100 families and 500 genera have cyanogenic properties, but the aglycone has only occasionally been characterized.[9] Thus, only about 40 cyanogenic glycosides have been identified. Cyanogens (substances that can release cyanide) also occur in the defense secretions of centipedes, millipedes, and moths.

Amygdalin

Amygdalin was first isolated from bitter almonds, the seeds of the tree *Prunus dulcis* var. *amara*. The sugar moiety in this compound is gentiobiose, typical for many members of Rosaceae, and trace amounts may be present in the fleshy parts of fruits, in bark, and in leaves.

Amygdalin is responsible for the bitterness and toxicity of the seeds of bitter almond and of apricots. An amygdalin-containing drug called laetrile has been used as an anticancer medicine, though its use is now restricted.[10]

Prunasin

This compound occurs in the leaves and bark of *Prunus* species, as well as some other vascular plants and some ferns, such as bracken fern (*Pteridium aquilinum*).[11] In small quantities, prunasin exhibits expectorant, sedative, and digestive properties. Prunasin is the main active principle of wild cherry bark (*Prunus serotina*), used as an expectorant, antitussive, and flavoring agent in cough syrups.

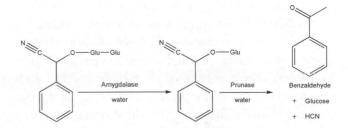

Fig. 4.13. Prunasin metabolism

Glucosinolates

The glucosinolates, also called isothiocyanates, are glycosides that are not toxic per se but release the volatile oils commonly known as mustard oils upon enzymatic hydrolysis. Release occurs when plant tissue is crushed, through the reaction of the glucosinolate with the enzyme thioglucosidase, which is always present in plants that contain glucosinolates. Glucosinolates are β-thioglucoside *N*-hydroxysulfates, which are primarily found in cruciferous vegetables, such as cabbage, broccoli, brussels sprouts, cauliflower, bok choy, and kale.

Chemically, glucosinolates are nitrogen-sulfur compounds with the same basic formula; one sulfur atom is bonded to glucose as the *S*-glucoside and the other sulfur is present as the oxygen-linked sulfate anion. About 80 glucosinolates are known. The majority of glucosinolates are aliphatic, and the remainder are benzyl or indole derivatives. The best-known aliphatic derivatives are sinigrin and glucocapparin. A typical benzyl derivative is sinalbin, and an indole derivative is glucobrassicin.[12]

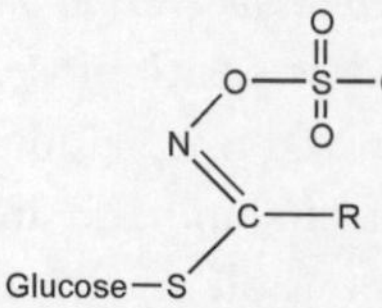

Fig. 4.14. Basic structure of a glucosinolate

Glucosinolates are characteristic constituents of the mustard family, Brassicaceae. They occur, for example, in cabbage, cauliflower, cress, mustard, rape, and turnip. These glycosides are also uniformly present in other families in the same order, Capparales, to which Brassicaceae belongs: Capparidaceae, Moringaceae, Resedaceae, Stegnospermataceae, and Tovariaceae. There are several unrelated occurrences, notably in the genera *Carica* (Caricaceae), *Limnanthes* (Limnanthaceae), and *Tropaeolum* (Tropaeolaceae). The seeds of these plants are often a rich source of glucosinolates, although the compounds are normally distributed throughout the plant.

The major function of glucosinolates in plants is to deter predators. However, specialist insects, such as the white cabbage butterfly, *Pieris rapae*, become adapted to their toxic effects and use the presence of mustard oils in host plants as feeding cues and oviposition guides. Regular dietary intake of quantities of glucosinolates causes toxic effects in farm animals, especially damage to the thyroid, liver, and kidneys. The same effects may occur in humans, although this has rarely been observed in practice.

Actions of Glucosinolates

When applied topically, mustard oils act as rubefacients, causing local vasodilation. Thus, mustard poultices are applied to break up congestion in the lungs and bronchioles, although care must be taken not to irritate the skin. Taken internally, the compounds serve as effective decongestants for sinus conditions and also stimulate digestion. Large doses may induce emesis.

As with all sulfur compounds, mustard oils exhibit some antibiotic effects. Glucosinolates depress thyroid function in animals; therefore, all plants in the genus *Brassica* are *potentially* goitrogenic. This action may be harnessed therapeutically in cases of hyperthyroidism.

Dietary intake of glucosinolates (in the form of broccoli, cabbage, cauliflower, or brussels sprouts) may have a protective effect against colon cancer. Experimental tumor production is greatly inhibited by pretreatment with isothiocyanates. The isothiocyanates interfere with the metabolism of carcinogens by enhancing the activity of several cytochrome P_{450} enzymes involved in the detoxification processes. They inhibit procarcinogen activation and induce phase II enzymes, such as NAD(P)H quinone reductase and glutathione-*S*-transferase, which detoxify the electrophilic metabolites capable of altering the structure of nucleic acids.[13]

Sinigrin

Sinigrin is common in the Brassicaceae—for example, in horseradish (*Armoracia rusticana*), mustard plants (*Brassica nigra*, *B. hirta*, and *B. juncea*), and cabbage (*B. oleracea* var. *capitata*). Sinigrin and its breakdown product, allyl isothiocyanate, which is formed during hydrolysis, are volatile, intensely pungent, and responsible for the biting taste of mustard.[14]

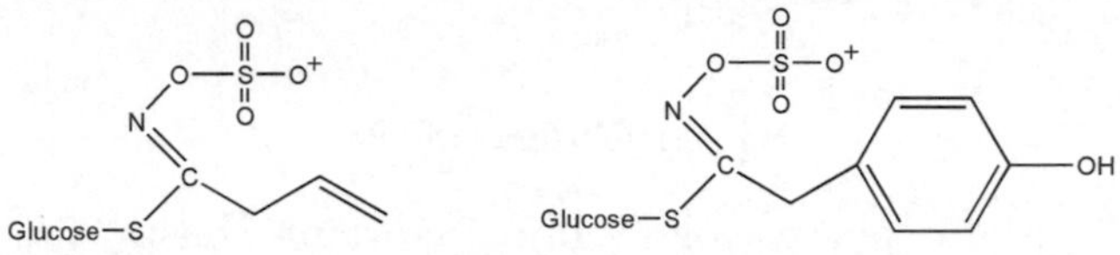

Fig. 4.15. Sinigrin and sinalbin

Indole-3-Carbinol

Indole-3-carbinol is a breakdown product of the glucosinolate glucobrassicin, also known as indole-3-glucosinolate.

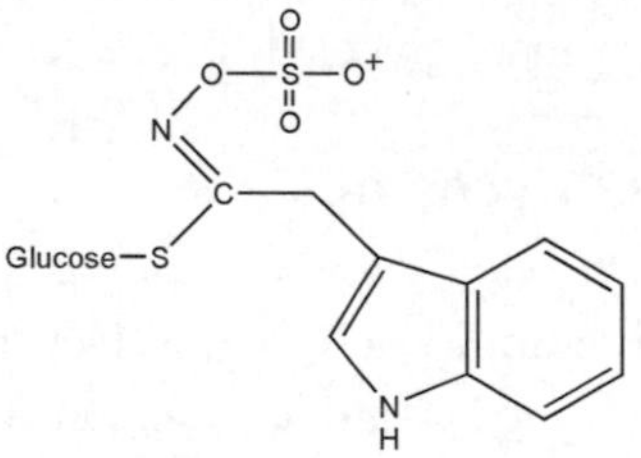

Fig. 4.16. Glucobrassicin

While glucosinolates themselves have minimal anticancer activity, indole-3-carbinol may have chemopreventive properties.[15] Indole-3-carbinol is produced from indole-3-glucosinolate via the action of the enzyme myrosinase (thioglucoside glucohydrolase). This enzyme is present in cruciferous vegetables and activated upon the breakup of the vegetables during cooking or the grinding action of teeth. Indole-3-carbinol may modulate estrogen metabolism.[16] It may also have antioxidant and antiatherogenic activities.

GUMS AND MUCILAGES

Gums, like acacia and tragacanth, and mucilages, such as those from flaxseed, psyllium seed, and marshmallow root, are found in many plants. They are usually formed from the cell wall or deposited on it in layers. They consist of monosaccharides and uronic acid units.

The term *mucilage* is loosely used, often interchangeably with *gum*. Chemically, mucilage is closely allied with gums and pectins, but differs in certain physical properties. While gums swell in water to form sticky, colloidal dispersions and pectins gelatinize in water, mucilages form slippery, aqueous colloidal dispersions that are optically active and can be hydrolyzed and fermented.

Mucilages are not pathological plant products, but are formed within the plant during normal growth by mucilage-secreting hairs, sacs, and canals. Gums, on the other hand, are deposited on the surface of plants as exudates, which are formed as a result of bacterial or fungal action after mechanical injury.

Mucilage is a naturally occurring organic plant constituent with a molecular weight of 200,000 or greater, the detailed structure of which is unknown. Mucilages occur in nearly all classes of plants in various plant parts, usually in relatively small percentages. They are often associated with other constituents, such as tannins. The most common sources are the root, bark, and seed, but they are also found in the flower, leaf, and cell wall.

Plants Containing Mucilage

Acacia senegal (acacia or gum arabic)
Althaea officinalis (marshmallow root and leaf)
Astragalus gummifer (tragacanth)
Chondrus crispus (carrageen)
Cyamopsis tetragonolobus (guar)
Cydonia oblonga (quince seed)
Plantago ovata, P. arenaria (psyllium seeds)
Sterculia urens (sterculia)
Symphytum officinale (comfrey root and leaf)
Trigonella foenum-graecum (fenugreek)
Tussilago farfara (coltsfoot leaves)
Ulmus rubra (slippery elm bark)

Any biological functions of mucilage within the plant are unknown, but it is thought that they may aid in water storage, decrease diffusion in aquatic plants, help in seed dispersal and germination, and act as membrane thickeners and food reserves.

The chief industrial sources of mucilages are Icelandic and Irish moss, flax or linseed, locust bean, slippery elm bark, and quince seed. They are usually extracted with water or a dilute sodium carbonate solution, purified by precipitation with alcohol or salt solutions from the aqueous solution, and marketed as powders. Mucilages are used in cosmetics, in medicine as laxatives and diuretics, as pharmaceutical emulsifying agents, and as materials that prevent precipitation of colloidal suspension.

Most mucilages are considered to be polysaccharides that contain the same group of sugars as gums and pectins; they commonly occur as salts. The cations are chiefly of calcium, magnesium, potassium, and sodium. The most common acids are uronic acids, such as mannuronic acid. Hydrolysis of mucilages yields pentoses and hexoses, the most common being arabinose, galactose, glucose, mannose, rhamnose, and xylose.

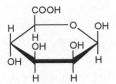

Fig. 4.17. *d*-mannuronic acid

The physical properties of mucilages are more important than their chemical properties. They are quite indigestible; however, even if polysaccharides were broken down in the digestive tract, the breakdown products, sugars and uronic acids, have little pharmacological effect and are generally regarded as inert. Whether or not this is the case in practice is not known.

Mucilage retains a large amount of water and hence maintains an elevated temperature, which progressively penetrates tissues. This makes mucilage useful in hot compresses—for example, linseed compresses. Mucilage also checks fermentation and bacterial growth, absorbs toxins, and assists the body in eliminating wastes. Like other water-soluble fibers, mucilage helps lower cholesterol, and its hydrophilic properties produce a sensation of fullness in the stomach without adding calories, making it useful for appetite suppression. In addition, a blood sugar–lowering effect has been observed in both diabetics and normal subjects.

Mucilage acts primarily as a local demulcent or emollient when it comes in direct contact with mucous membrane surfaces or skin. Here they produce a coating of "slime" that soothes and protects exposed or irritated surfaces of the gastrointestinal tract. They are used extensively in the management of inflammatory digestive disorders, especially when there is ulceration. Their relative indigestibility and hydrophilic properties have important influences on bowel behavior.

Laxative: The bulking effect of mucilage stimulates peristalsis.
Antidiarrheal: Small quantities of mucilage absorb excess water in the colon.

Gum Arabic

Gum arabic, or acacia gum, is the gum obtained from *Acacia senegal* and closely related species. *A. senegal* is a spiny tree up to 6 meters high that grows in the Sudan and Senegal. Harvesting starts with an incision through the bark to the cambium layer of the tree. The bark above and below the cut is removed so that an area of the cambium is laid bare. This injury stimulates the formation of gum as droplets in the cut, which dry to opaque balls with a crackled surface. The gum is collected 20 to 30 days after the incision is made.

Arabic acid, made up of calcium, potassium, and magnesium salts, is a major constituent of acacia gum. This acid is a branched-chain polysaccharide, the building blocks of which are D-galactose, L-arabinose, L-rhamnose, and D-glucuronic acid.[17]

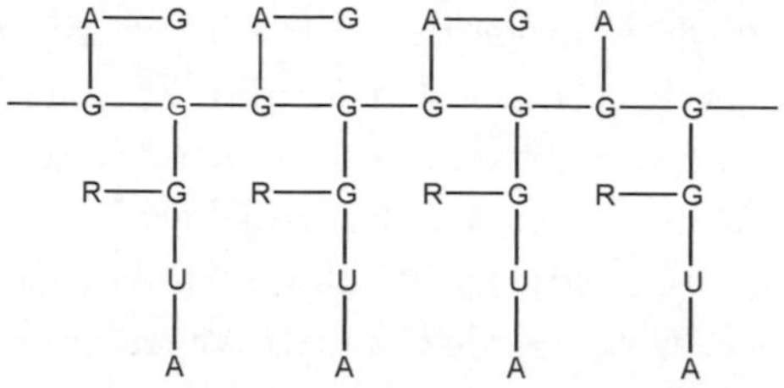

Fig. 4.18. General structure of arabic acid
(A = L-arabinose, R = L-rhamnose, G = D-galactose, U = D-glucuronic acid)

Gum acacia also contains oxidizing enzymes, such as peroxidases. For this reason, it should not be mixed with easily oxidized compounds. In pharmaceutical manufacturing, gum acacia is used as an emulsifier, as a constituent of suspensions, and in tablet production.

Tragacanth USP

Tragacanth is the gummy exudate from *Astragalus gummifer* and other Asiatic species of *Astragalus*.[18] When introduced into water, tragacanth absorbs a certain proportion of that liquid, swells greatly, and forms a soft adhesive paste, but does not dissolve. If agitated with water, this paste forms a uniform mixture, but in the course of one or two days most of the tragacanth separates out and is deposited, leaving a portion dissolved in the supernatant fluid. Several days should be allowed in order to obtain a uniform mucilage of the maximum gel strength. Tragacanth is wholly insoluble in alcohol.

Tragacanth powder is often used to stiffen a pill mass and render it adhesive. In glycerite form, it affords an excellent pill excipient. Tragacanth is also used as a suspending agent in lotions, mixtures, and various other preparations and prescriptions. It is used with emulsifying agents largely to increase consistency and retard creaming. The jellylike product formed when the gum is allowed to swell in water serves as the basis for pharmaceutical jellies, such as ephedrine sulfate jelly.

The constituent tragacanthin yields glucuronic acid and arabinose when hydrolyzed.

Guar Gum

Guar gum is obtained from the endosperm of the seed of *Cyamopsis tetragonolobus*, a plant cultivated in India, Pakistan, and the United States. Guar flour, milled from the seeds, contains about 86% water-soluble mucilage, which can be extracted by precipitation with ethanol. The main constituent is a galactomannan (with a molecular weight of about 220,000), a β-1,4-linked D-mannose linear polysaccharide with an α-1,6-linked D-galactose residue attached to every other D-mannose unit.

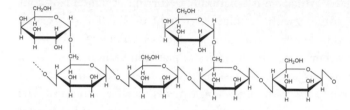

Fig. 4.19. Guar gum (partial structure)

Guar gum is used in pharmacy as a disintegrator in tablets, an emulsifier, and a thickener. It is also employed as a laxative. Taking guar gum before meals may lower blood glucose levels for diabetics. It also reduces the cholesterol level in blood serum, both in healthy people and in diabetics.[19]

Psyllium Seed and Husk

Psyllium seed is the ripe seed obtained from several *Plantago* species. The seeds are elliptical and 2 to 3 mm long, odorless, bland-tasting, and mucilaginous when chewed. The mucilages and hemicelluloses are located in the seed coat, or husk, making the husks about five times more active than the seeds. The mucilaginous husk of *P. ovata* separates fairly easily from the rest of the seed, so this is the species from which psyllium husk is derived.

To prepare psyllium for consumption, the whole seeds or husks are soaked in water for several hours; they are then taken with a large amount of liquid. The mucilage retains the moisture during gastrointestinal transit, promoting the passage of a soft stool after a transit time of 6 to 12 hours.

Agar

Agar (or agar agar) is a dried, hydrophilic, colloidal substance obtained from various species of red algae, including *Gelidium amansii*, *G. cartilagineum*, and *G. divaricatum*. The main constituents of the product are two polysaccharides:[20] *agarose*, a long-chain compound in which about 10% of the chains are esterified with sulfuric acid; and *agaropectin*, which differs from agarose in that significantly more chains are esterified with sulfuric acid.

Agar is sold commercially in the form of pale yellow strips or pieces or as a yellowish powder. Agar is indigestible and passes through the gastrointestinal tract almost unchanged. It undergoes little if any breakdown by intestinal microorganisms, which may account for its relatively low activity in the bowel. It acts solely through its ability to absorb water and swell within the intestine.

References

1. Behall KM, Scholfield DJ, Hallfrisch J. Effect of beta-glucan level in oat fiber extracts on blood lipids in men and women. *Journal of the American College of Nutrition* 1997; 16:46–51.

2. Estrada A, Yuri CH, Van Kessel A, et al. Immunomodulatory activities of oat beta-glucan in vitro and in vivo. *Microbiology and Immunology* 1997; 41:991–8.

3. Hallfrisch J, Scholfield DJ, Behall KM. Diets containing soluble oat extracts improve glucose and insulin responses of moderately hypercholesterolemic men and women. *The American Journal of Clinical Nutrition* 1995; 61:379–84.

4. Manzi P, Pizzoferrato L. Beta-glucans in edible mushrooms. *Food Chemistry* 2000; 68:315–18.

5. Borchers AT, Stem JS, Hackman RM, et al. Mushrooms, tumors, and immunity. *Proceedings of the Society for Experimental Biology and Medicine* 1999; 221:281–93.

6. Roberfroid MB, Delzenne NM. Dietary fructans. *Annual Review of Nutrition* 1998; 18:117–43.

7. Hauer J, Anderer FA. Mechanism of stimulation of human natural killer cytotoxicity by arabinogalactan from Larix occidentalis. *Cancer Immunology, Immunotherapy* 1993; 36:237–44.

8. Kelly GS. Larch arabinogalactan: clinical relevance of a novel immune-enhancing polysaccharide. *Alternative Medicine Review: A Journal of Clinical Therapeutic*. 1999; 4:96–103.

9. Harborne JB, Baxter H. *Phytochemical Dictionary: A Handbook of Bioactive Compounds from Plants*. London; Washington, DC: Taylor & Francis, 1993.

10. Ibid.

11. Ibid.

12. Ibid.

13. Thornalley PJ. Isothiocyanates: mechanism of cancer chemopreventive action. *Anticancer Drugs* 2002; 13(4):331–8.

14. Harborne JB, Baxter H. *Phytochemical Dictionary: A Handbook of Bioactive Compounds from Plants*. London; Washington, DC: Taylor & Francis, 1993.

15. Bradlow HL, Sepkovic DW, Telang NT, et al. Multifunctional aspects of the action of indole-3-carbinol as an anti-tumor agent. *Annals of the New York Academy of Sciences* 1999; 889:204–13.

16. Zeligs MA. Diet and estrogen status: the cruciferous connection. *Journal of Medicinal Food* 1998; 1:67–82.

17. Harborne JB, Baxter H. *Phytochemical Dictionary: A Handbook of Bioactive Compounds from Plants*. London; Washington, DC: Taylor & Francis, 1993.

18. Ibid.

19. Evans WC. *Trease & Evans' Pharmacognosy*, 13th edition. London: Baillere Tindall, 1989.

20. Harborne JB, Baxter H. *Phytochemical Dictionary: A Handbook of Bioactive Compounds from Plants*. London; Washington, DC: Taylor & Francis, 1993.

Suggested Reading

Bruneton J. *Pharmacognosy, Phytochemistry, Medicinal Plants*. Hampshire, UK: Intercept, 1999.

Evans WC. *Trease & Evans' Pharmacognosy*, 13th edition, London: Baillere Tindall, 1989.

Harborne JB, Baxter H. *Phytochemical Dictionary: A Handbook of Bioactive Compounds from Plants*. London; Washington, DC: Taylor & Francis, 1993.

5

_⁂_

LIPIDS

Lipids are a large and diverse class of organic molecules found in living systems. Most are insoluble in water but soluble in nonpolar solvents, such as alcohol. (This definition excludes the mineral oils and other petroleum products obtained from fossil material.) In a physiological sense, lipids are fundamentally important for both humans and plants.

Major classes of lipids include fatty acids, glycerol-derived lipids (including fats, oils, and phospholipids), the sphingosine-derived lipids (including ceramides, cerebrosides, gangliosides, and sphingomyelins), steroids and their derivatives, terpenes and their derivatives, certain aromatic compounds, and long-chain alcohols and waxes. Often lipids are found conjugated with proteins or carbohydrates, and the resulting substances are known as _lipoproteins_ and _lipopolysaccharides_. The fat-soluble vitamins can also be classified as lipids. The material in this chapter focuses on representative lipids found in medicinal plants.

Important Functions of Lipids

Among many other functions, lipids serve as the basis of cell membranes and as a form of fuel storage.

- Major structural components of all biological membranes
- Energy reserves and fuel for cellular activities
- Vitamins and hormones (lipids and lipid derivatives)
- Protective coatings with important immunological functions for cells
- Waterproof protective coverings in plants and some animals
- Blood-based carriers of fat-soluble vitamins such as A, D, E, and K

CLASSIFICATION OF LIPIDS

Any classification of lipids, whether by physical properties, chemistry, biological function, or occurrence, is arbitrary. The classification of lipids can be based on their physical properties, chemical structure, biological func-

tion, or occurrence. This makes the choice of classification arbitrary; ideally, it can be based on the interests of the classifier. Structural variations within each class are due to the different fatty acid residues that may be present.

Simple aliphatic (straight-chained) hydrocarbons act as structural backbones to which functional groups can be added to create various types of lipids. Those most often encountered within the creative cornucopia of plant cells include:

- Halogenated hydrocarbons
- Alcohols
- Sulfides
- Esters
- Fatty acids

Large, unsaturated hydrocarbons are common in plant waxes. As chain length and number of unsaturated bonds increase, the molecule becomes increasingly waxy and then solid at room temperature. In their functionalized forms, these are the lipids we know as fatty acids.

FATTY ACIDS

Fatty acids are C_{10} to C_{20} straight-chain compounds that have a single carboxyl radical. They play a profound nutritional role, supplying not only lipids to the diet but also vitamin F, the essential fatty acids used by the body to build and maintain membrane structures, among other functions.

The numbering of carbons in fatty acids begins with the carbon of the carboxyl group. Fatty acids that contain no carbon-carbon double bonds are termed _saturated fatty acids;_ those that contain double bonds are _unsaturated fatty acids_. The numbers used for fatty acids come from the number of carbon atoms, followed by the number of sites of unsaturation. For example, palmitic acid is a 16-carbon fatty acid with no unsaturation and is designated by 16:0. The site of unsaturation in a fatty acid is indicated by the symbol Δ and the number of the first carbon of the double bond. Thus, palmitoleic acid is a 16-carbon fatty acid

Most fatty acids come from the diet. However, the body can make all the various fatty acid structures needed, with two key exceptions. These are the highly unsaturated fatty acids linoleic acid and linolenic acid, which contain unsaturation sites beyond carbons 9 and 10. Because these two fatty acids cannot be synthesized from precursors in the body, they are known as *essential fatty acids*, as they must be provided in the diet. Since plants are capable of synthesizing linoleic and linolenic acid, humans can acquire these fats either by consuming a variety of plants or by eating the meat of animals that have consumed these plant fats.

Classification of Fatty Acids

In saturated fatty acids, all the bonds are filled. Unsaturated fatty acids contain double bonds, making such molecules more biochemically active. Cyclic monobasic fatty acids are less common, but include such clinically important molecules as chaulmoogric and hydnocarpic acids, which are discussed later in this chapter.

Table 5.1. Saturated Straight-Chain Acids

COMMON NAME	SYSTEMIC NAME	STRUCTURAL FORMULA
Butyric	n-tetranoic	$CH_3[CH_2]_2COOH$
Isovaleric	3-methy-butanoic	$[CH_3]_2CHCH_2COOH$
Caproic	n-hexanoic	$CH_3[CH_2]_4COOH$
Caprylic	n-hexanoic	$CH_3[CH_2]_6COOH$
Capric	n-octanoic	$CH_3[CH_2]_8COOH$
Lauric	n-decanoic	$CH_3[CH_2]_{10}COOH$
Myristic	n-tetradecanoic	$CH_3[CH_2]_{12}COOH$
Palmitic	n-hexadecanoic	$CH_3[CH_2]_{14}COOH$
Stearic	n-octadecanoic	$CH_3[CH_2]_{16}COOH$
Arachidic	n-eicosanoic	$CH_3[CH_2]_{18}COOH$

Structural Classification of Lipids

Fatty acids
- Saturated fatty acids
- Unsaturated fatty acids
- Branched-chain fatty acids
- Hydroxy fatty acids, including prostaglandins

Lipids containing glycerol
- Mono-, di-, and triacylglycerols (acylglycerols)
- Glyceryl ethers (alkoxydiglycerides)
- Glycosylmono- and glycosydiacyl-glycerols
- Phospholipids (phosphatides)
- Plasmalogens (acetal phosphatides)

Lipids containing sphingosine
- Sphingomyelins
- Ceramides
- Neutral glycosphingolipids (cerebrosides)
- Sialoglycosphingolipids (gangliosides)
- Sulfoglycosphingolipids (sulfatides)

Complex lipids
- Lipoproteins and proteolipids
- Lipopolysaccharides

Long-chain aliphatic alcohols and waxes

Hydrocarbons such as squalene and carotene

Sterols and related compounds such as vitamin D

with one site of unsaturation between carbons 9 and 10, and is designated by 16:1Δ9. Saturated fatty acids that contain fewer than eight carbon atoms are liquid at body temperature, whereas those containing more than 10 are solid. The presence of double bonds in fatty acids significantly lowers the melting point relative to that of saturated fatty acids.

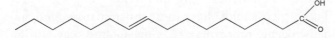

Fig. 5.1. Palmitoleic acid

Occurrence and Distribution

In plants, fatty acids occur mainly in bound form, esterified to glycerol, as fats or lipids. These lipids comprise up to 7% of the dry weight of leaves in higher plants, and are important as membrane constituents in chloroplasts and mitochondria. Considerable quantities of lipids also occur in the seeds or fruits of many plants, providing a stored form of energy to use during germination. Seed oils from

Table 5.2. Unsaturated Straight-Chain Acids

COMMON NAME	NUMBER OF UNSATURATED BONDS	STRUCTURAL FORMULA
Palmitoleic	1	$CH_3[CH_2]_5CH=CH[CH_2]_7COOH$
Oleic	1	$CH_3[CH_2]_7CH=CH[CH_2]_7COOH$
Linoleic	2	$CH_3[CH_2]_4CH=CHCH_2CH=CH-[CH_2]_7COOH$
Linolenic	3	$CH_3CH_2=CHCH_2CH=CHCH_2-CH=CH[CH_2]_7COOH$
Arachidonic	4	$CH_3[CH_2]_4CH=CHCH_2CH=CHCH_2-CH=CHCH_2CH=CH[CH_2]_3COOH$

plants such as olive, palm, coconut, soy, sunflower, rape, and peanut are exploited commercially as food fats, for soap manufacture, and in the paint industry. Plant fats, unlike animal fats, are rich in unsaturated fatty acids, and there is now abundant evidence that some of these are essential human dietary requirements.

Certain polyunsaturated fatty acids cannot be synthesized by humans and therefore must be supplied in food. These are the essential fatty acids, distinguished by double bonds beyond the one in the C-9 position (counted from the carboxyl end). Examples include omega-3 fatty acids (linoleic acid, linolenic acid, gamolenic acid, and *cis*-6, *cis*-9, and *cis*-12-octadecatrienoic acids) and the omega-6 fatty acid gamma linolenic acid.

Gamma-Linolenic Acid

Gamma-linolenic acid (GLA) is an unusual constituent of living matter that is found in very few plants. These include borage *(Borago officinalis)*, evening primrose *(Oenothera biennis)*, black currant *(Ribes nigrum)*, and hemp *(Cannabis sativa)*.[1]

GLA is an omega-6 (Ω-6) polyunsaturated fatty acid made up of 18 carbon atoms and three double bonds. It is a precursor in the synthesis of the beneficial series-1 prostaglandins. Through the synthesis of these prostaglandins, GLA can play a role in lowering blood pressure, making platelets less sticky, decreasing inflammation, and enhancing immune function. It may also help lower blood cholesterol and triglyceride levels.

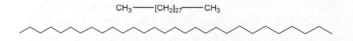

$$CH_3 —— [CH_2]_{27} —— CH_3$$

Fig. 5.2. Gamma-linolenic acid

Black Currant Seed Oil

Black currant seed oil, from the seeds of *Ribes nigrum*, contains about 15% to 20% GLA, making it a rich source of omega-6 fatty acids. Black currant seed oil also contains up to 20% of the omega-3 (Ω-3) polyunsaturated fatty acids alpha-linolenic (ALA) and linoleic acids. Research suggests that black currant oil has antithrombotic and anti-inflammatory actions. [2,3]

Borage Oil

Borage oil, from the seeds of *Borago officinalis*, is a rich source of GLA. The amount of GLA in borage oil, measured as the percentage of total fatty acid content, ranges from about 20% to 27%. Borage oil also contains approximately 10% alpha-linolenic acid (ALA).[4]

Evening Primrose Oil

Evening primrose oil, from the seeds of *Oenothera biennis*, contains approximately 7% to 14% GLA and about 10% linolenic acid.[5] According to research, evening primrose oil has demonstrated anti-inflammatory actions in some cases of rheumatoid arthritis. It may also be indicated in other inflammatory disorders, such as Sjogren's syndrome and ulcerative colitis.[6] It is approved in the United Kingdom as a pharmaceutical treatment for mastalgia and for atopic dermatitis, particularly to help with itching.[7]

Alpha-Linolenic Acid

Alpha-linolenic acid (ALA) is an omega-3 (Ω-3) polyunsaturated fatty acid containing 18 carbon atoms and three double bonds. ALA is metabolized to eicosapentaenoic acid (EPA), a precursor of the series-3 prostaglandins, the series-5 leukotrienes, and the series-3 thromboxanes. These eicosanoids have anti-inflammatory and antiatherogenic properties. ALA metabolites may also inhibit the production of the pro-inflammatory eicosanoids, prostaglandin E_2 and leukotriene B_4, as well as the pro-inflammatory cytokines, tumor necrosis factor-α, and interleukin β1.

The incorporation of ALA and its metabolites into cell membranes can affect membrane fluidity, which may play a role in the anti-inflammatory and antiplatelet actions of ALA. The Mediterranean diet, high in ALA, appears to lower the risk of coronary artery disease and certain types of cancer.[8]

Flaxseed Oil

Flaxseed oil, also known as flax or linseed oil, is made from the seeds of *Linum usitatissimum*. Flax is a very rich source of ALA, containing approximately 40% to 60% of this essential fatty acid. Linoleic acid and oleic acid are also present, but in smaller amounts (about 15% each). In addition, flaxseed oil contains secoisolariciresinol diglycoside, a type of phytoestrogen known as a lignan, in varying amounts. Flaxseed oil may have anti-inflammatory, antithrombotic, and antiproliferative activities.[9]

Chaulmoogric acid

Chaulmoogric acid, or *(S)*-13-(cyclopent-2-enyl) tridecanoic acid, is present in amounts of about 27% as the glyceride ester in chaulmoogra oil, extracted from seeds of *Hydnocarpus wightiana*. The ethyl ester has been used in the treatment of leprosy.[10]

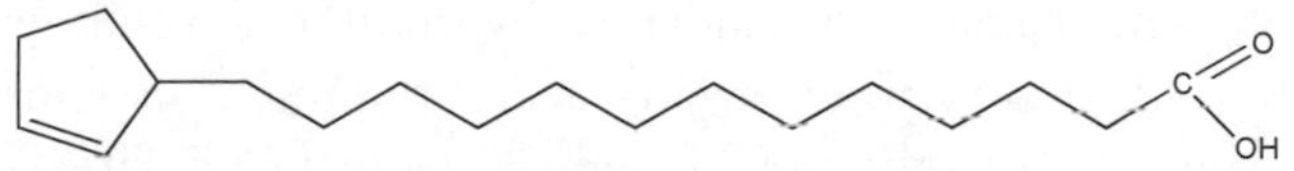

Fig. 5.3. Chaulmoogric acid

Prostaglandins

Prostaglandins can be regarded as derivatives of prostanoic acid. Prostanoic acid is not found in living tissue, so this is simply a chemical distinction. (Refer to chapter 9 for a detailed discussion on prostaglandin synthesis.)

All naturally occurring prostaglandins have a double bond in the *trans* configuration between C-13 and C-14. Additional double bonds in the *cis* configuration can occur between C-5 and C-6, as well as between C-17 and C-18. Depending on the substituents in the ring, prostaglandins are assigned to series E, F, D, and so on. According to the number of double bonds in the side chain, they are further divided into subgroups, such as E1, E2, F1, F2, and so on.

Prostaglandins occur in practically all tissues. However, they are not stored, but synthesized from the corresponding polyunsaturated C20 fatty acids only when needed. Depending on the organ, they show a variety of

physiological effects, discussed in detail in chapter 9. For example, PGE2 is a vasodilator and bronchodilator, and PGF2 is a vasoconstrictor and bronchoconstrictor.

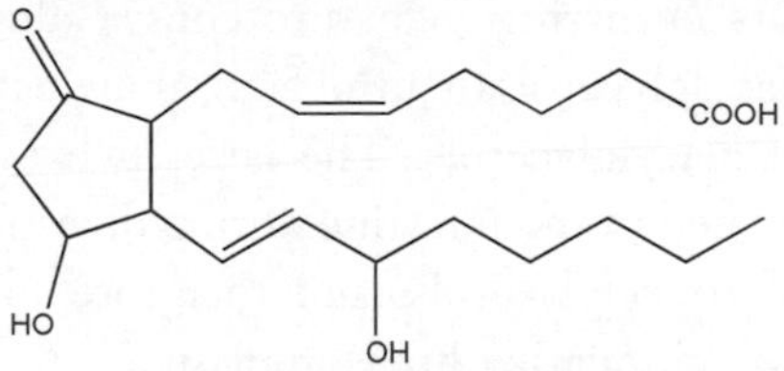

Fig. 5.4. Prostaglandin E2

Thromboxanes and prostacyclins are related to the prostaglandins. Thromboxane B2 is the metabolic product of the unstable thromboxane A2, which induces platelet aggregation. The prostacyclin (also known as prostaglandin PGI2) formed in the blood vessel wall, on the other hand, prevents platelet aggregation.

Fig. 5.5. Prostacyclin

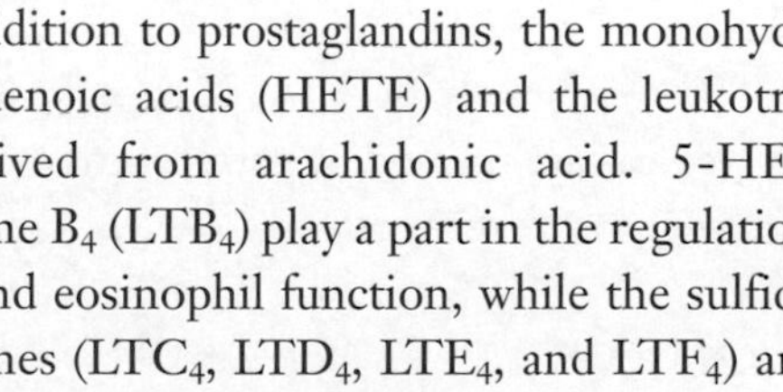

Fig. 5.6. Thromboxane B2

In addition to prostaglandins, the monohydroxy-(e)-icosatetraenoic acids (HETE) and the leukotrienes are also derived from arachidonic acid. 5-HETE and leukotriene B4 (LTB4) play a part in the regulation of neutrophil and eosinophil function, while the sulfidopeptide leukotrienes (LTC4, LTD4, LTE4, and LTF4) are important smooth muscle antispasmodics.

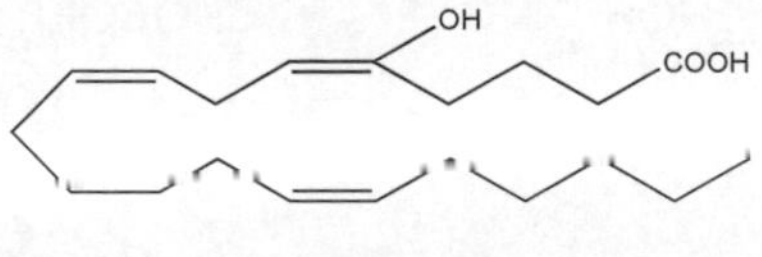

Fig. 5.7. 5-hydroxy-(e)-icosatetraenoic acid

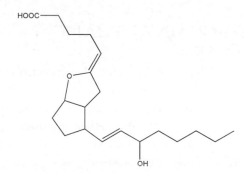

LIPIDS CONTAINING GLYCEROL

These lipids are composed of a glycerol backbone to which three fatty acids are esterified.

The fats occurring in nature consist almost exclusively of triacylglycerols (neutral fats), along with traces of mono- and diacylglycerols. The latter two esters, however, are formed in the intestine during digestion and absorption of triacylglycerols, and therefore may also be found among circulating lipids in plasma.

Natural fats may be solid or liquid at room temperature. At least 5 and up to 12 or more different fatty acids occur in these fats, which are a mixture of extremely diverse triacylglycerols. The fatty acids of most natural fats consist of mixtures of saturated and unsaturated acids. In general, the melting point of a fat increases with the proportion of saturated fatty acids it contains.

LONG-CHAIN ALIPHATIC ALCOHOLS

Aliphatic alcohols occur widely. Several alcohols belong to aroma compounds that play a role in environmental and food systems. They are found with normal, branched (mono- or isoprenoid), saturated or unsaturated chains of various length and sometimes with secondary or even tertiary alcohol functions.

Waxes

Waxes, strictly speaking, are esters of fatty acids with aliphatic straight-chain monohydric alcohols, usually cetyl alcohol and octadecyl alcohol, but frequently also with higher alcohols, up to C-30. Among the saturated fatty acids, cerotinic acid occurs most frequently; occasionally, hydroxy acids are also found. In many natural waxes, the fatty acid and alcohol components have the same chain length.

The epidermis of animals and plants excretes waxes as protective films against water loss or wetting. For example, the surface waxes of plants in very dry climates help the plants conserve water. In humid climates, the surface waxes of fruits and the lanolin found on the skin and in the hair of most furry animals repel excess moisture. In many zooplankton and other species of marine animals, waxes serve as energy reserve materials.

Urushiols (Alkylcatechols)

Urushiols have a side chain containing 15 or 17 carbon atoms; they may be saturated or unsaturated, with one to three double bonds.[11] These compounds, found in the oil of poison ivy and poison oak, produce contact dermatitis and are discussed in more detail in chapter 10.

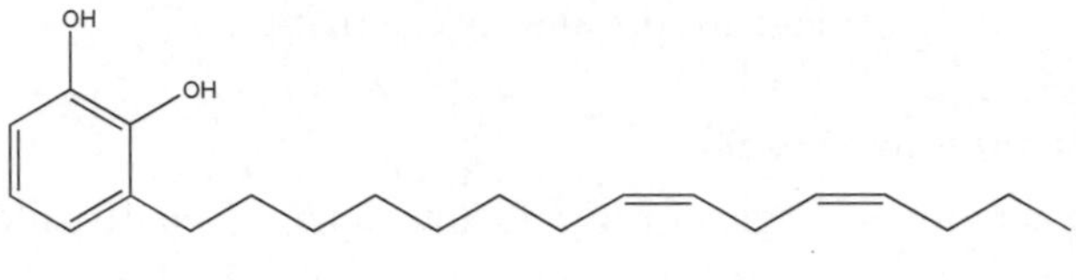

Fig. 5.8. Urushiol III

HYDROCARBONS

Straight-chained, or aliphatic, hydrocarbons resulting from decarboxylation of fatty acids are present in some plants. That is, they are thought to be metabolic breakdown products of fatty acids. They may be saturated or unsaturated, but unlike their fatty acid counterparts, they usually have an odd number of carbon atoms.

Turpentine is a rich source of saturated hydrocarbons

Acylglycerols

Acylglycerols are formed by esterification of glycerol with one, two, or three fatty acids, yielding a mono-, di-, or triacylglycerol, respectively.

CH_2OCOR	CH_2OH	CH_2OCOR^1	CH_2OCOR^1	CH_2OCOR^1
$\|$	$\|$	$\|$	$\|$	$\|$
$CHOH$	$CHOCOR$	$CHOCOR^2$	$CHOH$	$CHOCOR^2$
$\|$	$\|$	$\|$	$\|$	$\|$
CH_2OH	CH_2OH	CH_2OH	CH_2OCOR^3	CH_2OCOR^3
1-acylglycerol	2-acylglycerol	1,2-diacylglycerol	1,3-diacylglycerol	1,2,3-triacylglycerol
(α-monoacylglycerol)	(β-monoacylglycerol)	(α, β-diacylglycerol)	(α, α-diacylglycerol)	(triacylglycerol)

such as heptane. Turpentine is the volatile fraction distilled from the oleoresins of various pines, which is then further processed. Sources include *Pinus pinaster* and *P. hetero-phylla*.[12] See chapter 6 for a detailed discussion on these compounds.

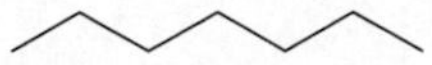

Fig. 5.9. Heptane

The primary source of saturated hydrocarbons in living plants is the waxy coating on some leaves and fruits. A common leaf wax constituent is nonacosone, found in the leaves of brussels sprouts *(Brassica oleracea* var. *gemmifera)*.

Unsaturated hydrocarbons play a pivotal role in plant metabolism. Ethylene is an important plant growth hormone, and isoprene is the building block of the whole gamut of terpenes, discussed in chapter 6.

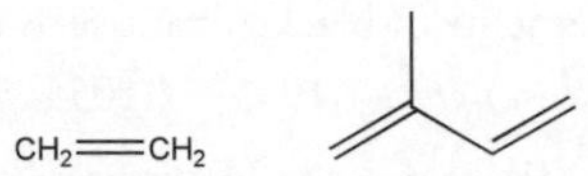

Fig. 5.10. Ethylene and isoprene

Polyacetylenes

These molecules contain a highly reactive triple bond, as found in the gas acetylene. They often contain additional functional groups, but can be conveniently classified here.

Many polyacetylenes are extremely toxic, such as the compound cicutoxin found in cowbane and water hemlock *(Cicuta virosa)*. Others, such as the antifungal compound wyerone found in broad beans *(Vicia faba)*, act as phytoalexins that protect the plant against fungal pathogens.

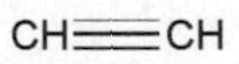

Fig. 5.11. Acetylene

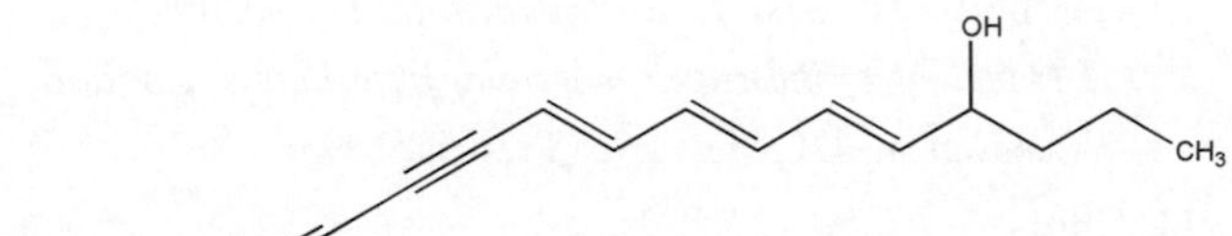

Fig. 5.12. Cicutoxin

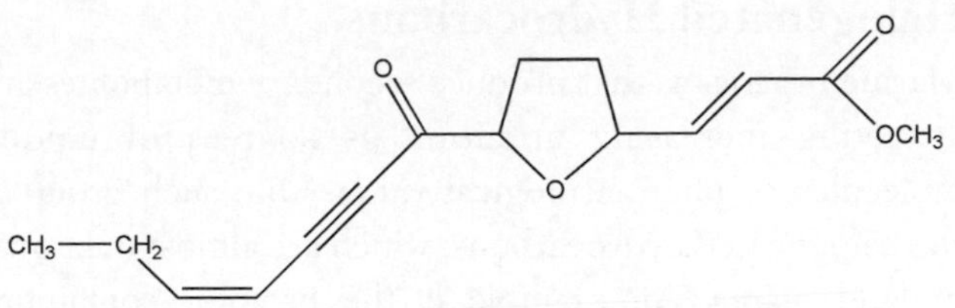

Fig. 5.13. Wyerone

Alkamides

There are more than 140 closely related alkamides, all of which have a more or less unsaturated aliphatic acid residue linked with different amine parts. Apart from a very few saturated derivatives from *Piper amalago*, the alkamides fall into two groups.

Compounds with purely alkene patterns. Purely alkene alkamides have been isolated from four plant families: Piperaceae, Aristolochiaceae, Rutaceae, and Asteraceae.

Compounds with alkene and alkyne linkages. Alkyne alkamides are restricted to the Asteraceae, and most are found in the Anthemideae and Heliantheae tribes. Eighty different acetylenic alkamides have been isolated from these tribes. This structural diversity stems from various combinations of 14 amine and 85 acid moieties. Such diversity provides valuable chemotaxonomic criteria.

Several alkamides, especially alkene isobutyl amides, are known for their insecticidal activity as well as for their pungent taste. They also produce local anesthesia of the mucous membranes, accompanied by profuse salivation. Plants that yield these substances have been used medicinally since ancient times, especially in cases of toothache. The position of double bonds and isomerism both play important roles in the physiological and insecticidal activities of the alkamides. A representative alkamide is affinin, which is found in the roots of the Mexican silagogue *Heliopsis longipes*.[13]

Most of the alkamides have been isolated from the Anthemideae and Heliantheae tribes of the family Asteraceae. Within these taxa, distribution is mainly confined to a few closely related genera.

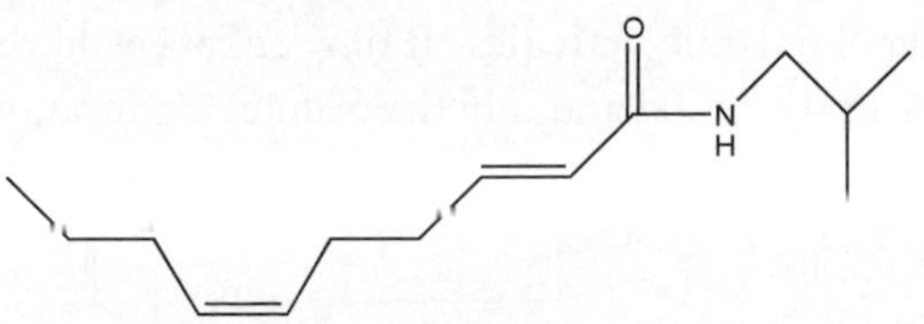

Fig. 5.14. Affinin.

Halogenated Hydrocarbons

Marine organisms that produce secondary metabolites are attracting increasing attention as sources of unique molecules of pharmacological value. One such group is the halogenated hydrocarbons, which are almost unknown in land plants. An example is the bromine-containing spirolaurenone from *Laurencia*, a genus of red algae.

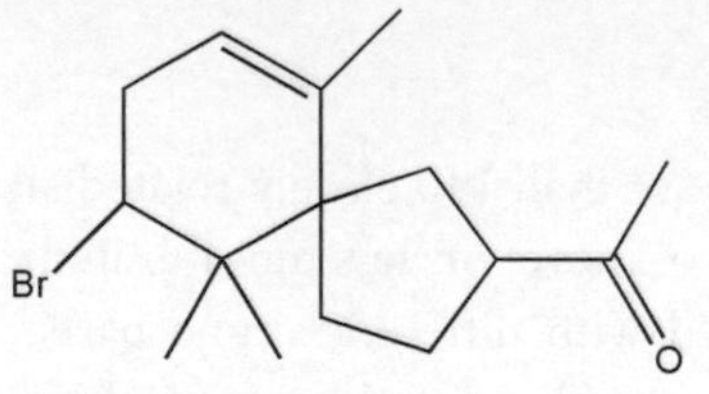

Fig. 5.15. Spirolaurenone

Alcohol Hydrocarbons

These are hydrocarbons that contain a hydroxyl group as part of the molecule. If biosynthetically derived from isoprene, alcohol hydrocarbons may be considered acyclic terpenes (for example, geraniol), which are discussed in chapter 6. A nonterpenoid example is octanol (caprylic alcohol). This volatile substance is a component of many orchid flower scents and is used in perfumery.

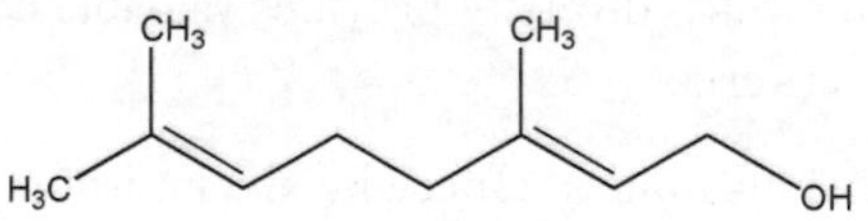

Fig. 5.16. Geraniol

Hydrocarbon Sulfides

Hydrocarbon sulfides are relatively uncommon in plants but of great importance in human diet and health care. These are odoriferous molecules (perhaps better termed *odious*, if one is English!) such as those found in garlic (*Allium sativum*) and skunk cabbage (*Symplocarpus foetidus*).

Allicin

The major odor principle of garlic, allicin is produced from the amino acid alliin by the enzyme alliinase when exposed to air. In both laboratory and clinical studies, allicin has demonstrated antidiabetic, antihypertensive, antibiotic, and hypolipidemic activities. It also enhances fibrinolytic activity in the blood and inhibits platelet aggregation.[14]

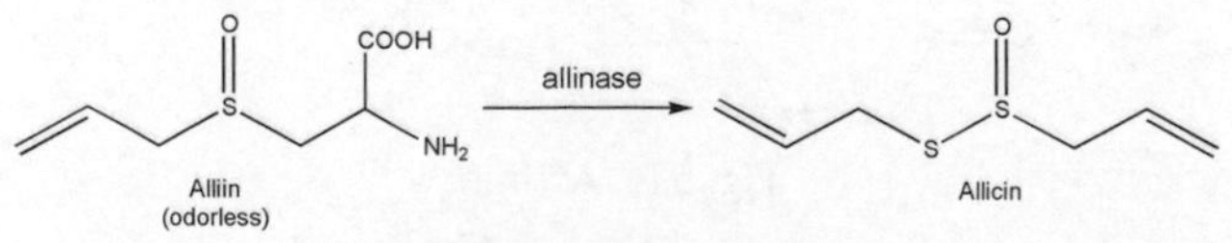

Fig. 5.17. Allicin

Hydrocarbon Esters

These condensation products of hydrocarbon alcohols and acids tend to have pleasant aromas. This reaction is fundamental to biochemistry, so a wide variety of esters exist. See chapter 6 for more information.

References

1. Evans WC. *Trease & Evans' Pharmacognosy*, 13th edition. London: Baillere Tindall, 1989.
2. Deferne JL, Leeds AR. Resting blood pressure and cardiovascular reactivity to mental arithmetic in mild hypertensive males supplemented with blackcurrant seed oil. *Journal of Human Hypertension* 1996; 10:531–7.
3. Watson J, Byars ML, McGill P, Kelman AW. Cytokine and prostaglandin production by monocytes of volunteers and rheumatoid arthritis patients treated with dietary supplements of blackcurrant seed oil. *British Journal of Rheumatology* 1993; 32:1055–58.
4. Evans WC. *Trease & Evans' Pharmacognosy*, 13th edition. London: Baillere Tindall, 1989.
5. Mills S, Bone K. *Principles and Practice of Phytotherapy: Modern Herbal Medicine*. Edinburgh: Churchill Livingstone, 1999.
6. Belch JJF, Hill A. Evening primrose oil and borage oil in rheumatologic conditions. *The American Journal of Clinical Nutrition* 2000; 71(suppl):352S–5S.
7. Huang Y-S, Mills DE, eds. *Gamma-linolenic Acid: Metabolism and Its Roles in Nutrition*. Champaign, IL: AOCS Press, 1996.
8. James MJ, Gibson RA, Cleland LG. Dietary polyunsaturated fatty acids and inflammatory mediator production. *The American Journal of Clinical Nutrition* 2000; 71(suppl):343S–48S.
9. Prasad K. Dietary flaxseed in prevention of hypercholesterolemic atherosclerosis. *Atherosclerosis* 1997; 132:69–76.
10. Harborne JB, Baxter H. *Phytochemical Dictionary: A Handbook of Bioactive Compounds from Plants*. London; Washington, DC: Taylor & Francis, 1993.
11. Ibid.
12. Evans WC. *Trease & Evans' Pharmacognosy*, 13th edition. London: Baillere Tindall, 1989.
13. Budavari S, ed. *The Merck Index*, 12th edition. Whitehouse Station, NJ: Merck, 1996.
14. Harborne JB, Baxter H. *Phytochemical Dictionary: A Handbook of Bioactive Compounds from Plants*. London; Washington, DC: Taylor & Francis, 1993.

Suggested Reading

Bruneton J. *Pharmacognosy, Phytochemistry, Medicinal Plants*. Hampshire, UK: Intercept, 1999.

Evans WC. *Trease & Evans' Pharmacognosy*, 13th edition. London: Baillere Tindall, 1989.

Harborne JB, Baxter H. *Phytochemical Dictionary: A Handbook of Bioactive Compounds from Plants*. London; Washington, DC: Taylor & Francis, 1993.

6

❧

TERPENES

The terpenes, also known as isoprenoids, are the largest group of secondary plant metabolites. More than 20,000 structures have been described.[1] The name *terpene* comes from *turpentine*, which in turn comes from the old French *ter(e)binth*, meaning "resin." They are all derived chemically from 5-carbon isoprene units assembled in different ways.

Terpenes of different sizes and composition are found throughout all classes of organisms. Larger terpenoid molecules are essential components of human metabolism and include the adrenal hormones, the membrane component cholesterol, and the lipid soluble vitamins A, E, and K. An even greater variety of terpenoid molecules exist as secondary metabolites in plants and fungi, as well as some bacteria and insects.

While not essential for viability, terpenes enable plants to prosper in their specific environments. They have a variety of natural functions. They may be flavors or scents or act as growth regulators, defense secretions, or pollinator attractants. Terpenes appear to have evolved quite separately within small groups of organisms, and therefore comprise a great diversity of structures capable of specific interactions with a range of biological receptors.

Plants with distinctive terpenes provide many of the compounds used as research leads for pharmaceutical, agricultural, and other commercial applications.

- Paclitaxel (taxol) from yew trees inhibits mammalian cell division and is used clinically in cancer treatment.
- α-santonin is one of the anthelmintic components of *Artemisia* spp.
- Artemisinin, from *Artemisia annua*, is active against malaria, including strains that have developed resistance to quinine derivatives.
- Pyrethrins from *Tanacetum cinerariifolium* provide biodegradable insecticides.
- Stevioside, a compound that is hundreds of times sweeter than sucrose, is a valuable sweetener.

CLASSIFICATION OF TERPENES

The molecules in this diverse group are all biosynthesized from the 5-carbon precursor isoprene, and so are also known as isoprenoids. The isoprene units can be assembled and modified in thousands of different ways, allowing plants to produce a seemingly endless number of chemical variations based on the simple unit. Most are multicyclic structures that differ from one another not only in functional groups, but also in their basic carbon skeletons. This group includes essential oils and resins, steroids, carotenoids, and rubber.[2]

Major Groups of Terpenoids

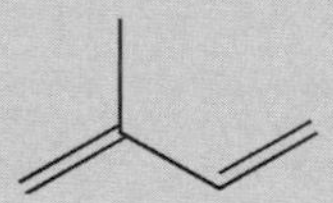

Fig. 6.1. Isoprene

NAME	NUMBER OF CARBONS	EXAMPLE
Monoterpenes	10 (2 x 5)	Volatile oils
Sesquiterpenes	15 (3 x 5)	Volatile oils
Diterpenes	20 (4 x 5)	Resins
Triterpenes	30 (6 x 5)	Saponins, sterols, steroids
Tetraterpenoids	40 (8 x 5)	Carotenoid pigments
Polyprenes	(N x 5)	Rubbers

MONOTERPENES

Monoterpenes, the C_{10} representatives of the terpenoid family, are derived from the union of two isoprene precursors joined head to tail. Monoterpenes and the related sesquiterpenes are important components of plant essential oils, or volatile oils. Monoterpenes tend to occur in members of certain plant families, such as Lamiaceae, Pinaceae, Rutaceae, and Apiaceae, from which many essential oils are commercially produced.[3] Some of these compounds, such as geraniol, are almost ubiquitous and can be found in small amounts in the volatile secretions of most plants.

Volatile oils occur in plants that have specialized secretory structures, such as oil cells, glandular hairs, and resin ducts. In plants, they are believed to help attract pollinators to flowers, defend green tissues from predation by herbivores, and protect against microbial infection.

Monoterpenes are volatile, aromatic, colorless, oily substances, although a few (such as camphor) are crystalline. They are not soluble in water, but some contain polar groups that facilitate the formation of emulsions in which the oil disperses in droplets.

Classification of Monoterpenes

Monoterpenes may be classified either by their structures or according to their functional groups.

Table 6.1. Functional Classification

FUNCTIONAL GROUP	EXAMPLE
Unsaturated hydrocarbons	Limonene
Alcohols	Linalool
Alcohol esters	Linalyl acetate
Aldehydes	Citronellal
Ketones	Carvone

Optical isomerism is a common feature of monoterpenes, and some compounds, such as carvone, can occur in more than one optically active form. Although any given plant rich in essential oils may have only a few major constituents, it may contain up to 50 other monoterpenes in smaller amounts.

In some plants, there may be considerable chemical variation within the species; different plant populations contain different mixtures of monoterpenes. Plants displaying these chemical variations are called *chemotypes*. For example, 13 different chemotypes of thyme have been recognized among populations growing in France.

Hydrocarbons

These are monoterpenes with a purely hydrocarbon-based functional group.

Limonene

(+)-Limonene is the main constituent of volatile oils from the fresh peel of *Citrus* fruits, such as lemon, tangerine, bitter orange, and sweet orange. It also occurs in neroli oil (orange flower oil, from *Citrus aurantium* var. *amara*) and in oils of caraway *(Carum carvi)* and dill *(Anethum graveolens)*. (-)-Limonene is present in oil of fir, made from the needles and young twigs of *Abies alba*, and in mint oils, from *Mentha* species.

Limonene has expectorant and sedative activities. Various essential oils containing limonene are used to flavor foods and beverages. In addition, this molecule has attracted much research attention as a representative monoterpene.[4] It has demonstrated potential cancer-preventive properties, antineoplastic activity in both pancreatic and breast cancer, and clinical application as a solvent of gallstones. [5,6,7] Pure limonene may be irritating to the skin.[8]

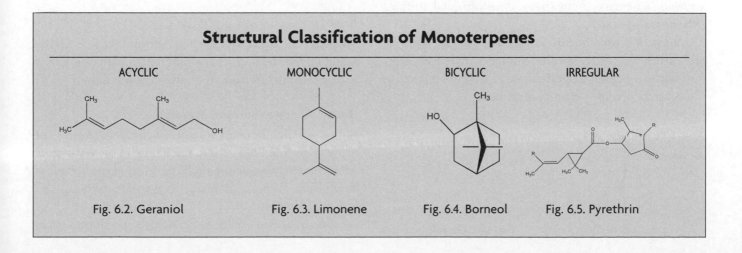

Structural Classification of Monoterpenes

ACYCLIC — Fig. 6.2. Geraniol

MONOCYCLIC — Fig. 6.3. Limonene

BICYCLIC — Fig. 6.4. Borneol

IRREGULAR — Fig. 6.5. Pyrethrin

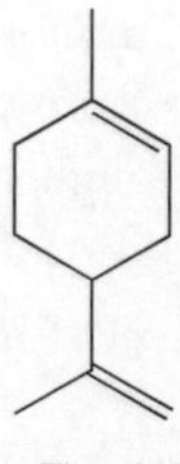

Fig. 6.6.
Limonene

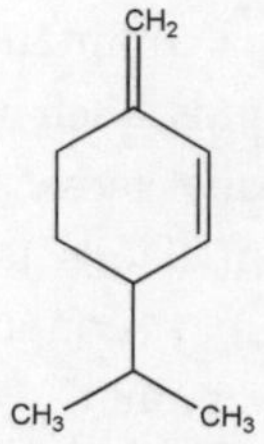

Fig. 6.7.
β-phellandrine

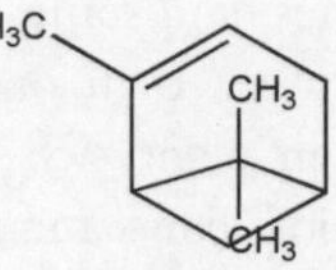

Fig. 6.8.
α-pinene

β-phellandrene

β-phellandrene is a very common constituent of essential oils. One isomeric form occurs in the volatile oils of several fir (*Abies*), spruce (*Picea*), and pine (*Pinus*) species, while another is the main constituent of the essential oil from the seeds of the water fennel (*Oenanthe aquatica*).[9] It has expectorant properties and is abundant in pharmaceutical pine needle oil.

α-pinene

This is an important constituent of many essential oils, especially oil of turpentine, which is distilled from the oleoresin of *Pinus palustris* and other *Pinus* species. Other examples include many oils from Pinaceae, Cupressaceae, Myrtaceae, and Lamiaceae and oils made from the peel of *Citrus* species.

Pinene is an irritant that can cause skin eruption, delirium, ataxia, and kidney damage.[10] It is used in the manufacture of camphor, insecticides, perfume bases, and synthetic pine oil.[11]

Alcohols

These are monoterpenes with a hydroxyl group attached.

Borneol

The (+) form of borneol is the main constituent of Borneo camphor, distilled from *Dryobalanops aromatica*, and is also present in oils of spike lavender (*Lavandula latifolia*), rosemary (*Rosmarinus officinalis*), and nutmeg (*Myristica fragrans*).

Borneol is used mainly for the manufacture of its esters, which are widely used in cosmetics. However, some free borneol is used in perfumery. It has toxic effects in the central nervous system of mammals.[12]

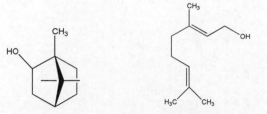

Fig. 6.9. Borneol

Fig. 6.10. Geraniol

Geraniol

Geraniol is the main constituent of a number of essential oils, including palmarosa oil (*Cymbopogon martinii*) and oils from allied species, such as lemongrass (*C. citratus*) and citronella (*C. nardus*). It is also found in oil or attar of rose from *Rosa centifolia*, *R. damascena*, and other roses.

Geraniol has strong antiseptic activity, which is seven times stronger than that of phenol. It has a sweet rose odor, and is used in perfumery and as an insect attractant in traps.[13]

Linalool

This is the main constituent of oil of coriander (*Coriandrum sativum*). It also occurs in lavender oils (from the flowering tops of *Lavandula* spp.), in oil of bergamot (*Citrus aurantium* ssp. *bergamia*), orange flowers (*C. aurantium* var. *amara*), and many other essential oils.

Linalool is antiseptic and fungistatic; it also has sedative properties.[14] It is used in perfumery as a substitute for bergamot and French lavender oils.[15]

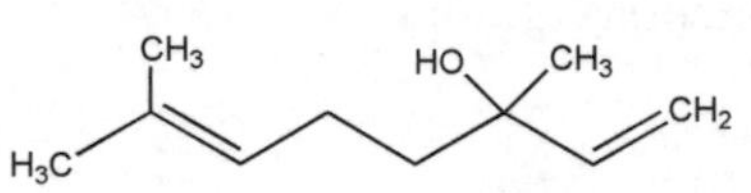

Fig. 6.11. Linalool

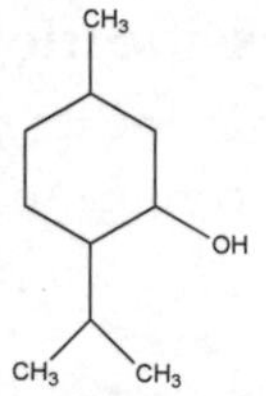

Fig. 6.12. Menthol

Menthol

Menthol occurs in both free and ester forms as the main constituent of peppermint oil, the steam-distilled volatile oil from *Mentha piperita* and other *Mentha* species.

Used as an inhalant, menthol helps to relieve symptoms of bronchial and nasal congestion, and acts as a carminative and gastric sedative when used internally. Applied topically, it has antipruritic, analgesic, and antiseptic effects.[16] However, it can give rise to rare hypersensitivity reactions, such as contact dermatitis.

Esters

Monoterpene esters have a general formula of R-C-O-R1. R and R1 may be the same or different, and may be either aliphatic (straight-chained) or aromatic (cyclic).

Bornyl Acetate (borneol acetate)

Bornyl acetate occurs in volatile oils from the needles of many pine and fir species, including *Pinus pinaster*, *P. sylvestris*, *Abies alba*, and *A. sibirica*, and also certain Lamiaceae plants, such as rosemary (*Rosmarinus officinalis*) and thyme (*Thymus vulgaris*).

Bornyl acetate smells like pine needles. Bornyl esters

of acetic, formic, and isovaleric acids occur in the volatile oil from the rhizome and root of valerian (*Valeriana officinalis*).

Pine needle oil has expectorant properties and is used as a bronchial and nasal inhalant. (+)-Bornyl isovalerate is sedative.[17]

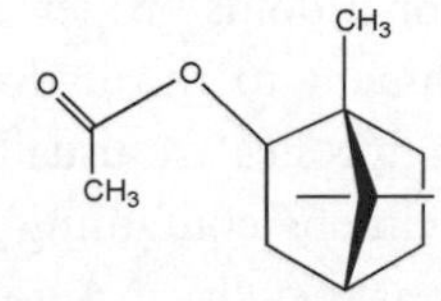

Fig. 6.13. Bornyl acetate

Aldehydes

Aldehydes are compounds that contain the carbonyl group CO, and in which the carbonyl group is bonded to at least one hydrogen. The general formula for an aldehyde is RCHO, in which R is hydrogen or an alkyl or aryl group. Low-molecular-weight aldehydes, such as formaldehyde and acetaldehyde, have sharp, unpleasant odors. Higher-molecular-weight aldehydes, such as benzaldehyde and furfural, have pleasant, often flowery odors and are found in essential oils.

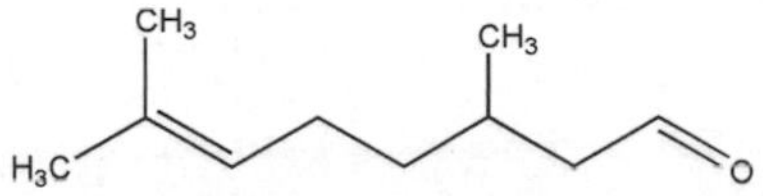

Fig. 6.14. Citronellal

Citronellal

Citronellal is the main constituent of citronella oil, made from the fresh leaves of *Cymbopogon nardus*. It also occurs in the volatile oils of *Eucalyptus* species, lemon balm (*Melissa officinalis*), lemon (*Citrus limon*), and various other plants.

Oil of lemon balm has antiseptic and sedative properties. It is used in soap, perfumes, and as an insect repellent.[18]

Ketones

Monoterpene ketones are compounds that contain the carbonyl group CO, and in which this carbonyl group is bonded only to carbon atoms. The general formula for a ketone is RCOR′.

Camphor

The (+) form of camphor is found in rectified or Japanese oil of camphor, made from the camphor tree (*Cinnamomum camphora*). The (-) form occurs in feverfew (*Tanacetum parthenium*) and various species of *Artemisia* and *Lavandula*.

Camphor is irritating to the skin and has been used as

a rubefacient. It is initially cooling to the skin and has mild anesthetic and antipruritic actions. It is used as a moth repellent and as a preservative in pharmaceuticals and cosmetics.[19]

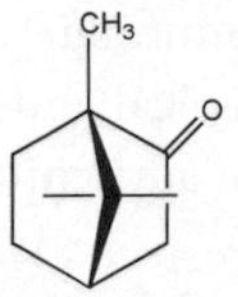

Fig. 6.15. Camphor 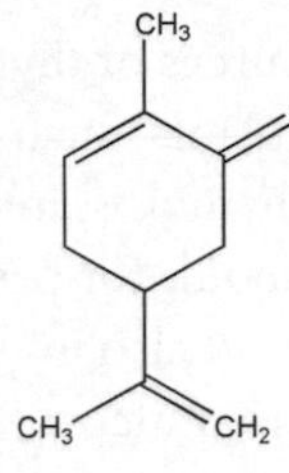   Fig. 6.16. Carvone

Carvone

Carvone is the main constituent in oil of spearmint (*Mentha spicata*), and (+)-carvone is the major constituent of oils of caraway and dill, from the dried ripe fruits of *Carum carvi* and *Anethum graveolens*, respectively. Carvone has carminative and antiseptic actions.[20] It is used in the manufacture of liqueurs, for flavoring confectioneries, and in perfumes and soaps.

Phenols

The isoprene units in monoterpene phenols are assembled so that there is a benzene ring in the molecule to which a hydroxyl group is attached.

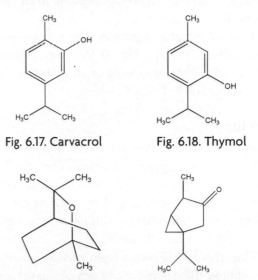

Fig. 6.17. Carvacrol   Fig. 6.18. Thymol

Fig. 6.19. 1,8-cineole   Fig. 6.20. Thujone

Carvacrol

This constituent is found in a number of oils from Lamiaceae plants, including oregano oil, distilled from the flowering tops of *Origanum vulgare*, and thyme oil, from the leaves and tops of *Thymus vulgaris*.

Carvacrol is strongly antiseptic, demonstrating one and a half times the activity of phenol. It also shows antifungal and anthelmintic properties. It is used commercially in mouthwashes.[21]

Thymol

The best sources of thymol are the essential oils of some Lamiaceae plants, such as *Thymus vulgaris* and *Monarda punctata*. Thymol is antiseptic and antifungal. It is used to destroy mold, for preserving botanical and biological specimens, and also in dentistry as an antiseptic.[22] It may irritate gastric mucosa.

1,8-cineole (eucalyptol, cajeputol)

This is the main constituent in oil of eucalyptus (*Eucalyptus globulus* and some other *Eucalyptus* spp.), oil of cajeput (*Melaleuca leucadendron* and other *Melaleuca* spp.), and many other essential oils. It has anthelmintic, expectorant, and antiseptic activities, and also shows cockroach-repellent activity.[23]

Thujone (thujan-3-one)

Thujone occurs as a mixture of two stereoisomers that differ in the stereochemistry of the 4-methyl group. It is found in many essential oils, such as white cedar oil from the leaves of *Thuja occidentalis*, tansy oil from the leaves and tops of *Tanacetum vulgare*, and, together with thujyl alcohol and acetate, in wormwood oil from the aerial parts of *Artemisia absinthium*.

Thujone is highly toxic; ingestion may cause convulsions.[24] (Please see chapter 10 for more information.) Wormwood oil has been used as an anthelmintic agent and cedar leaf oil as a rubefacient.

Iridoids

Iridoids are bitter-tasting monoterpenoid lactones derived from monoterpene precursors. They are found in about 70 families of flowering plants distributed in 13 orders.[25] They are characterized by a cyclopentanodihydropyran ring, shown below with the numbering system used in iridoid nomenclature.[26]

The term *iridoid* comes from *iridodial*, a compound first found in the defense secretions of the fire ant, *Irido myrmex*. Similar structures occur in the defense secretions of other ants, stick insects, and beetles.

There is no consensus on the classification of iridoids, of which more than 1,000 have been identified. In *The Dictionary of Natural Products*, three subcategories are described.[27]

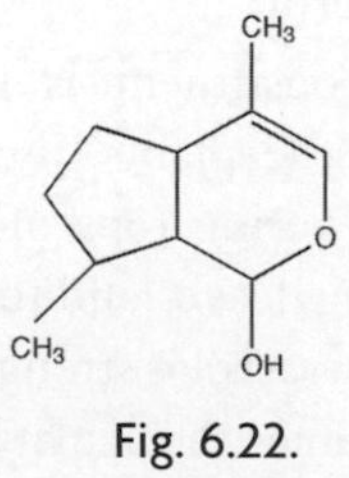

Iridoid Glycosides

Iridoid glycosides, or iridoids proper, are lactones, often with glucose attachment to the hydroxyl group of the lactone ring. The aglycones are usually highly unstable, and herbarium specimens containing iridoid glucosides also often turn dark as they dry.[28] A good example of this group is aucubin (below).

Simple Iridoids

Simple iridoids are volatile aglycones. An example is nepetalactone, the psychoactive constituent of catnip (*Nepeta cataria*), the plant so loved by members of the cat family.[29] The valepotriates, such as valtrate from *Valeriana officinalis*, also possess this action. These mainly nonglucosidic iridoids are sedatives.[30]

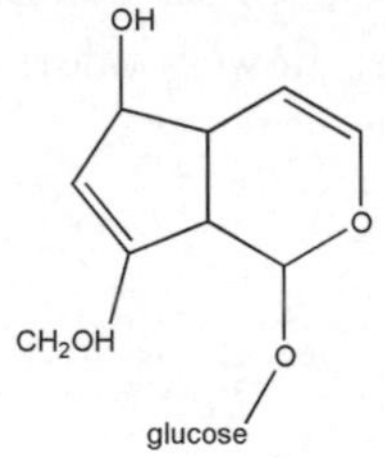

Fig. 6.23. Aucubin

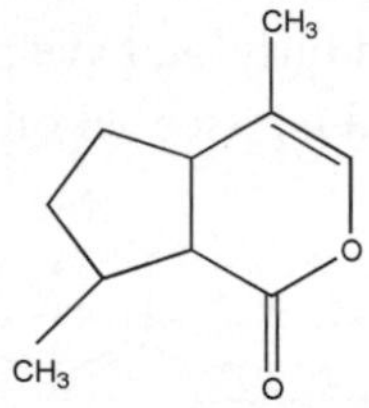

Fig. 6.24. Nepetalactone

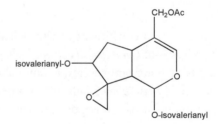

Fig. 6.25. Valtrate

Secoiridoids

Secoiridoids are distinguished by an open 5-membered ring. They are biosynthetic precursors of terpene alkaloids, and often occur with their related alkaloids. Gentiopicrin is a good example.[31]

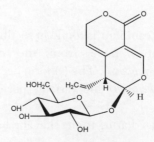

Fig. 6.26. Gentiopicrin

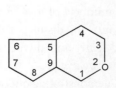

Fig. 6.21.
Cyclopentanodihydropyran
ring

Fig. 6.22.
Iridodial

Pharmacological Activity of Iridoids

Plants containing iridoids play a central role in herbalism, as they are often the basis of what is known as the *bitter principle*.[32] Iridoids are the bitterest of plant compounds, with a taste perceptible at a dilution as high as 1:50,000. Bitters are known to stimulate the release of gastrin in the gastrointestinal tract, leading to an increase in digestive secretions, including bile. Many are used as bitter tonics, such as bogbean *(Menyanthes trifoliata)*, and others as anti-inflammatory agents, including eyebright *(Euphrasia officinalis)*.

Iridoids that are found as glycosides, such as fulvo-plumierin and allamandin, have demonstrated antimicrobial or antileukemic activities in laboratory studies.[33] Aucubin and various other iridoid glucosides show laxative and diuretic properties, while the valepotriates are sedative. In large concentrations and in the presence of acids, iridoid glycosides are toxic.

Asperuloside

This compound is found in many species of the Rubiaceae family—for example, sweet woodruff *(Galium odorata)* and cleavers *(G. aparine)*. It has a laxative action.[34]

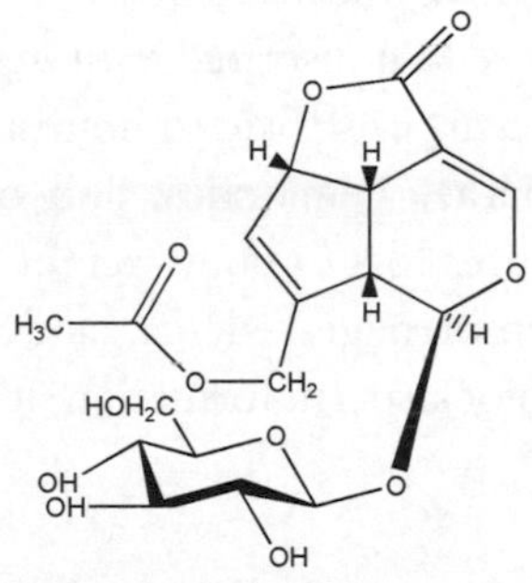

Fig. 6.27. Asperuloside

Aucubin

Common in many families of dicotyledons, aucubin has laxative and diuretic properties. The aglycone, aucubigenin, shows antimicrobial and antitumor activities, but is toxic to mammals.[35]

Gentiopicrin (gentiopicroside)

This is found in the roots of *Gentiana lutea* and in other plants of the Gentianaceae family. It has demonstrated antimalarial activity.[36]

Harpagoside

Found in the roots of devil's claw *(Harpagophytum procumbens)*, in the rhizomes of Chinese figwort *(Scrophularia buergeriana)*, and in some *Lamium* species, harpagoside demonstrates analgesic activity.[37] It is also extremely bitter.

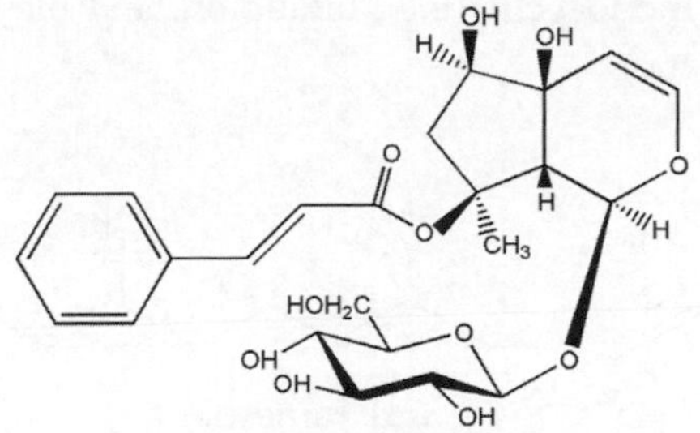

Fig. 6.28. Harpagoside

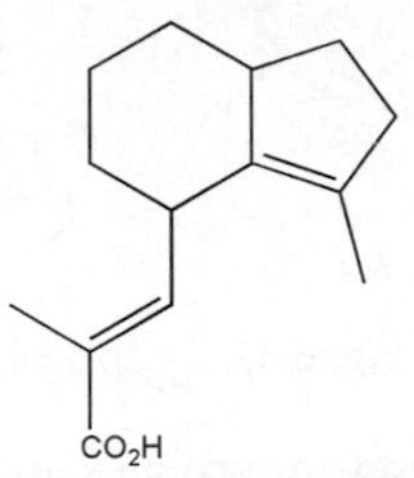

Fig. 6.29. Valerenic acid

Valerenic Acid

This compound is well known because of its occurrence in *Valeriana officinalis*, in which it contributes to the herb's antispasmodic activity.[38]

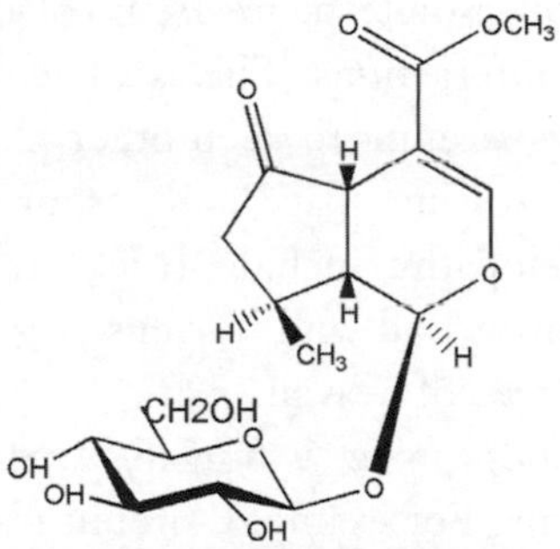

Fig. 6.30. Verbenalin

Verbenalin

Verbenalin is found in *Verbena officinalis*. Its activity weakly resembles that of ergot in promoting uterine contractions. It is also a mild parasympathomimetic agent, gently relaxing the autonomic nervous system.[39]

SESQUITERPENES

The sesquiterpenes are derived from three isoprene units. Based on biogenetic origin, there are more than 200 different structural types of sesquiterpenes, and several thousand such compounds are known.[40]

Classification of Sesquiterpenoids

These compounds can be conveniently classified into three main groups according to structure: acyclic (e.g., farnesol), monocyclic (e.g., bisabolol), and bicyclic (e.g., caryophylene).

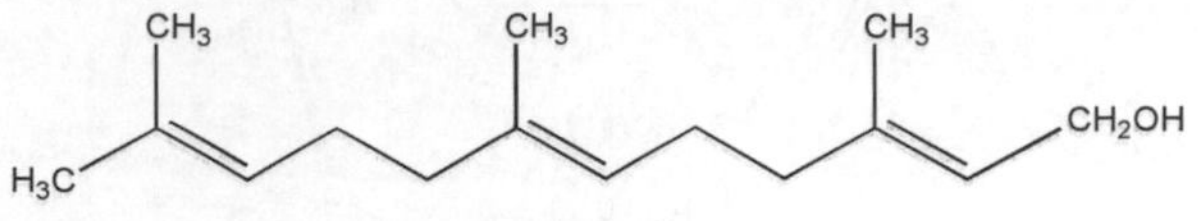

Fig. 6.31. Farnesol

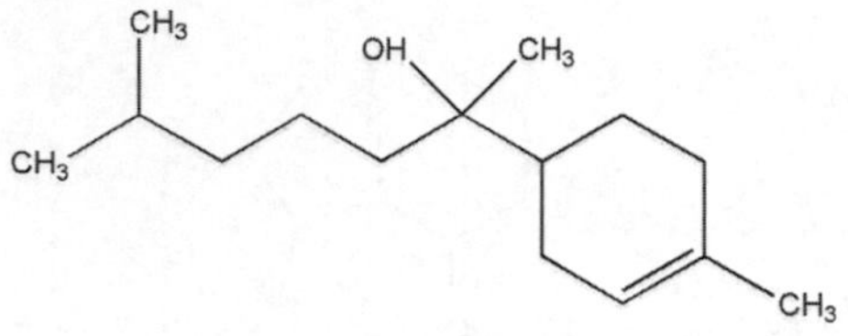

Fig. 6.32. Bisabolol

One large group of sesquiterpenes, made up of those with an additional lactone function, is discussed later in this chapter under the heading Sesquiterpene Lactones.

In addition to higher plants, sesquiterpenes are well represented in bryophytes, fungi, microorganisms, and some marine animals and insects. It appears that this class of molecules fulfills a number of ecological roles.

- A number of sesquiterpenes are involved in *allelopathic* plant-plant interactions. This is a chemical process by which plants attempt to keep other plants from competing for growing space and resources. Plants that employ allelopathy include black walnut, *Artemisia* species (wormwood and various sagebrushes), sunflower, and tree of heaven.
- Sesquiterpenes can act as fungal *pheromones*, or chemical attractants. For example, sirenin is involved in the attraction of gametes in fungi of the genus *Allomyces*. In addition, a number of sesquiterpenes have roles as pheromones in insects.
- Several sesquiterpenoid phytoalexins have been found, mostly in the Solanaceae family. *Phytoalexins* are formed as chemical responses to infection or infestation in plants.
- Many sesquiterpenes play a defensive role as allomones in plant-insect and plant-fungal interactions. *Allomones* are chemicals produced by one species that act on another species.

β-caryophylene

β-caryophylene occurs as a mixture of α-caryophylene and isocaryophylene in many essential oils, such as oil of clove, prepared from the dried flower buds of *Syzygium aromaticum*, and oil of copaiba, the oleoresin from species

of *Copaifera*. α-caryophylene is synonymous with humulene. β-caryophylene is widely used in perfumery.[41]

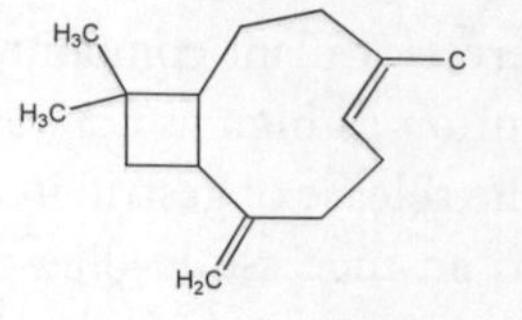

Fig. 6.33. Caryophylene

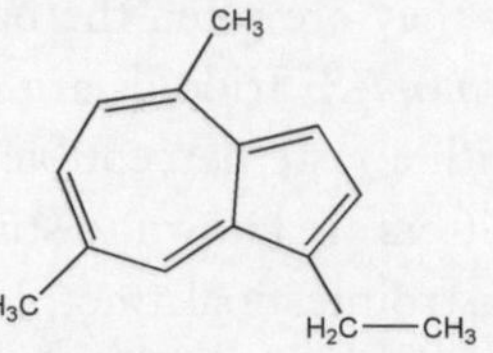

Fig. 6.34. Chamazulene

Chamazulene

Chamazulene is a component of the blue oil produced by steam distillation of chamomile (*Matricaria recutita*), wormwood (*Artemisia absinthium*), and yarrow (*Achillea millefolium*). In addition, sesquiterpene lactones found in these plants are converted to matricin and achillin during distillation. Chamazulene has anti-inflammatory and antipyretic activities.[42]

Gossypol

Gossypol occurs in a *racemic* form in the seeds of cotton (*Gossypium* spp.), meaning that it is a mixture of dextrorotatory and levorotatory isomers in such proportions that the mixture has no optical activity.

Gossypol has demonstrated antifungal and antitumor activities. However, it is toxic to nonruminant mammals, birds, insect larvae, nematodes, and other animals. In mammals, it causes loss of body weight, diarrhea, cardiac irregularity, hemorrhage, edema, and other ill effects. Because it can block sperm formation, it may act as a male contraceptive.[43]

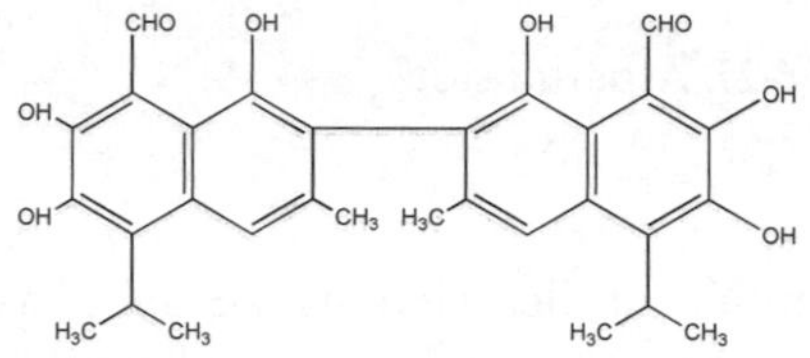

Fig. 6.35. Gossypol

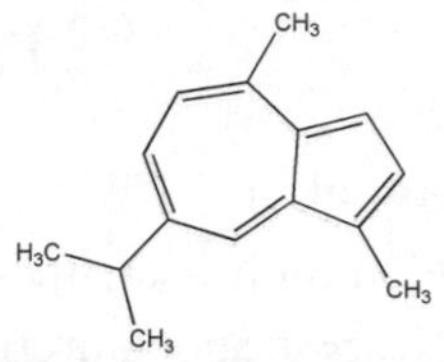

Fig. 6.36. Guaiazulene

Guaiazulene

Guaiazulene is a component of the blue oil produced during the steam distillation of chamomile (*Matricaria recutita*) and guaiac wood (*Guaiacum officinale* or *G. sanctum*), formed from structurally related substances present in these plants. It has anti-inflammatory activity.[44]

Humulene

This is a constituent of many essential oils, including hops (*Humulus lupulus*). Humulene is used in perfumery.[45]

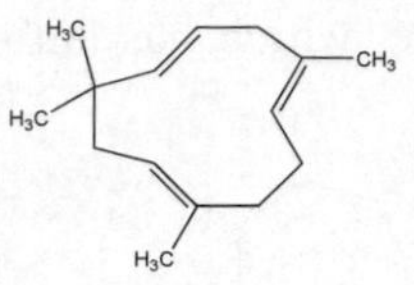

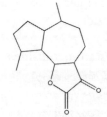

Fig. 6.37. Humulene 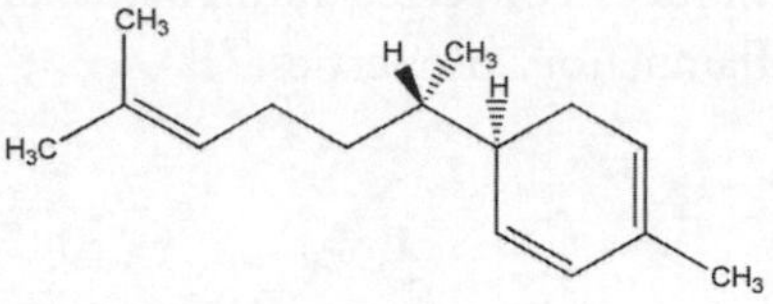   Fig. 6.38. Zingiberene

Zingiberene

Zingiberene occurs in the rhizomes of ginger (*Zingiber officinale*) and in the related *Curcuma* species. Oil of ginger has a carminative activity. It is used as a flavoring agent.[46]

SESQUITERPENE LACTONES

Sesquiterpene lactones are a class of natural sesquiterpenes, distinct from other members of the group because of the presence of an α-lactone system.

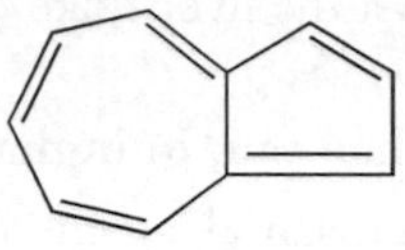

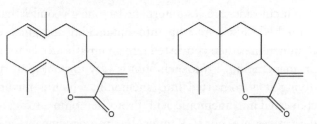

Fig. 6.39. Sesquiterpene lactone skeleton

Sesquiterpene lactones are biologically very active. Some are highly toxic to mammals, and others can cause allergic contact dermatitis in humans handling the plants in which they occur. Many have antitumor activity, but their considerable cytotoxicity has prevented any specific medicinal application.

At least 3,000 lactones have now been described. The great majority of these have been obtained from a single plant family, Asteraceae, in which they are characteristic constituents. Lactone constituents have been reported occasionally in plants from 16 other angiosperm families, most notably Apiaceae.[47]

In Asteraceae plants, sesquiterpene lactones are found mainly in the aerial parts of the plant (the leaves and flowering heads) in concentrations of about 5% of the dry weight. Certain species store large amounts of sesquiterpene lactones in glandular hairs called *trichomes*. When touched, the glands release the sesquiterpene lactones, which then elicit their various biological or pharmacological effects.

Sesquiterpene lactones are frequently present in mixtures of up to 15 components per plant species. Infraspecific variations can occur, notably in some *Artemisia* and *Ambrosia* species.

Classification of Sesquiterpene Lactones

Sesquiterpene lactones are classified into four major groups.

- Germacranolides, with a 10-membered ring (e.g., alatolide, the largest class)
- Eudesmolides, with two fused 6-membered rings (e.g., alantolactone)
- Guaianolides, with a 5-membered ring fused to a 7 and a methyl substituent at C-4
- Pseudoguaianolides, which have the same characteristics as guaianolides, but with a methyl substituent at C-5 (e.g., ambrosin)

Fig. 6.40. Germacranolide   Fig. 6.41. Eudesmanolide

Fig. 6.42. Guaianolide

Pharmacology and Uses

The antineoplastic activity of sesquiterpene lactones in the Asteraceae has led to the identification of structure-activity relationships that show that all cytotoxic, antileukemic, tumor-inhibiting, and immunostimulating sesquiterpene lactones have an α,β-unsaturated exocyclic lactone.[48]

Various sesquiterpene lactones exhibit antibacterial, antifungal, anthelmintic, antihyperlipidemic, and cardiovascular properties, and some show anti-inflammatory activity.[49] Judaicin, found in *Artemisia judaica*, has demonstrated potential as a digitalis-like cardioactive agent.

The migraine-preventive activity of feverfew has been attributed to its content of sesquiterpene lactones, of which parthenolide is the major component. Parthenolide comprises 85% of the total sesquiterpenes in feverfew. All of the feverfew sesquiterpenes that demonstrate anti-migraine activity are classified as germacranolide-type sesquiterpenes.

Toxicity

The sesquiterpene lactones are highly irritating to the nose, eyes, and gastrointestinal tract of sheep and goats. Plants that contain sesquiterpene lactones kill thousands of sheep each year in the United States. Among the toxic sesquiterpene lactones identified are tenulin in *Helenium amarum* (bitter sneezeweed) and hymenoxon in *Hymenoxys odorata* (bitter rubberweed). Mammalian toxicity has also been attributed to alantolactone from elecampane (*Inula helenium*).[50] For more information on the toxicity of sesquiterpene lactones, see chapter 10.

Ranunculosides

Ranunculosides are sesquiterpene lactone glycosides that, upon hydrolysis, split up into ranunculin and glucose. Ranunculin is then converted into an unsaturated lactone, protoanemonin. Protoanemonin is very unstable, but on drying it is converted into anemonin, which is further converted into anemonic acid. Protoanemonin is toxic; its derivatives are not.[51] Ranunculin, protoanemonin, and anemonin have medicinal properties; anemonic acid does not. Please refer to chapter 10 for a discussion about the toxicity of ranunculosides.

Plants Containing Ranunculosides

Christmas rose (*Helleborus niger*)
Field buttercup (*Ranunculus acris*)
Globe flower (*Trollius europaeus*)
Marsh marigold (*Caltha palustris*)
Pasqueflower (*Pulsatilla vulgaris*)
Wood anemone (*Anemone nemorosa*)

Absinthin (absinthiin)

This is the main bitter principle in wormwood, *Artemisia absinthium.*

Wormwood is used as an anthelmintic, as a bitter tonic, and for flavoring vermouth.[52]

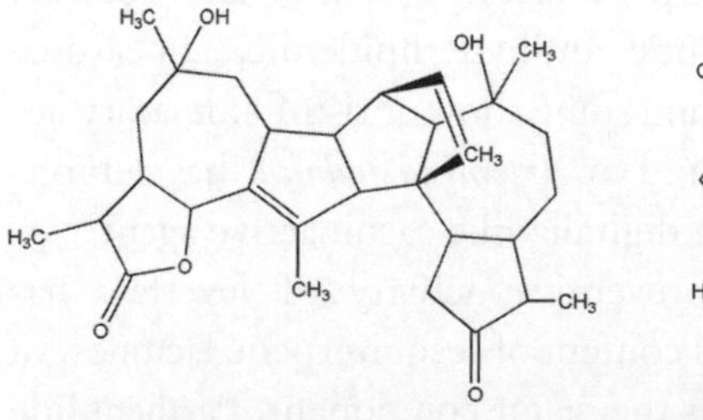

Fig. 6.43. Absinthin 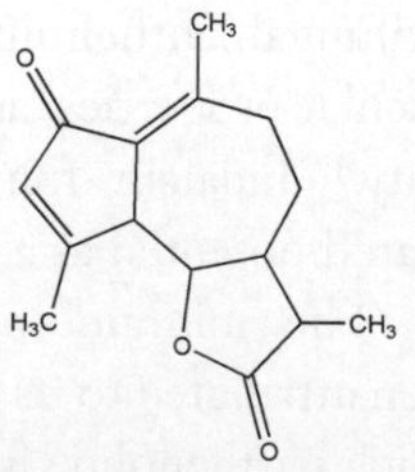   Fig. 6.44. Achillin

Achillin (santolin)

Achillin is found in yarrow (*Achillea millefolium* and other *Achillea* spp.) and in several *Artemisia* species. It functions as a plant growth inhibitor. During steam distillation, achillin is converted into chamazulene, which has anti-inflammatory properties.[53]

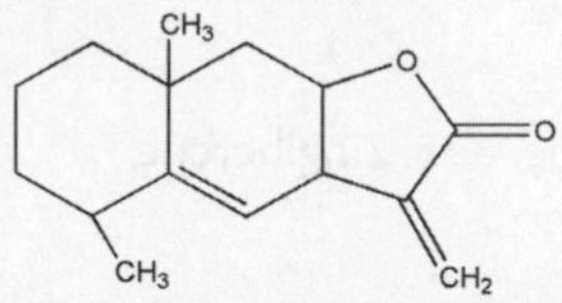

Fig. 6.45. Alantolactone 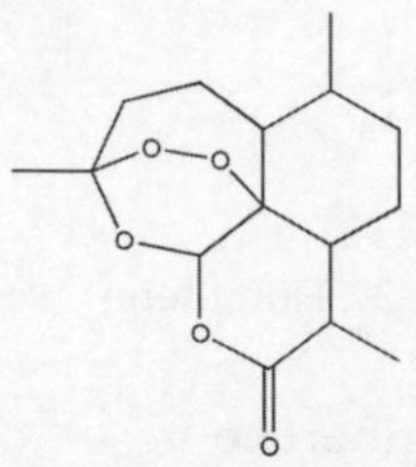   Fig. 6.46. Artemisinin

Alantolactone

Alantolactone occurs in oil of elecampane (*Inula helenium*) and other *Inula* species. Helenin (a mixture of alantolactone and isoalantolactone) has antibacterial and antifungal activities. Although alantolactone causes allergic contact dermatitis in humans, it has been employed as an expectorant, a cholagogue, and a urinary tract antiseptic. It has also been used to stimulate intestinal secretion and as a vermifuge against the liver fluke (*Fasciola hepatica*).[54]

Artemisinin (qing hau sau, quinghaosu)

Artemisinin, an antimalarial agent, occurs in *Artemisia annua* (*qing hau* or sweet Annie). It has demonstrated toxicity against chloroquine-resistant strains of various species of mosquito (*Plasmodium falciparum, P. vivax,* and *P. ovale*) in in vitro and in vivo tests. Artemisinin is used clinically in China for the treatment of malaria.[55] It also has potential as an anticancer agent.

Eupacunin

Eupacunin is found in the stems, leaves, and flowers of *Uncasia cuneifolia* and *Eupatorium lancifolium*. It has demonstrated cytotoxic and antitumor activities.[56]

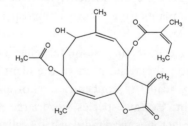

Fig. 6.47. Eupacunin

Inulicin

Occurring in *Inula japonica* (Japanese elecampane), inulicin has antiulcer actions as well as capillary-strengthening and diuretic properties. Inulicin also stimulates the activity of the central nervous system and the smooth muscles of the intestine.[57]

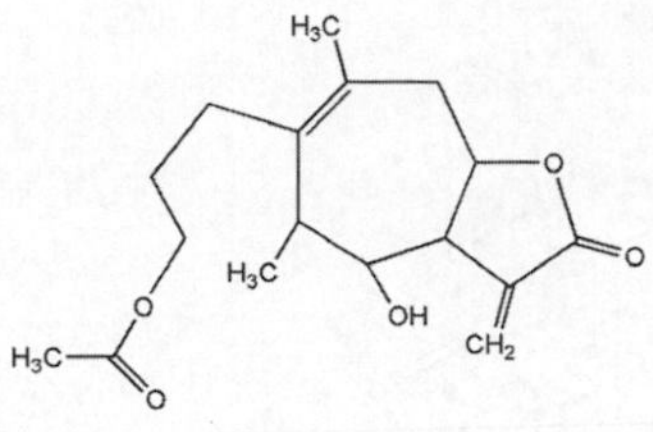

Fig. 6.48. Inulicin 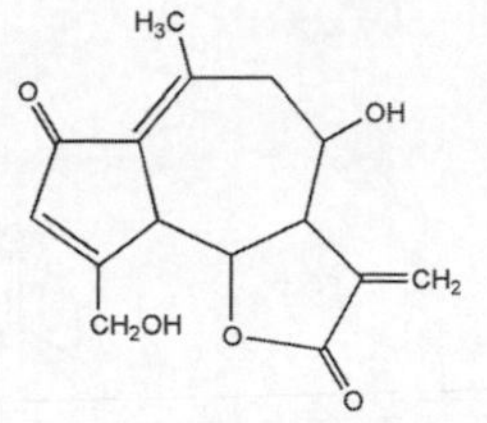   Fig. 6.49. Lactucin

macrocyclic substances. Many diterpenes have additional ring systems, which occur in side chains, in ester substitutions, or as epoxides. Some have 6-membered rings that have undergone aromatization, while others have fused 5- and 7-membered rings.

Lactucin

Lactucin occurs in various wild lettuce species, including *Lactuca serriola* and *L. virosa*, and in chicory *(Cichorium intybus)*. It demonstrates cytotoxic and antitumor activities.[58] Lactucin has a sedative action and is a bitter tonic.

Matricin

Matricin is found in chamomile *(Matricaria recutita)* and in several *Achillea* species. It is a precursor of chamazulene, an anti-inflammatory compound formed from matricin and achillin during steam distillation of the plant material.

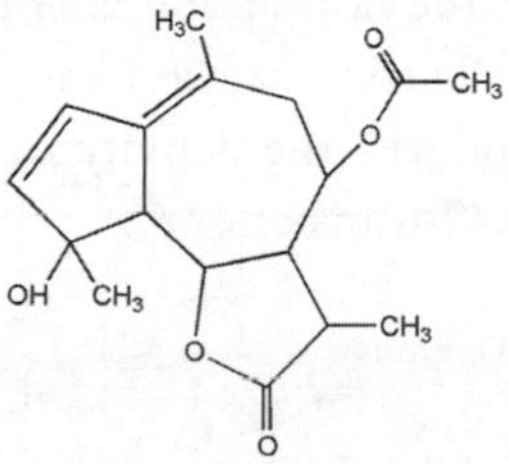

Fig. 6.50. Matricin 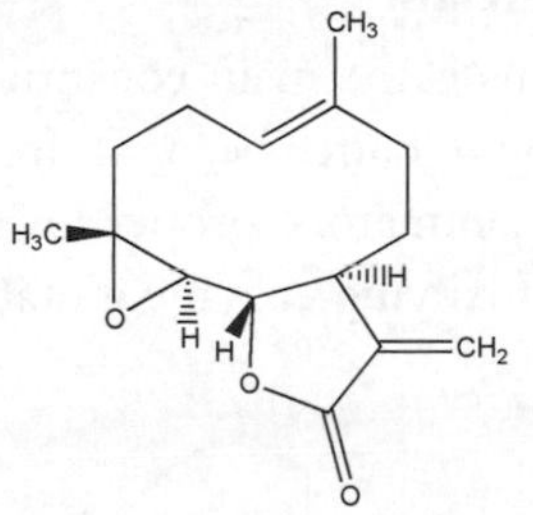   Fig. 6.51. Parthenolide

Parthenolide

This compound is found in glands on the leaf surface of feverfew *(Tanacetum parthenium)*, in several *Ambrosia* and *Arctotis* species, and in other members of the Asteraceae family.[59]

Parthenolide has demonstrated cytotoxic, antitumor, antibacterial, and antifungal activities. It is a primary active principle of feverfew, which is used in the treatment of migraine.

DITERPENOIDS

The diterpenoids are C_{20} molecules derived from four isoprene units, but modifications during the later stages of synthesis produce a wealth of different structures. Diterpenes share many chemical properties with sesquiterpenes, but are usually crystalline solids rather than liquids.

Classification of Diterpenes

Diterpenes are classified according to the number of ring systems present.[60] In addition, they form either acyclic or

Acyclic Diterpene

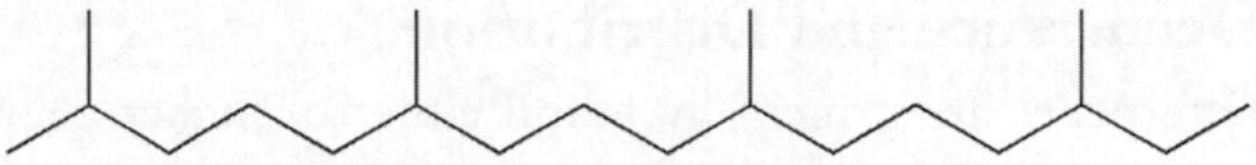

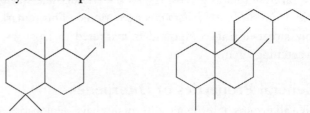

Fig. 6.52. Phytane

Bicyclic Diterpenes

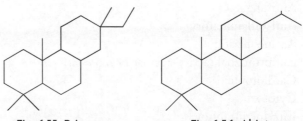

Fig. 6.53. Labdane   Fig. 6.54. Clerodane

Tricyclic Diterpenes

Fig. 6.55. Primarane 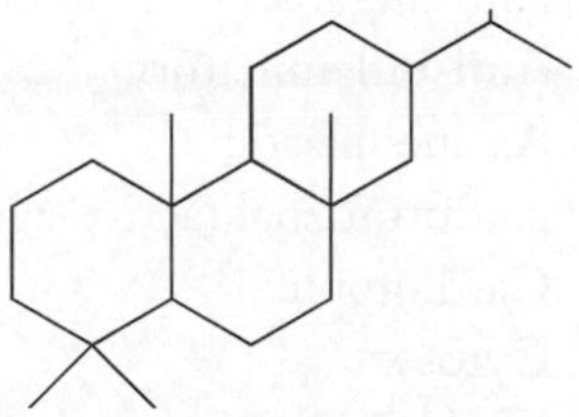   Fig. 6.56. Abiatane

Tetracyclic Diterpenes

Fig. 6.57. Kaurane   Fig. 6.58. Gibberellane

Macrocyclic Diterpenes

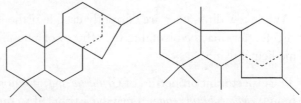

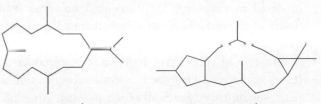

Fig. 6.59. Cembrane   Fig. 6.60. Lathyrane

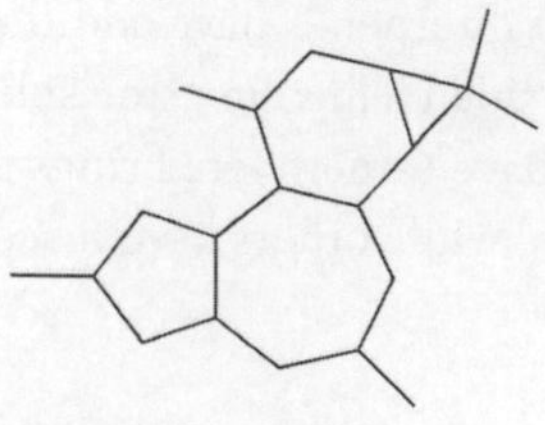

Fig. 6.61. Tigliane

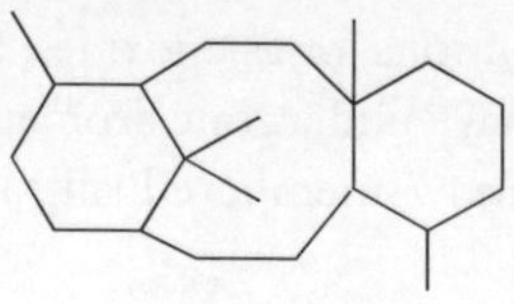

Fig. 6.62. Taxane

Occurrence and Distribution

Diterpenes are principally found either in higher plants or in fungi. Phytol is universal in higher plants, where it is associated with chlorophyll. Practically all other diterpenes, however, are of very restricted distribution. They are rarely found as glycosides, so the triglucoside stevioside, from *Stevia rebaudiana*, is exceptional. This remarkably sweet-tasting compound is marketed in Japan as a sweetening agent.

General Properties of Diterpenes

Like all groups of terpenes, diterpenes have demonstrated a range of pharmacological properties:[61,62]

- Analgesic
- Antibacterial
- Antifungal
- Anti-inflammatory
- Antineoplastic
- Antiprotozoal (active against *Leishmania*)
- Cardiotonic
- Cytotoxic
- Enzyme inhibitor
- Insecticidal
- Skin irritant
- Sweetening agents

While few diterpenes are currently used in orthodox medicine, they may be pivotal to the efficacy of a number of medicinal plants.

- The expectorant properties of *Grindelia* spp. and horehound (*Marrubium vulgare*) may be attributed to their diterpene content.
- A range of cardiovascular activities has been demonstrated for forskolin from *Coleus forskohlii*, as discussed in detail in chapter 9.[63] Diterpenoid quinones from *Salvia miltiorrhiza* have also demonstrated cardiovascular activities.
- A unique and very active hallucinogen found in the leaves of *Salvia divinorum* is a nonnitrogenous diterpene, salvinorin A. Since all other molecules that have this property contain nitrogen, this finding is very intriguing.

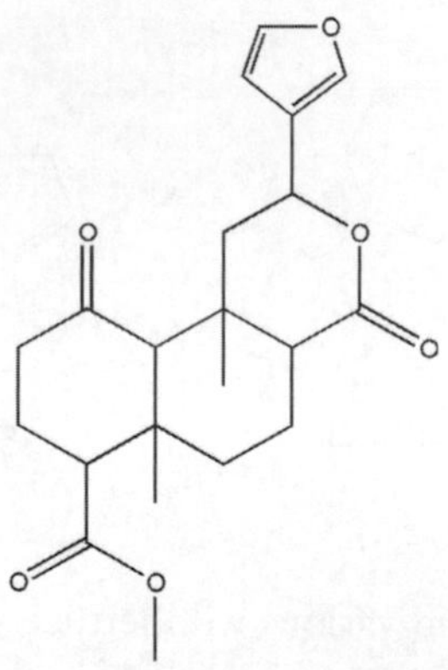

Fig. 6.63. Salvinorin A

A number of diterpenoids are very toxic, especially the tigliane-type phorbol esters of croton oil and *Euphorbia* latex, which are notable for their irritant and cocarcinogenic properties. The phorbol esters are being actively studied for insights that might be gained into the cancer process.[64]

Cafestol

This is the main constituent of the nonsaponifiable portion of coffee bean oil, from *Coffea* spp. Cafestol has anti-inflammatory properties and induces the activity of the detoxifying enzyme glutathione-*S*-transferase.[65]

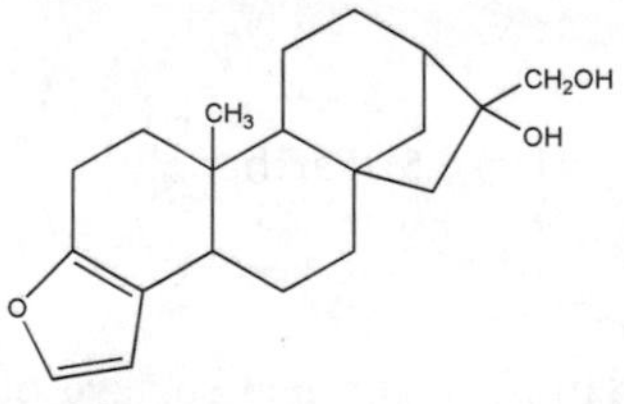

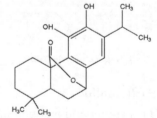

Fig. 6.64. Cafestol   Fig. 6.65. Carnosol

Carnosol

Carnosol is found in sage (*Salvia officinalis*) and in rosemary (*Rosmarinus officinalis*). It was traditionally used as an aromatic bitter.[66]

Coleonol

Coleonol, from the leaves of *Coleus forskohlii*, has demonstrated hypotensive activity.[67] (See chapter 9 for a detailed discussion of the cardiovascular properties of *Coleus forskohlii*.)

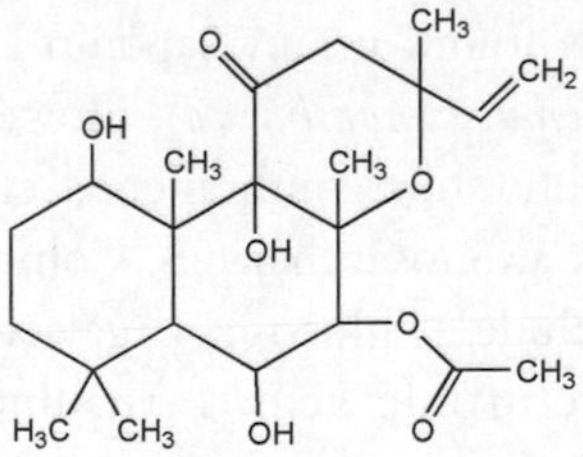

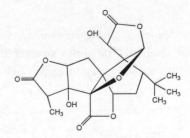

Fig. 6.70. Ginkgolide A

Fig. 6.66. Coleonol   Fig. 6.67. Columbin

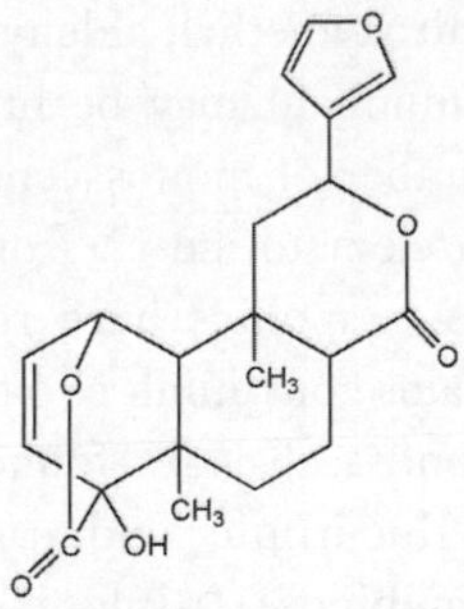

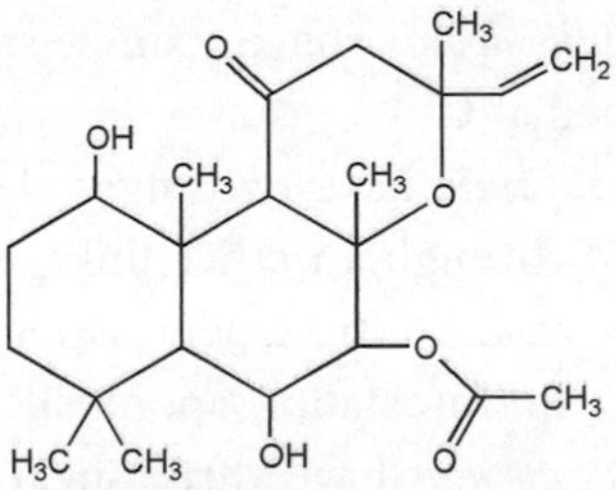

Fig. 6.68. Forskolin

Grindelic Acid

This labdane skeleton-based diterpene found in *Grindelia* spp. may be implicated in the herb's respiratory properties.

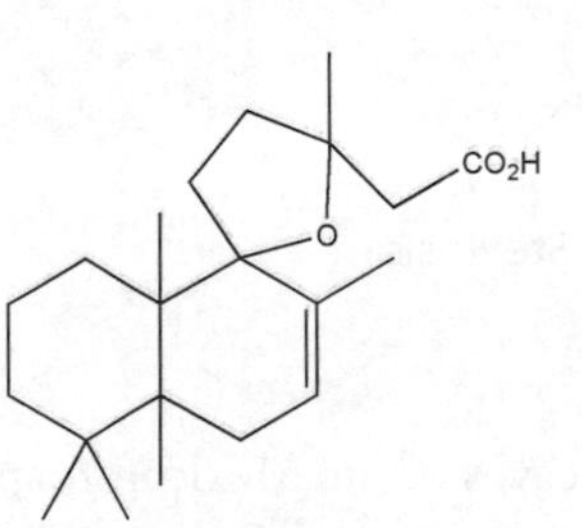

Fig. 6.71. Grindelic acid   Fig. 6.72. Marrubiin

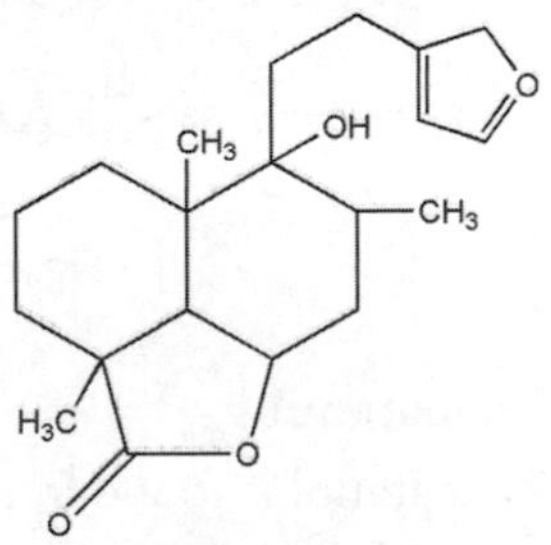

Columbin

This very bitter substance is found in columba root (*Jateorhiza palmata*). The roots of *J. palmata* are used for the preparation of a bitter tonic, called Radix Columba in various European pharmacopoeias.

Forskolin

Found in the roots of *Coleus forskohlii*, forskolin demonstrates cardiovascular activity.[68]

Geranylgeraniol

Found in flax or linseed oil (*Linum usitatissimum*), the diphosphate of geranylgeraniol is the biogenetic precursor of diterpenes.

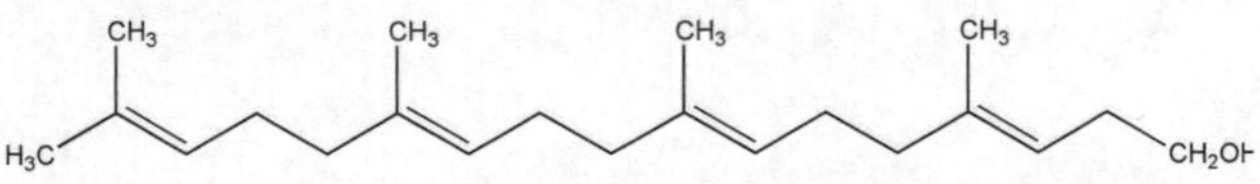

Fig. 6.69. Geranylgeraniol

Ginkgolide A

Found in the root bark and leaves of *Ginkgo biloba*, ginkgolide A and related ginkgolides are bitter substances with bronchodilating and antiasthmatic properties.[69]

Marrubiin

A bitter principle found in horehound (*Marrubium vulgare*), marrubiin is generated from premarrubiin as an artifact of the extraction process. *M. vulgare* is used as an expectorant.[70]

Phytol

Phytol occurs in all chlorophyll-containing plants as an ester of the propionic side chain of chlorophyll. Phytol is used in the preparation of vitamins E and K.[71]

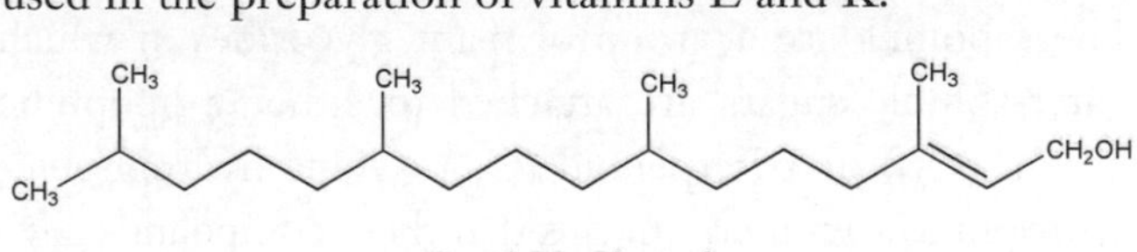

Fig. 6.73. Phytol

Premarrubiin

Premarrubiin, which occurs in horehound (*Marrubium vulgare*), is converted into marrubiin during the extraction process.

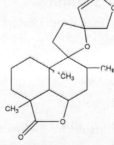

Fig. 6.74. Premarrubiin

Stevioside

Found in the leaves of *Stevia rebaudiana*, stevioside is a glycoside that is about 300 times sweeter than sucrose. The aglycone steviol shows a gibberellin-like growth hormone activity.[72]

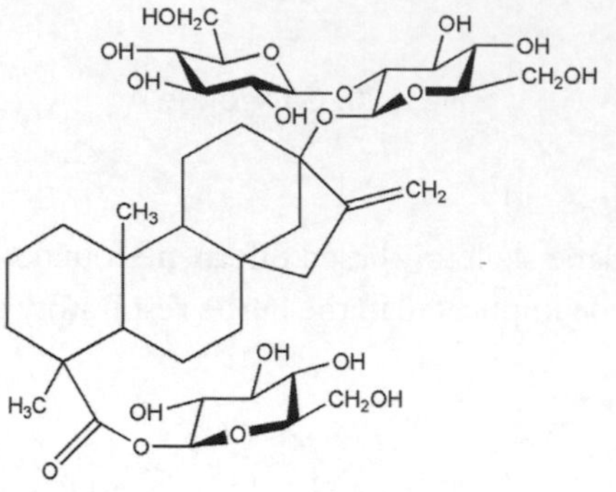

Fig. 6.75. Stevioside

Zoapatanol

Zoapatanol is found in the leaves of the Mexican zoapatle tree (*Montanoa tomentosa*). The compound possesses antifertility activity, and has been used in Mexico to prepare a tea to induce menses and labor.[73]

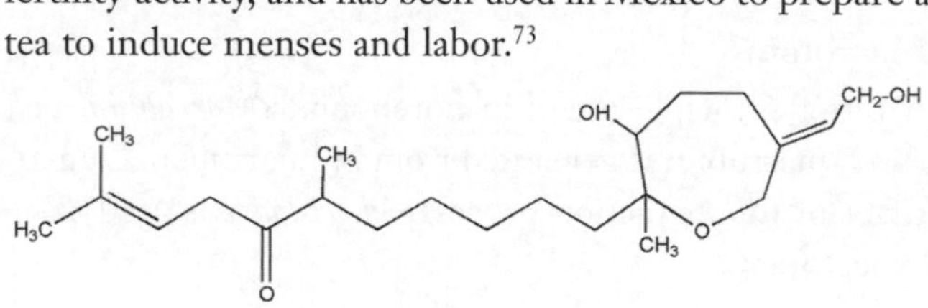

Fig. 6.76. Zoapatanol

SAPONINS

The saponins are a group of plant glycosides in which water-soluble sugars are attached to either a lipophilic steroid (C_{27}) or triterpenoid (C_{30}).[74] This hydrophobic-hydrophilic asymmetry means that these compounds have the ability to lower surface tension, and are soaplike. They form foam in aqueous solutions and cause hemolysis of blood erythrocytes in vitro. The aglycone portion of the saponin molecule is called the *genin* or *sapogenin*.

Classification of Saponins

Depending on the type of genin present, the saponins fall into three major classes.[75]

- Triterpene glycosides
- Steroid glycosides
- Steroid alkaloid glycosides

The aglycones normally have a hydroxyl group at C-3, and certain methyl groups are frequently oxidized to hydroxymethyl, aldehyde, or carboxyl groups. The sugar component may be linear or branched, and the largest number of monosaccharides found in any saponin is 11 (in clematoside C, from *Clematis manshurica*). However, most saponins have relatively short, unbranched sugar chains containing two to five monosaccharides. Common monosaccharides found include D-glucose, D-galactose, D-glucuronic acid, D-galacturonic acid, L-rhamnose, L-arabinose, D-xylose, and D-fructose.

The types of saponin glycosides are further classified as follows.

- *Monodesmosidic saponins* have a single sugar chain, normally attached at C-3.
- *Bidesmosidic saponins* have two sugar chains, often with one attached through an ether linkage at C-3 and an ester linkage at C-28 (triterpene saponins) or an ether linkage at C-26 (furostanol saponins).
- *Tridesmosidic saponins* have three sugar chains and are seldom found.

A striking feature of saponins is the great difference in the type of properties displayed by mono- and bidesmosidic saponins. The bidesmosides either lack or show much less activity than the corresponding monodesmosides. However, the surface activities of the saponins (their ability to lower surface tension) remain unchanged whether they are bidesmosides or monodesmosides.

Biosynthesis of Saponins

Saponins are built up of six isoprene units and have a common origin in that they are all derived from squalene. Other important classes of secondary metabolites, such as phytosterols, cardenolides, cucurbitacins, quassinoids, and limonoids, are also derived from squalene.[76]

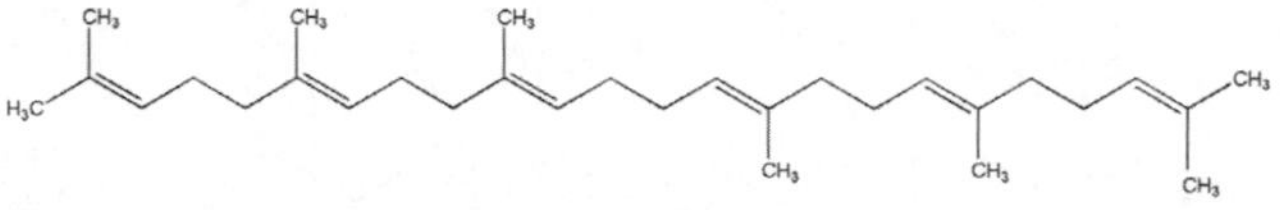

Fig. 6.77. Squalene

Herbs Containing Saponins

Achillea millefolium (yarrow)
Aralia nudicaulis (wild sarsaparilla)
A. racemosa (spikenard)
Arctium lappa (burdock)
Astragalus membranaceus (astragalus)
Calendula officinalis (calendula or pot marigold)
Caulophyllum thalictroides (blue cohosh)
Chionanthus virginicus (fringetree)
Codonopsis spp. (codonopsis)

Digitalis purpurea (foxglove)
Dioscorea villosa (wild yam)
Eleutherococcus senticosus (Siberian ginseng)
Gentiana lutea (gentian)
Glycyrrhiza spp. (licorice)
Panax ginseng (Korean ginseng)
P. quinquefolius (American ginseng)
Phytolacca americana (poke)
Polygala senega (Seneca snakeroot)
Rumex crispus (yellow dock)
Salvia officinalis (sage)
Smilax spp. (sarsaparilla)
Symphytum officinale (comfrey)
Taraxacum officinale (dandelion)
Verbascum thapsis (mullein)

Occurrence and Distribution

Saponins are extremely widely distributed in flowering plants and have been identified in more than 100 families.[77] They are found in many plants that are used as human food, including soybeans, chickpeas, peanuts, mung beans, broad beans, kidney beans, lentils, garden peas, spinach, oats, eggplant, asparagus, fenugreek, garlic, sugar beets, potatoes, green peppers, tomatoes, onions, tea, cassava, and yams. They also occur in leguminous forage species, such as alfalfa.

The actual saponin content of a plant depends on many factors, including the cultivar, age, physiological state, and geographical location of the plant. There can be considerable variation in the composition and quantity of saponins in plants growing in different places. Saponin distribution among the organs of a particular plant also varies considerably. The flowers of *Calendula officinalis* contain 3.57% saponins, and the roots 2.55% (dry weight). Ginsenoside levels in *Panax ginseng* are lowest in the leafstalks and stem (0.77%), higher in the main root (1.3%) and lateral roots (3.5%), and highest in the leaves (5.2%) and root hairs (6.1%).[78]

The fact that saponins are localized in organelles that have a high metabolic turnover rate implies that they are not simply ballast material, but may be physiologically significant constituents that play important regulatory roles in the metabolism and development of the organism.

There is not always a clear explanation for the high saponin content of some plants, which may consist of up to 30% saponins. One theory is that they serve as protection for the plant against fungal attack, as there is often an increase in saponin content in the part of the plant under microbial attack.

Researchers have proposed that bidesmosidic sapo-

nins, which are soluble in water but frequently lack some of the other typical properties of saponins, serve a transport function between the organs not at risk (e.g., leaves) and those parts of the plant (e.g., roots, bark, seeds) under attack by microorganisms. When plant tissue is damaged, the enzymes released act on the bidesmosidic saponins. Once transformed into their monodesmosidic derivatives, the saponins can provide a defense against microbial invasion at the threatened area.

General Properties of Saponins

The material that follows on general and more specific properties of this large group of secondary plant constituents was derived from two primary references: *Saponins*, by Hostettmann and Marston, and an extensive review of saponin research by Lacaille-Dubois and Wagner.[79,80] Refer to these works for more details.

Saponins have three common properties: bitter taste, hemolytic activity, and an ability to form stable foams when shaken in water. This latter surface-acting or "detergent" effect may be a key to their physiological properties. They are typical glycosides, with the aglycone (the sapogenin) occurring as a polycyclic ring.

Saponins have demonstrated numerous pharmacological properties. However, it is important to remember that the specific actions enumerated below do not occur in a vacuum, but rather are interrelated at the metabolic level in both the plant and the person. The list of biological activities associated with saponins is also very long. Some of these characteristics, such as fungicidal and piscicidal effects, have been known for many years, and new activities are continually being discovered. However, caution is needed when extrapolating from in vitro or in vivo studies to human applications.

Pharmacological and Biological Properties of Saponins

- Adaptogenic
- Alterative/tonic
- Anthelmintic
- Antifungal
- Anti-inflammatory
- Antimicrobial
- Antiulcerogenic
- Capillary-strengthening
- Cholesterol lowering
- Diuretic
- Expectorant
- Hemolytic
- Hepatoprotective

- Hormone-modulating
- Immunomodulating
- Molluscicidal
- Piscicidal
- Spermicidal and contraceptive

Pharmacological Properties

Local Effects

The detergent effect is important in understanding the actions of saponins upon skin and membranes. Many wound-healing herbs are rich in saponins, including *Calendula officinalis*. The expectorant and diuretic properties of saponin-rich herbs such as *Polygala senega* and *Primula* spp. may be related to the saponins' irritant effects on mucous membranes of the respiratory and urinary tracts.

Hemolytic Effects

Saponin aglycones can increase the permeability of membranes. They bring about hemolysis by destroying the membranes of red blood cells, thus releasing the hemoglobin. When saponins are taken orally, this effect is nullified in the stomach before the aglycones enter the bloodstream. Low concentrations of saponins are capable of destroying (lysing) erythrocyte membranes, causing a release of hemoglobin. This phenomenon occurs through a reduction of surface tension between the aqueous and lipid phases of the erythrocyte membrane, which causes emulsion of the lipids and their subsequent departure from the membrane. Na^+ and water are able to enter the cell through the holes in the membranes, while K^+ exits the cell. This flux occurs until the membrane ruptures and hemoglobin is shed into the plasma.

Cholesterol Metabolism

Saponins reach the human body in relatively large amounts as a result of the intake of foods rich in these glycosides. The cholesterol-lowering effects of saponins are well documented but poorly understood. One theory is that they form insoluble complexes with cholesterol in the gut, thus limiting assimilation. New research suggests that they may have an effect (or effects) upon systemic cholesterol metabolism.

Triterpene glycosides given to hens in their feed appear to decrease the amount of cholesterol in both blood and tissues. One possible explanation for this effect is that the triterpene glycosides form an insoluble complex with cholesterol in the digestive tract; this complex is subsequently eliminated from the body. It is also possible that the glycosides exert a direct effect on cholesterol metabolism.

Cardiovascular Activities

Saponins are able both to increase the permeability of cell plasma membranes and to cause positive inotropic effects in isolated cardiac muscles. Panaxatriol saponins from *Panax notoginseng* have demonstrated antiarrhythmic actions in rats and rabbits. The antihypertensive activity of some ginseng saponins is attributed to a vascular relaxant effect; they appear to block Ca^{2+} channels without affecting voltage-operated Ca^{2+} channels or Ca^{2+} release from the intracellular store. Crude saponins from *Panax notoginseng* have also shown vasodilatory effects.

Effects on the Adrenocorticotropic System

Many saponins can induce the release of adrenocorticotropic hormone (ACTH), but this is not considered to be a general property of triterpene saponins. The ginsenoside Rb1 both induces corticosterone release and stimulates ACTH secretion in cultures of pituitary cells.

Anti-Inflammatory Activities

Substances with anti-exudative and anti-edematous properties form a subgroup of anti-inflammatory agents in that they influence the earlier stages of inflammation. In some cases, the anti-inflammatory action of these substances seems to be independent of the pituitary-adrenal axis, while in other cases, the drugs appear to exert a direct action on the adrenal cortex (for example, glycyrrhetinic acid).

When given parenterally, the saponin mixture aescin, from horse chestnut (*Aesculus hippocastanum*), has been shown to be 600 times more effective than rutin in reducing rat paw edema. No effect was observed, however, after oral application.

Effects on Capillary Fragility and Venous Insufficiency

Saponins that decrease capillary fragility also have a beneficial effect on capillary permeability. Weakness of the blood vessels (especially veins) can lead to several complications. Enlarged veins can contribute to the development of hypertension. Increased blood vessel permeability can result in edema or reduced blood flow, increasing the risk of thrombosis. Related disorders include hemorrhoids and varicose veins.

Certain saponin-containing plants, such as horse chestnut (*Aesculus hippocastanum*), have capillary-protective properties that reduce capillary fragility.

Substances that affect the veins can be divided into three major categories of activity.

1. Substances that strengthen the veins by either reducing or increasing venous cross-sectional area
2. Diuretic agents
3. Agents that protect against edema, thus decreasing capillary permeability

Antiulcer Activity

Pharmacologically, the best known saponin-containing antiulcerogenic herbs is licorice *(Glycyrrhiza glabra)*, although we now know that active constituents other than glycyrrhizin also contribute to its antiulcer effects. These are flavonoids, such as licoflavonol, licoricone, and kumatekenin. Flavonoids do not inhibit gastric acid secretion, but are instead believed to exert their antiulcerogenic effects by promoting mucus formation, directly activating gastric membrane protective factors, or stimulating inherent protective mechanisms via irritation of the gastric mucosa.

Immunomodulation

Saponins belong to the classes of substances that have an effect on the human immune system. (Other important immunomodulators are lipids, lectins, polysaccharides, and fungal polysaccharides.) Immunomodulating saponins enhance both humoral and cellular immune responses; the immunostimulant effects of saponins used as adjuvant therapies do not depend solely on an increased uptake of antigen.

Saponins can form ordered, particulate structures around 35 mm in diameter (about the size of a virus particle) with the surface protein from enveloped viruses. These have been named *immunostimulating complexes* (ISCOMs). ISCOM vaccines have been developed against a number of viruses, including influenza, measles, Epstein-Barr, and HIV-1.[81]

Some of the nonspecific effects of immunostimulant saponins may occur as a result of their irritant properties. This so-called induction of paramunity can be provoked via the oral route or through the mucous membranes of the respiratory, digestive, and urogenital systems.

Since saponins taken by mouth have low bioavailability, it is unclear how they work to stimulate the immune system, whether through enhanced cell proliferation, induction of helper T cell activity, or B cell activation. One theory suggests that an initial impact on mucosal immune system components leads to secretion of immune system mediators, which then initiate a multitude of cellular events.

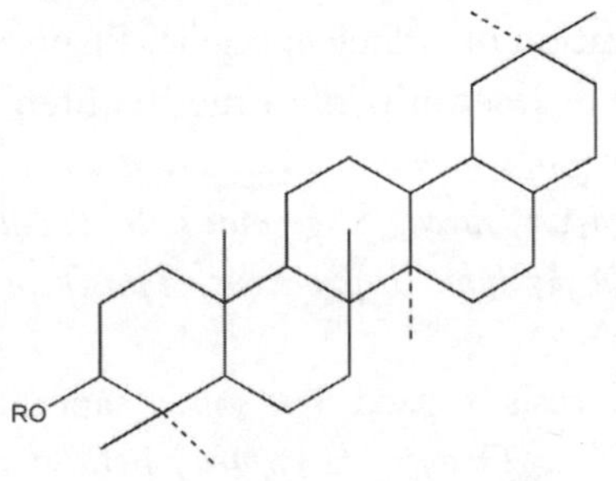

Fig. 6.78. Triterpene class

Expectorant and Antitussive Activities

Saponins possess a general and nonspecific ability to produce local irritation, especially of mucous membranes. This can take place in the nasal cavity, the throat, the bronchi, the lungs, and in kidney epithelia.

The expectorant activity of saponin-containing herbs such as *Polygala senega*, *Primula* spp., and *Glycyrrhiza glabra* is attributed at least in part to local irritation of mucous membranes, although their mechanism of action is not clear. The irritation of the throat and respiratory tract caused by these saponins may increase respiratory fluid volume by drawing more water into the bronchial

---

Immunomodulators

The category of agents known as *immunomodulators* includes *immunostimulants*, which boost the activity of an organism's immune system, and *immunosuppressive* factors, which block the activity of the immune system. Immunostimulants are employed during chemotherapy, in the treatment of infectious diseases, and to stimulate the immune response after vaccination. Immunosuppressive agents are used in the treatment of autoimmune diseases and allergies and to help prevent transplant rejections.

Immunomodulators can be further divided into two categories, *specific* and *nonspecific*. Specific immunomodulators are generally used as adjuvant therapy, while nonspecific immunostimulants are administered on their own in order to elicit a generalized state of resistance to pathogens or tumors.

Immunostimulants work by increasing phagocytosis by granulocytes and macrophages, activating helper T cells, and stimulating cell division and transformation in lymphocytes. Immunosuppressive agents activate suppressor cells and have cytotoxic effects on other cells.

secretions, thus diluting the mucus and reducing its viscosity. Alternatively, the surface activity of the saponins may render the sputum less viscid, making it more mobile and easier to eject. Another possibility is that the amphiphilic nature of saponins causes them to spread out as a monomolecular film at the back of the throat and subsequently aid elimination of mucus. Saponins are considered *amphiphilic* because one end of the molecule is hydrophilic (*water loving*, or polar) and the other is hydrophobic (*water hating*, or nonpolar).

Diuretic Activity

The diuretic action of many saponins can be traced back to local irritation of kidney epithelia. Plants with diuretic activity due at least in part to their content of saponins include *Astragalus membranaceus*, *Herniara glabra*, *H. hirsuta*, *Solidago virgaurea*, *S. gigantea*, *S. canadensis*, *Elymus repens*, *Betula pendula*, *B. pubescens*, *Equisetum arvense*, and *Viola tricolor*.

The diuresis caused by some saponin-containing plants, such as *Ononis*, *Herniara*, *Betula*, and *Solidago* species, is relatively mild. In these plants, the effect may originate from the combined influence of saponins, flavonoids, and essential oils.

Anthelmintic Activity

Some saponin preparations have a practical use as anthelmintics in traditional medicine systems. In fact, a large number of saponins exhibit anthelmintic activities, but many find no practical application because of the parallel irritation of mucous membranes.

Spermicidal and Contraceptive Activities

In the ongoing effort to find new sources of contraceptive agents, numerous medicinal plants have been investigated for antifertility effects. Saponins have a variety of important activities in this area, including spermicidal effects. The mechanism of action here probably involves a disruption of the spermatozoid plasma cell membrane, similar to the action of the commercially available spermicide nonoxynol-9.

Other Effects

Saponins may help protect the liver through some impact upon the Kupffer's cells, immune system cells found in the liver. Saponins from *Panax ginseng*, *Bupleurum falcatum*, licorice (*Glycyrrhiza* spp.), alfalfa (*Medicago sativa*), and soy (*Glycine max*) have all demonstrated this property.[82]

Saponins appear to have a profound yet little understood stimulating effect upon the reticuloendothelial system and the white cell macrophages of the mononuclear phagocyte system (MPS). In biochemical terms, the MPS removes a great deal of waste matter from the blood—in other words, it "cleanses" the blood. This sounds a bit like classic alterative activity! Some saponin-containing herbs have also been shown to stimulate the production of interferon in the body. In addition, examples of saponins with adaptogenic properties are found in *Eleutherococcus senticosus* and *Panax* species.

Saponins have a reputation for bitterness. For example, the seed coat of quinoa (*Chenopodium quinoa*) contains bitter saponins that must be removed before cooking. Similarly, partially acetylated soyasaponins are responsible for the bitter and astringent taste of soybeans (*Glycine max*). Saponins also impart a bitter taste to asparagus (*Asparagus officinalis*) so that the bottom cut must be discarded during processing. However, there are exceptions. For example, glycyrrhizin, the principal saponin in licorice, is about 50 times sweeter than sucrose.

Biological Effects

Molluscicidal Activity

Saponins have a pronounced action against mollusks. The mechanism of this toxicity is thought to involve the binding of the saponin to the gill membranes, which causes an increase in their permeability and a subsequent loss of important electrolytes. Saponins are also toxic to insects.

The toxicity of saponins to snails has stimulated great interest in their potential for controlling schistosomiasis, a tropical parasitic disease affecting approximately 250 million people worldwide. Snails are directly implicated in the transmission of this disease, as they act as intermediate hosts during the life cycle of the parasite.

Plants that contain saponins are among the most promising for large-scale application against the schistosomiasis parasite for a number of reasons.

- High molluscicidal activity
- Low oral toxicity
- Water soluble
- Widely distributed in the plant kingdom
- Frequently occur in large amounts in plants

Piscicidal Activity

The ability of some plants to act as fish poisons has been exploited for many hundreds of years. Death of fish results from damage to the gill capillaries. The gills not only are respiratory organs, but also play a crucial role in the regulation of ion balance and osmotic pressure.

Fungicidal Activity

The strongest fungicidal activities have been found in monodesmosidic saponins. Those with four or more sugars in the chain show the greatest degree of activity; shorter carbohydrate chains lead to lower water solubility and weaker antifungal activity. One mechanism proposed to explain the antifungal activity of saponins suggests that the saponins form complexes with sterols in the plasma membrane of the fungi, thus destroying the cellular semipermeability and leading to death of the cell. Another theory holds that the saponins themselves are inactive and comprise only water-soluble transport forms. The aglycone, or active membranolytic component, forms only in the presence of cell membrane glycosidases.

Triterpenoid Saponins

Triterpenoid sapogenins have 5-ring structures. Sugars are commonly attached at the 3-hydroxyl position. They are frequently present in plants as a complex mixture of closely related glycosides based on one or more triterpenoid sapogenins. They are usually found in all parts of the plant, with some concentration in root, foliage, or seed. Recently, triterpene saponins have been isolated from marine organisms.

Table 6.2. Pentacyclic Triterpenoid Saponin Herbs and Actions

HERB	ACTIONS
Aesculus hippocastanum (horse chestnut)	Vascular tonic, anti-inflammatory
Bupleurum falcatum (bupleurum)	Anti-inflammatory, antihepatotoxic
Calendula officinalis (calendula)	Vulnerary, lymphatic, anti-inflammatory
Glycyrrhiza glabra (licorice)	Anti-inflammatory, demulcent, expectorant, antiulcerogenic
Guaiacum officinale (guaiacum)	Anti-inflammatory, diaphoretic
Polygala senega (Seneca snakeroot)	Expectorant
Primula spp. (primrose)	Vary among species
Quillaja saponaria (quillaja)	Emulsifying agent

General Properties of Triterpenoid Saponins

Triterpenoid saponins share the general properties of saponins, with the addition of an ability to form complexes with cholesterol.

- Bitterness
- Hemolytic activity
- Decrease surface tension (i.e., form stable foams)
- Formation of complexes with cholesterol

Triterpene saponins (especially bidesmosides) have the ability to increase the solubility of water-insoluble compounds. In addition, the saponins of *Bupleurum falcatum* can be solubilized by ginseng saponins. Saikosaponin A is normally soluble at 0. 1 mg/ml in water, but when ginsenoside Ro is added, this increases to 3.4 mg/ml.

Biological and Pharmacological Properties of Triterpenoid Saponins

Antibacterial Activity

Although strongly antifungal, triterpene saponins have virtually no antibacterial activity.

Antiviral Activity

Some antiviral activity has been reported in in vitro studies. However, the therapeutic index is unfortunately low, limiting the usefulness of triterpene saponins as isolated constituents in humans.

Cytotoxic and Antitumor Activity

Cytotoxic activity has been documented in vitro for many triterpenoid saponins, but their high toxicity has inhibited their use in therapy. It must be remembered that there is a big difference between whole plant activity and research on isolated constituents. Please see chapter 9 for a discussion on the effects of plant constituents on cancer processes.

Aescin

Found in the seed of the horse chestnut (*Aesculus hippocastanum*), aescin is also the collective name for the complex mixture of more than 30 different saponins present in horse chestnut. The main component (shown on page 80) makes up about 20% of the saponin content of the complex.

Aescin has strong hemolytic activity and shows anti-inflammatory and anti-exudative actions. It also inhibits fungal growth and has demonstrated anticancer cancerostatic properties.[83]

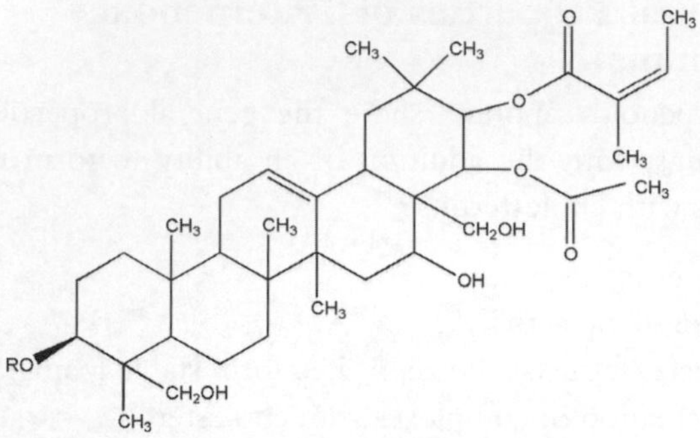

Fig. 6.79. Aescin

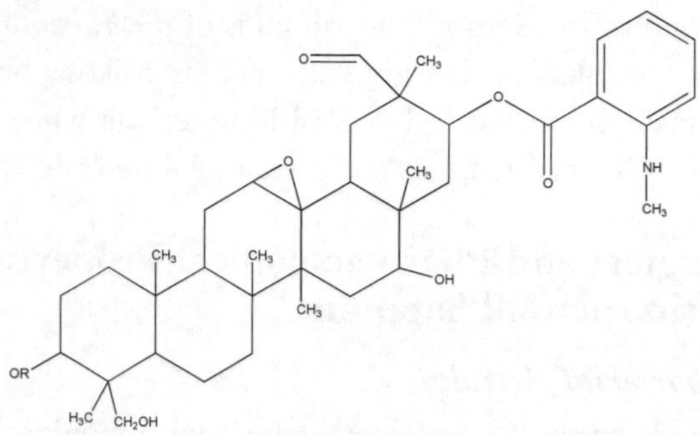

Fig. 6.80. Avenacin

Avenacin A-l

Avenacin A-l is found in oats (*Avena sativa*). It demonstrates hemolytic activity in animals and strongly inhibits pathogenic fungi in plants.

Cucurbitacin E

The cucurbitacins are triterpenoid saponins predominantly found in the Curcubitaceae family, but also present in the Begoniaceae, Brassicaceae, Scrophulariaceae, and others. They are a group of extremely bitter-tasting, oxygenated saponins derived from the cucurbitane skeleton. They cannot be considered steroidal, since the methyl from C-10 has moved to C-9. Pharmacological effects of the cucurbitacins and the plants containing them are very varied:[84]

• Antifertility (in female mice)
• Anti-inflammatory
• Bitter stimulant
• Cytotoxic, antitumor
• Hepatoprotective
• Purgative
• Stomachic

They may also play other biological roles as plant growth regulators and insect feedants or antifeedants.

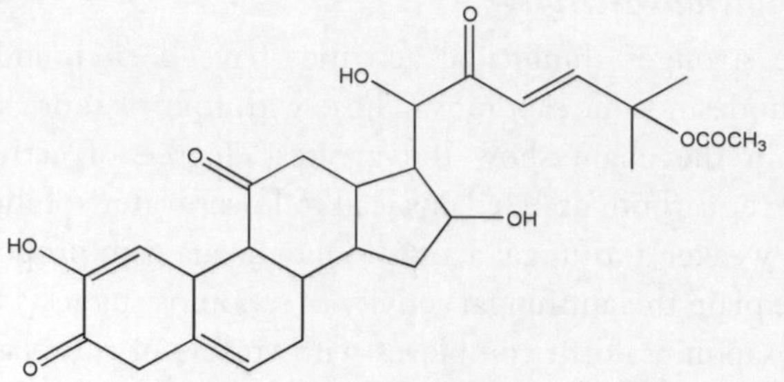

Fig. 6.81. Curcurbitacin E

Glycyrrhetic Acid

A sapogenin from the dried roots and rhizomes of licorice (*Glycyrrhiza glabra*), glycyrrhetic acid has anti-inflammatory and antiulcerogenic properties. It possesses mineralocorticoid action, which can result in increased renal sodium resorption, leading to an increase in blood pressure, hypokalemia, and water retention.[85]

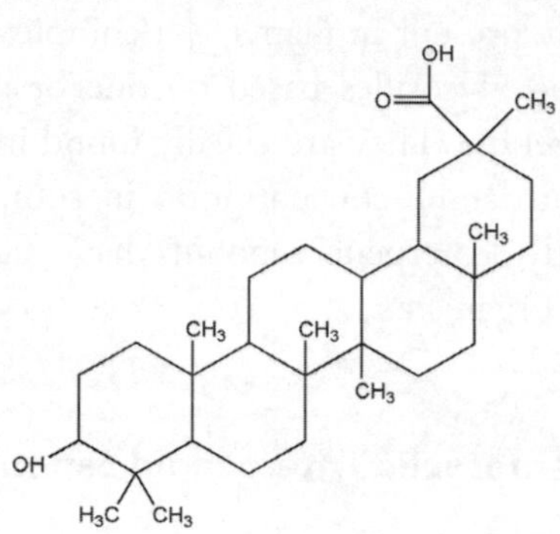

Fig. 6.82. Glycyrrhetic acid

Glycyrrhizin

This saponin from the roots and rhizomes of *Glycyrrhiza glabra* induces the activity of interferons. It is intensely sweet, with a taste about 50 times sweeter than sucrose. It also has antiulcerogenic and expectorant properties.[86]

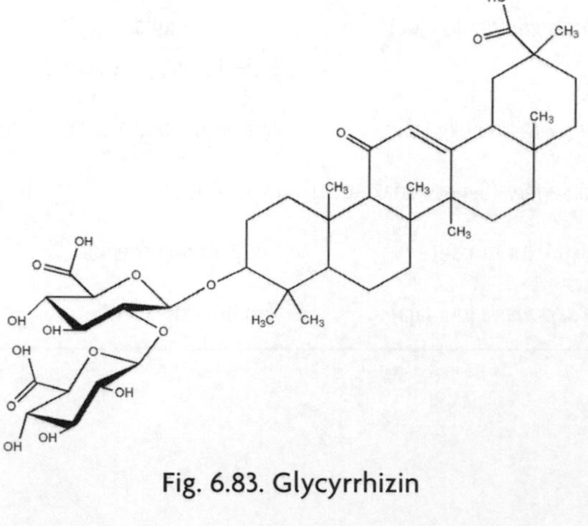

Fig. 6.83. Glycyrrhizin

Saikosaponin A

Saikosaponin A occurs in the roots of *Bupleurum falcatum* and *B. chinense*.

The saponin fractions of these herbs demonstrate anti-inflammatory and immunomodulatory activities.[87]

Senegin II

This compound is found in the roots of *Polygala senega*. A mixture of senegin II and related saponins from *P. senega* shows anticancer and expectorant activities.[88]

Steroid Saponins

These saponins are similar to the triterpenoid saponins in structure, biogenesis, and biological activity, but have four rings. They also bear structural similarities to the cardiac glycosides. The first natural source of steroid saponins was foxglove *(Digitalis purpurea)*, in which digitogenin co-occurs with the cardiac glycosides digitalin and digitoxin.

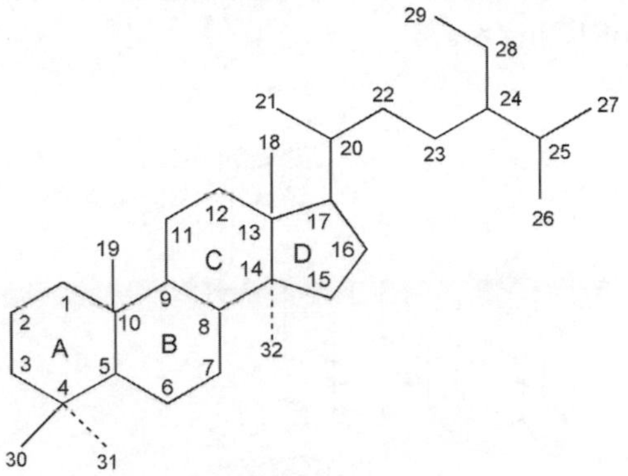

Fig. 6.84. Steroid structure
and numbering system

Occurrence and Distribution

Steroid saponins are present in the Agavaceae, Dioscoreaceae, Liliaceae, and Scrophulariaceae plant families. They resemble the triterpenoid saponins in the number and location of their sugar components. The glycosides can be difficult to purify, so sapogenins such as diosgenin and yamogenin are better known than the corresponding saponins. Diosgenin, isolated from *Dioscorea* roots, is a starting material for the partial synthesis of sex hormones used in contraceptive pills, but does not act as a precursor of "natural progesterone" in the human body—an important distinction.

Steroid saponins are used as detergents, as foaming agents in fire extinguishers, and as fish poisons. Their lack of human toxicity is apparent in the fact that such saponins occur in a number of food plants, such as asparagus.

Table 6.3. Industrial Sources of Steroidal Saponins

HERB	SOURCE MATERIAL FOR
Agave sisalana (sisal)	Saponins for pharmaceuticals
Dioscorea spp. (wild yam)	Saponins for pharmaceuticals
Glycine max (soy)	Phytosterols
Ruscus aculeatus (butcher's broom)	Cardiovascular, anti-inflammatory, vasoconstrictor drugs
Smilax spp. (sarsaparilla)	Saponins for pharmaceuticals
Trigonella foenum-graecum (fenugreek)	Anti-inflammatory, hypotensive drugs
Trillium erectum (beth root)	Saponins for pharmaceuticals*
Yucca spp. (yucca)	Saponins for pharmaceuticals

*Trillium erectum is unfortunately now an endangered species and should not be used.

Table 6.4. Sources of Cardioactive Saponins

HERB	ACTIONS
Convallaria majalis (lily of the valley)	Cardioactive, diuretic
Digitalis spp. (foxglove)	Cardioactive, diuretic
Helleborus niger (hellebore)	Cardioactive, diuretic
Nerium oleander (oleander)	Cardioactive, diuretic
Strophanthus kombe (strophanthus)	Cardioactive, diuretic
Urginea maritima (squill)	Expectorant, cardioactive, diuretic

General Properties of Steroidal Saponins

Many steroidal saponins share the core properties of the larger class of saponins:

• Antifertility
• Antihepatotoxic
• Anti-inflammatory
• Antimicrobial (fungicidal, antibacterial, antiviral)
• Capillary-strengthening
• Cytotoxic, antitumor
• Insecticidal and antifeedant
• Molluscicidal
• Piscicidal
• Plant growth inhibitors

Astragaloside III

This compound from the roots of *Astragalus membranaceus* has been shown to inhibit the formation of lipid peroxidase induced by intraperitoneal administration of adriamycin in rats. This suggests antioxidant activity.[89]

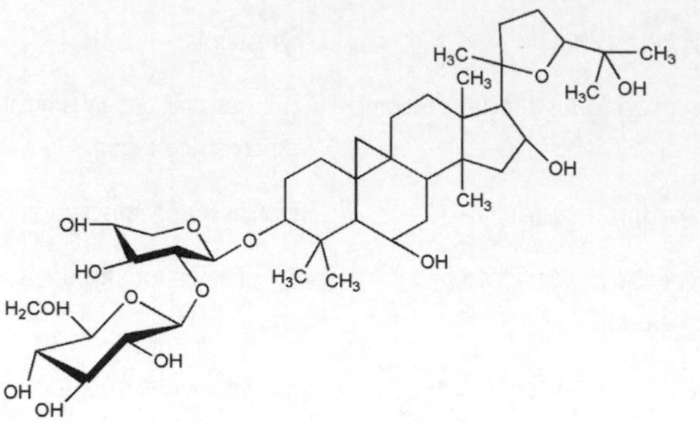

Fig. 6.85. Astragaloside III

Cimicifugoside

Found in some *Cimicifuga* spp., this has been found to be a potent and selective inhibitor of nucleoside transport at the plasma membrane site of mammalian cells in vitro.[90]

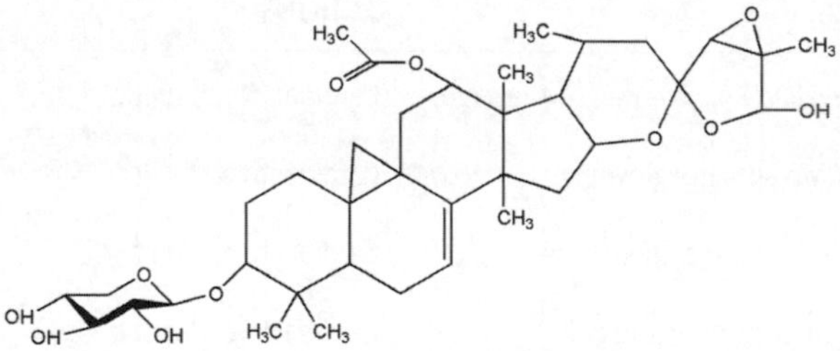

Fig. 6.86. Cimicifugoside

Diosgenin

Diosgenin is obtained through acid hydrolysis of many different saponins (for example, dioscin, deltonin, and gracillin), from *Dioscorea*, *Costus*, *Trillium*, and *Trigonella* species. It is used in the partial synthesis of hormones having a steroid structure, such as pregnenolone and progesterone.[91]

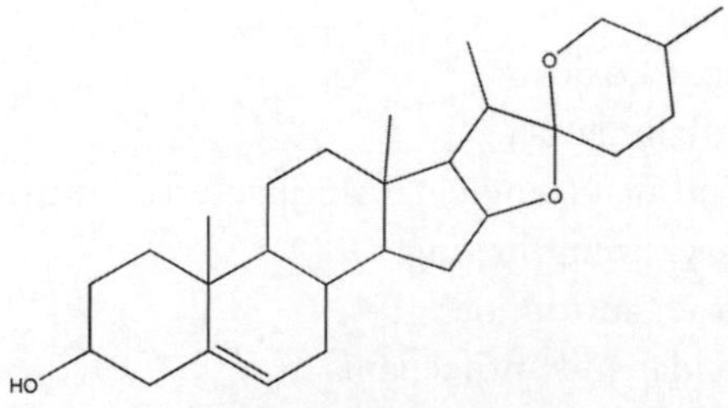

Fig. 6.87. Diosgenin

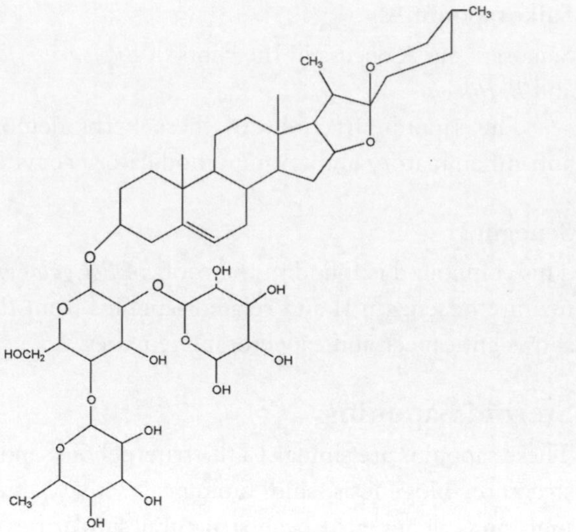

Fig. 6.88. Dioscin

Ginsenoside Re

Ginsenoside Re is found in *Panax pseudoginseng* and *P. ginseng*. Ginsenoside Re causes analgesic effects in mice at doses of 10 mg /kg.[92]

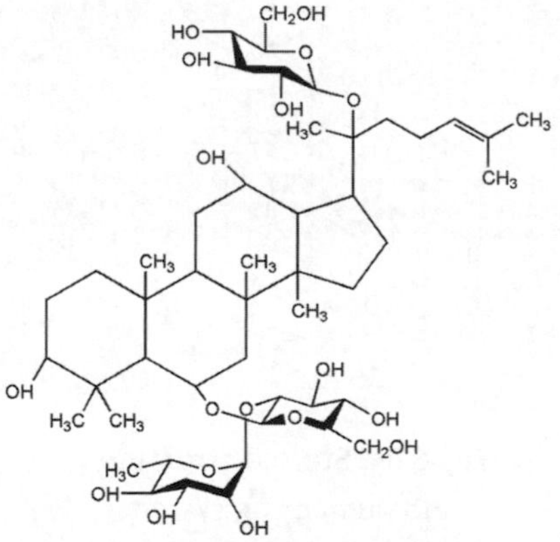

Fig. 6.89. Ginsenoside Re

Ginsenoside Rf

This is found in the roots of Korean ginseng (*Panax ginseng*).

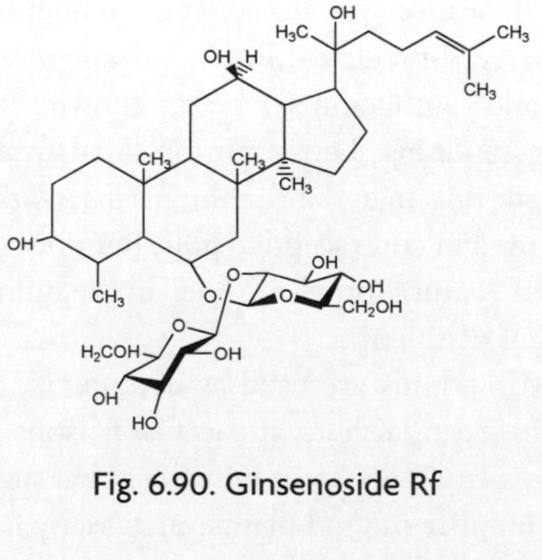

Fig. 6.90. Ginsenoside Rf

Ginsenoside Rg

This is another ginsenoside found in the roots of Korean ginseng (*Panax ginseng*).

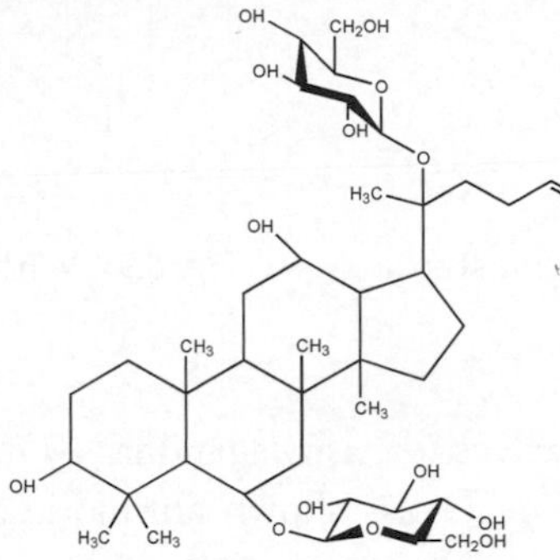

Fig. 6.91. Ginsenoside Rg

Ruscogenin

This compound, found in the rhizomes of butcher's broom (*Ruscus aculeatus*), is used in the treatment of hemorrhoids. Ruscosides A and B, partly identified glycosides of ruscogenin, decrease the cholesterol content of blood, reduce lipid deposition in the aorta, and lower liver arterial tension. They also show antiarteriosclerotic and hypotensive actions.[93]

CARDENOLIDES AND BUFADIENOLIDES

The cardenolides and bufadienolides are two related groups of C_{23} and C_{24} steroids of triterpenoid origin. The cardenolides are heart poisons that, when used in small doses, are extremely valuable clinically for controlling congestive heart failure.

Cardiac glycosides occur principally in the closely related families of the Apocynaceae and Asclepiadaceae.[94] In the milkweed genus, *Asclepias*, the compounds are secreted in the latex, and virtually every species that has been examined contains them. Cardiac glycosides are also found in a number of other dicotyledon families, such as Brassicaceae, Moraceae, and Scrophulariaceae (notably *Digitalis*), and in monocotyledon groups, especially Liliaceae. Cardenolides are remarkably nontoxic to lepidoptera. Some species of danaid butterflies store them in their bodies and wings to protect themselves from birds, as the cardenolides have an emetic effect on birds that prey on these butterflies.

Bufadienolides can be distinguished from cardenolides by the fact that the lactone ring substituting at C-17 in the steroid nucleus is 6-membered, rather than 5-membered. Bufadienolides were first identified in toad venom.

Convallatoxin

This is the major cardiac glycoside from the flowers and leaves of lily of the valley (*Convallaria majalis*). While it is very toxic to vertebrates, it has been used in minute doses as a cardiotonic.[95]

Digoxin

Digoxin is found in *Digitalis lanata* and *D. orientalis*. While toxic to vertebrates, derivatives of digoxin are used as cardiotonic agents.

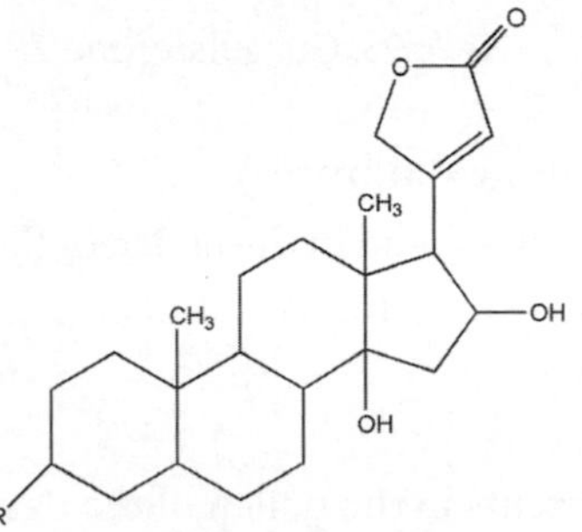

Fig. 6.92. Digitalin

PHYTOSTEROLS

Phytosterols are characterized by the presence of a hydroxyl group attached at C-3 and an extra methyl or ethyl substituent in the side chain, which is not present in animal sterols.[96] At one time, all sterols were believed to be animal products, but an increasing number of such compounds have been detected in plant tissues.

Three phytosterols are ubiquitous in higher plants, as they are all essential components of plant membranes: sitosterol, stigmasterol, and campesterol. These occur both in free form and as 3-glucosides.[97] A less common phytosterol is α-spinasterol, an isomer of stigmasterol found in spinach.

Occurrence and Distribution

In spite of the structural differences between plant and animal sterols, certain animal sterols have been found in plants. Estrone, for example, has been found in trace amounts in date palm seed (*Phoenix dactylifera*), while testosterone is present in the pollen of Scotch pine (*Pinus sylvestris*).[98] A large number of insect molting hormones have also been found in plants. These are known as *phytoecdysones*, and some 100 structures have been described. Ecdysone, the molting hormone of many insects, itself occurs in plants, but many of the other structures, such as prodecdysone B, are recorded only in the plant kingdom.

Commiphora mukul

Known as guggul in India, the resin contains steroids (called *guggulsterones*) that lower blood cholesterol and triglycerides via stimulation of thyroid function.[99]

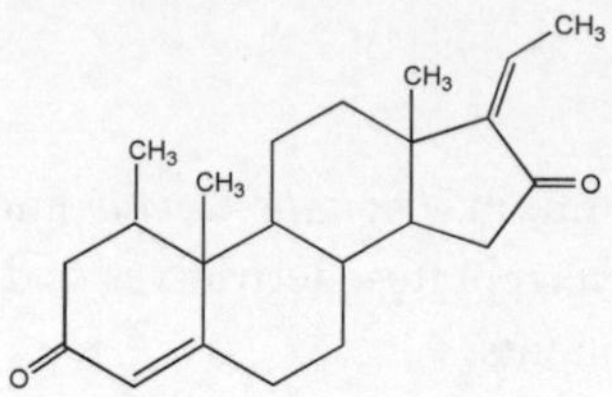

Fig. 6.93. Guggulsterone Z

Androstenedione (androtex)

This phytosterol is found in the pollen of Scotch pine, *Pinus sylvestris*. It has demonstrated androgenic activity.[100]

Cholesterol

Cholesterol occurs in the pollen of the date palm *(Phoenix dactylifera)* and in many marine red algae. It is a common sterol of animal tissues.

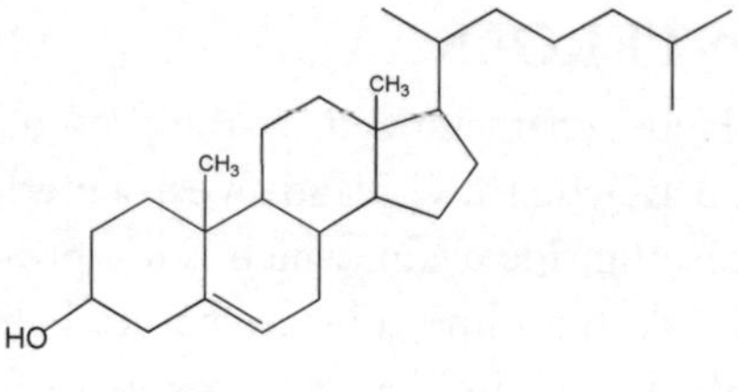

Fig. 6.94. Cholesterol

β-sitosterol

β-sitosterol has a widespread occurrence in higher plants. Among many others, it is found in wheat germ (*Triticum* spp.) and in corn (*Zea mays*). It is an essential component of plant cell membranes. β-sitosterol has shown anti-hyperlipoproteinemic activity.[101]

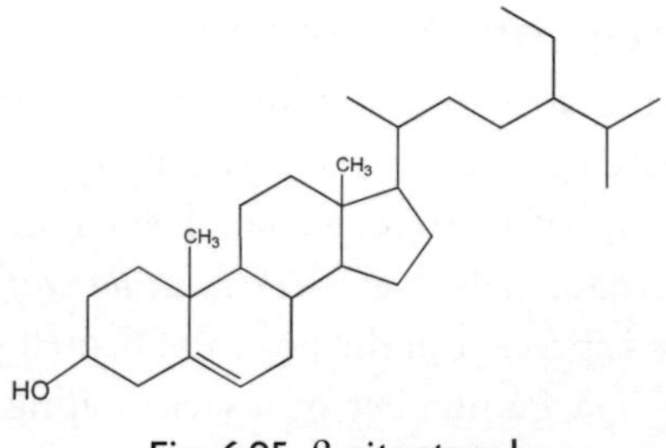

Fig. 6.95. β-sitosterol

Stigmasterol

Found in many higher plants, including soybeans (*Glycine max*), stigmasterol plays a vital structural role in plant cell membranes.

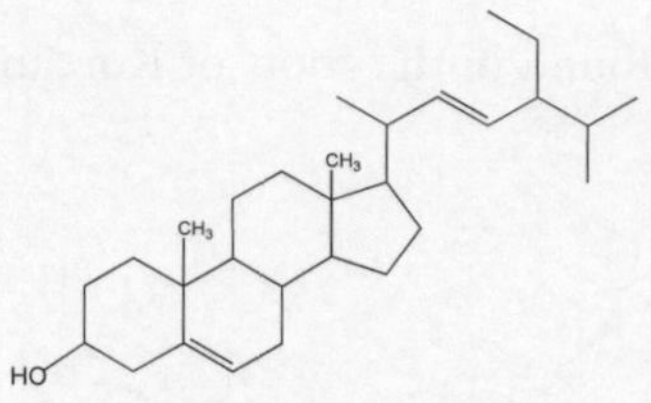

Fig. 6.96. Stigmasterol 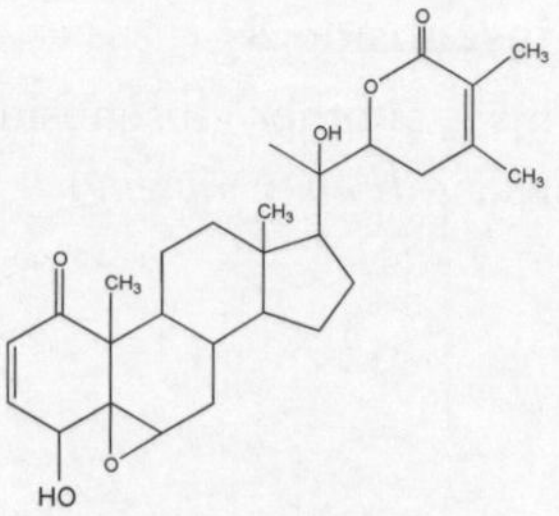   Fig. 6.97. Withanolide

Withanolide D

Found in the leaves of ashwagandha *(Withania somnifera)*, withanolide D has shown antibiotic and antitumor activities.[102]

NORTRITERPENOIDS

Nortriterpenoids are formed from triterpene precursors through oxidation and degradation, so they contain fewer than the 30 carbon atoms typically present in triterpenoids. There are two main groups: the limonoids (C_{26}) and the quassinoids (C_{20} and C_{19} triterpenoids).

More than 75 quassinoids have been described, all from the same plant family, Simaroubaceae, to which the genus *Quassia* belongs. Limonoids are also found in Simaroubaceae, but are more abundant in three related families: Rutaceae, Meliaceae, and Cneoraceae.[103]

Limonoids and quassinoids are notable for having very bitter tastes. Quassinoids have demonstrated antitumor activities in vitro, but none has yet been developed as an anticancer drug because of the toxicity. Some quassinoids show antiamoebic properties, and glaucarubin is used as a medicinal preparation for this purpose in France. Limonoids are of interest chiefly because of the need to counteract the bitter taste they impart to citrus drinks. However, they also hold commercial promise as the first members of a new generation of natural insecticides.

Limonin

Limonin is found in navel and Valencia oranges (*Citrus* spp.) during ripening. It is used to delay the development of bitterness in certain citrus fruit juices.[104]

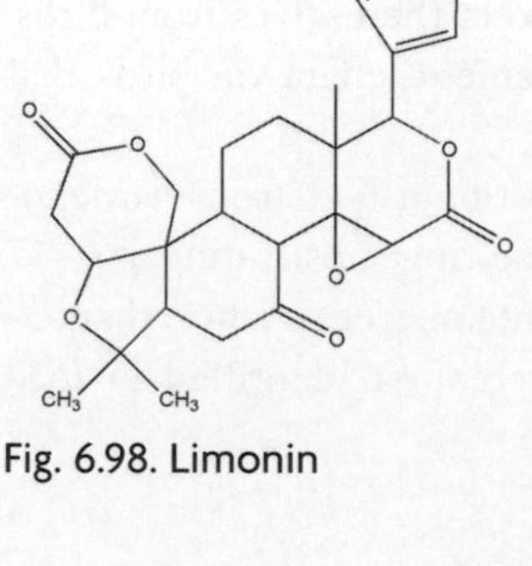

Fig. 6.98. Limonin 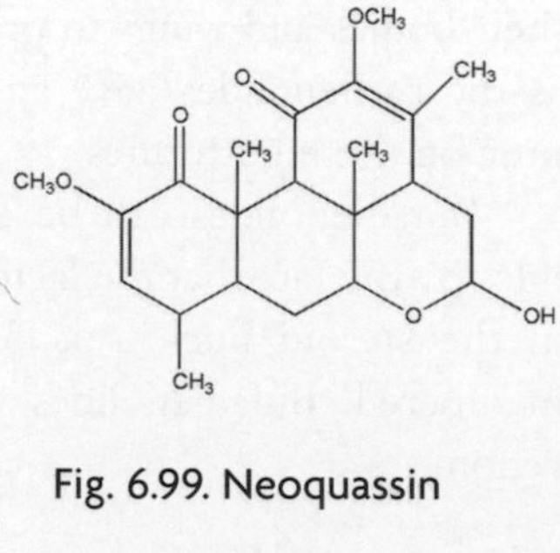   Fig. 6.99. Neoquassin

Neoquassin

This very bitter compound occurs in the wood of *Quassia amara* and in various *Picrasma* species. It may have potential as a natural insecticide.[105]

TETRATERPENOIDS

This class of molecules with 40 carbon atoms includes carotenes, xanthophylls, and retinoids. Here we will discuss the carotenoids.

Carotenoids

Carotenoids, C_{40} tetraterpenoids, are lipid-soluble pigments found in all plants. In animals, several carotenoids (especially β-carotene) are metabolized to vitamin A. Carotenoids appear to have two principal functions in plants: They supply accessory pigments during the process of photosynthesis and serve as coloring matter for flowers and fruits. In flowers, they mostly appear as yellow colors, as in daffodils, pansies, and marigolds. In fruits, they may be orange or red (for example, rose hips, tomatoes, and peppers). Dietary carotenoids also provide many brilliant animal colors, seen in flamingos, starfish, lobsters, and sea urchins.

Only a few carotenoids are common in higher plants.[106] Well-known carotenoids are either simple unsaturated hydrocarbons based on lycopene or oxygenated derivatives of unsaturated hydrocarbons known as xanthophylls. The chemical structure of lycopene consists of a long chain of eight isoprene units joined head to tail. This completely conjugated system of alternate double bonds becomes the *chromophore* that gives the compound its color, or the part of the molecule responsible for a given spectral band. The term arose in the dye industry and referred originally to the groups in the molecule that are responsible for a dye's color.

Capsanthin

Capsanthin occurs in the ripe fruits of sweet red pepper or paprika (*Capsicum annuum*) and in some barberries (*Berberis* spp.), and in the petals of orange lilies (for example, *Lilium pumilum*) and the anthers of other lilies, such as the tiger lily (*Lilium lancifolium*).

Capsanthin is used commercially to provide orange-red food colorings and as flavoring in sauces, salad dressings, sausages, and other foods.[107]

Carotene

β-carotene occurs in almost all green leaves of higher plants and in many lower plants, including ferns, mosses, and algae, as well as in fungi and some bacteria. It is widely found in roots, such as carrot (*Daucus carota*) and sweet potato (*Ipomoea batatas*), and in the yellow and orange flowers of many plants, including gorse (*Ulex* spp.). It also occurs in seeds, such as oats (*Avena sativa*) and fruits, including sweet red pepper (*Capsicum annuum*), yams (*Dioscorea* spp.), and rose hips (*Rosa* spp.).

β-carotene is the most important of the carotenoid vitamin A precursors. It is used commercially as a yellow food coloring for fats (for example, margarine) and as a sunscreen agent to prevent the photosensitivity reaction of erythropoietic protoporphyria.

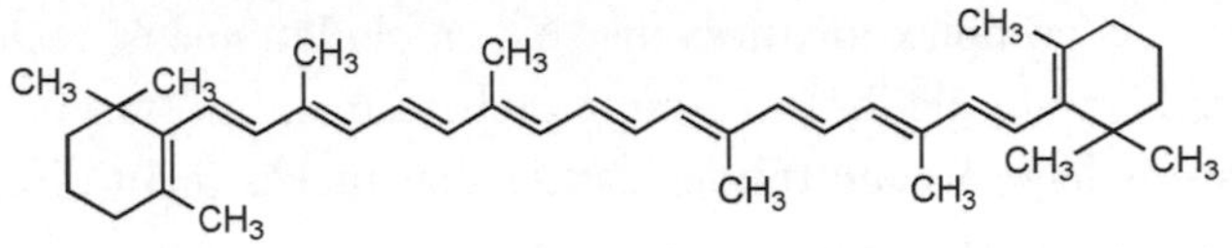

Fig. 6.100. β-carotene

Lycopene

Lycopene occurs in the ripe fruits of tomatoes (*Lycopersicon esculentum*), *Citrus* species, persimmon (*Diospyros kaki*), dog rose (*Rosa canina*), and numerous other fruits and berries. It also occurs in the petals of many orange flowers (for example, *Calendula officinalis*), in very large amounts in the ripe seeds of bitter melon (*Momordica charantia*), in rutabagas (*Brassica napus*), and in red varieties of carrot (*Daucus carota*).[108]

Dietary intakes of tomatoes and products containing lycopene are associated with decreased risk of chronic illnesses such as cancer and cardiovascular diseases.[109] Serum and tissue lycopene levels have also been shown to be inversely related to the risk of lung and prostate cancers. Lycopene is a potent antioxidant, which is clearly one of its major mechanisms of action. As an antioxidant, lycopene traps singlet oxygen and reduces mutagenesis in the Ames test.

PLANT EXUDATES

Plant exudates are chemically complex, solid or semisolid mixtures of vegetable origin, such as balsams, gums, oleoresins, and resins. The proportions of their constituents vary with climate, season of the year, and other factors.

Resins

A resin is a natural or synthetic organic compound consisting of a noncrystalline or viscous liquid substance. Most natural resins are exuded from trees, especially pines and firs. Resin forms in response to injury to the bark from wind, fire, lightning, or other cause. The secretion usually loses some of its volatile components through evaporation, leaving a soft, initially soluble residue that becomes insoluble as it ages.

Resins are characteristically insoluble in water and mostly soluble in alcohol; because of their chemical complexity, they often will not crystallize, but instead soften or melt at moderate heat. They are usually the oxidized terpenes of volatile oils, and, because they are insoluble in water, have little taste. When pure, resins are generally transparent, but when water is added they become opaque and lose their hard or brittle qualities. They do not conduct electricity, but when rubbed do become negatively charged.

As complex mixtures that may include lignans, resin acids, resin alcohols, resinotannols, esters, and resenes, resins have an amorphous nature that makes them difficult to classify. They may occur in mixtures with other plant constituents, as in gum resins, oleogum resins, and glycoresins.

One way in which to classify natural resins is to determine whether they are alcohol- or oil-soluble. Among the alcohol-soluble resins are balsams, long popular as healing agents; turpentines, used as solvents; and mastic, dragon's blood, damar, sandarac, and lac, all used as components of varnishes. The oil-soluble resins include rosin, derived along with turpentine from the long-leaf pine; copal, used in varnishes; amber, the hardest natural resin, which is fabricated into jewelry; and cashew nutshell oil.

In addition, a distinction must be made among natural resins, prepared resins, and synthetic resins.

A *natural resin* is one that occurs as a plant exudate. Mastic, formerly an official medicine in *The United States Pharmacopoeia*, is a good example.

A *prepared resin* can be made by exhausting a drug that owes its activity to resinous constituents with alcohol—in other words, by pouring the concentrated alcoholic percolate into water and collecting, washing, and drying the precipitate. The resin made from *Podophyllum* is an example of this class. A prepared resin may also be derived from a natural oleoresin by driving off the volatile oil with heat, as in Rosin NF.

Synthetic resins are polymeric substances that are formed either by condensation or by the addition of readily available common chemicals. Phenol and formaldehyde serve as examples. These compounds interact initially to produce hydroxybenzyl alcohols, which then condense to yield a large series of phenol-formaldehyde (Bakelite) resins. These and many other synthetic resins constitute the foundation of the modern plastics industry.

Table 6.5. Herbs Containing Resins

HERB	COMMON USES
Boswellia serrata (frankincense)	Perfumery
Cinnamomum camphora (camphor)	Rubefacient
Commiphora molmol (myrrh)	Antimicrobial, vulnerary, rubefacient
Daemonorops draco (dragon's blood)	Antimicrobial
Eriodictyon californicum (yerba santa)	Expectorant
Grindelia spp. (grindelia)	Relaxing expectorant, anti-inflammatory
Guaiacum officinale (guaiacum)	Anti-inflammatory, diaphoretic
Ipomoea purga (jalap)	Powerful cathartic
Turnera diffusa var. *aphrodisiaca* (damiana)	Nervine

Rosin

Rosin, also called colophony, is a type of resin used for varnish and in manufacturing many products. It becomes sticky when warm and has a faint pinelike odor. Gum rosin is the residue produced through distillation of the oleoresin from pine trees, the volatile component of which is spirit of turpentine. Wood rosin, obtained by solvent extraction of stumps, is usually a darker color. Rosin and its chemical derivatives are used chiefly in the manufacture of soaps, varnishes, sealing wax, printing inks, dryers, size for paper, adhesives, binders, soldering fluxes, gloss oils for paints, and pitch for casks.

Guaiac

This resin from the wood of *Guaiacum officinale* or *G. sanctum* is reported to contain about 70% α- and β-guaiaconic acids; 11% guaiacic acid, related compounds, and guaiaretic acid; and 15% vanillin, guaiac yellow, and guaiac saponin. It is insoluble in water but freely soluble in alcohol, chloroform, ether, creosote, and alkali.

In medicine, it is used as a reagent in tests for occult (hidden) blood. It is also employed to test for the presence of oxidizing enzymes or cyanogenetic glycosides in various materials.

Oleoresins

Oleoresins are liquid preparations that consist of natural volatile oils and resins extracted from plants by percolation with a menstruum of acetone, alcohol, or ether. As with resins, a distinction must be made between natural and prepared oleoresins.

Natural oleoresins are mixtures of volatile oils and resin, generally obtained by incising the trunks of trees in which they occur. Turpentine and copaiba are natural oleoresins formerly recognized as official preparations in the National Formulary of the United States.

Prepared oleoresins are concentrated liquid preparations made by percolating drugs that contain both volatile oils and resin with an appropriate solvent (acetone, ether, or alcohol), and concentrating the percolate until the solvent dissipates.

Balsams

Balsams are aromatic resinous plant exudates that consist of a resin dispersed in benzoic or cinnamic acid esters. Balsams are difficult to distinguish from oleoresins, which are resins dissolved in essential oils, but in general, oleoresins are slightly more fluid. Examples include Peru balsam, a true balsam from a tropical tree (*Myroxylon balsamum* var. *pereirae*), which provides a fragrant, thick, deep brown or black fluid used in perfumery; and Tolu balsam, an even thicker brown balsam used in cough syrups and lozenges. The latter, made from *Myroxylon balsamum* var. *balsamum*, becomes solid over time.

Gum Resins

These are natural mixtures of gum and resin, usually obtained as exudations from plants, such as myrrh.

Myrrh

Myrrh is the air-dried oleo-gum resin obtained from *Commiphora molmol* and closely related species, trees native to northeast Africa and Arabia. Myrrh contains 2% to 10% essential oil, 25% to 45% alcohol-soluble resins, and 30% to 60% a water-soluble gum. The essential oil is thick, with a yellow- to reddish brown color. Myrrh resin collects in canals in the inner bark of the tree. It is secreted through fissures, wounds, or incisions made in the bark. Ground myrrh quickly loses its essential oil and cakes easily due to moisture absorption, so it should be stored in a sealed container.

References

1. Harborne JB, Baxter H. *Phytochemical Dictionary: A Handbook of Bioactive Compounds from Plants*. London; Washington, DC: Taylor & Francis, 1993.
2. Ibid.
3. Ibid.
4. [No authors listed] d-limonene. *IARC monographs on the evaluation of carcinogenic risks to humans* 1999; 73:307–27.
5. Crowell PL, Gould MN. Chemoprevention and therapy of cancer by d-limonene. *Critical Reviews in Oncogenesis* 1994; 5(1):1–22.
6. Crowell PL, Siar Ayoubi A, Burke YD. Antitumorigenic effects of limonene and perillyl alcohol against pancreatic and breast cancer. *Advances in Experimental Medicine and Biology* 1996; 401:131–6.
7. Igimi H, Tamura R, Toraishi K, et al. Medical dissolution of gallstones. Clinical experience of d-limonene as a simple, safe, and effective solvent. *Digestive Diseases and Sciences* 1991 Feb; 36(2):200–8.
8. Budavari S, ed. *The Merck Index,* 12th edition. Whitehouse Station, NJ: Merck, 1996.
9. Harborne JB, Baxter H. *Phytochemical Dictionary: A Handbook of Bioactive Compounds from Plants*. London; Washington, DC: Taylor & Francis, 1993.
10. Ibid.
11. Budavari S, ed. *The Merck Index*, 12th edition. Whitehouse Station, NJ: Merck, 1996.
12. Ibid.
13. Harborne JB, Baxter H. *Phytochemical Dictionary: A Handbook of Bioactive Compounds from Plants*. London; Washington, DC: Taylor & Francis, 1993.
14. Ibid.
15. Budavari S, ed. *The Merck Index*, 12th edition. Whitehouse Station, NJ: Merck, 1996.
16. Eccles R. Menthol and related cooling compounds. *The Journal of Pharmacy and Pharmacology* 1994 Aug; 46(8):618–30.
17. Harborne JB, Baxter H. *Phytochemical Dictionary: A Handbook of Bioactive Compounds from Plants*. London; Washington, DC: Taylor & Francis, 1993.
18. Budavari S, ed. *The Merck Index*, 12th edition. Whitehouse Station, NJ: Merck, 1996.
19. Goodman LS, Gilman A. *The Pharmacological Basis of Therapeutics*, 7th edition. New York: Macmillan, 1985.
20. Budavari S, ed. *The Merck Index*, 12th edition. Whitehouse Station, NJ: Merck, 1996.
21. Ibid.
22. Matthijs S, Adriaens PA. Chlorhexidine varnishes: a review. *Journal of Clinical Peridontology* 2002 Jan; 29(1):1–8.
23. Harborne JB, Baxter H. *Phytochemical Dictionary: A Handbook of Bioactive Compounds from Plants*. London; Washington, DC: Taylor & Francis, 1993.

24. Ibid.

25. Ibid.

26. Bianco A. The chemistry of iridoids. In: Atta-Ur Rahman HEJ, ed. *Studies in Natural Products Chemistry*, vol. 7. Amsterdam: Elsevier, 1990.

27. Buckingham J. *Dictionary of Natural Products*. London; New York: Chapman & Hall, 1994.

28. Harborne JB, Baxter H. *Phytochemical Dictionary: A Handbook of Bioactive Compounds from Plants*. London; Washington, DC: Taylor & Francis, 1993.

29. Robles M, Aregullin M, West J, et al. Recent studies on the zoopharmacognosy, pharmacology and neurotoxicology of sesquiterpene lactones. *Planta Medica* 1995 Jun; 61(3):199–203.

30. Houghton PJ. *Valerian*. Amsterdam: Harwood Academic Publishers, 1997.

31. Harborne JB, Baxter H. *Phytochemical Dictionary: A Handbook of Bioactive Compounds from Plants*. London; Washington, DC: Taylor & Francis, 1993.

32. Evans WC. *Trease & Evans' Pharmacognosy*, 13th edition. London: Baillere Tindall, 1989.

33. Harborne JB, Baxter H. *Phytochemical Dictionary: A Handbook of Bioactive Compounds from Plants*. London; Washington, DC: Taylor & Francis, 1993.

34. Ibid.

35. Mackenzie MA, et al. The influence of glycyrrhetinic acid on plasmol cortisol and cortisone levels in healthy young volunteers. *The Journal of Clinical Endocrinology and Metabolism* 1990; 70:1637–43.

36. Budavari S, ed. *The Merck Index*, 12th edition. Whitehouse Station, NJ: Merck, 1996.

37. Harborne JB, Baxter H. *Phytochemical Dictionary: A Handbook of Bioactive Compounds from Plants*. London; Washington, DC: Taylor & Francis, 1993.

38. Houghton PJ. *Valerian*. Amsterdam: Harwood Academic Publishers, 1997.

39. Harborne JB, Baxter H. *Phytochemical Dictionary: A Handbook of Bioactive Compounds from Plants*. London; Washington, DC: Taylor & Francis, 1993.

40. Ibid.

41. Ibid.

42. Ibid.

43. Coutinho EM. Gossypol: a contraceptive for men. *Contraception* 2002 Apr; 65(4):259–63.

44. Harborne JB, Baxter H. *Phytochemical Dictionary: A Handbook of Bioactive Compounds from Plants*. London; Washington, DC: Taylor & Francis, 1993.

45. Ibid.

46. Ibid.

47. Bruneton J. *Pharmacognosy, Phytochemistry, Medicinal Plants*. Hampshire, UK: Intercept, 1999.

48. Robles M, Aregullin M, West J, et al. Recent studies on the zoopharmacognosy, pharmacology and neurotoxicology of sesquiterpene lactones. *Planta Medica* 1995 Jun; 61(3):199–203.

49. Hausen BM. Sesquiterpene lactones. In: DeSmet, ed. *Adverse Effects on Herbal Drugs*, vol 1. Berlin: Springer-Verlag, 1992.

50. Ibid.

51. Lovell CR. *Plants and the Skin*. Oxford, Boston: Blackwell Scientific Publications, 1993.

52. Harborne JB, Baxter H. *Phytochemical Dictionary: A Handbook of Bioactive Compounds from Plants*. London; Washington, DC: Taylor & Francis, 1993.

53. Ibid.

54. Ibid.

55. Frederich M, Dogneacute JM, Angenot L, et al. New trends in anti-malarial agents. *Current Medicinal Chemistry* 2002 Aug; 9(15):1435–56.

56. Harborne JB, Baxter H. *Phytochemical Dictionary: A Handbook of Bioactive Compounds from Plants*. London; Washington, DC: Taylor & Francis, 1993.

57. Ibid.

58. Ibid.

59. Bruneton J. *Pharmacognosy, Phytochemistry, Medicinal Plants*. Hampshire, UK: Intercept, 1999.

60. Hanson JR. Diterpenoids. *Natural Product Reports* 1998; 1:93–106.

61. Alcarez MJ, Rios JL. Pharmacology of diterpenoids. In: Harborne JB, Toma-Barberan FA, eds. *Ecological Chemistry and Biochemistry of Plant Terpenoids*. Oxford: Clarendon Press, 1991.

62. Singh M, Pal M, Sharma RP. Biological activity of the labdane diterpenes. *Planta Medica* 1999 Feb; 65(1):2–8.

63. de Souza NJ, Dohadwalla AN, Reden J. Forskolin: a labdane diterpenoid with antihypertensive, positive inotropic, platelet aggregation inhibitory, and adenylate cyclase activating properties. *Medicinal Research Reviews* 1983 Apr–Jun; 3(2):201–19.

64. Evans FJ. *Naturally Occurring Phorbol Esters*. Boca Raton, FL: CRC Press, 1986.

65. Harborne JB, Baxter H. *Phytochemical Dictionary: A Handbook of Bioactive Compounds from Plants*. London; Washington, DC: Taylor & Francis, 1993.

66. Ibid.

67. Ibid.

68. de Souza NJ, Dohadwalla AN, Reden J. Forskolin: a labdane diterpenoid with antihypertensive, positive inotropic, platelet aggregation inhibitory, and adenylate cyclase activating properties. *Medicinal Research Reviews* 1983 Apr–Jun; 3(2):201–19.

69. Harborne JB, Baxter H. *Phytochemical Dictionary: A Handbook of Bioactive Compounds from Plants*. London; Washington, DC: Taylor & Francis, 1993.

70. Ibid.

71. Ibid.

72. Ibid.

73. Ibid.

74. Lacaille-Dubois MA, Wagner H. A review of the biological and pharmacological activitities of saponins. *Phytomedicine: International Journal of Phytotherapy and Phytopharmacology* 1996; 2(4):363–86.

75. Hostettmann K, Marston A. *Saponins*. Cambridge, New York: Cambridge University Press, 1995.

76. Ibid.

77. Ibid.

78. Ibid.

79. Ibid.

80. Lacaille-Dubois MA, Wagner H. A review of the biological and pharmacological activitities of saponins. *Phytomedicine: International Journal of Phytotherapy and Phytopharmacology* 1996; 2(4):363–86.

81. Watanabe, et al. Solubilizing of saponins of Bupleuri radix with ginseng saponins: cooperative effect of dammarane saponins. *Planta Medica* 1988; 54:405–9.

82. Sjolander A, Cox JC, Barr IG. ISCOMs: an adjuvant with multiple functions. *Journal of Leukocyte Biology* 1998 Dec; 64(6):713–23.

83. Harborne JB, Baxter H. *Phytochemical Dictionary: A Handbook of Bioactive Compounds from Plants*. London; Washington, DC: Taylor & Francis, 1993.

84. Miro M. Cucurbitacins and Their Pharmacological Effects. *Phytotherapy Research* 1995; 9:159–68.

85. Harborne JB, Baxter H. *Phytochemical Dictionary: A Handbook of Bioactive Compounds from Plants*. London; Washington, DC: Taylor & Francis, 1993.

86. Ibid.

87. Ibid.

88. Ibid.

89. He K, Wang HK. Recent development of chemical studies on some medicinal plants of Astragalus spp. *Yao Xue Xue Bao* 1988 Nov; 23(11):873–80.

90. Lacaille-Dubois MA, Wagner H. A review of the biological and pharmacological activitities of saponins. *Phytomedicine: International Journal of Phytotherapy and Phytopharmacology* 1996; 2(4):363–86.

91. Hostettmann K, Marston A. *Saponins*. Cambridge, New York: Cambridge University Press, 1995.

92. Harborne JB, Baxter H. *Phytochemical Dictionary: A Handbook of Bioactive Compounds from Plants*. London; Washington, DC: Taylor & Francis, 1993.

93. Ibid.

94. Ibid.

95. Ibid.

96. Ibid.

97. Ibid.

98. Ibid.

99. Satyavati G. Guggulipid: a promising hypolipidaemic agent from gum guggul (*Commiphora wightii*). In: Wagner H, Farnsworth NR, *Economic and Medicinal Plant Research*, vol.5. San Diego: Academic Press, 1991.

100. Harborne JB, Baxter H. *Phytochemical Dictionary: A Handbook of Bioactive Compounds from Plants*. London; Washington, DC: Taylor & Francis, 1993.

101. Ibid.

102. Ibid.

103. Ibid.

104. Ibid.

105. Ibid.

106. Ibid.

107. Duke JA. Promising phytomedicinals. In: Janick J, Simon JE, eds. *Advances in New Crops*. Portland, OR: Timber Press, 1990.

108. Harborne JB, Baxter H. *Phytochemical Dictionary: A Handbook of Bioactive Compounds from Plants*. London; Washington, DC: Taylor & Francis, 1993.

109. Heber D, Lu QY. Overview of mechanisms of action of lycopene. *Experimental Biology and Medicine (Maywood)* 2002 Nov; 227(10):920–3.

Suggested Reading

Bruneton, J. *Pharmacognosy, Phytochemistry, Medicinal Plants*. Hampshire, UK: Intercept, 1999.

Evans WC. *Trease & Evans' Pharmacognosy*, 13th edition. London: Baillere Tindall, 1989.

Harborne JB, Baxter H. *Phytochemical Dictionary: A Handbook of Bioactive Compounds from Plants*. London; Washington, DC: Taylor & Francis, 1993.

7

❧

POLYPHENOLS

About 8,000 naturally occurring plant phenolics have been identified, and about half of these are flavonoids. There are many structurally simple phenols, such as phenolic acids, phenylpropanoids, and phenolic quinones. Several important groups of plant polymeric materials are phenolic: the lignins, melanins, and tannins. Finally, phenolic groups are occasionally found in alkaloids and terpenoids.[1]

Phenolics contribute significantly to the color, taste, and flavor of many herbs, foods, and drinks. Some flavonoids are valued pharmacologically for their anti-inflammatory activities (such as quercetin) or antihepatotoxic properties (for example, silybin).[2] Certain isoflavonoids, such as genistein and daidzein, are phytoestrogens, while others are insecticidal or piscicidal. The anthocyanins have a clearly defined function in flowers and fruits in attracting pollinators and as seed dispersal agents. Many of these phenolic molecules are also effective antioxidants and free radical scavengers, especially the flavonoids. As discussed later, they are also the basis of most flower colors.

Major Functions of Polyphenols

Polyphenols have in common an aromatic benzene ring bearing one or more hydroxyl groups.

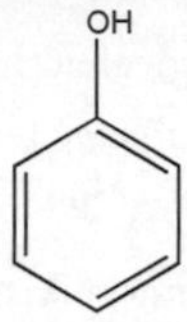

Fig. 7.1. Phenol

The majority of polyphenols are water-soluble; they usually occur naturally as glycosides, located within the plant cell in the central vacuole. Other phenolics are lipophilic and are present in the cell cytoplasm or at the surface of plants in waxes and bud exudates.

CLASSIFICATION OF PHENOLICS

Phenolics are classified according to their structure or biosynthetic origin, but no ideal system is available. Their great diversity makes simple classification extremely

Table 7.1. Major Classes of Phenolics in Plants

NUMBER OF C ATOMS	BASIC SKELETON	CLASS	EXAMPLE
6	C_6	Simple phenolics	Arbutin 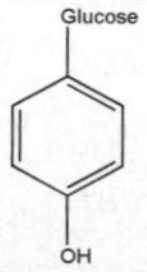
7	C_6-C_1	Phenolic acids	Salicylic acid 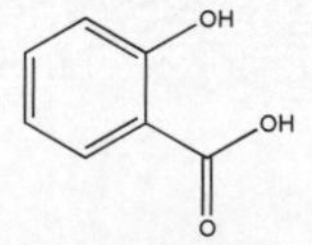
8	C_6-C_2	Benzofurans	Usnic acid 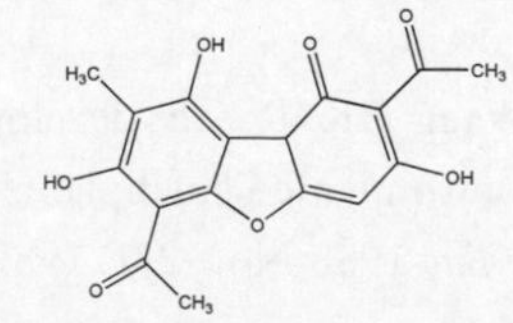

NUMBER OF C ATOMS	BASIC SKELETON	CLASS	EXAMPLE	
9	C_6-C_3	Cinnamic acids	Caffeic acid	
		Phenylpropenoids	Myristicin	
		Coumarins	Umbelliferone	
10	C_6-C_4	Naphthoquinones	Juglone	
13	$C_6-C_1-C_6$	Xanthones	Mangiferin	
14	$C_6-C_2-C_6$	Stilbenoids	Resveratrol	
		Anthraquinones	Emodin	
15	$C_6-C_3-C_6$	Flavonoids	Kaempferol	
18	$(C_6-C_3)_2$	Lignans	Dihydroguaiaretic acid	
30	$(C_6-C_3-C_6)_2$	Biflavonoids	Ginketin	
n	$(C_6-C_3)_n$	Lignins		
	$(C_6-C_3-C_6)_n$	Flavolans (condensed tannins)		

problematic. What follows is a system that proves most relevant to the needs of the herbalist.

SIMPLE PHENOLS AND PHENOLIC ACIDS

Phenolic acids (C_6-C_1) are ubiquitous among plants, but free phenols (C_6) are rare. The pharmacological properties of these widely found constituents are probably best demonstrated by the urinary tract antimicrobial arbutin and the anti-inflammatory salicylates. A property shared by all phenols is antimicrobial activity. In fact, phenol itself was the first antiseptic used in surgery.

Hydroquinone is probably the most widely distributed of the simple phenols, occurring in a number of plants as the glucoside arbutin. Simple phenols with side chains are often skin irritants, such as urushiol III from the poison ivy plant. Urushiol III may be classified as a phenol or a terpene, depending upon the focus of interest.

Table 7.2. Herbal Activities Related to Content of Simple Phenolics

HERB	ACTIVITY
Arctostaphylos uva-ursi (bearberry)	Antimicrobial, diuretic
Capsicum spp. (cayenne)	Food, circulatory stimulant, rubefacient, analgesic
Cynara scolymus (artichoke)	Digestive bitter, cholagogue
Dryopteris filix-mas (male fern)	Anthelmintic
Filipendula ulmaria (meadowsweet)	Anti-inflammatory, analgesic
Gaultheria procumbens (wintergreen)	Anti-inflammatory, analgesic
Salix spp. (willow)	Anti-inflammatory, analgesic
Solidago virgaurea (goldenrod)	Anticatarrhal, diuretic
Vanilla planifolia (vanilla)	Food, perfumery
Viburnum prunifolium (black haw)	Antispasmodic

Arbutin

Found in the leaves of *Arctostaphylos uva-ursi* (bearberry), *Vaccinium myrtillus* (bilberry), and *Origanum majorana* (marjoram), arbutin demonstrates diuretic, antitussive, and urinary antimicrobial properties. It is easily hydrolyzed into hydroquinone and glucose; however, the gallotannins in simple plant extracts prevent hydrolysis, preserving the effectiveness of such extracts.[3]

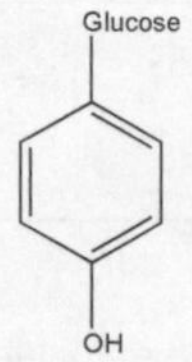

Fig. 7.2. Arbutin

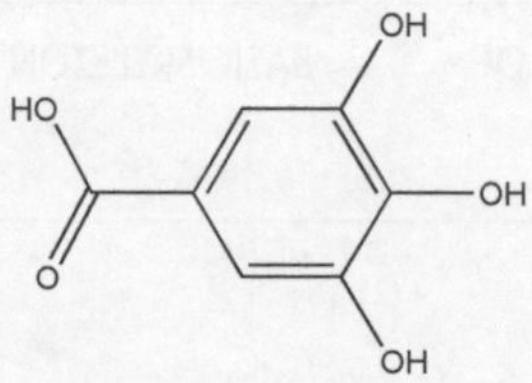

Fig. 7.3. Gallic acid

Gallic Acid

This phenolic acid is the parent compound of the gallotannins and is relatively widespread. Gallic acid is well known for astringent properties, but has demonstrated many other activities in vitro, including antibacterial, antiviral, antifungal, anti-inflammatory, antitumor, anti-anaphylactic, antimutagenic, choleretic, and bronchodilatory actions. It also inhibits insulin degradation and promotes smooth muscle relaxation.[4]

Guaiacol

Guaiacol occurs in creosote made from beechwood tar, in guaiac resin, and in various plant oils and saps—for example, celery seed oil (*Apium graveolens*). Guaiacol is used as an expectorant in veterinary practice, mostly in the form of esters. In humans, it has been applied externally to treat eczema and other skin diseases.[5]

Salicin and Salicylates

This widely distributed group of simple phenolics appear to play a defensive role in plant ecology.[6] The type example of the class, salicin, was first identified in the bark of willow (*Salix* spp.). This class of simple phenolics is widely distributed in flowering plant families, including Salicaceae (*Populus* spp. and *Salix* spp.), Rosaceae (*Filipendula ulmaria),* and Caprifoliaceae (*Viburnum prunifolium*). Salicin and salicylates have a long history of use in folk medicine for relief of headaches and musculoskeletal pain.

Properties of Salicin and Salicylates

- Analgesic
- Antipyretic
- Anti-inflammatory

Salicin does not demonstrate the anticlotting effect that is seen with aspirin. On the other hand, aspirin has a well-known tendency to cause gastric ulceration and hemorrhage, and there is no evidence that salicin-containing herbs have the same adverse effects.

Hydroquinone

Upon hydrolysis in the body, arbutin releases a diphenol, which is immediately oxidized to hydroquinone. For this release of antiseptic properties, an alkaline environment in the urine is needed. It has antibacterial, antitumor, antimitotic, and hypertensive actions.[7]

Salicin

Salicin occurs in the bark of poplar (*Populus* spp.) and willow (*Salix* spp.), and in the female flowers of *Salix* species. It is also found in the root bark of black haw (*Viburnum prunifolium*) and the aerial parts of meadowsweet (*Filipendula ulmaria*). Salicin is used as an analgesic, anti-inflammatory, and antirheumatic agent.[8]

Fig. 7.4. Hydroquinone 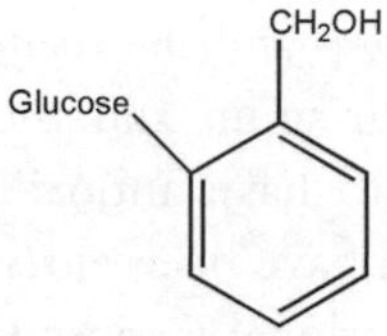   Fig. 7.5. Salicin

Δ^9-tetrahydrocannabinol

This compound occurs in the resin and the tips of shoots of *Cannabis sativa*. This, the active principle of marijuana, demonstrates anti-inflammatory, antiemetic, and hallucinogenic properties.[9]

Vanillin

Vanillin is widespread in plants, but is generally found in small amounts. It is commercially important and is present in the pods of the tropical orchid *Vanilla planifolia*, where it occurs with its glucoside, vanilloside. Vanillin also occurs in the sprouts of *Asparagus* spp. and in the essential oils of *Ruta* and *Spirea* species. It is antifungal.[10]

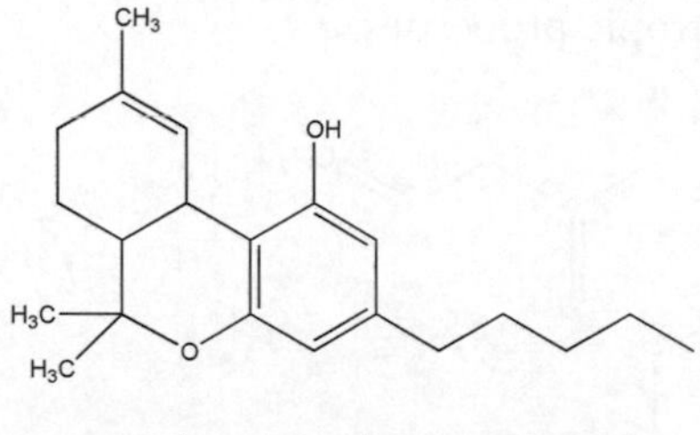

Fig. 7.6. Δ^9-tetrahydrocannabinol 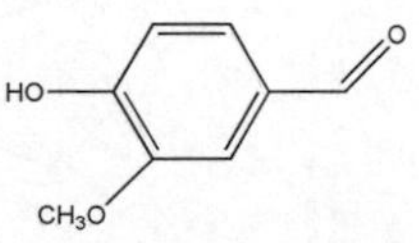   Fig. 7.7. Vanillin

Benzofurans

The benzofuran nucleus (C_6-C_2), in which a benzene ring and a furan ring are fused, is present in many secondary plant metabolites, some of which are classified as coumarins and flavonoids.

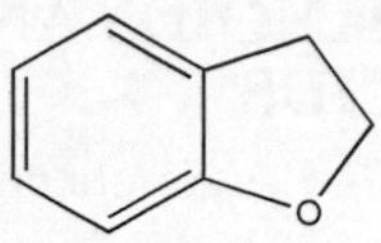

Fig. 7.8. Benzofuran nucleus

The simple benzofurans, such as usnic acid, have two benzene rings fused on either side of a central furan ring. They are characteristically present in lichens. A biological property many benzofurans share is antifungal activity. Antifungal substances may either occur naturally in the plant or as phytoalexins formed after plants have suffered microbial infection. Other benzofurans are toxic to insects, fish, cattle, and humans.

Lithospermic Acid

Lithospermic acid is found in the roots of various plants in the Boraginaceae family, including *Lycopus europaeus*, *L. virginicus*, *Lithospermum ruderale*, *L. officinale*, and *Symphytum officinale*. There have been unconfirmed reports of contraceptive properties in humans.[11]

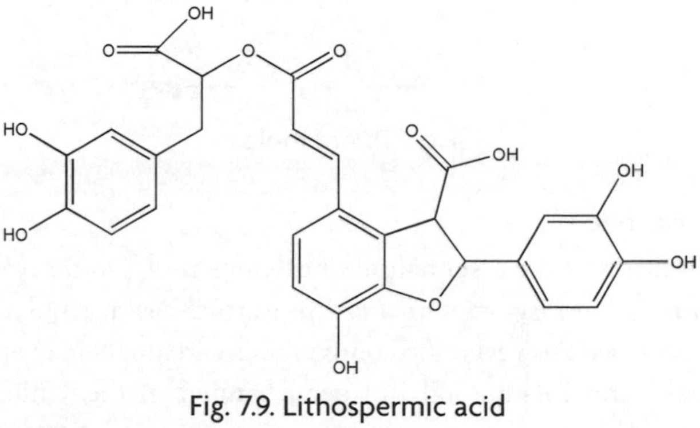

Fig. 7.9. Lithospermic acid

Usnic Acid

Usnic acid is found in a number of lichens—for example, *Usnea*, *Ramalina*, *Evernia*, *Parmelia*, *Lecanora*, and *Cladonia* species. Usnic acid demonstrates antibacterial activity, especially against the tuberculosis bacterium, *Mycobacterium tuberculosis*.[12]

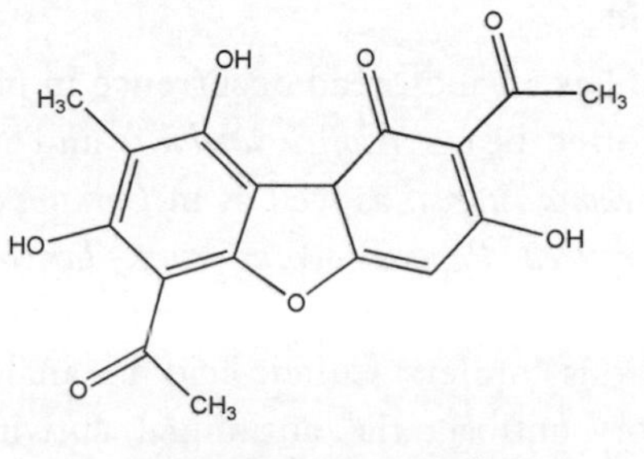

Fig. 7.10. Usnic acid

PHENYLPROPANOIDS AND CINNAMIC ACIDS

Phenylpropanoids (C_6-C_3) are phenolic compounds that have an aromatic ring to which a 3-carbon side chain is attached. The most widespread are the hydroxycinnamic acids, such as *p*-coumaric acid and caffeic acid. Another group in this class is made up of the phenylpropenes, which contribute to the volatile flavors and odors of plants (for example, anethole). Glycosides of some phenylpropanoids have been shown to inhibit the enzymes cAMP-specific phosphodiesterase, aldose reductase, and 5-lipoxygenase. The lignins, random polymers that contribute universally to the structure and rigidity of plant cell walls, are also phenylpropanoid in origin.

Anethole

Anethole is found in essential oils of plants such as anise *(Pimpinella anisum)* and fennel *(Foeniculum vulgare)*. Anethole demonstrates spasmolytic activity and has been shown to stimulate hepatic regeneration in rats.[13]

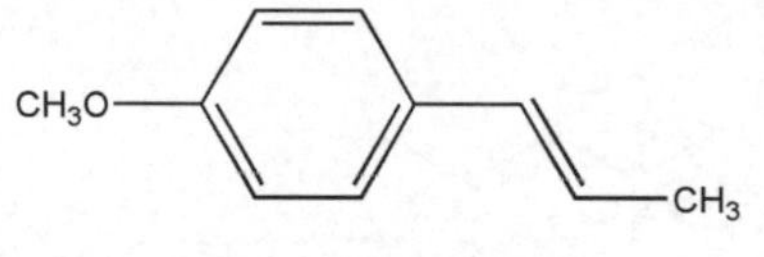

Fig. 7.11. Anethole

β-asarone

Occuring in the essential oil of calamus root *(Acorus calamus)* and in *Piper angustifolium*, β-asarone has spasmolytic properties. However, the compound is carcinogenic in animals, and calamus oil has been banned in the United States.[14]

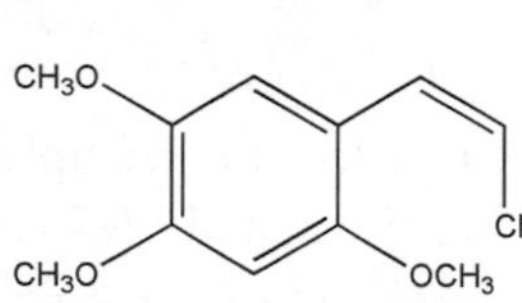

Fig. 7.12. β-asarone

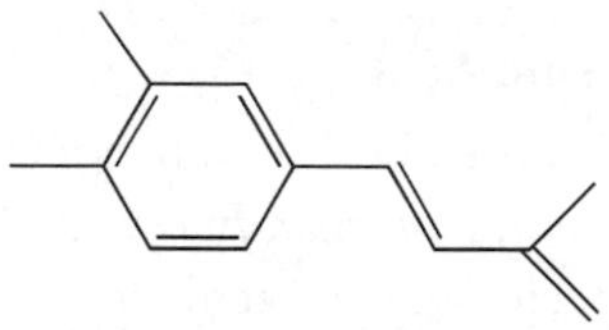

Fig. 7.13. Caffeic acid

Caffeic Acid

Caffeic acid has a widespread occurrence in plants and is found in coffee beans *(Coffea arabica)* and in the root bark of *Cinchona cuprea*, as well as in *Conium maculatum*, *Digitalis purpurea*, *Papaver somniferum*, *Taraxacum officinale*, *Chamaemelum nobile*, *Achillea millefolium*, and the resin of various conifers. Caffeic acid has analgesic, anti-inflammatory, antibacterial, antifungal, antiviral, and antioxidant properties. It also demonstrates antihepatotoxic and antiulcerogenic activities.[15]

p-coumaric Acid

p-coumaric acid has a very widespread occurrence in the plant world. It shows antifungal and antihepatotoxic activities, and some cytotoxicity in vitro.[16]

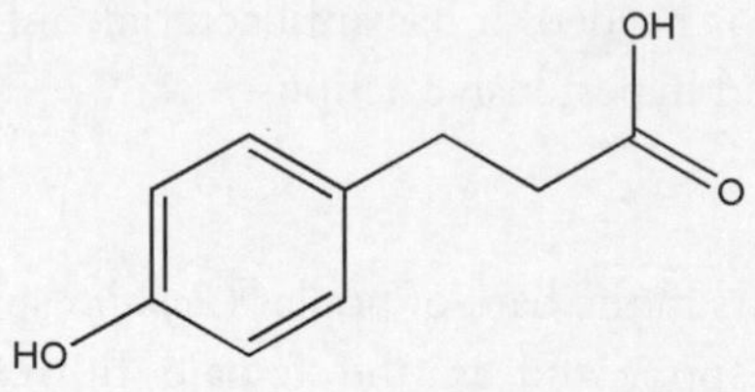

Fig. 7.14. *p*-coumaric acid

Curcumin

Curcumin is found in the roots of certain tropical spice plants in the Zingiberaceae family, including turmeric *(Curcuma longa)* and the related *C. aromatica* and *C. xanthorrhiza*. Curcumin and the other curcuminoids have been found to have antioxidant and anti-inflammatory activities and have been entered into Phase I clinical trials by the National Cancer Institute to investigate their cancer-preventive activities.[17]

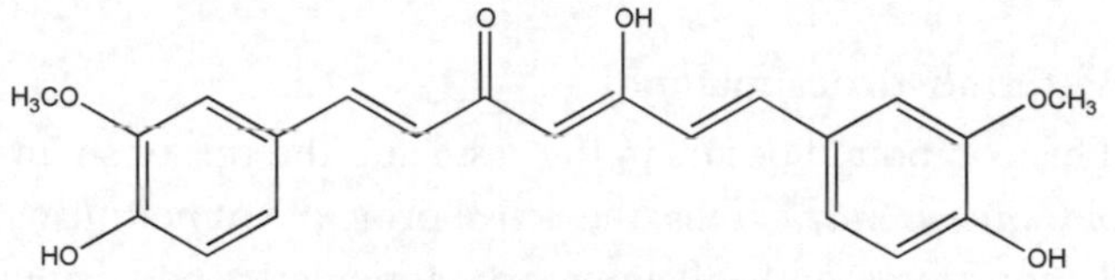

Fig. 7.15. Curcumin

Myristicin

Myristicin is found in essential oils made from the seeds of nutmeg *(Myristica fragrans)*, celery *(Apium graveolens)*, parsley *(Petroselinum crispum)*, and carrot *(Daucus carota)* and the bark of cinnamon *(Cinnamomum glanduliferum)*. In vitro studies have shown that myristicin inhibits monoamine oxidase and platelet aggregation in rabbit blood.[18] It has psychotropic properties.

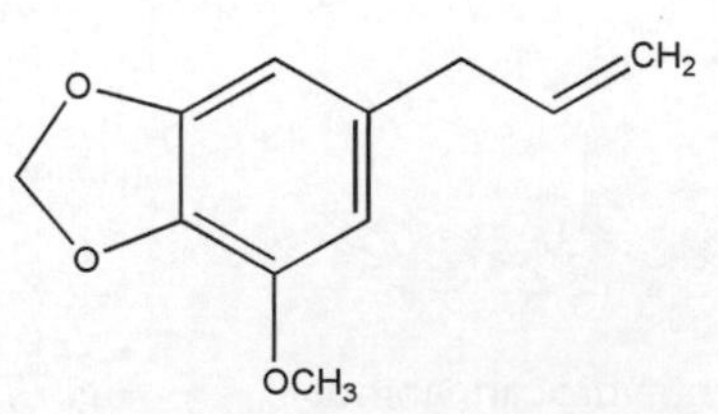

Fig. 7.16. Myristicin

Coumarins

The 700 or more plant coumarins (C_6-C_3) are derived from the parent compound coumarin, which has a characteristic odor of freshly mown hay. The compound occurs widely in plants, usually in bound form. Coumarin has been found in 150 plant species in more than 30 families. The richest sources of coumarin itself are sweet clover or melilot (*Melilotus* spp.), tonka bean (*Dipteryx odorata*), and sweet woodruff (*Galium odoratum*).

The name *coumarin* is derived from the French vernacular name for tonka bean. The word *tonka* comes from the language spoken by the indigenous peoples of the former French West Africa colony, now the independent Republic of Guinea. Another language of the same region, Tupi, gave rise to the old genus name, *Coumarouna*, from their name for the tonka tree, *kumarú*. This led to the derivation of the name of tonka's main constituent, *coumarin*.

In almost all cases, with coumarin itself serving as an exception, coumarins have a hydroxyl group in position 7, according to the structural substitution system delineated here.

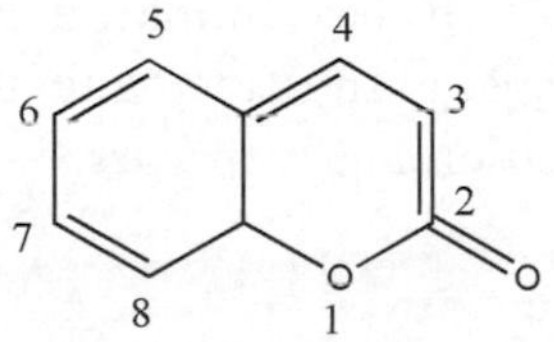

Fig. 7.17. Coumarin structure

Based upon structural substitutions, there are three major classes of coumarins:

- Simple *hydroxycoumarins*, such as umbelliferone and esculetin
- *Furanocoumarins*, typified by angelicin
- *Pyranocoumarins*, such as psoralen

Simple hydroxycoumarins and their glucosides, prevalent in higher plants, have been identified in about 100 families. The furano- and pyranocoumarins, which usually occur in a free state in fruits and roots, are mainly restricted to the Apiaceae and Rutaceae families.

Most simple coumarins are substituted with OH or OCH_3 at positions C-6 and C-7. They often occur in glycosidic form; for example, aesculin is the glycoside of aesculetin. Furanocoumarins, also called furocoumarins, have a furan ring at C-6 and C-7 (psoralen) or C-7 and C-8 (angelicin) of the coumarin ring system; however, these are not phenolic in structure.

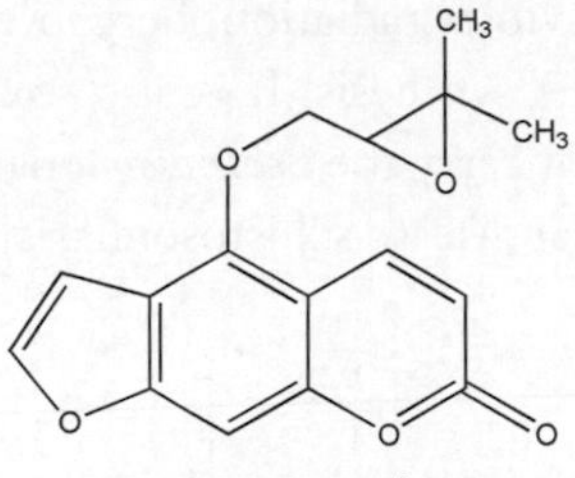

Fig. 7.18. Psoralen

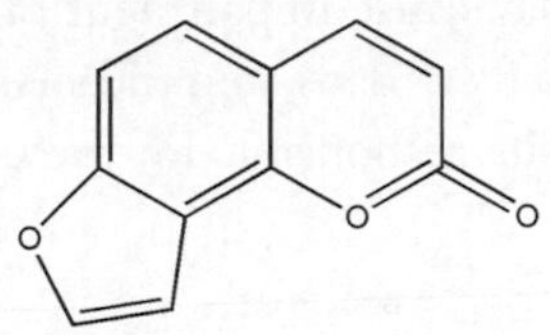

Fig. 7.19. Angelicin

The furanocoumarins psoralen and bergapten have photosensitizing properties that are exploited in treatments for vitiligo and psoriasis in which the patient is concurrently exposed to solar radiation. This is discussed in more detail in chapter 10. Such coumarins are found in *Ammi majus*, *Angelica archangelica*, *Ruta graveolens*, and *Citrus* species.

The furanochromone khellin is the active constituent of khella (*Ammi visnaga*), an herb used for its antispasmodic and antiasthmatic properties in North African traditional medicine. Pyranocoumarins, which contain a pyran ring fused at C-7 and C-8, are also present in *Ammi visnaga*.

The International Agency for Research on Cancer (IARC), part of the World Health Organization, found coumarin itself to be noncarcinogenic in humans. For humans, the most dangerous coumarins are the hepatotoxic aflatoxins and the substance dicoumarol, a potent anticoagulant. Please refer to chapter 10 for more information.

Table 7.3. Herb Activities Related to Coumarin Content

HERB	ACTIVITY
Aesculus hippocastanum (horse chestnut)	Anti-inflammatory, vascular tonic
Ammi visnaga (khella)	Antispasmodic, coronary vasodilator
Angelica archangelica (angelica)	Antispasmodic
Melilotus officinalis (sweet clover)	Anti-inflammatory, anti-edematous, vascular tonic

Bergapten

Bergapten is widespread among plants in the Rutaceae family, such as bergamot (*Citrus aurantium* ssp. *bergamia*). It is also common in Apiaceae plants, including *Ligusticum*, *Angelica*, *Ammi*, *Levisticum*, *Pimpinella*, and *Petroselinum*. While less effective than psoralen, bergapten is also used in the treatment of vitiligo and psoriasis.

In combination with ultraviolet radiation, bergapten may cause impairment of DNA synthesis. It is also toxic to fish, toads, and the snails that carry the *Schistosoma* parasite responsible for the tropical disease schistosomiasis.[19]

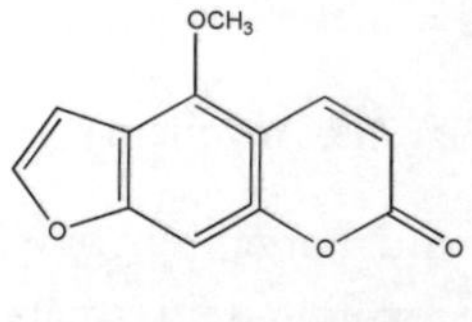

Fig. 7.20. Bergapten 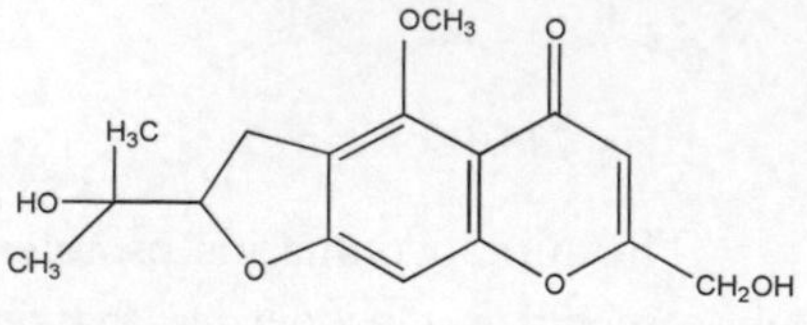   Fig. 7.21. Cimicifugin

Cimicifugin

Cimicifugin occurs in the roots and rhizomes of *Cimicifuga* species, such as *C. racemosa*, and as a glucoside in *Angelica japonica*. The compound demonstrates hypotensive activity in animals; it has been shown to increase coronary blood flow in isolated guinea pig hearts.[20]

Coumarin

One of the most widespread of all coumarins, coumarin is present in most families of angiosperms. In gymnosperms, it is found in Pinaceae, and, among ferns, in Polypodiaceae. It often occurs in glucosidic form; free coumarin is released during tissue damage. Coumarin has hemorrhagic effects and for this reason is used as a rat poison; it also causes liver damage in rats and dogs. In addition, it has piscicidal, antifungal, and antitumor properties.[21]

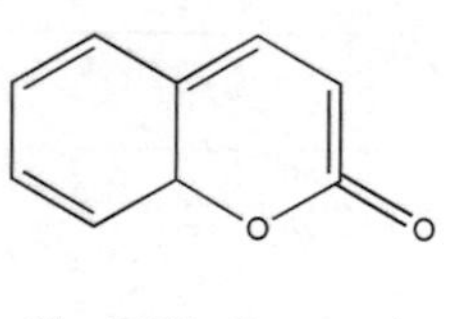

Fig. 7.22. Coumarin 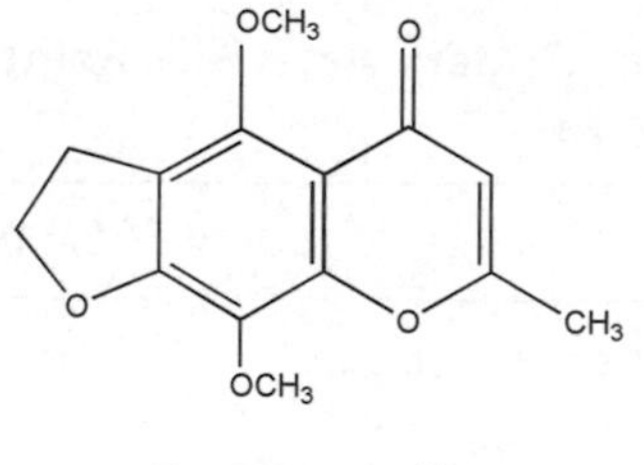   Fig. 7.23. Khellin

Khellin

This coumarin, found in the seeds of khella (*Ammi visnaga*), exhibits antiviral phototoxicity. This is an intriguing property by which the molecule kills viruses when activated by certain wavelengths of ultraviolet light. Khellin is a vasodilator and phosphodiesterase inhibitor; it has also demonstrated anthelmintic, antispasmodic, antiarteriosclerotic, antiasthmatic, bronchodilatory, antidiabetic, and antiulcerogenic properties.[22]

Psoralen

Psoralen, which occurs in the seeds of *Psoralea* species, possesses photosensitizing activity. This constituent is an essential component of PUVA treatment of psoriasis and vitiligo. In PUVA, a combination treatment used in dermatology, the patient takes psoralen (P) and then exposes the skin to long-wave ultraviolet radiation (UVA). Psoralen is also active against *Mycobacterium tuberculosis*, the pathogen that causes tuberculosis. In the presence of ultraviolet light, psoralen impairs DNA synthesis.[23]

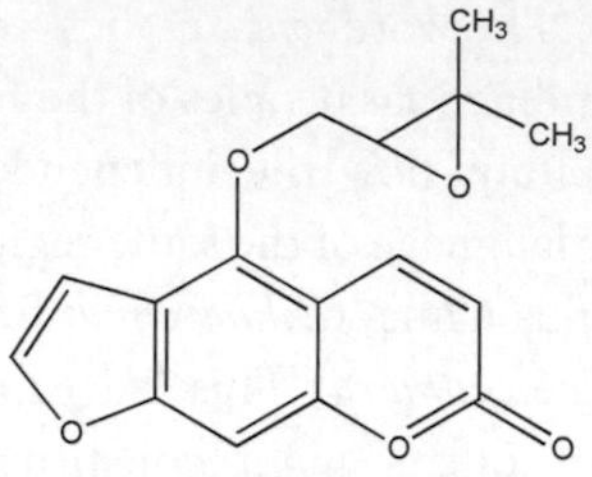

Fig. 7.24. Psoralen 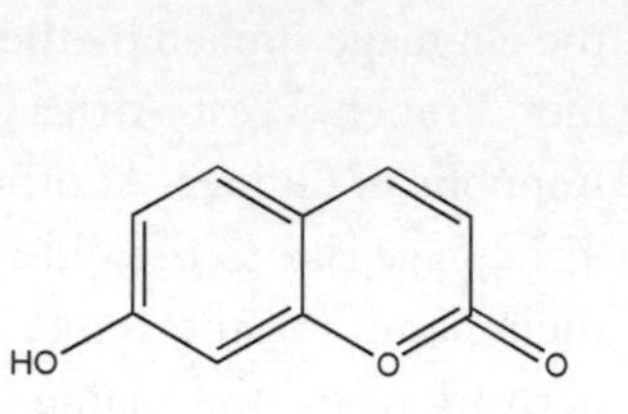   Fig. 7.25. Umbelliferone

Umbelliferone

Umbelliferone is widespread in the resin of various Apiaceae plants, including *Ferula*, *Apium*, *Pimpinella*, and *Heracleum* species. It has antifungal and antibacterial properties. It is used in sunscreen lotions and creams because of its UV-adsorbing properties.[24]

QUINONES

Quinones, of which at least 1,200 have been identified, provide pigments that range in color from yellow to almost black, but most are yellow, orange, or red. Although many quinone-containing plants have been used as dyes, they actually contribute little to plant color. They are usually hidden in bark, heartwood, or roots, or else occur in tissues where their colors are masked by other pigments.

Among quinones that have been used as dyes, madder root (*Rubia tinctorum*) contains anthraquinones that are the source of the orange-red pigment alizarin, and alkanet (*Alkanna tinctoria*) contains the naphthoquinone red dye alkannin.

Quinones are classified into three groups according to increasing molecular size: benzoquinones, naphthoquinones, and anthraquinones. Many are substituted by isoprenyl groups and hence are lipophilic. Others are hydroxylated, with phenolic properties, and may occur both in free form and as glycosides. Here are representative structures with the numbering system used for each type.

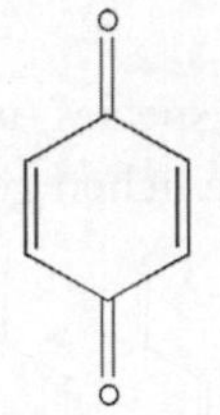

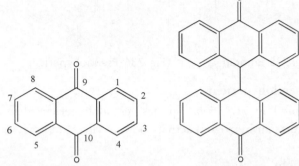

Fig. 7.26. Quinone structure

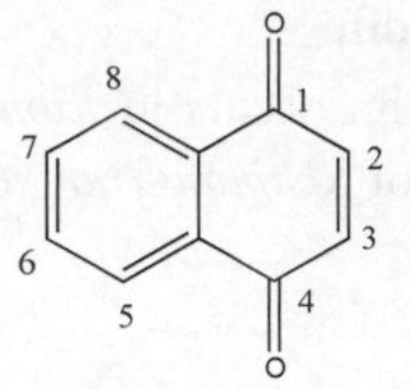

Fig. 7.27. Naphthoquinone structure

Fig. 7.28. Anthraquinone structure

Fig. 7.29. Naphthodianthone structure

Naphthoquinones

Naphthoquinones (C_6-C_4) are dark yellow pigments with a range of pharmacological properties. The dye henna is derived from the plant *Lawsonia inermis*, which contains the naphthoquinone lawsone as a glycoside. Other naphthoquinones have antimicrobial and antifungal properties, including juglone from walnut *(Juglans regia)* and butternut *(J. cineraria)*. Juglone is a laxative and vermifuge.

Other naphthoquinones with antimicrobial properties are plumbagin from sundew *(Drosera rotundifolia)* and lapachol from pau d'arco *(Tabebuia* spp.).

Table 7.4. Herb Activities Related to Naphthoquinone Content

HERB	ACTIVITY
Drosera rotundifolia (sundew)	Antispasmodic, antitussive
Juglans regia (walnut)	Antiparasitic, astringent
Lawsonia inermis (henna)	Dye plant

Juglone

Juglone, found in the stem bark of *Juglans nigra*, is the allelopathic agent of the walnut tree, meaning that the tree releases the chemical into the soil to prevent other plants from growing too close. Juglone demonstrates activity against fungi, mollusks, and herpes simplex virus type 1.[25] It also has sedative properties in fish and mammals.

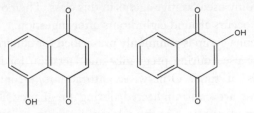

Fig. 7.30. Juglone

Fig. 7.31. Lawsone

Lawsone (henna)

Lawsone occurs in the leaves of *Lawsonia inermis*, the henna plant. It is used as a cosmetic and hair dye, and also as a sunscreen agent because of its UV-adsorption properties.[26]

Plumbagin

Found in the roots of *Plumbago europaea* and in various species of carnivorous plants, including sundew *(Drosera rotundifolia)*, plumbagin enhances the phagocytotic activity of human granulocytes in vitro. It is cytotoxic at high doses and immunostimulating at low doses.[27] In addition, it has molluscicidal properties.

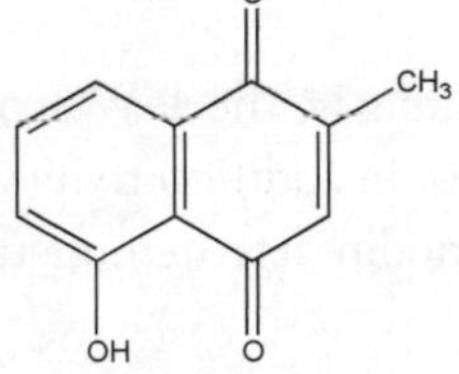

Fig. 7.32. Plumbagin

Anthraquinones

Anthraquinones (C_6-C_2-C_6) constitute the largest group of naphthoquinones, and are often red or purple, rather than yellow. They are widely distributed in plants, especially in the families Fabaceae *(Senna)*, Liliaceae *(Aloe)*, Polygonaceae *(Rheum)*, and Rhamnaceae *(Rhamnus)*. The anthraquinone class contains many important laxative compounds, including aloe-emodin and emodin, from *Aloe* species. Dimeric anthraquinones, also known as anthrones, include such compounds as cassiamin C, sennoside A, and the bianthraquinone hypericin, from St. John's wort *(Hypericum perforatum)*.

Among anthraquinone-containing laxatives, the gentlest-acting compounds belong to the buckthorns *(Rhamnus catharticus* and *R. frangula)* and Chinese rhubarb *(Rheum palmatum)*. These herbs are aged for at least one year, during which the more irritant anthraquinones are converted to milder compounds. The presence of tannins in these plants also tends to moderate the laxative effect. *Aloe* and *Senna* species are the other commonly used laxative agents in this class. Their onset of action occurs around eight hours after ingestion.

Senna syrup is commonly prescribed for children and may be used during pregnancy and lactation for limited periods of time. Otherwise, anthraquinone-containing laxatives are contraindicated during pregnancy. Due to the stimulant effect of these laxatives, they are also contraindicated in spastic colon conditions. A slight overdose can produce griping, which can be counterbalanced with carminatives, such as peppermint and coriander oils. All the anthraquinone-containing laxatives can lead to dependency. These important herbs are discussed in more depth in chapters 10 and 13.

Herbal Laxatives Containing Anthraquinones

Aloe spp. (aloe)
Rhamnus cathartica (purging buckthorn)
R. frangula (buckthorn)
R. purshiana (cascara sagrada)
Rheum spp. (Chinese rhubarb)
Senna alexandrina (senna)

Aloe-emodin

Aloe-emodin is found in the leaves of *Aloe*, *Senna*, and some *Rheum* species. In addition to its well-known cathartic action, aloe-emodin has demonstrated antileukemic activities.[28]

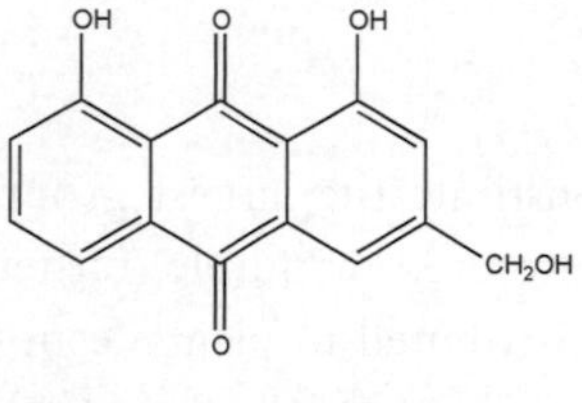

Fig. 7.33. Aloe-emodin

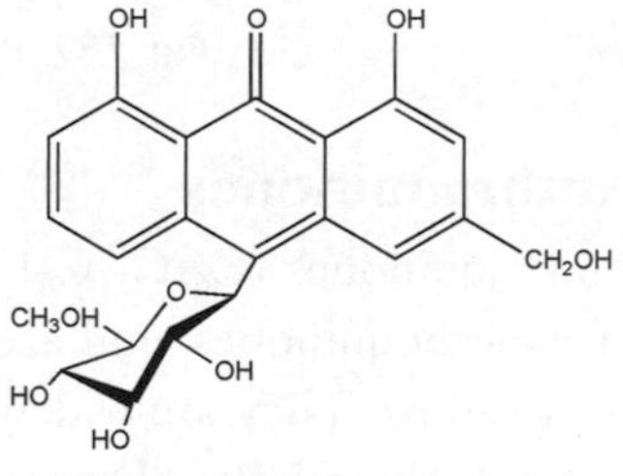

Fig. 7.34. Barbaloin

Barbaloin

This C-glucoside of aloe-emodin occurs in the leaves of several *Aloe* species cultivated as medicines, including *A. vera*, *A. ferox* and *A. perryi*. It is used commercially as a purgative.[29]

Emodin

Emodin occurs in *Rumex* and *Rheum* species, in the root bark of *Rhamnus frangula*, and in some lichen genera.[30]

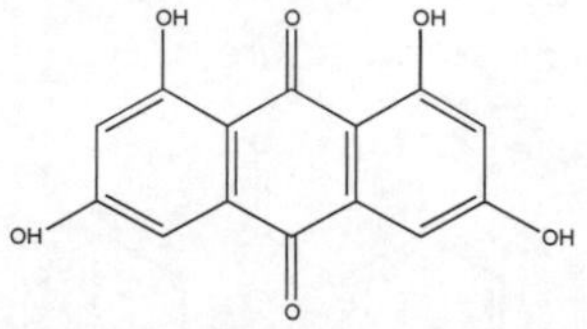

Fig. 7.35. Emodin

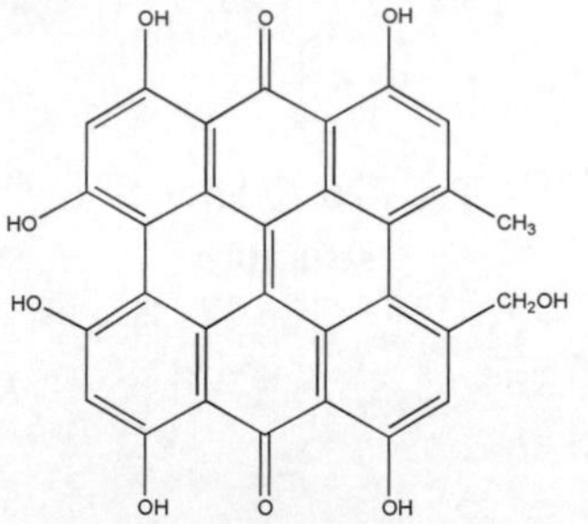

Fig. 7.36. Pseudohypericin

Pseudohypericin

Found in *Hypericum* species, pseudohypericin demonstrates antiretroviral activity both in vitro and in vivo.[31]

Rhein

Rhein is found in all parts of *Scrophularia nodosa* and in the roots of *Rumex*, *Rheum*, and *Senna* species. Rhein displays moderate antifungal activity against dermatophytes.[32]

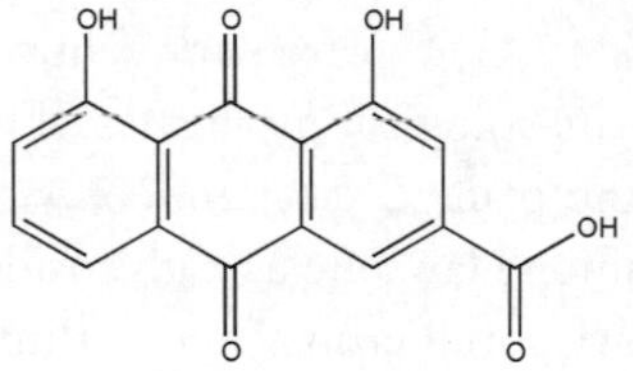

Fig. 7.37. Rhein

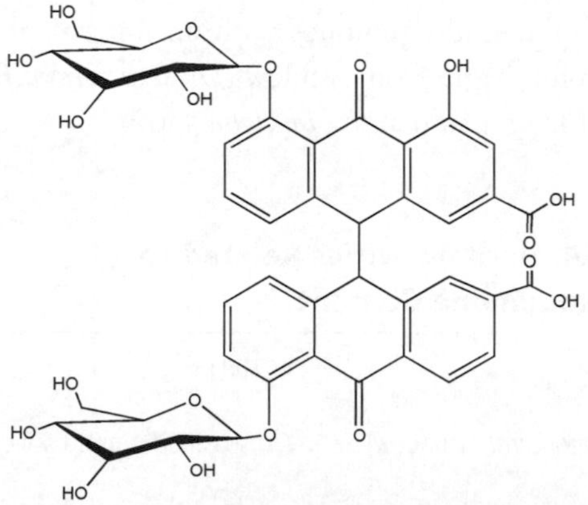

Fig. 7.38. Sennoside A

Sennoside A

Sennoside A is found in the leaves of *Senna*, where it is formed during drying, as well as in the fruit of *S. alexandrina* and in rhizomes of *Rheum palmatum*. This cathartic agent is used for the treatment of chronic constipation, and is found in many stimulating herbal laxatives.[33]

Hypericin

Found in St. John's wort (*Hypericum perforatum*) and other *Hypericum* species, hypericin shows activity against retroviruses in vitro and in vivo.[34] The compound is photosensitizing and may have antidepressant effects in mammals, although it is unlikely that hypericin is the constituent responsible for the herb's mild antidepressant effects.[35]

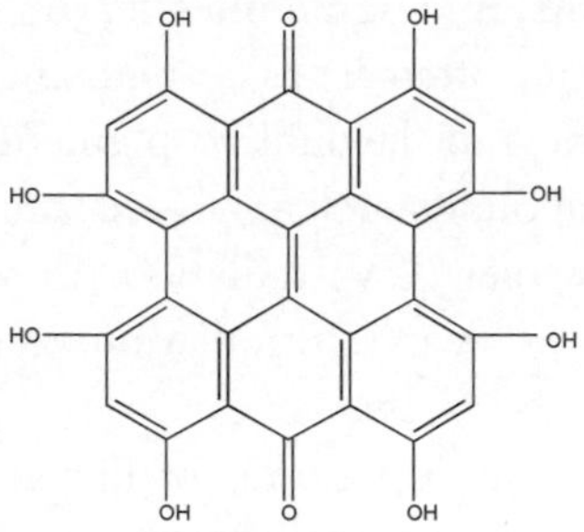

Fig. 7.39. Hypericin

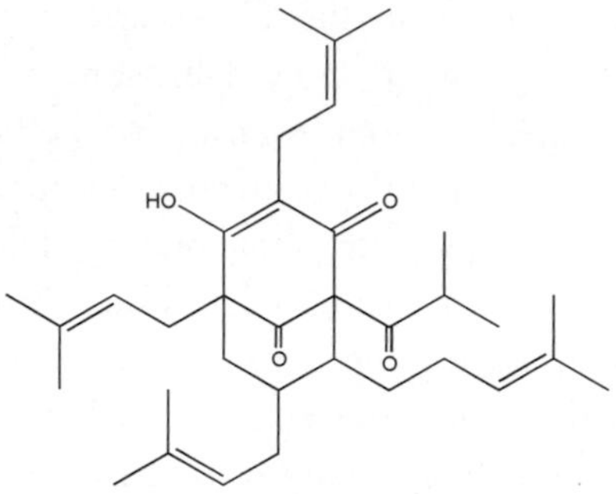

Fig. 7.40. Hyperforin

Hyperforin

This is a derivative of phloroglucinol found in the flowers and fruits of St. John's wort (*Hypericum perforatum*). Currently, hyperforin is thought to be pivotal to the mild antidepressant properties of this herb.

XANTHONES

Xanthones are related to flavonoids, as they share precursors, but xanthones have a single carbon bridge (C_6-C_1-C_6) instead of the 3-carbon bridge of the flavonoids. A biologically active yet taxonomically restricted group, xanthones demonstrate a range of effects in living organisms. Compounds such as bellidifolin inhibit monoamine oxidase activity, while psorospermin exhibits both cytotoxic and antitumor properties. Many other xanthones are recorded as having antimicrobial, insecticidal, anti-inflammatory, or tuberculostatic effects. They are found in herbs such as gentian (*Gentiana lutea*), swertia (*Swertia* spp.), and mango (*Mangifera indica*).

Gentisein

Gentisein is found in the roots of *Gentiana lutea*, and is considered antibacterial and antitubercular.[36]

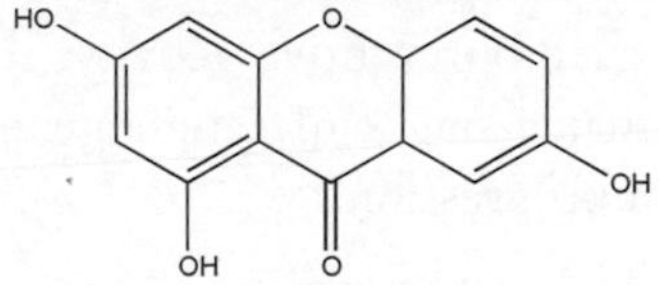

Fig. 7.41. Gentisein

STILBENOIDS

This group of compounds is based on a structure of two benzene rings bridged by a chain of two carbons. Limited in distribution, they are common in the Orchidaceae family and also found in liverworts. They are constituents of the heartwood of both gymnosperm and angiosperm trees. Stilbenoids have been found in plants in the free state, as glycosides, and as oligomers. Many are strongly antifungal and serve as phytoalexins.[37]

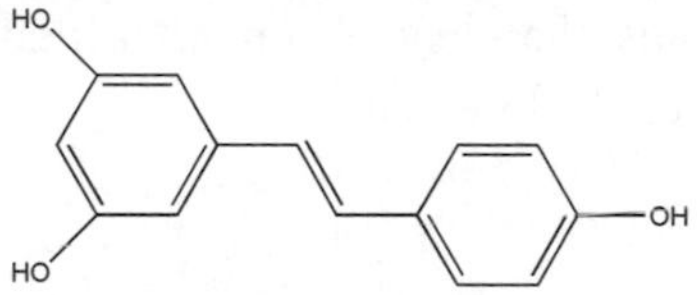

Fig. 7.42. Resveratrol

Resveratrol (*trans*-3,5,4'-trihydroxystilbene)

Found in many plants as a phytoalexin, resveratrol is abundant in the skins of red grapes (*Vitis vinifera*). It has been suggested that resveratrol underlies the phenomenon known as the "French paradox," which is discussed in more detail later in this chapter. Wine is the most notable dietary source of this compound; a fluid ounce of red wine contains an average of 160 µg of resveratrol.[38]

Physiological concentrations of resveratrol can modulate multiple molecular pathways thought to be associated with the development and progression of cardiovascular disease and cancer, including Phase II drug metabolism, cyclooxygenase, lipid metabolism, nitric oxide, DNA synthesis, inflammation, cell survival, cell death, and cell division cycle pathways.[39]

Research highlights a number of resveratrol effects relevant to the cardiovascular system:

- Antioxidant[40]
- Inhibits peroxidation of low-density lipoprotein (LDL)[41]
- Reduces platelet aggregation[42]

Resveratrol has also been shown to function as a cancer chemopreventive agent. Such agents reduce the incidence of tumorigenesis by intervening at one or more of the stages of carcinogenesis.[43] In research, resveratrol demonstrated chemopreventive activity in assays representing three major stages of carcinogenesis: initiation, promotion, and progression.[44,45]

Initiation: antioxidant and antimutagenic effects; induced Phase II drug-metabolism enzymes
Promotion: inhibited cyclooxygenase and hydroperoxidase
Progression: induced human pro-myelocytic leukemia cell differentiation; inhibited the growth of leukemia cells in vitro

FLAVONOIDS

The term *flavonoid* describes all the polyphenolic plant pigments that have a C_6-C_3-C_6 skeleton analogous to that of the flavones—that is, two substituted benzene rings connected by a 3-carbon chain. All of the approximately 4,000 flavonoids that have been identified possess this same basic structural makeup.

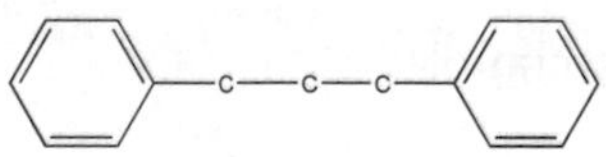

Fig. 7.43. Flavonoid core structure

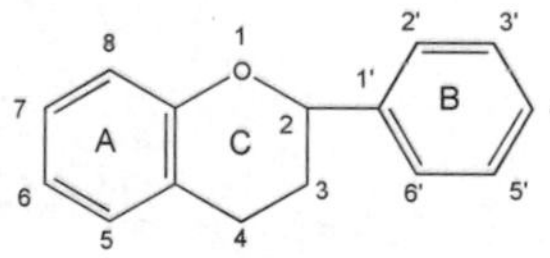

Fig. 7.44. Flavonoid structure

However, as an example of the many subtleties that can prove so confusing in phytochemistry, flavone, the parent substance of the flavonoids, occurs naturally but is not itself a phenolic compound, as it lacks a hydroxyl group.

Taxonomic Distribution

Molecules in this group are very widely distributed in higher plants as components of leaves and pigments in flowers. No flavonoids have been found in algae, but some are common in Bryophytes. In Pteridophytes, the Psilotales and Selaginellales are characterized by the presence of biflavonoids, and Equisetales by proanthocyanins.

Anatomical Distribution of Flavonoids

Flavonoid glycosides are water-soluble and accumulate in plant cell vacuoles. Depending on the species, they either concentrate in the leaf epidermis or are dispersed in both the epidermis and the mesophyll. In flowers, they are concentrated in epidermal cells. Whenever flavonoids are present in the leaf cuticle, they are almost always free aglycones, made even more lipophilic by the partial or total methylation of their hydroxyl groups.

Plant Pigmentation

Flavonoids are plant pigments, responsible for the color of flowers, fruits, and sometimes leaves. When not directly visible, they often act as co-pigments. For example, colorless flavone and flavonol co-pigments protect plant tissues and compounds such as anthocyanins against damage from ultraviolet (UV) radiation. In some cases, the molecule absorbs near-UV radiation, and this color is perceived only by insects.

Names of many categories of flavonoids have their roots in Greek or Latin color terms; the word *flavone* itself comes from *flavus*, the Latin word for "yellow." *Anthocyanin* comes from the Greek *anthos* (flower) and *kyanos* (blue). The word is used broadly, as in "anthocyanin pigments," without regard for whether they are glycosides (anthocyanins) or aglycones (anthocyanidins).

Anthocyanins generate petal colors; red flower colors are usually based on cyanidin and blue on delphinidin. The yellow *anthochlor* pigments, chalcones and aurones, are so named because the color of yellow flowers that contain these pigments changes to red when the flowers are fumed with ammonia. (Yellow flowers containing only carotenoids are unchanged after this treatment.)

Chalcones are readily oxidized both in vivo and in vitro to aurones, and both classes of pigment are often found together in yellow flowers. The word *chalcone* is derived from the Greek words *chalcos*, meaning copper, and *aurone*, from the Latin *aurum*, meaning gold. The obsolete name *leucoanthocyanin* was once used to denote all substances that could be converted into anthocyanins when heated with mineral acid.

While flavonoids are responsible for most plant pigments, pigments may also be provided by members of some, but not all, families of the Caryophyllidae, in which betalain alkaloids contribute color. These families include the Phytolaccaceae, Cactaceae, Chenopodiaceae, and Amaranthaceae.

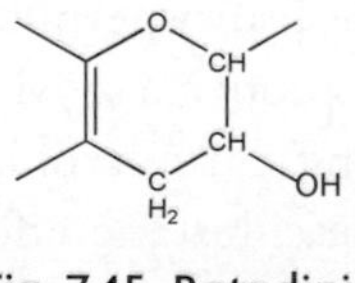

Fig. 7.45. Betadinin

Variations in the structure of anthocyanins generate the wonderful diversity of hue and tone in the colors of flowers and fruits. A number of factors are believed to contribute to this kaleidoscopic abundance of color:

- Differences in electron charge
- Number of methoxyl and hydroxyl groups
- Number and type of sugars attached to the aglycone
- Presence of metal ions
- Presence of other pigments

Acertaining the specific effects of anthocyanin structure on plant color is not straightforward. For example, when anthocyanins are heated, they may become either paler in color or more stable in structure, as heating may cause them to polymerize. Anthocyanins are generally colorless in neutralized pH, redder in an acid medium, and bluer in an alkaline medium and in certain other circumstances—for example, when they form complexes with metals.

Classification of Flavonoids

Numerous variations on the basic C_6-C_3-C_6 structure occur in flavonoids, which has led to the development of various systems for classifying this diverse and abundant group of secondary metabolites. Unfortunately, these systems do not always correlate with one another, and unless this fact is recognized, much confusion may result. Of the systems described here, that based on degree of oxidation is the one uscd throughout this discussion.

The sugar most likely to be present is D-glucose, but L-rhamnose, D-galactose, L-arabinose, and D-xylose are also found. This means that for every aglycone, there may be many different glycosidic combinations. Structural variability expands further in glycosides formed with a disaccharide or a trisaccharide, in which a linear or branched structure may be seen.

Each class of flavonoids contains molecules with different substituents on the structural skeleton that they have in common. In addition, each flavonoid may be present as a glycoside or as a simple aglycone. To facilitate nomenclature, a numbering system that describes variants in each class has been developed.

REPRESENTATIVE CLASSES OF FLAVONOID AGLYCONES

Flavones and Flavonols

In these molecules, which represent about 80% of known flavonoids, ring A is substituted by two hydroxyl groups at C-5 and C-7. These groups may be free, etherified, or linked glycosidally. However, other substitutions are also possible.

Flavones and flavonols are universally distributed in plants, but some of the substitution patterns are restricted to certain families or groups of families—hence their interest to chemotaxonomists. They often occur as pigments associated with anthocyanins in petals and leaves of higher plants. They are found most frequently in the form of glycosides, but they may also be present as

Flavonoid Classification Systems

Degree of Saturation

Two major categories encompass flavonoids in which the central heterocyclic ring is either saturated or unsaturated. If saturated, as in flavanols, the molecule will be planar, and thus non-optically active. Flavonoids with unsaturated rings, such as flavones, are defined by stereoisomerism.

Biosynthetic Origin

In this classification scheme, one group of flavonoids includes those that are both intermediate steps in biosynthesis and end products, such as chalcones and flavanones. The other flavonoids constitute a second group in that they are known only as end products. These include anthocyanins and flavonols.

Molecular Size

This scheme differentiates among monomeric, dimeric, trimeric, and polmeric flavonoid structures.

Conjugates

Flavonoids normally exist in conjugate or combined forms, also known as glycosylflavonoids. These conjugates are commonly glycosides, in which a bond (-C-O-C-) is formed between a hydroxyl of the flavonoid and a sugar. The bond may be established with any of the hydroxyl groups on the aglycone, but the groups involved are generally the hydroxyls in the 7-position of the flavones and in the 3-position of the flavonols. The sugar may be a mono-, di-, or trisaccharide.

Table 7.5. Flavonoid Categories

CLASS	STRUCTURE OF CENTRAL C-3 UNIT	EXAMPLE
Catechins (flavan-3-ols)		Catechin
Dihydrochalcones		Phloretin
Chalcones		Butein
Flavanones (dihydroflavones)		Naringenin
Flavones		Apigenin
Isoflavones		Genistein
Anthocyanidins		Pelargonidin
Aurones		Sulfuretin
Flavanols		Taxifolin
Flavonols		Quercetin

aglycones on leaf surfaces, in fruits, and in bud exudates. Flavones differ from flavonols in that they lack a 3-hydroxyl substitution, which changes their spectroscopic properties. Apigenin and luteolin are the only common flavones.

Several hundred flavone and flavonol aglycones are known, but only three are common: kaempferol, quercetin, and myricetin. Quercetin has the widest distribution in nature of all phenolic compounds, and 135 different glycosides of quercetin have been described. The most common is quercetin-3-rutinoside, commonly known as rutin, which is used in the treatment of capillary fragility.

Many different saccharides may serve as the sugars in flavone and flavonol glycosides. Ten monosaccharides are known: D-apiose, L-arabinose, L-rhamnose, D-xylose, D-allose, D-galactose, D-glucose, D-mannose, and D-galacturonic and D-glucuronic acids. Disaccharides are associated with flavones; rutinose is particularly widespread. Trisaccharides, linear or branched, are also known, and one branched tetrasaccharide has been identified.

In addition, there are a number of flavones with various other substituents. Among the flavones with isoprene substitution, the linkage is generally observed at the C-6 and/or C-8 position of the flavone. About 100 flavone and flavonol sulfates and some flavone alkaloids have also been reported.

Oxidation or Substitution

Here the various classes of flavonoids are distinguished by the degree of oxidation of the C-3 chain. This is the system used throughout the discussion of flavonoids in this chapter. The following illustrates the hierarchy of flavonoids according to increasing degree of oxidation.

catechins—›
    dihydrochalcones—›
       proanthocyanidins—›
         flavanones—›
           flavanols—›
             flavones—›
               anthocyanidins—›
                 flavonols

Kaempferol (3,5,7,4'-tetrahydroxyflavone)

Kaempferol is very widespread, both free and in glycosides.[46]

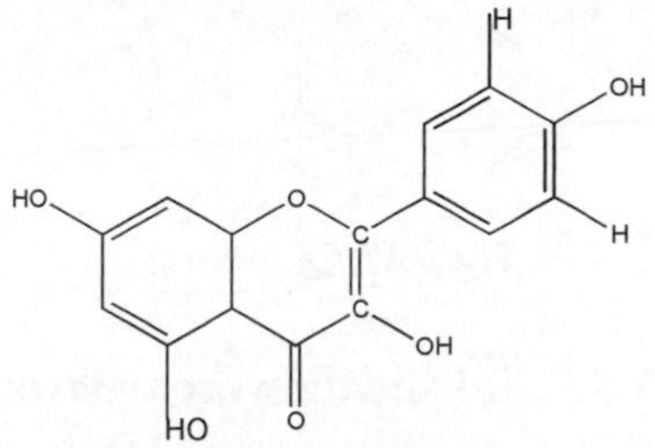

Fig. 7.46. Kaempferol

Consider table 7.6, which lists commonly used plants that are sources of kaempferol.

Table 7.6. Plant Sources of Kaempferol

PLANT	PLANT PART
Allium cepa (onion)	Bulb
Althaea officinalis (marshmallow)	Leaf
Anethum graveolens (dill)	Seed
Calendula officinalis (calendula)	Whole plant
Camellia sinensis (tea)	Whole plant
Centella asiatica (gotu kola)	Whole plant
Equisetum arvense (horsetail)	Whole plant
Eupatorium perfoliatum (boneset)	Whole plant
Ginkgo biloba (ginkgo)	Leaf
Harpagophytum procumbens (devil's claw)	Root
Lactuca sativa (lettuce)	Whole plant
Matricaria recutita (chamomile)	Whole plant
Ocimum basilicum (basil)	Leaf
Passiflora incarnata (passionflower)	Whole plant
Sambucus nigra (black or European elder)	Flower
Silybum marianum (milk thistle)	Seed
Thymus vulgaris (thyme)	Whole plant
Viola odorata (sweet violet)	Whole plant

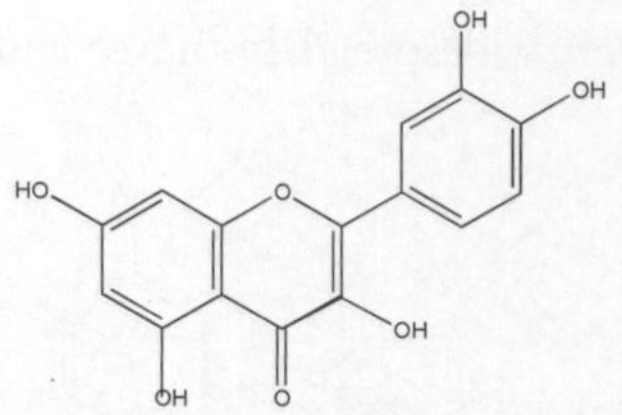

Fig. 7.47. Quercetin

Quercetin (3,5,7,3',4'-pentahydroxyflavone)

This is the flavonoid most commonly found in higher plants, usually in one of its many glycosidic forms. However, it may also occur in free form in Asteraceae, Passifloraceae, Rhamnaceae, and Solanaceae plants.[47]

Table 7.7. Plant Sources of Quercetin

PLANT	PLANT PART	AMOUNT
Oenothera biennis (evening primrose)	Leaf	91,000–207,000 ppm
Podophyllum peltatum (mayapple)	Resin, sap	50,000 ppm
Allium cepa (onion)	Bulb	0–48,100 ppm
Camellia sinensis (tea)	Leaf	10,000 ppm
Azadirachta indica (neem)	Flower	1,000 ppm
Helianthus annuus (sunflower)	Flower	100–400 ppm
Malus domestica (apple)	Pericarp	58–263 ppm
Vaccinium macrocarpon (cranberry)	Fruit	100–250 ppm

The Use and Abuse of Quercetin

Quercetin has gained the attention of the supplement industry, and is now widely promoted as a natural anti-inflammatory and antioxidant magic bullet. This has the effect of confusing both the public and practitioners as to the difference between whole plant and active ingredient herbalism. An acknowledgment of the role of an isolated constituent in health maintenance should emphasize the importance of the many herbal and dietary sources of the compound, rather than focus on "natural magic bullets" available only in dietary supplement form.

Quercetin affects a whole array of enzyme systems. There appears to be a theme of involvement in inflammatory processes that partially explains the anti-inflammatory action of many quercetin-containing plants.

Enzyme Systems Modified by Quercetin[48]

Transport ATPases
Protein kinases
Cyclic nucleotide phosphodiesterases
Catechol-*O*-methyl-transferase
Phospholipase A_2
Cyclooxygenase

Lipoxygenase
Aldose reductase
Xanthine oxidase
Hyaluronidase
Histidine decarboxylase
Estrogen synthetase

There are a number of specific indications typically given for quercetin, but they do not always take into account the richness of the compound's therapeutic possibilities when it is used in the bio-evolved complex of its herbal sources. Quercetin finds its main use as a safe systemic anti-inflammatory, indicated in most cases of allergy or inflammation-based pathology.[49] This application stems from the impact of quercetin on the biochemical processes that influence these physiological responses in the body. Such therapeutically valuable responses will, of course, also occur when the flavonoid is taken in the form of a whole plant preparation.

Growing evidence indicates that quercetin has antiviral activity, both in vivo and in vitro, most markedly against herpes simplex type 1, parainfluenza type 3, polio virus type 1, and respiratory syncytial virus.[50] It is interesting to note that boneset *(Eupatorium perfoliatum)* is both a rich source of quercetin and a traditional treatment for flu. Quercetin may also play a role in tumor inhibition.[51] Please see chapter 9 for more details on the anticancer effects of flavonoids.

PLANT	PLANT PART	AMOUNT
Allium sativum (garlic)	Bulb	200 ppm
Brassica oleracea var. *capitata* (cabbage)	Leaf	2–100 ppm
Capsicum annuum (cayenne)	Fruit	63 ppm
Brassica oleracea var. *acephala* (kale)	Leaf	7–50 ppm
Pyrus communis (pear)	Pericarp	28 ppm
Brassica oleracea var. *gemmifera* (brussels sprouts)	Axillary bud	25 ppm
Brassica oleracea var. *gongylodes* (kohlrabi)	Shoot	20 ppm
Spinacia oleracea (spinach)	Leaf	19 ppm

Isorhamnetin

This flavonol has a very widespread occurrence, both free and in the form of glycosides.

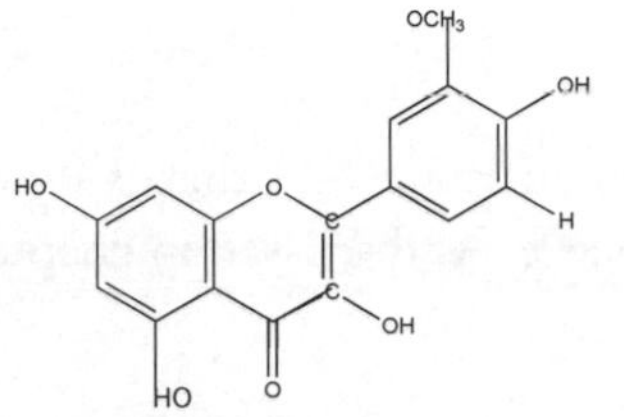

Fig. 7.48. Isorhamnetin 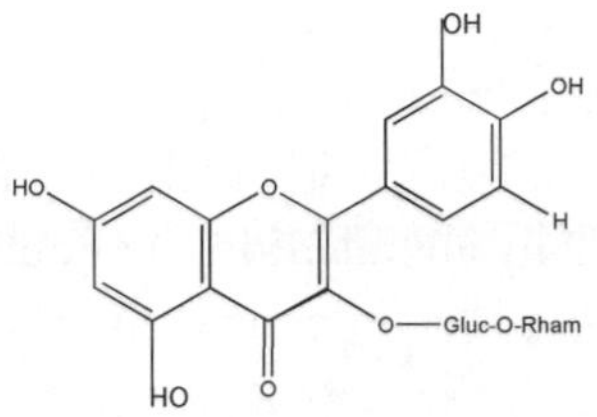   Fig. 7.49. Rutin

Rutin (quercetin-3-rutinoside)

First isolated from rue *(Ruta graveolens)*, rutin is widespread in higher plants. It demonstrates many of the general actions of quercetin and other flavones and flavonols. (Please see chapter 9 for more information.) Rutin has anti-inflammatory activity because of an ability to inhibit the action of the enzyme lipoxygenase. It is specifically recognized as a free radical scavenger and has been used clinically against capillary fragility and varicosities. In vitro studies show that it also has antiviral and antibacterial properties.[52]

Table 7.8. Herbs Containing Rutin

HERB	PLANT PART
Achillea millefolium (yarrow)	Whole plant
Agathosma betulina (buchu)	Leaf
Allium cepa (onion)	Bulb
A. sativum (garlic)	Whole plant
Apium graveolens (celer)	Whole plant
Artemisia absinthium (wormwood)	Whole plant
Asparagus officinalis (asparagus)	Root
Azadirachta indica (neem)	Leaf
Calendula officinalis (calendula)	Flower
Camellia sinensis (tea)	Leaf
Capsella bursa-pastoris (shepherd's purse)	Whole plant
Coriandrum sativum (coriander)	Fruit
Crataegus laevigata (hawthorn)	Leaf
Erythroxylum coca (coca)	Leaf
Eschscholzia californica (california poppy)	Flower
Eupatorium perfoliatum (boneset)	Plant
Filipendula ulmaria (meadowsweet)	Plant
Foeniculum vulgare (fennel)	Fruit
Hypericum perforatum (St. John's wort)	Plant
Ilex paraguariensis (maté)	Leaf
Leonurus cardiaca (motherwort)	Whole plant
Matricaria recutita (chamomile)	Whole plant
Mentha piperita (peppermint)	Whole plant
Passiflora incarnata (passionflower)	Whole plant
Pimpinella anisum (anise)	Seed
Rheum officinale (chinese rhubarb)	Root
Ruta graveolens (rue)	Whole plant
Salix alba (white willow)	Bark
Sambucus nigra (black elder)	Flower, leaf
Solidago virgaurea (goldenrod)	Leaf
Spinacia oleracea (spinach)	Leaf
Viola odorata (sweet violet)	Flower
V. tricolor (pansy)	Flower

Apigenin

The aglycone of apigenin is occasionally found on leaf surfaces and on fern fronds. Many glycosides are known. Research has shown that it has anti-inflammatory, antibacterial, diuretic, and hypotensive properties.[53]

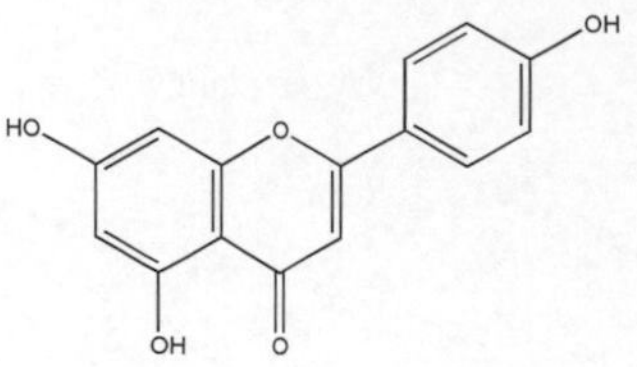

Fig. 7.50. Apigenin

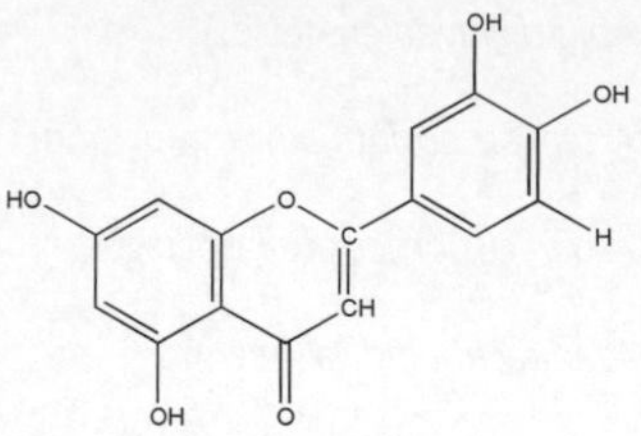

Fig. 7.51. Luteolin

Luteolin

This aglycone is common, especially in leaf exudates. Luteolin often occurs as the 7-glucoside and 7-glucuronide.[54]

Anthocyanins and Anthochlors

There are two main classes of flavonoid pigments that provide flower color:

Anthocyanins (red to blue colors)
Anthochlors, including *chalcones* and *aurones* (yellow petal colors)

The most common anthocyanidin (anthocyanin aglycone) is cyanidin. The other 15 known anthocyanidins, 6 of which are widely distributed, differ only in the number and position of methoxyl or hydroxyl groups. The glycosidal anthocyanins are incredibly numerous; cyanidin alone is found in 76 different glycosidic combinations.[55]

Anthocyanidin pigments are responsible for the wide array of pink, scarlet, red, mauve, violet, and blue colors in flowers, leaves, fruits, fruit juices, and wines. They are also responsible for the astringent taste of fruit and wines. Genera that contain yellow anthochlor pigments include *Dianthus*, *Dahlia*, *Potentilla*, and *Antirrhinum*.

Cyanidin

Cyanidin is found in glycosidic form in nearly all green plants. Elderberries and red cabbage, which each contain many different cyanidin glycosides, are potential sources of natural red food colorings.[56]

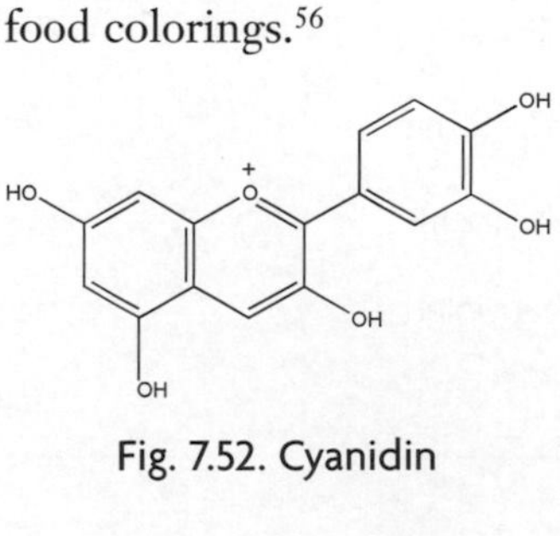

Fig. 7.52. Cyanidin

ISOFLAVONOIDS

The more than 600 isoflavonoids are divided into subclasses according to the oxidation level of the central pyran ring. They differ from other flavonoids in that they display greater structural diversity and are usually present in the free state, rather than as glycosides. *Isoflavones* are the most abundant subclass; other subclasses include *isoflavanones*, *pterocarpans*, *coumestans*, *isoflavans*, *rotenoids*, and *neoflavonoids*.

Isoflavones are isomeric with the more widely occurring flavones. They are more restricted in distribution than flavones and flavonols, found regularly in only one subfamily of Fabaceae, the Papilionoideae. Widely occurring isoflavones include daidzein, genistein, formononetin, and biochanin A, which are noted for their estrogenic properties.

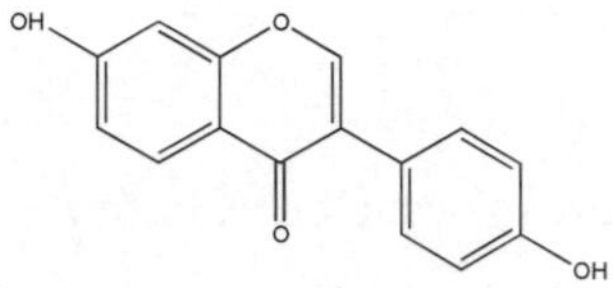

Fig. 7.53. Daidzein

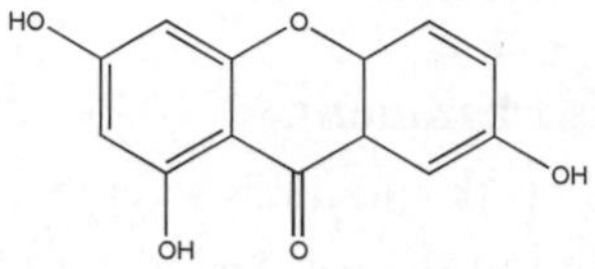

Fig. 7.54. Genistein

Daidzein

Daidzein is a widely distributed isoflavone that is especially abundant in the Lamiaceae. As discussed in chapter 9, it is an effective phytoestrogen.

Table 7.9. Plants Containing Daidzein

PLANT	PLANT PART
Genista tinctoria (dyer's broom)	Shoot
Glycine max (soy)	Seed
Phaseolus coccineus (scarlet runner bean)	Whole plant
Psoralea corylifolia (babchi)	Root
Pueraria lobata, P. phaseoloides (kudzu)	Root
Trifolium pratense (red clover)	Flower
Ulex europaeus (gorse)	Aerial parts

Genistein

This isoflavone occurs in clover (*Trifolium* spp.), soy (*Glycine max*), and many other Fabaceae plants, as well as in the wood of *Prunus* species.[57]

Table 7.10. Herbs Containing Genistein

HERB	PLANT PART
Baptisia tinctoria (wild indigo)	Leaf
Cytisus scoparius (Scotch broom)	Flower
Genista tinctoria (dyer's broom)	Flower
Glycine max (soy)	Seed
Glycyrrhiza glabra (licorice)	Shoot
Lupinus albus (white lupine)	Hypocotyl
Medicago sativa (alfalfa, lucerne)	Leaf
Phaseolus coccineus (scarlet runner bean)	Whole plant
P. lunatus (butter bean, lima)	Leaf
P. vulgaris (kidney bean)	Fruit
Pisum sativum (garden pea)	Shoot
Prunus cerasus (sour cherry)	Fruit
Pueraria lobata (kudzu)	Leaf
P. phaseoloides (kudzu)	Root
Stellaria media (chickweed)	Whole plant
Trifolium pratense (red clover)	Leaf
T. repens (white clover)	Leaf
Vigna angularis (adzuki bean)	Seed

Pterocarpans

Pterocarpans are significantly antifungal and are found in the heartwood of many legume trees, but are also induced as phytoalexins in some plants in response to fungal infection. The rotenoids have a common tetracyclic ring system, as in rotenone, and are distinguished by their insecticidal and piscicidal properties.

Rotenone inhibits the electron transport pathway in mitochondria and is therefore toxic to all forms of life. However, it can be used safely as a fish poison because the oral toxicity in humans is very low. Powdered derris root contains rotenone and is a well-known insecticidal dust.

Rotenone (tubotoxin)

Major sources of rotenone include derris root (*Derris elliptica*) and Jamaica dogwood (*Piscidia erythrina*). It is also found in the leaves of mullein (*Verbascum thapsus*). Rotenone demonstrates insecticidal and antiprotozoal activity. It is toxic, with an intraperitoneal LD_{50} in mice of 2.8 mg/kg. While the toxicity in humans is low, it is more toxic when inhaled than when ingested.[58]

Minor Flavonoids

Harborne and Baxter use the term *minor flavonoid* to describe flavonoids that have a limited distribution (as opposed to the more widespread anthocyanins, flavones, and flavonols) and a central pyran ring at a higher level of oxidation.

- Flavanones
- Dihydrochalcones
- Dihydroflavonols (flavan-3-ols)
- Flavan-3,4-diols

The best-known minor flavonoids are the *flavanones* and the *flavanon-3-ols* or *dihydroflavonols*.

Flavanones

Two flavanones, naringenin and eriodictyol, are relatively common. Flavanone glycosides are often notable for their taste; naringin and eriocitrin contribute to bitterness in citrus fruits. However, not all flavanones are bitter. Some are sweet; for example, neohesperidin dihydrochalcone, a compound related to neohesperidin, is used in the food industry as a nonsugar sweetener.

Naringenin

This compound has a widespread occurrence in plants, especially in the Asteraceae family (for example, *Artemisia* spp.). Naringin, the glycoside of naringenin, is widely distributed in Rutaceae. Naringenin has antibacterial, antifungal, antihepatotoxic, antioxidant, antispasmodic, and antiulcerogenic properties.[59]

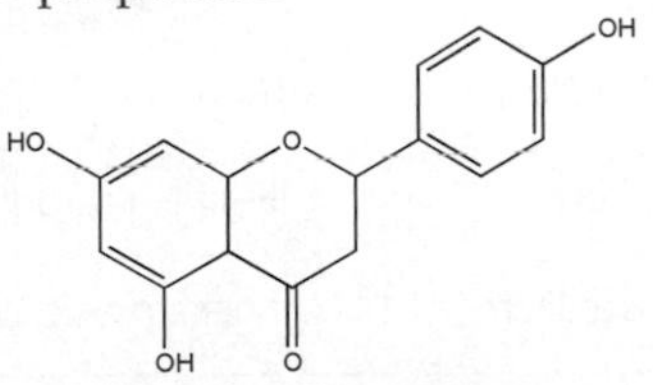

Fig. 7.55. Naringenin

Dihydrochalcones

Flavonoids in this group have an open central ring. They are structurally related to the flavanones, but are not as widely distributed.

Phloretin

Phloretin occurs as a glycoside, especially in Rosaceae and Ericaceae. The compound demonstrates antibacterial and anti-inflammatory actions.[60]

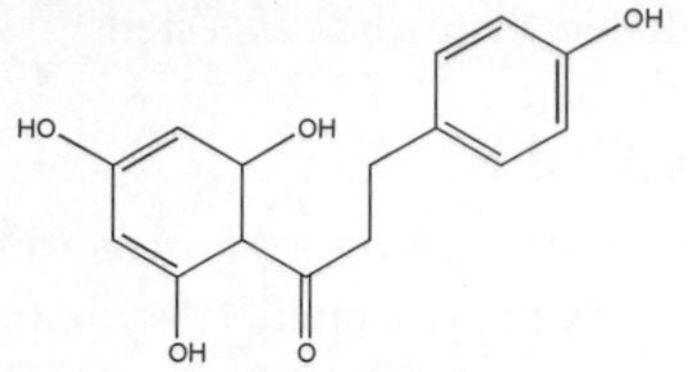

Fig. 7.56. Phloretin

Dihydroflavonols

Here, the molecule has a closed central ring. These relatively common compounds are also known as flavan-3-ols.

Catechin, a dihydroflavonol, and silybin, a flavolignan from milk thistle *(Silybum marianum)*, are used therapeutically because of their anti-inflammatory and antihepatotoxic properties. Many of these structures have antimicrobial activity, and several are phytoalexins.

(+)-Catechin

Catechin is very widespread, especially in woody plants. Examples of medicinal plants that contain this dihydroflavonol are provided in table 7.11.

Table 7.11. Catechin-Rich Herbs and Actions

HERB	ACTION
Agrimonia eupatoria (agrimony)	Bitter, astringent
Crataegus laevigata (hawthorn)	Cardiotonic, hypotensive
Humulus lupulus (hops)	Bitter, hypnotic, antispasmodic
Leonurus cardiaca (motherwort)	Relaxing nervine, antispasmodic
Quercus alba (white oak)	Astringent
Salix alba (white willow)	Anti-inflammatory, analgesic
Vaccinium myrtillus (bilberry)	Antihepatotoxic, antioxidant

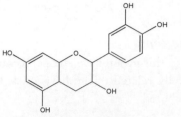

Fig. 7.57. Catechin

Silybin

Silybin occurs in the seeds of milk thistle *(Silybum marianum)* as a component of "silymarin," a complex of *S. marianum* flavanolignans that possess antihepatotoxic activity. Silybin was formerly called silymarin.[61]

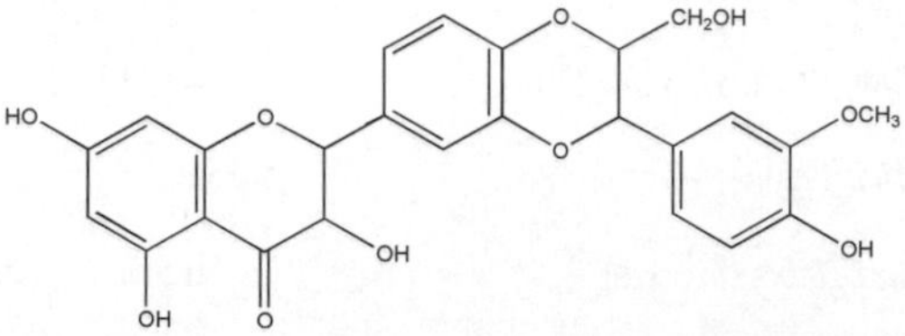

Fig. 7.58. Silybin

Biflavonoids

Another variant in the flavone series is the biflavonyl. These dimeric compounds are formed by carbon-carbon or carbon-oxygen couplings between two flavone units (usually apigenin). Methyl ethers are common, for example, ginkgetin, which occurs in the autumnal leaves of *Ginkgo biloba*. Biflavonyls occur almost exclusively in gymnosperms.

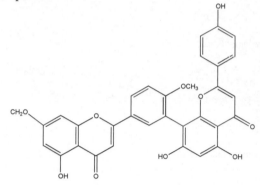

Fig. 7.59. Ginkgetin

Ginkgetin

This dimethyl ether of amentoflavone occurs in autumnal leaves of *Ginkgo biloba*.[62]

PHARMACOLOGY AND THERAPEUTIC POTENTIAL OF FLAVONOIDS

Flavonoids have become the focus of much attention within the research community. Both in vitro and in vivo studies attest to their potential in modern medicine.[63] However, this potential simply mirrors the therapeutic strengths of the whole plants, long recognized in traditional herbal medicine and its modern manifestation, phytotherapy.

While new research that points to potential applications for isolated flavonoids is exciting, it should not deflect the attention of the practitioner from the therapeutic cornucopia offered by the plants themselves.[64] Traditional herbal and naturopathic protocols, often the cues that inspired the research in the first place, have great inherent value based on generations of observation and use. This is a time to affirm their value, not to belittle their lack of statistical validity or bemoan the dearth of double-blind, placebo-controlled studies. After all, where is the controlled study that validates *Vis Medicatrix Naturae* (the healing power of nature)?

Flavonoids have many properties, but to individually list the physiological effects of isolated chemicals can obscure the fact that they work in complex, synergistic ways. It is vital to differentiate between effects of whole plants and research on specific molecules. In the case of herbs used in phytotherapy, it is generally inappropriate to speak of "flavonoid-containing herbs," because while flavonoids probably contribute to the activity of drugs, they only rarely act alone. Essential oils, other phenolic compounds, minerals, and saponins, to name just a few, are also essential components of their activity.

From a traditional herbal perspective, many links can be made between research-based reports of flavonoid activity and the well-known actions of plants in our materia medica. The following list highlights some of these correlations.

Actions of Flavonoids

- Antioxidant
- Hypoglycemic
- Stabilize capillary permeability
- Anti-inflammatory
- Immunomodulatory
- Antihepatotoxic
- Antineoplastic
- Hypotensive
- Regenerate connective tissue
- Sedative
- Regulate cardiac function
- Weakly estrogenic
- Antimicrobial
- Antispasmodic
- Diuretic
- Cholagogue

Because these ubiquitous phytochemicals have a gentle impact on a whole range of organs, tissues, and physiological processes, they are sometimes described as *biological response modifiers*. The heart, blood vessels, liver, immune system, connective tissue, adrenal glands, kidneys, musculature, and nervous system may all benefit from herbs containing these constituents.

The following material focuses largely on research on specific chemicals. It is important to remember that the specific effects enumerated below do not occur in isolation, but are interrelated at the metabolic level in both plants and people. Not all flavonoids or plants that contain them demonstrate all of the properties discussed here and, similarly, this is far from a complete listing of reported effects.

A comprehensive review by Middleton and Kandaswami of the impact of flavonoids on immune system function and the inflammatory response illuminated a wide range of effects.[65] Please refer to this review for complete citations.

- Flavonoids have profound effects on immune system and inflammatory cells.
- Certain flavonoids, depending on structure, can affect (usually inhibit) secretory processes, mitogenesis, and cell-cell interactions, including effects on adhesion molecule expression and function.
- The effects of flavonoids on secretory processes suggest that they may influence the function of cytoskeletal elements, supporting cellular health and activity through some positive effect on the microfilaments that make up the elements of the cytoskeleton.
- Certain flavonoids may affect gene expression and the activity of cytokines and cytokine receptors.
- Flavonoids can stimulate or inhibit protein phosphorylation and thereby regulate cell function.
- Flavonoids are recognized antioxidants and free radical scavengers.
- Resting cells are not significantly affected by flavonoids, but once activated by a physiological stimulus may generate a flavonoid-sensitive substance. The interaction of flavonoids with that substance dramatically alters the outcome of the activation process.

Possible Biological Response Modification Mechanisms

Flavonoids appear to modify the body's reaction to other substances, such as allergens, viruses, and carcinogens, as evidenced by their anti-inflammatory, antiallergenic, antiviral, and anticancer properties. As antioxidants, flavonoid molecules are unique in that they are active against a wide variety of oxidants and free radicals. Among their effects is an ability to increase vitamin C levels within cells, decreasing breakage and leakage of small blood vessels, protecting against free radical damage, and supporting joint structures. Many flavonoids modulate prostaglandin synthesis and are powerful enzyme inhibitors. These properties have profound physiological implications.

Flavonoids as Enzyme Inhibitors

As a general rule, flavonoids are enzyme inhibitors in vitro. Several flavonoids (such as cirsiliol and hypolaetin) are potent inhibitors of 5-lipoxygenase; therefore, they inhibit the production of the leukotrienes that mediate inflammation and allergic reactions. In addition, several flavonoids (luteolin, apigenin, and chrysin) inhibit cyclooxygenase and platelet aggregation. These properties, which have been demonstrated in vitro, may in part explain the anti-inflammatory and antiallergic properties commonly attributed to various drugs known to contain flavonoids.[66]

Absorption of Flavonoids in the Gastrointestinal Tract

The absorption of flavonoid glycosides is poor, although trace amounts of intact glycosides can sometimes be detected in bile or urine. Usually, the glycosides are initially broken down to their aglycones and, subsequently, to ring fission products. Flavonol aglycones, free flavones, and flavonols, such as quercetin, tend to be poorly absorbed, but the more saturated flavonoids, such as flavonones and flavonols like (+)catechin, are more readily absorbed. The exposure of gastric mucosa to glycosides may raise levels of cytoprotective prostaglandins, which may help explain how glycosides exert their protective effects on gastrointestinal mucosa. Flavonoids are metabolized by a variety of cells, especially liver cells, and since the metabolites are excreted in urine, there is no accumulation of metabolites in the body.

Flavonoids and the French Paradox

Red wine is a rich source of flavonoids, and regular red wine consumption is associated with a decreased risk of coronary heart disease (CHD). French epidemiological studies show an association between increased wine consumption and reduction in death from heart disease. This phenomenon has come to be known as "the French paradox," as the French diet is characteristically high in animal fats and other factors associated with heart disease.[67]

Investigators have now concluded that wine and fruit consumption both correlate with reduced mortality from heart disease.[68] Several mechanisms have been suggested to explain the protective effect of wine, of which the best known is the ability of alcohol to alter blood lipid levels by lowering total cholesterol and raising levels of high-density lipoprotein (HDL). However, if the findings concerning fruit are taken into account, other mechanisms must be considered.

Wine is rich in flavonoids. Phenolics are well known for the sensory subtleties they impart to wine, and for this reason, French researchers have been investigating their chemistry for decades. Since they are antioxidants, these substances are at the foundation of the long aging process undergone by some wines. Wines low in flavonoids, such as white wines, rarely age gracefully.

Might phenolic antioxidants influence the development of atherosclerosis in humans? A study at the University of California, Davis, showed that they inhibit the oxidation of low-density lipoprotein (LDL) in vitro. If this effect occurs in vivo, it could slow the development of arterial plaque. In addition, since the aggregation of platelets (thrombosis) is an important factor in precipitating a heart attack, compounds that reduce platelet aggregation could also lower CHD mortality. Wine flavonoids have been shown to decrease platelet aggregation, apparently by inhibiting oxygenase enzymes.

Wine is not the only dietary source of phenolic compounds. Fresh fruits are a rich source, and fruit consumption correlates highly with reduced CHD mortality. Tea is another source of phenolics, but green and black tea have quite different compositions. Green tea contains mainly monomeric catechins—for example, epigallocatechin 3-gallate—while black tea possesses oligomeric and polymeric forms.

The results of a Finnish study on the association between dietary flavonoid intake and subsequent CHD mortality suggest that people with very low intakes of flavonoids have higher risks of heart disease.[69] Taken together, this combination of epidemiological and laboratory research clearly suggests that flavonoids are beneficial nutrients that can reduce CHD mortality.[70]

Anti-Inflammatory Actions

Many different mechanisms may contribute to the anti-inflammatory properties of flavonoids, including effects on prostaglandin synthesis and arachidonic acid metabolism, enzyme inhibition, and antioxidant activities. The effects of flavonoids on collagen and on the function of immune cells may also play a role.

Effects on Prostaglandin Synthesis

The well-recognized anti-inflammatory actions of many flavonoids are due in part to their ability to modulate prostaglandin synthesis. Some flavonoids inhibit prostaglandin synthesis, while others stimulate the production of prostaglandins. Research on flavonoids with the ability to inhibit prostaglandin synthetase (PGS) has identified certain common structural features.

However, inhibition of PGS is only a partial answer as to why flavonoids suppress inflammation. Leukotrienes, products of arachidonic acid produced by the 5-lipoxygenase pathway, are also involved in the inflammatory process, and some flavonoids, such as quercetin, can inhibit lipoxygenase.

Flavonoids appear to have an important advantage over nonsteroidal anti-inflammatory drugs (NSAIDs) in that they are largely free of adverse effects. NSAIDs work in part by inhibiting the synthesis of prostaglandins, not only those that cause inflammation, but also the cytoprotective prostaglandins that help prevent ulceration of the gastric mucosa. Thus, by inhibiting prostaglandin formation, NSAIDs also cause gastric ulceration.

Flavonoids do not cause gastric ulceration and, as a class, are remarkably free of side effects. Why flavonoids do not damage gastric tissues is not fully understood, but it may be because their anti-inflammatory actions are based on several mechanisms rather than on a single mechanism, like inhibition of prostaglandin synthesis.

Effects on Arachidonic Acid Metabolism

Flavonoids, particularly quercetin, are inhibitors of allergic, IgE-mediated release of histamine and other chemicals from mast cells and basophils, via inhibition of lipoxygenase and other enzymes involved in the metabolism of arachidonic acid in cells. Quercetin exhibits both allergic-mediator release activity and selective inhibition of the biosynthesis of pro-inflammatory arachidonic acid metabolites, which may help explain its antiallergic and anti-inflammatory actions.[71] Animal studies have demonstrated that endogenous prostaglandins are involved in mucosal injury produced by absolute ethanol and that quercetin has antiulcer and cytoprotective properties in such situations.[72]

Antioxidant Effects

Active oxygen species, or free radicals, cause considerable damage in inflammation. These include hydrogen peroxide, hypochlorous acid, hydroxyl radicals, and possibly other species, such as singlet oxygen and hydroperoxy radicals. These species are derived from superoxide anions liberated from stimulated phagocytic cells. Many flavonoids are powerful antioxidants and scavengers of free radicals. In addition to removing free radicals, they may also suppress their formation, since many flavonoids have the ability to bind heavy metal ions that are known to catalyze the production of free radicals.

Inhibition of Enzymes

One enzyme that is strongly inhibited by flavonoids is phosphodiesterase, which catalyzes the breakdown of cyclic adenosine monophosphate (cAMP). Cyclic AMP is a fundamentally important regulatory molecule in cellular activity. As discussed in detail in chapter 9, cAMP can trigger a range of intracellular effects by activating various enzymes. High cAMP levels are anti-inflammatory, since cAMP tends to decrease the secretion from cells of destructive agents, such as lysosomal enzymes and prostaglandins. In the presence of inflammation, drugs that elevate intracellular cAMP levels have some anti-inflammatory action, which is probably related to the rise in cAMP. Thus the anti-inflammatory action of flavonoids may be due in part to the fact that they inhibit the breakdown of cAMP.

Effects on Collagen

Many flavonoids have a beneficial effect on collagen, which is responsible for maintaining the integrity of the ground substance in connective tissue. Collagen is destroyed during inflammatory processes that occur in rheumatoid arthritis, gout, and other conditions involving bones, joints, cartilage, and other connective tissue. Anthocyanidins and other flavonoids affect collagen metabolism in many ways:[73]

- Cross-link collagen fibers, reinforcing the collagen matrix of connective tissue (ground substance or cartilage)
- Prevent free radical damage with potent antioxidant and free radical scavenging actions
- Inhibit destruction of collagen structures by enzymes secreted during inflammation

• Prevent the release and synthesis of compounds that promote inflammation, such as histamine

Overall Antioxidant Activities

Flavonoids can inhibit formation of superoxide anions and the generation of hydroxyl radicals. With the new insights concerning the role of free radicals in aging, autoimmune diseases, and many other health issues, the antioxidant potential of flavonoid-containing herbs suggests exciting therapeutic possibilities. Perhaps more important, this is simply the affirmation of traditional herbal practice, which makes extensive use of many flavonoid-rich herbs.

Flavonoids are potent antioxidants, free radical scavengers, metal chelators, and inhibitors of lipid peroxidation. The structural requirements for these functions include a hydroxyl group in carbon position 3, a double bond between carbon positions 2 and 3, a carbonyl group in carbon position 4, and polyhydroxylation of the A and B aromatic rings.

These structural features prevent the formation of free radicals and the leukotrienes that promote inflammation. In a general sense, many polyphenols scavenge reactive chemical radicals formed under various circumstances (for example, anoxia, inflammation, and lipidic autoxidation). Normally, the cascade of reactions involved in the inflammatory response is interrupted by enzymic systems, such as superoxide dismutases, catalase, and glutathione peroxidase, which reduce peroxides, and, later on, hydroperoxides.

Many polyphenols and flavonoids react with free radicals to prevent the degradation caused by the intense activity of these pro-oxidants on membrane phospholipids. It has been hypothesized that the capacity of flavonoids to modify membrane-dependent processes, such as free-radical-induced membrane lipid peroxidation, is related not only to their structural characteristics, but also to their ability to interact with and penetrate the lipid bilayers.[74]

Researchers have begun to elucidate the antioxidant mechanisms underlying the clinical applications of oligomeric procyanidins (OPCs) as vascular protective agents. (For more information on OPCs, see the discussion on Tannins later in this chapter.) Studies have shown that OPCs inhibit xanthine oxidase (a generator of free radicals) and the activity of the lysosomal enzyme system. This system governs the release of enzymes that can damage the connective tissue surrounding capillary walls.[75] In these studies, OPCs demonstrated a wide range of antioxidant abilities, summarized below.

Antioxidant Effects of OPCs

• Trap hydroxyl free radicals
• Trap lipid peroxides and the free radicals that initiate their formation
• Markedly delay the onset of lipid peroxidation
• Chelate free iron molecules, preventing iron-induced lipid peroxidation
• Inhibit production of free radicals by inhibiting xanthine oxidase
• Inhibit the damaging effects of enzymes (e.g., hyaluronidase, elastase, collagenase) that can degrade connective tissue structures

Effects on Immunological Processes

No doubt can remain that flavonoids have profound effects on the function of immune and inflammatory cells, as confirmed by a large number and variety of observations from in vitro and some in vivo studies. That these ubiquitous dietary chemicals may have significant in vivo effects on homeostasis within the immune system and on the behavior of secondary cell systems that comprise the inflammatory response seems highly likely, but more work is required to strengthen this hypothesis.

Evidence also indicates that certain flavonoids may affect gene expression and the elaboration and effects of cytokines and cytokine receptors. How all of these effects are mediated is not yet clear, but one important mechanism may be the capacity of flavonoids to stimulate or inhibit protein phosphorylation and thereby regulate cell function.[76]

LIGNANS AND NEOLIGNANS

These are dimeric compounds in which phenylpropane (C_6-C_3) units are linked to form three-dimensional networks.[77] Dimers are molecules formed from two similar constituents, called monomers. They are chemically related to the polymeric lignins that make up the plant cell wall and are found mainly in woody tissues.[78]

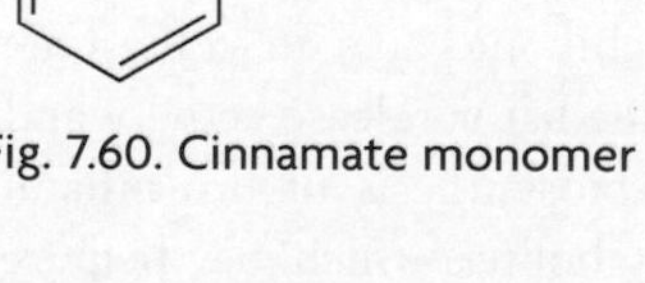

Fig. 7.60. Cinnamate monomer

The Five Structural Classes of Lignans[79]

- Simple lignans
- Lignanolides with lactone substitution
- Monoepoxylignans
- Diepoxylignans
- Cyclolignans

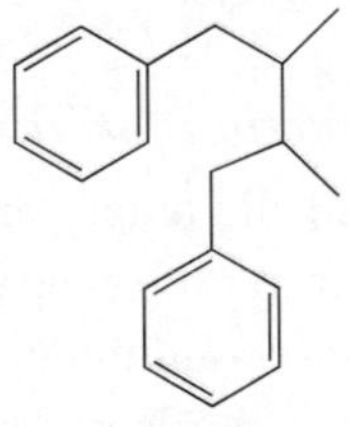

Fig. 7.61. Simple lignan

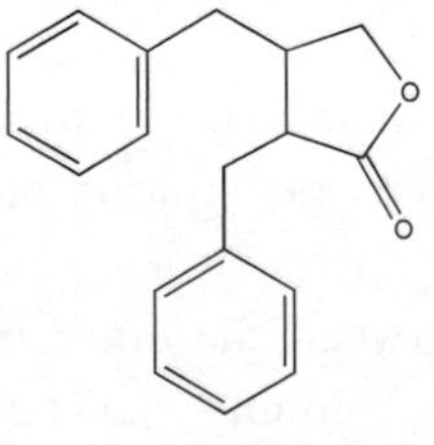

Fig. 7.62. Lignanolide

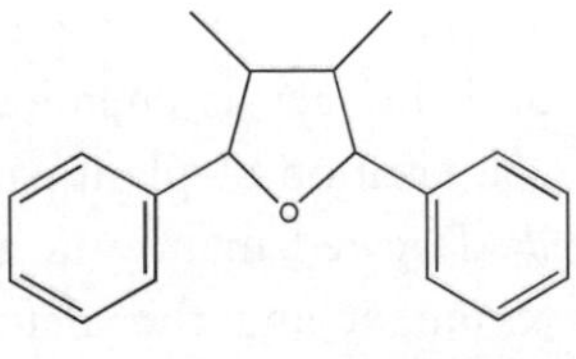

Fig. 7.63. Monoepoxylignan

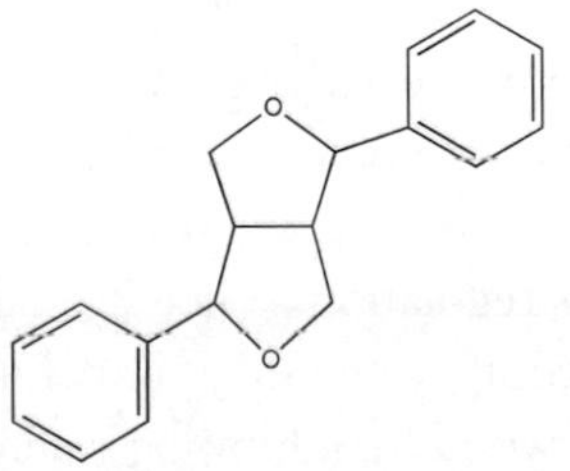

Fig. 7.64. Diepoxylignan

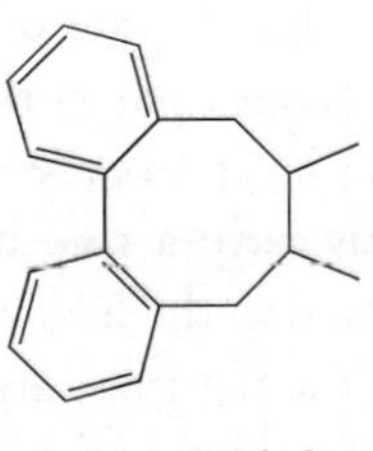

Fig. 7.65. Cyclolignan

There is also a small group of related neolignans formed by asymmetrical carbon-carbon links in the side chains.

Lignans occur widely in the wood of gymnosperm trees, and they have also been recorded in some 50 angiosperm families, where they can be found in both the wood and the bark. The majority of the more than 200 naturally occurring lignans are found in the free state in the heartwood of trees. Some have been isolated from other plant parts, where they may be present as glycosides. In plants, lignans have antibacterial, antifungal, and antifeedant properties.

Lignans have attracted the attention of the research community because they have shown antitumor and antiviral activities, among many other actions. Some cyclolignans and lignolides have cytotoxic and antimitotic properties, although toxicity has limited their therapeutic application.

Flavolignans of milk thistle (*Silybum marianum*) and the schisandrins from *Schisandra chinensis* have valuable hepatoprotective attributes. Schisandrins reverse destruction of liver cells by inducing cytochrome P_{450} activity.[80]

For more information on the hepatoprotective activity of milk thistle flavolignans, see chapter 9.

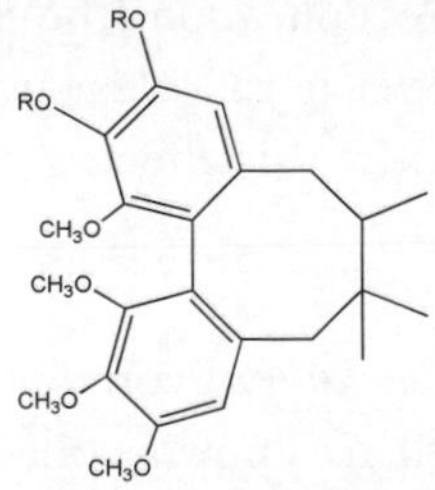

Fig. 7.66. Schisandrin

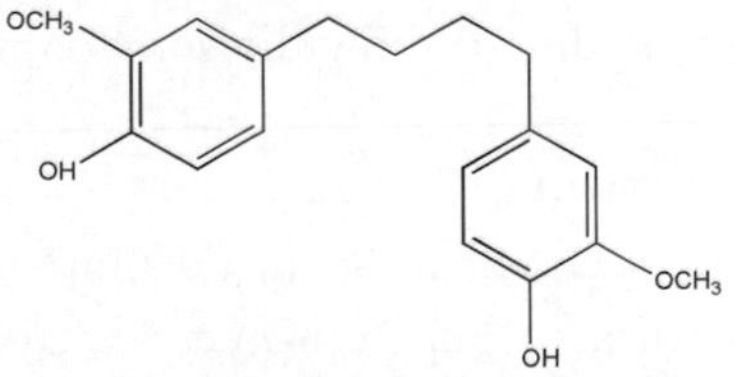

Fig. 7.67. Dihydroguaiaretic acid

Dihydroguaiaretic acid from chaparral (*Larrea* spp.) is a potent antioxidant, and other lignans display allergenic, cathartic, and cardiovascular effects. Lignans such as enterolactone, matairesinol, and enterodiol are excreted in human urine, and are believed to be formed through bacterial degradation of dietary plant lignans in the gut. These lignans are phytoestrogens that appear to exert weak effects on estrogen receptors, improving female menstrual function. The overall cancer risk reduction may also work through this mechanism. A role for lignans has also been proposed in colon cancer prevention.[81]

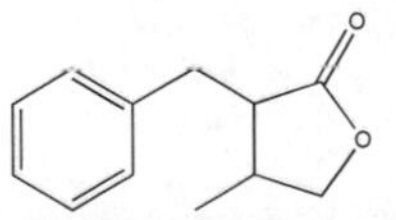

Fig. 7.68.
Enterolactone

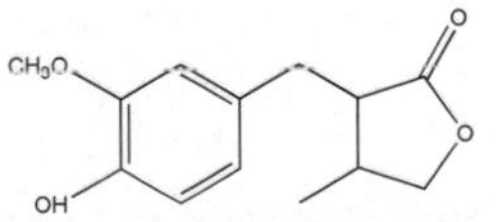

Fig. 7.69.
Matairesinol

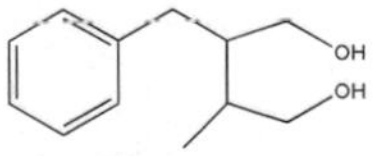

Fig. 7.70.
Enterodiol

Podophyllotoxin

Podophyllotoxin (podofilox) and its derivatives, etoposide and teniposide, are all antimitotic glucosides.

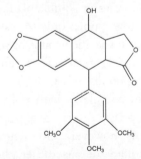

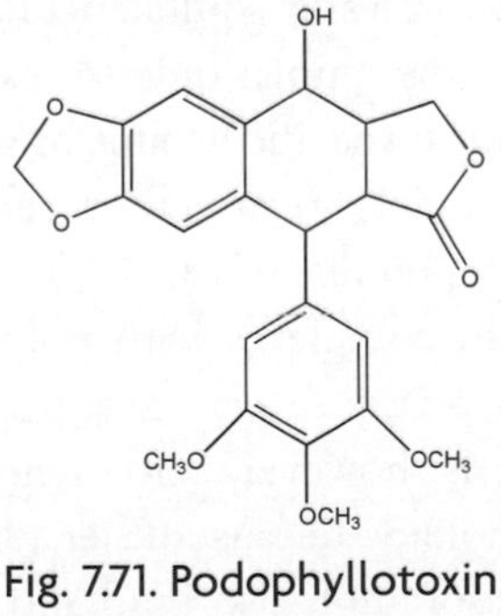

Fig. 7.71. Podophyllotoxin

Podofilox is an extract of mayapple (*Podophyllum peltatum*), which generally acts as a poison to cells undergoing mitosis. Podofilox itself is not used as a chemotherapy agent; instead, it is applied as an ingredient in creams for the treatment for genital warts. Genital warts, which are caused by the human papillomavirus (HPV), have been associated with squamous cell carcinomas of the genital organs.

The synthetic analogues etoposide and teniposide

block the cell cycle in two specific places: between the last cell division and the start of DNA replication (the G1-phase) and at the beginning of DNA replication (the S-phase). However, researchers do not yet have a clear understanding of how the compounds exert this effect.

Silymarin

The seeds of milk thistle *(Silybum marianum)* contain a mixture of hepatoprotective flavolignans known collectively as silymarin. Silybin is the major component; other flavolignans in the mixture include silychristin and taxifoline. The pharmacology of hepatoprotection is discussed in chapter 9.

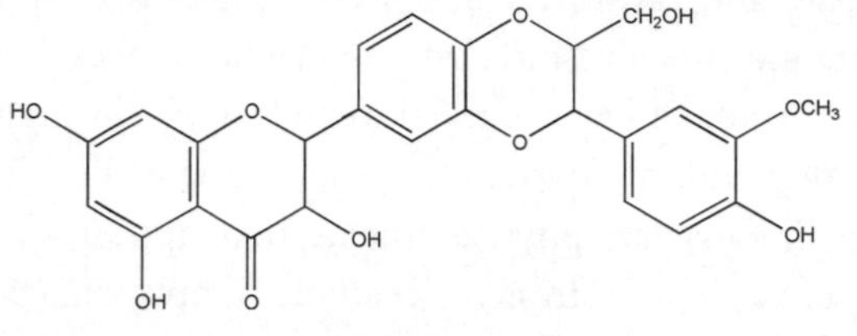

Fig. 7.72. Silybin

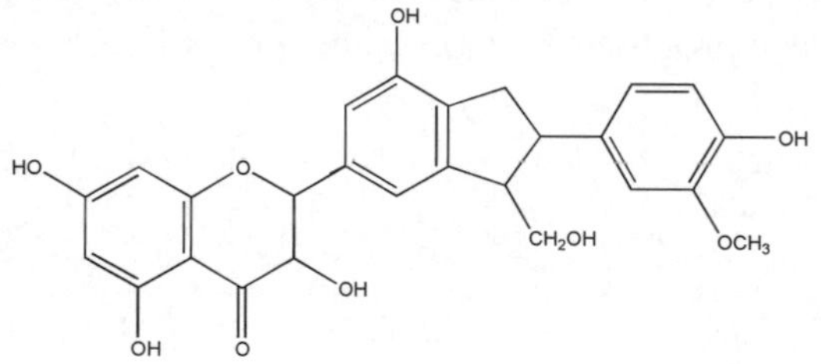

Fig. 7.73. Silychristin

TANNINS

The word *tannin* has long been used to describe organic substances present in water-soluble plant extracts that are capable of converting animal hide to leather. The application of the term to specific groups of structurally characterized chemicals is relatively recent. Tannins are polyphenolic compounds $(C_6-C_3-C_6)$n that precipitate proteins and form complexes with polysaccharides, and are composed of a very diverse group of oligomers and polymers. There is, however, some degree of confusion about the terminology, because other phenolics, such as pyrogallol and resorcinol, also bind and precipitate proteins. In addition, not all polyphenols precipitate proteins or form complexes with polysaccharides.

A technical definition in current use describes a tannin as any phenolic compound that has a sufficiently high molecular weight and contains enough hydroxyls and other suitable groups to form strong complexes with protein and other macromolecules under the particular environmental conditions being studied.

Tannins are widely distributed among plants and are common in both gymnosperms and angiosperms, although they are more frequently found in dicotyledons than in monocotyledons. They are sequestered in various plant tissues so that they do not interfere with normal plant metabolism. Only after cell breakdown and death do they exert their metabolic effects.

Occurrence and Functions of Tannins in Plants

Buds: Most common in the outer part of the bud, tannins are probably present to protect against freezing.

Leaves: Tannins are most common in the upper epidermis; however, in evergreen plants, they are evenly distributed in all leaf tissues, protecting against predation by reducing palatability.

Roots: Most commonly found in the hypodermis, tannins probably act as chemical barriers to penetration and colonization by plant pathogens.

Seeds: Located mainly in a layer between the outer integument and the aleurone layer, tannins may help maintain dormancy and provide allelopathic and bactericidal protection.

Stems: Tannins are often found in the active growth areas of trees, such as the secondary phloem and xylem and the layer between epidermis and cortex, where they may have a role in growth regulation. They are also found in the heartwood of conifers and may contribute to the natural durability of wood by inhibiting microbial activity.

There are two main types of tannin, condensed (proanthocyanidins) and hydrolyzable tannins. These are unevenly distributed in plants; the condensed tannins occur almost universally in ferns and gymnosperms and are widespread among angiosperms, especially trees and shrubs. By contrast, hydrolyzable tannins are limited to dicotyledonous plants. Both types of tannin can occur together in the same plant.

Hydrolyzable Tannins

Hydrolyzable tannins are soluble in water and alcohol. There are two types, based on either gallic or epigallic acids. In the presence of acids or enzymes, proanthocyanidins (condensed tannins) do not hydrolyze.

Gallotannins hydrolyze to gallic acid and glucose.

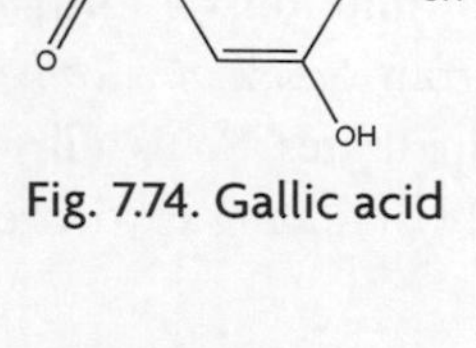

Fig. 7.74. Gallic acid

The phenolic groups in gallotannins are sometimes dimers or higher oligomers of gallic acid; each single monomer is called a galloyl. Gallotannins are found in rhubarb (*Rheum* spp.), cloves (*Syzygium aromaticum*), petals of red roses (*Rosa* spp.), bearberry (*Arctostaphylos uva-ursi*), witch hazel (*Hamamelis virginiana*), sweet chestnut (*Castanea sativa*), and maple (*Acer* spp.).

Ellagitannins hydrolyze to ellagic acid and glucose.

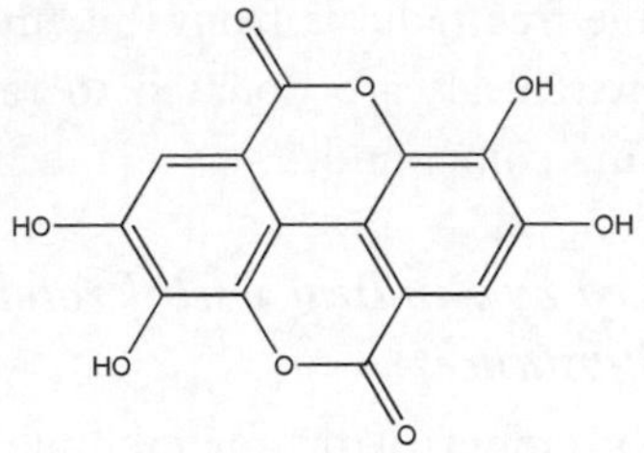

Fig. 7.75. Ellagic acid

The phenolic groups in ellagitannins consist of hexahydroxydiphenic acid, which spontaneously dehydrates to ellagic acid. They are found in pomegranate (*Punica granatum*), eucalyptus leaves (*Eucalyptus* spp.), kousso (*Brayera anthelmintica*), sweet chestnut (*Castanea sativa*), oak bark (*Quercus* spp.), and agrimony (*Agrimonia* spp.). An example is agrimoniin from *Agrimonia eupatoria*.

Ellagic acid is one of the products of ellagitannin hydrolysis, which occurs upon storage, drying, extraction, or digestion of plants containing ellagitannins. Therefore, ellagic acid is taken in by everybody who ingests ellagitannin-containing plants as foods or drugs, although ellagic acid itself is not usually present in living plants.

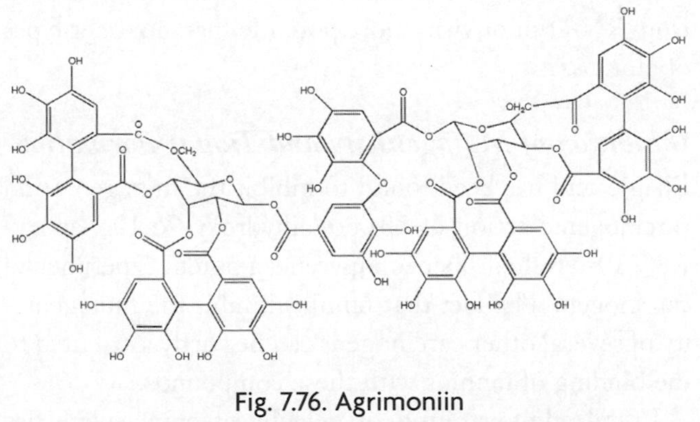

Fig. 7.76. Agrimoniin

Condensed Tannins (Proanthocyanidins)

Condensed tannins, or flavolans, are formed biosynthetically by the condensation of flavan-3-ols, such as catechin and epicatechin, into dimers and then higher oligomers. The name *proanthocyanidin* is used alternatively for condensed tannins because, on treatment with hot acid, some of the carbon-carbon linking bonds are broken, and anthocyanidin monomers may be formed.

When two proanthocyanidin molecules are linked together, the result is called a *dimer*; a linkage of three forms is a *trimer* and four a *tetramer*. Collectively, mixtures of proanthocyanidin dimers, trimers, tetramers, and larger molecules are known as *oligomeric procyanidins* (OPCs).

Fruit-bearing plants are high in oligomeric procyanidins, and heartwood and bark are rich sources of unusual proanthocyanidins. OPCs, called "pycnogenols" in the commercial supplement market, are available in extracts of grape seeds and the bark of the maritime pine.[82] It should be noted that the word *pycnogenol* is a commercial term and not an accepted chemical descriptor.

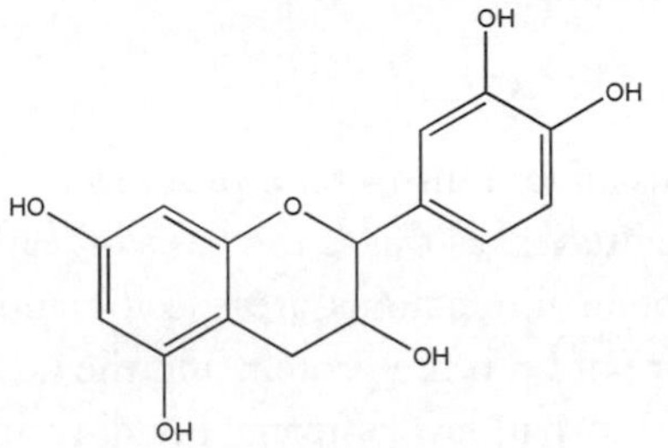

Fig. 7.77. (-)-Epicatechin

Proanthocyanidins are more widely distributed than are hydrolyzable tannins. The commonest anthocyanidins produced are cyanidin (from procyanidin) and delphinidin (from prodelphinidin). Proanthocyanidins may contain 2 to 50 or more flavonoid units; proanthocyanidin polymers have complex structures because the flavonoid units can differ for some substituents and because the sites for interflavan bonds vary.

Interactions with Other Macromolecules

Tannins have a major impact on animal nutrition because of their ability to form complexes with numerous types of molecules.[83] These molecules include but are not limited to:

- Carbohydrates
- Proteins
- Polysaccharides
- Bacterial cell membranes
- Enzymes involved in protein and carbohydrate digestion

Carbohydrates

Both starch and cellulose are complexed by tannins. Tannin-carbohydrate interactions are increased in the presence of carbohydrates with high molecular weight, low solubility, and conformational flexibility. These interactions are probably based on hydrophobic and hydrogen linkages.

Starch-tannin interaction: Starch has the ability to form hydrophobic cavities that allow inclusion complexes with tannins and many other lipophilic molecules. The hydrophobic molecules are, in effect, encapsulated in the cavity formed by the complexes.

Cellulose-tannin interaction: Cellulose has a direct surface interaction with tannins.

Cell-wall carbohydrate-tannin interaction: This association is less understood. One explanation is that tannins associate with plant cell walls in a manner similar to that of lignin. However, it is also possible that this association occurs as an artifact when tannins are isolated from nonliving cells.

Proteins

The capacity of tannins to bind proteins has been recognized for centuries, as this is the basis of leather tanning. Tannin-protein interactions are specific and depend on the structure of both the protein and the tannin. Protein characteristics that favor strong bonding include large molecular size, open and flexible structures, and a high content of proline. Tannin characteristics that favor strong bonding are high molecular weight and high conformational mobility.

Properties of Tannins

One of the most important properties attributed to tannins is astringent action. Astringents cause contraction of tissue, blanching and wrinkling of mucous membranes, and diminished exudations. When applied to wounds, they form a thin protective surface, cutting down on the secretion of exudates. Precipitation of surface proteins and/or polysaccharides results in hardening of the epidermis, which lessens the absorption of toxins and protects against irritants. Tannins also display antimicrobial properties. Many are able to constrict blood vessels, thereby reducing bleeding.

Applications of Tannins

- Protect inflamed mucous membranes
- Exert a drying effect on mucous membranes, reducing hypersecretion
- Reduce the inflammation and swelling that accompany infection
- Prevent bleeding from small wounds
- Reduce uterine bleeding (for example, in menorrhagia)
- Relieve symptoms of diarrhea or dysentery through binding effects in the gut
- Used externally for astringent action in douches, snuffs, and eyewashes

Biological and Other Activities of Isolated Tannins

Since tannins are polyphenols, and are fairly large molecules containing several phenolic hydroxyl groups located mostly on the molecule surface, phenolic groups have a strong influence on the properties and biological activities of tannins.[84] Radical scavenging is an important activity of tannins. This kind of activity is due to the formation of stable free radicals from the tannin molecules after hydrogen radicals are donated to radicals formed from a coexisting compound.

Effects Induced by Binding with Protein and Other Substances

The binding of tannins with, for example, proteins and other large molecules or basic compounds is thought to be key to the various biological activities of tannins. Such binding plays a role in the antidiarrhetic activity of tannins (one of the most widely exploited effects of tannin-containing medicinal plants) by protecting digestive organs from injurious attack. It also contributes to the antihemorrhagic effects of tannin-rich drugs.

Effects on Enzymes

At relatively high concentrations, tannins usually inhibit the activity of enzymes, but at low concentrations they often stimulate enzyme activity. The extent of inhibition and stimulation varies, depending on the enzyme and the structure and concentration of the tannin. Oligomeric hydrolyzable tannins inhibit reverse transcriptase isolated from RNA tumor virus more potently than do other types of tannins.[85]

Inhibition of Mutagenicity and Tumor Formation

Ellagic acid has been found to inhibit the mutagenic and carcinogenic action of 7β-,8α-dihydroxy-9α,10α-epoxy-7,8,9,10-tetrahydrobenzo[a]pyrene, a potent experimental carcinogen. The fact that tannins inhibit the mutagenicity of several other carcinogens can be partly attributed to the binding of tannins with these compounds.

Oral administration of epigallocatechin gallate has been found to inhibit duodenal cancer induced by *N*-ethyl-*N*'-nitro-*N*-nitrosoguanidin, suggesting that oral administration may be useful for the treatment of duodenal tumors.[86]

Inhibition of Viruses

Although the inhibitory actions of tannins against bacteria and fungi are not strong, researchers have observed remarkable inhibition of certain viruses by several tannins and related polyphenols.[87] In studies, tannins inhibited the replication of human immunodeficiency virus (HIV) and herpes simplex viruses (HSV).

Procyanidin B₄ (catechin-(4α-8)-epicatechin)

Procyanidin B_4 has a widespread occurrence in plants. It is found, for example, in the leaves of the raspberry *(Rubus idaeus)*. An infusion of raspberry leaves containing procyanidin B_4 and hydrolyzable tannins is used as a gargle and for treating wounds and ulcers.[88]

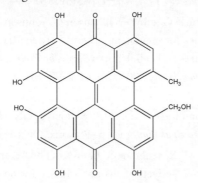

Fig. 7.78. Procyanidin B₄

References

1. Harborne JB, Baxter H. *Phytochemical Dictionary: A Handbook of Bioactive Compounds from Plants.* London; Washington, DC: Taylor & Francis, 1993.

2. Haslam, et al. Traditional herbal medicines—the role of polyphenols. *Planta Medica* 1989; 55:1–8.

3. Dombrowicz, et al. Phenolic acids in leaves of Arctostaphylos uva ursi L., Vaccinium vitis-idaea L. and Vaccinium myrtillus L. *Pharmazie* 1991; 46(9): 680–1.

4. Harborne JB, Baxter H. *Phytochemical Dictionary: A Handbook of Bioactive Compounds from Plants.* London; Washington, DC: Taylor & Francis, 1993.

5. Ibid.

6. Ibid.

7. Ibid.

8. Ibid.

9. Ibid.

10. Ibid.

11. Ibid.

12. Ibid.

13. Reddy BS. Chemoprevention of colon cancer by minor dietary constituents and their synthetic analogues. *Preventive Medicine* 1996 Jan–Feb; 25(1):48–50.

14. Harborne JB, Baxter H. *Phytochemical Dictionary: A Handbook of Bioactive Compounds from Plants.* London; Washington, DC: Taylor & Francis, 1993.

15. [No authors listed] Caffeic acid *IARC Monographs on the Evaluation of Carcinogenic Risks to Humans* 1993; 56:115–34.

16. Harborne JB, Baxter H. *Phytochemical Dictionary: A Handbook of Bioactive Compounds from Plants.* London; Washington, DC: Taylor & Francis, 1993.

17. Kawamori T, Lubet R, Steele VE, et al. Chemopreventive effect of curcumin, a naturally occurring anti-inflammatory agent, during the promotion/progression stages of colon cancer. *Cancer Research* 1999; 59:597–601.

18. Hallstrom H, Thuvander A. Toxicological evaluation of myristicin. *Natural Toxins* 1997; 5(5):186–92.

19. Harborne JB, Baxter H. *Phytochemical Dictionary: A Handbook of Bioactive Compounds from Plants.* London; Washington, DC: Taylor & Francis, 1993.

20. Ibid.

21. Ibid.

22. Ibid.

23. Ibid.

24. Mann J. *Secondary Metabolism.* Oxford; New York: Oxford University Press, 1993.

25. Harborne JB, Baxter H. *Phytochemical Dictionary: A Handbook of Bioactive Compounds from Plants.* London; Washington, DC: Taylor & Francis, 1993.

26. Ibid.

27. Ibid.

28. Ibid.

29. Ibid.

30. Ibid.

31. Ibid.

32. Ibid.

33. Ibid.

34. Ibid.

35. Ibid.

36. Ibid.

37. Ibid.

38. Chanvitayapongs S, Draczynska-Lusiak B, Sun AY. Amelioration of oxidative stress by antioxidants and resveratrol in PC_{12} cells. *Neuroreport* 1997; 8:1499–1502.

39. Roemer K, Mahyar-Roemer M. The basis for the chemopreventive action of resveratrol. *Drugs Today* 2002 Aug; 38(8):571–80.

40. Frankel EN, Waterhouse AL, Kinsella JE. Inhibition of human LDL oxidation by resveratrol. *Lancet* 1993; 341:1103–4.

41. Belguendouz L, Fremont L, Gozzelino MT. Interaction of transresveratrol with plasma lipoproteins. *Biochemical Pharmacology* 1998; 55:811–16.

42. Rotondo S. Effect of trans-resveratrol, a natural polyphenolic compound, on human polymorphonuclear leukocyte function. *British Journal of Pharmacology* 1998; 123:1691–9.

43. Bhat KP, Pezzuto JM. Cancer chemopreventive activity of resveratrol. *Annals of the New York Academy of Sciences* 2002 May; 957:210–29.

44. Jang M, Cai L, Udeani GO, et al. Cancer chemopreventive activity of resveratrol, a natural product derived from grapes. *Science* 1997 Jan 10; 275(5297):218–20.

45. Tsan MF, White JE, Maheshwari JG, Chikkappa G. Anti-leukemia effect of resveratrol. *Leukemia & Lymphoma* 2002 May; 43(5):983–7.

46. Harborne JB, Baxter H. *Phytochemical Dictionary: A Handbook of Bioactive Compounds from Plants.* London; Washington, DC: Taylor & Francis, 1993.

47. Ibid.

48. Formica JV, Regelson W. Review of the biology of Quercetin and related bioflavonoids. *Food and Chemical Toxicology* 1995 Dec; 33(12):1061–80.

49. Hertog MG, Hollman PC. Potential health effects of the dietary flavonol quercetin. *European Journal of Clinical Nutrition* 1996 Feb; 50(2):63–71.

50. Chu CK, Cutler HG. *Natural Products as Antiviral Agents.* New York: Plenum, 1992.

51. Boik J. *Cancer & Natural Medicine: A Textbook of Basic Science and Clinical Research.* Princeton, MN: Oregon Medical Press, 1996.

52. Harborne JB, Baxter H. *Phytochemical Dictionary: A Handbook of Bioactive Compounds from Plants.* London; Washington, DC: Taylor & Francis, 1993.

53. Ibid.

54. Ibid.

55. Harborne JB, Williams CA. Anthocyanins and other flavonoids. *Natural Product Reports* 2001 Jun; 18(3):310–33.

56. Harborne JB, Baxter H. *Phytochemical Dictionary: A Handbook of Bioactive Compounds from Plants.* London; Washington, DC: Taylor & Francis, 1993.

57. Ibid.

58. Ibid.

59. Ibid.

60. Ibid.

61. Ibid.

62. Ibid.

63. Middleton E. The flavonoids as potential therapeutic agents. In: Kimball SE, ed. *Immunopharmaceuticals.* Boca Raton, FL: CRC Press, 1995.

64. Hertog MG. Epidemiological evidence on potential health properties of flavonoids. *The Proceedings of the Nutrition Society* 1996 Mar; 55(1B):385–97.

65. Middleton E, Kandaswami C. Effects of flavonoids on immune and inflammatory cell functions. *Biochemical Pharmacology* 1992 Mar 17; 43(6):1167–79

66. Depeint F, Gee JM, Williamson G, Johnson IT. Evidence for consistent patterns between flavonoid structures and cellular activities. *The Proceedings of the Nutrition Society* 2002 Feb; 61(1):97–103.

67. Adzet T, Camarasa J. Pharmacokinetics of polyphenolic compounds. In: Craker LF, Simon JE, eds. *Herbs, Spices and Medicinal Plants,* vol 3. Phoenix: Oryx Press, 1988.

68. Bohm M, Rosenkranz S, Laufs U. The "French Paradox"—effects of alcohol, wine and wine polyphenols on the heart. *Deutsche medizinische Wochenschrift* 2002 Dec; 127:51–52, 2748–56.

69. de Lorgeril M, Salen P, Paillard F, et al. Mediterranean diet and the French paradox: two distinct biogeographic concepts for one consolidated scientific theory on the role of nutrition in coronary heart disease. *Cardiovascular Research* 2002 Jun; 54(3):503–15.

70. Knekt, et al. Flavonoid intake and coronary mortality in Finland: a cohort study [see comments]. *British Medical Journal* 1996; 312 (7029):478–81.

71. Hertog MG, Feskens EJ, Hollman PC, et al. Dietary antioxidant flavonoids and risk of coronary heart disease: the Zutphen Elderly Study. *Lancet* 1993 Oct 23; 342(8878):1007–11.

72. Welton AF, Tobias LD, Fiedler-Nagy C, et al. Effect of flavonoids on arachidonic acid metabolism. *Progress in Clinical and Biological Research* 1986; 213:231–42.

73. Alarcon de la Lastra C, Martin MJ, Motilva V. Antiulcer and gastroprotective effects of quercetin: a gross and histologic study. *Pharmacology* 1994; 48:56–62.

74. Haslam E, Lilley TH. Interactions of natural phenols with macromolecules. *Progress in Clinical and Biological Research* 1986; 213:53–65.

75. Saija A, Scalese M, Lanza M, et al. Flavonoids as antioxidant agents: importance of their interaction with biomembranes. *Free Radical Biology & Medicine* 1995; 19(4):481–6.

76. Facino RM, et al. Free radicals scavenging action and anti-enzyme activities of procyanidines from Vitis

vinifera. A mechanism for their capillary protective action. *Arzneimittel-Forschung* 1994; 44:592–601.

77. Middleton E, Kandaswami C. Effects of flavonoids on immune and inflammatory cell functions. *Biochemical Pharmacology* 1992; 43(6):1167–79.

78. Ayres DC, Loike JD. *Lignans: chemical, biological, and clinical properties.* Cambridge, UK; New York: Cambridge University Press, 1990.

79. Harborne JB, Baxter H. *Phytochemical Dictionary: A Handbook of Bioactive Compounds from Plants.* London; Washington, DC: Taylor & Francis, 1993.

80. Ward RS. Lignans, neolignans and related compounds. *Natural Product Reports* 1999; 1:75–96.

81. Ghisalberti EL. Cardiovascular activity of naturally occurring lignans. *Phytomedicine: International Journal of Phytotherapy and Phytopharmacology* 1997; 4(2):151–66.

82. Adlercreutz H, et al. Lignan and isoflavonoid conjugates in human urine. *The Journal of Steroid Biochemistry and Molecular Biology* 1995; 52(1):97–103.

83. Masquelier J, et al. Flavonoids and pycnogenols. *International Journal for Vitamin and Nutrition Research* 1979; 49:307–11.

84. Haslam E, Lilley TH. Interactions of natural phenols with macromolecules. *Progress in Clinical and Biological Research* 1986; 213:53–65.

85. Chung KT, Wong TY, Wei CI, Huang YW, Lin Y. Tannins and human health: a review. *Critical Reviews in Food Science and Nutrition* 1998 Aug; 38(6):421–64.

86. Namba T, Kurokawa M, Kadota S, Shiraki K. Development of antiviral therapeutic agents from traditional medicines. *Yakugaku Zasshi* 1998 Sept; 118(9):383–400.

87. Fukuchi K, Sakagami H, Okuda T, et al. Inhibition of herpes simplex virus infection by tannins and related compounds. *Antiviral Research* 1989 Jun–Jul; 11(5–6):285–97.

88. Harborne JB, Baxter H. *Phytochemical Dictionary: A Handbook of Bioactive Compounds from Plants.* London; Washington, DC: Taylor & Francis, 1993.

Suggested Reading

Bruneton J. *Pharmacognosy, Phytochemistry, Medicinal Plants.* Hampshire, UK: Intercept, 1999.

Evans WC. *Trease & Evans' Pharmacognosy*, 13th edition. London: Baillere Tindall, 1989.

Harborne JB, Baxter H. *Phytochemical Dictionary: A Handbook of Bioactive Compounds from Plants.* London; Washington, DC: Taylor & Francis, 1993.

8

❧

ALKALOIDS

Alkaloids are organic compounds with at least one nitrogen atom in a heterocyclic ring. Their definition is problematic, as they do not represent a homogeneous group of compounds from any standpoint, whether chemical, biochemical, or physiological. Except for the fact that they are all nitrogen-containing compounds, no general definition fits all alkaloids. They display great structural diversity and physiological activity. More than 10,000 have been identified, and about one new alkaloid is described in the scientific literature every day.

Despite the difficulty in defining alkaloids, they do share some physical and chemical properties. They are usually insoluble or sparingly soluble in water, and their salts are sparingly soluble. Most alkaloids are crystalline solids, although a few are amorphous. A few that lack oxygen in their molecules (coniine, nicotine, and sparteine) are liquids. Most, but not all, are alkaline, owing to the presence of an amino nitrogen, and many possess physiological activity.

Much has been written about why alkaloids occur in plants and what functions they may serve.

Postulated Functions of Alkaloids
- Poisonous agents that protect the plant against insects and herbivores
- End products of detoxification reactions that sequester compounds that might otherwise harm the plant
- Regulatory growth factors
- Reserves of nitrogen or other elements necessary to the plant

OCCURRENCE AND DISTRIBUTION

Although found in some animals, such as fire ants and toads, most alkaloids occur in flowering plants, with 40% of plant families containing at least one alkaloid-bearing species. Alkaloids accumulate in 15% to 20% of vascular plants, mostly dicotyledons, but also in the monocot families Liliaceae, Amaryllidaceae, and Poaceae. Their distribution is uneven: They are universal in some families (for example, Papaveraceae), common in others (Amaryllidaceae and Rutaceae), and rare in others (Apiaceae). They occur only rarely in gymnosperms, club mosses, and horsetails, and although uncommon in fungi, there are exceptional cases, such as the ergot fungus (*Claviceps*) and "magic" mushrooms (*Psilocybe* spp.).[1]

In general, annual plants contain larger amounts of alkaloids than do perennials. Trees tend to have small amounts of alkaloids, usually of simpler structure. The compounds may be present throughout the plant or restricted to certain tissues, such as root or bark. Concentration can vary from a small fraction of 0.01% to as much as 12% of the dry weight of a plant. Any plant that accumulates more than 0.05% dry weight of alkaloids is considered an alkaloid-bearing plant.

Alkaloid content can vary among members of a given plant species, and also changes depending upon where the plant is growing. Cultivated varieties of wild plants contain different proportions of alkaloids than their wild counterparts, but the alkaloids found in the parent plant are usually present in the cultivar. The alkaloid content of different parts of an individual plant varies also. For example, nicotine is produced in the root of the tobacco plant but accumulates in the leaves, so more alkaloid will be found in the leaves.

CLASSIFICATION AND NOMENCLATURE

Classification of alkaloids is usually based on the type of ring system present (for example, pyrrolidine or piperidine) and on their biosynthetic origin from one or another of the protein amino acids. Some structures fit into more than one category, making a rigid hierarchical classification inappropriate. Some groups are defined by their chemistry, such as the peptide, pyrrolizidine, quinolizidine, and tropane classes. Some groups are partly terpenoid in origin, and others are defined by their botanical distribution.

Common names for alkaloids, such as *nicotine*, usually

terminate in -ine. Many of these names are derived from the plant genus in which the alkaloid occurs, such as atropine from *Atropa*, or from the plant species, such as cocaine from *Erythroxylum coca*. Other alkaloid names are derived from the name of a plant drug (for example, ergotamine from ergot) or from a physiological activity (emetine, named for its emetic effects). Occasionally a name is coined to commemorate the person who discovered the compound, such as lobeline, named after the French botanist L'Obel. All alkaloids also have scientific names derived by the systematic nomenclature rules of organic chemistry.

Table 8.1. Major Classes of Alkaloids

CLASS OF ALKALOID	STRUCTURAL TYPE
Pyrrole	
Pyrrolidine	
Piperdine	
Tropane	
Pyrollizidine	
Isoquinoline	
Indole	
β-carboline	
Quinoline	
Quinolizidine	

PHARMACOLOGICAL PROPERTIES

Alkaloids pose major cultural issues because of their properties. This group of constituents provides humanity with challenges such as nicotine, heroin, and cocaine, as well as the profound gift of visionary entheogens, such as psilocybin and mescaline. Some alkaloids are extremely toxic, such as coniine and strychnine, while others, including atropine, codeine, morphine, and vincristine, are used as pharmaceuticals.

While not all alkaloids have a major impact on the functioning of the body, the diverse array of pharmacological actions demonstrated by various alkaloids includes analgesia, local anesthesia, cardiac stimulation, respiratory stimulation and relaxation, vasoconstriction, muscle relaxation, and toxicity, as well as antineoplastic, hypertensive, and hypotensive properties.

Morphine and codeine are analgesics and narcotics, and cocaine is a central nervous system stimulant. Atropine has mydriatic effects, while physostigmine is miotic. Ephedrine causes a rise in blood pressure, but reserpine decreases blood pressure. Some alkaloids are *entheogens*, psychoactive plants or chemical substances taken to facilitate the religious experience—for example, peyote cactus as used by the Native American Church.

Without claiming to be comprehensive, the following table provides examples of the reported effects of various alkaloids on enzymes. The scientific literature cites effects on a range of cellular membrane transport processes, subcellular structures, and nucleic acids, as well as various components of protein synthesis. Effects on numerous neuroreceptors have also been reported, including cholinergic, adrenergic, opiate, and serotonergic receptors. Inhibition or activation of enzymes is also common, as illustrated in table 8.2.[2]

Table 8.2. Reported Effects of Alkaloids on Enzymes

ALKALOID	ENZYME
Theophylline	Alkaline phosphatase
Protoberberines	Liver alcohol dehydrogenase
Colchicine	Various phosphatases
Mimosine	Pyridoxal phosphate enzymes
Quinidine	Several glycolytic enzymes
Isoquinolines	Tyrosine hydroxylase
d-Tubocurarine	Several dehydrogenases
Indolizidines	α-mannosidase
Methylated xanthines	Xanthine oxidase

PYRROLIDINE AND PIPERIDINE ALKALOIDS

The nitrogen atom of a pyrrolidine alkaloid is in a 5-membered ring and piperine alkaloids have 6-membered rings. Indolizidine alkaloids, those with a nitrogen atom shared between a 5- and a 6-membered ring, are also included in this category.

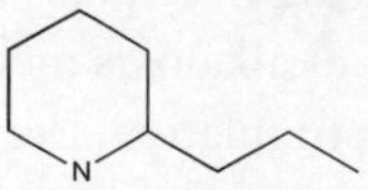

Fig. 8.1. Piperidine 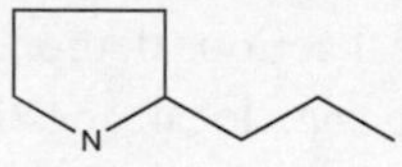   Fig. 8.2. Pyrrolidine

Piperidine alkaloids are identified by their saturated heterocyclic ring (the piperidine nucleus). Pyrrolidine alkaloids are similar to piperidine alkaloids except that the heterocyclic-ringed, nitrogen-containing nucleus is unsaturated. Perhaps the best-known piperidine alkaloids are the poisons in *Conium maculatum*, commonly known as poison hemlock.

Betonicine

Found in *Stachys officinalis, S. sylvatica, Marrubium vulgare*, and *Achillea millefolium*, betonicine demonstrates anti-inflammatory activity.[3]

Coniine

Coniine occurs in the leaves and seeds of poison hemlock (*Conium maculatum*), and is produced by the carnivorous pitcher plant (*Sarracenia flava*) to paralyze insect prey. This extremely toxic compound, which causes paralysis of motor nerve endings, occurs in all parts of the plant as a colorless oil with a mild pepper odor and a burning taste. It reportedly causes teratogenic effects.[4]

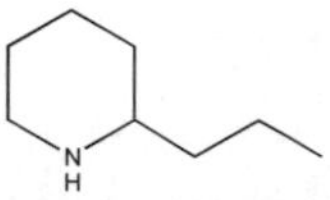

Fig. 8.3. Coniine 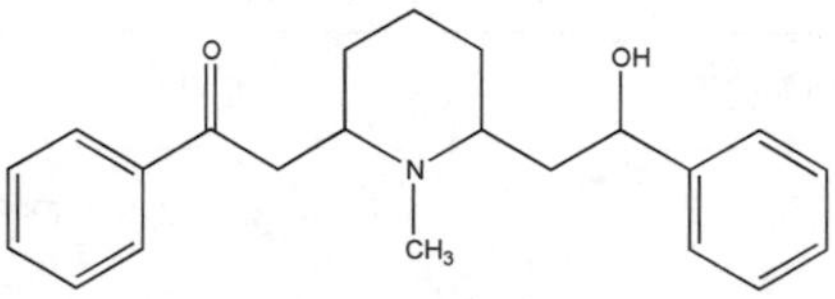   Fig. 8.4. Lobeline

Lobeline

The alkaloid lobeline, found in *Lobelia inflata, L. nicotinaefolia*, and *L. hassleri*, is similar to nicotine.[5] The racemate, known as lobelidine, is an analeptic. *Lobelia inflata* contains 14 alkaloids, of which lobeline is the most important. Lobeline produces pharmacological effects similar to but weaker than those of nicotine on peripheral circulation, neuromuscular junctions, and the central nervous system. It stimulates the respiratory center and induces coughing.

Lobelia inflata is a relaxant and bronchodilator and is used in phytotherapy to treat asthmatic conditions. Because lobeline is similar to nicotine, *Lobelia* has been added to commercial preparations intended to help with tobacco withdrawal.

Nicotine

Found in the tobacco plant (*Nicotiana tabacum*) and other *Nicotiana* species, nicotine has tranquilizing properties and is the addictive component of tobacco. It is also extremely toxic, causing respiratory paralysis at high doses. As the major source is *Nicotiana tabacum*, nicotine and related structures are referred to as "tobacco alkaloids." Anabasine is a tobacco alkaloid in which a pyridine ring is linked to a piperidine rather than a pyrrolidine nucleus.[6]

Nicotine is a ganglion (nicotinic) cholinergic-receptor agonist with complex pharmacological actions, including effects mediated by binding to receptors in the autonomic ganglia, the adrenal medulla, the neuromuscular junction, and the brain.

Nicotine is lethal to all animal life; it is commonly used as a horticultural insecticide. The fatal human dose is about 50 mg.[7] A small amount of nicotine stimulates breathing, but a larger amount depresses respiration. Death from overdose results from respiratory failure. Addiction to tobacco smoking (and to nicotine) can be addressed to some extent by taking the piperidine derivative lobeline.

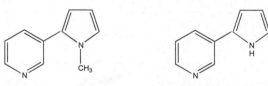

Fig. 8.5. Nicotine   Fig. 8.6. Anabasine

TROPANE ALKALOIDS

These condensed derivatives of pyrrolidine-piperidine alkaloids include atropine, hyoscyamine, and scopolamine. Highly toxic, they are found in Solanaceae plants, such as thornapple and jimsonweed (*Datura stramonium*), angel's trumpets (*Brugmansia* spp.), henbane (*Hyoscyamus niger*), belladonna or deadly nightshade (*Atropa belladonna*), and European mandrake (*Mandragora officinarum*). A prominent feature of the tropane alkaloids is their ability to produce hallucinations and delirium.

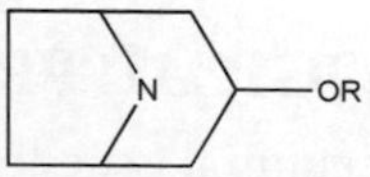

Fig. 8.7. Tropane

A second family rich in tropanes is Erythroxylaceae, which includes coca *(Erythroxylum coca)*, the major source of cocaine. Tropane alkaloids have a limited occurrence in at least eight other unrelated plant families: Convolvulaceae, Brassicaceae, Dioscoreaceae, Elaeocarpaceae, Euphorbiaceae, Orchidaceae, Proteaceae, and Rhizophoraceae. They occur rarely in algae.[8]

Atropine and scopolamine compete with acetylcholine at the postganglionic synapse of the parasympathetic nervous system. Clinically useful properties include antispasmodic effects, employed principally in the treatment of spastic colitis, gastroenteritis, and peptic ulcer to relieve spasms of the bowel. They also have antisecretory effects and are used to reduce respiratory secretions in patients undergoing anesthesia, suppress gastric secretions during peptic ulcer therapy, and decrease nasal and sinus secretions caused by the common cold and allergies. In addition, their mydriatic (pupil-dilating) effects help prevent adhesions between the iris and lens of the eye in cases of iritis. Toxicity symptoms that can occur during the therapeutic use of atropine, scopolamine, or belladonna tincture include skin rash and flushing, mouth dryness, difficult urination, eye pain, blurred vision, and light sensitivity.

The name *Atropa* alludes to the toxicity of the herb; it is derived from *Atropos*, the name of the Greek Fate who cuts the thread of life. *Belladonna* comes from the Italian *bella*, meaning beautiful, and *donna*, meaning lady. (When placed in the eyes, the juice of the berry causes dilation of the pupils, affording a striking appearance.)

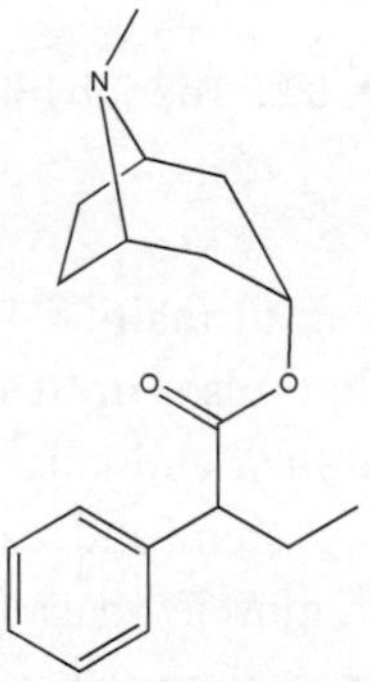

Fig. 8.8. Atropine

Atropine

Atropine is a highly toxic compound that occurs in *Atropa belladonna*, *Datura stramonium*, and other Solanaceae plants, especially in the roots.[9] As figure 8.9 shows, atropine is a structural rearrangement of hyoscyamine.

Atropine demonstrates anticholinergic activity, causing blurred vision, suppressed salivation, vasodilation, excitement, and delirium. It is used in anesthesia and as an antidote in cases of poisoning caused by cholinesterase inhibitors, such as physostigmine and organophosphate insecticides. The lethal dose in humans is 100 mg.

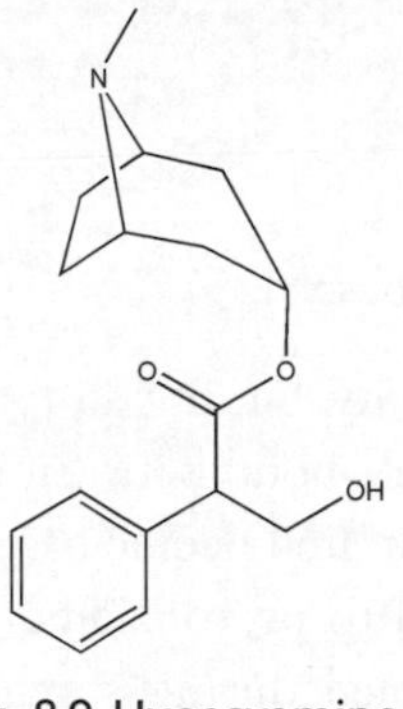

Fig. 8.9. Hyoscyamine 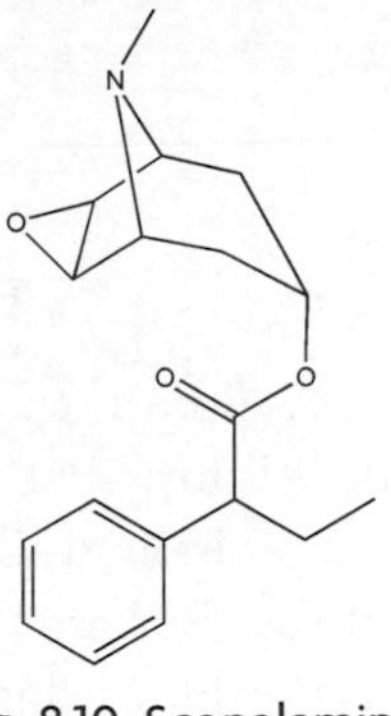   Fig. 8.10. Scopalamine

Hyoscyamine

Hyoscyamine is an anticholinergic agent that helps control gastric secretions, visceral spasms, hypermotility in spastic colitis, and abdominal cramps. In Parkinson's disease, it is used to reduce rigidity and tremors.[10]

Scopolamine

Scopolamine, also called hyoscine, occurs along with hyoscyamine in members of the Solanaceae family. Scopolamine is widely used to help prevent motion sickness.

Cocaine

This alkaloid, obtained from coca *(Erythroxylum coca)*, a shrub native to the Andean highlands of South America, exerts a stimulant effect on the central nervous system. Do not confuse coca with cacao *(Theobroma cacao)*, the plant from which chocolate is made.

PYRROLIZIDINE ALKALOIDS

The chemical class of pyrrolizidine alkaloids (PAs) contains about 200 structurally related compounds present in more than 350 species of the plant families Apocynaceae, Asteraceae, Boraginaceae, Celastraceae, Euphorbiaceae, Fabaceae, Orchidaceae, Poaceae, Ranunculaceae, Rhicophoraceae, Santalaceae, Sapotaceae, and Scrophulariaceae. Among these are a variety of plants used for medicinal purposes, including *Tussilago farfara*, *Petasites* spp., *Senecio* spp., *Alkanna tinctoria*, *Eupatorium* spp., and *Symphytum* spp.[11]

Chemically, the pyrrolizidines are readily distinguished by the presence of a fused two 5-membered ring system, with a nitrogen in position 4, a hydroxymethyl group in position 9, and a hydroxy group in position 7. This structure is called the necine base.

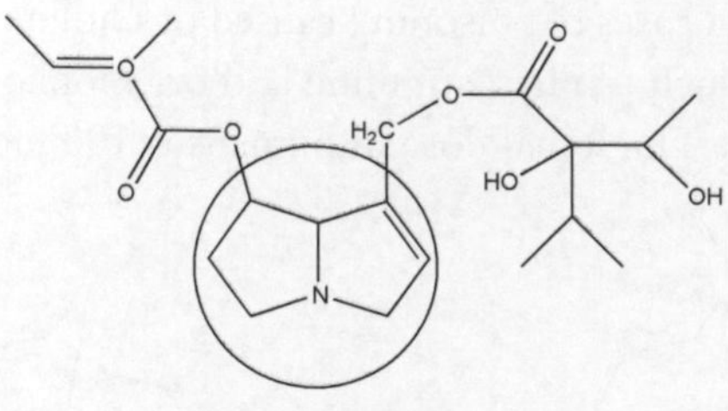

Fig. 8.11. Necine base

PAs have a reputation for toxicity, but not all PAs are toxic. All toxic PAs contain a double bond between the 1 and 2 position, while PAs with saturated necine bases are nontoxic. PAs are readily oxidized to pyrrolizidine alkaloid-N-oxides, which can be formed during storage of PA-containing plants but are also present in fresh plant material. The N-oxides are much more water-soluble than the parent PAs and are better extracted from plant material during the preparation of herbal teas.

Because PAs are often the toxic but not the biologically active principles of many herbal medicines, methods have been developed to eliminate PAs from crude plant extracts. Removal of PAs is accomplished by treating alcoholic plant extracts with cation-exchange resins.

Medicinal plants that contain only nontoxic saturated PAs are *Arnica montana* and *Echinacea* species. Toxic PAs, those with an unsaturated necine base, are hepatic and genetic toxins; some are also respiratory toxins. The toxicology of PAs and the plants that contain them are discussed in greater detail in chapter 10.

Symphytine

Found in comfrey *(Symphytum officinale)*, Russian comfrey *(S. x uplandicum)*, *S. orientale*, and the water forget-me-not *(Myosotis scorpioides)*, symphytine has hepatotoxic properties.[12]

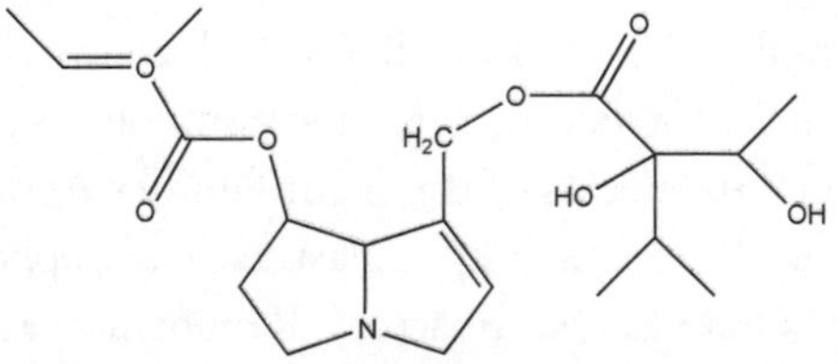

Fig. 8.12. Symphytine

PURINE ALKALOIDS

Purines, which include nucleic acids, are a group of compounds found in both plants and animals. Xanthine, a purine that occurs as a breakdown product of nucleic acid metabolism, is itself oxidized in the body to uric acid.[13]

Three important methylxanthines—caffeine, theobromine, and theophylline—all have stimulating effects on the central nervous system.

Caffeine

Caffeine occurs in a number of botanically unrelated species, including coffee *(Coffea* spp.), tea *(Camellia sinensis)*, maté *(Ilex paraguariensis)*, guarana *(Paullinia cupana)*, and kola *(Cola acuminata)*.

Caffeine is bound to chlorogenic acid in raw coffee beans. The roasting process liberates the caffeine and other compounds that contribute to the aroma of coffee. Caffeine is a diuretic and has stimulant effects on the respiratory, cardiovascular, and central nervous systems. It is incorporated in many proprietary aspirin and acetaminophen preparations to enhance analgesic activity.

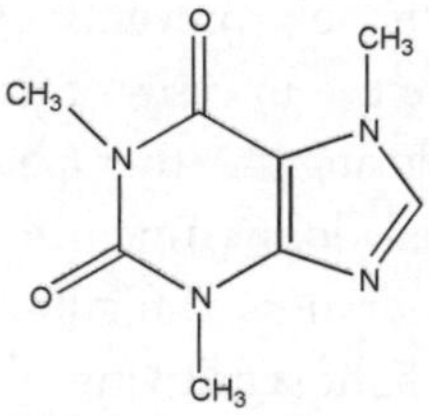

Fig. 8.13. Caffeine

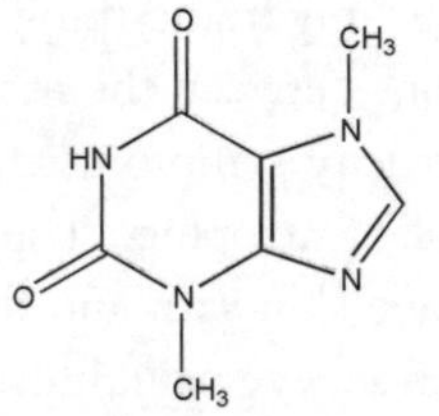

Fig. 8.14. Theobromine

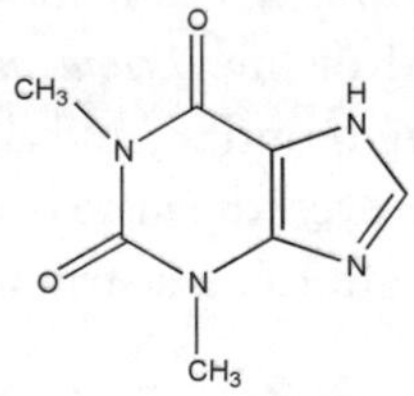

Fig. 8.15. Theophylline

Theobromine

This alkaloid is found mainly in the cocoa plant *(Theobroma cacao)*, but also in tea *(Camellia sinensis)*, guarana *(Paullinia cupana)*, and kola *(Cola acuminata)*.[14] It is a central nervous system and cardiac stimulant, vasodilator, and smooth muscle relaxant, and is used mainly as a diuretic and bronchial muscle relaxant.

Theobromine is isomeric with theophylline; however, its central nervous system effects are much less potent than those shown by caffeine and theophylline, the two other alkaloids in this class.

Theophylline

Theophylline is present in small amounts in tea *(Camellia sinensis)* and guarana *(Paullinia cupana)*. It is a short-acting diuretic and a cardiac stimulant that demonstrates only slight central nervous system stimulation.[15]

Structurally, theophylline resembles caffeine; however, it lacks a methyl group in the 5-carbon ring. Although it occurs naturally in the tea plant, it is synthesized from caffeine for use in medicine. The effects of theophylline on the cardiovascular and central nervous systems are similar to but milder than those of caffeine, while the diuretic activity is more pronounced. Theophylline relaxes involuntary muscles, and is employed mainly as a bronchial smooth muscle relaxant in the treatment of asthma, emphysema, and chronic bronchitis. It is the basis of the drug aminophylline, used as a diuretic and asthma medicine.

ISOQUINOLINE ALKALOIDS

This is the largest group of alkaloids, derived from the amino acids phenylalanine and tyrosine. Isoquinoline alkaloids characteristically contain a phenylethylamine structure in an isoquinoline ring system. They are common in the Magnoliaceae, Ranunculaceae, Papaveraceae, Fumariaceae, Cactaceae, Fabaceae, and Rutaceae families. Many isoquinolines are found in Papaveraceae, especially in the genera *Papaver*, *Chelidonium*, and *Sanguinaria*.[16]

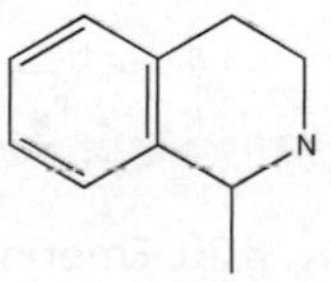

Fig. 8.16. Isoquinoline structure

A subgroup of isoquinolines is made up of the morphinan alkaloids, including morphine, codeine, and heroin, all of which are derived from opium, the dried latex of the opium poppy *(Papaver somniferum)*. Opium has two primary narcotic properties: hypnotic (inducing sleep) and analgesic (blunting pain). Initial stimulation by opium is followed by dream-filled sleep.

Only about 15 minutes are required for a small dose of morphine hydrochloride to induce sleep and dull pain, and the effect lasts about six hours. Heroin, a morphine derivative, has similar properties but is more addictive. Codeine, the methyl ether of morphine, is approximately one tenth as strong a narcotic as morphine. Since its effect on the respiratory center is less potent than that of morphine, codeine has been used in cough suppression. In the body, codeine is demethylated to morphine.

Table 8.3. Pharmacological Properties of Isoquinoline Alkaloids

ACTION	EXAMPLE
Analgesic	Morphine
Antibacterial	Sanguinarine
Antidepressant	Glaziovine
Antifungal	Latrorrhizine
Anti-inflammatory	Fetidine
Antimalarial	Tliacorine
Antimicrobial	Oxyacanthine
Antioxidant	Oxyacanthine
Antiprotozoal	Emetine
Antispasmodic	Papaverine
Antitrypanosomal	Obaberine
Antitubercular	Cepharanthine
Antitumor	Berbamine
Antitussive	Codeine
Antiviral, cholagogue, expectorant	Emetine
Enzyme inhibitor	Sanguinarine
Hemostatic	Hydrastine
Hepatoprotective	Boldine
Hypertensive	Mecambrine
Hypotensive	Canadine
Insecticidal	Annonaine
Muscle relaxant	Isochondrodendrine
Nematocidal	Bocconine
Oxytocic	α-allocrytopine

Berberine

Berberine is found in 23 genera spanning seven plant families. The most important berberine-containing herbal medications are derived from *Berberis vulgaris* and *Mahonia aquifolium* of the Berberidaceae; *Hydrastis canadensis*, *Coptis chinensis*, *C. trifolia*, and *C. teeta* of the Ranunculaceae; *Sanguinaria canadensis* of the Papaveraceae; and

Phellodendron amurensis of the Rutaceae. In some of these plants, berberine and co-occurring alkaloids have equally potent physiological effects. For example, in the well-known herbs *Hydrastis canadensis* and *Sanguinaria canadensis*, the pharmacological effects are not caused by berberine alone.

Berberine is found in highest concentration (about 6.1%) in the root bark of *Berberis vulgaris*, with smaller amounts in the aboveground stem bark and just 0.4% in the woody portion of the root. Only traces of berberine are present in the leaves, and the alkaloid is absent from the flowers, fruit pulp, and seeds.[17] It is present, however, in the seeds of some other species in this genus.

Other alkaloids in *B. vulgaris* include berbamine, berberrubine, bervulcine, columbarnine, isotetrandine, jatrorrhizine, oxycanthine, palmatine, and vulcracine.[18] In addition to berberine, *Mahonia aquifolium* is reported to contain the alkaloids aromoline, berbamine, columbarnine, corytuberine, isoboldine, isocorydine, isotentrandine, jatrorrhizine, magnoflorine, obanegine, oxyberberine, oxycanthine, and palmatine.[19]

Berberine has demonstrated amoebicidal, antibacterial, antifungal, antimalarial, antitumor, cytotoxic, and hepatoprotective actions. It also acts as a bitter and a cholagogue and inhibits tyramine and elastase. Berberine has been shown to have antiarrhythmic actions and a negative inotropic effect that markedly reduces atrial rate. It is moderately toxic, with a 27.5 mg/kg LD_{50} in humans, and can cause cardiac damage, dyspnea, and hypotension.

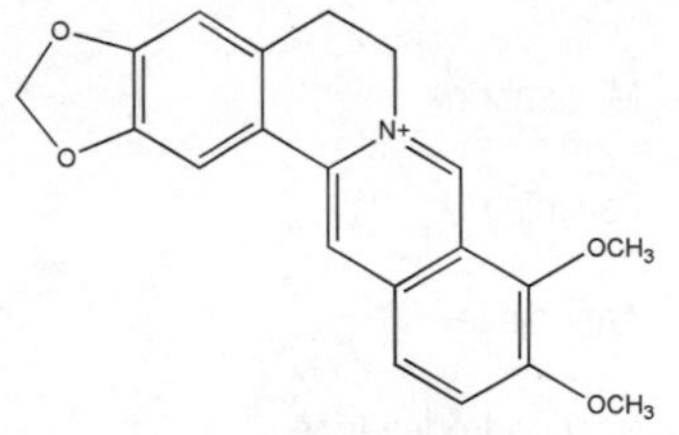

Fig. 8.17. Berberine

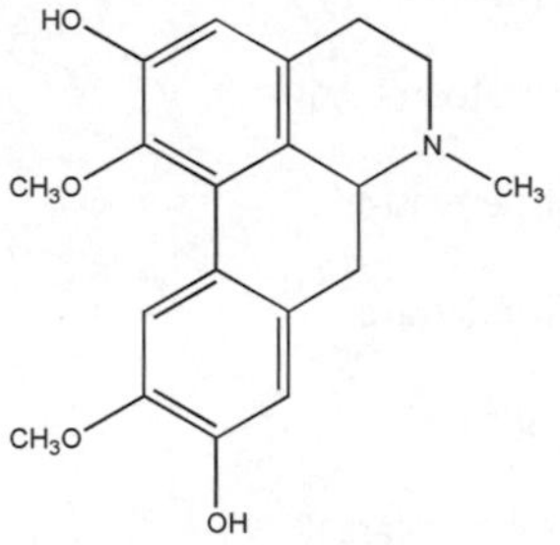

Fig. 8.18. Boldine

Boldine

Boldine occurs in the leaves of *Peumus boldus*, *Sassafras albidum*, and in members of the plant families Annonaceae, Magnoliaceae, Rhamnaceae, and Atherospermataceae.[20] It is choleretic and diuretic.

Cephaeline

After emetine, this is the most important alkaloid in the roots of *Cephaelis ipecacuanha*. It has emetic, expectorant, and antiamoebic activities.[21]

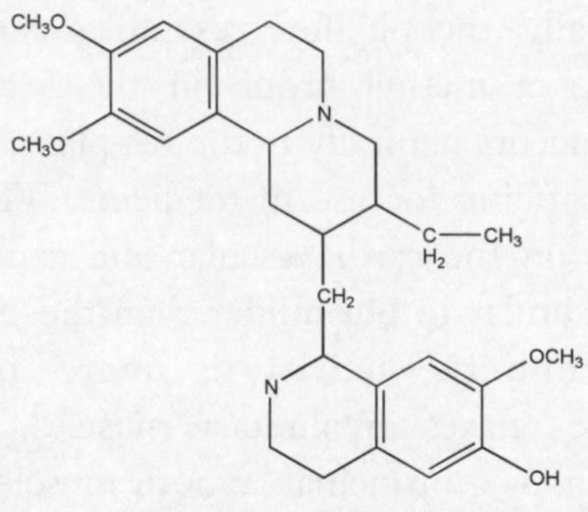

Fig. 8.19. Cephaeline

Codeine

Codeine, from the dried latex of the opium poppy (*Papaver somniferum*), has spasmolytic, narcotic analgesic, and antitussive properties. It is used in the management of pain and diarrhea and as a cough suppressant.[22]

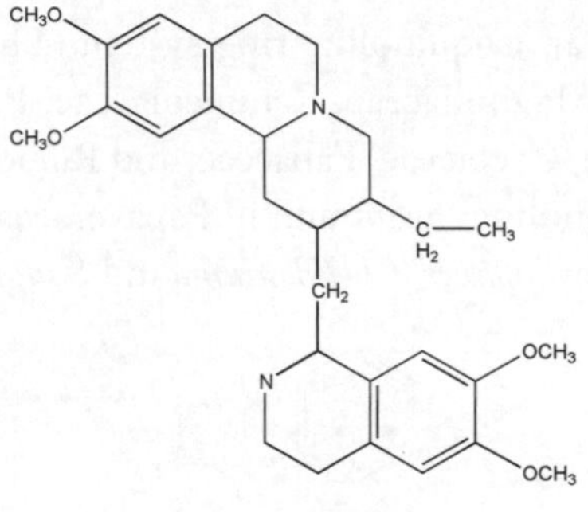

Fig. 8.20. Emetine

Emetine

Occurring in all ipecacuanhas, including *Cephaelis ipecacuanha*, and *C. acuminata*, emetine has expectorant, emetic, antiamoebic, and cytotoxic properties. It also demonstrates antiviral and anticancer activities, probably due to its inhibition of DNA and other components of the transcription process.

Emetine is indicated in chronic bronchitis, but at higher doses acts as an emetic. Ipecac, extract of *C. ipecacuanha* in the form of a tincture or syrup, is typically used as an emetic to induce vomiting when a toxic substance has been ingested. Emetine is toxic to *Entamoeba hystolytica*, the organism that causes amoebic dysentery, and emetine hydrochloride is used in medicine as an antiprotozoal agent.[23]

Hydrastine

Hydrastine is a major alkaloid of goldenseal (*Hydrastis canadensis*). It is hemostatic and antiseptic and has been used to treat uterine hemorrhage. Hydrastine also demonstrates emetic, expectorant, and antiamoebic activities.[24]

Morphine

Found in the opium poppy *(Papaver somniferum)*, morphine is a powerful analgesic, antispasmodic, narcotic, sedative, and antitussive. Prolonged use leads to habituation. The lethal dose in humans lies between 1 and 10 mg.[25]

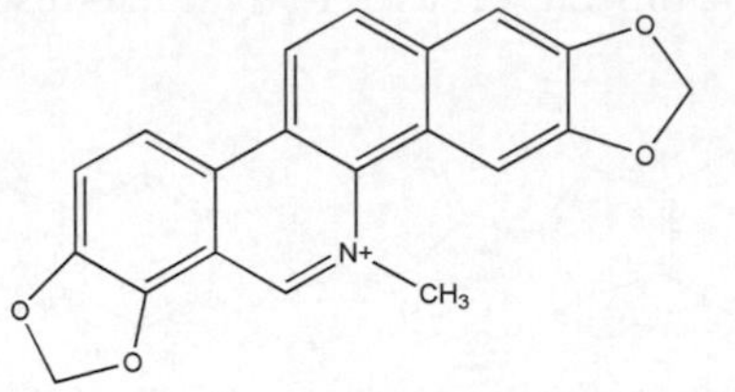

Fig. 8.21. Sanguinarine

Sanguinarine

This alkaloid is widespread among plants in the families Papaveraceae (including *Papaver somniferum, Sanguinaria canadensis,* and *Chelidonium majus*) and Fumariaceae (for example, *Fumaria officinalis*). Sanguinarine is antibacterial, cytotoxic, and anti-inflammatory. Because it demonstrates antiplaque activity, it is used in toothpastes and mouthwashes. It is positively inotropic and inhibits various enzymes, including adenosine triphosphate (ATP), diamine oxidase, and some aminotransferases.

Sanguinarine is toxic, with an LD_{50} in mice of 19.4 mg/kg. At high doses taken over a prolonged period of time, it may cause glaucoma.[26]

INDOLE ALKALOIDS

Indole alkaloids constitute the second largest group of alkaloids. They are derived from the amino acid tryptophan, which has a basic structure containing a pyrrole ring fused to a benzene ring. There are a small number of simple indoles, such as harman, but the majority are derived from tryptophan and a terpenoid precursor, secologanin.[27] Indoles all share a common core structure, but different metabolic pathways result in different configurations.

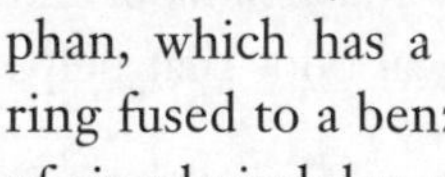

Fig. 8.22. Indole

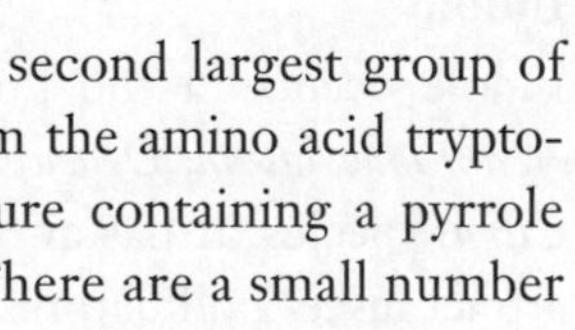

Fig. 8.23. Tryptophan

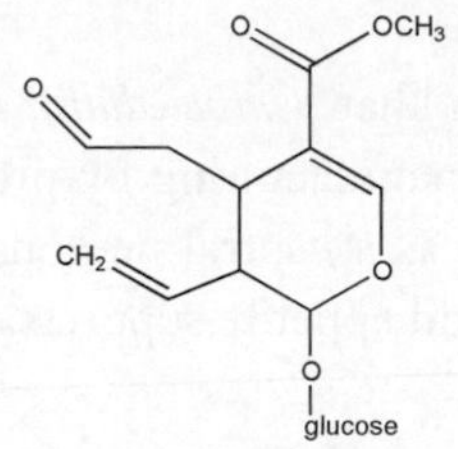

Fig. 8.24. Secologanin

Indole alkaloid structures typically involve multiple ring systems and are often complex in character. They form the basis of several pharmaceutical drugs, some potent hallucinogens, and a number of poisonous compounds, such as strychnine. The majority of indole alkaloids used in medicine and pharmacy are found in members of the family Apocynaceae (including *Rauvolfia, Vinca, Catharanthus,* and *Alstonia* spp.). Indole alkaloids are also found in fungi, such as ergot *(Claviceps* spp.) and *Psilocybe* species.

Some indole alkaloids are widely distributed; the harman alkaloids have been detected in more than 10 families. The Madagascar periwinkle *(Catharanthus roseus)* contains more than 60 indole alkaloids, including vinblastine and vincristine. These compounds are used in chemotherapy as treatments for Hodgkin's disease, lymphosarcoma, and reticulum cell sarcoma. Important classes of indole alkaloids include the ergot alkaloids and β-carbolines.

Ergot Alkaloids

The ergot alkaloids are the basis for lysergic acid as well as other compounds. Indoles of ergot include ergometrine, used to relax the uterine muscle during childbirth, and ergotamine, which relieves symptoms of migraine. Gelsemine and sempervirine, two indole alkaloids from the roots of the yellow jasmine *(Gelsemium sempervirens)*, depress the activity of the central nervous system.

Bufotenine

This is a hallucinogenic alkaloid that occurs in the plants of the genus *Piptadenia*, in fungi such as *Amanita citrina*, and in secretions from the skin of the toad *Bufo vulgaris*.[28]

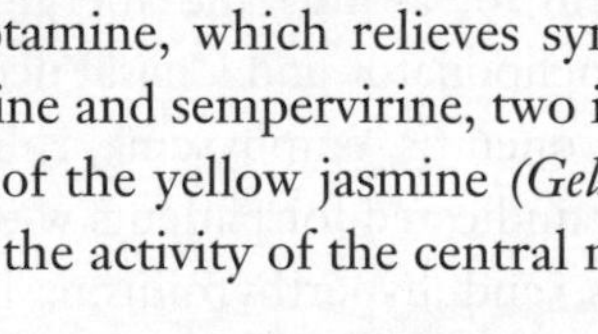

Fig. 8.25. Bufotenine

D-cathine

D-cathine occurs in khat *(Catha edulis)*, and is derived from *Ephedra* spp. as a manufacturing by-product of ephedrine production. It acts as a central nervous system stimulant, mild euphoriant, and appetite suppressant.

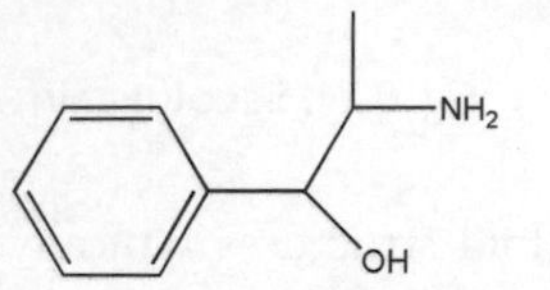

Fig. 8.26. Cathine

N,N-dimethyltryptamine

Found in the leaves of *Prestonia amazonica*, the flowers of the reed *Arundo donax*, the seeds and leaves of *Piptadenia peregrina*, and leaves, stems, and seeds of *Mucuna pruriens*, *N,N*-dimethyltryptamine demonstrates entheogenic activity.[29] It also causes hypertension and pupillary dilation.

L-ephedrine

L-ephedrine is found in the leaves and stems of ma huang, or *Ephedra* species (*E. sinica, E. equisetina, E. gerardiana*, and others), where it occurs with the D-isomer pseudoephedrine. It possesses sympathomimetic activity, with direct and indirect effects on both α- and β-adrenergic receptors, and produces peripheral vasoconstriction and elevated blood pressure. It is also a central nervous system stimulant. L-ephedrine is used as a bronchodilator and respiratory stimulant in asthma and as a vasoconstrictor of mucous membranes in rhinitis and sinusitis. Pseudoephedrine is broadly similar in activity.

In Western herbal medicine, *Ephedra* is considered a reliable treatment for asthma and allergic conditions. As it is both a bronchodilator and a nasal decongestant, it is useful also in bronchitis, emphysema, rhinitis, and influenza. It is contraindicated for patients with hypertension, angina pectoris, and hyperthyroidism; in those taking monoamine oxidase inhibitor drugs (MAO inhibitors); and also during pregnancy.

β-carboline Alkaloids

β-carbolines are a widely distributed class of indole alkaloids found in 23 angiosperm plant families, 3 fungi genera, and a variety of animal tissues.[30] They are structurally similar to and biosynthetically derived from the amino acid L-tryptophan. Trypophan derivatives are very important in central nervous system function and include the neurotransmitter serotonin, the pineal metabolite melatonin, the potent hallucinogen dimethyl tryptamine (DMT), and the monoamine oxidase inhibitors known as β-carbolines.

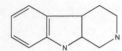

Fig. 8.27. β-carboline structure

Harmaline

Harmaline occurs in the seeds of *Peganum harmala, Banisteria caapi*, and *Passiflora incarnata*. It has entheogenic properties. At one time, it was used to treat Parkinson's disease.[31]

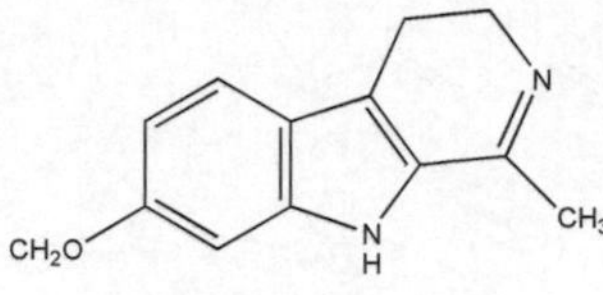

Fig. 8.28. Harmaline

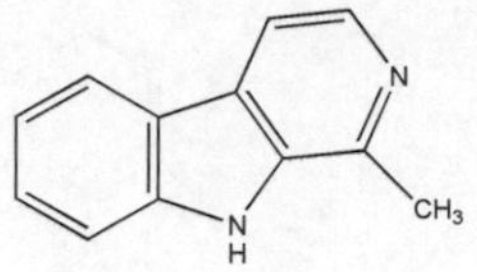

Fig. 8.29. Harman

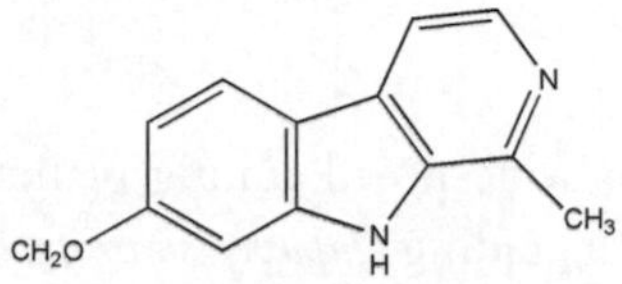

Fig. 8.30. Harmine

Harman

Harman occurs in passionflower *(Passiflora incarnata)*. At low doses, it depresses motor function in animals; it causes convulsions at high doses.[32]

Harmine

Found in *Peganum harmala, Banisteria caapi*, and passionflower *(Passiflora incarnata)*, harmine is a central nervous system stimulant that is entheogenic at high doses.[33]

Indole

Indole occurs in the flowers of *Sauromatum guttatum, Arum maculatum, Dracunculus vulgaris*, and *Jasminum* and *Citrus* species. It has an unpleasant fecal odor that helps attract insect pollinators.

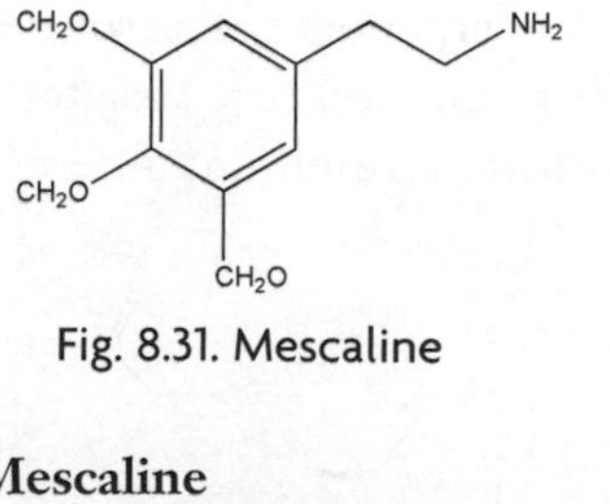

Fig. 8.31. Mescaline

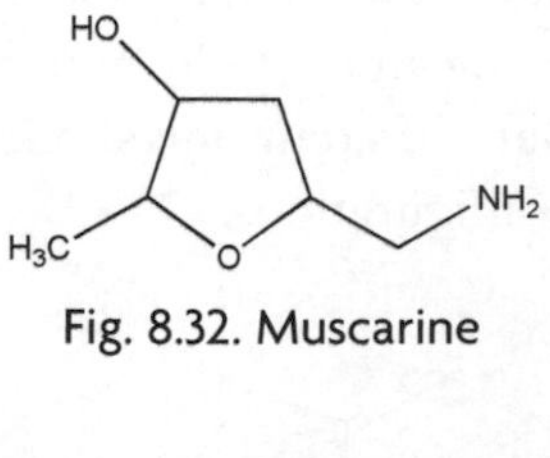

Fig. 8.32. Muscarine

Mescaline

Found in the flowering heads of peyote *(Lophophora williamsii)* and other cacti, including *Trichocereus pachanoi*, mescaline is entheogenic.

Muscarine

This alkaloid occurs in the fly agaric mushroom (*Amanita muscaria*) and some species of *Inocybe* and *Clitocybe*. Muscarine is a cholinergic agent that acts at the muscarinic receptors. Symptoms of poisoning occur within 30 to 120 minutes of ingestion and can include blurred vision; contraction of the pupils; and increased perspiration, salivation, and lacrimation (discharge of tears). Other symptoms of poisoning include bradycardia, hypotension, and dyspnea. The LD_{50} in mice is 0.23 mg/kg (IV).[34]

Psilocin

Psilocin occurs in the sacred mushroom, teonanacatl (*Psilocybe mexicana*), and other blue-staining *Psilocybe* species. Psilocin is entheogenic, causing sensations of intellectual and physical relaxation and perceptual distortions of time and space. The alkaloid is readily oxidized to a blue pigment when the mushroom is bruised.[35]

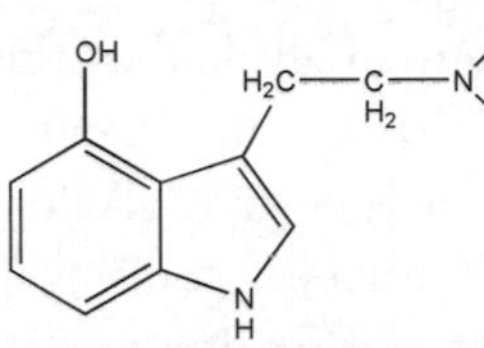

Fig. 8.33. Psilocin

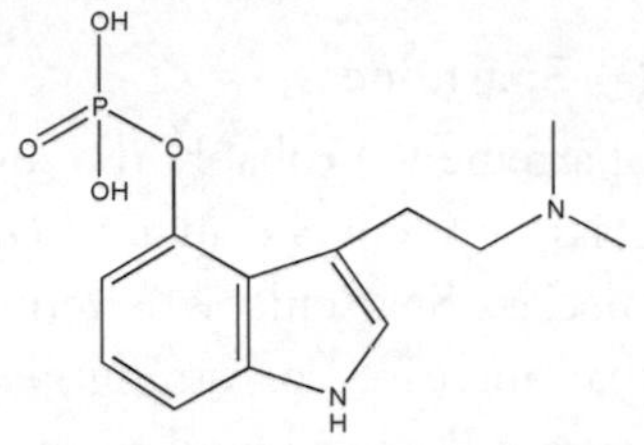

Fig. 8.34. Psilocybin

Psilocybin

Psilocybin is found in the same mushrooms as psilocin. Its properties are similar to those of psilocin, which is converted into psilocybin through phosphorylation.[36]

Reserpine

Present in *Rauvolfia serpentina*, *R. vomitoria*, and many other species and genera of the family Apocynaceae, reserpine is used clinically as an antihypertensive agent and tranquilizer. However, about 15% of people treated with reserpine for hypertension develop depression.

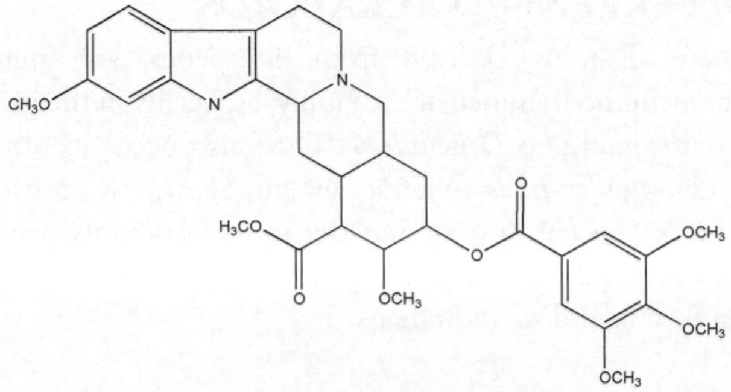

Fig. 8.35. Reserpine

Serotonin

Serotonin is found in bananas (*Musa* spp.), tomatoes (*Lycopersicon esculentum*), and the stinging hairs of the nettle (*Urtica dioica*). It acts as a neurotransmitter in the central nervous system but does not pass the blood-brain barrier, so a precursor, 5-hydroxytryptophan, is used clinically to treat depression.

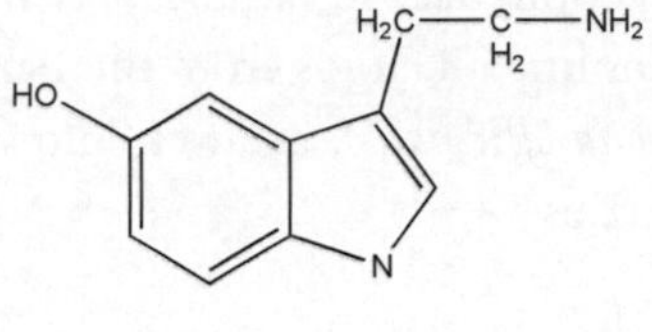

Fig. 8.36. Serotonin

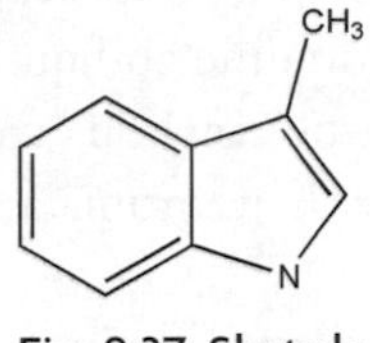

Fig. 8.37. Skatole

Skatole

Skatole is found in *Arum* species, in which it contributes to the unique (vile!) odor of these plants, and in beets (*Beta vulgaris*). Skatole is also responsible for the characteristic odor of feces.[37]

Vinblastine

This is an important compound found in the leaves of the Madagascar periwinkle (*Catharanthus roseus*). Its antitumor activity has led to widespread clinical use in the treatment of leukemia and Hodgkin's disease.

Vincristine

Found in the Madagascar periwinkle (*Catharanthus roseus*), vincristine is an antitumor agent used especially for acute childhood lymphocytic leukemia.

Yohimbine

Yohimbine is a major alkaloid in yohimbe bark (*Pausinystalia yohimbe*). Two stereoisomers, α- and β-yohimbine, occur in the same plant. It is an α-adrenergic blocking agent, a serotonin antagonist, and a mydriatic.[38]

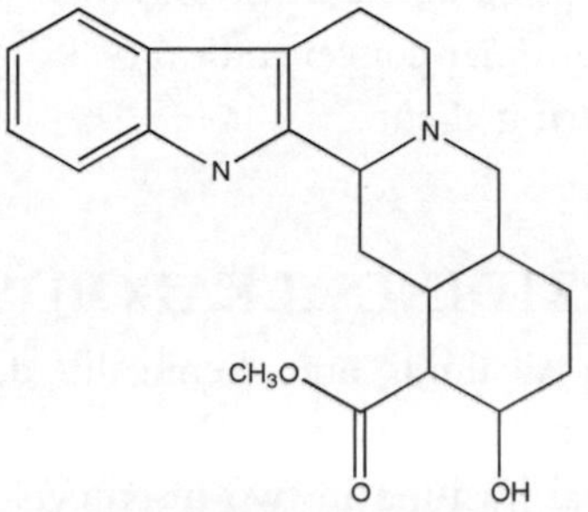

Fig. 8.38. Yohimbine

QUINOLINE ALKALOIDS

Quinoline alkaloids are based on a bicyclic system in which a benzene and a pyridine ring are fused together. Most of them occur in the plant family Rutaceae, especially rue *(Ruta graveolens)*, from which 30 quinoline alkaloids have been isolated. Quinoline alkaloids have also been identified in members of the Acanthaceae, Malvaceae, Saxifragaceae, and Zygophyllaceae families.[39] Cinchonidine and quinine, quinoline alkaloids from the bark of the cinchona tree *(Cinchona officinalis)*, are well known for their antimalarial properties.

Camptothecin

Occurring in the fruits, stem wood, and bark of *Camptotheca acuminata*, camptothecin is highly toxic to both animals and humans. It has antitumor and antileukemic activities and is used in China for the treatment of various forms of cancer.[40]

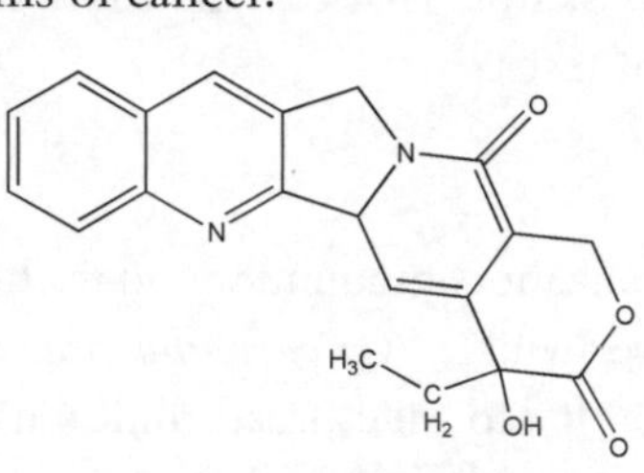

Fig. 8.39. Camptothecin

Quinine

Quinine is found in the bark of *Cinchona officinalis* and other *Cinchona* species, in which it occurs together with its stereoisomer, quinidine. Both isomers are antimalarials used against *Plasmodium flaccarpum*, which is usually drug-resistant.[41]

Quinine is a weak cardiac depressant and is occasionally used in clinical practice as an antiarrhythmic agent. It has abortifacient and spermicidal properties and is used as a bitter, analgesic, and antipyretic in veterinary practice.[42]

Quinine is one of the most bitter substances known, detectable at a molar concentration of 1×10^{-5}. It is used in food as a bittering agent.

QUINOLIZIDINE ALKALOIDS

Quinolizidine alkaloids are chemically defined by the presence of a structural unit in which a nitrogen atom occupies a central position in two fused cyclohexane rings, as in lupinine. These are also referred to as lupine alkaloids, as they were first discovered in *Lupinus* species.[43] Important quinolizidine alkaloids include sparteine, found in Scotch broom *(Cytisus scoparius)* and greater celandine *(Chelidonium majus)*, and cytisine, from lupine.

Quinolizidine alkaloids occur primarily in Fabaceae. There are about 170 quinolizidine alkaloids in this family, and these are readily classified according to the number of rings present. A typical bicyclic structure is lupinine. Angustifoline is a good example of a tricyclic structure and sparteine of a tetracyclic compound.

Structurally related but distinctly different quinolizidine alkaloids occur in *Lycopodium* and are known as lycopodium alkaloids.

Although universally present in *Lupinus*, a genus of some 200 species, quinolizidine alkaloids are found in more than 40 related genera of legumes. Consumption of these plants, particularly their seeds, has been responsible for much accidental poisoning in sheep, cattle, and humans. Cytisine and anagyrine are more acutely toxic than lupinine and sparteine; they harm livestock through teratogenic effects.

(-)-Sparteine

Sparteine is probably the most common alkaloid of this class, present in many *Baptisia*, *Cytisus*, and *Lupinus* species. Sparteine is a tetracyclic, oxygen-free alkaloid that increases or strengthens the heartbeat, causing a greater flow of blood to the kidneys and resulting in increased urine production. Sparteine has proved valuable in treating certain cases of cardiac fibrillation. It acts as a peripheral vasoconstrictor and, because it demonstrates ergotlike oxytocic effects (inducing contractions of uterine muscle), it has been used as a substitute for ergot drugs. It binds strongly to muscarinic receptors and less strongly to nicotinic receptors.[44]

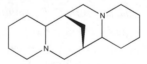

Fig. 8.40. Sparteine

DITERPENOID ALKALOIDS

These alkaloids, derived from diterpenes, are found mainly in the Ranunculaceae family, especially in the genera *Aconitum* and *Delphinium*. They also occur in other plants, such as *Inula* (Asteraceae) and *Spiraea* (Rosaceae). *Aconitum* species are among the most poisonous plants known, and 2 to 5 mg of a pure *Aconitum* alkaloid extract can be a fatal dose in humans.

Aconitine

This toxic alkaloid occurs in the roots of *Aconitum napellus*, but all parts of the plant are poisonous due to the presence of other alkaloids. Aconitine is a potent and quick-acting poison that slows the heart rate and lowers blood pressure. Several *Aconitum* species are used in China, after processing, for various purposes. Absorption of aconitine through the skin can be fatal.[45]

Ryanodine

Found in *Ryania speciosa*, ryanodine inhibits the binding of calcium to muscle protein and retards circulation by vascular constriction.[46] It is used as an insecticide.

STEROID ALKALOIDS

Steroid alkaloids have been found in approximately 250 species of plants in the Solanaceae and Liliaceae families. They occur mostly as glycosides that have properties similar to those of saponins. Some are very toxic, causing severe, even fatal, gastroenteritis.[47]

Solanine was the name given to the first alkaloidal glycoside found in *Solanum*. Now solanine is known to consist of six different glycosides; each hydrolyzes to the sugar peculiar to its particular glycoside and to the aglycone solanidine, a steroidal alkaloid.

Steroid alkaloids have a fairly complex nitrogen-containing nucleus. Two important classes are the solanum type and the veratrum type.

Solanum-Type Alkaloids

Solanum-type alkaloids are found in plants in the form of glycosides of steroid alkaloids, known as glycoalkaloids. They occur primarily in Solanaceae family plants. One example is solanidine, a steroid alkaloid that is the aglycone for two glycoalkaloids, solanine and chaconine, which can manifest as poisons in potatoes. They have the same aglycone, solanidine, but the structure of their carbohydrate side chains is different. Other plants in the Solanaceae, including various nightshades and tomatoes, also contain solanum-type glycoalkaloids.

The production of these alkaloids is favored by the same conditions that promote the development of chlorophyll, such as exposure to sunlight. In potatoes, the concentration of glycoalkaloids is highest in sprouts and green skins, and in tomatoes, highest in vines and green fruit. Care should be taken to avoid exposing potatoes to sunlight, to prevent the production of the toxic alkaloids. These alkaloids are not destroyed by cooking or drying at high temperatures. New potato varieties may not be introduced unless they contain less than 20 mg/100 g glycoalkaloids.

The glycoalkaloids are more poisonous than the aglycones. However, glycoalkaloids are poorly absorbed by the gastrointestinal tract of mammals, and an appreciable amount of solanum-type glycoalkaloids is hydrolyzed in the gut of mammals to the less toxic aglycones, which are then rapidly excreted. In potatoes, solanum-type glycoalkaloids cause a bitter taste in concentrations higher than 14 mg/100 g, and a burning sensation in the mouth and throat in concentrations higher than 20 mg/100 g.

Veratrum-Type Alkaloids

There are more than 50 veratrum alkaloids, such as veratramine, that occur in plants of the *Veratrum* genus. These are the alkaloids that make hellebores, such as the white hellebore (*Veratrum album*), highly toxic.

MISCELLANEOUS ALKALOIDS

These are alkaloids with rare structures that are difficult to classify elsewhere, including the oxazoles and the pyrazines (for example, aspergillic acid). In addition, some 14 alkaloids with flavonoid substituents are known—for example, ficine, found in the wild fig (*Ficus pantoniana*).[48]

Some alkaloids in this group are very toxic, such as taxine A from the yew (*Taxus* spp.). This is also true of mycotoxins such as verruculotoxin, which can get into the human food chain via the peanut. However, several of these alkaloids have promising anticancer activity, notably cephalotoxine, cryptopleurine, harringtonine, and taxol.

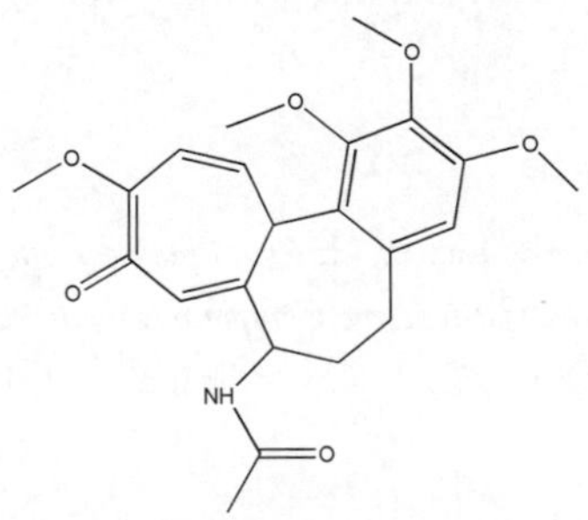

Fig. 8.41. Colchicine

Colchicine

Found in *Colchicum autumnale* and other *Colchicum* species, colchicine is highly toxic, with a lethal dose of 10 mg in humans. It is also irritant, carcinogenic, and teratogenic, but has been used in minute doses to relieve the pain of acute gout. Plant scientists use it to induce polyploidy in plants. (Plant cells are polyploid if they contain more than two sets of chromosomes. This is very common in plants, especially in angiosperms. Between 30% and 70% of today's angiosperms are thought to be polyploid.

Species of coffee with 22, 44, 66, and 88 chromosomes are known.)

Harringtonine

Harringtonine occurs in *Cephalotaxus harringtonia, C. fortunei*, and *C. hainensis*. This alkaloid shows antitumor activity and has been used clinically to treat acute myelocytic leukemia. It inhibits the biosynthesis of DNA and proteins.[49]

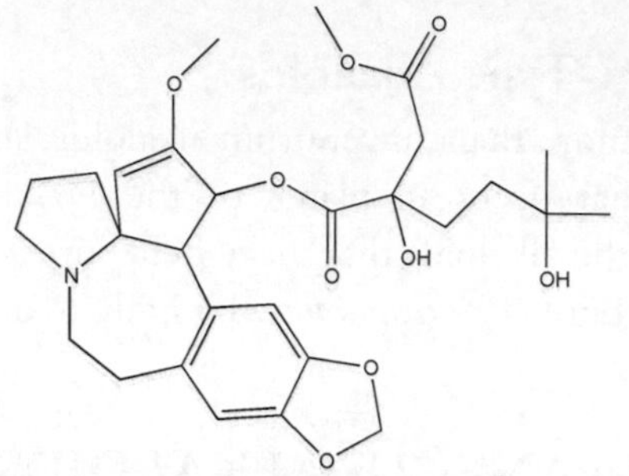

Fig. 8.42. Harringtonine

Taxol

Found in the stem bark of *Taxus brevifolia* and *T. cuspidata*, taxol is also present in trace amounts in other *Taxus* species, including *T. baccata*. Following much laboratory and clinical research, taxol (Paclitaxel) was approved by the FDA for use in a number of protocols investigating the treatment of metastatic carcinoma of the ovary, non–small cell lung cancer, and AIDS-related Kaposi's sarcoma, as well as adjuvant treatment of node-positive breast cancer. Taxol is toxic, with an oral LD_{50} of 9 mg/kg in dogs.

References

1. Harborne JB, Baxter H. *Phytochemical Dictionary: A Handbook of Bioactive Compounds from Plants*. London; Washington, DC: Taylor & Francis, 1993.

2. Ibid.

3. Ibid.

4. Ibid.

5. Ibid.

6. Ibid.

7. Ibid.

8. Ibid.

9. Ibid.

10. Ibid.

11. Smith LW, Culvenor CCJ. Plant sources of hepatotoxic pyrrolizidine alkaloids. *Journal of Natural Products* 1981; 44:129–52.

12. Harborne JB, Baxter H. *Phytochemical Dictionary: A Handbook of Bioactive Compounds from Plants*. London; Washington, DC: Taylor & Francis, 1993.

13. Ibid.

14. Ibid.

15. Ibid.

16. Ibid.

17. Etcu P, Goina T. Neue Methoden zur Extrahierung der Alkaloide aus Berberis vulgaris. *Planta Medica* 1970; 18:372–75.

18. Dopke W. Neue Alkaloide aus Berberis vulgaris L. *Die Naturwissenschaften* 1963; 50:595.

19. Gruenwald J, et al. *PDR for Herbal Medicines*. Montvale, NJ: Medical Economics Company, 1998.

20. Harborne JB, Baxter H. *Phytochemical Dictionary: A Handbook of Bioactive Compounds from Plants*. London; Washington, DC: Taylor & Francis, 1993.

21. Ibid.

22. Ibid.

23. Ibid.

24. Ibid.

25. Ibid.

26. Ibid.

27. Ibid.

28. Ibid.

29. Ghosal S, Singh S, Bhattacharya SK. Alkaloids of Mucuna pruriens, chemistry and pharmacology. *Planta Medica* 1971; 19:279.

30. Schultes RE, Hofmann A. *The Botany and Chemistry of Hallucinogens*. Springfield, IL: Charles C. Thomas, 1980.

31. Ibid.

32. Ibid.

33. Ibid.

34. Ibid.

35. Ibid.

36. Ibid.

37. Harborne JB, Baxter H. *Phytochemical Dictionary: A Handbook of Bioactive Compounds from Plants*. London; Washington, DC: Taylor & Francis, 1993.

38. Ibid.

39. Ibid.

40. Ibid.

41. Ibid.

42. Barnes K, Durrheim D, Blumberg L. Quinine as unofficial contraceptive—concerns about safety and efficacy. *South African Medical Journal* 1998; 88(10):1280, 1282.

43. Harborne JB, Baxter H. *Phytochemical Dictionary: A Handbook of Bioactive Compounds from Plants*. London; Washington, DC: Taylor & Francis, 1993.

44. Ibid.

45. Ibid.

46. Ibid.

47. Ibid.

48. Ibid.

49. Ibid.

Suggested Reading

Bruneton J. *Pharmacognosy, Phytochemistry, Medicinal Plants*. Hampshire, UK: Intercept, 1999.

Evans WC. *Trease & Evans' Pharmacognosy*, 13th edition. London: Baillere Tindall, 1989.

Harborne JB, Baxter H. *Phytochemical Dictionary: A Handbook of Bioactive Compounds from Plants*. London; Washington, DC: Taylor & Francis, 1993.

Schultes RE, Hofmann A. *The Botany and Chemistry of Hallucinogens*. Springfield, IL: Charles C. Thomas, 1980.

9

PHARMACOLOGY

Pharmacology is the branch of science that studies therapeutic agents in all of their aspects. Such agents are usually called drugs. This can cause some confusion when discussing herbal medicines, as the general public tends to differentiate between herbs and drugs, viewing herbs as natural and drugs as synthetic. However, both herbs and drugs contain chemical compounds that affect the body in various ways, so an understanding of pharmacology is relevant to both.

It is worth noting that the word *drug* is derived from the middle English *drogge*, which in turn is thought to come from the middle Dutch word *droge*, meaning "dry." Thus, our modern word *drug* refers to the use of dry plants in medicine. In other words, *drug* is an herbal word!

The word *pharmacology* itself is derived from the Greek words *pharmakon* (drug) and *logos* (word). This branch of science is very extensive and is divided into numerous subspecialties.

Pharmacodynamics is the study of the physiological or biochemical mechanisms by which drug actions are produced, which involves identifying effects produced and the sites and mechanisms of their actions in the body.

Pharmacokinetics investigates factors that modify the effects of a drug, such as routes of administration, rates of absorption, differential distribution, and mechanisms of excretion and detoxification.

Toxicology is the study of effects that are unfavorable to health.

Pharmacognosy deals with the identification and analysis of plant and animal tissues from which drugs may be extracted.

Pharmacy is concerned with the art and science of the preparation, compounding, and dispensing of drugs.

PHARMACOLOGY AND PHYTOTHERAPY

Pharmacology addresses important questions about herbal medicines and their therapeutic indications. Consider the following, which have been grouped into pharmacological subject categories.

Absorption and Distribution

- How do the physicochemical properties of the herb's constituents impact the bioavailability of the herb and thus patient outcomes?
- Are the most medically relevant constituents of the herb water-soluble?

Site of Action

- Which organs are impacted by the actions of the herb, and how?
- What mechanism of activity is involved?
- Are there specific receptors that mediate this action?

Metabolism and Excretion

- What impact does herbal treatment have on hepatocyte activity and biotransformation?
- Are metabolites of herbal constituents cleared by the kidneys or in the gastrointestinal tract?

Toxicity and Adverse Effects

- How does the therapeutic dose compare with the potentially toxic dose (i.e., what is the therapeutic index)?
- Are there reports of resistance or unusual reactions?
- What is the treatment for an overdose?

Drug Interactions

- Does the combination of the herb with another therapeutic agent cause any synergism, antagonism, or changes in the effect of the herb or its metabolism?
- Will the herb affect the actions or metabolism of the other therapeutic agent?
- Are certain combinations contraindicated?

PHARMACODYNAMICS

Both the therapeutic and toxic effects of a substance occur as a result of its interactions with molecules in the body. An important aspect of pharmacology is determining whether a drug effect is due to a specific structural component of the molecule or is a result of a *nonspecific* drug action. In most instances, drugs act by associating with specific molecules in ways that alter their biochemical or biophysical activity, in which case they are known as *specific* drugs.

Nonspecific Drugs

The activity of nonspecific compounds is often related to their solubility in lipids, which determines their ability to interact with and alter cellular membrane function. Inhalation anesthetics and some disinfectants are examples of drugs that work through this type of nonspecific activity.

Characteristics of Nonspecific Drugs

- Do not specifically bind with a particular biological structure
- Are active only in relatively high doses
- Have similar activities but vastly different chemical structures
- Show largely similar activity after chemical modification

Specific Drugs

Specific drugs are usually more potent than nonspecific drugs; their effects are evident at lower drug concentrations. Activity is highly dependent on chemical structure, including the shape, size, and stereochemical configuration of the molecule, as well as the position of functional groups and charge distribution. Small structural changes can result in profound changes in pharmacological activity.

Table 9.1. Mechanisms of Action for Specific Drugs

MECHANISM	EXAMPLES
Receptor interaction	
Stimulate receptors	Apigenin from *Matricaria recutita* is a ligand for certain benzodiazepine receptors that exerts anxiolytic and slight sedative effects but no anticonvulsant or myorelaxant actions.[1]
	Chrysin confers anxiolytic actions without inducing sedation or muscle relaxation; it may be a partial agonist of benzodiazepine receptors.[2] Chrysin is found in species of *Passiflora* and *Scutellaria*.
Block receptors	The furanocoumarin phellopterin, from the roots of *Angelica dahurica*, strongly inhibits the binding of diazepam to central nervous system benzodiazepine receptors in vitro.[3]
	Some extracts inhibit contraction of the rabbit aorta induced by histamine and serotonin in vitro. Xanthones from *Garcinia mangostana* interact with various receptors. α-mangostin acts as a histamine H_1 receptor antagonist, and γ-mangostin is a 5-HT_{2a} receptor antagonist.[4]
Alter cellular transport processes	
Block ion channels	Alkaloids from Oregon grape *(Mahonia aquifolium)*, corytuberine, magnoflorine, isothebaine, and isocorydine, inhibit the influx of calcium into cells of the rat aorta.[5]
Alter carrier-mediated transport	Loop diuretics inhibit $Na^+,K^+,2Cl^-$ carrier. Thiazides inhibit Na^+,Cl^- cotransport.
Interfere with active transport	Cardiac glycosides inhibit $Na^+,K^+,$ATPase. Antidepressants inhibit reuptake of monoamines or serotonin.
Change enzyme functions	
Inhibit enzymes	Tannins inhibit the activity of protein kinases (PK).[6] Some hydrolyzable tannins are selective inhibitors of various protein kinases, such as cAMP-dependent PK and calcium and phospholipid-dependent PK. Herbal ACE inhibitors inhibit angiotensin-converting enzyme.[7]
Activate enzymes	Forskolin activates adenylate cyclase. Metal ions, like Mg, Ca, Zn, Cu, and Mn, also activate enzymes.

Characteristics of Specific Drugs

- Interact with specific receptors
- Open or block ion channels
- Modify transport systems
- Inhibit or activate enzymes
- Interfere with particular aspects of biosynthesis in microorganisms

ENZYMES

A range of clinically relevant effects are mediated via plant constituent interactions with enzymes. The cell is the site of tremendous metabolic activity, processes that go on continually in living organisms. These activities include the buildup of new tissue, replacement of old tissue, conversion of food to energy, disposal of waste materials, and reproduction—in short, all of the activities undertaken by cells to maintain life.

However, all of this takes place in the face of a paradox. Biochemical reactions do not occur spontaneously, but are facilitated by catalysis. *Catalysis* is the acceleration of a chemical reaction by some substance that itself undergoes no permanent chemical change. The catalysts of biochemical reactions are enzymes, which are responsible for almost all chemical reactions that occur in living organisms.

Without enzymes, of which nearly 2,000 are known in humans, these reactions would take place too slowly for the needs of life processes. Because of their central role in cellular processes, deficiency, excess, or improper regulation of enzymes can result in a variety of diseases. An important aspect of enzyme function is that it can be regulated.

The Chemical Nature of Enzymes

All known enzymes are proteins. They are high molecular weight compounds made up principally of chains of amino acids linked together by peptide bonds. Their molecular weights range from 10,000 to 2,000,000 and control the amount of metabolites and the rate at which they move through metabolic pathways. As biological catalysts, they speed the rate of attainment of chemical equilibrium by lowering the energy barrier between substrate and products. In other words, a catalyst will increase the rate of a reaction, but will not affect the position of the reaction equilibrium.

Enzymes are unique in that the enhancements they cause are on an order of magnitude greater than those of most other catalysts. A typical enzyme will convert about 1,000 molecules of substrate to product in one second. Some will convert as many as one million. Unlike most other catalysts, enzymes work at ambient temperature, atmospheric pressure, and usually in a narrow, near-neutral pH-range. However, there are exceptions, such as pepsin, which operates in the stomach in a pH range of 2.0 to 5.0.

Specificity of Enzymes

One of the unique properties of enzymes is their specificity. In general, there are four distinct types of specificity.

Absolute specificity: The enzyme will catalyze only one reaction.

Group specificity: The enzyme will act only on molecules that have specific functional groups, such as amino, phosphate, and methyl groups.

Linkage specificity: The enzyme will act on a particular type of chemical bond regardless of the rest of the molecular structure.

Stereochemical specificity: The enzyme will act on a particular steric or optical isomer.

Many enzymes require the presence of other compounds, called cofactors, before they become active. This entire active complex is known as the *holoenzyme* and is made up of an *apoenzyme* (protein portion) plus the *cofactor* (a coenzyme, prosthetic group, or metal ion activator).

Apoenzyme + Cofactor = Holoenzyme

Enzyme Terminology

Except for some of the first-studied enzymes, such as pepsin, rennin, and trypsin, most enzyme names end in *-ase;* however, there are many exceptions to this rule. The International Union of Biochemistry (IUB) created a systematic naming scheme for enzymes.[8] Enzymes are classified and named according to the type of reaction catalyzed. The enzyme is assigned a four-number classification and a two-part name, or systematic name. A shorter version, called the recommended name, is suggested for everyday use. There are six major categories of enzymes.

Oxidoreductases

Oxidoreductases catalyze oxidation reduction reactions between two substrates through the transfer of electrons. They are responsible for the production of heat and energy. Many of these enzymes are present in mitochondria.

- *Dehydrogenases* catalyze the removal of hydrogen from a substrate.
- *Oxidases* activate oxygen so that it will readily combine with a substrate.

- *Catalases* catalyze the decomposition of hydrogen peroxide to water and oxygen.
- *Peroxidases* catalyze the decomposition of organic peroxides to hydrogen peroxide and water.

Transferases

Transferases catalyze reactions involving the transfer of groups from one molecule to another. Trivial names for the transferases often include the prefix *trans*.

- *Transglycosidases* catalyze the transfer of monosaccharides.
- *Transphosphorylases* and *phosphomutases* catalyze the transfer of phosphate groups.
- *Transaminases* catalyze the transfer of amino groups.
- *Transacetylases* catalyze the transfer of acetyl groups.

Hydrolases

Hydrolases catalyze reactions in which the cleavage of bonds is accomplished by the addition of water. They are named for the substrate upon which they act.

- *Carbohydrases* catalyze the hydrolysis of carbohydrates into simple sugars.
- *Esterases* catalyze the hydrolysis of esters into acids and alcohols.
- *Proteinases* hydrolyze proteins to peptides.
- *Peptidases* hydrolyze polypeptides to amino acids.
- *Nucleases* catalyze the hydrolysis of nucleic acids.

Lyases

Lyases catalyze the removal of groups by means other than hydrolysis, usually involving the formation of carbon-carbon double bonds.

- *Fumarases* catalyze the change of fumaric acid to L-malic acid in the Krebs cycle.
- *Decarboxylases* catalyze the removal of a molecule of carbon dioxide from a carboxylic group.
- *Deaminases* catalyze the removal of amino groups from compounds.

Isomerases

Isomerases catalyze intramolecular rearrangements; that is, they catalyze the interconversion of optical, geometric, or structural isomers.

- *Epimerases* catalyze the inversion of asymmetric carbon atoms.
- *Mutases* catalyze the intramolecular transfer of functional groups.

Ligases

Ligases catalyze the formation of bonds between two substrate molecules—specifically, through the hydrolysis of the pyrophosphate bond in adenoside triphosphate (ATP) or another triphosphate. The energy is always supplied by ATP hydrolysis. The names of many ligases include the term *synthetase*. Several other ligases are called *carboxylases*. One of these is fundamental to life processes.

- *Ribulose bisphosphate carboxylase/oxygenase* (rubisco) is the plant enzyme that facilitates the formation of organic carbon from the inorganic carbon dioxide in the air; rubisco helps generate phosphoglycerates.

ENZYMES AND HERBS

A number of herbal constituents affect metabolic processes by modulating the activity of specific enzymes in various ways, including activating or inhibiting enzyme functions. Enzyme activation and inhibition both can be harnessed for specific therapeutic effects.

Forskolin and the Activation of Adenylate Cyclase

Coleus forskohlii, a plant used in ayurvedic medicine, is the source of a compound of unique biological importance. A screening of medicinal plants by the Indian Central Drug Research Institute revealed the presence of a hypotensive and spasmolytic component in *C. forskohlii*, a labdane diterpene named forskolin.

Forskolin works by activating adenylate cyclase, an enzyme that raises levels of cyclic adenosine monophosphate (cAMP) in cells.[9] Cyclic AMP is a vital cell-regulating compound involved in a variety of cellular functions. Normally, cAMP is formed when a stimulatory hormone (for example, epinephrine) binds to a receptor site on the cell membrane and stimulates the activation of adenylate cyclase. This enzyme is incorporated into all cellular membranes and only the specificity of receptors determines which hormone will activate the enzyme in a particular cell.

Forskolin appears to bypass this need for direct hormonal activation of adenylate cyclase via transmembrane activation. As a result of this transmembrane activation, intracellular cAMP levels rise.

Physiological and Biochemical Effects of Elevated Intracellular cAMP

- Inhibition of platelet activation and degranulation
- Inhibition of mast cell degranulation and histamine release
- Increased force of heart muscle contraction
- Relaxation of the arteries and other smooth muscles
- Increased insulin secretion
- Increased thyroid function
- Increased lipolysis

Forskolin possesses additional properties, such as inhibition of membrane transport proteins and channel proteins through a mechanism that does not involve the production of cAMP. The outcome is again a transmembrane signaling that results in activation of other cellular enzymes. Forskolin also inhibits platelet-activating factor (PAF) by interfering with PAF binding to receptor sites. PAF inhibition is discussed later in this chapter.

Thus, the therapeutic potential of *C. forskohlii* is great, as there are many conditions in which a decreased intracellular cAMP level may be a major factor in the development of the disease process. These include eczema, asthma, psoriasis, angina, and hypertension.

Inhibition of Enzymes

Pharmacologically speaking, there are a number of types of enzyme inhibitors, which are differentiated by the specific mechanism involved at the molecular level. A complete discussion of different types of enzyme inhibitors, however, is beyond the scope of this book. Instead, we shall consider a number of enzyme inhibitory mechanisms that are relevant to modern phytotherapy.

Acetylcholinesterase Inhibitors

Agents that inhibit the enzyme cholinesterase have attracted attention as therapeutic agents for the treatment of Alzheimer's disease. These agents have effects on the parasympathetic nervous system, which regulates processes responsible for energy assimilation and storage. They operate when the body is at rest, decreasing heart activity and relaxing respiratory processes. Among their many roles, cholinesterase inhibitors facilitate the digestive process, increasing secretory activity and peristalsis and decreasing sphincter tone.

The most important neurotransmitter in this system is acetylcholine (ACh). Reduced ACh levels are observed in various forms of dementia, and therapeutic approaches have been developed to facilitate cholinergic replacement. ACh is inactive if taken orally as a medicine, so other methods have been developed to achieve therapeutically meaningful elevations.

Levels of synaptic acetylcholine can be readily increased by using centrally acting inhibitors of acetylcholinesterase (AChE), the enzyme that catabolizes ACh. Tacrine is currently the only drug approved for Alzheimer's disease in the United States. While an effective AChE inhibitor, it has a number of other sites of action and may cause hepatotoxicity.[10] Among other AChE inhibitors under development is the alkaloid huperzine A, from *Huperzia serrata*, a club moss used in traditional Chinese medicine.

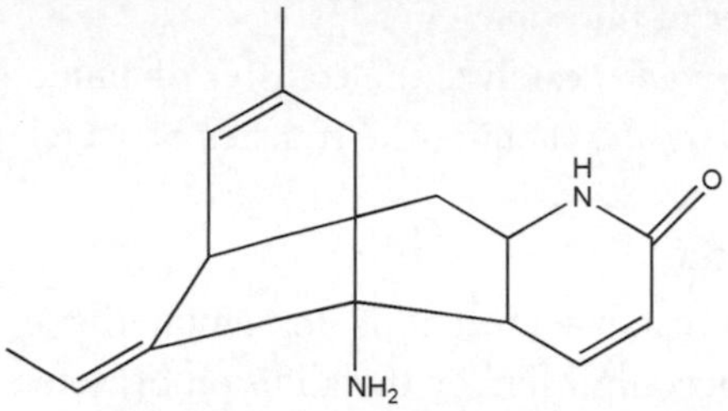

Fig. 9.1. Huperzine A

The club moss *Huperzia serrata* is the Chinese folk medicine *qing ceng ta*. This herb is found chiefly in southern China, where it grows in moist places in hilly regions. A decoction of the dried whole plant has been used to treat trauma, fractures, scalds, hematuria, and infections of the skin and subcutaneous tissues. The herb is a component of a tea administered to elderly patients in China. Huperzine A and its cogener, huperzine B, were isolated from the moss, identified, and shown to be potent AChE inhibitors.[11]

5-α-reductase Inhibition

Benign prostatic hyperplasia (BPH) is believed to be caused by accumulation of testosterone in the prostate. However, once in the prostate, testosterone is converted to dihydrotestosterone (DHT). DHT, a more potent hormone than testosterone, acts on the prostate gland and other sexual organs.

DHT is produced from testosterone by the enzyme 5-α-reductase, and is necessary for the normal growth and development of the prostate. Its presence is also necessary for the pathologic enlargement of the prostate that occurs in BPH. Thus, one therapeutic approach to treating this condition is to reduce the formation of DHT by blocking the enzyme 5-α-reductase. *Serenoa repens* (saw palmetto) has this effect, and may also possess receptor site–binding effects.

RECEPTORS

One way of explaining the action of herbal constituents on the body is through their specific interactions with receptors. Such receptor interactions initiate a chain of biochemical events that lead to the observed effects. Cellular activity is coordinated by the transmission of signals, chemical or electrical, between cells.

The ability of a cell to respond to an extracellular signal depends on the presence of specific receptor proteins on its surface or in the cytoplasm. The receptors bind the chemical signal, triggering a mechanism that modifies the behavior of the cell. Cells contain an array of specific receptors, allowing them to respond to a variety of chemical signals. The nature of these intracellular events differs according to the type of receptor. The same molecular signal may cause different responses in different types of cell.

Thus, receptors have a dual function. They detect a ligand signal by forming a ligand-receptor complex and they conduct and translate the signal, leading to the pharmacological effect.

The Molecular Nature of Receptors

Most receptors are proteins, presumably because their structures provide both the diversity and the specificity of shape and electrical charge. They are present in only small amounts in cells, ranging from about 0.001% of total soluble protein in aldosterone receptors to 0.1% in progesterone receptors. The actual quantities vary in response to stimuli, and their properties change with physiologic conditions. When a hormone or neurotransmitter is present in excess, the number of active receptors generally decreases (a process known as *down regulation*), while a deficiency of the chemical messenger causes an increase in the number of active receptors, or *up regulation*.

Antagonism and Agonism

An *antagonist* is a compound that will bind to the receptor but not activate it. In contrast, an *agonist* has both an affinity for the receptor and the ability to trigger the response. Antagonists exert their effects by preventing agonists from binding to and activating receptors. They are divided into two classes, depending on whether or not they reversibly compete with agonists for binding to receptors.

Antagonism can be *competitive* (reversible), meaning that the antagonist competes for the receptor and so requires a higher concentration of the agonist in order to achieve the same effect as would the agonist alone.

Alternately, antagonism can be *noncompetitive* (irreversible), a situation in which the antagonist's affinity for the receptor is so high that for practical purposes the receptor is unavailable for binding by the agonist.

Receptors and Hormonal Control of Gene Expression

Receptor sites are complex assemblages of molecules with subunits that change shape in response to various messengers, all in a finely tuned way. From one perspective, their study is revealing a window into how "fearfully and wonderfully" made we human beings are (Ps. 139:14).

To explore the concept of receptor interactions, we will discuss hormones and their receptors. Hormones transmit information from one cell to another to coordinate a whole range of homeostatic adaptations, growth, development, and reproduction. Hormone receptors are found throughout the cell, including the outer membrane. When hormones are released into the blood as a result of some stimulus, they circulate throughout the body and bind to these receptors.

Once bound, the receptors and their lipid-soluble ligands traverse the membrane and enter the nucleus, where they directly exert their effects by binding to special enhancers (called *hormone-responsive elements*) and by stimulating the transcription of certain genes.

The mechanism used by hormones to regulate gene expression has two therapeutically important consequences.

- All of these hormones produce their effects after a characteristic lag period of three minutes to several hours—the time required for the synthesis of new proteins.
- Their effects can persist for hours or days after their concentration has been reduced to zero.

The interactions of steroid hormones with receptors starts as the hormones arrive via the blood. Blood transports steroids either bound to a blood protein or unbound. Binding of the steroid to its receptor molecule results in conformational change, an alteration of the three-dimensional structure of the receptor from an inactive to an active form.

This activated receptor-steroid complex has an affinity for specific binding sites on DNA, resulting in activation or transcription of the gene to produce messenger RNA (mRNA). The mRNA is translated on cytoplasmic ribosomes to produce the code for protein. Once the receptor-hormone complex has interacted with a gene, the protein undergoes reactions that result in the reestablishment of unoccupied receptors and elimination of the steroid from the cell.

Hormone + Receptor ◄──► Hormone-Receptor Complex
Inactive   Active

The basic structure of receptor proteins comprises three domains: one for hormone binding, another for binding to DNA, and one immunologic domain. Receptor proteins can adopt various conformational forms, but when bound to a hormone take on the active shape. While a receptor that is not attached to a hormone can bind to DNA, it will not activate transcription unless the hormone is also bound.

Mechanisms exist to facilitate the transmission of the chemical signal across the barrier posed by the plasma membrane. Each mechanism has evolved distinctive receptor families that transduce many different signals. These receptors are found on the cell surface and within the cell, as well as in enzymes and other components that generate, amplify, coordinate, or terminate post-receptor signaling by chemical second messengers in the cytoplasm.

There are four basic mechanisms by which signals are transmitted across membranes:

1. A lipid-soluble molecule crosses the membrane passively and acts on an intracellular receptor.
2. Intracellular activity is regulated by a molecule that binds to an extracellular site on a receptor protein whose structure crosses the membrane (examples include receptors for insulin, low-density lipoprotein, growth hormone, and cytokines).
3. A transmembrane ion channel is induced to open or close by the binding of a molecule (examples include receptors for nicotine, GABA, and glycine).
4. A transmembrane receptor protein stimulates a G protein that in turn generates an intracellular secondary messenger. This intricate process can facilitate many interactions with exogenous molecules.

G Proteins and Second Messengers

Guanine nucleotide binding proteins, or G proteins, are membrane proteins that link the activation of a membrane receptor to the subsequent activation of its cellular second messenger. Receptors coupled to G proteins are structurally related to one another, comprising a family of *serpentine receptors*, so called because the receptor polypeptide chain crosses the plasma membrane seven times.

Receptors for adrenergic amines, serotonin, acetylcholine, many peptide hormones, odors, and visual receptors in the retinal rod and cone cells are all serpentine. The amino and carboxyl terminals of each of these receptors are located on the extracellular and cytoplasmic sides of the membrane, respectively.

Within the membrane, a G protein binds to an exogenous molecule, causing a conformational change and activating a cascade of reactions that produce various second messengers. No matter which pathway is activated, the result is a change in the functioning of the affected cell in response to the original message-bearing molecule.

Phytoestrogens and Receptors

As an example of the role of receptor interactions in herbal activity, consider the phytoestrogens. It has been estimated that more than 300 species of plants have some degree of demonstrable estrogen activity.[12] The concept of *phytoestrogens* originally came from toxicology, but it has since taken on a more positive aspect, as epidemiology has uncovered many clues about the role of dietary phytoestrogens. See chapter 10 for more information on the toxicity of phytoestrogens.

Health-Protective Effects of Phytoestrogens

• Epidemiological studies reveal low mortality from hormone-dependent cancer in both Japanese women and men consuming a traditional diet, which may be related to the high intake of phytoestrogens in soybeans and other foods.[13]

• Dietary intake of soy is associated with a decreased risk of both hormone-dependent and hormone-independent cancers, and it has been suggested that genistein, the predominant isoflavone in soy foods, is responsible for this effect.[14]

• The low mortality from prostate cancer in Japanese men may be associated with their isoflavone-rich traditional diet.[15]

• Consumption of a plant-based diet can prevent the development and progression of chronic diseases that are associated with extensive neovascularization.[16]

• Researchers suggest that human cancer mortality rates could be markedly reduced by supplementing human diets with certain soybean products shown to suppress carcinogenesis in animals.[17]

• Because many Western diseases are hormone-dependent cancers, it has been postulated that the typical Western diet, compared with a vegetarian or semi-vegetarian diet, may alter hormone production, metabolism, or action at the cellular level.[18]

Classification of Hormones

Hormones can be grouped into classes based upon the method by which they are transmitted.

Group 1 Hormones

Lipid-soluble steroidal hormones cross the cell membrane and act upon an intracellular receptor. Steroid hormones exert effects at all levels of biological organization, using similar mechanisms to produce the same general effects (the induction of RNA and protein synthesis). The major classes of steroid hormones, all derived from cholesterol, are *progestins*, *corticosteroids*, *estrogens*, and *androgens*. Several signal molecules are lipid-soluble enough to cross the plasma membrane and act on intracellular receptors. One of these is a gas, nitric oxide (NO), that acts by stimulating an intracellular enzyme, guanylyl cyclase, which produces cyclic guanosine monophosphate (cGMP).

Group 2 Hormones

These hormones are water-soluble and thus do not use blood transport proteins. They bind to cell-surface receptors, which then use secondary messengers to relay their message to the nucleus. This transmembrane signaling system has three components:

- The hormone is specifically detected by a cell-surface receptor.
- The receptor triggers the activation of a G protein located on the cytoplasmic face of the plasma membrane, which changes the activity of an effector element, usually an enzyme or ion channel.
- This element then changes the concentration of the intracellular second messenger.

The type of secondary messenger determines the subclasses of Group 2 hormones.

GROUP 2A HORMONES

The secondary messenger for Group 2A hormones is cyclic adenosine monophosphate (cAMP), which mediates such hormonal responses as mobilization of stored energy, vasopressin-mediated conservation of water by the kidneys, Ca^{2+} homeostasis, and rate and contractile force of the heart muscle. It also regulates the production of adrenal and sex steroids, the relaxation of smooth muscle, and many other endocrine and neural processes. A stimulator of intracellular cAMP is forskolin, a diterpene from *Coleus forskohlii* that acts as an adenylate cyclase activator to increase intracellular cAMP by stimulating its biosynthesis.[19]

GROUP 2B HORMONES

The secondary messenger for Group 2B hormones is cyclic guanosine monophosphate (cGMP). cGMP has signaling roles in only a few types of cells.

GROUP 2C HORMONES

The secondary messengers here are calcium, phosphoinositides, or both, which act through a transmembrane ion channel that can be induced to open or close by the binding of a ligand. Some of the hormones, neurotransmitters, and growth factors that trigger this pathway bind to receptors linked to G proteins, while others bind to tyrosine kinase receptors.

GROUP 2D HORMONES

The secondary messenger for this group of hormones, including insulin, prolactin, and growth factor, is unknown.

The average sperm count in men has been consistently declining since the Second World War, apparently because of exposure to xenoestrogenic environmental pollutants. The environmental science literature actually talks about the fact that we live in a "sea of estrogens." We have to recognize that estrogenic plant effects, even though they are important and we herbalists have an attachment to them, occur in the context of total exposure to estrogens.

Type II Estrogen–Binding Sites and Estrogen Antagonism

In addition to nuclear-bound estrogen receptor (Type I sites), a second estrogen-binding site is found in nuclei of various tissues. These Type II nuclear estradiol–binding sites are located on the nuclear matrix. One event stimulated by exposure to estrogen is an increase in the number of Type II estrogen–binding sites. Nuclear Type II receptors are occupied by an endogenous ligand that appears to be an inhibitor of cell proliferation.

PHYTOESTROGENS

A remarkable diversity of naturally occurring and synthetic compounds mimic the biological effects of β-estradiol, indicated in the laboratory by their ability to bind to the nuclear estrogen receptor, activate transcriptional response, and promote growth of estrogen-dependent MCF7 cells in culture.[20]

The most important of these appear to be isoflavones, coumestans, lignans, and phytosterols. In the diet, the precursors of the biologically active compounds

---

A Closer Look at "Estrogens"

Estrogen

There is no chemical called "estrogen." *Estrogen* is a term that describes an effect, not a particular chemical. We really should talk about *estrogens*, the spectrum of molecular structures that share this effect. These are various natural or synthetic substances that possess the biological activity of estrus-producing hormones. *Estrus* is the period in a female mammal during which ovulation occurs and she is receptive to mating. This is an important point, because the periodicity and the receptive time frame vary from one mammalian species to another. Most of the research on plant estrogens has utilized rodents, and rats and mice have very different estrous cycles than humans—starting with the fact that they do not menstruate.

This raises many questions about how to extrapolate data from rat studies to therapeutic applications in humans. Estrogens are synthesized from androgens, primarily in the ovaries, and, to a lesser extent, in the adrenal cortex. These hormones can also be produced in the testes of males. The major estrogen, β-estradiol, is synthesized from testosterone.

Phytoestrogens

A *phytoestrogen* is a plant constituent that possesses estrogenic activity. However, to say that something possesses estrogenic activity does not mean that all estrogens have the same degree of estrogenic activity, nor does it mean they all possess the whole spectrum of effects that human estrogens have. It is also important to understand that phytoestrogens are not precursors of human hormones, but instead interact with human estrogen receptors to elicit various responses.

Xenoestrogens

Xenoestrogens are environmental estrogens, usually synthetic pesticides such as DDT and hormones in our diet. One source is residual hormones that make their way into dairy products after having been originally fed to cows. DDT, PCB, and many other synthetic pesticides are estrogens. In fact, they work in part by disrupting the reproductive cycle of the animal they are designed to deter. Without making too much of a point of xenoestrogens, it should be noted that quantitatively, environmental pollutant estrogens appear to have far more of an effect on humans than do plant estrogens.

originate in soybean products (which contain mainly isoflavones but also lignans in smaller amounts) as well as in whole grain cereals and seeds. The phytoestrogens in berries and nuts are believed to be mainly lignans.[21]

Coffee has phytoestrogenic effects, as do beer, bourbon, mescaline, and *Cannabis*. Actually, it is quite amazing how many substances that cause social issues also have estrogenic effects. Coffee extracts, unlike tea and cocoa, actively compete with estradiol for uterine cytosol binding sites.[22]

Isoflavones

A number of phytoestrogens belong to chemically related classes of flavonoids, including chalcones, flavanones, flavones, flavonols, and isoflavones. The most active of these, the isoflavones, represent a structural variant of the flavonoid family of plant phenolics and are only found regularly in one subfamily of the Fabaceae, the Papilionoideae. They have been recorded occasionally in a few other families, such as Asteraceae, Iridaceae, Myristicaceae, and Rosaceae. It is possible that they are more widespread, but the lack of a satisfactory method of screening for their presence makes the search difficult.[23]

Widely occurring isoflavones include daidzein, genistein, formononetin, and biochanin A. A study of relative estrogenic activities for some isoflavones identified a range of potencies. In order of decreasing potency, the most active was zearalenone, followed by β-zearalenol, coumestrol, genistein, daidzein, phloretin, formononetin, and biochanin A. The hormonal activity of these compounds was specific for the estrogen receptor and sensitive to inhibition by 4-hydroxytamoxifen.[24]

In laboratory studies, genistein inhibited the proliferation of human tumor cell lines in vitro, constrained endothelial cell proliferation and angiogenesis, and inhibited the proliferation of various other types of tumor cells.[25, 26] It also inhibited the activity of purified topoisomerase II in vitro, and the production of reactive oxygen ions that can lead to tissue damage and DNA modification. Additionally, genistein acts as a weak estrogen, modifies cellular differentiation, modulates cell cycle events, and may precipitate apoptosis.[27]

Lignans

Lignans are dimers that are chemically related to the lignins of plant cell walls; they are found mainly in woody tissues. Some have been isolated from other plant parts, such as roots, leaves, and flowers, and in such cases they may be found in glycosidic combinations. The active molecular forms of lignans are produced only after they are metabolized by the gut flora, pointing yet again to the fundamental importance of digestive tract health.

The lignan enterolactone is a moderate inhibitor of human estrogen synthetase. This lignan binds to or near the active site of the P_{450} enzyme.[28] Research suggests that the high concentration of lignans seen in vegetarians may play a protective role against estrogen-dependent cancers by serving as antipromotional compounds, inhibiting aromatase in peripheral or cancer cells, and lowering estrogen levels.[29]

Phytosterols

At one time, sterols were considered to be mainly animal products, but an increasing number of such compounds have been detected in plant tissues. Indeed, three phytosterols are ubiquitous in higher plants: β-sitosterol, stigmasterol, and campesterol. Phytosterols are structurally distinct from animal sterols in that they have an extra methyl or ethyl radical in the side chain. An example is β-sitosterol, a common constituent in flowering plants.

Interactions of Phytoestrogens with Receptors

Two important interactions are mediated via sex hormone binding globulin (SHBG) and Type II estrogen binding sites in the nucleus. Lignans and isoflavones may affect the uptake and metabolism of sex hormones by helping to regulate SHBG levels, although phytoestrogens bind only weakly to SHBG.[30] They also compete with estradiol for binding to unfilled cytoplasmic estrogen receptors or unfilled nuclear Type II estrogen receptor sites, which may be the mechanism by which they inhibit cancer cell growth.[31] Bound nuclear receptors are then processed in a manner that rapidly decreases the total number of cellular estrogen receptors.

Research Conclusions

Not all phytoestrogens are created equal; they display a range of actions and different potencies. This variability points out how important it is to fully characterize each phytoestrogen in terms of its sites of action, balance of agonistic and antagonistic properties, natural potency, and short- and long-term effects.[32] Thus, a plethora of variables are encountered when drawing conclusions about phytoestrogens.

Phytosterols, lignans, and isoflavones have all been shown to possess both estrogenic and antiestrogenic activity.[33] This apparent contradiction results from the array of assays used to identify estrogenicity, each of which evaluates distinct responses in the spectrum of estrogenic activities. The reasons behind the differences in activity can be grouped into three broad categories:

- Variability in potency and activity among different specific phytoestrogens[34]
- Variability in response among different test animals and humans[35]
- Variability based on dosage, timing, and route of administration[36]

What it comes down to is that no specific generalizations can actually be made about phytoestrogenic constituents, because each has a different spectrum of effects. However, consider the following research conclusions.

- It is clear that there is a significant number of structurally diverse secondary plant metabolites that contribute to human estrogen exposure, and these phytoestrogens have estrogenic effects at dietary levels.[37]
- Dietary macro- and micronutrients play an important role in estrogen metabolism.[38]
- Lignans and isoflavones have been shown to influence not only sex hormone metabolism and biological activity, but also intracellular enzymes, protein synthesis, growth factor action, and malignant cell proliferation, differentiation, and angiogenesis, making them strong candidates as natural cancer-protective compounds.[39]
- In two thirds of reviewed studies on the effect of phytoestrogen-rich soy materials in animal models of cancer, the risk of cancer (incidence, latency, or number of tumors) was significantly reduced.[40]
- Greater dietary incorporation of isoflavone-rich foods may be a safe and effective means of reducing cancer risk.[41]
- It has been suggested that some of the 400 plants used as galactagogues work via phytoestrogenic stimulation of prolactin production, which then stimulates breast milk production.[42]

Implications for Phytotherapy

With the wealth of new data flowing from the research community, it is not easy to come to conclusions relevant to phytotherapy. However, it can be stated with some degree of confidence that phytoestrogens act predominantly as weak partial agonists in Type I estrogen receptors and as weak partial antagonists in Type II estrogen receptors.

From this, some broad clinical guidelines can be deduced.

- During the child-bearing years, the impact of phytoestrogens will be minimal. This is because of their relative lack of potency when compared with endogenous estrogens.
- During the menopausal and postmenopausal years, this potency disparity becomes less important because of changing levels of endogenous hormones, and as such, phytoestrogens may have much to offer in the treatment of menopausal discomforts. This observation underscores the phytotherapist's experience of traditional herbal efficacy in such cases.
- Epidemiological studies of Japanese women eating a traditional diet reveal that they have a lower incidence of osteoporosis. Western research has not yet confirmed a link between consumption of dietary phytoestrogens and prevention of bone loss, but a prudent practitioner would do well to consider them in the development of treatment programs for women.
- The risk of estrogen-sensitive carcinomas may be reduced by intake of dietary phytoestrogens. The main area in which confusion has arisen concerns therapeutic conclusions about the treatment of breast cancer. In general, estrogens are all potentially carcinogenic. This is one of the real problems with synthetic hormone replacement therapy. However, some herb books caution against the use of phytoestrogen-containing plants because estrogens can stimulate the development of tumors in the breast. To the contrary, human research has made it clear that phytoestrogens act as weak estrogen antagonists in Type II estrogen receptors in the breast, and so might actually help reduce the risk of breast cancer related to estrogens.

PHARMACOKINETICS

Pharmacokinetics is the study of factors that modify the effects of drugs, including:

- Administration
- Absorption
- Distribution (biotranslocation)
- Biotransformation
- Elimination from or storage in the body

To illustrate what happens to a therapeutic substance after it is administered, the following diagram tracks an essential oils on its journey through the body.

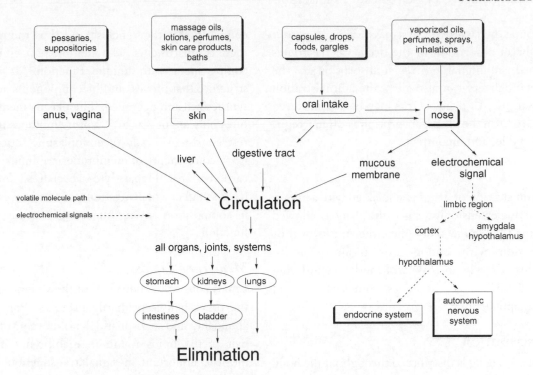

Fig. 9.2. Pharmacokinetic pathways of volatile oils in the body

Administration and Absorption

Absorption refers to mechanisms by which molecules pass from the point of entry into the bloodstream. When administering any herbal preparation, one must select:

- A route of administration
- A dose
- A dosage form (liquid, tablet, capsule, or injection)

A constituent's site of action is often remote from its point of entry into the body. The best route of administration is usually determined by the physical characteristics of the substance, the speed of absorption, and the occasional need to bypass hepatic metabolism. The right dosage form will ensure herbal efficacy at the site of action by providing a pharmacologically effective concentration, and will also maintain the concentration for an adequate period of time.

Oral Administration

Herbal medicines are commonly taken by mouth. To be effective, the remedy must be in a form that is soluble and stable in stomach fluid, able to enter the intestine and cross the lining of the intestine, and thus able to enter the bloodstream. Because they are already in solution, herbs taken in liquid form tend to be absorbed more rapidly than those given in tablet or capsule form. The rate of absorption of herbs taken in solid form is limited by the rate at which the solid dissolves and by the specific chemistry of constituents.

Oral administration is a convenient route, but the constituents are subject to extensive biotransformation in the gastrointestinal wall and liver. Constituents absorbed from the gastrointestinal tract enter the bloodstream by going directly to the liver via the portal vein. Once there, they may be metabolized rapidly, possibly inactivating constituents before they can reach the intended site of action. This *first-pass effect* is responsible for the fact that some drugs, such as morphine, are active when injected but much less active when taken by mouth. Absorption after oral administration may be slowed by concurrent ingestion of food, mucilage-rich herbs, or antacids. Fast absorption implies rapid onset of effects.

Other Routes of Administration

Routes of administration other than oral may improve the pharmacological efficacy of the substance at a particular site or reduce toxicity.

Inhalation

Inhalation delivers large amounts of drug directly to the lungs, useful in cases of respiratory disease.

Mucous Membranes

Occasionally, drugs are administered through the mucous membranes of the mouth or nose, from which sites the drug can be directly absorbed into the bloodstream. Administration by *buccal* (through the mouth), *sublingual* (under the tongue), nasal, rectal, or *transdermal* (through the skin) routes bypasses the first-pass effect to permit quick and direct absorption of the drug. Of the routes just described, sublingual and rectal absorption are the fastest. Rectal delivery can also allow the administration of larger quantities of drug. Herbs may be administered in suppository form; however, absorption is often irregular, unpredictable, and incomplete.

Topical

Topical administration of drugs is associated with a higher incidence of hypersensitivity, since the drug is allowed adequate time to become allergenic either on its own or in combination with endogenous tissue proteins. However, this is rarely an issue with herbs, considering the long and safe use of poultices, fomentations, and other topical applications.

Drug Distribution

Once absorbed, a drug is distributed throughout the body by the circulating blood, passing across various barriers to reach its site of action. At any given time, only a very small portion of the total amount of a drug in the body is in contact with its receptors. Most of the administered drug will be found in areas of the body that are remote from the site of action.

For example, in the case of a psychoactive drug, most of the drug circulates outside the brain and therefore does not contribute directly to its pharmacological effect. This wide distribution often accounts for drug *side effects*, or results that are different from the primary, or therapeutic, effect for which the drug is taken.

Bioavailability

The percentage of a drug that is absorbed and actually reaches the systemic circulation is an expression of its *bioavailability*. Because drugs are metabolized and eliminated from the body, the level of drug in the body will decrease with time after a single dose.

To achieve a more constant serum level, multiple doses are given at fixed time intervals. In general, shorter intervals lead to more constant serum levels. Once in the bloodstream, the drug must penetrate the cells of the target organs in order to exert its therapeutic action. Thus the extent and rate of absorption and penetration depend on the ability of the drug to pass through lipid-rich cell membranes—in other words, its lipid solubility.

Transport through a Cell Membrane

Cell and organelle membranes are not passive barriers. They control the structures and environments of the compartments they enclose and thus the metabolism of these compartments. The membrane itself is a metabolic compartment with unique functions. It is a dynamic structure that moves, and its components are continually synthesized and degraded. The plasma membrane constitutes only about 2% to 5% of membranes in the cell; the rest consist primarily of endoplasmic reticula. The primary components of membranes are lipids, proteins, and carbohydrates. Hepatocytes specialized for metabolism have a higher concentration of membranes. Differences in composition among membranes reflect differences in function.

Membrane Lipids

Lipids constitute about half of the weight of membranes; the other half is primarily proteins. Phospholipids are abundant, and phosphatidylcholine constitutes roughly half of the lipids found in membranes. Phosphatidylinositol, important in signal transduction, is present in smaller amounts. Other membrane lipids include sphingomyelin, glycosphingolipid, and cholesterol.

Membrane Proteins

Proteins associated with membranes are asymmetrical. They are different on the outside from on the inside, and are integrated into the membrane in only one orientation relative to the inside of the cell. These proteins fulfill a number of vital functions:

- Catalytic enzymes
- Receptors for signals such as hormones
- Transport systems
- Structural components

Membrane Carbohydrates

Carbohydrates are bonded to proteins or lipids as glycoproteins or glycolipids. Typical sugars present include glucose, galactose, mannose, fructose, and nitrogenated sugars, such as *N*-acetylglucosamine, *N*-acetylgalactosamine, and *N*-acetylneuraminic acid (sialic acid). Membrane sugars are pivotal in cell interactions as a means of identification and recognition.[43] They are found only on the outside of the plasma membrane or on the inside of vesicles.

Membrane Structure

A membrane can be viewed as a lipid bilayer composed of phospholipid and cholesterol along with various proteins. Integral proteins are embedded, while peripheral proteins may be loosely attached to the surface of the membrane.

Membranes separate and maintain the chemical environments on both sides of the membrane. Proteins and lipids diffuse in the membrane, but ions are found at different concentrations on either side of the cell membrane, creating an ion gradient. Membranes maintain these gradients by preventing ion diffusion, necessitating active transport of ions from one side of the plasma membrane to the other.

Nonpolar molecules are *lipophilic* (lipid-loving) and polar molecules are *hydrophilic* (water-loving). Lipophilic molecules pass readily through membranes because they dissolve in the hydrophobic, nonpolar portion of the lipid bilayer. Although permeable to water, the nonpolar lipid bilayer of cell membranes is impermeable to many other polar molecules, necessitating specific transport systems.

Passive Diffusion

Some substances can cross membranes by a process of passive diffusion, which involves no energy expenditure. Water and small lipophilic organic compounds can cross in this way, but charged compounds and large molecules, such as proteins, cannot. In passive diffusion, the molecule will only move down the concentration gradient—that is, from a higher to a lower concentration.

Protein Channels

Protein channels transport specific ions. For example, ion channels exist for the movement of Na+, K+, and Ca++. The protein forms a gate that opens and closes under the control of the membrane potential. Ion movement through channels is always down the concentration gradient.

Mediated Transport

Transport of molecules across membranes by molecular carriers is termed *mediated transport*. These carriers are variously called *porters, porting systems, translocases, transport systems*, and *pumps*.

Membrane Receptors

Cell-cell communication is achieved by chemical messengers that interact with the cell in one of two ways, either by entering the cell by diffusion through the cell membrane or by binding to a receptor on the plasma membrane.

Distribution in the Body

After crossing the transport barrier, a molecule remains in the interstitial spaces between cells, which are filled with water and loose connective tissue. The molecule can enter the bloodstream directly via blood capillaries or indirectly via lymphatic capillaries. The amount of the drug that may be found in various tissues is affected by many factors.

Solubility of the Drug

The greater the solubility of the drug in a tissue, the greater will be its concentration.

Size of the Organ

More drug is required to achieve therapeutic relevant concentrations in larger organs than in smaller organs.

Lymphatic Drainage

Lymphatic capillaries are minute vessels, located in the interstitial spaces, in which one end is closed and the other drains into larger lymphatic vessels. The walls of these capillaries are composed of endothelial tissue with loose junctions between cells, and as a result are more porous than blood capillaries. Plasma proteins and excess fluid in the interstitial spaces enter the lymphatic capillaries, flowing back to the heart via the lymphatic system.

Blood Flow to an Organ

The rate at which drugs move to the various tissues of the body depends largely on the rate of blood flow. In the average-size adult, the heart pumps approximately 5 liters of blood each minute, an amount roughly equal to the total volume of blood in the circulatory system. Thus, the entire blood volume circulates in the body about once every minute. Therefore, once a drug is absorbed into the bloodstream, it is rapidly distributed throughout the circulatory system.

Protein Binding

Some molecules reversibly bind to proteins present in the blood plasma. As proteins are too large to cross the capillary wall, such bound chemicals are confined in the bloodstream and not readily distributed to the tissues. Molecules bound to plasma proteins have lower concentrations in tissues than do those not bound to plasma proteins.

Anatomic Barriers

Barriers in certain organs limit the distribution of some molecules. The *blood-brain barrier* consists of tight capillary walls around which glial cells are wrapped, a situation unique to the capillaries in the brain. Molecules must diffuse through these two barriers to get from blood to the nerve cells of the brain.

The blood-brain barrier blocks the passage of proteins and most water-soluble chemicals, but water, most lipid-soluble molecules, oxygen, and carbon dioxide diffuse through it readily. It is slightly permeable by electrolytes, but is poorly permeable by large molecules. The blood-brain barrier is the reason behind the fact that the ions of some highly water-soluble metals, such as mercury and lead, are nontoxic to adult brains. However, because the blood-brain barrier is less well developed in children, their brains are more sensitive to the toxicity of lead.

Another barrier is the *blood-testis barrier*, which limits the passage of large molecules like proteins and polysaccharides, medium-sized molecules like galactose, and some water-soluble molecules from the blood into the seminiferous tubules of the testis. However, water and very small water-soluble molecules, like urea, can pass through the barrier.

Placenta membranes are unique. They separate two distinct human beings with different genetic compositions, physiological responses, and sensitivities to drugs. The fetus obtains essential nutrients and eliminates metabolic waste products through the placenta without help from its own organs, many of which are not yet functional.

This dependence of the fetus upon the mother, however, places the fetus at the mercy of the placenta when foreign substances appear in the mother's blood. The placental barrier between mother and fetus is the leakiest barrier of all and is a very poor block to chemicals. The placenta is composed of several layers of cells that act as a barrier to the diffusion of substances between the maternal and fetal circulatory systems. Lipid- and water-soluble molecules can cross readily, while the transfer of large-molecular-weight molecules is limited.

Biotransformation

The extent of pharmacological activity of a substance depends on the ability of the body to metabolize the chemical involved. This process is called *biotransformation*, defined as the structural modification of a chemical by enzymes in the body. Biotransformation occurs in several organs, including the kidneys, lungs, skin, intestines, placenta, and, most important, the liver. At the subcellular level, the enzymes responsible for biotransformation are located in the endoplasmic reticula, mitochondria, cytosol, lysosomes, or even the nuclear envelope or plasma membrane.

Chemicals absorbed in the gastrointestinal tract must pass through the liver, where they may be biotransformed and eliminated before they get distributed to other parts of the body. However, biotransformation is not synonymous with inactivation. Some drugs must be metabolized before they become active, whereas others produce a toxic metabolite, an additional active metabolite, or both. Intestinal microorganisms in the colon (the gut flora) are capable of many biotransformation reactions. In addition, molecules may be metabolized by gastric acid, digestive enzymes, or enzymes in the wall of the intestine.

Primary Objectives of Biotransformation

- To alter a chemical substance in order to change its biologic effects
- To transform the chemical into a more polar, and therefore more water-soluble, species that is more easily eliminated from the body

These reactions occur in the cytoplasm and endoplasmic reticula of all cells, although cells near major entry points for xenobiotic substances contain larger quantities of biotransformative enzymes. Biotransformation pathways may be grouped as either Phase I or Phase II reactions. In Phase I, the molecule is modified by the addition of a functional group. This modification allows Phase II, the conjugation or joining of the drug molecule with one found naturally in the body, to take place. In most cases, the major end product is a more water-soluble chemical that is easily excreted.

Phase I Reactions

These are reactions in which a functional chemical group is attached to the molecule, oxidizing or reducing it to another oxidation state. Such mechanisms are necessary to increase molecular polarity, which facilitates more efficient urinary excretion because the more lipophilic molecule can be reabsorbed in the renal tubules.

Oxidation

Oxidation is the addition of oxygen and/or the removal of hydrogen. Most oxidation steps occur in the endoplasmic reticulum. Common reactions include:

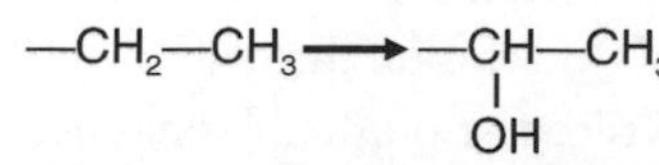

$$-CH_2-CH_3 \longrightarrow -\underset{\underset{OH}{|}}{CH}-CH_3$$

Fig. 9.3. Alkyl group into an alcohol

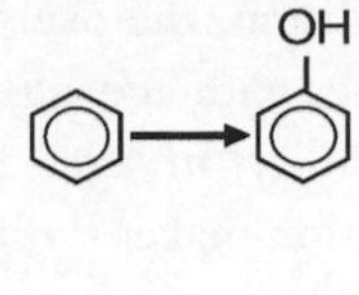

Fig. 9.4. Aromatic ring into a phenol

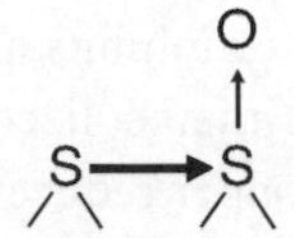

Fig. 9.5. Oxidation at S or N

Reduction

Reduction reactions involve the addition of hydrogen and/or the removal of oxygen. For example, azo (-N = N-) or nitro groups ($-NO_2$) are converted to amines ($-NH_2$) through reduction.

Hydrolysis

Hydrolysis describes an addition of water facilitated by enzymatic action, which causes the breakdown of a molecule.

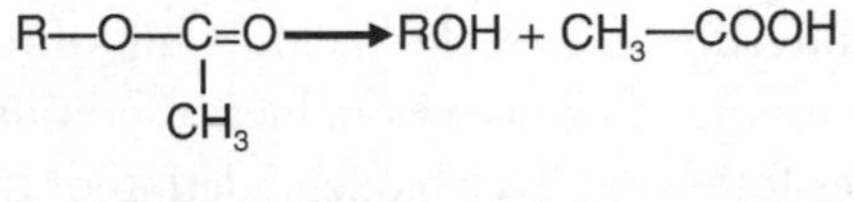

Fig. 9.6. Esters into an alcohol and an acid

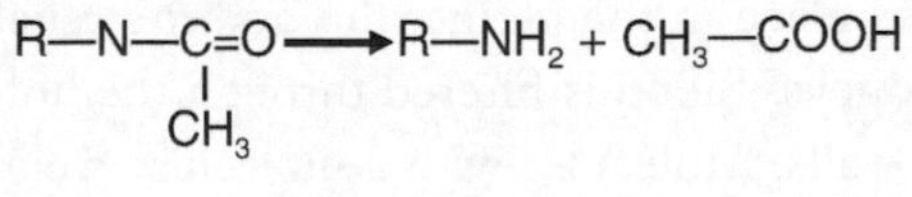

Fig. 9.7. Amides to an amine and an acid

Phase II

Phase II reactions, also known as *conjugation reactions*, increase the size and weight of a molecule by adding a chemical group. Several enzyme systems catalyze Phase II reactions, including:

- Glucuronyl transferase
- Glutathione-*S*-transferase
- *N*-acetyltransferase
- Sulfotransferase

Conjugation reactions bind the exogenous chemical with an endogenous molecule, leading to the formation

of a final product that is usually more water-soluble and thus more easily excreted. These reactions involve the addition of molecules naturally present in the body to the drug molecule, which may first have undergone a Phase I reaction.

The Cytochrome P_{450} Enzyme System

Cytochrome P_{450} enzymes comprise the most important enzyme system for drug biotransformation and metabolism. Interactions between a drug and the enzymes that metabolize it largely determine whether that drug will be active, ineffective, toxic, or carcinogenic.

Cytochrome P_{450} enzymes catalyze most Phase I metabolism, which transforms lipophilic molecules to more polar compounds that can be excreted by the kidneys.[44] The metabolites are usually less active than the parent compound, although some drugs must undergo biotransformation in order to become pharmacologically active agents. In some cases, the metabolites are toxic.

The cytochrome P_{450} system is made up of a family of very versatile enzymes responsible for catalyzing a range of different reactions. A single hepatocyte can contain a variety of cytochrome P_{450} enzymes. An individual enzyme may be capable of metabolizing many different drugs, but one specific enzyme may be required to metabolize a particular drug.

Reactions Catalyzed by Cytochrome P_{450} Enzymes
- Oxidative reactions
- Hydrolysis of esters and amides
- Reduction reactions
- Conjugation reactions

At least twelve cytochrome P_{450} gene families have been identified in humans, although three particular families are responsible for the majority of drug biotransformations. These are the cytochrome P_{450} 1, 2, and 3 families (CYP_1, CYP_2, and CYP_3).[45] These groupings are based on amino acid sequence similarities, and can be further separated into subfamilies.

Variability in the Cytochrome P_{450} System

This system can be altered by a number of mechanisms, and the efficiency of the system varies significantly among individuals, leading to variability in both the efficacy and the toxicity of drugs. Induction and inhibition of P_{450} enzymes are the most common causes of variability. Induction increases the rate of biotransformation, thus decreasing drug concentration and pharmacological effect.

Inhibition of cytochrome P_{450} enzymes results in an increased concentration of the drug, prolonged pharmacological effects, and increased incidence of drug-induced toxicity.

Drugs can bind irreversibly or reversibly with the heme-binding site of the enzyme and thus inhibit other drugs from binding. Irreversible (or mechanism-based) inhibition occurs when drugs are metabolized by the cytochrome P_{450} system to active metabolites that bind to the enzyme and cause irreversible loss of function.[46] Activity can be restored only through the synthesis of new enzymes, which may take several days.

Irreversible inhibitors are bound to enzymes by covalent bonds. Reversible inhibitors are bound to enzymes by weaker, noncovalent forces. Herbs have been shown to possess both reversible and irreversible enzyme inhibition properties. Extracts of *Fraxinus excelsior, Populus tremula*, and *Solidago virgaurea* in a combination of 1:3:1 (v/v/v) were found to have actions similar to those of a variety of synthetic nonsteroidal anti-inflammatory drugs because they reversibly inhibit dihydrofolate reductase.[47]

Genetic Polymorphisms

Genetic polymorphisms commonly cause variations in biotransformation. A *polymorphism* is the presence within a population of at least two groups of people with distinctly different abilities to metabolize drugs.[48] Individuals can be characterized as extensive (rapid) or poor (slow) metabolizers. Poor metabolizers often have an increased incidence of adverse effects.

Pathology

A disease state may alter metabolism by modifying absorption, distribution, and/or excretion; altering nutritional states; or changing the rate of blood and oxygen delivery to the liver, among other factors. Impaired liver function decreases biotransformation. Pathologies that impair liver function include hepatitis, alcoholic liver disease, biliary cirrhosis, and hepatocarcinoma. Diabetes has a mixed effect, either increasing or decreasing metabolism depending on the individual. Infection may also alter biotransformation. Phagocytosis, which occurs during bacterial infections, releases a factor that depresses biotransformation in adjacent hepatocytes.[49]

Age

Infants do not develop a competent P_{450} system for more than two weeks after birth. The elderly have age-related decreases in liver mass, hepatic enzyme activity, and hepatic blood flow. In addition, the overall metabolic capacity of the liver decreases with age, although the considerable individual variability in age- and disease-related changes in organ function makes it difficult to generalize.

Nutrition

A low-protein diet decreases xenobiotic metabolism, while fasting enhances or inhibits metabolism, depending on the chemical to be metabolized. Deficiencies of calcium, zinc, iron, and copper reduce metabolism, as do deficiencies of vitamins C, A, and E. Hormone levels also have an impact. Adrenocorticotropic and growth hormones increase metabolism. Metabolism is enhanced by thyroxine and decreased by thyroidectomy. Both glucocorticoids and anabolic steroids enhance metabolism.

Excretion and the Termination of Drug Action

Potential damage from a chemical is minimized by excretion, biotransformation, or both. The main routes through which drugs leave the body are the kidneys, the lungs, and the bile. Excretion through the lungs occurs only with highly volatile or gaseous agents, such as general anesthetics, and, in small amounts, alcohol and garlic oils. Drugs that are passed through the bile and into the intestine are usually reabsorbed into the bloodstream from the intestine. Thus, the major route of drug elimination from the body is via kidney excretion of drug metabolites following liver biodegradation of the drug.

Elimination by the Kidneys and Liver

Urinary excretion, the most common pathway of elimination, takes place in the glomerulus and the renal tubules of the kidneys. Blood is filtered through the holes in the capillary walls. Molecules with a molecular weight lower than 60,000 end up in the filtrate, while red blood cells, large proteins, and chemicals bound to plasma proteins are not filtered.

Chemical exchange also takes place along the renal tubule. As the filtrate flows down the renal tubule, essential molecules, such as amino acids and glucose, are reabsorbed by active transport in the first portion of the tubule (the proximal tubule). Chemicals in the filtrate are also reabsorbed by active transport if they resemble these essential molecules. Lipid-soluble chemicals are reabsorbed in the renal tubule, and so only water-soluble chemicals are excreted to a significant extent.

Because drugs are small particles, they are filtered into the kidneys and then reabsorbed into the bloodstream. As the drug is concentrated inside the nephrons (a result of water reabsorption), the drugs are reabsorbed into plasma. Thus, the kidneys alone cannot eliminate drugs from the body. Some other mechanism must overcome this process of drug reabsorption. This occurs through the process of hepatic biotransformation, in which fat-soluble molecules are converted into water-soluble metabolites that are poorly reabsorbed once they are filtered into the renal tubules.

The second major excretory route is via bile, which is formed in the liver and flows into the intestinal tract. The liver does not filter chemicals, but secretes them into bile for eventual elimination in the feces. However, biliary excretion of a chemical does not necessarily result in its elimination from the body. Chemicals in the bile may be reabsorbed by the intestine and in turn reenter the liver via the portal vein. This cycling of a chemical (the *enterohepatic cycle*) can continue for a long time, keeping the chemical in the body.

Other Routes of Elimination

Excretion of drugs into sweat, saliva, and tears is small. Elimination by these routes is dependent mainly upon diffusion of the nonionized, lipid-soluble form of drugs through the epithelial cells of the glands; it is also pH dependent. Reabsorption of nonionized drugs from the primary secretion probably also occurs in the ducts of the glands, and active secretion of drugs across these ducts may also occur.

The composition of sweat is similar to that of plasma, except that sweat does not contain proteins. Sweat is a filtrate of plasma containing electrolytes and metabolic wastes. After secretion, it moves through the sweat ducts, where salt and water are reabsorbed. Because sweat resembles plasma, water-soluble chemicals, including some drugs and metal ions, can be found in sweat. However, sweat is not a major route of excretion.

Drugs excreted in the saliva enter the mouth, where they are usually swallowed. The concentration of some drugs in saliva parallels that in plasma. Saliva may therefore be a useful biological fluid with which to determine drug concentrations when it is difficult or inconvenient to obtain blood. Excretion of drugs into hair and skin is minimal.

Breast milk is a potential route of excretion, but, more important, it is a potential means of chemical exposure for breast-fed infants. Most chemicals enter milk by diffusion, and so only the nonionized, lipid-soluble forms of organic chemicals are found to any significant extent. Chemicals with a molecular weight less than 200 that are present in plasma unbound to proteins are likely to be found in milk. Because of the lipid content, highly lipid-soluble chemicals may concentrate in milk. Therefore, milk can be a significant route of excretion for highly lipid-soluble chemicals in lactating women.

Variability in Responses to Drugs

Even healthy people may show large variations in their abilities to absorb and metabolize drugs, leading to variable outcomes in different individuals. The way a drug affects an individual may be influenced by age, sex, body weight, temperament, race, the environment, the presence of the drug or other drugs, and other (often unpredictable) factors, including diurnal cycles, temperature, pregnancy, menstruation, and disease.

There may be little relation between an individual's sensitivity to the desired effects of a drug and sensitivity to the toxicity of a drug. A combination of substances may result in *synergy*, in which the total effect is greater than the sum of the combination, or *antagonism*, in which the total effect is less than the sum of the combined effects. Other factors include prior hypersensitivity to this or a related drug and any tolerance developed through prior exposure to the drug.

Tachyphylaxis

Tachyphylaxis indicates a rapid development of tolerance to the action of a drug. For example, tyramine produces its effect indirectly, by causing the release of stored catecholamines that have biologic activity; as soon as endogenous stores of catecholamines are depleted, however, the drug no longer has an effect.

Drug Disposition Tolerance

Drug disposition tolerance is a tolerance that develops because of increased metabolism of the drug. This type of tolerance is characterized by a faster-than-normal drop in blood levels of the drug after a given dose, indicating a decreased half-life for blood levels of the drug.

Desensitization

An additional complication is *desensitization*, a phenomenon in which an initial application of a high concentration of an agonist serves to depress the effect of that agonist upon subsequent administration. The specific mechanism involved varies with drug and receptor, but would suggest that the occurrence of some temporary chemical or conformational change subsequently blocks receptor response.

Pharmacodynamic Tolerance

Pharmacodynamic tolerance indicates desensitization to a drug that causes changes in a particular drug-induced body function. This type of tolerance is characterized by decreased action or lowered potency of the drug at any given serum concentration.

PHARMACOLOGICAL ACTIONS

Pharmacological research into the activity of herbs and their constituents is taking place all over the world. In the following sections, we will review research on some important herbal actions. This is far from a comprehensive review of modern herbal research; rather, these are examples meant to serve as insights into the research endeavor.

IMMUNOMODULATORS

A wide range of plants and phytochemicals appears to impact the functioning of the immune system. There is still far too little research in this area to allow broad generalization, but this should not be taken to mean that the herbs themselves lack value as immunomodulatory agents.

In a comprehensive review, Wagner and Proksch grouped identified immunostimulant constituents according to whether they are high- or low-molecular-weight compounds.[50]

Low-Molecular-Weight Compounds

A range of low-molecular-weight plant constituents have been shown to be immunomodulators. Because of their diverse chemistry, a similar diversity of mechanisms is probably involved.

Alkaloids and Other Nitrogen-Containing Compounds

A number of these compounds demonstrate immunological activity of some kind. However, the effects described by the umbrella term *immunomodulation* are generally subtle, and on the whole, bioactive alkaloids are not subtle! An example is aristolochic acid from serpentary or birthwort *(Aristolochia clematitis)*, which shows anti-inflammatory, antifertilty, and antimicrobial activity, but can be carcinogenic to mammals.

Terpenes

Important sesquiterpene immunostimulants include helenalin and tenulin, found in species of *Helenium*, and eupahyssopin from *Eupatorium hyssopifolium*. Many saponins, especially triterpenes, are considered *immunoadjuvants* and are used as such in Japan, either in the form of the plant source or as the extracted chemical.

Phenolics

A number of phenolic molecules demonstrate immunological effects. The simple phenolic acids are ubiquitous among flowering plants, fruits, and vegetables. Ferulic acid, named after asafoetida *(Ferula foetida)*, increases phagocytosis in mice. Anethol, found in aniseed oil *(Pimpinella anisum)*, increases the leukocyte count in the blood; the widely found pseudotannin catechol stimulates granulocytes. The more complex lignans, with a range of effects including stimulation of phagocytic activity in polymorphonuclear granulocytes, cytotoxicity, and induction of interferon, are also proving to be important.

Flavonoids

The flavonoids, a subgroup of plant phenolics, have been shown to possess immunomodulatory activity. This may be due to their antioxidant or free radical–scavenging

Lack of Evidence or Lack of Research?

All too often, a lack of research is taken to mean that the herb in question lacks activity. This is self-evidently absurd. The studies undertaken by Asian scientists to investigate the pharmacology of their traditional remedies are contributing greatly to the field of immunology. However, the same attention is rarely given to traditional European or North American herbs. This is because of a lack of research funding, not because the plants themselves lack inherent value. Perhaps if nettles *(Urtica dioica)* were given the same quality of attention garnered by *Astragalus,* we might have the immunological "proof" we need to draw conclusions about its profound effects.

properties. In addition, the oligomeric procyanidins possess immunological activity.

High-Molecular-Weight Compounds

High-molecular-weight lectins (glycoproteins) and polysaccharides are important immunomodulators. It has been suggested that their impact is predicated upon some interaction with the membranes of immunocompetent cells.

Lectins

These are sugar-binding, carbohydrate-specific proteins that agglutinate some cells, such as erythrocytes, and precipitate some molecules. When originally found in plants, they were called *phytohemagglutinins*; however, they have since been found in bacteria, fungi, invertebrates, and vertebrates. Some well-known plant toxins are lectins, such as ricin from castor bean *(Ricinus communis)*.

A range of lectin effects has been demonstrated in the laboratory, including stimulation of lymphocyte mitosis, inhibition of protein synthesis in bacteria, and agglutination of malignant cells by tumor-specific lectins. Lectin-containing plants familiar to the herbalist are poke *(Phytolacca americana)* and mistletoe *(Viscum album)*. Research shows that the well-known North American antimicrobial plant wild indigo *(Baptisia tinctoria)* contains active glycoproteins.[51]

Polysaccharides

Polysaccharides are often pivotal to the immunomodulating effects of herbs. Laboratory studies have revealed a range of impressive results:

- General improvement of many immune-response measures
- T-lymphocyte activation
- Antitumor activity
- Increase in certain serum proteins
- Nonspecific activation of the complement system
- Stimulation of interferon production
- Increased phagocytosis

An important group of active polysaccharides is the mycopolysaccharides found in medicinal fungi. Their principal bioactive substances are believed to be the β-D-glucans, usually simply called β-glucans. These are indigestible polysaccharides found in grains, yeast, bacteria, algae, and fungi. It is likely that the activities of the mycopolysaccharides depend on chemical characteristics such as their molecular weight, branching patterns, solubility in water, and tertiary structure.

Edible mushrooms rich in β-glucans include shiitake *(Lentinus edodes)*, maitake *(Grifola frondosa)*, himematsutake *(Agaricus blazei)*, button mushrooms *(Schizophyllum commune* and *Sclerotina sclerotiorum)*, wood ear *(Auricularia auricula)*, tremella *(Tremella fuciformis)*, poria *(Wolfporia cocos)*, and enoki *(Flammulina velutipes)*. Huitlacoche *(Ustilago maydis)* is another edible fungus that is also rich in β-glucans. Nonedible mushrooms rich in β-glucans include reishi *(Ganoderma lucidum)* and the coriolus mushroom *(Coriolus versicolor)*.

The most studied mushroom β-glucans are lentinan, from *Lentinus edodes;* grifolan, from *Grifola frondosa;* schizophyllan, from *Schizophyllum commune;* sclerotan, from *Sclerotinia sclerotiorum;* and polysaccharide krestin and polysaccharide peptide, from *Coriolus versicolor.*[52] Lentinan and schizophyllan are approved in Japan for the treatment of cancer.

Based upon in vitro, in vivo, and some human studies, the mycopolysaccharides appear to have immunomodulatory, antitumor, antimicrobial, lipid-lowering, and glucose-regulating properties. However, after ingestion, there is virtually no digestion of β-glucans in the small intestine, as there are no β-glucosidases among the digestive enzymes. These enzymes are essential for the metabolism of the β-glucans.

Some digestion of myco-β-glucans may occur in the small intestine, and some digestion takes place in the large intestine via the action of bacterial β-glucans. Some oligosaccharides that are produced via bacterial β-glucosidases may be absorbed, as may a large percentage of the ingested myco-β-glucosidases. However, a large percentage of ingested myco-β-glucans is excreted in the feces.

Lentinan is a particularly well-studied β-glucan that demonstrates a range of properties, including antitumor activity. However, lentinan is typically administered parenterally and appears to show little antitumor activity after oral administration. In studies, parenterally administered lentinan has demonstrated various immunomodulatory activities. It stimulated macrophages, monocytes, and neutrophils, as well as natural killer (NK) and lymphokine-activated killer (LAK) cells.[53] Stimulation of these cells by lentinan may release a number of different cytokines, including tumor necrosis factor (TNF), and interleukin 2 α and 6 α (IL 2 α and IL 6 α). Lentinan may also stimulate the production of nitric oxide (NO) in macrophages. These effects may result in antimicrobial and antitumor activities. Grifolan, schizophyllan, and sclerotan have been shown to have similar effects when used parenterally.

The possible immunomodulatory effects of orally

administered mushroom β-glucans remain unclear. They may exert immunological actions by virtue of their interaction with gut-associated lymphoid tissue (GALT). When activated by contact with mushroom or other β-glucans in the gut, immune cells associated with GALT may migrate to other tissues and exert immunomodulatory effects there. In addition, substances in mushrooms other than β-glucans may have immunomodulatory activities.[54] In any case, the possible antitumor and antimicrobial activities of the myco-β-glucans are thought to be accounted for, in large part, by their immunomodulatory properties.[55]

The mycopolysaccharides may have anticarcinogenic, immune-modulating, antimicrobial, anti-inflammatory, cardioprotective, hepatoprotective, nephroprotective, hypoglycemic, and anticaries effects.[56] For species-specific findings, please see the references cited above, but for examples, consider the herbs listed in table 9.2. Sources are listed in Wagner and Proksch.[57]

Table 9.2. Influence of Polysaccharide Fractions on Phagocytosis

HERB	ENHANCEMENT OF PHAGOCYTOSIS
Arnica montana	44%
Echinacea purpurea	45%
Eleutherococcus senticosus	52%
Eupatorium cannabinum	22%
E. perfoliatum	37%
Matricaria recutita	31%
Serenoa repens	36%

INFLAMMATION AND ANTI-INFLAMMATORY AGENTS

Inflammation is the complex response of living, vascularized tissue to injury. Inflammation is a classic "double-edged sword" that is essential for life and preservation of function, but also causes significant tissue damage and loss of function. The inflammatory response is triggered whenever tissues are injured. The cardinal signs of acute inflammation are redness (erythema), swelling (edema), pain, and heat; the word itself is derived from the root *inflamm*, meaning "to set on fire." Inflammation prevents the spread of damaging agents to nearby tissues, disposes of cell debris and pathogens, and initiates the tissue repair processes. It is nonspecific, occurring in response to many different causes.

Inflammation is initiated by the release of chemical mediators into the extracellular fluid. Sources of these mediators include injured tissue cells, phagocytes, lymphocytes, mast cells, and blood proteins, the most important of which are histamine, kinins, prostaglandins, complement, and lymphokines. They are all vasodilators, and as blood flow to the area increases, local blood congestion occurs, accounting for the redness and heat.

These mediators also increase capillary permeability, so that an exudate containing proteins, such as clotting factors and antibodies, seeps from the bloodstream to the interstitial fluid. This exudate causes local edema, which in turn presses on adjacent nerve endings, causing pain. (Other sources of pain include the release of bacterial toxins, lack of nutrition to injured cells, and hypersensitivity caused by the release of prostaglandins and kinins.)

Edema dilutes any harmful substances present, increases oxygenation, supplies nutrients necessary for healing, and facilitates the entry of clotting proteins. These form a fibrin mesh in the interstitial spaces that isolates the injured tissue, prevents the spread of harmful agents, and also forms a matrix for tissue repair.

After the initiation of the inflammatory response, phagocytic white blood cells, neutrophils, and macrophages migrate to the area. If pathogens are present, complement is activated and lymphocytes and antibodies invade the injured site, mounting an immune response. Leukocytosis is a characteristic sign of inflammation. Leukocytosis-inducing factors released by injured cells promote a rapid release of neutrophils from bone marrow, and the number of neutrophils in the bloodstream increases four- to fivefold. Neutrophils usually migrate randomly, but are attracted to inflammatory chemicals, termed *chemotactic* agents, at the site of the injury.

The outpouring of fluid from the blood into the injured area slows blood flow in the region, and neutrophils begin to cling to the inner walls of the capillaries, a phenomenon known as *margination* or *pavementing*. Neutrophils squeeze through the capillary walls, moving toward the site of inflammation, and within an hour of initiation of the inflammatory response, neutrophils are active at the injury site. Neutrophils are followed by monocytes entering from the bloodstream. Monocytes are poor phagocytes, but within 8 to 12 hours after entering the tissues, they swell, develop large numbers of lysosomes, and become macrophages. Macrophages, which predominate at sites of chronic inflammation, facilitate the final disposal of cell debris as acute inflammation subsides.

A creamy, yellow pus may accumulate in the wound. This is a mixture of dead or dying neutrophils, dead tissue cells, and living and dead pathogens. If the inflammatory mechanism fails to clear the area of debris, the sac of pus may be walled off by collagen fibers to form an abscess. Surgical drainage of the abscess may be necessary before healing can occur.

Mediators of Inflammation

Many symptoms associated with disease are caused not directly by a pathogen, but rather by the body's response to the pathogen or by the release of chemical mediators. This class of substances encompasses a wide range of compounds, produced by many different tissues, that have profound pharmacological effects in very small quantities.

Vasoactive Amines

Produced by mast cells, basophils, and platelets, vasoactive amines are stored ready for release and act via histamine receptors. Vascular smooth muscle is particularly responsive in tissues that are subject to allergic responses. Histamine possesses immediate but transient effects that promote vasodilation of arterioles and increased permeability of capillaries, thus permitting the formation of exudate.

There are three major types of vasoactive amines.

- H1 increases vascular permeability, contraction of smooth muscle, pulmonary vasoconstriction, chemokinesis of leukocytes, and prostaglandin production in the lungs.
- H2 promotes gastric and mucous secretions, elevates cAMP levels, increases chemokinesis of leukocytes, and activates suppressor T cells.
- H3 inhibits the synthesis and release of histamine.

Procyanidins from *Hypericum perforatum* antagonize histamine-induced arterial contractions.[58] Inhibition of cellular phosphodiesterase might be involved in the underlying mechanism of action. In addition to its role as a neurotransmitter, serotonin (5-hydroxytryptamine) is present in platelets and is released after platelet aggregation. It has inflammatory properties similar to those of histamine.

Complement and Complement Fragments

The complement system is made up of 20 proteins and their cleavage products, all of which are found in blood plasma. (These cleavage products are proteins designated as C1 through C8 and factors B, D, and P.) They lead to lysis of microbes, but also play a role in inflammation by increasing vascular permeability and vasodilation; enhancing leukocyte adhesion, chemotaxis, and activation; and promoting phagocytosis.

The complement pathway can be activated in two ways, by either classic or alternate pathways. The classic pathway is initiated by the binding of an antigen-antibody complex to the C1 fragment, whereas the alternate pathway is directly activated by bacterial endotoxins, complex polysaccharides, or aggregated globulins.

Kinins

Kinins are highly bioactive peptides found in the pancreas and a variety of other body tissues. (The word *kinin* comes from the Greek *kallikreas*, meaning "pancreas.") The two primary groups of kinins, kallidin and bradykinin, are derived from precursors called *kininogens*. They can cause vasodilation of small arteries, but tend to constrict large arteries and most veins regardless of size. They also increase capillary permeability, edema, and bronchial and intestinal smooth muscle contractions. Kinins are powerful pain producers; their release may have a role in the pathophysiology of migraines.

Arachidonic Acid Metabolites (Eicosanoids)

Because they are derived from the polyunsaturated eicosanoic (C_{20}) fatty acid known as arachidonic acid, these compounds—thromboxanes, prostaglandins, epoxygenases, leukotrienes, and lipoxins—are collectively known as *eicosanoids*.

The eicosanoids are local mediators of receptor-dependent events in a range of physiologic processes and in a diverse group of human pathologies, including bronchial asthma, inflammation, and coronary disease. Arachidonic acid is derived from animal fats or through conversion of linoleic acid from plants. It is bound to cell membrane phospholipids and released by the action of cellular phospholipases, which are activated by mechanical, chemical, and physical stimuli.

Platelet-Activating Factors

Platelet-activating factors (PAF) have a remarkably broad range of effects throughout the body. They are produced in response to specific stimuli by a variety of cell types, including neutrophils, basophils, platelets, and endothelial cells. Several molecular types of PAF have been identified. They cause platelet aggregation, release of vasoactive amines (histamine and serotonin), vasoconstriction, bronchoconstriction, vasodilation (at low concentrations), enhanced venule permeability, increased leukocyte adhesion to endothelia, and leukocyte chemotaxis.

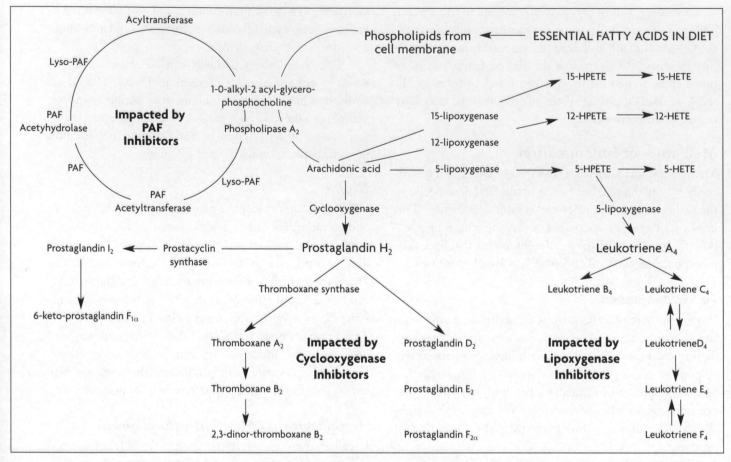

Fig. 9.8. The inflammation cascade

They also stimulate the synthesis of prostaglandins and leukotrienes.

Oxygen-Derived Free Radicals

Reactive oxygen metabolites are released from neutrophils and macrophages after exposure to chemotactic agents, immune complexes, or a phagocytic challenge. Their release leads to endothelial cell damage and increased vascular permeability. These reactive oxygen metabolites are inactivated by serum antioxidants, such as superoxide dismutase (SOD).

Nitric Oxide

Nitric oxide (NO) is a soluble free radical gas generated by nitric oxide synthases. NO relaxes vascular smooth muscle, leading to vasodilation. Nitric oxide interacts with superoxide anions to produce potent peroxynitrite ions that cause oxidative damage. As nitric oxide and peroxynitrite are bactericidal, the ability of macrophages to produce NO is important in their ability to defend against some infections. Epigallocatechin-3-gallate, a catechin contained in green tea, reduces NO production.[59]

Cytokines

Inflammatory responses are coordinated by cytokines derived from various leukocytes and tissue cells. These polypeptides function as "cellular hormones" or locally acting cell-to-cell mediators that participate in intricate networks in order to achieve their effects. Some elicit early permeability changes in microvasculature, but most are involved in coordinating the activities of cells essential to inflammation and repair, including chemoattraction, activation, secretion, phagocytosis, and proliferative actions. As examples of the significance of cytokines, consider the pro-inflammatory cytokines interleukin 1 and tumor necrosis factor (TNF).

Interleukin 1 (IL1)

- Activates prostaglandin production in the hypothalamus
- Mediates pain and fever
- Potently activates mast cells, T cells, and endothelia
- Induces hepatic acute phase protein secretion
- Induces endothelial surface adhesion molecules for leukocytes
- Induces chemokines for leukocyte recruitment

- Induces NO generation by macrophages
- Produces microvascular injury and hypotensive effects

Tumor Necrosis Factor (TNF)
- Exerts effects similar to those of interleukin 1 and acts synergistically with it

- Stimulates a variety of cells, including endothelial cells
- Induces synthesis of cell adhesion molecules
- Induces creation of gaps between endothelial cells
- Induces synthesis and release of prostacyclin I_2 (PGI_2) and PAF
- Increases thrombogenesis in endothelia

Pathways of Arachidonic Acid Metabolism

Arachidonic acid is metabolized via two metabolic pathways.

Cyclooxygenase Pathway

Cyclooxygenase converts arachidonic acid into prostaglandin intermediates, which in turn lead to the formation of prostaglandins, prostacyclin, and thromboxanes. *Prostaglandins* are lipids first isolated from prostate secretions in seminal fluid. *Prostacyclin* and *thromboxanes* are related substances derived from the same intermediate compound. These compounds are produced by most tissues of the body, but are found primarily in the brain, gastrointestinal tract, kidney, lung, pancreas, uterus, and human menstrual blood. Nonsteroidal anti-inflammatory drugs (NSAIDs) inhibit all products of the cyclooxygenase pathway. Prostaglandins are divided into groups designated D_1, D_2, E_1, E_2, and so on, on the basis of their ring structures.

- *Thromboxane A_2:* Produced by platelets, thromboxane A_2 is essential for platelet aggregation and functions as a vasoconstrictor.
- *Prostaglandin D_2:* This prostaglandin constricts the pulmonary veins but dilates renal vasculature.
- *Prostaglandin E_2:* This is a potent vasodilator that lowers blood pressure. It generates fever, causes pain by sensitizing nerve endings, and exerts cytoprotective effects in the gastric mucosa. It is also a bronchodilator. Prostaglandin E_2 increases luteal progesterone secretion; it constricts the muscles of the pregnant uterus, but relaxes the nonpregnant uterus.
- *Prostacyclin:* This prostaglandin intermediate is released by vascular endothelial cells and exerts its influence via cAMP. It inhibits platelet aggregation, elicits vasodilation, and antagonizes the effects of thromboxane A_2.

Isozymes, or isoenzymes, are chemically distinct forms of an enzyme that perform the same biochemical function. Two isozymes of cyclooxygenase are known.

- COX-1: Constitutive cyclooxygenase is found in a variety of tissues, including the stomach mucosa.
- COX-2: Inducible cyclooxygenase is released from inflammatory cells only during the inflammatory response. Glucocorticoids block the induction of this enzyme.

Lipoxygenase Pathway

Lipoxygenase metabolizes arachidonic acid into compounds that are the basis of leukotrienes. Leukotrienes are mediators derived from arachidonic acid through a different pathway than that used in prostaglandin synthesis. A number of plant anti-inflammatory agents appear to work this way.[60] They are released primarily by anaphylactic mechanisms from mast cells and other inflammatory cells, especially in the lung. Like prostaglandins, leukotrienes are synthesized as needed.

NSAIDs inhibit the cyclooxygenase but not the lipoxygenase pathway. Their use may, therefore, lead to increased or preferential synthesis of leukotrienes, which could be the basis for the condition known as aspirin-induced asthma.

- Induces systemic effects of inflammation, such as fever
- Contributes to the hypotension of septic shock

New technology has allowed for detailed studies on the interactions of herbs with cytokines. In a study investigating the immunomodulating and antitumor effects of saponins from *Solidago virgaurea*, the compounds demonstrated mitogenic effects on murine spleen and thymus cells, as well on human mononuclear cells in vitro. Mice treated with virgaureasaponin E showed phagocytosis of bone marrow cells and proliferation of spleen and bone marrow cells. In addition, TNF-α concentration in blood increased in treated mice, compared with the control group.[61]

In another in vitro study, levels of IL1 and TNF produced by cultured rat Kupffer's cells were increased in the presence of an extract of *Cordyceps sinensis*.[62] Polysaccharides from *Panax notoginseng* induced the production of a significant amount of TNF-α in cell cultures.[63] The lectin known as *Viscum album* agglutinin-I induced expression of interleukin 1 α, interleukin 1 β, interleukin 6, TNF-α, interferon-γ, granulocyte-monocyte colony stimulating factor, and interleukin 10 genes.[64]

Cell Adhesion Molecules

A number of membrane glycoproteins promote cell attachment and participate in the inflammatory response. Lectin cell adhesion molecules, or *selectins*, are expressed on the surface of endothelia, leukocytes, and platelets. They influence leukocyte-endothelial adhesion at sites of inflammation. *Integrins* are adhesion molecules involved in regulation of cell-matrix and cell-cell adhesion. They are transmembrane in structure, thus linking or "integrating" exterior or surface stimuli to the internal cell cytoskeleton. Baicalein, a flavonoid from *Scutellaria baicalensis*, inhibited interleukin 1 β and TNF-α and induced endothelial leukocyte adhesion molecule-1 (ELAM-1) and intercellular adhesion molecule-1 (ICAM-1) expressions.[65]

Interferon

Lacking the cellular machinery to synthesize proteins, viruses invade cells and take over metabolic processes in order to reproduce themselves. The infected cells help protect uninfected cells by secreting small proteins called interferons. Interferon molecules diffuse to nearby cells, stimulating synthesis of other proteins that inhibit or interfere with viral replication in those cells. The protection conferred by interferons is not virus specific, but rather host specific. Thus, mouse interferons have little or no antiviral activity in humans.

Interferon is a group of proteins, each of which has different physiological effects. Lymphocytes secrete interferon-γ, but most other leukocytes produce interferon-α. In addition to being antiviral, all interferons activate macrophages, and interferon-γ mobilizes natural killer cells.

While macrophages and natural killer cells act directly against malignant cells, interferons are assumed to have some anticancer role. In a study, mistletoe extract, derived from *Viscum album* grown on pine trees, stimulated peripheral mononuclear cells in blood from healthy donors. An increase of interferon-γ and interleukin 2 was also observed.[66]

ANTI-INFLAMMATORY AGENTS

As can be seen from the brief discussion above, the term *inflammation* covers a complex series of reparative and protective responses to tissue injury, whether caused by infection, autoimmune stimuli, or mechanical injury. Anti-inflammatory substances must address similar mechanisms, but compounds differ in their specific mechanisms of activity because their actions focus upon different inflammatory mediators.

Currently used anti-inflammatory agents, such as NSAIDs, inhibit cyclooxygenase and therefore prostaglandin synthesis. These also have antipyretic activity, since prostaglandins are implicated in the mediation of fever. Free radical–scavenging agents also play a role in inflammation, because liberation of such radicals damages tissue during the inflammatory process. Flavonoids and other phenolics are thought to act by preventing either the generation or the action of free radicals. Studies have shown that quercetin inhibits the action of lipoxygenase on arachidonic acid, the release of histamine from mast cells and basophils, and the generation of superoxide anion.

Phospholipid-Derived Inflammatory Mediators as Biological Targets

The level of free arachidonic acid at the site of inflammation is regulated by phospholipases, which hydrolyze phospholipids, but also by re-esterification catalyzed by acyl-CoA transferases. The released arachidonic acid may be metabolized oxidatively by several different enzymatic routes.

Prostaglandin endoperoxide synthases catalyze the production of prostaglandin endoperoxides, which can be converted to prostaglandins, thromboxanes, and prostacyclin. These inflammatory mediators are completely or partially responsible for increased blood vessel permeability, dilation of vessels, chemotaxis of granulocytes, degradation of cartilage, and proliferation of B- and T-lymphocytes. Arachidonic acid is further metabolized by monooxygenases to hydroxy acids and epoxides.

The three main groups of lipoxygenases (15-, 12-, and 5-lipoxygenases) specifically introduce molecular oxygen into arachidonic acid and form the hydroperoxy acids. 5-lipoxygenase also converts 5-hydroperoxy acid to leukotriene A_4, an intermediate in the biosynthesis of leukotrienes and lipoxins. The leukotrienes are very potent inducers of granulocyte chemotaxis and are involved in inflammatory conditions such as asthma.

Upon hydrolysis of membrane-bound phospholipids by phospholipase A2 (PLA2), lysophospholipids are liberated, forming the precursor to yet another inflammatory mediator, PAF. At the cellular level, PAF causes contraction of smooth muscle and an increase in vascular permeability and platelet aggregation. It also stimulates *exocytosis* in both platelets and leukocytes, the secretory process by which substances contained in vesicles are discharged from cells by a fusion of the vesicle membrane with the cell membrane.

Nonsteroidal substances with different biosynthetic origins have been isolated from plants and shown to demonstrate inhibitory activity against the target enzymes cyclooxygenase and 5-lipoxygenase. The most potent cyclooxygenase inhibitors are found among the flavonoids, phenolic phenylpropane derivatives, naphthoquinones, alkylamides, diaryl heptane derivatives, and tannins.

Among several classes of 5-lipoxygenase inhibitors, a number of substances with antioxidant properties have been described, the most dominant of which are phenolic substances with catechol structures. Another group consists of arachidonic acid analogs and substances related to long-chain unsaturated fatty acids.

Many potent natural products belonging to different subclasses have been shown to affect PAF, including the neolignan kadsurenone, the diterpene group of ginkgolides, and the sesquiterpene manoalide.[67]

CANCER AND PLANT CONSTITUENTS

Cancer is a term applied to malignant diseases that affect many different parts of the body. These diseases are characterized by a rapid and uncontrolled formation of abnormal cells, which may mass together to form a growth or tumor, or proliferate throughout the body, initiating abnormal growth at other sites. If the process is not ar-

---

Natural Products with Influence on Phospholipid-Derived Mediators

Cyclooxygenase Inhibitors
- Flavonoids
- Phenolic phenylpropane derivatives
- Naphthoquinones
- Alkyl amides
- Tannins

5-lipoxygenase Inhibitors
- Phenolic structures
- Arachidonic acid analogs
- Long-chain unsaturated fatty acids

Dual Inhibitors
- Diaryl heptanoids, such as falcarindiol[68]

PAF Antagonists
- Ginkgolides
- Lignans and neolignans

---

rested, it may progress until it causes the death of the organism. Cancer is encountered in all higher animals, and plants also develop growths that resemble cancer.

Carcinogenicity, the process that leads to cancer, is a complex course of abnormal cell growth and differentiation. At least two stages are recognized: initiation and promotion. In initiation, a normal cell undergoes irreversible changes. During promotion, initiated cells are stimulated to progress to cancer. Chemicals can act as both initiators and promoters of cancerous changes.

The initial neoplastic transformation results from the mutation of the cellular genes that control normal cell functions. The mutation may lead to abnormal cell growth, and may cause loss of suppressor genes that usually restrict abnormal cell growth. Many other factors may also be involved, including growth factors, immune suppression, and hormones.

Research is revealing the chemical basis for the reputations of many well-known anticancer remedies and suggesting new possibilities for other plants.[69] The phytochemical examination of plants with a history of traditional use for cancer often results in the isolation of principles with antitumor activity. An important survey lists more than 1,400 genera of plants with a history of use in cancer treatments.[70,71]

One group of important plant materials used clinically are the alkaloids of Madagascar periwinkle (*Catharanthus roseus*).[72] Research was stimulated by its traditional use in the treatment of diabetes, but the susceptibility of the treated test animals to bacterial infection led the researchers to look for possible immunosuppressive effects. Alkaloids with antileukemic activity were found, and vinblastine and vincristine are now used, either alone or in combination with other therapies, for cancer treatment. Differences exist among the kinds of tumors that respond to these alkaloids. Vinblastine is mainly useful in the treatment of Hodgkin's disease, a cancer affecting the lymph glands, spleen, and liver, while vincristine is used for childhood leukemia.

Cytotoxic agents target cells that are dividing rapidly, and since cancer cells proliferate faster than most normal cells, such agents can be toxic to the cancer cells. A wide variety of phytochemicals are cytotoxic. For example, many cytotoxic alkaloids have been described, including aconitine, acronycine, bisindole, camptothecine, colchicine, ellipticine, emetine, maytansine, and pyrrolizidines, as well as alkaloids from *Taxus*. Other secondary metabolites demonstrating cytotoxicity include cardenolides, coumarins, coumarolignans, diterpenes, flavonoids, iridoids, lignans, monoterpenes, quinones, sesquiterpenes, sesquiterpene lactones, and saponins.

The Cell Cycle

To appreciate phytochemical-cell interactions, the various stages in the life cycle of cells must be taken into account, including proliferation, differentiation, and cell death. The cell cycle is an ordered set of events, culminating in cell growth and division into two daughter cells. The cell cycle has four phases: G1, S, G2, and M. The S-stage stands for *synthesis*. This is the stage in which DNA replication occurs. The M-stage stands for *mitosis*, and is when nuclear chromosomes separate and cytoplasmic division (cytokinesis) occurs.

G1 is a time period of quiescence that varies in duration. During this stage, the cell carries out its normal role in supporting the life of the organism. If there is a commitment to proliferation, then purines and pyrimidines (building blocks for DNA synthesis) must be produced.

The cell enters the active reproductive phase of the cell cycle in the later part of G1, at which time nucleotides and enzymes are synthesized. In the S-phase, DNA synthesis occurs, replicating DNA for the new cell. An enzyme of this system that is particularly vulnerable to plant chemicals is topoisomerase, which separates the daughter DNA strands. In the next phase, G2, the cell

prepares other structures needed for mitosis. The M phase is mitosis itself, in which two daughter cells, which will subsequently enter the cycle themselves, are produced.

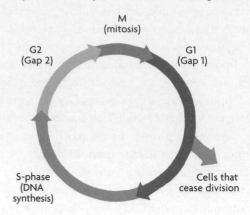

Fig. 9.9. The cell cycle

In a given tissue or tumor, the fraction of cells that are currently proliferating in the M- or S-phase is called the *growth fraction*. The higher the growth fraction, the faster the tissue is growing. Normal proliferative tissues have growth fractions of 20% to 30%, whereas the growth fractions of tumors range from 20% to 70%. The higher the growth fraction, the more susceptible the tumor is to chemotherapy. Larger tumors have smaller growth fractions, one of the reasons they are harder to combat with chemotherapy.

Cytotoxics target cells with a high growth fraction, and since cancer cells proliferate faster than most normal cells, they are the ones most affected. Normal cells with a high proliferation rate (such as hair follicles, the lining of the gastrointestinal tract, and bone marrow) suffer the same consequences, accounting for chemotherapy side effects such as hair loss, nausea, digestive impairment, immunosuppression, and hematologic complications.

Most flavonoids induce G1 arrest in human cancer cells, and the isoflavone genistein specifically inhibits their cell cycle at the G2- through M-phases. Apigenin (a flavone) was found to inhibit the proliferation of B104 rat neuronal cells by arresting their cell cycle at G2- through M-phases.[73]

Cell cycle–specific agents interrupt the cell cycle during either the synthesis or the mitosis phase. The tumor must be growing in order for them to be effective, as they depend on the presence of cell proliferation to exert their actions. Thus, S-phase drugs affect DNA synthesis. M-phase drugs affect mitosis or the mitotic spindle, and are used primarily against rapidly proliferating cancers, such as leukemias, since cells from these cancers enter the S- or M-phases more frequently than do cells of slow-growing cancers. (The *spindle* in a cell is a structure composed of microtubules along which chromosomes move during cell division.)

Cell cycle–nonspecific agents interrupt the cell cycle regardless of which phase the cell is in. They directly damage DNA and so do not depend on cell proliferation to exert their effects. Although they can kill any cell, they still have the greatest effect on proliferating cells, and are used primarily against slow-growing cancers, such as most solid tumors.

The Stages of Metastasis

Metastasis is the process by which cancer cells spread to sites distant from the primary tumor. The process requires that the cancer cells enter the vascular system—in other words, the lymphatic vessels, veins, and arteries. Once within the system, the cancer cells are transported passively to distant sites. In the lymph system, they are trapped in lymph nodes, which may serve as temporary barriers. They may enter the blood vessels by extension from lymph nodes or, more rarely, by passing directly through the connective tissue sheath surrounding the lymph nodes. The cancer cells are eventually entrapped in the smallest branches of blood vessels, the capillaries. Cancer cells thus trapped are the "seeds" from which larger colonies of tumor cells grow into secondary sites, called metastases.

Cell Detachment and Intravasation

Once detached from the primary tumor, cancer cells contact a blood vessel and enzymatically digest the basement membrane. Tumor cells then slip between vascular endothelial cells to enter the vessel. This process, called *intravasation*, is expedited by the weak basement membranes and fragile capillaries that develop during neovascularization. Thus, an intact basement membrane is a barrier to intravasation.

Detachment may be stimulated by decreased expression on the cell's surface membrane of adhesion molecules, which mediate cell-cell and cell-matrix interactions. Examples are cell-surface lectins and lectin-binding polysaccharides. Polysaccharides may inhibit neoplasia by directly affecting these adhesion molecules.

Cell Arrest

Cancer cells leave the bloodstream by attaching to a capillary wall, a process known as *cell arrest*. Cell arrest is promoted by the denuding of the basement membrane, tumor cell aggregation, platelet aggregation, and thrombus formation, processes that might be impacted with herbs.

Differentiation

Cancer cells can be thought of as cells that regain the ability to proliferate. Much work has been done to identify oncogenes and tumor suppressor genes that are thought to control this abnormal proliferative state. One approach to therapy has been to try to induce cells to differentiate into more specialized cells that will therefore stop proliferating.

CHEMOTHERAPEUTIC AGENTS

A number of underlying mechanisms have been identified to explain the activity of chemotherapeutic agents, whether synthetic or of plant origin.

DNA-Interactive Agents and Topoisomerase II Inhibitors

These alter DNA structure and interfere with its functions in a number of different ways. One mechanism involves inhibition of the enzyme topoisomerase II. Chromosomal DNA exists in a dynamic, three-dimensional arrangement known as its *topologic state*. The topoisomerases regulate this topologic state, facilitating the unwinding of the coiled DNA molecules and playing a critical role in the regulation of DNA replication and transcription.

Topoisomerase I catalyzes the relaxation of supercoiled DNA by briefly severing one of the two DNA strands. Topoisomerase II mediates the passage of one double-strand DNA segment through another by the formation of a temporary "gate" through both strands of one segment.

Etoposide and teniposide are semisynthetic lignan derivatives of podophyllotoxin from the mayapples *Podophyllum hexandrum* and *P. peltatum*. Although not used clinically, podophyllotoxin is an antimitotic agent that binds to tubulin. Its derivatives, known as epipodophyllotoxins, do not affect microtubular assembly at pharmacological concentrations, but act as inhibitors of topoisomerase II, stabilizing DNA double-strand breaks. Cells are prevented from progressing beyond G2. Etoposide is used in the treatment of small-cell lung cancer and testicular cancer, and teniposide in pediatric cancers.

The isoflavone genistein decreases the incidence and number of tumors in animal models of cancer.[74] Proposed mechanisms include inhibition of angiogenesis, interaction with steroid hormone receptors, inhibition of tyrosine kinase, inhibition of radical oxygen species formation, and interaction with topoisomerase.[75,76,77] Research suggests that genistein stabilizes the enzyme-DNA complex in such a way that both strands are nicked and DNA breaks occur. This leads to altered gene expression and cell differentiation, with an associated decrease in cell proliferation.[78]

Microtubules and Tubulin-Interactions

Some molecules damage the cellular machinery necessary for cell division. Tubulin is a protein that polymerizes to form microtubules, structural components that are critical to spindle and aster formation during mitosis, but that also help maintain cell shape, cellular motility, attachment, and intracellular transport.[79] Inhibition of tubulin polymerization into microtubules leads to the disappearance of the spindle.

The target site of action for the vinca alkaloids and the "taxoids" (natural and synthetic analogs of *Taxus* alkaloids) is microtubule formation. The vinca alkaloids vinblastine and vincristine, from the Madagascar periwinkle (*Catharanthus roseus*), promote microtubule disassembly by binding to tubulin, stopping mitosis at the metaphase.[80] Taxol (Paclitaxel) is extracted from the bark of the Pacific yew (*Taxus brevifolia*), as well as the needles and stems of other yews. The semisynthetic docetaxel is derived from baccatin III, found in the needles of the English yew (*Taxus baccata*).

Cells treated in vitro with Paclitaxel form disorganized bundles of microtubules in all phases of the cell cycle. Cells are either arrested in mitosis or in the G- or S-phase.[81] Taxoids are used in ovarian, breast, and non-small-cell lung cancer. Response rates have varied from 30% to 70%.[82]

Hormonal Agents

These inhibit the growth of endocrine-responsive neoplastic tissues, either directly through specific receptor interactions or indirectly through modulation of endogenous hormone metabolism. A variety of hormone agonists and antagonists are used to hamper the growth of tumors that have not yet lost their hormone response mechanisms. Some flavonoids and isoflavonoids reversibly inhibit the growth of certain cancer cells that contain Type II estrogen-binding sites. The affinity of flavonoids for these binding sites correlates with their growth-inhibiting activity.[83]

Biological Response Modifiers

Biological response modifiers directly or indirectly utilize the immune system to counter cancer or minimize the side effects of many treatments. They represent an attempt to repair, stimulate, or enhance the immune system's natural anticancer function. Theoretically, biological response modifiers may offer ways to make cancer cells more susceptible to destruction by the immune response. They may also alter the growth patterns of cancer cells to promote behavior similar to that of healthy cells, block or reverse cancer activity, enhance the body's ability to repair cells damaged by chemotherapy or radiation, or prevent metastases.

A variety of biological response modifiers are being used clinically. Mycopolysaccharides are currently used in Japan as biological response modifiers in the treatment of cancer.

Cytokines and Cancer

Cytokines are regulatory proteins that are released by cells of the immune system to act as intercellular mediators of the immune response. They are thus intimately involved in all cancer stages.

Interleukins

Many interleukins, or regulatory cytokines, have been identified; interleukin 2 has been the most studied in cancer treatment. It stimulates the growth and activities of immune cells that destroy cancer cells, such as lymphocytes. In one study, the flavonoid baicalein, from *Scutellaria baicalensis*, inhibited endothelial leukocyte adhesion molecule-1 and intercellular adhesion molecule-1 (ICAM-1), the production of which are induced by IL1β and TNF-α.[84]

Tumor Necrosis Factor

Tumor necrosis factor (TNF) damages tumor cells and blood vessels within tumors. Although TNF has antitumor activity in laboratory studies, the dose needed for a clinical effect is extremely toxic. *Taraxacum officinale* has been shown to inhibit the production of TNF-α from rat astrocytes.[85]

Colony-Stimulating Factors

Colony-stimulating factors (CSF) promote bone marrow cell activity. They have the potential to protect or restore hematopoietic activity in bone marrow after damage caused by chemotherapy or radiation. This may stimulate immune system components and enhance the antitumor activity of other therapies. CSFs are often used in combination with high-dose chemotherapy. In a study of the CSF-inducing activity of Amazonian plants, isoflavone glycosides from *Dalbergia monetaria* produced significant effects.[86]

Interferons

Interferons have an array of immunomodulating, anti-neoplastic, and antiviral properties. They are small, soluble proteins generated by cells when infected by RNA- or DNA-containing viruses. They may act directly on cancer cells by inhibiting their growth or by promoting their development into cells with more normal behavior. It appears that some interferons also may stimulate B and T cells, strengthening the immune system's overall anti-cancer function.

The medical use of interferons has been limited by their associated toxicity. However, another approach involves stimulating the natural cellular sources of interferons. A number of medicinal plants and constituents have been shown to stimulate the release of interferons. Garlic is one such plant, but also one with a role in the treatment and prevention of cancer that goes far beyond this single mechanism.[87]

Agents That Interfere with Cell Arrest

Treatment of endothelial cells with cytokines induces the expression of specific leukocyte adhesion molecules on cell surfaces. A number of flavonoids inhibit cytokine-induced endothelial cell adhesion protein gene expression. Since interfering with this process of adhesion may constitute a therapeutic target, flavonoid-rich plants may hold promise as cancer treatments.[88]

Natural Agents That Induce Differentiation

Some flavonoids can promote the differentiation of un-differentiated malignant cells into mature phenotypes. For example, the isoflavone genistein stimulates mouse erythroleukemia cells to synthesize hemoglobin.[89] Isoflavones have been shown to inhibit proliferation, promote differentiation, and exert chemopreventive effects.[90] Genistein and daidzein are differentiation inducers and tyrosine protein kinase inhibitors.

Some malignancies may progress because of a block in differentiation activity; induction of differentiation may be useful in treating such malignancies. Both plant extracts and constituents can induce differentiation in human leukemia, melanoma, colon carcinoma, bladder carcinoma, and brain cancer, as well as in a variety of mouse cancer cell lines.[91] When these cells are exposed to differentiating agents, they may develop into normal cells, losing the ability to proliferate.

Necrosis and Apoptosis

It appears that the primary mechanism by which most chemotherapeutic agents induce cell death is by causing damage, especially genetic damage. Death of cancer cells may occur either as a result of necrosis or of apoptosis.

Necrosis is the process of cell death that occurs in response to external events, such as hypoxia (oxygen deprivation), chemical exposure, and radiation injury. Cells swell, become vacuolated, and are finally digested either by their own enzymes or by the enzymes of neutrophils. Necrosis generally occurs in contiguous cells and is accompanied by an inflammatory response. Many currently available cancer treatments induce necrosis.

In contrast to necrosis, *apoptosis* is defined as programmed cell death, a process that triggers rapid DNA damage, condensation of chromatin, and fragmentation of DNA. Apoptosis is an orderly method for removing old, damaged, or otherwise unwanted cells. The word is derived from the Greek *apo*, meaning "apart," and *ptosis*, meaning "fallen."

In apoptosis, the cell fragments and is phagocytized by macrophages or neutrophils without causing inflammation, and so adjacent cells are not damaged. Several chemotherapeutic agents that cause DNA damage also lead to apoptosis, and it is possible that natural agents may facilitate this process. Defects in apoptosis may be implicated in both the initiation and the proliferation of cancer cells. One possible cause of cancer is that apoptosis fails to remove cells with damaged DNA, allowing them to survive long enough to progress from the initiation stage to the promotion and proliferation stages.[92]

Plants That Induce Apoptosis

The ability of plants to arrest the proliferation of cancer cells by influencing apoptosis has been the topic of much research.[93] Agents that have been found to induce apoptosis include extracts of plants like mistletoe (*Viscum album*) and *Semecarpus anacardium*. Isolated compounds like bryonolic acid, crocin (from saffron), and allicin have also been found to induce apoptosis and thereby arrest proliferation. The discovery that *Panax ginseng* prevents irradiation-induced apoptosis in hair follicles may have important therapeutic implications. Soy, garlic, ginger, green tea, and other herbs suggested by epidemiological research to reduce the incidence of cancer may do so by inducing apoptosis.

Apoptosis is a highly conserved mechanism of self-defense that has also been observed to occur in plants. It is natural to assume that they must contain chemicals that regulate programmed cell death in their own tissues. Thus, plants are likely to prove to be important sources of agents able to modulate programmed cell death in humans.

Mistletoe and Apoptosis

The European mistletoe *(Viscum album)*, used as adjuvant cancer therapy, has immunostimulant and cytotoxic effects. While polysaccharides are immunostimulant, lectins, such as those in mistletoe, are cytotoxic. Lectins are proteins that cause agglutination of cells. In vitro studies show that mistletoe lectins inhibit tumor growth and cause the DNA in the tumor cells to fragment, as would be expected in apoptosis.[94] There is evidence that these lectins cause membrane damage that leads to necrosis as well as DNA damage indicative of apoptosis.[95]

Angiogenesis

A growing tumor induces the development of its own blood supply, a process called *angiogenesis*. Angiogenesis facilitates tumor growth by supplying the tumor with oxygen and nutrients and providing ready access to the blood circulation, thus assisting metastasis. This process is not limited to malignant tumors, as it also occurs in benign tumors, some non-neoplastic diseases, and healthy tissue during wound healing, ovulation, menstruation, and pregnancy.

Numerous angiogenic compounds are found throughout the body, which stimulate angiogenesis only under specific, but poorly understood, circumstances. Two ginseng saponins have been shown to possess the ability to inhibit the metastasis of tumor cells to the lungs. The researchers hypothesized that the mechanism for this antimetastatic effect involved antiangiogenic activity as well as inhibition of adhesion and invasion of tumor cells.[96]

Anticarcinogens

A review published in 1992 cites more than 200 studies that correlate fruit and vegetable intake with protective effects against various cancers.[97] Although the vitamins and minerals in these foods are a factor, nonnutritive constituents are believed to also play a significant anticarcinogenic role.

Two mechanisms have been suggested by which such dietary components may inhibit carcinogenesis: by blocking the action of carcinogens or tumor promoters and by suppressing the evolution of initiated cells.[98] Blocking agents act by at least four mechanisms:

1. Inhibit the metabolism of noncarcinogenic compounds into carcinogenic compounds
2. Induce enzyme systems that detoxify carcinogens
3. Scavenge free radicals
4. Prevent tumor promoters from reaching or reacting with their cellular targets

Brassica and *Allium* species contain a variety of anticarcinogenic substances. Regular consumption of cruciferous vegetables (such as cabbage and broccoli) is associated with reduced rates of colon, lung, and other cancers in humans. This has led to the hypothesis that cancer may be a disease of maladaptation to diets that lack a rich variety of these compounds.[99]

ANTIVIRAL AGENTS

The term *antiviral* is used in many ways, depending on what endpoint criteria are used. In theory, an antiviral compound can work in one of several different manners. Some exert a direct virucidal effect, inhibiting viral replication in the infected host. This method of action encompasses virucidal agents that kill viruses extracellularly, as well as the so-called true antivirals that interfere with specific steps in the viral replication process.

An antiviral compound may also work by interfering with the virus replication cycle directly, at some stage between viral adsorption and the emergence of progeny viruses from the infected cell. Finally, some agents protect cells from subsequent virus infection through an interferon-like induction of host antiviral mechanisms.

The effects of a given antiviral compound might be specific to one virus or have more general activities. No standard assay for evaluating the antiviral properties of plants has been developed, and most of the methods in current use come from chemists; these procedures yield chemical data without taking bioactivity into account. Any useful antiviral should be noncytotoxic at effective concentrations, although cell cultures vary tremendously in their sensitivities to some compounds, making extrapolation difficult.

Plant Extracts with Antiviral Activity

Ethnobotany is bringing many potential antiviral plants to the attention of the research community. For example, one study reported on the antiviral activity of 40 different species used by the Australian Aboriginal people. They were tested at noncytotoxic concentrations for activity against human cytomegalovirus (HCMV), Ross River virus (RRV), and poliovirus type 1. The plants most active against poliovirus were the aerial parts of *Pterocaulon sphacelatum* and the roots of *Dianella longifolia*. *Euphorbia australis* and *Scaevola spinescens* were the most active against HCMV. *Eremophila latrobei* and *Pittosporum phylliraeoides* exhibited activity against RRV.[100]

A range of plant constituents that inhibit different stages in the replication cycle of viruses has been identified. A recent review of those that impact replication of human immunodeficiency virus (HIV) highlighted the following constituents.[101]

Table 9.3. Plant Constituents That Inhibit HIV

STEP IN VIRAL REPLICATION	CONSTITUENT TYPES
Viral adsorption	Chromone alkaloids
	Isoquinoline alkaloids
	Sulfated polysaccharides
	Sulfated polyphenolics
	Flavonoids
	Coumarins
	Phenylpropenoids
	Tannins and triterpenes
Virus cell fusion	Lectins
	Triterpenes
Reverse transcription	Alkaloids
	Coumarins
	Flavonoids
	Phloroglucinols
	Lactones
	Tannins
	Iridoids
	Triterpenes
Integration	Coumarins
	Depsidones
	O-caffeoyl derivatives
	Lignans
	Phenolics
Proteolytic cleavage (protease inhibition)	Saponins
	Xanthones
	Coumarins
Glycosylation	Indolizidine alkaloids
	Piperidines
	Pyrrolizidines
Assembly/release	Naphthodianthrones
	Photosensitizers
	Phospholipids

ANTIOXIDANTS AND FREE RADICAL SCAVENGERS

Although oxygen is essential for life, breathing pure oxygen at atmospheric pressure for longer than 48 hours will lead to respiratory distress and death. This toxicity is not caused by oxygen per se, but rather by highly reactive ions produced from oxygen. Under normal conditions, these reactive molecules are produced by the body (and indeed are part of normal metabolism), but their rate of production does not exceed the capacity of cells to catabolize them. When their production exceeds the capacity of the body's natural defenses, a variety of diseases can occur, such as cancer, stroke, and neurodegeneration.

Of course, animals are not the only living beings that utilize antioxidants. The enzyme ascorbate peroxidase, for example, prevents oxidative damage in plants, especially in nitrogen-fixing root nodules, by scavenging cellular hydrogen peroxide. The growing root nodules of alfalfa (*Medicago sativa*) contain elevated levels of this antioxidant, as well as its corresponding mRNA transcript and substrate. High levels of antioxidants found in these nodules are indicative of their role in plants and animals.[102]

Thus, the fact that antioxidant compounds can be expected to be present in plants has led to much research activity. As an example, a 1995 paper reported on the results of testing for superoxide anion–scavenging effects in 65 plant extracts. Of these, horse chestnut (*Aesculus hippocastanum*) and witch hazel (*Hamamelis virginiana*) were found to have strong scavenging and protective activities against cell damage induced by active oxygen, leading the researchers to propose potential applications for these plants as antiaging or antiwrinkle treatments for the skin.[103]

Chemical reactions involving radicals are central to the maintenance of homeostasis. They play a fundamental role in physiological processes, such as oxidative transformation reactions mediated by cytochrome P_{450}, enzymatic oxidation reactions, oxidative phosphorylation, smooth muscle tone regulation, and elimination of microorganisms. However, excessive generation of free radicals can damage tissue, so cells have a range of biochemical defense systems designed to safeguard them against such damage. When the generation of pro-oxidants overwhelms the capacity of antioxidant systems, *oxidative stress* ensues. This in turn may cause tissue damage and subsequent pathophysiological events.

Free Radicals

A free radical is an atom or molecule that contains a single unpaired electron. This condition makes the molecule extremely reactive and causes the formation of molecular links that normally would not occur.

The term *reactive oxygen species* (ROS) describes oxygen-centered radicals, such as superoxide (O_2) and hydroxyl (OH), as well as nonradical species derived from oxygen, such as hydrogen peroxide (H_2O_2), singlet oxygen, and hypochlorous acid (HOCl). The concept of *species* in chemistry has nothing to do with the biological use of that term, but refers instead to a chemical entity, such as a radical, ion, molecule, or atom.

Damage done by free radicals in the body includes peroxidation of membrane lipids, oxidative damage to nucleic acids and carbohydrates, and oxidation of susceptible groups in proteins. They also appear to initiate and promote carcinogenesis. An involvement of ROS in aging and in many chronic diseases has been proposed.

Causes of Free Radical Production in the Body

- Cellular respiration
- Trace element metabolism
- Radiation
- Pollution
- Cell death and tissue injury
- Toxins
- Xenobiotics (chemical pollutants)
- Immune system activation
- Inflammation
- Reperfusion injury
- Metabolism
- Diet

Lipids

Lipids are hydrophobic compounds, some of which are integral to the structure of membranes and the regulation of membrane fluidity. Unsaturated fatty acids are particularly susceptible to attack by hydroxyl free radicals, a process that generates the formation of *lipid peroxides*. Peroxidation of unsaturated fatty acids alters the structure of the cell membrane, thereby disturbing normal membrane function.

Protein oxidation enhances the metabolic breakdown of membranes and has major deleterious effects on normal function, especially if oxidation occurs at a crucial area of structure, such as the active site of the enzyme molecule. Thus, the defense provided by antioxidant systems is critical to survival.

MECHANISMS OF ANTIOXIDANT PROTECTION

A number of mechanisms diminish the harmful effects of oxidants in the cell. These mechanisms are generally sufficient to maintain homeostasis, because free radicals are fairly easily controlled under normal conditions. However, when these defense mechanisms are overwhelmed and the cell enters a state of oxidative stress, a wide variety of diseases can result. Detoxification of ROS in the cell is provided by both enzymic and nonenzymic systems that constitute the antioxidant defense systems. A third important antioxidant system is the body's use of metal chelators to block the formation of free radicals.

Enzymic Systems

Some enzymic systems, such as superoxide dismutase (SOD) and catalase, act specifically against ROS, while certain other enzyme systems reduce the sulfur-containing thiols.

Superoxide dismutase is present in cytosol and mitochondria.
Catalase, a highly reactive enzyme found in peroxisomes, breaks down hydrogen peroxide to oxygen and water.
Glutathione peroxidase (one of the few enzymes found in humans that require selenium for its activity) occurs in the mitochondria and cytosol and reduces organic hydroperoxides and hydrogen peroxide.

Sulfhydryl Compounds and Glutathione

Many thiols exist in the body, either in a free state, as free dimers, or covalently linked to a protein. Thiols, including sulfhydryl compounds and glutathione, are very efficient reducing agents.

Glutathione (g-glutamylcysteinylglycine, or GSH) is a sulfhydryl antioxidant, antitoxin, and enzyme cofactor found ubiquitously in living systems. Adequate cellular concentrations of glutathione maintain a strong reducing environment. GSH detoxifies hydrogen peroxide in a reaction catalyzed by glutathione peroxidase and also participates in the transport of amino acids across cell membranes.

Nonenzymic Systems

Nonenzymic antioxidants are less specific and may be water-soluble or lipid-soluble, depending on their sites of action in the cell membranes. These compounds react with free radicals without generating further radical production, and so scavenge and quench various other radicals in addition to ROS. A variety of such antioxidants with a range of different structures exist.

Vitamin C

Ascorbic acid, or vitamin C, is an essential compound for human health and is a universal component of plant cells. It is a reducing agent, involved in hydroxylation reactions and other redox (oxidation-reduction) reactions, and is capable of chelating metals. Ascorbic acid protects other antioxidants, such as vitamin A, vitamin E, and essential fatty acids, from oxidative damage.

Vitamin C and flavonoids coexist in plants and are eaten together in the diet. Flavonoids possess antioxidant-dependent, vitamin C–sparing activities. They are also known to increase the absorption of vitamin C.

Flavonoids and Polyphenols

Many plant constituents scavenge free radicals. Polyphenols, especially flavonoids, are very efficient radical scavengers. As discussed in chapter 7, flavonoids consist of structurally similar compounds that differ only in the degree of ring substitution, the type of substitution, and the type and degree of glycosylation.

Phagocytic white blood cells, such as monocytes, neutrophils, eosinophils, and macrophages, all generate ROS. Radical production by phagocytes is an important part of their bactericidal and antitumor functions, as phagocytosis is accompanied by an increase in oxygen consumption (called the *respiratory burst*) with an attendant production of oxygen ions. These highly reactive oxygen metabolites promote inflammation, causing tissue damage. In addition to scavenging radicals, flavonoids can inhibit the formation of these oxygen ions.

Dietary exposure to flavonoids is significant. The average diet in the United Kingdom and the United States may contain up to 1 gram of mixed flavonoids per day, far exceeding the content of vitamin E, a monophenolic antioxidant, and of β-carotene. Chemically, they are typical phenolics that act as potent metal chelators, free radical scavengers, and powerful antioxidants.

Antioxidant Functions of Flavonoids

- Metal chelators and reducing agents
- Scavengers of ROS
- Chain-breaking antioxidants
- Quenchers of singlet oxygen formation

Enzyme Systems Modified by Flavonoids[104]

Aldose reductase
Aromatase
Cyclooxygenase
Cytochrome P_{450}
Dependent mixed-function oxidases
Epoxide hydrolase
Glutathione
Lipoxygenases
Myeloperoxidase
Nicotinamide adenine dinucleotide phosphate (NADPH) oxidase
Nucleotide phosphodiesterases
Ornithine decarboxylase
Phospholipase A_2
Phospholipase C
Protein kinase C
Protein tyrosine kinase
Reverse transcriptase
Several adenosine triphospatases (ATPases)
Sialidase
Transferase
Various other kinases
Xanthine oxidase

Some of these enzyme systems are pivotal to immune function, the cell cycle, tumor growth, and cancer cell metastasis. The antioxidant function and enzyme-modifying actions of flavonoids may account for many of their pharmacological activities.

Coenzyme Q_{10}

Coenzyme Q_{10} (also called *ubiquinone* because it is ubiquitous in all biological systems) is an essential part of the cellular respiratory chain, the components of which are physically located in the inner membrane of the mitochondrion.

Vitamin A and Related Compounds

Vitamin A is formed in the intestine from its precursor, β-carotene. β-carotene and the carotenoids as a whole are abundant in green plants, carrots, and other orange and yellow vegetables. Vitamin A and other carotenoids are effective radical scavengers. The carotenoids lutein and lycopene are both found in tomatoes, but lycopene also occurs in the florets of *Calendula officinalis*.

Vitamin E

Vitamin E is made up of a group of eight naturally occurring compounds called tocopherols. Tocopherols are highly active free radical scavengers that protect unsaturated membrane lipids from oxidation.

Metal Chelators

The third approach to protecting against oxidative damage is to try to prevent the formation of free radicals in the first place. Metals such as iron and copper can cause the formation of free radicals. However, if these metals are bound, which effectively removes them from solution, radical formation can be prevented. In the body, iron is stored as *ferritin* and is transferred around the body as *transferrin* or *lactoferrin*. Iron is also associated with other proteins (hemoglobin, myoglobin, ferredoxin) and is always tightly bound. Copper is transported around the body as *ceruloplasmin*.

Exogenous Antioxidants in Food

Free radical production also occurs outside of the body. Free radicals in food can destroy vitamins, reducing their nutritional value; damage pigments, causing bleaching; and change aromas and flavors. The addition of antioxidants to foods to prevent rancidity and prolong shelf life has long been common practice. A variety of antioxidants are used in foods, but tertbutylhydroxyanisole (BHA) and tertbutylhydroxytoluene (BHT) are two of the most common.

PLANTS AND THE CARDIOVASCULAR SYSTEM

The green world furnishes many important cardiovascular medicines. A 1998 review describes more than 700 secondary plant metabolites known to exhibit some kind of cardiovascular activity.[105]

The cardiac glycosides digoxin and lanatoside C from *Digitalis* and ouabain from *Strophanthus* have a positive inotropic effect on the heart and are the drugs of choice for congestive heart failure. The anticoagulants dicoumarol and other coumarin derivatives were developed from plant sources. The alkaloid ergotamine is a vasoconstrictor used in the treatment of severe vascular headache; alkaloids from *Veratrum* and *Rauvolfia* species are antihypertensive; and tannins, which occur in many plant species, are hemostatic. Quinidine, from *Cinchona* bark, was the main antifibrillatory agent in clinical practice until the advent of modern antiarrhythmic drugs and is still used today.

A substance may effect the activity of the heart in a variety of different ways. Table 9.4 correlates some of these actions with the characteristic actions of plant compounds. Some classes of substances, like cardiac glycosides, sympathomimetics, and beta-blockers, appear several times, as they exert several different types of activities on the heart.

Table 9.4. Cardiovascular Activities of Plant Compounds

ACTIVITY	DEFINITION	CONSTITUENT
Positive inotropic	Increase contractility	Cardiac glycosides
Negative inotropic	Decrease contractility	Beta-blockers
Positive chronotropic (sympathomimetics)	Increases cardiac frequency	Ephedrine
Negative chronotropic	Decrease cardiac frequency	Cardiac glycosides
Positive dromotropic (sympathomimetics)	Increases flow rate	Caffeine
Negative dromotropic	Decrease flow rate	Cardiac glycosides
Antiarrhythmic	Eliminates cardiac arrhythmias	Quinidine
Coronary dilating	Dilate coronary arteries	Flavonoids, theophylline

Cardiac Glycosides

Cardiac glycosides improve the efficiency of the heart muscle without increasing its need for oxygen. This enables the heart to pump adequate amounts of blood around the body and ensures that no fluid builds up in the lungs or extremities. That sounds wonderful, as indeed it is, but there is a drawback. Because the solubility and removal rates of cardiac glycosides tend to be low, the possibility exists for high levels of glycosides to accrue in the body. This is the main disadvantage with foxglove (*Digitalis* spp.) and explains why it is potentially poisonous unless used with appropriate skill and knowledge concerning monitoring of blood levels.

Cardiac glycosides appear to be confined to angiosperms. Cardenolides are the most common and are particularly abundant in Apocynaceae and Asclepiadaceae. The bufanolides occur in some Liliaceae plants, such as squill *(Urginea maritima)*, and in some Ranunculaceae.

Table 9.5. Plants Containing Cardiac Glycosides

PLANT FAMILY	GENERA
Apocynaceae	*Acocanthera, Adenium, Apocynum, Carissa, Cerbera, Nerium, Strophanthus, Thevetia, Urechites*
Asclepiadaceae	*Asclepias, Calotropis, Cryptostegia, Menabea, Pachycarpus, Periploca, Xysmalobium*
Liliaceae	*Bowiea, Convallaria, Ornithogalum, Rhodia, Urginea*
Ranunculaceae	*Adonis, Helleborus*
Moraceae	*Antiaris, Antiaropsis, Castilla*
Brassicaceae	*Cheiranthus, Erysimum*
Sterculiaceae	*Mansonia*
Tiliaceae	*Corchorus*
Celastraceae	*Euonymus*
Fabaceae	*Coronilla*
Scrophulariaceae	*Digitalis*

The pharmacological effect of cardiac glycosides is dependent on both the aglycones and the sugar attachments. The inherent activity resides in the aglycones, but the sugars render the compounds more soluble and increase the power of fixation of the glycosides to the heart muscle.

The number of different effects produced by the *Digitalis* glycosides complicates our understanding of their overall action, and their exact mode of action on myocardial muscle is still under investigation. *Digitalis* probably competes with potassium ions for specific receptor enzyme (ATPase) sites in the cell membranes of cardiac muscle and is particularly successful during the depolarization phase of the muscle, when there is an influx of Na ions.

The clinical effect of digitalis glycosides in cases of congestive heart failure is increased force of myocardial contraction. Because of their vagus effects, the digitalis glycosides are also used to control atrial arrhythmias. The diuretic action of *Digitalis* arises from the improved circulatory effect.

Nonsteroidal Cardioactive Plant Constituents

Although orthodox medicine makes much use of cardiac glycosides of plant origin, the search continues for new active substances that provide either better therapeutic indices or different types of activity. In addition to plants such as hawthorn *(Crataegus* spp.) and garlic *(Allium sativum)*, in vitro studies suggest other remedies new to the West.

The isolation of forskolin from *Coleus forskohlii* shows that the plant kingdom continues to offer medicine new

Cardiotonic or Cardioactive?

In a strictly technical sense, the pharmacological term *cardiotonic* is synonymous with "positive inotropic." In pharmacology, the word *cardiotonic* is used not only to describe agents that increase contractility, but also to indicate an increase in frequency, an increase in the beat volume, or a general increase in cardiac performance.

In the phytotherapeutic literature, however, slightly different terminology is used. Here, *cardioactive* plants are those that owe their effects on the heart to cardiac glycosides or other very active substances; they thus possess both the strengths and the drawbacks of these constituents. An example is *Digitalis* (foxglove). *Cardiotonic* plants, on the other hand, are those that have an observable beneficial action on the heart and blood vessels but contain no cardiac glycosides, such as *Crataegus* (hawthorn). The mechanisms behind their actions are obscure and constitute a subject of considerable pharmacological debate.

and potent cardiac agents. Forskolin is a labdane diterpenoid with antihypertensive, positive inotropic, antiplatelet, and adenylate cyclase-activating properties. As discussed earlier in this chapter, the activation of adenylate cyclase results in increased levels of intracellular cyclic AMP (cAMP).

Coleus forskohlii and forskolin lower blood pressure and improve the contractility of the heart muscle, making this herb relevant in the treatment of hypertension, congestive heart failure, and angina. These actions are related to an increase in cAMP levels throughout the cardiovascular system, which results in relaxation of the arteries and increased force of contraction. The net effect is an improvement in many cardiovascular functions.

Several studies suggest that forskolin may significantly lower blood pressure. In one clinical study involving seven patients with dilated cardiomyopathy, forskolin improved left ventricular function, primarily by reducing pre-load, without raising metabolic costs.[106] (*Pre-load* is the tension in the heart muscle at the end of the diastolic phase, just before the contraction.) The study also showed that forskolin increased the contractile force of heart muscle. These results indicate that forskolin may best be used in congestive heart failure in combination with other cardiotonic botanicals, such as *Crataegus*.

A number of classes of nonsteroidal substances with cardiovascular effects have been identified, including phenylalkylamines, indole derivatives, tetrahydroisoquinolines, imidazoles and purines, diterpenes, sesquiterpenes, flavonoids, and other phenolic compounds. Here we shall focus briefly on those found in the primary cardiovascular herbal remedies.

Phenalkylamines

This class of alkaloids was the model for the development of sympathomimetic drugs. The main representative is L-ephedrine, first found in ma huang (*Ephedra sinica*). Since ephedrine has other, more prominent activities, its action on the heart is often considered a side effect. Ephedrine and its relatives have been found in plants in the families Portulacaceae, Rutaceae, Cactaceae, Amaryllidaceae, Moraceae, Musaceae, and Rosaceae. These include numerous food plants, such as citrus fruits, bananas (*Musa* spp.), and purslane (*Portulaca oleracea*). Synephrine occurs in the fruit of the mandarin orange (*Citrus reticulata*). Cathinone, from khat (*Catha edulis*), shows strong positive inotropic activity, contributing to the cardiac stimulant activity of khat leaves.

Phenylethylamines, which constitute a subgroup of phenylalkylamines, are widely distributed in Cactaceae,

Rosaceae, Rutaceae, and Fabaceae. The prototype of this group is tyramine, which at high concentrations shows positive inotropic activity. Strong positive inotropic activity is also displayed by *N*-methyltyramine, hordenine, and *p*-methoxyl-β-phenethylamine, all of which have been found in hawthorn flowers. This group is also found in night-blooming cereus (*Selenicereus grandiforus*), a favorite remedy of the early American Eclectic and Physiomedicalist physicians for cardiac insufficiency and angina pectoris. The cardiovascular action of *Viburnum* species may also be related to the presence of tyramine, which has been found in *V. odoratissimum* and *V. opulus*. Tyramine and *p*-methoxyl-β-phenethylamine have also been found in *Viscum album*.

Other Nitrogen-Containing Compounds

Methylcanadine from prickly ash (*Zanthoxylum* spp.) and sanguinarine from bloodroot (*Sanguinaria canadensis*) possess positive inotropic activity. The lupine alkaloid sparteine possesses specific antiarrhythmic activity and is found in Scotch broom (*Cytisus scoparius*).

Cyclic AMP also possesses inotropic properties and is widely distributed in the plant kingdom. In view of the low concentrations of cAMP found so far in plants, pharmacologists exclude a cardiotonic role for cAMP-containing plant extracts. Such conclusions might stem from a too narrow interpretation clouded by a "magic bullet" perception of biochemistry. From a synergistic perspective, all the constituents in a plant work together to produce its healing effects.

Flavonoids and Other Phenolics

Comprehensive investigations and reviews have been published on the cardioactivity of *Crataegus*. The main active principles in this plant are thought to be flavonoids and procyanidin oligomers. The evidence suggests that the flavonoids impact the heart via inhibition of cellular phosphodiesterase and elevation of cellular cAMP concentration, as well as by affecting the permeability of cell organelles to calcium ions. Please see chapter 14 for more information on this remarkable plant.

Phosphodiesterase-inhibitory action is not limited to flavonoids. Some lignans are potential phosphodiesterase inhibitors, and the cardiotonic action of mistletoe (*Viscum album*) can probably be attributed to lignan content.

Cholesterol- and Lipid-Lowering Activity

High serum levels of cholesterol and triglycerides (a condition known as *hyperlipidemia*) are important risk factors in the development of coronary heart disease (CHD).

Cholesterol is an essential component of cell membranes and a metabolic intermediate in the synthesis of steroid hormones and bile salts. Some cholesterol is obtained from the diet (about 25%) and the rest is manufactured by the liver. However, elevated levels in serum may be a result of high dietary intake, a condition known as *exogenous hyperlipidemia*, or secondary hyperlipidemia.

Endogenous hyperlipidemia, also called primary or familial hyperlipidemia, is a disorder of cholesterol metabolism that may be caused by genetic factors. This is much less common than exogenous hyperlipidemia. Diseases such as diabetes mellitus, gout, hypothyroidism, obstructive jaundice, cirrhosis of the liver, and renal failure can cause secondary hyperlipidemia.

Fat from the diet is absorbed into the bloodstream and transported in the form of lipoproteins. These are classified according to their density, for example, low density lipoprotein (LDL) or high density lipoprotein (HDL). Triglycerides are saturated fatty acids that are found in the bloodstream with normal blood levels between 10 and 150 milligrams per deciliter. Their levels in serum used to classify primary hyperlipidemias. Elevated serum cholesterol *per se* is not the only indicator of atherosclerosis. In certain disorders, cholesterol levels may remain fairly normal while triglyceride levels rise. It is preferable, therefore, to always measure levels of each lipoprotein fraction, especially LDL, all of which contain cholesterol.

The mechanisms of action of drugs used to treat primary and secondary hyperlipidemia may involve inhibition of cholesterol synthesis in the liver. Some drugs, such as bezafibrate, suppress endogenous cholesterol and triglyceride synthesis and stimulate catabolism via systemic lipoprotein and hepatic lipases. The omega-3 polyunsaturated fatty acids found in fish and flaxseed oils act by increasing lipoprotein lipase activity as well as by inhibiting the synthesis of very low density lipoprotein (VLDL) in the liver. VLDL is a lipoprotein that acts as a carrier for cholesterol and fats in the bloodstream. Elevation of VLDL in the bloodstream is associated with an increased risk of atherosclerosis and coronary artery disease.

Food and medicinal plants are both important in the dietary control of hyperlipidemia. Garlic (*Allium sativum*) is one plant that might be described as both food and medicine. Another herbal food that lowers serum cholesterol is fenugreek seed (*Trigonella foenum graecum*), which is used as a condiment. Other naturally occurring hypolipidemics include khellin, from *Ammi visnaga*, and guggulsterone, from *Commiphora mukul*.

Several clinical studies have shown that complex carbohydrates, such as oat bran, guar gum, and carob gum, also lower serum cholesterol levels; however, these conclusions are now being questioned, because diets that contain these substances are also usually low in fat. Complex carbohydrates may work by inhibiting fat absorption rather than through a direct pharmacological effect. Antioxidants with free radical scavenging ability, such as flavonoids, have demonstrated cholesterol-lowering activities in models of experimental hyperlipidemia. The mechanism of action here is due in part to inhibition of lipid peroxidation, but other factors that affect cholesterol control mechanisms may also be involved.

Hypertension and Hypotensive Agents

More than 35 million Americans have *hypertension*, or high blood pressure. For unknown reasons, the occurrence of the disorder is twice as high in African Americans as Caucasians. While hypertension is a common problem in our culture, it is rare in those that remain relatively untouched by the western lifestyle. Lifestyle plays a major role in causing and perpetuating hypertension. Thus, dietary, psychological, and social factors must all be addressed before any real change can occur.

A distinction must be made between elevated blood pressure with no obvious medical cause, known as *primary* or *essential hypertension*, and hypertension caused by an underlying pathology, such as kidney, endocrine, or cerebral disease, which is called *secondary hypertension*. For the purposes of this discussion, we will focus on essential hypertension.

Hypertension typically causes no symptoms until complications arise, in which case symptoms can include dizziness, flushed face and skin, headache, fatigue, epistaxis (nosebleed), and nervousness. These symptoms may all be caused by other conditions as well, making it difficult to diagnose hypertension by symptoms alone.

Diagnosis must be based on a finding that both systolic and diastolic blood pressure are usually (but not always) higher than normal, and other causes of symptoms must be excluded. In general, hypertension is indicated by a blood pressure measurement higher than 140/90 mm Hg. However, "normal" blood pressure varies among individuals, and thus normal should always be viewed in terms of a range, as opposed to a specific measurement. Observable changes in retinal blood vessels are diagnostic indicators of the degree of damage caused to the body by the hypertension.

Screening for antihypertensive effects in traditional medicines has been performed over many years, and several animal models have been utilized.[107]

Calcium Channel Blockers

Calcium (Ca) antagonistic drugs are widely used in the treatment of cardiovascular disorders, such as angina pectoris, myocardial infarction, atherosclerosis, and hypertension. Even though currently used calcium channel blockers have different chemical structures and sites of action, they all inhibit the transmembrane influx of calcium ions (Ca^{2+}) through voltage-dependent Ca channels. These are transmembrane ion channels whose permeability to ions is extremely sensitive to the transmembrane voltage difference. This action reduces smooth muscle contractility and vascular resistance, resulting in lowered blood pressure.

Ca antagonists influence many functions, including muscle contraction, gland secretion, platelet cell activity, changes in gene expression, and the release of transmitters. However, their main therapeutic influence is on the function of the heart and blood circulation. Ca channel blockers are coronary artery dilators that reduce peripheral vascular resistance and hence reduce the cardiac workload. They inhibit Ca^{2+} influx through voltage-sensitive Ca^{2+} channels and may therefore slow the early rise in cytosolic Ca^{2+}. They are energy-sparing drugs that slow the rate of ATP exhaustion, and may also protect against lipid peroxidation.

The three main groups of prescription Ca channel blockers are dihydropyridines, benzodiazepines, and phenylalkylamines. These include many common compounds used in therapy, such as nifedipine, diltiazem, and verapamil.

In recent years, various plant constituents have shown apparent Ca channel–blocking activity in in vitro screening models.[108] A recent review of Ca antagonists isolated from plants suggests that many have activity comparable to that of compounds currently used in therapy.[109] However, even though ion channel modulators are important drugs, they appear to constitute a neglected area as far as natural product screening is concerned.

Table 9.6. Plant Sources of Calcium Channel Blockers

CONSTITUENT TYPE	EXAMPLE
Terpenoids	
Monoterpenes	Menthol, menthofuran
Sesquiterpene lactones	Gossypol, santonin
Hydrocarbon derivatives	
Garlic compounds	Allicin
Phenolic ketones	Eugenol, apiol
Coumarins	
Hydroxycoumarins	Coumarin, umbelliferone
Furanocoumarins	Bergapten, psoralen
Pyranocoumarins	Visnadin
Chromones	Khellin
Naphthoquinones	Juglone, plumbagin
Lignans	Eudesmin
Alkaloids	Sanguinarine

ACE Inhibitors

Inhibition of angiotensin-converting enzyme (ACE) is another important option in the control of hypertension. ACE is a hydrolase enzyme that cleaves biologically inactive angiotensin I to form active angiotensin II. Angiotensin II causes contraction of vascular smooth muscle and thus raises blood pressure and stimulates aldosterone release from the adrenal glands. Drugs that inhibit ACE are used to treat hypertension and congestive heart failure. The renin-angiotensin system, which consists of renin, ACE, and angiotensin II, is pivotal to renal and cardiovascular homeostasis. Renin is an enzyme produced in the kidney that acts on angiotensinogen to form angiotensin I. ACE is believed to be the rate-limiting step in angiotensin II formation by the renin-angiotensin system.

Two kinds of renin-angiotensin systems exist.

1. A circulating endocrine renin-angiotensin system is responsible for short-term cardio-renal homeostasis.
2. Local renin-angiotensin systems are present in many tissues and exert influences on local functions. The tonic control of vascular resistance and local tissue function (e.g., in the kidney) is influenced by the intrinsic tissue renin-angiotensin system.

An in vitro assay for the detection of ACE inhibitors in plant extracts has been developed. Researchers have identified a number of plants that contain such compounds, including *Allium ursinum*, *Amelanchier ovalis*, *Cistus clusii*, and *Lespedeza capitata*.[110] They have also isolated three classes of compounds with potential ACE-inhibitory activity: flavonoids, procyanidins, and peptides.[111]

However, the presence of a strong ACE inhibitor does not necessarily imply that a plant is a potent antihypertensive drug. For example, some flavonoids show activity in vitro because they generate chelate complexes within the active center of ACE.[112] It is also important to remember that a negative screen for ACE-inhibitory action does not mean that the plant species will not work as an antihypertensive drug, as compounds that influence other hypotensive mechanisms could well be present.

Inhibition of cAMP Phosphodiesterase

Another approach to finding new antihypertensive agents looks for substances that inhibit levels of intracellular cAMP. Such compounds mediate cardiac contractility by increasing the levels of cAMP or by inhibiting its metabolism. These include β-adrenergic agonists, adenylate cyclase activators (such as forskolin from *Coleus forskohlii*), and phosphodiesterase inhibitors.

When stimulated, the adenylate cyclase enzyme converts adenosine triphosphate (ATP) into cAMP. This second messenger initiates a series of phosphorylation reactions by protein kinases, which mediate the influx of extracellular Ca^{2+} and the release of stored calcium ions by the sarcoplasmic reticulum. A phosphodiesterase III enzyme then inactivates cAMP by converting it into the inert 5'adenosine monophosphate (5'AMP). It is likely that increases in intracellular cAMP may be the result of increases in levels of prostacyclin.

A number of lignans inhibit cAMP phosphodiesterase activity. In studies of structure-activity relationships, three classes of lignans have received the most attention: dibenzylbutyrolatones, tetrahydrofurans, and furanofurans. Furanofuran lignans with this activity have been isolated from olive (*Olea* spp.), ash (*Fraxinus* spp.), and the traditional Chinese tonic herb *Eucommia ulmoides*.

Platelet Function and Cardiovascular Disease

Platelets (anuclear cells present in large numbers in the blood) are involved in a range of cardiovascular diseases. Inactivated platelets do not adhere to one other or to vascular endothelium. However, they adhere to subendothelial surfaces (adhesion) and to each other (aggregation) at sites of vascular injury. During the process of activation, platelets secrete various substances, such as adenosine diphosphate (ADP) and thromboxane A_2, which cause further aggregation and accelerate the coagulation process. Unfortunately, adhesion, aggregation, and secretion,

the primary events in the arrest of bleeding, can also lead to the deposition of platelet thrombi in blood vessels and on heart valves.

It is now generally accepted that blood platelets are involved in the genesis of many cardiovascular diseases, including stroke, myocardial infarction, diabetic vascular disorders, and atherosclerosis.

Platelet Aggregation

When platelets interact with certain substances, or when they adhere to a damaged vessel wall, aggregation may occur. Initially reversible, aggregation may progress to a second, irreversible aggregation, during which various active substances are released. Platelets may be activated through exposure to a number of substances, including:

- Hormones (such as adrenaline and vasopressin)
- Autacoids, including adenosine diphosphate (ADP)
- Serotonin (5-hydroxytryptamine)
- Eicosanoids
- Platelet activating factor (PAF)
- Blood coagulation and complement factors (thrombin and plasmin)
- Vascular proteins (collagen, elastin, and others)

These stimuli interact with receptor sites on the platelet and activate intracellular metabolic pathways. Secondary messenger systems involving cyclases, protein kinase C, and calcium channels result in liberation of arachidonic acid from membrane phospholipids and ultimately cause platelet aggregation and thrombus formation. Arachidonic acid metabolism is pivotal in platelet activation and is an intrinsic part of the inflammatory response.

Platelet-Activating Factor

Platelet-activating factor (PAF) is a potent lipid pro-inflammatory mediator with effects in many body systems; it is of particular importance in the cellular immune response. PAF, or 1-O-alkyl-2-O-acetyl-sn-glycero-3-phosphorylcholine, exists endogenously as a mixture of molecules that have slight structural variations. In addition to platelet aggregation, PAF also activates basophils, endothelial cells, eosinophils, lymphocytes, macrophages, mast cells, monocytes, and neutrophils. These cells not only respond to PAF, but also produce and release it themselves.

PAF induces a number of responses, including phagocytosis, exocytosis, superoxide production, chemotaxis, aggregation, proliferation, adhesion, eicosanoid generation, degranulation, and calcium mobilization, as well as diverse morphological changes in cells. Thus the activity of PAF extends well beyond platelet activation and it is thought to be involved in anaphylactic shock, inflammation, hypertension, allergic responses, and respiratory and cardiovascular disorders. PAF antagonists displace PAF from its receptor binding site, in most cases without initiating any response of their own.

Physiologically, local levels of certain cytokines are major controlling factors in blood platelet hemostasis. Among other activities, prostacyclin has been shown to be a potent vasodilator and inhibitor of platelet activation. It is largely produced as an arachidonate metabolite in endothelial cells and excreted into the blood, where it modulates platelet reactivity and acts as a vasodilatory agent. The enzymes, receptors, and various other macromolecules involved in this *arachidonic acid cascade*, as well as those involved in the recognition and reaction of the platelet to cytokines, provide potentially important sites of action for antiplatelet compounds, or PAF antagonists.

Natural Products with Antiplatelet Activity

According to their effects on platelet aggregation, release reaction, and signal transductions, antiplatelet plant constituents have been tentatively classified into eight groups:[113]

- Platelet-activating factor (PAF) antagonists
- Collagen-receptor antagonists
- Thromboxane-receptor antagonists
- ADP-receptor agonists
- Inhibitors of phosphoinositide breakdown
- Inhibitors of thromboxane formation
- Agents that increase cyclic nucleotides
- Protein kinase C activators

New pharmacological agents derived from medicinal plant sources may provide leads for the development of effective new cardiovascular drugs. However, from the herbal perspective, it might be more useful to consider the chemical groups involved.

Organosulfur Derivatives

A number of sulfur compounds from plants in the genus *Allium*, such as garlic and onion, have antiplatelet activity. These compounds work by a number of mechanisms, including direct inhibition of enzymes in the arachidonic cascade, inhibition of metabolite uptake by platelets, and direct inhibition of platelet phospholipase activity.

Antiplatelet Compounds in *Allium*
Ajoene
Alliin
Allicin
Allylmethyltrisulphide
2-Vinyl-1,3-dithiene
1-Propylmethyldisulphide

Flavonoids

The impact of flavonoid constituents on platelet activity must be seen in the context of the whole gamut of pharmacological effects discussed earlier in this chapter and in chapter 7. They have been shown to affect both aggregation and adhesion. Inhibition of phosphodiesterase has also been implicated.

Antiplatelet Flavonoids
Apigenin
Chrysin
Hispidulin
Phloretin
Quercetin

Coumarins

Coumarins inhibit aggregation but are relatively weak. An example of a coumarin with antiplatelet activity is disenecioyl-*cis*-khellactone.

Sesquiterpene Lactones

Parthenolides from feverfew (*Tanacetum parthenium*) inhibit both platelet aggregation and the release of serotonin from platelets.

Diterpenes

As discussed earlier, forskolin is a diterpene isolated from the roots of *Coleus forskohlii*. It stimulates adenylate cyclase activity in many tissues, which appears to be the action responsible for its antiplatelet activity.

Ginkgolides

PAF is dramatically inhibited by ginkgolides from *Ginkgo biloba*.

PAF and the Respiratory System

The most numerically important disorders of the respiratory system, excluding infections, are the allergic conditions asthma and hay fever. In both conditions, IgE antibodies attach to mast cells, and renewed exposure to antigen causes their degranulation. Also, inflammatory damage to the endothelium of the airways causes the underlying muscle to become supersensitive to external irritants and inflammatory mediators, including histamine, leukotrienes, thromboxanes, PAF, and chemotactic agents.[114] When this process occurs mainly in the nose, eyes, and throat, the result is hay fever. Bronchospasm, mucosal edema, and excessive mucus production lead to the coughing and wheezing that characterize asthma.

Occasionally, massive release of mediators leads to anaphylaxis, a life-threatening condition triggered by allergens. Anaphylaxis, which involves severe bronchospasm, edema in the nose and throat, and cardiovascular collapse, is treated with intravenous adrenaline, antihistamines, and corticosteroids.

Mast cell stabilizers play an important role in treatments used in orthodox medicine to prevent anaphylaxis; the main one is sodium cromoglycate. This drug was developed from khellin, a chromone from *Ammi visnaga*. Khellin derivatives relax bronchial smooth muscle, but cromoglycate also protects the tissue from the effects of bronchoconstrictors, such as histamine and acetylcholine. Its mechanism of action is unclear, but it appears to reduce the influx of calcium into antigen-sensitized mast cells, preventing the release of histamine.[115]

In the lung, PAF activates the arachidonic acid cascade with a dose-dependent generation of thromboxane. Formation of PAF in the lungs may also contribute to histamine release in anaphylaxis.[116] The most relevant PAF antagonists at present are of natural origin.

Ginkgolides

These C_{20} diterpenes suppress PAF-induced bronchoconstriction and airway hyperreactivity in humans and animals. They exert a protective effect against antigen-induced bronchial provocation tests in asthmatic patients. Ginkgolide B is the most potent member of the ginkgolide family of PAF antagonists; it inhibits PAF-induced platelet aggregation, chemotaxis, and adhesion. It is orally effective against PAF-induced bronchospasm.

Lignans

Kadsurenone, a neolignan found in *Piper futukadsura*, is a potent PAF inhibitor, and also inhibits degranulation of neutrophils while antagonizing other PAF-induced phenomena. Other lignans of interest as PAF antagonists include burseran, from *Bursera microphylla*, and the nectandrins A and B, from *Nectandra rigida*.

Gliotoxins

These are piperazine alkaloids produced by a wide range of fungi. Gliotoxin itself is a relatively weak PAF inhibitor, but various derivatives have been shown to inhibit PAF-induced bronchoconstriction in rats.

Forskolin

Asthma is characterized by a relative decrease in cAMP in the bronchial smooth muscle that causes mast cells to degranulate and smooth muscle cells to contract. Excessive levels of PAF are also present in asthma. Current drug therapy for asthma is largely designed to increase cAMP levels through the use of substances that either stimulate adenylate cyclase (for example, corticosteroids) or inhibit phosphodiesterase, which breaks down cAMP (for example, methyxanthines). *Coleus forskohlii* may be particularly useful in asthma, as it increases cellular levels of cAMP, resulting in relaxation of bronchial muscles and relief of symptoms.

HERBS AND THE LIVER

Conventional medicine does not provide many remedies for hepatitis, cirrhosis, biliary tract disorders, or liver damage by toxins. Patients with liver disorders are usually given supportive treatment, which may include dietary change and elimination of toxins (for example, paracetamol, alcohol, or other drugs) as opposed to active therapy. In both Western and Asian medical systems, herbs have long been utilized for liver problems, and pharmacological and clinical experiments have proved their efficacy. *Silybum marianum* (and its complex of flavolignans, known as silymarin) is perhaps the best known of these herbs.

Hepatoprotection and Phytotherapy

The main causes of liver disease are viral infection and hepatotoxic chemicals such as ethyl alcohol, peroxides (particularly peroxidized edible oils), toxins in food (especially aflatoxins), pharmaceuticals, and environmental pollutants. The liver has the ability to regenerate, but this innate ability is impaired or stops altogether when the liver is infected or damaged by alcohol or other drugs.

Hepatotoxin-induced liver lesions may be reversed in the early stages, but they cannot be healed simply by removal of the toxins after critical periods of exposure. This highlights the need for effective remedies for liver diseases.

In the face of the toxic challenge presented by modern life, the green world has help to offer.

A number of herbs long used for liver disorders in

traditional medicine have revealed their unique potential to pharmacological investigation. Research on these plants has resulted in the isolation of a number of anti-hepatotoxic (or hepatoprotective) constituents. Anti-hepatotoxic agents appear to work through a combination of two main mechanisms:

- Alteration of cell membranes, so that only small amounts of toxins may penetrate into the cell
- Acceleration of protein synthesis, with a subsequent stimulation of cell regeneration

A number of plants and secondary metabolites have been shown to possess antihepatotoxic activity. Of these, *Silybum marianum* is the best known and studied, but many others are coming to light.

- *Bidens pilosa* and *B. chilensis*, Taiwanese traditional medicines, are hepatoprotective against various toxins and have demonstrated potential as broad-spectrum antihepatotoxic agents.[117]
- *Scutellaria rivularis* improved pathological hepatic lesions caused by a number of liver toxins, and compared well to the standard antihepatotoxics glycyrrhizin and silymarin.[118]
- In an in vitro study of immunological liver injury to rat hepatocytes, all saponins from the roots of *Pueraria lobata* tested demonstrated hepatoprotective action.[119]

Natural compounds that elevate levels of biotransformation enzymes or reduce levels of activating enzymes can be considered good candidates for cancer-protective actions as well as generally beneficial effects for the liver. The sulfur-containing constituents characteristic of *Allium* species have attracted much attention. In one rat study investigating modulation of hepatic drug-metabolizing enzymes, the *Allium* compounds induced both Phase I and Phase II enzyme systems.[120] In addition, the alkyl sulfides demonstrated a possible inhibitory effect on the first step of carcinogenesis via modulation of enzymes involved in carcinogen metabolism. In both in vitro and in vivo studies, zeaxanthin and zeaxanthin dipalmitate were shown to be the hepatoprotective components of *Lycium chinense*.[121]

Functions of the Liver

The liver, the largest solid organ in the body and one of the most complex, has a wide range of vital functions:

- Metabolizes protein (amino acid degradation, synthesis of clotting factors, urea and plasma proteins)
- Metabolizes carbohydrates
- Stores glycogen
- Metabolizes lipids, including the synthesis of cholesterol and bile acids
- Initiates the formation of bile
- Engages in the transport of bilirubin
- Biotransforms waste, toxins, and drugs
- Produces blood-clotting factors and other blood proteins (including albumin, certain enzyme inhibitors, cholesterol and other lipoproteins, transport proteins, transferrin iron, and vitamin B_{12})

Glucose is combined with phosphate in the liver cells and is either transported to peripheral tissues for metabolic purposes or stored in the hepatocyte as glycogen. The liver plays a central role in metabolizing fat by converting stored fatty acids to their energy-releasing form, acetyl-coenzyme A, when hepatic glucose and glycogen stores are exhausted or unavailable for metabolic purposes. The liver also synthesizes the cell membrane component phospholipid and the lipoproteins that carry lipids in the blood. Hepatocytes can convert certain amino acids and products of glucose metabolism into glucose through gluconeogenesis. Reticulo-endothelial cells (the Kupffer's cells) play a role in immunity.

The liver is able to regenerate itself after injury or disease. However, if a disease progresses beyond the tissue's capacity to regenerate new cells, the body's entire metabolism will be severely affected. Any number of disorders can affect the liver and interfere with the blood supply or the functioning of bile ducts, Kupffer's cells, and other hepatic cells.

Silybum marianum and Silymarin

Milk thistle (*Silybum marianum*) was historically used in Europe as a liver tonic, and modern phytotherapy indicates its use in a range of liver and gallbladder conditions, including hepatitis and cirrhosis. A wealth of European research has produced data showing that milk thistle seeds can reverse toxic liver damage as well as protect against damage from hepatotoxins. As American physicians became interested in phytotherapy, this herbal antihepatotoxic gained a solid clinical reputation in the United States as well.[122]

The extraordinary actions of *Silybum* on the human liver are dramatically demonstrated by its hepatoprotective effects against the life-threatening damage caused by the death cap mushroom, *Amanita phalloides*, which contains the toxins phalloidin and α-amanitin. This remarkable herb also has therapeutic effects in liver disease. Clinical trials have confirmed its ability to reverse many liver disorders, from acute viral hepatitis to cirrhosis, by stimulating hepatocytes to replace diseased tissue.

Laboratory Studies

A number of specific phytochemicals in *Silybum* seed have been shown to protect liver cells. They are primarily flavolignans and are grouped together in a complex known as silymarin. The silymarin complex makes up between 1.5% and 3% of milk thistle seeds and includes silybin, silychristin, silydianin, and isosilybin.

In laboratory studies, silymarin has demonstrated a range of effects:

- Protected against carbon tetrachloride-induced liver damage in rats[123]
- Reduced prolongation of hexobarbital-induced sleeping time produced by carbon tetrachloride[124]
- Prevented inhibition of hepatic metabolism of *p*-oxyphenylpyruvic acid caused by carbon tetrachloride[125]
- Diminished increases in serum levels of enzymes (including glutamic-oxaloacetic transaminase, glutamic-pyruvic transaminase, and sorbitol dehydrogenase) raised by experimental treatment with carbon tetrachloride[126]
- Protected against the development of acute hepatitis (similar to viral hepatitis in humans) in rats treated with the liver toxin D-galactosamine[127]
- Partially counteracts alcohol damage to the liver; almost completely prevents mitochondrial changes caused by ethanol[128]
- Reduced death rate and prolonged life span in mice challenged by administration of α-amanitin; antagonized the toxicity of phalloidin[129]

- Enhanced RNA synthesis as a result of the stimulation of DNA-dependent RNA-polymerase A[130]
- Increased the activity of both superoxide dismutase and glutathione peroxidase, which may explain the protective effect of the herb against free radicals[131]

In another mouse study, silymarin also demonstrated protective effects against UVB radiation–induced nonmelanoma skin cancer. Silymarin treatment reduced tumor incidence by 20% to 40% and tumor volume per mouse by 66% after the tumor-initiation phase of the study. During UVB-induced tumor promotion, silymarin treatment reduced tumor incidence from 60% to 100% and tumor volume per mouse by 90%. In experimental UVB-induced complete carcinogenesis, silymarin reduced tumor incidence from 25% to 100% and tumor volume per mouse by 97%. Application of silymarin also resulted in a statistically significant inhibition of UVB-induced sunburn, apoptotic cell formation, skin edema, depletion of catalase activity, and induction of COX activities. The researchers concluded, "Silymarin can provide substantial protection against different stages of UVB-induced carcinogenesis, possibly via its strong antioxidant properties."[132]

Clinical Studies

Numerous human studies confirm that the effects demonstrated by *Silybum* and the silymarin complex in the laboratory are borne out in clinical practice.[133] The MedLine database contains references to 627 papers discussing silymarin and 41 clinical trials. The material that follows has been abstracted from an excellent review by Michael Murray, N.D.[134]

One study involved 129 patients and a control group of 56 for a period of about one month. Their conditions included toxic metabolic liver damage, fatty degeneration of the liver due to various causes, and chronic hepatitis. Treatment with milk thistle extract markedly improved both subjective and objective symptoms of liver and digestive disorders and normalized enzyme activities. The investigators reported a 50% regression in pathological symptoms in the group receiving milk thistle treatment, compared with 25% in controls; enlarged livers also diminished substantially in volume in the treated group. No intolerance, side effects, or allergic reactions were observed.

In another placebo-controlled study, researchers compared levels of a number of important markers of liver function in 28 patients treated with silymarin with 29 patients treated with a placebo. After only five days of treatment, the silymarin-treated subjects showed greater improvements in levels of aspartate transaminase (AST), alanine transaminase (ALT), and serum bilirubin, and after three weeks, the number of patients who attained normal values was also higher in the silymarin-treated group.

Long-term treatment with silymarin of chronic hepatopathies caused by psychopharmaceuticals resulted in significant improvements in liver function parameters such as AST, ALT, and BSP. (The BSP parameter is a measurement of the retention of the chemical sulfobromophtalein.) This helps investigators assess the efficiency of drug clearance by the liver.

In two additional studies involving patients with liver disease, those treated with silymarin demonstrated marked improvements in various liver parameters. In the first, 106 patients with liver disease (mostly alcohol-induced) were selected on the basis of elevated serum transaminase levels and randomly allocated into active and control groups. Decreases of serum ALT and AST in the treated group were statistically significantly higher than those of the controls.

In the second study, which involved patients with chronic liver disease, silymarin prevented decreases in seralbumin beginning at three months and continuing to the end of the study. Histopathological findings related to focal necrosis and fibrosis were also much improved. Overall, silymarin proved beneficial in parameters of parenchymal disorders, intralobular mesenchymal reactions, and fibrosis.

Diabetic patients with cirrhosis require insulin treatment because of insulin resistance. As chronic alcoholic liver damage is partly caused by peroxidation of hepatic cell membranes, antioxidants may be useful in treating or preventing such damage. A 1997 study investigated the effects of long-term treatment with silymarin in diabetic patients with cirrhosis. The results suggested that treatment with silymarin may reduce both lipid peroxidation of cell membranes and insulin resistance. In the study, silymarin also significantly decreased endogenous insulin overproduction and the need for exogenous insulin administration.[135]

Cisplatin is an active cytotoxic agent used in the treatment of testicular cancer. Its use, however, is associated with significant side effects, including ototoxicity, neurotoxicity, and nephrotoxicity. A clinical study evaluated the effects of the milk thistle compound silibinin in ameliorating drug-induced alterations in renal glomerular and tubular function and tubular morphology. Results showed that silibinin totally or partly ameliorated all of these effects. Thus, silibinin appears to also function as a nephroprotectant agent; the researchers suggested that it may have beneficial effects on the kidney in clinical settings.[136] This exciting data led to a randomized clinical trial to investigate the protective effects of silibinin against cisplatin-associated nephrotoxicity in patients with testicular cancer.[137]

HYPOGLYCEMIC AGENTS

More than 1,123 plant species have been used traditionally or experimentally to treat symptoms of diabetes mellitus.[138] These represent 725 genera in 183 families of plants. In addition, more than 200 compounds from plants have been reported to lower blood glucose.[139] Table 9.7 provides a summary of the chemical classes in which these compounds can be found.

The diversity represented here suggests that a variety of mechanisms must be involved in the glucose-lowering activities of plant compounds. Some of these compounds may have therapeutic potential, while others produce hypoglycemia as a side effect of their toxicity.

Table 9.7. Natural Products with Hypoglycemic Activity[140]

CHEMICAL CLASS	NUMBER ACTIVE
Alkaloids	38
Carbohydrates	66
Coumarins	4
Cyanogenic glycosides	1
Flavonoids	7
Glycopeptides	20
Inorganic salts	3
Iridoids	4
Lipids	6
Peptides and amines	15
Phenolics (simple)	4
Phenylpropanoids	1
Steroids	7
Stilbenes	1
Sulfur compounds	2
Terpenoids	17
Vitamins	2
Xanthenes	1

There are many plant extracts with proven hypoglycemic activity. No isolated compounds from these plants have yet been developed for clinical use, but all are used in traditional or complementary medicine to treat diabetes mellitus. Many of those that are dietary components have been tested in human diabetics and found to be hypoglycemic.

Plant Extracts with Hypoglycemic Activity

Allium cepa (onion)

A. sativum (garlic)

Momordica charantia (bitter gourd or melon)

Nelumbo nucifera (sacred lotus)

Opuntia ficus-indica (prickly pear)

Panax ginseng (ginseng)

Psidium gujava (guava)

Syzygium cumini (jambul)

Trigonella foenum-graecum (fenugreek)

Vernonia amygdalina (bitter leaf)

Testing of plants for hypoglycemic properties is based on inducing diabetes in animals with toxins (such as alloxan) and evaluating the hypoglycemia or glucose tolerance produced by a plant extract compared with that of a standard, such as tolbutamide. Alloxan causes selective necrosis of the pancreatic islet β cells. The experimental severity of the disease can be increased or decreased by varying the dose of alloxan.

Glycans from the mushroom *Ganoderma lucidum* produce significant hypoglycemia in alloxan-induced diabetes in animals. They appear to operate through a unique mechanism, probably affecting glycogen or glucose metabolism.[141] Ganoderan B, one of these glycans, has been shown to elevate plasma insulin levels and increase the activities of hepatic glucokinase, phosphofructokinase, and glucose-6 phosphate dehydrogenase. It also decreases the activities of hepatic glucose-6 phosphatase and glycogen synthetase and lowers hepatic glycogen content.

Momordica charantia, commonly known as bitter gourd, is a traditional remedy of the Pacific and Indian Ocean islands for diabetes mellitus. A controlled clinical trial involving 100 people with moderate noninsulindependent diabetes examined the effects of the herb on fasting and postprandial serum glucose levels. (Postprandial levels were measured two hours after oral intake of 75 gm of glucose.) Drinking the herb in the form of an aqueous homogenized suspension of pulp led to significant reductions in both fasting and postprandial serum glucose levels. This hypoglycemic action was observed in 86% of subjects.[142]

In another study, polypeptides from bitter gourd seeds stimulated lipogenesis and inhibited corticotropin-induced lipolysis in vivo, activities similar to those of insulin. The researchers suggested that the mechanism of action behind these effects involved interaction of the peptides with β-adrenergic or corticotropin receptors.[143] Inhibition of glucose uptake by intestinal fragments was also observed in this study, and was attributed to a glycosidic constituent of the fruit extract. This suggests that constituents of *M. charantia* have both pancreatic and extra-pancreatic effects and offer therapeutic potential for diabetic patients.

Madagascar periwinkle *(Catharanthus roseus)* has also been employed traditionally in the treatment of diabetes. In modern research, six alkaloids from this plant, including catharanthine, have demonstrated mild hypoglycemic activity.[144]

The major hypoglycemic principles of onion *(Allium cepa)* and garlic *(A. sativum)* are the sulfur-containing compounds, allyl propyl disulfide and allicin. They are thought to work via competitive interaction with insulin, which also has a disulfide bond.

Coumarin causes profound hypoglycemia in normal and alloxan-induced diabetic rats, probably because of its hepatotoxicity. Coumarin is hepatotoxic in rats and dogs, in which it is metabolized through 3-hydroxycoumarin to reactive quinone metabolites that bind to microsomal proteins. In humans, however, coumarin is metabolized through 7-hydroxycoumarin to a glucuronide conjugate that is rapidly excreted, and no hepatotoxicity occurs.[145]

Seeds of a number of species of Fabaceae plants (for example, *Trigonella foenum-graecum*, or fenugreek) are traditional treatments for diabetes. In addition to direct hypoglycemic effects, dietary effects are also important. In clinical studies, people eating a diet high in legumes showed improvements in many indices of blood glucose control. Beans are high in complex carbohydrates, which are more slowly digested than other types of starch. Noncellulosic types of dietary fiber (such as carob gum, guar gum, and high-molecular-weight galactomannans from *Ceratonia siliqua* and *Cyamopsis tetragonolobus*) reduce intestinal absorption of glucose by slowing gastric emptying and by thickening the water layer adjacent to the intestinal villi.[146]

A variety of glucans and heteroglycans from plants used in Asian traditional medicine have shown remarkable hypoglycemic activity when administered intraperitoneally to mice.[147] Panaxans A through E, glycans of *Panax ginseng*, demonstrate different mechanisms of action despite their similar structures. Panaxans A and B stimulate hepatic glucose utilization by increasing the activity of glucose-6-phosphate dehydrogenase, phosphorylase-a, and phosphofructokinase.

Panaxan A decreases the activity of glucose-6-phosphatase but does not affect hepatic glycogen content. Panaxan B has no effect on glucose-6-phosphatase, but decreases glycogen synthetase activity and hepatic glycogen content.[148] Panaxan A does not affect plasma insulin levels or insulin sensitivity, but panaxan B elevates the plasma insulin level by potentiating insulin secretion from pancreatic islets. It also enhances insulin sensitivity by increasing insulin binding to receptors.[149]

Ginseng also contains other hypoglycemic constituents with different mechanisms of action. Adenosine, from a water extract of ginseng rhizomes, was shown to enhance lipogenesis and the accumulation of cAMP in adipocytes, which possess specific adenosine receptors. Some of the panaxosides inhibited adrenocorticotropin-induced lipolysis and, at the same doses, suppressed insulin-stimulated lipogenesis, while others stimulated the release of insulin from cultured islets.[150,151]

Intracellular cAMP also acts as a secondary messenger in the β-cells. Increasing intracellular cAMP concentration potentiates cholecystokinin and glucose-stimulated insulin release. As mentioned earlier, forskolin from *Coleus forskohlii* is an adenylate cyclase activator that increases intracellular cAMP by stimulating its biosynthesis.[152] Theophylline and other methylxanthenes from *Camellia sinensis* and papaverine from *Papaver somniferum* are phosphodiesterase inhibitors that increase levels of intracellular cAMP by preventing its breakdown.

References

1. Viola H, Wasowski C, Levi de Stein M, et al. Apigenin, a component of Matricaria recutita flowers, is a central benzodiazepine receptors-ligand with anxiolytic effects. *Planta Medica* 1995; 61(3):213–16.

2. Wolfman C, Viola H, Paladini A, et al. Possible anxiolytic effects of chrysin, a central benzodiazepine receptor ligand isolated from Passiflora coerulea. *Pharmacology, Biochemistry, and Behavior* 1994; 47(1):1–4.

3. Bergendorff O, Nielsen M, et al. Furanocoumarins with affinity to brain benzodiazepine receptors in vitro. *Phytochemistry* 1997; 44(6):1121–24.

4. Furukawa K, Chairungsrilerd N, Ohta T, et al. Novel types of receptor antagonists from the medicinal plant Garcinia mangostana. *Nippon Yakurigaku Zasshi (Japanese Journal of Pharmacology)* 1997; 110(suppl 1):153P–58P.

5. Sotnikova R, Kettmann V, Kostalova D, Taborska E. Relaxant properties of some aporphine alkaloids from Mahonia aquifolium. *Methods and Findings in Experimental and Clinical Pharmacology* 1998; 19(9):589–97.

6. Polya GM, Wang BH, Foo LY. Inhibition of signal-regulated protein kinases by plant-derived hydrolysable tannins. *Phytochemistry* 1995; 38:307–14.

7. Hansen, et al. In vitro screening of traditional medicines for anti-hypertensive effect based on inhibition of the angiotensin converting enzyme (ACE). *Journal of Ethnopharmacology* 1995; 48(1):43–51.

8. Webb EC. *Enzyme Nomenclature 1992: Recommendations of the Nomenclature Committee of the International Union of Biochemistry and Molecular Biology*. San Diego: Academic Press, 1997.

9. Seamon KB, Daly JW. Forskolin: a unique diterpene activator of cyclic AMP-generating systems. *Journal of Cyclic Nucleotide Research* 1981; 7(4):201–24.

10. Freeman SE, Dawson RM. Tacrine: A pharmacological review. *Progress in Neurobiology* 1991; 36:257–77.

11. Jia Sen, et al. Study of the chemistry of huperzine A and B. *Acta Chimica Sinica* 1986; 44:1035–104.

12. Price KR, Fenwick GR. Naturally occurring oestrogens in foods—a review. *Food Additives and Contaminants* 1985; 2:73–106.

13. Adlercreutz H, Honjo H, Higashi A, et al. Urinary excretion of lignans & isoflavonoid phytoestrogens in Japanese men & women consuming a traditional Japanese diet. *The American Journal of Clinical Nutrition* 1991 Dec; 54(6):1093–100.

14. Barnes S, Peterson TG. Biochemical targets of the isoflavone genistein in tumor cell lines. *Proceedings of the Society for Experimental Biology and Medicine* 1995; 208(1):103–8.

15. Adlercreutz H, Markkanen H, Watanabe S. Plasma concentrations of phyto-oestrogens in Japanese men. *Lancet* 1993 Nov 13; 342(8881):1209–10.

16. Fotsis T, Pepper M, Adlercreutz H, et al. Genistein, a dietary ingested isoflavonoid, inhibits cell proliferation and in vitro angiogenesis. *The Journal of Nutrition* 1995 Mar; 125(3 suppl):790S–97S.

17. Kennedy AR. The evidence for soybean products as cancer preventive agents. *The Journal of Nutrition* 1995 Mar; 125(3 suppl):733S–43S.

18. Herman C, Adlercreutz T, Goldin BR, et al. Soybean phytoestrogen intake and cancer risk. *The Journal of Nutrition* 1995 Mar; 125(3 suppl):757S–70S.

19. Seamon KB, Padgett W, Daly JW. Forskolin: unique diterpene activator of adenylate cyclase in membranes

and in intact cells. *Proceedings of the National Academy of Sciences of the United States of America* 1981; 78(6):3363–7.

20. Miksicek RJ. Commonly occurring plant flavonoids have estrogenic activity. *Molecular Pharmacology* 1993 Jul; 44(1):37–43.

21. Herman C, Adlercreutz T, Goldin BR, et al. Soybean phytoestrogen intake and cancer risk. *The Journal of Nutrition* 1995 Mar; 125(3 suppl):757S–70S.

22. Kitts DD. Studies on the estrogenic activity of a coffee extract. *Journal of Toxicology and Environmental Health* 1987; 20(1–2):37–49.

23. Miksicek RJ. Estrogenic flavonoids: structural requirements for biological activity. *Proceedings of the Society for Experimental Biology and Medicine* 1995 Jan; 208(1):44–50.

24. Miksicek RJ. Interaction of naturally occurring non-steroidal estrogens with expressed recombinant human estrogen receptor. *The Journal of Steroid Biochemistry and Molecular Biology* 1994 Jun; 49(2–3):153–60.

25. Barnes S. Effect of genistein on in vitro and in vivo models of cancer. *The Journal of Nutrition* 1995 Mar; 125(3 Suppl):777S–83S.

26. Fotsis T, Pepper M, Adlercreutz H, et al. Genistein, a dietary ingested isoflavonoid, inhibits cell proliferation and in vitro angiogenesis. *The Journal of Nutrition* 1995 Mar; 125(3 Suppl):790S–97S.

27. Peterson G. Evaluation of the biochemical targets of genistein in tumor cells. *The Journal of Nutrition* 1995 Mar; 125(3 Suppl):784S–89S.

28. Adlercreutz H, Bannwart C, Wahala K, et al. Inhibition of human aromatase by mammalian lignans and isoflavonoid phytoestrogens. *The Journal of Steroid Biochemistry and Molecular Biology* 1993 Feb; 44(2):147–53.

29. Ibid.

30. Adlercreutz H, Mousavi Y, Clark J, et al. Dietary phytoestrogens and cancer: in vitro and in vivo studies. *The Journal of Steroid Biochemistry and Molecular Biology* 1992; 41(3–8):331–7.

31. Martin PM, Horwitz KB, Ryan DS, McGuire WL. Phytoestrogen interaction with estrogen receptors in human breast cancer cells. *Endocrinology* 1978 Nov; 103(5):1860–7.

32. Whitten PL, Lewis C, Russell E, Naftolin F. Potential adverse effects of phytoestrogens. *The Journal of Nutrition* 1995 Mar; 125(3 Suppl).:771S–76S.

33. Molteni A, Brizio-Molteni L, Persky V. In vitro hormonal effects of soybean isoflavones. *The Journal of Nutrition* 1995 Mar; 125(3 Suppl.):751S–56S.

34. Whitten PL, Russell E, Naftolin F. Influence of phyto-

estrogen diets on estradiol action in the rat uterus. *Steroids* 1994 Jul; 59(7):443–9.

35. Whitten PL, Russell E, Naftolin F. Effects of a normal, human-concentration, phytoestrogen diet on rat uterine growth. *Steroids* 1992 Mar; 57(3):98–106.

36. Levy JR, Faber KA, Ayyash L, Hughes CL Jr. The effect of prenatal exposure to the phytoestrogen genistein on sexual differentiation in rats. *Proceedings of the Society for Experimental Biology and Medicine* 1995 Jan; 208(1):60–6.

37. Miksicek RJ. Interaction of naturally occurring non-steroidal estrogens with expressed recombinant human estrogen receptor. *The Journal of Steroid Biochemistry and Molecular Biology* 1994 Jun; 49(2–3):153–60.

38. Adlercreutz H, Hockerstedt K, Bannwart C, et al. Effect of dietary components, including lignans and phytoestrogens, on enterohepatic circulation and liver metabolism of estrogens and on sex hormone binding globulin (SHBG). *Journal of Steroid Biochemistry* 1987; 27(4–6):1135–44.

39. Herman C, Adlercreutz T, Goldin BR, et al. Soybean phytoestrogen intake and cancer risk. *The Journal of Nutrition* 1995 Mar; 125(3 Suppl):757S–70S.

40. Barnes S. Effect of genistein on in vitro and in vivo models of cancer. *The Journal of Nutrition* 1995 Mar; 125(3 Suppl):777S–83S.

41. Molteni A, Brizio-Molteni L, Persky V. In vitro hormonal effects of soybean isoflavones. *The Journal of Nutrition* 1995 Mar; 125(3 Suppl):751S–56S.

42. Bingel AS, Farnsworth N. Higher plants as potential sources of Galactagogues. In: *Economic and Medicinal Plant Research*, vol. 6. San Diego: Academic Press, 1995.

43. Elliot T. T Cell recognition of glycosylated peptides. *Science and Medicine* 1994; 5(3):44–53.

44. Spatzenegger M, Jaeger W. Clinical importance of hepatic cytochrome P_{450} in drug metabolism. *Drug Metabolism Reviews* 1995; 27:397–417.

45. Benet LZ, Kroetz DL, Sheiner LB. Biotransformation of drugs. In: Hardman JG, Limbird LL, Molinoff PB, et al., eds. *Goodman and Gilman's The Pharmacological Basis of Therapeutics*, 9th edition. New York: McGraw-Hill, 1996.

46. Murray M. P_{450} enzymes. Inhibition mechanisms, genetic regulation, and effects of liver disease. *Clinical Pharmacokinetics* 1992; 23:132–46.

47. Strehl E, Schneider W, Elstner EF. Inhibition of dihydrofolate reductase activity by alcoholic extracts from Fraxinus excelsior, Populus tremula and Solidago virgaurea. *Arzneimittel-Forschung* 1995 Feb; 45(2):172–73.

48. Poulsen HE, Loft S. The impact of genetic polymorphisms in risk assessment of drugs. *Archives of Toxicology. Supplement* 1994; 16:211–22.

49. Peterson TC, Renton KW. Depression of cytochrome P$_{450}$ dependent drug biotransformation in hepatocytes after the activation of the RES by dextran sulphate. *The Journal of Pharmacology and Experimental Therapeutics* 1984; 229:299–304.

50. Wagner H, Proksch A. Immunostimulatory drugs of fungi and higher plants. In: *Economic and Medicinal Plant Research*, vol. 1. San Diego: Academic Press, 1985.

51. Beuscher N, Kopanski L. Immunologically active glycoproteins of Baptisia tinctoria. *Planta Medica* 1989 Aug; 55(4):358–63.

52. Manzi P, Pizzoferrato L. Beta glucans in edible mushrooms. *Food Chemistry* 2000; 68:315–18.

53. Ladanyi A, Timar J, Lapis K. Effect of lentinan on macrophage cytotoxicity against metastatic tumor cells. *Cancer Immunology, Immunotherapy* 1993; 36:123–26.

54. Kidd P. The use of mushroom glucans and proteoglycans in cancer treatment. *Alternative Medicine Review: A Journal of Clinical Therapeutic* 2000; 5:4–27.

55. Borchers AT, Stem JS, Hackman RM, et al. Mushrooms, tumors, and immunity. *Proceedings of the Society for Experimental Biology and Medicine* 1999; 221:281–93.

56. Wasser SP, Weis AL. Therapeutic effects of substances occurring in higher Basidiomycetes mushrooms: a modern perspective. *Critical Reviews in Immunology* 1999; 19:65–96.

57. Wagner H, Proksch A. Immunostimulatory drugs of fungi and higher plants. In: *Economic and Medicinal Plant Research*, vol.1. San Diego: Academic Press, 1985.

58. Melzer R, Fricke U, Holzl J. Vasoactive properties of procyanidins from Hypericum perforatum L. in isolated porcine coronary arteries. *Arzneimittel-Forschung* 1991 May; 41(5):481–83.

59. Chan MM, Fong D, Ho CT, Huang HI. Inhibition of inducible nitric oxide synthase gene expression and enzyme activity by epigallocatechin gallate, a natural product from green tea. *Biochemical Pharmacology* 1997 Dec 15; 54(12):1281–86.

60. Kumar S, Ziereis K, Wiegrebe W, Muller K. Medicinal plants from Nepal: evaluation as inhibitors of leukotriene biosynthesis. *Journal of Ethnopharmacology* 2000 Jun; 70(3):191–95.

61. Plohmann B, Bader G, Hiller K, Franz G. Immunomodulatory and antitumoral effects of triterpenoid saponins. *Pharmazie* 1997 Dec; 52(12):953–57.

62. Liu P, Zhu J, Huang Y, Liu C. Influence of Cordyceps sinensis (Berk.) Sacc. and rat serum containing same medicine on IL-1, IFN and TNF produced by rat Kupffer cells. *Chung Kuo Chung Yao Tsa Chih* 1996 Jun; 21(6):367–69.

63. Gao, et al. Immunostimulating polysaccharides from Panax notoginseng. *Pharmaceutical Research* 1996 Aug; 13(8):1196–200.

64. Hajto T, Hostanska K, Fischer J, Saller R. Immunomodulatory effects of Viscum album agglutinin-I on natural immunity. *Anticancer Drugs* 1997 Apr; 8 (Suppl 1):S43–S46.

65. Kimura Y, Matsushita N, Okuda H. Effects of baicalein isolated from Scutellaria baicalensis on interleukin 1 beta- and tumor necrosis factor alpha-induced adhesion molecule expression in cultured human umbilical vein endothelial cells. *Journal of Ethnopharmacology* 1997 Jun; 57(1):63–7.

66. Stein GM, Berg PA. Mistletoe extract-induced effects on immunocompetent cells: in vitro studies. *Anticancer Drugs* 1997 Apr; 8 (Suppl. 1):S39–S42.

67. Rolfsen WNA. PAF antagonists from natural products. *Drugs of the Future* 1990; 15:597–603.

68. Zschocke S, Lehner M, Bauer R. 5-Lipoxygenase and cyclooxygenase inhibitory active constituents from Qianghuo (Notopterygium incisum). *Planta Medica* 1997 Jun; 63(3):203–6.

69. Cassady Douros. *Anticancer Agents Based on Natural Product Models*. New York: Academic Press, 1980.

70. Hartwell JL. Plants used against cancer. A survey. *Lloydia* 1967; 30:379–436.

71. Hartwell JL. Plants used against cancer. A survey. *Lloydia* 1971; 32:204–55.

72. Taylor WI, Farnsworth NR. *The Catharanthus Alkaloids*. London: Marcel Dekker, 1975.

73. Sato F, Matsukawa Y, Matsumoto K, et al. Apigenin induces morphological differentiation and G2-M arrest in rat neuronal cells. *Biochemical and Biophysical Research Communications* 1994; 204: 578–84.

74. Barnes S. Effect of genistein on in vitro and in vivo models of cancer. *The Journal of Nutrition* 1995; 125:777S–83S.

75. Fotis T, Pepper M, et al. Genistein, a dietary ingested isoflavonoid, inhibits cell proliferation and in vitro angiogenesis. *The Journal of Nutrition* 1995; 125:790S–97S.

76. Peterson G. Evaluation of the biochemical targets of genistein in tumor cells. *The Journal of Nutrition* 1995; 125:784S–89S.

77. Barnes S, Peterson TG. Biochemical targets of the isoflavone genistein in tumor cell lines. *Proceedings of the Society for Experimental Biology and Medicine* 1995; 208:109–15.

78. Conctantinou A, Huberman E. Genistein as an inducer of tumor cell differentiation: possible mechanisms of action. *Proceedings of the Society for Experimental Biology and Medicine* 1995; 208:109–15.

79. Rowinsky EK, Cazenave LA, Donehower RC. Taxol: A novel investigational antimicrotubule agent. *Journal of the National Cancer Institute* 1990; 82:1247–59.

80. Salmon SE, Sartorelli AC. Cancer chemotherapy. In: Katzung BG, ed. *Basic and Clinical Pharmacology*. Norwalk, CT: Appleton and Lange, 1989.

81. Pazdur R, Kudelka AP, et al. The taxoids: paclitaxel (Taxol®) and docetaxel (Taxotere®). *Cancer Treatment Reviews* 1993; 19:351–86.

82. Runowicz CD, Wiernik PH, et al. Taxol in ovarian cancer. *Cancer* (Suppl.) 1993; 71:1591–96.

83. Ranelletti FO, et al. Growth-inhibitory effect of quercetin and presence of type-II estrogen-binding sites in human colon-cancer cell lines and primary colorectal tumors. *International Journal of Cancer* 1992; 50:486.

84. Kimura Y, Matsushita N, Okuda H. Effects of baicalein isolated from Scutellaria baicalensis on interleukin 1 beta- and tumor necrosis factor alpha-induced adhesion molecule expression in cultured human umbilical vein endothelial cells. *Journal of Ethnopharmacology* 1997 Jun; 57(1):63–67.

85. Kim, et al. Taraxacum officinale inhibits tumor necrosis factor-alpha production from rat astrocytes. *Immunopharmacol Immunotoxicol* 2000 Aug; 22(3):519–30.

86. Kawaguchi, et al. Colony stimulating factor-inducing activity of isoflavone C-glucosides from the bark of Dalbergia monetaria. *Planta Medica* 1998 Oct; 64(7):653–5.

87. Lamm DL, Riggs DR. Enhanced immunocompetence by garlic: role in bladder cancer and other malignancies. *The Journal of Nutrition* 2001 Mar; 131(3 suppl):1067S–70S.

88. Gerritsen, et al. Flavonoids inhibit cytokine-induced endothelial cell adhesion protein gene expression. *American Journal of Pathology* 1995; 147:278–92.

89. Watanabe T, et al. Inhibitors for protein-tyrosine kinase, ST638 and genistein, induce differentiation of mouse erythroleukemia cells in a synergistic manner. *Experimental Cell Research* 1989; 183:335.

90. Waxman S. Structural requirements for differentiation-induction and growth-inhibition of mouse erythroleukemia cells by isoflavones. *Anticancer Research* 1995; 15:1147–52.

91. Breitman TR. The role of prostaglandins and other arachidonic acid metabolites in the differentiation of HL-60. *Prostaglandins in Cancer Research*. Berlin: Springer-Verlag, 1987.

92. Schwartzman RA, Cidlowski JA. Apoptosis: The biochemistry and molecular biology of permanent cell death. *Endocrine Reviews* 1993; 14(2):133–45.

93. Thatte U, Bagadey S, Dahanukar S. Modulation of programmed cell death by medicinal plants. *Cellular and Molecular Biology (Noisy-le-Grand, France)* 2000 Feb; 46(1):199–214.

94. Janssen O, Scheffler A, Kabelitz D. In vitro effects of mistletoe extracts and mistletoe lectins. *Arzneimittel-Forschung* 1993; 43:1221–27.

95. Bussing A, Suzart K, et al. Induction of apoptosis in human lymphocytes treated with Viscum album L. is mediated by the mistletoe lectins. *Cancer Letters* 1996; 99:59–72.

96. Mochizuki, et al. Inhibitory effect of tumor metastasis in mice by saponins, ginsenoside-Rb2, 20(R)- and 20(S)-ginsenoside-Rg3, of red ginseng. *Biological & Pharmaceutical Bulletin* 1995 Sept; 18(9):1197–202.

97. Block G, Patterson B, Subar A. Fruit, vegetables and cancer prevention: a review of the epidemiological evidence. *Nutrition and Cancer* 1992; 18(1):1–29.

98. Wattenberg LW. Inhibition of carcinogenesis by minor dietary constituents. *Cancer Research* (suppl) 1992; 52:2085–91.

99. Steinmetz KA, Potter JD. Vegetables, fruit and cancer. *Cancer Causes Control* 1991; 2(6):427–42.

100. Semple, et al. Screening of Australian medicinal plants for antiviral activity. *Journal of Ethnopharmacology* 1998; 60(2):163–72.

101. Vlietinck, et al. Plant-derived leading compounds for chemotherapy of human immunodeficiency virus (HIV) infection. *Planta Medica* 1998; 64(2):97–109.

102. Dalton DA, et al. Antioxidant defenses in the peripheral cell layers of legume root nodules. *Plant Physiology* 1998 Jan; 116(1):37–43.

103. Masaki, et al. Active-oxygen scavenging activity of plant extracts. *Biological & Pharmaceutical Bulletin* 1995; 18(1):162–6.

104. Kandaswami C, Middleton E. Free radical scavenging and antioxidant activity of plant flavonoids. In: Armstrong D, ed. *Free Radicals in Diagnostic Medicine*. New York: Plenum Press, 1994.

105. Ghisalberti, et al. Survey of secondary plant metabolites with cardiovascular activity. *Pharmaceutical Biology* 1998; 36(4):237–79.

106. Lindner E, Dohawalla AN, Bhattacharya BK. Positive inotropic and blood pressure lowering activity of a diterpene derivative isolated form coleus forskohli: forskolin. *Arzneimittel-Forschung* 1978; 28:284–9.

107. Villar, et al. Plants with anti-hypertensive action. *Fitoterapia* 1986; 57:131–45.

108. Neuhaus-Carlisle K, Vierling W, Wagner H. Screening plant extracts and plant constituents for calcium-channel blocking activity. *Phytomedicine: International Journal of Phytotherapy and Phytopharmacology* 1997; 4(1):67–69.

109. Vuorela, et al. Calcium channel blocking activity: Screening methods for plant derived compounds. *Phytomed* 1997; 4:167–81.

110. Elbl G, Wagner H. A new method for the in vitro screening of inhibitors of angiotensin converting emzyme (ACE), using the chromophore- and fluorophore-labelled substrate, dansyltriglycine. *Planta Medica* 1991; 57:137–41.

111. Wagner H. Leading structures of plant origin for drug development. *Journal of Ethnopharmacology* 1993; 38:105–12.

112. Wagner, et al. Evaluation of natural products as inhibitors of angiotensin I converting enzyme (ACE). *Pharmaceutical and Pharmacological Letters* 1991; 1:15–18.

113. Teng CM, Ko FN. Antiplatelet agents isolated from medicinal plants. *Research Communications in Molecular Pathology and Pharmacology* 1998 Dec; 102(3):211–25.

114. Barnes PJ, et al. Inflammatory mediators and asthma. *Pharmacological Reviews* 1988; 40:49–84.

115. Gould MK, Raffin TA. Pharmacological management of acute and chronic bronchial asthma. *Advances in Pharmacology* 1995; 32:169–204.

116. Summers JB, Albert DH. Platelet activating factor antagonists. *Advances in Pharmacology* 1995; 32:67–168.

117. Chin HW, Lin CC, Tang KS. The hepatoprotective effects of Taiwan folk medicine ham-hong-chho in rats. *The American Journal of Chinese Medicine* 1996; 24(3–4):231–40.

118. Lin CC, Shieh DE, Yen MH. Hepatoprotective effect of the fractions of Ban-zhi-lian on experimental liver injuries in rats. *Journal of Ethnopharmacology* 1997 May; 56(3):193–200.

119. Arao T, Udayama M, Kinjo J, Nohara T. Preventive effects of saponins from the Pueraria lobata root on in vitro immunological liver injury of rat primary hepatocyte cultures. *Planta Medica* 1998 Jun; 64(5):413–16.

120. Siess MH, Le Bon AM, Canivenc-Lavler MC, Suschetet M. Modification of hepatic drug-metabolizing enzymes in rats treated with alkyl sulfides. *Cancer Letters* 1997 Dec 9; 120(2):195–201.

121. Kim HP, Kim SY, Lee EJ, et al. Zeaxanthin dipalmitate from Lycium chinense has hepatoprotective activity. *Research Communications in Molecular Pathology and Pharmacology* 1997 Sep; 97(3):301–14.

122. Flora K, Hahn M, Rosen H, Benner K. Milk thistle (Silybum marianum) for the therapy of liver disease. *The American Journal of Gastroenterology* 1998 Feb; 93(2):139–43.

123. Vogel G, Trost W, Braatz R, et al. Studies on pharmacodynamics, site and mechanism of action of silymarin, the antihepatotoxic principle from Silyburn marianurn (L.) Gaert. *Arzneimittel-Forschung* 1975; 2(5):179–85.

124. Wagner H. Plant constituents with antihepatotoxic activity. In: Beal JL, Reinhard E eds. *Natural Products as Medicinal Agents*. Stuttgart: Hippokrates-Verlag, 1981.

125. Ibid.

126. Ibid.

127. Ibid.

128. Valenzuela A, Lagos C, Schmidt K, Videla LA. Silymarin protection against hepatichpid peroxidation induced by acute ethanol intoxication in the rat. *Biochemical Pharmacology* 1985; 34:2209–12.

129. Vogel G, Trost W, Braatz R, et al. Studies on pharmacodynamics, site and mechanism of action of silymarin, the antihepatotoxic principle from Silyburn marianurn (L.) Gaert. *Arzneimittel-Forschung* 1975; 2(5):179–85.

130. Sonnenbichler J, Goldberg M, Hane L, et al. Stimulatory effect of silibinin on the DNA synthesis in partially hepatectornized rat livers: non-response in hepatoma and other malignant cell lines. *Biochemical Pharmacology* 1986; 35:538–41.

131. Wellington K, Jarvis B. Silymarin: A review of its clinical properties in the management of hepatic disorders. *Biodrugs* 2001; 15(7):465–89.

132. Katiyar, et al. Protective effects of silymarin against photocarcinogenesis in a mouse skin model. *Journal of the National Cancer Institute* 1997 Apr 16; 89(8):556–66.

133. Saller R, Meier R, Brignoli R. The use of silymarin in the treatment of liver diseases. *Drugs* 2001; 61(14):2035–63.

134. Murray Michael. *Healing Power of Herbs*. Rocklin, CA: Prima, 1992.

135. Saller R, Meier R, Brignoli R. The use of silymarin in the treatment of liver diseases. *Drugs* 2001; 61(14):2035–63.

136. Gaedeke, et al. Cisplatin nephrotoxicity and protection by silibinin. *Nephrology, Dialysis, Transplantation* 1996 Jan; 11(1):55–62.

137. Bokemeyer, et al. Silibinin protects against cisplatin-induced nephrotoxicity without compromising cisplatin or ifosfamide anti-tumour activity. *British Journal of Cancer* 1996 Dec; 74(12):2036–41.

138. Neef H, et al. Hypoglycaemic activity of selected European plants. *Phytotherapy Research: PTR* 1995; 9(1):45.

139. Perl M. The biochemical basis of the hypoglycemic effects of some plant extracts. In: Cracker LE, Simon JE, eds. *Herbs, Spices and Medicinal Plants*, vol. 3. Phoenix: Oryx Press, 1988.

140. Marles RJ, Farnsworth NR. Antidiabetic plants and their active constituents. *Phytomedicine: International Journal of Phytotherapy and Phytopharmacology* 1995; 2:137–89.

141. Hikino H, et al. Mechanisms of hypoglycemic activity of ganoderan B: a glycan of Ganoderma lucidum fruit bodies. *Planta Medica* 1989; 55:423–28.

142. Ahmad N, Hassan MR, Halder H, et al. Effect of Momordica charantia (Karolla) extracts on fasting and postprandial serum glucose levels in NIDDM patients. *Bangladesh Medical Research Council Bulletin* 1999; 25(1):11–3.

143. Ng T, et al. Insulin-like molecules in Momordica charantia seeds. *Journal of Ethnopharmacology* 1986 Jan; 15(1):107–17.

144. Singh S, Vats P, Suri S, et al. Effect of an antidiabetic extract of Catharanthus roseus on enzymic activities in streptozotocin induced diabetic rats. *Journal of Ethnopharmacology* 2001 Aug; 76(3):269–77.

145. Cohen AJ. Critical review of the toxicology of coumarin with special reference to interspecies differences in metabolism and hepatotoxic response and their significance to man. *Food and Cosmetics Toxicology*. 1979 Jun; 17(3):277–89.

146. Karlstrom B, et al. Effects of leguminous seeds in a mixed diet in non-insulin-dependent diabetic patients. *Diabetes Research* 1987; 5(4):199–205.

147. Perl M, Hikino H. Effect of some hypoglycemic glycans on glucose uptake and glucose metabolism by inverted intestinal fragments. *Phytotherapy Research: PTR* 1989; 3(5):433–35.

148. Suzuki Y, Hikino H. Mechanisms of hypoglycemic activity of panaxans A and B, glycans of Panax ginseng roots: effects on the key enzymes of glucose metabolism in the liver of mice. *Phytotherapy Research: PTR* 1989; 3(1):15–19.

149. Suzuki Y, Hikino H. Mechanisms of hypoglycemic activity of panaxans A and B, glycans of Panax ginseng roots: Effects on plasma level, secretion, sensitivity and binding of insulin in mice. *Phytotherapy Research: PTR* 1989; 3:20–4.

150. Waki I, Kyo H, Yasuda M, Kimura M. Effects of a hypoglycemic component of Ginseng radix on insulin biosynthesis in normal and diabetic animals. *Journal of Pharmacobio-dynamics* 1982; 5:547–54.

151. Ng TB, Yeung HW. Hypoglycemic constituents of Panax ginseng. *General Pharmacology* 1985; 16:549–52.

152. Ammon HP, Muller AB. Forskolin: from an ayurvedic remedy to a modern agent. *Planta Medica* 1985 Dec; (6):473–77.

Suggested Reading

Boik J. *Cancer & Natural Medicine: A Textbook of Basic Science and Clinical Research*. Princeton, MN: Oregon Medical Press, 1996.

Hardman JG, Limbird LE, eds. *Goodman & Gilman's the Pharmacological Basis of Therapeutics*. New York: McGraw-Hill, 2001.

Mutschler E. *Drug Actions: Basic Principles and Therapeutic Aspects*. Stuttgart: Medpharm Scientific; Boca Raton, FL: CRC Press, 1995.

10

Ꙭ

TOXICITY, CONTRAINDICATIONS, AND SAFETY

Recent years have seen profound cultural changes that are transforming the sociopolitical environment within which the practice of herbalism is flowering. The dominant culture has moved to embrace herbalism, and it is no longer seen as fringe. Within this brave new world, the phytotherapy community faces both wonderful opportunities and profound challenges. One of the thorniest of these concerns the safety, toxicity, and contraindications of herbs.

Today, much is being written about herbs and herbalism that has little to do with plants or patients and everything to do with the belief system and dogma of the writer. The herbal "true believers" deny any problems that might exist with herbs because herbs are natural, while summarily denouncing synthetic drugs. On the other hand, some supposedly objective scientists can make even hawthorn sound as dangerous as crack cocaine. Some critical thinking is needed to traverse this maze of information and misinformation, evangelism and bigotry.

In general, statements about the toxicity of a plant may be based on any of a number of factors.

Observation of actual cases. These may be published reports on individual responses to herbs or may come from published research on therapeutic trials in which research subjects were either healthy volunteers or undergoing treatment for a health condition.

Extrapolation from chemical effects to whole plant effects. Knowing the effects of a specific plant constituent provides little basis for conclusions about effects of the whole plant. An example here is a contraindication for salicylate-containing herbs in cases of peptic ulcer based on the fact that aspirin will aggravate peptic ulcer. While this may sound appropriate in theory, in reality the salicylate-rich plant meadowsweet *(Filipendula ulmaria)* works as an effective anti-inflammatory and vulnerary in such conditions—and causes none of the side effects of aspirin.

Extrapolation from animal evidence to humans. For example, the statement that St. John's wort *(Hypericum perforatum)* causes photosensitivity is based on observance of phototoxicity reactions in light-colored range animals that graze on the plant.

Traditional knowledge, or belief based on experience with extensive use, is another potential source of information about risks and contraindications for herbs. However, this information must also be carefully considered. For example, feverfew is traditionally used for the prophylaxis of migraine in the form of a fresh leaf chewed daily, which may cause canker sores (aphthous ulcers). However, this often-repeated risk does not apply when the leaf is swallowed or when the herb is taken in tablet and tincture forms, which cause no buccal irritation.

Subjective opinion or belief system. Subjective statements from those considered experts in the field are often unquestioningly accepted as insightful, considered opinions. But who are the experts in these situations?

Consider the following quotation from *The Honest Herbal,* by Professor Varro Tyler. Charles C. Bennett, vice president of Public Education for the Arthritis Foundation, has suggested that inquiries concerning yucca be answered

". . . by saying that there is no proper scientific evidence that yucca tablets are helpful in treating rheumatoid arthritis or osteoarthritis; that they are probably harmless; and that the real danger would be in taking yucca tablets instead of following proper and proven treatment procedures, which could lead to irreversible joint damage and possible disabilities." Nothing need be added to this statement.[1]

I beg to differ. This statement turns the opinion of Mr. Bennett about treatment advisability into a statement about a plant. The statement is about patient choice, and yucca has nothing to do with it. There needs to be a recognition here of two distinct issues. First, herbs are medicinal substances. Second, phytotherapy is a valid therapeutic modality, and the skills and clinical experience of its practitioners must be recognized.

EVALUATING CAUSALITY IN ADVERSE EVENTS

Correct identification of the herbs involved in any adverse reaction is critical to the development of reliable data on herb safety, toxicity, and interactions. Too often, herbal products have been associated with adverse events because of mislabeling, which in turn results from either intentional or accidental substitution of botanical ingredients. The following quotation from DeSmet and D'Arcy may prove enlightening.

> When such reports of reactions and interactions, as are available, are carefully analyzed, it becomes obvious that many of these cases where herbal products have been associated with actual human poisoning were not in fact caused by herbs alleged to be in the product, but resulted from substitution or contamination of the declared ingredients, intentionally or by accident, with a more toxic botanical, a poisonous metal, or a potent non-herbal drug substance.[2]

When evaluating causality of adverse events, a number of questions must be answered.

- Are the effects consistent with the known pharmacology of the substance?
- Is there is a reasonable temporal relationship between the use of the substance and the observed effect?
- Is there evidence of overdose or misuse of the substance?
- Did the effects disappear when use of the substance was discontinued?
- Did the effects reappear on rechallenge?

An evaluation of approximately 3,000 adverse drug reports (ADRs) related to veterinary medicines received in one year revealed some interesting conclusions:

- Only 1% of reports could definitely be associated with the product.
- 31% of reports were probably associated with a given product.
- 45% of reports were possibly associated with a given product.
- 12% were definitely not related to the product.
- 11% lacked adequate information to evaluate possible causality.

In the material that follows, we shall explore the basis for assessing toxicity. But first I would like to take this opportunity to voice some concerns about the use of potentially toxic herbs by the phytotherapeutic community. The issues are threefold.

My first concern is pharmacological. When dealing with plants that contain constituents with a potentially major impact on the human body, the concerns of the toxicologist become relevant. It is a challenge to accurately assess levels of such constituents in whole plants or extracts without some form of standardization or batch-by-batch chromatographic analysis. Levels of secondary plant metabolites can vary with the phase of the moon, diurnal changes, soil conditions, atmospheric conditions, and humidity, as well as the drying and extracting processes.

This is of no consequence when we are using plants for gentle effects, such as *Urtica dioica*, but with a plant like *Atropa belladonna*, knowledge and understanding of such variations is critical to safe prescribing. Similarly, the use of drop measurements when dosage levels are critical borders on malpractice. The quantitative measurement of a drop varies with the diameter of the hole in the dropper, the roughness of the edge, the viscosity of the liquid being dispensed, the force of pressure applied to the bulb, and, finally, elevation above sea level. In other words, a drop in Boulder, Colorado, will be different in size from a drop in Santa Cruz, California (and it's not just the surf!).

Taken together, all of these factors create a huge potential for variability—enough that I would not chance using these herbs for the pharmacological effects of their constituents, as controlling dosage becomes very challenging.

The second concern is an educational and ethical one. Teachers may be trained to a sufficient level of competence to use these tinctures, but to discuss their use without ensuring that students have a similar broad framework of knowledge raises some worrying questions. We need to recognize the current state of knowledge and experience in the general herbal community in the United States. I am saying nothing about intelligence, commitment, caring, or innate healing compassion, but simply acknowledging the shortcomings of the educational environment bequeathed to us by the carnage of the Flexner report.

The Flexner report of 1911 is considered by many to mark the beginning of modern orthodox medical education. However, its legacy also serves as a de facto definition of medicine as a science-based endeavor. Here is not the place to debate the pros and cons of this report, but simply to acknowledge that in its wake, herbal medicine, among other therapeutic modalities, suffered immensely. The report led to the closing of the Eclectic medical schools, and thus the virtual disappearance of academic centers of herbal excellence.

In short, I feel that phytotherapists who teach must recognize the need for comprehensive, basic herbal education to provide a framework of understanding within which herbalists can cope safely with issues like this one. A little bit of knowledge is a dangerous thing, but it is potentially lethal if the recipient does not know just how little it is.

The third concern is more of a philosophical one. We are blessed with a diversity of therapeutic approaches within the community of medical herbalists. The practitioner, the educator, and students are all faced with ongoing choices as to the therapeutic context within which they should use their materia medica. But just because we have plants with certain effects at our disposal, should we use them? The application of effectors as strong as *Atropa* is very similar in nature and reasoning to an allopathic approach.

There is nothing wrong with this in itself, but such an approach must be a conscious choice rather than an intellectual delusion. My reasons for not using herbs that can be seen simply as drug delivery systems, such as *Atropa*, is that we herbalists cannot do it safely, and I see no reason to use such herbs within the context of a holistic practice. If powerful chemicals are indicated, then I suggest that prescription medications are safer. Let me clarify this. I do not mean that phytotherapists should turn to prescription medications. I am simply suggesting we acknowledge that the unique and wonderful strength of phytotherapy lies in the use of nurturing, toning, gentle plants.

Is Comfrey Safe?

Herb safety issues are complex, extending far beyond the realm of the reliable, objective scientific method. The questions raised and the answers given often need to be deconstructed in the light, when assessing not only the toxicological facts, but also the political and sociological context within which the discussion is occurring.

As an example, consider comfrey *(Symphytum officinale)*, an herb with a very long history of traditional use. Comfrey has been used both internally (as a demulcent) and externally (as a vulnerary). The herb has become a topic of considerable debate, as it contains pyrrolizidine alkaloids (PAs), which have been shown to pose a real risk of hepatotoxicity.

There can be no question about the concerns posed by PAs to humans.[3] However, it must be remembered that we cannot demonize a naturally occurring substance simply because it is inappropriate for human consumption. PAs play vital roles in the ecology of many butterflies.[4] Several species feed on PA-containing plants. The butterflies incorporate the PAs into their tissues and thus become unpalatable to predators.[5] In the tropical danaid butterflies, PAs serve as essential precursors to pheromones that act as oviposition stimulants for females.[6]

However, comfrey is not simply a vehicle for the pharmacological effects of a specific constituent. The herb's pharmacological impact is far more complex than that. The only time an herb can be viewed solely as an "organic drug delivery system" is when it contains pharmacologically active levels of potent constituents that override any potential whole plant effects. The fact that PAs pose risks cannot be simply used by extension to imply that comfrey is an unsafe herb. A recent, well-balanced review by Dorena Rode on toxicological findings concerning comfrey sheds considerable light on this subject.[7]

To address the question of whether or not comfrey is safe for therapeutic use, a range of issues must be considered, and not all of these involve toxicology. *Webster's Revised Unabridged Dictionary* defines the word *safe* as meaning:

> Free from harm, injury, or risk; untouched or unthreatened by danger or injury; unharmed; unhurt; secure; whole; as, safe from disease; safe from storms; safe from foes.

Unfortunately, there is a common assumption that might be paraphrased as "Herbs are natural, and therefore safe." This is clearly not the case. Cliffs are natural and yet people fall off them, water is natural and yet people drown, arsenic is natural and yet it is lethally toxic. To put this in the crudest terms, we are all going to die, and that too is natural!

Thus, if "safe" is taken to mean completely risk-free, then the answer must be no, comfrey is not safe. For example, as with all herbs and drugs, there is a small chance that an allergic response will occur. As is discussed later in this chapter, it is more meaningful to consider the concepts of *hazard* and *risk* than "safety." When these concepts are applied to comfrey, we see that the hazard it poses is its potential to cause an adverse effect, and the risk it poses is the statistical probability that the hazard will occur under specific exposure conditions.

All substances (including herbs) and all activities (including taking herbs internally) carry risks. The core therapeutic issue is whether the benefits outweigh the dangers. This *therapeutic index* is discussed in more detail later in this chapter. However, it should be noted here that determining a risk-benefit relationship depends on the informed judgment of the clinician, not an absolute of pharmacology. Many very risky pharmaceuticals are prescribed because the clinician believes that the benefits outweigh the risks.[8]

To compound matters, questions of herb safety are posed in very divergent contexts and lead to similarly divergent answers. The assumptions, expectations, belief system, knowledge, and experience of both the person who asks the question and the person who responds will affect the outcome. A bureaucrat given the responsibility of regulating the herbal marketplace is not likely to consider the crucial risk-benefit complexities that a phytotherapist takes into account when reaching clinical decisions about a unique patient.

When the reports on comfrey toxicity are reviewed, some interesting points can be made. The following quotation comes from Dorena Rode, author of an insightful review on comfrey toxicity.

> One might expect that new toxicity research or an unacceptable number of adverse reactions prompted these recent actions, but neither is the case.[9]

The very few specific reports of human toxicity related to comfrey all come from the period between 1980 and 1990, when a number of cases of veno-occlusive disease were reported.[10] There is no question about the diagnoses. However, it is important to note that in these cases, the connection with comfrey was not considered in the context of other contributing factors. For example, concomitant illness, the use of prescription or over-the-counter hepatotoxic drugs (like acetaminophen, for example), and impaired nutritional status clearly increase the likelihood that PA-containing herbs will cause hepatotoxicity.

With minimal epidemiological data, what insights can be garnered from the laboratory research into toxicity? As with many statements about herbal toxicity, the evidence proffered comes primarily from rodent studies that utilized high levels of purified PAs. No systematic toxicity testing or clinical trials of comfrey have been performed. Although PA poisoning in humans does occur, it is most commonly a consequence of consuming plants other than comfrey.[11]

Such reliance on animal experimentation data and toxicity reports about other plants gives us little insight into the risks and therapeutic benefits of the human use of comfrey. Rode enumerates four limitations of the published research.

Not all PAs have similar toxicity. As discussed in chapter 8 and later in this chapter, this group of alkaloids do not pose a uniform risk. Based on structure-toxicity studies, it can be concluded that the PAs in comfrey (such as symphytine, a retronecine monoester) are less toxic than those present in the plants *Senecio*, *Crotolaria*, and *Heliotropium*. These have actually caused human toxicity (for example, senecionine, a macrocyclic retronecine diester).[12]

Not all animals are susceptible to PA toxicity. As with most substances, responses to PAs among different animals vary greatly. Pigs, chickens, and rats are highly sensitive to poisoning by *Senecio*, whereas mice and sheep are resistant. However, and more significant, the response of one species to *Senecio* might not reflect its susceptibility to other PAs.[13] In addition, the route of administration can dramatically affect the toxic response. For example, rabbits are relatively resistant to chronic feeding of *Senecio*, but are killed by a single injection of the purified alkaloids.[14]

Although theoretically sensitivity to PAs, pigs readily accept comfrey as a food and show no adverse effects, even when comfrey represents 40% of their diet. Rats, however, appear to be very sensitive to the same PAs. When eating large amounts of comfrey or injected with comfrey PAs, rats develop the hepatic lesions indicative of PA poisoning.[15] This calls into question the validity of using rodent animal models as indicators of human response to PAs.

Comfrey species vary in PA content. Between 85% and 97% of the PAs in *Symphytum officinale*, the comfrey commonly grown in American gardens, are built around the less toxic retronecine monoester. However, Russian comfrey (*Symphytum* x *uplandicum*), contains higher levels of the diester, which is known to have a greater toxicity.[16] Bearing in mind the differences in toxicity among various PAs, and the variable distribution of PAs in different comfrey species and varieties, we might conclude that extrapolations of research results from one species to another may be unreliable.

Effects of isolated PAs might not be representative of whole plant use. As with many herbs, it is problematic to assume that the pharmacology of a specific constituent can be used to predict the pharmacology of the whole plant. Veterinary studies have shown that the formation of toxic PA metabolites is reduced by concurrent administration of the sulfur-containing amino acid methionine or cysteine.[17] Similarly, protein-deficient diets enhance the toxicity of PAs.[18]

Most toxicity studies used purified PAs, ignoring the potential protective effects of co-occurring nutrients present in the whole plant. This suggests that studies using purified PAs probably overstate the health risks associated with comfrey extracts or the whole plant.

So what can be concluded about the safe use of comfrey? Again, the clinical concept of comfrey's therapeutic index must be invoked. As discussed later in this chapter under Toxicology, the therapeutic index compares the therapeutically effective dose to the toxic dose of a substance. This gives an indication of the relative safety of a drug or herb by providing a ratio of the dose that produces toxicity to the dose needed to bring about the desired therapeutic response. According to *The Merck Manual*, the term describes "informed clinical judgment," but who are the relevant clinicians in the case of comfrey?

All of this might lead one to the conclusion that toxicologists' statements about the safety of comfrey may be based on inadequate data. Unless benefits are compared with risks, we have only conjecture. Consider, for example, the case of nonsteroidal anti-inflammatory drugs (NSAIDs). NSAIDs include such readily available medicines as aspirin and ibuprofen, as well as stronger prescription drugs like Celebrex, Indocin, and Vioxx. Such medications can play an undeniably beneficial role in the control of arthritic inflammation, for example. But are they safe?

More than 30 billion NSAIDs are consumed annually in the United States. The major effect of all NSAIDs is to decrease the synthesis of prostaglandins by reversibly inhibiting cyclooxygenase, an enzyme that catalyzes the formation of prostaglandins from the precursor arachidonic acid. Prostaglandins enhance the inflammatory response, but also renal blood flow and cytoprotection of gastrointestinal mucosa. The 1998 report from the American Association of Poison Control Centers (AAPCC) documents 52,751 toxic exposures to ibuprofen alone, of which 13,519 were treated in health care facilities. Four deaths were reported. For the same year, the AAPCC also reports a high rate of complications arising from therapeutic use of NSAIDs, specifically, 100,000 toxic exposures resulting in hospitalization and 10,000 resulting in fatality.[19]

In the face of such toxicological data, it may seem strange that ibuprofen is considered safe enough for non-prescription use. However, the benefits are believed to outweigh the risks. Thus, the toxicity data are seen in the context of the therapeutic benefits. The phytotherapist would say that the same process must be applied to comfrey before conclusive statements can be made. Thus, an assessment of comfrey's safety must take into account more than the real and theoretical risks posed by PAs:

- How does the toxicity of a whole plant preparation compare with that of the actual PAs present?
- How does the toxicity of comfrey PAs compare to that of the well-studied PAs contained in toxic plants from the genus *Senecio*?
- How does the hazard posed by comfrey PAs relate to the risk of using comfrey in herbal teas and tinctures?
- What real risks are posed and what therapeutic benefits are offered by the use of comfrey?
- How do the benefits compare with the risks?

Unless the knowledge and experience of clinical phytotherapists are taken into account, the lack of mainstream clinical experience with comfrey might suggest it offers no therapeutic benefits. However, in this book, the reader will discover that comfrey is suggested for inclusion in many treatment protocols. For more details on its safe use, please refer to the comfrey entry in chapter 26 and to specific body system chapters in part 2 of this book.

Factors to Consider When Assessing Herb Safety

In general, a number of broad factors must be taken into account:

- Has traditional use of the plant revealed any knowledge of toxicity?
- Does the plant contain constituents with established toxicity?
- Are there inherent risks unique to the form in which the herb is administered? (For example, does topical use of comfrey pose a different level of risk than internal use?)
- Does objective data for both toxicity and efficacy exist? Are the research results valid enough to form some basis for approximate risk assessment?
- How does the science compare with the *perceived* risk expressed by the FDA, practitioners of orthodox medicine, or herbalists?

Based on the context in which the herb is being prescribed, selected, or purchased, what might be called *iatrogenic* risks arise—in other words, inadvertent risks introduced through mistakes, lack of knowledge, or other such factors. If use of comfrey was suggested by a clinician, did this clinician understand the parameters for safe

Safety Guidelines for Phytotherapists

How do we create a bridge between the knowledge and experience of a well-trained phytotherapist and the unique perspective and language of the scientific method? The plethora of issues concerning safety and toxicity is an area in which I am trying to find meaningful corollaries, and, as a simple-minded herbalist, make sense of all of this. In this time of rapid change, I want to sound a plea for traditional protocols. Here are some provisional guidelines.

Don't jump to unwarranted conclusions about therapeutic indications and contraindications from research findings if:

- *They are derived from animal experiments.* This is partly a moral position, but there are also profound doubts about the validity of extrapolations from animal studies to human research applications. For example, does a specific animal model actually test what the interpretation suggests it tests? Much of the basic research on phytoestrogens uses a laboratory test that assesses estrogen-induced thickening of the uterine wall in rodents. This is all well and good, but to use results of such tests to arrive at human therapeutic protocols is absurd. The mere fact that rodents do not menstruate calls into question the validity of such extrapolation. This alone should inform us that the actual situation is much more complex than the one the test is designed to investigate.

- *The studies utilized isolated constituents, not whole plants.* Even if we don't invoke the biochemical synergy that may play a role in the actions of whole plant preparations, the stupendous number of potential interactions should make us wary of easy conclusions.

- *They disagree with established phytotherapeutic experience and protocols.* As our modality has inherent value (a statement that is obviously a reflection of my own belief system, not statistical data), we should not reject protocols or plants because of lack of research on their mechanisms of action.

use? At the other end of the spectrum, was the herb self-selected by a consumer under the influence of commercial hype?

The complex of issues concerning substance interactions must also be assessed. As discussed later in this chapter, the nature of interactions varies. One must consider the ways in which an herb might interact with prescription or over-the-counter drugs, other herbs, or even other modalities.

Sociopolitical risks must also be evaluated. From certain cultural perspectives, the use of herbs by anyone outside of a professional elite poses some unique concerns. The informed use of therapeutic plants empowers people. However, in this context, any lessening of people's dependence on the professional elite (or financial indebtedness to the industrial-medical complex) can be seen as a potential threat to the power structure of the dominant hierarchy. The more people develop their own relationship with nature, the less power the dominators will have. Just as attempts are made to discourage people about the green movement by labeling it "ecoterrorism," the scare tactic used against herbs is often the issue of safety.

Of course, determining how to use herbs safely is a real issue, but it is one that can also be used for political ends. This does not necessarily imply a conscious political effort, but is more often simply the expression of the belief system in which the person is embedded. "Expert status" is a mutually supportive addiction that often invokes a reflexive response.

In mainstream culture, herbal expertise is rarely recognized as existing outside the walls of academia. However, if becoming an expert involves some form of culturally recognized academic achievement, how is this to be obtained in a culture that offers no Ph.D. programs in herbalism? By this I mean clinical phytotherapy programs, not ethnobotany. In a cultural milieu in which the knowledge, skills, and experience of the herbalist are devalued or ignored, how can our expertise be recognized?

HERB CONTRAINDICATIONS AND INTERACTIONS

I have come to the conclusion that is it too soon in the development of modern phytotherapy to authoritatively define contraindications. Similarly, the interactions of herbs and even common foods with the various components of orthodox medicine have not been explored in enough depth or with a large enough patient population to reach reliable conclusions. Ideas abound, but consensus is rare. Specifics about individual herbs can be found in chapter 26.

TYPES OF INTERACTIONS

People are normally exposed to several chemicals at a time, rather than to one isolated chemical. Medical treatment and environmental factors both generally consist of multiple exposures at a time. Normally, the toxicity of a specific drug is determined by the study of animals exposed to only one chemical at a time. Researchers rarely test mixtures of substances for toxicity, since it is usually impossible to predict possible combinations of chemicals that might be present in multiple-chemical exposures.

All of this makes the process of predicting interactions very challenging. Medicines taken simultaneously may act independently; however, the presence of one chemical may drastically affect the body's response to another chemical. The toxicity of a combination of chemicals may be less or more than might be expected based on the known effects of individual chemicals.

It is important to have a conceptual context within which to place any discussion of herb-drug interactions. The following categories are based on two sources, the important work of Brinker and of DeSmet.[20,21] Interactions may be pharmacokinetic or pharmacodynamic in nature, and may not be uniformly negative. However, as is often the case, the complexities of real life may produce multiple or mysterious interactions between herbs and drugs.

Pharmacokinetic Interactions

Pharmacokinetic interactions may take a variety of forms and cause a range of different effects, some negative and some, as we shall see, potentially positive.

Interactions Leading to a Decrease in Drug Bioavailability

An herb may affect drug pharmacokinetics by altering drug absorption. Examples of herbs that may have such an effect include those that contain dietary fiber, mucilages, or tannins (for example, marshmallow, psyllium, and tea). Herbs may also cause changes in the rate of drug elimination. Examples include all laxative herbs and caffeine-containing herbs, such as coffee, kola nut, maté, and guarana.

Interactions Causing an Increase in Drug Bioavailability

Drug bioavailability may be enhanced by herbs that increase the rate of absorption, such as cayenne and black pepper, or by those that slow metabolism, such as citrus and licorice.

Interactions That Protect Against Adverse Effects

Several herbs, such as milk thistle, may afford protection against the adverse effects of drugs. This is discussed in greater detail in chapter 9.

Pharmacodynamic Interactions

Pharmacodynamic interactions between herbs and orthodox drugs may occur if they work via similar mechanisms. As the pharmacology of many herbs is still unclear, it should be assumed that if an herb predictably produces a certain outcome, there is a chance that interactions will occur with drugs that produce similar outcomes.

Enhancement of Drug Effects

Drug effects may be enhanced if an herb works by a mechanism different from that of the drug. For example, hawthorn may enhance the activity of digoxin, a medication used to treat arrhythmias (irregular heart rhythms).

Additive Effects

An agonistic combination of two or more substances may result in a cumulative effect that reflects the sum of the expected individual responses. This is the most common and most potentially toxic type of drug interaction, and may occur when the herb and drug have similar mechanisms of activity, such as *Ginkgo* and PAF inhibitors.

Antagonistic Effects

Here, an exposure to one medicine may diminish the effect of the other. This might be a physiological antagonism: For example, a severe drop in blood pressure resulting from a barbiturate overdose can be reversed by administration of a vasopressor to increase blood pressure.

TOXICOLOGY

Toxicology is the study of adverse effects of chemical or physical agents on living organisms. The material that follows provides a brief overview of the issues to consider when assessing toxicity and its attendant risks. The terms *toxicant*, *toxin*, and *poison* are often used interchangeably; however, there are subtle differences in meaning.

- *Toxicants* are substances that produce adverse biological effects of any kind; they may be chemical or physical in nature.
- *Toxins* are specific proteins produced by living organisms (for example, mushroom and tetanus toxins); most exhibit immediate effects.
- *Poisons* are toxicants that cause immediate death or illness upon exposure to very small amounts.

- A *toxic agent* is anything that produces an adverse biological effect; it may be chemical, physical, or biological in nature.

Systemic Toxic Effects

Toxicity may effect only one site in the body, or a *target organ*, or multiple sites, in which case it is called *systemic toxicity*. The timing of onset of symptoms can be important. Acute toxicity occurs within hours or days of an exposure. An acute exposure is generally a single dose or a series of doses received within a 24-hour period. Subchronic toxicity results from repeated exposure over the course of several weeks or months. This is the usual exposure pattern when medicinal plants are implicated.

Chronic toxicity results from cumulative damage to specific organ systems and may take many months or years to become recognizable, as is the case with pyrrolizidine alkaloids. Damage due to subclinical exposure may go unnoticed, but with repeated exposure, the effects slowly build up until they can be detected.

Developmental Toxicity

Toxic effects can impact the fetus, and can result from exposure of either parent before conception or of the mother and her developing fetus after conception. Developmental toxicity may manifest in failure to conceive, spontaneous abortion or stillbirth, growth retardation or delayed growth of specific organs, or *teratogenicity* (permanent birth defects).

Genetic Toxicity

Damage to DNA causes altered genetic expression. In this process, known as *mutagenesis*, the specific genetic change constitutes a *mutation*, and the agent that causes the change is a *mutagen*. If the mutation occurs in a germ cell, the effect may be inherited, in which case it causes no harm to the exposed person but is passed on to future generations. If the mutation occurs in a somatic cell, it can cause altered cell growth or cell death in the exposed person.

Organ-Specific Toxic Effects

The toxicity of a given substance may be confined to a particular body system or organ.

Blood and Cardiovascular Toxicity

Toxicity to the blood or cardiovascular system is caused by the direct impact of a toxin on cells in the blood, bone marrow, or heart. Examples include hypoxia (oxygen deficiency) caused by the binding of carbon monoxide to hemoglobin, which prevents the transport of oxygen, and leukemia caused by benzene damage of bone marrow cells.

Dermal Toxicity

Dermal toxicity may result either from direct contact of a substance with the skin or from internal distribution of the substance to the skin. Effects can range from mild irritation to severe injury or change, such as corrosion, hypersensitivity, or skin cancer.

Eye Toxicity

Eye toxicity may be caused by direct contact of a toxin with the eye or by internal distribution of the toxin to the eye. Conjunctivitis and corneal erosion may be observed after exposure to chemicals. Chemicals in the circulatory system distributed to the eye can result in corneal opacity, cataracts, and retinal and optic nerve damage.

Hepatotoxicity

The liver is particularly susceptible to toxicity because of its large blood supply and important role in metabolism, both of which expose the organ to potentially high doses of toxic metabolites. Hepatotoxicity can take many forms.

Table 10.1. Types of Hepatotoxicity

EFFECT	DEFINITION
Chemical hepatitis	Inflammation of the liver
Cirrhosis	Chronic fibrosis
Hepatic cancer	Cancer of the liver
Hepatic necrosis	Death of hepatocytes
Hypersensitivity	Immune reaction resulting in hepatic necrosis
Intrahepatic cholestasis	Backup of bile salts into liver cells
Steatosis	Lipid accumulation in hepatocytes

Immunotoxicity

Damage to the immune system can take several forms, including hypersensitivity, immunodeficiency, and uncontrolled cell proliferation.

Nephrotoxicity

The kidney is highly vulnerable to toxicity, because of both the great volume of blood that flows through it and the fact that the kidney filters large quantities of toxins, which can concentrate in the kidney tubules. Nephrotoxicity can result in systemic toxicity, leading to decreased ability to excrete body wastes, inability to maintain body fluids and electrolyte balance, and reduced synthesis of hormones, such as erythropoietin.

Neurotoxicity

Neurotoxicity involves damage to cells of the central nervous and peripheral nervous systems:

- Neuronopathy (neuron injury)
- Axonopathy (axon injury)
- Demyelination (loss of axon insulation)
- Interference with neurotransmission

Reproductive Toxicity

Specific reproductive organs and the developing fetus both represent potential sites of reproductive toxicity:

- Decreased libido or impotence
- Infertility
- Interrupted pregnancy (abortion, fetal death, or premature delivery)
- Infant death or childhood morbidity
- Altered sex ratio and multiple births
- Chromosome abnormalities and birth defects
- Childhood cancer

Respiratory Toxicity

Respiratory toxicity can take the form of pulmonary irritation, asthma, bronchitis, reactive airway disease, emphysema, allergic alveolitis, fibrotic lung disease, pneumoconiosis, or lung cancer.

DOSE

The toxicity of a substance is determined mainly by the dose at which the effect occurs. Toxicity is therefore not an independent characteristic of a substance, but a function of the quantity of the substance absorbed. Whether or not a toxic effect will appear is determined by the dose. When evaluating the toxicity of substances, both acute and chronic data must be taken into account, since short-term exposure to high concentrations generally causes symptoms different from those caused by long-term exposure to relatively low concentrations.

A dose is the amount of a substance administered at one time, but this is not the only parameter that must be taken into account when characterizing toxicity. Also important are the number of doses, frequency, and total duration of treatment. The total dose, harmful if received all at once, may be nontoxic when administered over a period of time. For example, 30 mg of strychnine swallowed all at once could be fatal to an adult, whereas 3 mg of strychnine swallowed each day for 10 days would not be fatal. The reason is that the body is often able to repair damage caused by subtoxic doses if sufficient time passes before the next dose.

The clinical and toxic effects of a dose are both related to age and body size, so one way to compare efficacy and toxicity is to consider the amount of a substance administered on the basis of body weight. A common dose measurement is mg/kg, which stands for milligrams (mg) of substance per kilogram (kg) of body weight. Some chemicals are toxic in much smaller amounts, so smaller fractions of the gram are used, such as a microgram (μg).

Table 10.2. Intensity of Toxic Effects

INTENSITY OF EFFECT	ORAL DOSAGE*
Extremely toxic	Micrograms
Very toxic	Milligrams
Moderately toxic	Hundreds of milligrams
Slightly toxic	Grams

*Per kilogram of body weight

Effective dose (ED) is a term used to indicate the efficacy of a substance. Normally, "effective dose" refers to a beneficial effect, but it can also stand for a harmful effect, so the specific endpoint must be indicated. *Toxic dose* (TD) indicates a dose that can be expected to cause adverse toxic effects.

Relative effective doses are generally described as follows.

ED_0: effective in 0% of the population
ED_{10}: effective in 10% of the population
ED_{50}: effective in 50% of the population
ED_{90}: effective in 90% of the population

Significance of the LD_{50}

A commonly used dose estimate for acute toxicity is the LD_{50}, in which LD stands for *lethal dose*. This is a statistically derived dose at which 50% of the individuals can be expected to die after administration of a given substance. Other dose estimates also may be used. LD_0 represents the dose at which no individuals are expected to die. This is just below the threshold for lethality. LD_{10}

refers to the dose at which 10% of the individuals will die, and so on.

The LD_{50} is merely a statistical expression that describes the lethal effect of a substance on a particular population under certain circumstances, not a fundamental property of the substance. More specifically, LD_{50} is a measure of the lethality of a substance under experimental circumstances. It is used, for example, to compare the relative toxicity of different substances and to classify substances according to the potential hazards they pose.

Although determination of the LD_{50} under well-described circumstances can provide valuable information, it concerns only one aspect of overall toxicity, namely lethality. Of much greater importance are, for example, the effects and the rate at which they occur and the pathological symptoms. Bear in mind also that it is difficult to extrapolate the LD_{50} of a substance for a particular population of one animal species to other populations of that species under slightly different conditions. Extrapolation to a different species altogether will lead to extremely uncertain results. In addition, comparison of LD_{50} values determined in various laboratories often shows that there are large variations in results from different laboratories.

Therapeutic Index

The *therapeutic index* (TI) is used to compare the therapeutically effective dose to the toxic dose. The TI is a statement of the relative safety of a drug, and represents a ratio of the dose producing toxicity to the dose needed to bring about the desired therapeutic response.

The usual method of deriving the TI is through the use of 50% dose-response points. For example, if the LD_{50} is 200 mg and the ED_{50} is 20 mg, the resulting ratio of 200:20 gives us a TI of 10. A clinician would consider a drug with a TI of 10 safer than one with a TI of 3. Thus, the higher the TI, the safer the drug and the larger the therapeutic window of opportunity. The greatest benefit of the concept of the TI is that it provides some indication of the probability that toxic adverse effects will be encountered.

The use of the ED_{50} and LD_{50} doses to derive the TI can be misleading. Another term used to denote the safety of a drug is the *margin of safety* (MOS). The MOS is usually calculated as the ratio of the dose that is just within the lethal range (LD_{01}) to the dose that is 99% effective (ED_{99}). ($MOS = LD_{01}/ED_{99}$.) A physician must use caution in prescribing a drug in which the MOS is lower than 1.

To put this important concept into a practical context, consider this quotation from *The Merck Manual*, which uses the phrase "benefit-to-risk ratio" instead of "therapeutic index."

> In every therapeutic endeavor, risks must be weighed against benefits for each particular clinical situation and patient. Drug therapy is justified only if the possible benefits outweigh the possible risks after considering the qualitative and quantitative impact of the use of a drug and the likely outcome if drug therapy is withheld. This decision depends on adequate clinical knowledge of the patient, knowledge of the disease and its natural history, and knowledge of the drugs pertinent to the specific situation. Although the term benefit-to-risk ratio is convenient and often used for individual patients, numerical predictions of benefit or risk do not exist and the mathematical division (to obtain a ratio) is never performed. The term is used to describe informed clinical judgment.[22]

Dose Response

The dose-response relationship correlates exposures and the spectrum of induced effects. Generally, the higher the dose, the more severe the response. Knowledge of the dose-response relationship is important for a number of reasons:

- Establishes *causality*, that the chemical has in fact induced the observed effects
- Establishes the lowest dose at which an induced effect may occur, or the *threshold effect*
- Determines the rate at which injury builds up, or the *slope* for the dose response

A threshold for toxic effects occurs at the point at which the body's ability to detoxify a xenobiotic substance or repair toxic injury has been exceeded. Most organs have a reserve capacity, so that some loss of organ function does not cause a significant decrease in performance. For example, the development of cirrhosis in the liver may not result in a clinical effect until more than 50% of the liver has been replaced by fibrous tissue.

ANIMAL TESTING FOR TOXICITY

I find the degree of animal testing in the world of pharmacology to be pornographic. However, in the overview of herbal science that makes up the first part of this book, it proved essential to refer to animal studies, because at present, bioscience is largely dependent on this research method. In any case, here is not the place to enter the debate about vivisection. The material that follows is intended to inform the reader, not serve as advocacy for animal testing.

Animal tests for toxicity are conducted prior to human clinical investigations. For pesticides and industrial chemicals, human testing is rarely conducted, so animal test results are used to predict toxicity in humans. Methods to evaluate toxicity exist for a wide variety of toxic effects. Some procedures for routine safety testing have been standardized.

To be standardized, a test procedure must have scientific acceptance as the most meaningful assay for the toxic effect. Toxicity tests can be very specific for a particular effect, such as dermal irritation, or may be general, such as a test for unknown chronic effects. Species selection varies with the toxicity test to be performed, as there is no single species that is appropriate for all tests. In some cases, it may not be possible to use the most desirable animal for testing because of animal welfare concerns or cost considerations. For example, monkeys and dogs are restricted to special cases, even though their reactions to such testing may most closely represent human reactions.

Testing should duplicate the potential exposure of humans as closely as possible. Thus, the route of exposure should simulate that of human exposure. In addition, the age of test animals should relate to that of humans likely to be exposed to the substance. For most routine tests, both genders are used. Gender differences in toxic responses are minimal, except for toxic substances with hormonal properties. Dose levels are normally selected in order to determine the toxic threshold as well as dose-response relationship.

Problems with Animal Testing

Apart from the overriding moral and ethical concerns with animal experimentation, there are a number of scientific concerns.

Inter- and Intraspecies Differences in Sensitivity

There may be considerable differences in sensitivity to a toxic substance among different species and among individuals. Mice are more sensitive than rats to the carcinogenic effects of 1,3-butadiene, a chemical used in the production of synthetic rubber and other resins that is one of the 189 hazardous air pollutants identified in the Clean Air Act amendments.[23]

Butadiene causes cancer through its conversion in the body to more-toxic metabolites, butadiene monoepoxide and butadiene diepoxide. Studies on the livers of rats, mice, and humans indicate that humans and rats metabolize butadiene in a similar manner, and rats are relatively resistant to the cancer-causing effects of this chemical. Mice produce significantly more butadiene monoepoxide than rats, as well as large quantities of butadiene diepoxide. This is important, as butadiene diepoxide is about 100 times more damaging to DNA than butadiene monoepoxide. The high levels of these epoxides produced by mice probably explains why they are so sensitive to the carcinogenic effects of butadiene.[24]

Interspecies Variations in Anatomy and Body Size

Small animals have a relatively large body-surface-to-body-volume ratio. This means that exposure to a substance via the skin surface can lead to the absorption of a relatively large quantity. The ratio also indicates that the animal's metabolic rate is relatively high, so it will ingest more food. If the food happens to be contaminated, a relatively high dose of the substance will be ingested.

Selective Toxicity Due to Physiology

An extreme example of this phenomenon is the difference between animals and plants. The toxicity of many insecticides is dependent on their effects on the nervous system. Plants, therefore, are relatively insensitive to the effects of insecticides. On the other hand, animals are relatively insensitive to most herbicides, many of which affect physiological mechanisms characteristic of plants, such as photosynthesis.

FACTORS AFFECTING TOXICITY IN HUMANS

Genetic Differences

Sensitivity may depend on genetic variability in enzyme activity. Individuals with a glucose-6-phosphate dehydrogenase deficiency in their red blood cells are hypersensitive to oxidative substances, such as aromatic nitro substances, chlorates, antimalarial agents, and glycosides from broad beans.

Age

Babies are more sensitive to the toxic effect of nitrates than adults. Their sensitivity is ascribed to a transient deficiency in NADH-methemoglobin reductase. Hence, in this case, babies constitute a high-risk group.

Dietary Habits and Lifestyle

Diet appears to be of great significance in the development of cancer. In the body, many carcinogenic substances are activated to become reactive metabolites under the influence of biotransformation enzymes.

Internal Absorption versus External Exposure

Often, the crucial factor is not the amount of a substance to which an individual is exposed, but its subsequent concentration in the body, specifically in the target organ or organs. This is the concentration to which the individual is actually exposed internally. If the absorption rate of a substance exceeds the rate of excretion and biotransformation, accumulation may take place, and the total amount of the substance in the body (the body burden) will increase. Distribution throughout the body will depend on the properties of the substance and tissue. For example, DDT is found mainly in adipose tissue.

HAZARDS AND RISKS

Hazard refers to the potential toxicity of a substance in an actual situation; how one deals with the substance in that particular situation determines the risk. Risk differs from hazard in that it cannot usually be determined experimentally. It may be inferred from epidemiological data or it may be predicted from mathematical models, but rarely can it be measured. Instead, a more qualitative approach to identifying risk must be adopted. The following terms are routinely used in risk assessments:

Hazard is the capability of a substance to cause an adverse effect, although the term can also be applied to physicochemical properties, such as flammability and explosiveness.

Risk is a statistical term that indicates the probability that the hazard will occur under specific exposure conditions.

Risk assessment is the process by which hazard, exposure, and risk are determined.

Risk management is the process of selecting the most appropriate action based on the results of risk assessment and social, economic, and political concerns.

There are four basic steps in the risk assessment process.

Hazard identification: the characterization of the innate adverse effects or toxicity of an agent

Dose-response assessment: the characterization of the relationship between doses and incidences of adverse effects in exposed populations

Exposure assessment: measurement or estimation of the intensity, frequency, and duration of human exposures to agents

Risk characterization: an estimation of the incidence of health effects under the various conditions of human exposure

Hazard Identification

In order to determine whether a substance is toxic when present in a large enough amount, several types of information are used. The most conclusive information comes from observation of cases in which humans are exposed to the substance, in either clinical or epidemiological studies. In the absence of information from human studies, inferences are drawn from animal studies, from in vitro studies using living cells, or from comparisons to similar substances that pose known hazards.

As the source of the information moves farther from actual human studies, the uncertainty becomes greater. One or more toxic hazards may be identified, but the primary hazard of concern will be one that can cause a serious health consequence at a lower dosage than required by other substances that cause serious toxic effects.

Risk Factors

What factors determine the risk from exposure to a toxic substance? Not all individuals are subject to the same health risk. For this reason, the term *high-risk group* was coined. The term *situational risk* refers to the risk inherent in a particular situation in which there is a high chance of exposure. Quite often, a distinction will be made between situational risks and increased individual sensitivity to a certain substance. People who live in the vicinity of an industry that pollutes the environment have a greater chance of coming into contact with the emissions of that industry than do others. If the same people also work in these industries, their risks are even higher.

Some people are at high risk because they have a greater sensitivity to one or more substances than do others in the population. People with chronic nonspecific lung disease, who have a comparatively high sensitivity to substances that irritate the airways, provide a good example. Small children constitute a high-risk group, not only because they have a higher inherent sensitivity to some potential hazards, but also because of their behavior. For example, they may be exposed to toxic substances present in the soil, a means of exposure that is far less likely for adults.

Certain hobbies can increase the risk of exposure to toxic substances. Pregnant women and their unborn children can be considered to be at higher risk from exposure to all kinds of substances. The same is true for elderly people. As age increases, the functional capacity of various organs, such as the liver and kidneys, starts to decline. Changes in metabolic and eliminative functions can cause significant changes in the toxicity of various substances. In addition, the reserve capacity of various organs is often severely reduced in the elderly, which may mean that seemingly small toxic exposures can have severe consequences.

HERB TOXICITY

An excellent review of the adverse effects of herbs by DeSmet cites a number of causes.[25] All concerned with these issues should refer to this book and its subsequent volume.

Eight categories of causes are given; these are discussed in more depth later:

- Poisonous plants
- Adulteration of commercial products
- Self-collection of medicinal plants
- Microorganisms and microbial toxins
- Pesticides and fumigation agents
- Radioactivity
- Toxic metals
- Environmental pollution

THE NATURE OF POISONOUS PLANTS

Poisonous plants contain physiologically active or toxic substances in sufficient amounts to cause harmful effects in animals and humans. The poisonous nature of a plant may be due to the presence of any of several kinds of substances:

- Substances that are themselves toxic
- Substances that are in themselves harmless, but which may decompose to form toxic products either before or soon after they are eaten, such as the nontoxic glucoside amygdalin, produced in the wild cherry, which hydrolyzes to form hydrogen cyanide
- Substances formed by the action of microorganisms on plants or plant products; for example, under certain conditions, fungi produce mold in hay or silage that in turn forms decomposition products, some of which may be toxic
- Substances absorbed directly from the soil and stored in harmful quantities in the tissues of certain plants, including selenium in certain species of locoweeds and potassium nitrate in oats and amaranth

PLANT TOXINS

Of course, it is plant chemistry that makes certain plants toxic. Here, I will discuss the toxicity of certain groups of secondary plant constituents. More information on phytochemistry can be found in chapters relevant to specific groups of compounds.

Oxalic Acid

Oxalic acid is a dicarboxylic acid. It may occur as an acid or as salts of the acid, such as calcium oxalate, potassium oxalate, and sodium oxalate. The leaves, stems, and roots of many plants contain oxalates, and plants of some species can accumulate large amounts. Rhubarb leaves contain up to 1% soluble sodium and potassium oxalates; these soluble oxalates are readily absorbed from the gastrointestinal tract.[26]

Systemic formation of calcium oxalate may produce hypocalcemia, while precipitation of insoluble salts in the renal system can lead to kidney dysfunction and electrolyte imbalance. Other plants that contain high levels of insoluble calcium oxalates in their leaves include *Dieffenbachia*, *Philodendron*, and sorrel (*Rumex* spp.). Insoluble calcium oxalate crystal needles are contained in *raphides*, bundles of needlelike crystals in plant cells.

Ingestion of a small amount of plant material with a high oxalate concentration usually causes only mild irritation of the mouth and esophageal mucosa. More pronounced gastrointestinal effects may follow ingestion of large amounts of soluble oxalate. Ingestion of oxalic acid can lead to extensive renal damage and even death. The lethal dose of oxalic acid for adults is 15 g to 30 g. Chronic consumption of oxalates is a risk factor for the development of certain types of stones (calculi). An estimated 66% of renal calculi and 75% of bladder calculi are composed of calcium oxalate. However, such stones may be caused by pathologies unrelated to the consumption of plants.

Interestingly, research has revealed that certain constituents, such as the triterpene saponin lupeol, have potential value in the prevention and treatment of oxalate-based stones.[27]

Only a few plants contain sufficient amounts of sodium and potassium oxalate to be considered toxic. Moreover, ruminants that consume these plants develop increasing levels of tolerance to oxalate. An oxalate-degrading anaerobic microorganism has been isolated from pure culture of rumen bacteria. This organism, *Oxalobacter formigens*, uses oxalate as a sole energy source and produces carbon dioxide and formate as end products. This ability is extremely rare among anaerobic bacteria, and therefore this organism occupies a unique niche in the microflora of the rumen. The ability of the ruminant to adapt to and tolerate a diet high in oxalates directly depends on the presence of oxalate-degrading microorganisms.

Terpenes

The terpenes are an enormous family of chemicals that are reviewed in chapter 6. Some are therapeutically important, and many appear to have no activity in humans, but some are toxic. These are briefly discussed here.

Thujone

Thujone is a terpene of widespread occurrence that is found in many essential oils. It occurs in some evergreens of the Cupressaceae family, including *Thuja occidentalis*, *Chamaecyparis thyoides*, *Juniperus sabina*, and several species of *Cupressus*. Thujone also is found in Asteraceae in *Achillea millefolium*, *Artemisia absinthium*, and *Tanacetum vulgare*, and in Lamiaceae in *Salvia officinalis*.

Wormwood oil, derived from *Artemisia absinthium*, was the principal flavoring of absinthe, and the hallucinogenic compound in absinthe was thujone. A dose of 30 mg of thujone per kilogram of body weight can produce convulsions and lesions of the cortex of the brain. The toxicity is cumulative.

Ranunculosides

Ranunculosides are lactone glycosides that on hydrolysis give ranunculin and glucose. Ranunculin is then converted into protoanemonin. Protoanemonin is toxic; its derivatives are not. (For a more detailed discussion on the chemistry of ranunculosides, see chapter 6.)

Anyone collecting or handling plants of the Ranunculaceae family with bare hands should be careful not to hold them for long periods of time, as the sap irritates the skin and can cause blistering. The sap of any plant of this family has a burning taste and may produce reddening and swelling on contact with the skin. If swallowed in large quantities, the sap can cause gastritis, which may develop into colic followed by extreme gastroenteritis and diarrhea mixed with blood. Large quantities of mucilage are required for treatment of such a reaction.

Plants Containing Ranunculosides

Christmas rose (*Helleborus niger*)
Field buttercup (*Ranunculus acris*)
Globe flower (*Trollius europaeus*)
Marsh marigold (*Caltha palustris*)
Pasqueflower (*Pulsatilla vulgaris*)
Wood anemone (*Anemone nemorosa*)

Sesquiterpene Lactones

Sesquiterpene lactones are a class of natural sesquiterpenoids that are chemically distinct from other members of the group through the presence of a lactone system. (For more information on the chemistry of sesquiterpene lactones, see chapter 6.)

Some lactones formed in plants are very toxic to animals, while others serve a protective function in removing harmful breakdown products of metabolism.

Many sesquiterpene lactones have antitumor activity, but their considerable cytotoxicity has limited their medicinal application as isolated constituents. They are biologically active; some are toxic to mammals, while others are responsible for allergic contact dermatitis in humans.

Sesquiterpene lactones are highly irritating to the nose, eyes, and gastrointestinal tract. In addition, the potential for sesquiterpene lactones in species of Asteraceae, Lauraceae, Magnoliaceae, and Jubulaceae to cause allergic contact dermatitis is well known. More than 80 sesquiterpene lactones possess allergenic properties.

Sensitive people tend to develop cross-reactions to related molecules when they come in contact with other species containing sesquiterpene lactones. Anyone who has acquired a delayed hypersensitivity (for example, contact dermatitis) to sesquiterpene lactone–containing plants should strictly avoid further contact with any other species or extracts containing sesquiterpene lactones in order to avoid new reactions.

Sesquiterpene lactones can induce this delayed type of hypersensitivity only when applied to the skin. When taken orally or administered by another route, they usually produce no allergic effects.

Glycosides

Glycosides hydrolyze to form sugar molecules (glycones) and various other nonsugar components (aglycones). Any toxicity caused by glycosides is due to the aglycones, not the glycones. Toxic glycosides include cyanogenic, coumarin, cardiac, saponin, protoanemonin, and anthraquinone glycosides, as well as glycosinolates, which produce the volatile oils known as mustard oils.

Cyanogenic Glycosides

Cyanogenic glycosides are found in more than 800 plant species in 80 families. The hydrolysis of these glycosides releases the sugar, the aglycone and hydrocyanic acid

(HCN), also known as prussic acid. The most common plants containing toxic cyanogenic glycosides are in the Rosaceae and Fabaceae families and in the genus *Sorghum* in Poaceae. An exception is cassava *(Manihot esculenta)* from Euphorbiaceae, which is used as a food plant in tropical regions after the toxic hydrocyanic acid is removed. The formation of cyanogenic glycosides in plants is often a response to damage from drought. See chapter 4 for a detailed discussion on the distribution and chemistry of cyanogenic glycosides, including amygdalin, the cyanogenic glycoside found in bitter almonds *(Prunus dulcis* var. *amara)*.

Ruminant animals are particularly susceptible to hydrocyanic acid poisoning because the enzymes of their bacterial flora contribute to rapid hydrolysis of cyanogenic glycosides. HCN is rapidly absorbed through the walls of the rumen into the blood. HCN inhibits enzymes active in cellular respiration, primarily the terminal enzyme in the electron transport chain of the mitochondria, thereby halting the generation of adenosine triphosphate (ATP) and oxygen utilization. The cells die from lack of oxygen, even though oxygen is plentiful.

Glucosinolates (Goitrogenic Glycosides)

Glucosinolates are characteristic of plants in the Brassicaceae, including cabbage *(Brassica oleracea* var. *capitata)*, field mustard *(B. campestris)*, and rape *(B. napus)*. They are found also in the closely related families Capparadaceae, Moringaceae, and Resedaceae, as well as Caricaceae, Limnanthaceae, and Tropaeolaceae.

More than 100 different glucosinolates are known, all of which contain a common structure with a variable side chain R (for example, sinigrin). Their major role in the plant appears to be defensive. When the plant is attacked by pests, an enzyme called myrosinase is released, which hydrolyzes the glucosinolate to release β-D-glucose and the aglycone. For more information on the chemistry of glucosinolates, see chapter 4.

When glucosinolate-containing plants are bruised, the compounds released are hydrolyzed by the enzyme thioglucosidase, which is always found in such plants. In all cases, the freed aglycone is unstable and is chemically restructured to an isothiocyanate. Isothiocyanates have a pungent odor and taste and are irritating to both the skin and the mucous membranes that line the gastrointestinal tract. They may also cause liver and kidney damage.

Isothiocyanates inhibit the uptake of iodine in the thyroid. However, the small amounts of isothiocyanates consumed in cabbage and related edible plants are not believed to cause thyroid problems in humans.

Saponin Glycosides

The pharmacology of the large, complex, and therapeutically important group of compounds known as saponins, which usually occur in plants as glycosides, presents some unique toxicity concerns. Because saponins are characteristically toxic to cold-blooded animals, plants containing them have been used as fish poisons around the world. Sap from crushed plants, agitated in a pond or stream, stuns fish, which float to the surface. The toxin acts on the respiratory organs of fish without affecting their edibility. Saponins are comparably nontoxic to warm-blooded animals. For more information on this varied group of compounds, please see the discussions in chapters 4 and 6.

Cardiac Glycosides

Although of fundamental importance to medicine, the cardiac glycosides are exceedingly toxic. Cardiac glycosides may be either bufadienolides or the more abundant cardenolides, two related groups of steroidal saponins of triterpenoid origin. The assumed mechanism of action involves inhibition of Na⁺, K⁺-ATPase, resulting in increased intracellular sodium and, subsequently, intracellular calcium, leading to enhanced muscle contraction in cardiac tissue. For a more detailed discussion of this group of compounds, see chapter 6.

Among the approximately 400 plants that contain cardiac glycosides, genera used therapeutically include *Digitalis*, *Urgenia*, *Convallaria*, *Nerium*, *Strophanthus*, and *Asclepias*. The entire *Digitalis* plant is toxic. Symptoms of poisoning include dizziness, vomiting, irregular heartbeat, and delirium or hallucinations. Digitonin, a cardenolide, is derived from *Digitalis purpurea*.

Polyphenolics

In general, this very large group of secondary plant constituents has minimal toxicity. However, as might be expected, there are some important exceptions.

Coumarin Glycosides

Coumarins and their glycosides are widely distributed. Coumarol (a coumarin glycoside) and the enzyme that causes its hydrolysis are constituents of sweet clover, *Melilotus* species. When cut as hay, sweet clover is easily contaminated with molds, especially when the foliage is lush or it is cut or cured when conditions are wet.

Molds such as *Penicillium nigricans*, *P. jensi*, and *Aspergillus* metabolize the coumarin into 4-hydroxy-coumarin, which reacts with formaldehyde in the spoiled hay to produce dicoumarol. Dicoumarol is similar in structure to vitamin K, and when unintentionally eaten it inhibits vitamin K production. Vitamin K is necessary for the activation of prothrombin. When tissue is damaged, thromboplastin is released and converts prothrombin to thrombin. Thrombin alters the solubility of fibrinogen in the blood and causes it to clot and seal the damage. Dicoumarol prevents this process.

Warfarin is a synthetic chemical derived from coumarol. It is used in rodenticides and acts as a vitamin K inhibitor to block the blood-clotting process and provoke hemorrhage.

Constituents in the plant may undergo chemical transformation by contaminating microorganisms. For example, mold in dried sweet clover (Melilotus officinalis) can result in serious hemorrhagic activity. It contains coumarin, 3,4-dihydrocoumarin, O-coumaric acid, O-hydroxycoumaric acid, and the O-glycoside of O-coumaric acid (melilotoside). Drying leads to the formation of the enzymatic glycoside hydrolysis, and the resulting O-coumaric acid is spontaneously transformed to coumarin, so the dried herb strongly smells of coumarin (the characteristic aroma of new-mown hay).[28]

Coumarin is devoid of anticoagulant effects in humans because a structurally essential characteristic for the anticoagulant potential of coumarin derivatives is absent.[29,30] However, the transformation product dicoumarol has potent anticoagulant effects.[31] While poisoning by molded sweet clover occurs almost exclusively in cattle, there was a report of abnormal clotting function and mild clinical bleeding in a woman who had been drinking large amounts of a herbal tea prepared from sweet clover and other coumarin-containing ingredients.[32] The chemistry of coumarins is discussed in more detail in chapter 7.

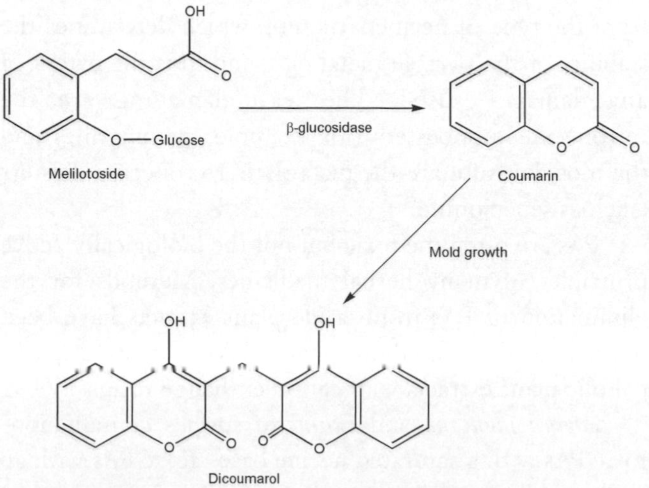

Fig. 10.1. Formation of coumarin and dicoumarol

Furocoumarin Glycosides

The furocoumarins are discussed under Photosensitivity, starting on page 210.

Gossypol

Gossypol is a polyphenol found mainly in the pigment glands of cotton, Gossypium species. Gossypol may exist free or bound, but free gossypol is considered the toxic form. The bound form is nontoxic because it is irreversibly bonded to proteins.

Gossypol has potential as a male contraceptive.[33] Its antifertility activity came to light in a somewhat circuitous manner. A group of farmers in rural areas of China developed fatigue and burning sensations on their faces, hands, and other exposed parts of the body; epidemiologists discovered that they had consumed homemade cottonseed oil containing gossypol. Many couples from these areas were found to be infertile. The women had amenorrhea and the men had low levels or complete absence of living sperm. It has since been determined that after three months the use of 50 mg of gossypol a week results in abrupt decreases in sperm counts, which are sometimes recoverable.[34] Hyperkalemia due to renal potassium loss has also been seen with clinical use of gossypol.[35]

Anthraquinone Glycosides

Anthraquinone aglycones are stimulant laxatives that act on the large intestine; they are discussed in more detail in chapters 7 and 13. At high doses, they are gastrointestinal irritants, causing symptoms that can include nausea, vomiting, bloody diarrhea, dizziness, abdominal pain, and, in severe cases, kidney damage.

Anthraquinones are found in the bark of cascara sagrada (Rhamnus purshiana) and other species in the Rhamnaceae family and in the leaves of Aloe vera (not the mucilaginous gel). They also occur in the root of Chinese rhubarb (Rheum officinale) but not common rhubarb (R. rhaponticum), and in the seeds and leaves of senna (Cassia spp.). Cascara bark from Rhamnus purshiana is stored for a year before it is processed. This delay allows for oxidation of the anthrones and dianthrones to anthraquinones, which tempers their potential griping effects.

Tannins

As discussed in chapter 7, tannins are complex polyphenols that form complexes with proteins, thus inhibiting enzyme activity. The toxicology of tannins has been extensively studied because of their potential deleterious effects on livestock. The primary sites of impact are the mouth, where proteins and carbohydrates get exposed to tannins, and the lumen of the gastrointestinal tract. Here, unbound tannins form complexes with both dietary proteins and metabolic proteins.

The major effect of tannins in the human diet appears to be a decrease in the efficiency of nutrient assimilation. Certain cancers, such as esophageal cancer, have been theoretically associated with the consumption of tannin-rich foods, such as betel nuts and herb teas. However, other studies, both epidemiological and clinical, indicate that tannin-rich black and green teas have anticarcinogenic properties. The anticarcinogenic and antimutagenic potential of tannins may be related to their antioxidant properties; tannins inhibit the generation of superoxide radicals. In the laboratory, tannins also inhibit the growth of many fungi, yeasts, bacteria, and viruses.[36]

Alkaloids

The group of compounds known as alkaloids contains many substances that are potentially toxic to humans, although not all alkaloids are toxic. In general, alkaloids are not toxic to plant cells, although purified forms can cause damage when applied to plant tissues, even those of the plant that produced the alkaloid. Plants may avoid alkaloid toxicity by accumulating them in certain ways—for example, in the vacuoles of the cells. Morphine is accumulated in the latex cells that occur throughout the opium poppy *(Papaver somniferum)*. These latex tubes are lacking in the parts of the pods where the seeds are formed, however, and thus do not affect the developing embryos. For a detailed discussion of the chemistry of alkaloids, see chapter 8.

Pyrrolizidine Alkaloids

Pyrrolizidine alkaloids (PAs) have become a major concern in the world of herbal medicine. The issues they raise encompass chemistry, pharmacokinetics, pharmacodynamics, toxicology, and phytotherapeutic clinical practice. Some of these are discussed here and in chapter 9. In addition, the interested reader should consult a major 1995 review of the science of PAs by Röder.[37]

Pyrrolizidine alkaloids consist of about 200 structurally related compounds contained in more than 350 species of the families Apocynaceae, Asteraceae, Boraginaceae, Celastraceae, Euphorbiaceae, Fabaceae, Orchidaceae, Poaceae, Ranunculaceae, Rhicophoraceae, Santalaceae, Sapotaceae, and Scrophulariaceae. A number of these plants are used medicinally, including *Tussilago farfara*, *Petasites* species, *Senecio* species, *Alkanna tinctoria*, *Eupatorium* species, and *Symphytum* species.[38]

Their structure is based on two 5-membered rings with a nitrogen in position 4, a structure called the necine base. PAs with saturated necine bases are nontoxic. All toxic PAs, on the other hand, contain a double bond between the 1 and 2 positions.

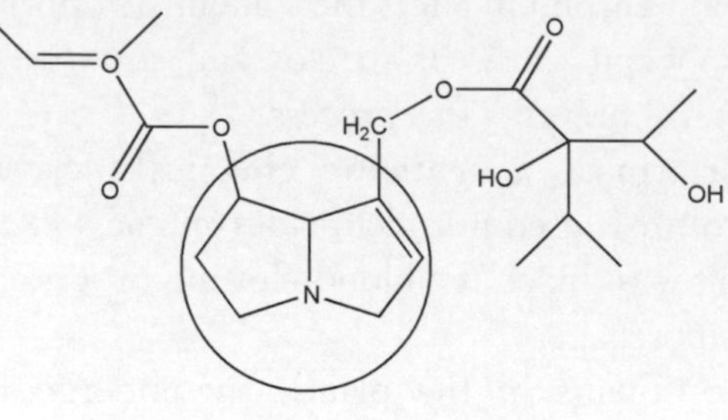

Fig. 10.2. Necine base

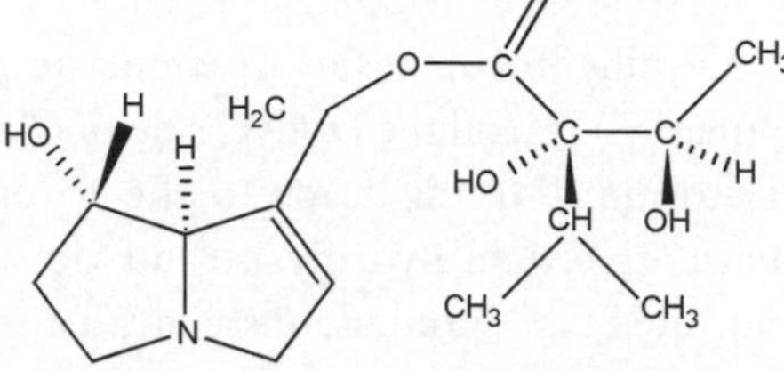

Fig. 10.3. A retronecine monoester

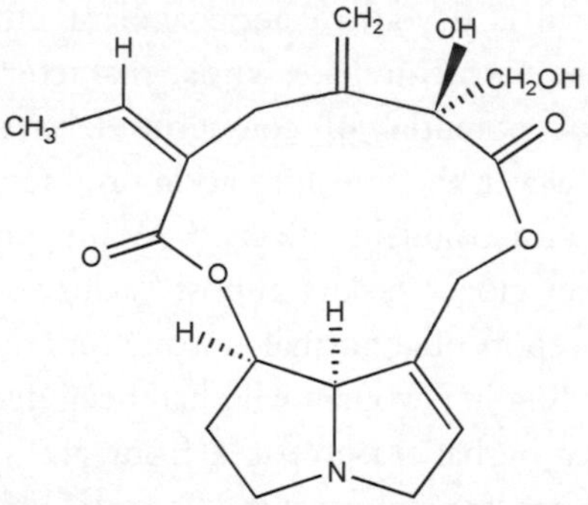

Fig. 10.4. A macrolytic retronecine diester

Additional variability in the toxicity of PAs results from the type of necine structure, which determines the stability of the pyrrole metabolite and thus the extent of any damage caused. The least damaging are the retronecine monoesters (for example, symphytine) and the most harmful are the macrolytic retronecine diesters (such as senecionine).

PAs are often the toxic but not the biologically active principles of many herbal medicines. Methods for the elimination of PAs from crude plant extracts have been developed. These methods remove PAs by treating the alcoholic plant extracts with cation exchange resins.[39]

Arnica montana and *Echinacea* species contain nontoxic PAs with a saturated necine base. Toxic PAs with an unsaturated necine base, such as those listed below, are hepatic and genetic toxins, and some are respiratory toxins.

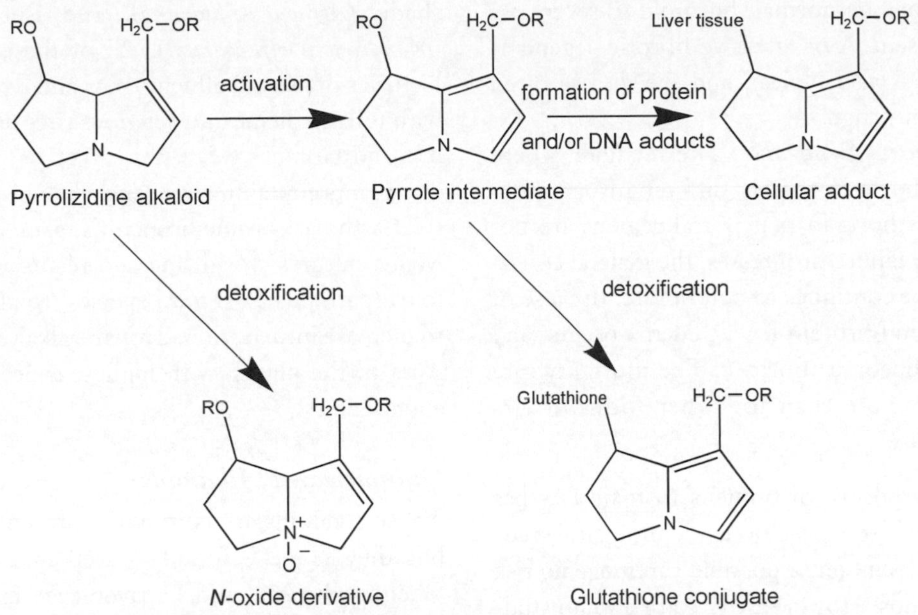

Fig. 10.5. Activation and detoxification of pyrrolizidine alkaloids

Plants Containing Toxic PAs

Alkanna tinctoria (alkanet)

Borago officinalis (borage)

Cynoglossum officinale (hound's tongue)

Eupatorium cannabinum (hemp agrimony)

Heliotropium spp. (e.g., common heliotrope)

Lithospermum officinale (gromwell)

Petasites spp. (e.g., butterbur)

Pulmonaria spp. (e.g., lungwort)

Senecio spp. (e.g., groundsel, ragwort)

Symphytum spp. (e.g., comfrey)

Tussilago farfara (coltsfoot)

PAs are absorbed from the intestine and reach the liver via the portal vein, where they are metabolized by esterase enzymes that release the free necine base. These reactions occur with both saturated and unsaturated PAs and are not part of the toxic reactions. On the contrary, they lead to a detoxification of toxic PAs.

Liver enzymes are also able to transform PAs to less toxic forms by increasing their water solubility. However, oxidative reactions catalyzed by oxidases lead to pyrrole-like intermediates, which are the ultimate toxic metabolites of the PAs (figure 10.5). These derivatives generate linkages (adducts) to proteins, RNA, and DNA. This mechanism is the basis for the hepatotoxicity of the PAs. However, detoxification may occur either via oxidation of the nitrogen or conjugation with glutathione.

There is no doubt that pyrrolizidine alkaloids are toxic to humans. Many cases have been reported in which individuals, hundreds of people, or even thousands of people have been intoxicated by the intake of PAs in the form of herbal remedies or foods. (For example, the seeds of *Crotalaria* species may contaminate grain foods.) In almost all cases of severe or fatal intoxication, the patients developed liver damage with cirrhosis and ascites (accumulation of fluid in the peritoneal cavity). This type of liver damage, called veno-occlusive disease, is the key syndrome associated with PA intoxication. When definitely caused by PAs, the condition may be referred to as *seneciosis*. The estimated daily intakes of certain PAs leading to fatal intoxication range from 0.5 mg/kg to 3.3 mg/kg.[39]

The symptoms of liver damage due to PA poisoning can be differentiated into three clinical stages.[40]

Acute Veno-Occlusive Syndrome: This stage is typically characterized by severe abdominal pain accompanied by vomiting and diarrhea. The liver is enlarged, and ascites is often present. Generalized edema is observed, and the patient may appear jaundiced. In some cases, the disease progresses dramatically and the patient dies a few weeks after the first symptoms occur. If the patient survives, complete remission may be possible, but the condition may also progress to subacute and chronic phases.

Subacute Veno-Occlusive Syndrome: This stage is characterized by an enlargement of the liver and sometimes the spleen. Other clinical symptoms are often absent.

Liver function may be normal, but mild to severe ascites may be present. A progressive fibrotic degeneration of the liver is also typical, and the disease often passes to a chronic stage.

Chronic Veno-Occlusive Syndrome: The key finding here is cirrhosis of the liver that is different from other forms of liver cirrhosis in that portal regions are not involved. As liver failure progresses, the general condition of the patient continues to deteriorate. Because of a decrease in serum protein levels, edema occurs, and the patient may become anorexic. The mortality rate is usually higher here than for other forms of cirrhotic liver disease.

Although the exposure of humans to toxic PAs has occurred many times in the past, no epidemiological studies are available to document a possible carcinogenic risk from these compounds. However, there are also no studies to demonstrate the absence of such a risk. Because of the positive results of animal carcinogenicity studies, together with the in vitro findings about the genotoxicity of unsaturated PAs, the possibility that PAs have a carcinogenic effect in humans must be taken into consideration.

There is no absolutely safe dose for genotoxic carcinogens. Extrapolations of dose-response curves from high to low concentrations are of questionable reliability, and animal experiments may not be applicable to humans. Nevertheless, such calculations are made to get crude information about the carcinogenic risk posed by certain compounds. The German Federal Ministry of Health recommends an allowable upper limit of toxic PAs in herbal remedies of 0.1 to 0.2 ppm. The daily intake should not exceed 30 g (senecionine) or 700 g (symphytine) per day.

Piperidine Alkaloids

The piperidine alkaloid coniine is the most important alkaloid in poison hemlock (*Conium maculatum*). This colorless, strongly basic oil has a mild pepper odor and a burning taste and occurs in all parts of the plant. Four other piperidine alkaloids are also found in poison hemlock. Coniine is lethal to all forms of animal life.

Tropane Alkaloids

Tropane alkaloids are found in many plants in the Solanaceae family, and include a number of important molecules, such as atropine, hyoscyamine, and scopolamine. Plants containing these substances include thornapples (*Datura* spp.), angel's trumpets (*Brugmansia* spp.), henbane (*Hyoscyamus niger*), belladonna or deadly nightshade (*Atropa belladonna*), and European mandrake (*Mandragora officinarum*). All of these plants have long histories of use as hallucinogens and have been connected with folk medicine and religious rites dating back to 1500 B.C. and Homer's *Odyssey*.

Plants containing tropane alkaloids have been used to treat asthma, chronic bronchitis, pain, and flu symptoms. Many cultures worldwide add plants with tropane alkaloids (particularly *Datura* species) to alcoholic beverages to increase intoxication. Tropane alkaloids are found in all parts of the plants, with highest concentrations in roots and seeds.

Quinolizidine Alkaloids

These alkaloids are commonly present in the Fabaceae, but they may be found as well in the Berberidaceae, Chenopodiaceae, and Papaveraceae families. Sparteine, from Spanish broom (*Spartium junceum*), increases or strengthens the heartbeat, causing a greater flow of blood to the kidneys and increasing urine production. Sparteine has been used in treating certain cases of cardiac fibrillation. Cytisine, found in Scotch broom (*Cytisus scoparius*), is known to be toxic, and in Great Britain, *Laburnum* is considered the second most toxic plant for animals after the yew, *Taxus*. Other sources of these lupine-type alkaloids are lupines (*Lupinus*) and wild indigo (*Baptisia*).

Pyridine Alkaloids

Nicotine is lethal to all forms of animal life. Small amounts stimulate breathing, but absorption of larger amounts depresses the respiratory rate. Death from nicotine poisoning results from respiratory failure. Humans are able to smoke tobacco only because the body is capable of breaking down and eliminating this alkaloid instead of accumulating it. Nicotine is used as an insecticide in agriculture and in home gardens.

Indole Alkaloids

Ergot alkaloids are found in the sclerotial bodies produced by the ergot fungus (*Claviceps purpurea*) and in the seeds of the morning glory (*Ipomoea tricolor*). Two indole alkaloids, gelsemine and sempervirine, that occur particularly in the roots of yellow jasmine (*Gelsemium sempervirens*) depress the central nervous system. The psychoactive alkaloids of the mescaline and psilocybin groups are considered toxic by the U.S. Drug Enforcement Administration, but this is very much a matter of opinion.

Isoquinoline Alkaloids

Isoquinoline alkaloids are found in many plant families, including the Ranunculaceae, Rubiaceae, Berberidaceae, Fumariaceae, and Papaveraceae. The *Chelidonium*, *Papaver*, and *Sanguinaria* genera of the Papaveraceae contain a large number of alkaloids. The largest number of alkaloids obtained from a single species in this family comes from *Papaver somniferum*, the opium poppy, which contains the morphinan alkaloids morphine and codeine. Heroin is synthesized from morphine.

Steroid Alkaloids

Steroid alkaloids, found in approximately 250 species of plants in the families Solanaceae and Liliaceae, occur mostly as glycosides with the properties of saponins. They are found in the tomato (*Lycopersicon*) as well as in the potato and other plants in the genus *Solanum*. Some are very toxic, causing severe gastroenteritis that may be fatal.

Species of *Solanum* contain solanine, which occurs in highest concentrations in areas that have a high metabolic rate, such as sprouts, green skin, and stems, and in lowest concentrations in ripe fruit. Solanine consists of six different glycosides; each hydrolyzes to the sugar peculiar to its particular glycoside and to the aglycone solanidine, a steroidal alkaloid.

Diterpenoid Alkaloids

These alkaloids are some of the most toxic chemicals found in plants. For example, aconitine, found in monkshood (*Aconitum*), has an LD_{50} of 0.12 mg/kg in mice. Another example is delphinine, from larkspur (*Delphinium*). In humans, 2 to 5 mg constitutes a lethal dose.

Polypeptides

These compounds are rarely toxic, although some of the poisons in the freshwater blue-green algae are polypeptides. However, the most notable exceptions are the toxins of the mushrooms in the genus *Amanita*, which are also polypeptides.

Amanita Toxins

All of the toxins found in the *Amanita* mushrooms are peptides. Amatoxins and phallotoxins are found in *A. bisporigera*, *A. ocreata*, *A. phalloides*, *A. phalloides* var. *alba*, *A. suballiacea*, *A. tenuifolia*, *A. virosa*, and some other mushrooms. Ibotenic acid is found in *A. cothurnata*, *A. muscaria* var. *formosa*, *A. muscaria* var. *muscaria*, and *A. pantherina*. The cap is the deadliest part of these mushrooms.

There are nine amatoxins:

α-amanitin
β-amanitin
γ-amanitin
ε-amanitin
Amanin
Amanin amide
Amanullin
Amanullinic acid
Proamanullin

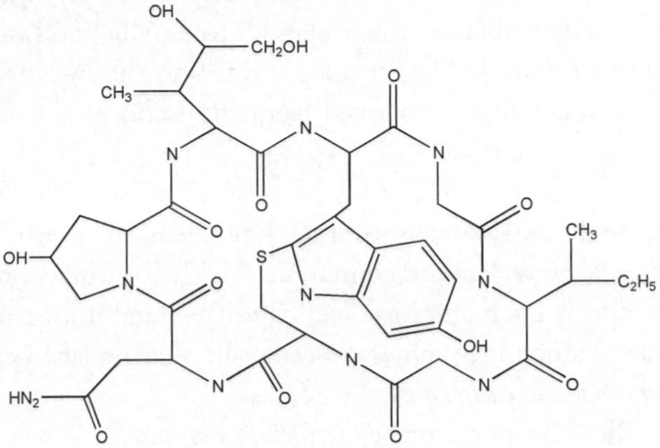

Fig. 10.6. α-amanitin

Amatoxins are responsible for fatal human responses to *Amanita* mushrooms. They are taken up by the liver, where they begin to cause damage. They are then secreted by the bile into the blood, where they are taken up by the liver again in a cycle of damage and excretion. In the liver, amatoxins inhibit RNA-polymerase II. The liver is slowly destroyed and is unable to repair itself due to the inactivation of the RNA-polymerase. Thus, the liver slowly dissolves with no hope of repair. However, rapid treatment with silymarin helps alleviate the toxicity of amatoxins.

There are seven naturally occurring phallotoxins:

Phallacidin
Phallacin
Phallisacin
Phallisin
Phalloidin
Phalloin
Prophalloin

Phallotoxins destroy liver cells by disturbing the equilibrium of hepatocyte membrane structure. This renders the cell susceptible to deformity in the face of changes in pressure of blood flowing through the liver. This is followed by loss of potassium ions and cytoplasmic enzymes, leading in turn to depletion of ATP and glycogen, which causes the final downfall of the liver.

Lectins

Lectins are glycoproteins that cause red blood cells to agglutinate (clump). The terms *phytohemagglutinins* and *lectins* are used interchangeably. Lectin-containing plants are found in many botanical groups, but most frequently occur in Fabaceae and Euphorbiaceae.

The interaction of lectins with carbohydrates is very specific—as specific, in fact, as enzyme-substrate and antigen-antibody interactions. Lectins may bind with free sugar or with sugar residues of polysaccharides, glycoproteins, or glycolipids, which may be free or bound (as in cell membranes). The term *lectin* refers to the specificity of this reaction; it is derived from the Latin root *legere*, meaning "to choose."

Lectins can impair growth, cause diarrhea, and interfere with nutrient absorption. The seeds of precatory bean (*Abrus precatorius*) contain the highly toxic glycoprotein abrin. Even less toxic lectins can be fatal if ingested in large amounts, such as concanavalin A from jack bean (*Concanavalia ensiformis*).

Ricin, from castor bean (*Ricinus communis*), is one of the most toxic natural substances known. It inhibits protein synthesis by inactivating ribosomes, and is a potent cytotoxin but a weak hemagglutinin. Castor bean seeds are poisonous to people, animals, and insects. When beaded into necklaces, these highly toxic seeds cause skin irritation at contact points. If the seed is swallowed without chewing, it will most likely pass harmlessly through the digestive tract if there has been no damage to the seed coat. However, if it is chewed or broken and then swallowed, the ricin toxin will be absorbed by the intestines. Children are more sensitive than adults to fluid loss from vomiting and diarrhea, and can quickly become severely dehydrated and die.

SKIN REACTIONS CAUSED BY PLANTS

By far the commonest plant-related problems experienced by people occur through skin contact. Such problems can take many forms and involve a number of physiological processes, as illustrated in table 10.3.

Contact Urticaria

The term *urticaria*, also known as hives, describes reddening and swelling of the skin. This reaction is short-lived, causes much itching, and clears without trace. If urticaria develops within an hour of exposure to an agent at the site of contact, the condition is called *contact urticaria*.

Table 10.3. Types of Skin Reactions to Plants and Plant Products[41]

REACTION	SIGNS AND SYMPTOMS
Contact urticaria	Immediate reaction (within minutes of contact) Itching, erythema, and/or edema
Irritant contact dermatitis	Skin dry and possibly itchy, often with fissures Usually restricted to areas of skin contact Typically follows prolonged or extensive exposure to irritant Cactus glochids, in particular, may cause an extensive pruritic eruption simulating scabies
Phytophotodermatitis	Erythematous, streaky eruption that may be vesicular or bullous, occurring within 2 days of plant contact Reaction occurs precisely at sites of contact in sun-exposed areas Brown hyperpigmentation, which persists for several weeks or months, is present at the same site Common in children
Allergic contact dermatitis	Pruritic, often streaky, erythema, sometimes vesicular Starts at areas of contact but may spread outward Develops, often progressively, within 3 days of exposure Recurrent episodes lasting several days each are typical and are usually followed by scaling; each episode may be worse than the last Minimal, if any, hyperpigmentation Airborne contact dermatitis typically affects face, neck, forearms, and hands, simulating photosensitivity

Contact urticaria may be caused by pharmacological mechanisms, such as the eruption induced by *Urtica dioica*, the stinging nettle, from which the term *urticaria* (literally, "nettle rash") is derived. In immunological urticaria, a Type I hypersensitivity to a specific component of the plant develops. Sensitized people develop a response within minutes after contact. Repeated exposure to such stimuli may lead to a persistent eczema-like condition.

Urticaria Due to Injection of Toxins

Some plants possess sharp hairs on the surface of leaves and stems that inject a mix of irritant chemicals into the skin or mucous membranes upon contact. This is thought to serve as a defense against browsing animals. Some caterpillars employ a similar strategy to avoid predation. A brush against the nettle plant shears off a cap from the hairs, revealing a sharp, beveled, hollow structure that resembles a hypodermic needle. From this structure, an irritant liquid enters the skin; this liquid contains inflammatory mediators such as histamine, acetylcholine, and 5-hydroxytryptamine. These chemicals cause the immediate reaction, but stinging can continue for more than 12 hours, even after features of urticaria have disappeared. This suggests the presence of other substances capable of inducing a secondary release of inflammatory mediators.

The nettle is less likely to cause stinging if squeezed firmly than if touched gently. Vigorous massage or application of cold compresses will often reduce symptoms of nettle-induced urticaria. However, reactions to some nettle plants may be more severe. *Urtica gigas* has caused death in horses in New Zealand and *U. ferox* has caused death in humans.

Immunological Contact Urticaria

An immediate Type I contact reaction can occur in anyone who has previously become sensitized to a particular substance. Molecules of the contact sensitizer penetrate the epidermis, and then react with specific immunoglobulin E (IgE) bound to mast cells, leading to release of vasoactive mediators. Histamine is the major mediator, but prostaglandins, kinins, leukotrienes, and others may amplify the inflammatory response.

Irritant hairs on the surface of some plants enhance penetration of the antigen. A good example is tumbleweed (*Salsola kali*), which possesses sharp bracts that cause an irritant reaction. Some people become sensitized to the effects of such plants and subsequently develop contact urticaria.

Irritant Contact Dermatitis

Irritant contact dermatitis describes an inflammatory response to physical or chemical injury that is not immunologically mediated. Severity of the response depends on the barrier function of the skin as well as the potency and duration of the irritant stimulus. It may be caused by more than one factor. For example, physical trauma caused by handling narcissus bulbs may enhance chemical trauma from oxalate crystals contained in the bulbs.

The severity of such reactions can range from irritation with erythema and possible fissuring to a severe response that renders the individual unable to work. The eruption affects areas of contact, especially where the stratum corneum is thinner, such as on the fingertips and back of the hands, under the free edge of fingernails, and between the fingers. Skin damage by irritants increases the individual's susceptibility to subsequent allergic sensitization.

Mechanical Irritants

Penetration of the skin by hairs, spines, or thorns can produce a papular irritant eruption. Many plants have glandular hairs (trichomes) on stems or leaves. Several members of the Boraginaceae family are covered in such coarse, stiff hairs, including borage itself (*Borago officinalis*). Other irritant plants of this family include forget-me-not (*Myosotis* spp.), hound's tongue (*Cynoglossum* spp.), comfrey (*Symphytum officinale*), and lungwort (*Pulmonaria officinalis*). American dogwoods (*Cornus* spp.) have T-shaped hairs that cause erythema and urtication when the leaf is rubbed on the skin in the direction of its long axis. In addition to its obvious spines, the pads and fruit of the prickly pear (*Opuntia ficus-indica*), cultivated for its edible fruit, bear tufts of shorter, hooked hairs called *glochids*, which may appear innocuous but can cause mechanical injury. These glochids may be transferred to clothing and to any part of the skin, particularly softer areas, such as the genitalia and between the fingers.

Table 10.4. Irritant Plants

INJURY	EXAMPLE
Mechanical/physical	
Blunt trauma	Falling branches, nuts
Thorns	Rose family (Rosaceae)
Sharp-edged leaves and leaf hooks	Holly, *Agave*, *Yucca*
Spines and glochids	Cacti, especially *Opuntia*
Stem/leaf hairs	Boraginaceae, Asteraceae
Irritant fibers	Rose hips, tulip bulbs
Chemical	
Stinging hairs	*Urtica*
Irritant sap/latex	Euphorbiaceae, Ranunculaceae
Calcium oxalate crystals	Bulbs

Chemical Irritants

A number of plants contain chemical irritants that may exacerbate the mechanical irritation caused by hairs or spines. A common chemical irritant is crystalline calcium oxalate, but a wide range of other chemicals dissolved or suspended in latex or housed in specific organelles may also cause chemical irritation. Many bulbs and some other plants, notably *Dieffenbachia* and rhubarb, contain calcium oxalate. This water-insoluble salt forms bundles of needle-like crystals (raphides), which are surrounded by a mucilaginous liquid and held in cells. After contact with water, the cell ejects the crystals into the skin or mucosa. These crystals may help the plant maintain ionic equilibrium, dispose of waste products, or protect against foraging animals. Some cacti, such as *Cephalocereus senilis*, contain up to 85% calcium oxalate by dry weight.[42]

There are many structural types among irritant constituents, including alkaloids, glycosides, proteolytic enzymes, saponins, phenolic compounds, and anthraquinones. Plants of the Ranunculaceae family, discussed earlier, contain the chemical irritant protoanemonin.

Allergic Contact Dermatitis

Allergic contact dermatitis is a specific immunological response to an external substance. Unlike immunologically mediated contact urticaria, this is a manifestation of delayed immunity. An allergic reaction can occur only in an individual who is already sensitized to the antigen, and classically the reaction is restricted to sites of exposure.

Allergic contact dermatitis displays the clinical and histological features of eczema. The exogenous substance, or hapten, is typically of low molecular weight, enabling it to penetrate the epidermis. It binds with molecules in the skin (for example, keratins) or directly binds to collagen bundles. The antigenic complex is then recognized by a specific lymphocyte. These cells migrate from the skin via lymphatic drainage to lymph nodes, where they proliferate and differentiate. The resultant sensitized effector and memory cells are distributed to the rest of the body through blood vessels.

When next exposed to the allergen, the sensitized individual develops an eczematous response at the site of contact. Further stimulation of memory cells occurs, causing increasingly severe responses on repeated exposure. For some people, frequent reexposure to small doses of the allergen may induce immunological tolerance, and it is possible to reduce sensitivity through oral dosing with the allergen, notably poison ivy.

Poison Ivy and Poison Oak

The Anacardiaceae genus *Toxicodendron* includes poison ivy, poison oak, and poison sumac. There are many related cross-reacting species, as well as several unrelated genera that cross-react with *Toxicodendron* species. Such cross-reactions are due to the presence of similar allergenic constituents in the various species of plants.

Table 10.5. Anacardiaceae Family and Cross-Reacting Plants

GENUS *TOXICODENDRON*	RELATED AND CROSS-REACTING CULTIVARS
Poison ivy	
T. radicans	Cashew (*Anacardium occidentale*)
T. rydbergdii	Ginkgo (*Ginkgo biloba*) Grevillea robusta
Poison oak	
T. diversilobum	Indian marking nut (*Semecarpus anacardium*)
T. toxicarium	Japanese lacquer (*Rhus verniciflua*)
Poison sumac	
T. vernix	Mango (*Mangifera indica*)
Entire *Toxicodendron* genus	African poison ivy (*Smodingium argutum*)

Contained in the oil of most members of Anacardiaceae is urushiol, an irritant mixture of pentadecylcatechols (PDCs). The base molecule of PDC has a completely saturated side chain at position 3. Unsaturation of the side chain leads to greater allergenicity. The name *urushiol* is derived from the Japanese word for sap, *kiurushi*.

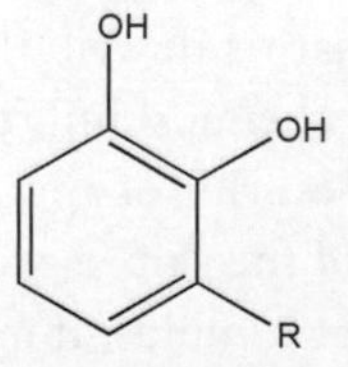

Fig. 10.7. Pentadecylcatechol skeleton

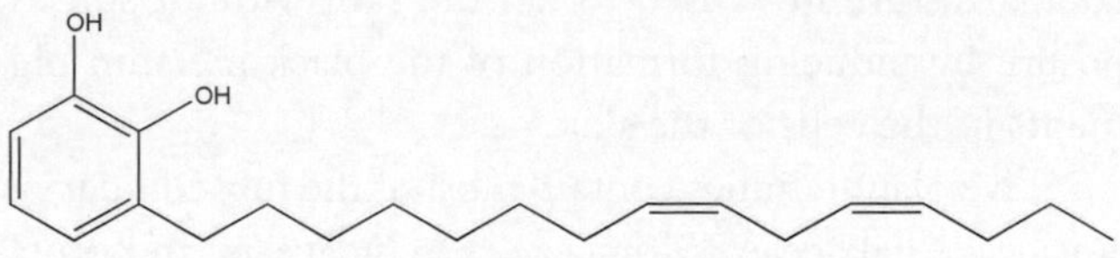

Fig. 10.8. Urushiol

Members of the Anacardiaceae family contain PDCs with mixtures of C-15 and C-17 side chains that have 1, 2, 3, or no double bonds. For example, poison ivy contains mainly C-15 side chains; poison oak, C-17; and poison sumac, C-13.

PHOTOSENSITIVITY

Phytophotodermatitis constitutes a specific pattern of phototoxic skin reaction in which delayed erythema, blistering, and hyperpigmentation are the major features. However, less obvious phototoxic reactions and photoallergy may also occur.

Photosensitization is a process by which a reaction to normally innocuous radiation is induced by the introduction of a specific radiation-absorbing component, known as the *photosensitizer*. In biological systems, the term *photosensitization* is generally understood to describe a process by which harmless doses of UVA or visible radiation are absorbed by a "foreign" molecule present at non-damaging concentrations. Reactions result from the involvement of cell and tissue constituents in the dissipation of the absorbed energy.

Psoralens appear to cause photosensitization via UVA light–induced binding of the psoralen molecule to nuclear DNA. This produces bonds, called photo-adducts, that cross-link with pyrimidine bases in the DNA.

Clinical Features

The characteristic eruption of a phototoxicity reaction is composed of linear dusky red lesions, often bullous or vesicular (blisterlike, containing a clear liquid) and associated with brown hyperpigmentation. Most such reactions occur in mid- to late summer, when the level of psoralens are highest in plants and the skin is unprotected by clothing. The eruption may be misdiagnosed as poison ivy or poison oak dermatitis; however, the phototoxic reaction is confined to the sites of contact and sun exposure. It is painful, but not pruritic, and may be followed by hyperpigmentation. In contrast, allergic contact dermatitis is pruritic; the eruption will often continue to evolve after presentation, and pigmentary changes are rare.

Table 10.6. Major Patterns of Phototoxicity Reactions

SKIN REACTIONS	PHOTOSENSITIZERS OR DISEASES
Type 1	
Prickling or burning during exposure	Coal tar
Immediate erythema	Pitch
Edema/urticaria with higher doses	Anthraquinone-based dyes
Sometimes, delayed erythema/hyperpigmentation	Benoxaprofen Chlorpromazine Erythropoietic protoporphyria
Type 2	
Exaggerated sunburn	Drugs such as chlorpromazine, chlorthiazides, quinine
Type 3	
Late-onset erythema	Psoralens (furocoumarins)
Blisters with slightly higher doses	Phytophotodermatitis
Hyperpigmentation only with low exposures	*Berloque* dermatitis
Type 4	
Increased skin fragility; skin blisters with trauma	Nalidixic acid Frusemide Tetracycline Naproxen

In Europe, the most common cause of phototoxic reactions is brushing against rue. The typical streaklike pattern of the reaction also occurs when application of rue to the skin as an insect repellent is followed by sun exposure. It is also seen among individuals who are working with parsley, parsnip, or celery plants during the summer.

Many molecules naturally present in biological systems can act as photosensitizers. Well-known examples include chlorophyll, iron-free porphyrins, and flavins, like riboflavin. The list of endogenous sensitizers includes bilirubin, tryptophan, nicotinamide adenine dinucleotide phosphate (NADPH), pyridoxine, quinones (present in respiratory chains), all-trans retinal (the pigment produced in the retina in response to light), and many proteins containing these compounds, including lipofuscin (the so-called age pigment) and melanin.

Table 10.7. Plant-Derived Substances Causing Unintentional Color Change to Skin

REACTION	EXAMPLE
	Essential oils
Red discoloration by terpenes	Juniper
	Lemon
	Lime
	Orange
	Perfume ingredients
Post-inflammatory depigmentation	Benzyl alcohol
	Benzyl salicylate
	Cananga oil
	Cinnamic alcohol
	Geraniol
	Hydroxycitronellal
	Jasmine absolute
	Lavender oil
	Methoxycitronellal
	Sandalwood oil
Pigmented cosmetic dermatitis	Ylang-ylang oil

There are also many naturally occurring exogenous photosensitizers.[43] Plants make photosensitizers, most likely in order to protect their surfaces against viruses, bacteria, fungal spores, yeasts, and small arthropods and their eggs, and probably also against insects. Photosensitizers found in plants include furanocoumarins, pterocarpans, isoquinolines, lignans, sesquiterpenes, hypericins, and curcumins.

Chemistry of the Furocoumarins

A common furocoumarin (or furanocoumarin) is psoralen; the name is derived from the genus *Psoralea*. Furocoumarins cause photosensitization and poisoning in humans and domestic animals but have been used medicinally as well. For more than 3,000 years, practitioners of Eastern medicine have applied poultices of plant juices containing furocoumarins to the whitened patches of skin seen in the disorder known as leukoderma or vitiligo. This condition is an inherited tendency that occurs in about 2% of the world's population. Synthetic furo-

coumarins are now used to tan the skin without sun exposure by inducing formation of the black melanin pigments in the cells of the skin.

Five plant families contain most of the furocoumarins: Apiaceae, Fabaceae, Moraceae, Orchidaceae, and Rutaceae. These compounds are also found in Asteraceae in yarrow (*Achillea millefolium*) and in Convolvulaceae in field bindweed (*Convolvulus arvensis*).

Two forms of furocoumarins occur. Linear furocoumarins, known as psoralens, are named for *Psoralea corylifolia*.

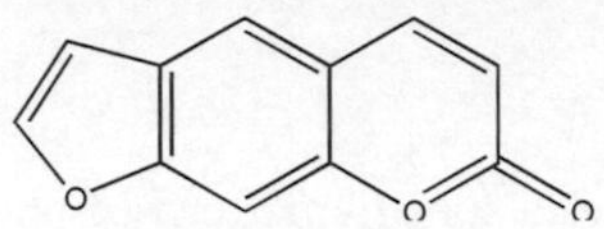

Fig. 10.9. Psoralen

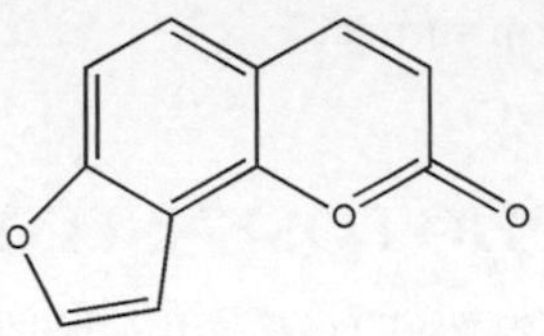

Fig. 10.10. Angelicin

Angular furocoumarins, known as *angelicins*, are related to the angelicin (isopsoralen) obtained from *Angelica archangelica*.

Not all furocoumarins are phototoxic. Their phototoxic potential varies with the shape of the molecule, and linear forms are more potent than angular. The degree and nature of substituent components of the molecule constitute another variable, which in psoralens decrease the phototoxic potential but in angelicins may increase it. Severe, acute phytophotodermatitis reactions are associated with psoralen itself and its derivatives, 8-methoxypsoralen (such as xanthotoxin from celery), 5-methoxypsoralen (bergapten), and, possibly, the angelicin pimpinellin.

Bergapten, a component of bergamot oil from *Citrus aurantium* ssp. *bergamia*, is the phototoxic component of lime peel extract and essential oil. The components of *Ammi majus*, used in the treatment of vitiligo, include both 8- and 5-methoxypsoralen along with imperatorin (8-isopentenyloxypsoralen).

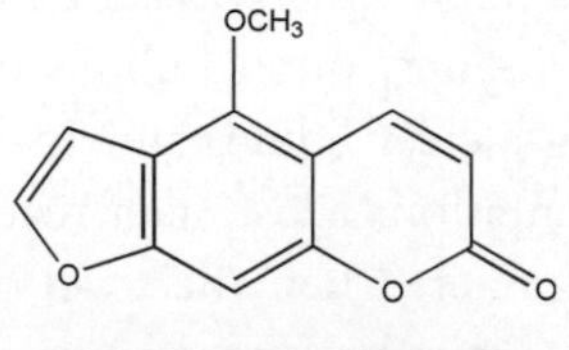

Fig. 10.11. Xanthotoxin

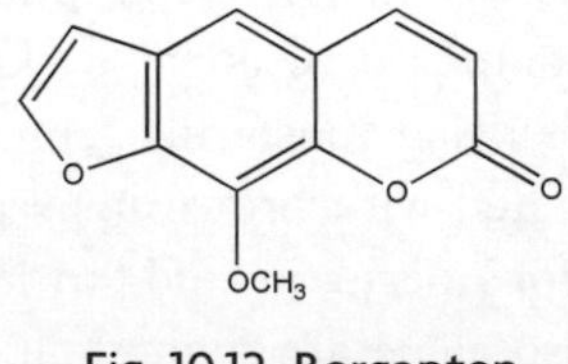

Fig. 10.12. Bergapten

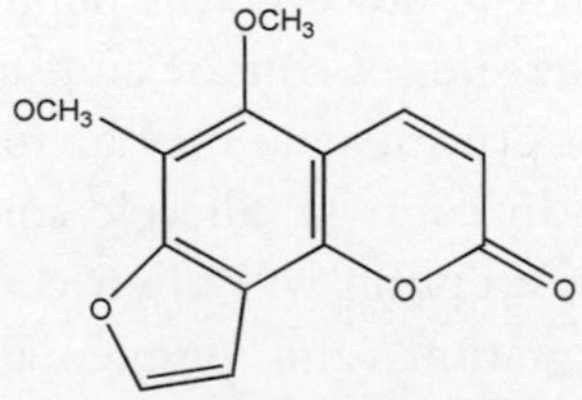

Fig. 10.13. Pimpinellin

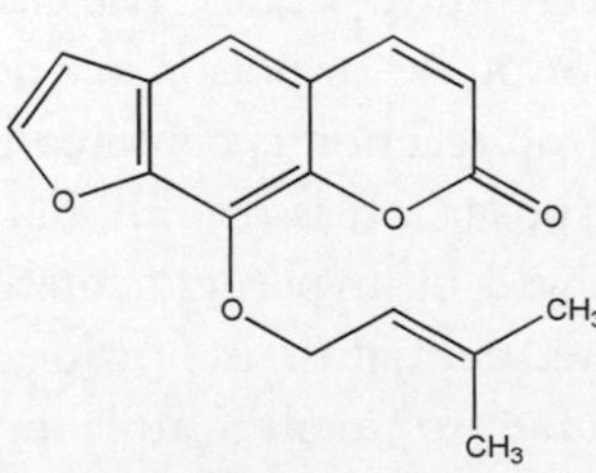

Fig. 10.14. Imperatorin

Levels of furocoumarins increase in response to fungal attack. Fresh celery (*Apium graveolens*) contains 10 to 100 µg/g wet weight of total psoralens. However, levels of furocoumarins as high as 320 µg/g have been measured in specimens infected with fungi. The development of disease-resistant cultivars of celery has led to an increased natural furocoumarin content in these plants. Similar increased exposure to phototoxic compounds may occur with other vegetables, such as parsnips.

As little as 1 µg of 8-methoxypsoralen per square centimeter of skin can produce blistering after exposure to artificial UVA equivalent to approximately 10 minutes of exposure to summer sunlight in the United Kingdom. In one unusual case of phytophotodermatitis, a patient who ingested large quantities of celery soup before using a UVA sun bed developed classic symptoms.

HERB TOXICITY UNRELATED TO CONSTITUENTS

There are situations in which toxicity stemming from herb use has nothing to do with the herb itself. These may be related to adulteration, spoiling, or pollution, which is usually unintentional, but, strange as it sounds, may also be intentional.

Adulteration of Commercial Products

Herb dealers may deviate from pharmacopoeial specifications for botanical identity for various reasons. Occasionally, if an officinal plant species is not available, it may be replaced by an equivalent related species. For instance, it has become difficult to obtain real goldenrod (*Solidago virgaurea*), but this species can be justifiably substituted with the related *S. gigantea* or *S. canadensis*.

In addition, a deliberate substitution of medicinal herbs by inferior or cheaper species may also be made. Some years ago, a Belgian consumer organization reported that the majority of locally purchased peppermint products did not contain *Mentha piperita* at all, but rather the much cheaper species *M. crispa*. Likewise, most samples of linden flower did not come from *Tilia cordata* or *T. platyphyllos* but instead from *T. argentea*.

Careless gathering, storage, or distribution of medicinal plant material may result in accidental substitution or contamination with another botanical. Inexpert or negligent herb dealers may fail to recognize such problems in time.

Self-Collection of Medicinal Plants

People who collect their own herbs must be absolutely certain of the identity of the plants they are harvesting. A serious *Digitalis* poisoning due to accidental substitution of foxglove for comfrey was reported in Great Britain. The patient was an elderly man, and he needed intensive care treatment to recover.

Microorganisms and Microbial Toxins

Commercially produced herbs may be contaminated by pathogenic microorganisms, like *Salmonella*, or microbial toxins, such as bacterial endotoxins. Toxic substances may also be formed through microbial transformation of botanical constituents. In short, herbal materials pose the same microbial health risks as other pharmaceuticals:

- Infection by pathogenic microorganisms
- Microbial transformation of botanical constituents into more toxic compounds
- Production of microbial toxins, such as bacterial endotoxins and mycotoxins

No official regulatory guidelines on microbial contamination of herbs exist. However, the requirements for the microbial purity of nonsterile medicines proposed by the Committee of Official Laboratories and Control Services of the *Federation Internationale Pharmaceutique* provide the following figures for assessing the microbial status of dried herbal materials:[44]

- An aerobic bacterial count between 102 and 108 colony-forming units per gram (CFU/g), mostly >104 CFU/g
- A coliform bacterial count between <102 and 104 CFU/g
- A yeast and mold count between 102 and 106 CFU/g

Extraction of herbs with an alcohol-based solution will reduce the number of microorganisms because of direct contact with the alcohol. Extraction with boiling water will also have a decontaminating effect.

Keeping heat-extracted herbal teas for longer than 24 hours is not advisable, because spore-forming species are not effectively eliminated by boiling water.[45] This is even more essential when an herbal tea has been prepared by cold infusion, as cold water has no decontaminating effect. When there are phytochemical considerations or other reasons to choose cold over hot extraction, each dose should be freshly prepared at the time of use. As a rule of thumb, cold infusions that are more than four hours old should be discarded.

Mycotoxins

Mycotoxins are toxic metabolites produced by fungi and molds. Over 300 mycotoxins have been identified, and it is thought that many more are yet to be discovered. Known classes of mycotoxins include:

- Aflatoxins
- Ochratoxins
- Rubratoxins
- Trichothecenes
- Zearalenone

Mold growth can occur at any time, from herb harvest until consumption. Mold spores are everywhere, and they lay dormant until conditions are right for them to sporulate and grow. The type and amount of mycotoxin produced depends on factors such as temperature, pH, relative humidity, drought stress, and insect or mechanical damage to the herb in which the mold is growing. Mold growth depends largely on the moisture content of the dried herb: the more moisture, the more mold, and the greater the risk of contamination with mycotoxins.

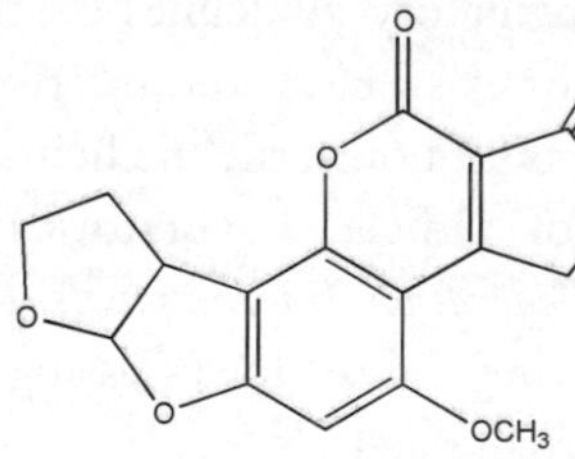

Fig. 10.15. Aflatoxin B1

There is clear evidence from animal studies that aflatoxins are carcinogenic, producing tumors primarily of the liver, colon, and kidneys. The primary route of human exposure is ingestion of contaminated food. Americans may consume up to an estimated 0.15 to 0.50 µg of aflatoxins daily. The Environmental Protection Agency (EPA) regulates aflatoxins under the Resource Conservation and Recovery Act, which designates aflatoxins as hazardous constituents of waste. The EPA's Carcinogen Assessment Group considers aflatoxins to be potentially carcinogenic. The Food and Drug Administration has established enforcement levels for aflatoxins of 0.5 ppb in milk and 20 ppb in other food products. Aflatoxins can be found in a wide range of food products due to contamination in the field, manufacturing process, or storage. Corn, peanuts, and cottonseed pose the highest risks.

Toxic Metals

There are two major reasons why it has become necessary to monitor levels of toxic metals in herbs. First, contamination of the general environment with toxic metals has increased. Second, exotic herbal remedies, particularly those of Asian origin, have been repeatedly reported to contain toxic levels of heavy metals or arsenic.

Studies on levels of toxic metals in medicinal herbs have been conducted in Germany. Considerable variation was found among levels of pollutants in the same species collected from different habitats.

The decoction of herbs can affect the metal content. One study compared lead and cadmium levels in 120 sam-

Table 10.8. Lead and Cadmium in Wild-Grown Herbs*

METAL	PLANT	HABITAT	Total	Flower	Leaf	Stem	Root
LEAD							
	Achillea millefolium	Median strip	8.41	4.66	23.73	1.34	4.59
		Roadside	2.37	2.33	8.90	1.25	4.16
	Hypericum perforatum	Median strip	11.97	5.77	17.82	2.32	4.57
		Roadside	1.77	1.85	5.96	1.05	5.06
CADMIUM							
	Achillea millefolium	Median strip	0.34	0.13	0.78	0.33	0.44
		Roadside	1.48	0.89	2.17	1.33	2.57
	Hypericum perforatum	Median strip	0.37	0.38	0.54	0.32	0.85
		Roadside	5.62	6.97	~7.43	3.74	3.30

LEVEL OF CONTAMINATION (MG/KG)

*Variation in levels of lead and cadmium by plant part and habitat in wild-grown *Achillea millefolium* and *Hypericum perforatum*[46]

ples of 19 herbs and in finished teas prepared from these samples.[47] Passage of metals into the tea was higher than 50% in only 12% of the lead assays and 8% of the cadmium tests. The majority of the tea samples (67% and 71%, for lead and cadmium, respectively) demonstrated a relatively low extraction of metals, 25% or less. Individual extraction values ranged from 0.1% to 87% for lead and from 1% to 68% for cadmium.

These large variations may well be connected to the different ways in which the samples were contaminated. When an herb is contaminated on its surface, it is likely that a relatively large proportion of the contaminant will dissolve in the hot water. Little will enter the tea if the metal ions are bound in the plant cell.

Toxic Metals in Asian Remedies

Reports of unacceptable levels of toxic metals in herbal remedies regularly appear in the literature. One report described arsenic poisoning in Singapore, and other reports attribute lead poisoning to the use of an Asian herbal medicine. Aside from the herbs themselves, potential sources of contamination include lead-releasing brewing pots, grinding weights, and other metal utensils.[48,49] However, in Asian remedies, the possibility exists that toxic metals found are not contaminants, as several Chinese herbal formulas contain arsenic and mercury salts as intentional ingredients.

Table 10.9. Relative Passage of Heavy Metals into Medicinal Teas*

CRUDE DRUG (NUMBER OF SAMPLES)	RELATIVE PASSAGE (MEAN VALUES IN %)	
	LEAD	CADMIUM
Aerial parts		
Achillea millefolium (5)	15	24
Equisetum arvense (13)	22	23
Hypericum perforatum (5)	12	19
Thymus vulgaris (6)	9	28
Leaves		
Betula alba (9)	16	15
Cassia angustifolia (8)	33	50
Melissa officinalis (1)	15	19
Mentha piperita (8)	20	28
Leaves and flowers		
Crataegus (1)	9	8
Flowers		
Crataegus (4)	9	6
Malva (4)	13	13
Matricaria recutita (16)	36	18
Tilia (1)	11	19
Fruits		
Carvum carvi (4)	73	25
Foeniculum (6)	40	16
Pimpinella anisum (10)	29	19

*Relative passage of heavy metals from crude herbal drugs into medicinal teas prepared by extraction with boiling water.[50]

References

1. Tyler VE. *The Honest Herbal: A Sensible Guide to the Use of Herbs and Related Remedies.* Binghamton, NY: The Haworth Press, 1993.

2. DeSmet PAGM, D'Arcy PF. Drug interactions with herbal and other non-orthodox remedies. In: D'Arcy PF, McElnay JC, Welling PG, eds. *Mechanisms of Drug Interactions.* New York: Springer-Verlag, 1996.

3. Röder E. Medicinal plants in Europe containing pyrrolizidine alkaloids. *Pharmazie* 1995; 50:83–98.

4. Mann J, Davidson RS, Hobbs JB, et al. *Natural Products: Their Chemistry and Biological Significance.* Harlow, UK: Longman Scientific & Technical; New York: Wiley, 1994.

5. Rothschild M, Edgar JA. Pyrrolizidine alkaloids from *Senecio vulgaris* sequestered and stored by *Danaus plexippus. Journal of Zoo and Wildlife Medicine* 1978; 186:347–9.

6. Schneider D, Boppré M, Schneider H, et al. A pheromone precursor and its uptake in male *Danaus* butterflies. *Journal of Comparative Physiology* 1975; 97:245–56.

7. Rode D. Comfrey toxicity revisited. *Trends in Pharmalogical Sciences* 2002; 23:497–9.

8. Beers MH, Berkow R, eds. *The Merck Manual of Diagnosis and Therapy.* Whitehouse Station, NJ: Merck Research Laboratories, 1997.

9. Rode D. Comfrey toxicity revisited. *Trends in Pharmalogical Sciences* 2002; 23:497–9.

10. Stickel F, Seitz HK. The efficacy and safety of comfrey. *Public Health Nutrition* 2000; 3:501–8.

11. Cheeke PR. Pyrrolizidine alkaloids. In: *Natural Toxicants in Feeds, Forages, and Poisonous Plants*, 2nd edition. Danville, IL: Interstate Publishers, 1998.

12. Ibid.

13. Rode D. Comfrey toxicity revisited. *Trends in Pharmalogical Sciences* 2002; 23:497–9.

14. Pierson ML, et al. Resistance of the rabbit to dietary pyrrolizidine (Senecio) alkaloid. *Research Communications in Chemical Pathology and Pharmacology* 1977; 16:561–4.

15. Stickel F, Seitz HK. The efficacy and safety of comfrey. *Public Health Nutrition* 2000; 3:501–8.

16. Muetterlein R, Aimold CG. Investigations concerning the content and the pattern of pyrrolizidine alkaloids in *Symphytum officale L.* (comfrey). *Pharmazeutische Zeitung* 1993; 138:119–25.

17. Cheeke PR. Pyrrolizidine alkaloids. In: *Natural Toxicants in Feeds, Forages, and Poisonous Plants*, 2nd edition. Danville, IL: Interstate Publishers 1998.

18. Schoental, R. Toxicology and carcinogenic action of pyrrolizidine alkaloids. *Cancer Research* 1968; 28:2237–46.

19. 1998 TESS Annual Report. *American Journal of Emergency Medicine* 1999; 17(5):435–87.

20. Brinker F. *Herb Contraindications and Drug Interactions.* Sandy, OR: Eclectic Medical Publications, 2001.

21. DeSmet PAGM, D'Arcy PF. Drug interactions with herbal and other non-orthodox remedies. In: D'Arcy PF, McElnay JC, Welling PG, eds. *Mechanisms of Drug Interactions.* New York: Springer-Verlag, 1996.

22. Beers MH, Berkow R, eds. *The Merck Manual of Diagnosis and Therapy.* Whitehouse Station, NJ: Merck Research Laboratories, 1997.

23. Himmelstein MW, Turner MJ, Asgharian B, et al. Comparison of blood concentrations of 1,3-butadiene and butadiene epoxides in mice and rats exposed to 1,3-butadiene by inhalation. *Carcinogenesis* 1994; 15(8):1479–86.

24. Medinksy MA, et al. In vivo metabolism of butadiene by mice and rats: A comparison of physiological model predictions and experimental data. *Carcinogenesis* 1994; 15(7):1329–40.

25. DeSmet P, et al. *Adverse Effects of Herbal Drugs*, vol. 1. New York: Springer-Verlag, 1992.

26. Woolf A. Oxalates. *Clinical Toxicology* 1993; 16:1–2.

27. Anand R, et al. Antioxaluric and anticalciuric activity of lupeol derivatives. *Indian Journal of Pharmacology* 1995; 27:265–68.

28. Vulto AG, DeSmet PAGM. Drugs used in non-orthodox medicine. In: Dukes MNG, ed. *Meylers Side Effects of Drugs*, 11th edition. Amsterdam: Elsevier, 1988.

29. Ritschel WA, Brady ME, Tan HSI, et al. Pharmacokinetics of coumarin and its 7-hydroxymetabolites upon intravenous and peroral administration of coumarin in man. *European Journal of Clinical Pharmacology* 1977; 12:457–61.

30. Reilley O. Anticoagulant, antithrombotic, and thrombolytic drugs. In: Goodman LS, Gilman A, eds. *The Pharmacological Basis of Therapeutics*, 6th edition. New York: Macmillan 1980.

31. Cheeke PR, Shull LR. *Natural Toxicants in Feeds and Poisonous Plants.* Westport, CT: AVI Pub. Co., 1985.

32. Hogan RP. Hemorrhagic diathesis caused by drinking an herbal tea. *JAMA: The Journal of the American Medical Association* 1983; 249:2679–80.

33. Hong CY, Huang JJ, Wu O. The inhibitory effect of gossypol on human sperm motility: relationship with time, temperature and concentration. *Human Toxicology* 1989; 8:49–51.

34. Coutinho EM. Gossypol: a contraceptive for men. *Contraception* 2002 Apr; 65(4):259–63.

35. Wu D. An overview of the clinical pharmacology and therapeutic potential of gossypol as a male contraceptive agent and in gynaecological disease. *Drugs* 1989; 38:333–41.

36. Chung KT, et al. Tannins and human health: a review. *Critical Reviews in Food Science and Nutrition* 1998 Aug; 38(6):421–64.

37. Röder E. Medicinal plants in Europe containing pyrrolizidine alkaloids. *Pharmazie* 1995; 50:83–98.

38. Mauz JC. Vorkommen und Genotoxizitat von Pyrrolizidinalkaloiden in Petasites hybridus L. und die Entfernung der Alkaloide aus Arzneipflanzenextrakten. *Dissertation Eidgenossische Technische Hochschule Zurich* No. 8246; 1987.

39. Mattocks AR. Toxicity of pyrrolizidine alkaloids. *Nature* 1968; 217:723–28.

40. Datta DV, Khuroo MS, Mattocks AR, et al. Herbal medicines and veno-occlusive disease in India. *Postgraduate Medical Journal* 1978; 54:511–15.

41. Lovell CR. *Plants and the Skin.* Oxford; Boston: Blackwell Scientific Publications, 1993.

42. Cheavin WVS. The crystals and crystoliths found in plant cells: part 1, Crystals. *Microscope* 1938; 2:155–58.

43. Downum KR. Light-activated plant defense. *The New Phytologist* 1992; 122:401.

44. Schilcher H. Ruckstande und Veruntreinigungen bei Drogen und Drogenzubereitungen. 19. Mitteilung: Zur Wertbestimmung und Qualitatsprufung von Drogen. *Planta Medica* 1982; 44:65–77.

45. Lenoble M, Fourniat I, Bourlioux P, et al. Controle de la qualité microbiologique dechantillons de Mentha piperita de diverses origines geographiques. *Annales Pharmaceutiques Françaises* 1980; 38:333–42.

46. Schilcher H, Peters H, Wank H. (1986) Pestizide und Schwermetall in Arzneipflanzen und Arzneipflanzen-Zubereitungen. *Drug Development and Industrial Pharmacy* 1987; 49:203–11.

47. Ali SL. Bestimmungder Pestiziduckstande und toxischen Schwermetallspuren in Arzneidrogen und deren Teeaufgussen. *Pharmazeutische Zeitung* 1985; 132:633–8.

48. Chia BL, Leng CK, Hsii FP, et al. Lead poisoning from contaminated opium. *British Medical Journal* 1973; 1:354.

49. Yu ECL, Yeung CY. Lead encephalopathy due to herbal medicine. *Chinese Medical Journal* 1987; 100:915.

50. Ali SL. Bestimmungder Pestiziduckstande und toxischen Schwermetallspuren in Arzneidrogen und deren Teeaufgussen. *Pharmazeutische Zeitung* 1985; 132:633–8.

Suggested Reading

Brinker F. *Herb Contraindications and Drug Interactions*. Sandy, OR: Eclectic Medical Publications, 2001.

DeSmet P, et al. *Adverse Effects of Herbal Drugs*, vols. 1–3. New York: Springer-Verlag 1992–97.

Harborne JB, et al. *Dictionary of Plant Toxins*. Chichester; New York: Wiley, 1996.

McGuffin M, et al., eds. *American Herbal Products Associations' Botanical Safety Handbook*. Boca Raton, FL: CRC Press, 1997.

Mitchell, J. *Botanical Dermatology: Plants and Plant Products Injurious to the Skin*. Vancouver, Canada: Greenglass, 1979.

11

THE FORMULATION AND PREPARATION OF HERBAL MEDICINES

A unique aspect of the art of phytotherapy is that the practitioner must know how to choose the dosage form and the preparation technique most appropriate for achieving optimum therapeutic benefits with a particular herb for a particular condition. Over the centuries, herbal practitioners have developed various preparation methods appropriate for releasing the healing properties of different plants. Thus, after having chosen the most appropriate herbs for the patient, the practitioner must select the best way to prepare them. A number of methods are available that release the biochemical constituents needed for healing without insulting the integrity of the remedy by isolating fractions of the whole plant.

Twenty-first-century herbal medicine making, or *phytopharmacy*, is a rich blend of the old and the new. On one hand, there has been a revival of the traditional skills with which all herbalists should be familiar. On the other, the herbal community has embraced technologies developed by the pharmaceutical industry, which has led to the use of extraction and formulation methods that are indistinguishable from those of that industry.

In fact, there is a rapidly growing phytopharmaceutical industry that is often driven more strongly by financial concerns than by the health of consumers. Phytopharmaceutical manufacturers may focus, for example, on unique methods of extract standardization in efforts to secure patent protection for their products. However, effective extraction of the medicinal properties of herbs need not depend on modern technology. There is a place and a need for both the traditional and the modern in herbal medicine. Even as attempts are made to improve modern phytopharmaceutical methods, it is important to remember the contributions of the long traditions of herbalism to herbal medicine making.

If one sees herbal medicine as "people's medicine," as I do, there remains an important place in health care for what might be called the folk method of preparing herbal remedies. These methods are simple, effective, and empowering. The work of a number of today's herbalists epitomizes the modern expression of the ancient skills of the herbal medicine maker, including Rosemary Gladstar, James Green, Christopher Hobbs, Kathi Keville, and Mindy Green. Refer to Suggested Reading at the end of this chapter for the titles of their books.

In addition, I cannot overstate the importance of the work of pharmacists, both eclectic and orthodox, in the nineteenth and early-twentieth centuries. Much of the material that follows relies on examples taken from their writings, published in the standard reference texts of their day. These are pharmacopoeias and formularies that describe herbs, drugs, chemicals, and preparation methods officially recognized for use in medicine.

Pharmacopoeias are issued by officially recognized authorities to serve as standards for the preparations of remedies. In many countries of the world, the officially recognized authority is a governmental body, but the situation is different in the United States. The United States Pharmacopoeia (USP) is a nongovernmental organization that establishes standards for prescription and nonprescription drugs. USP standards are currently published together with NF standards in a single official reference volume.

The references I cite most often in the text are indicated by the following acronyms. Please refer to Suggested Reading for complete publication information for these volumes.

BHP: *The British Herbal Pharmacopoeia*

BP: *The British Pharmacopoeia*

BPC: *British Pharmaceutical Codex*

NF: *The National Formulary* (U.S.)

Remington's: Remington's Pharmaceutical Sciences

USD: *The Dispensatory of the United States of America*

USP: *The United States Pharmacopoeia*

In the material that follows, many of the remedies used as examples are described in a strange form of Latin known as *pharmaceutical Latin*. This pharmaceutical name is usually derived from the Latin botanical name of the herb, and consists of a term indicating the part of the plant that is used followed by the genus name. For example, dandelion leaf would be described as "Taraxacum Folium." Refer to appendix 4 for abbreviations and translations of these Latin pharmacy terms.

UNDERSTANDING THE OPTIONS

In addition to knowing how to select the most appropriate herbs, the skilled herbal practitioner must understand the relevance of the plethora of medicinal choices available. Therapeutic specifics are discussed in part 2 of this book, but here are some important preliminary issues that must be considered when selecting dosage forms and methods of preparation for herbal remedies.

Route of administration. As discussed in chapter 9, medicines ingested are distributed throughout the body in a variety of ways. The practitioner must be able to determine what route of administration will provide the most effective delivery of desired herb constituents, whether oral, rectal, topical, or some other route. These considerations affect the choice of dosage form used.

Dosage form. There are many ways to formulate and prepare herbs for delivery into the body, each of which has its own benefits and drawbacks. Choice of dosage form must be based on the needs of the patient. Will a tablet form be as readily bioavailable as a liquid preparation? Would a suppository be more efficient than an oral dosage form in delivering medicinal effects to the desired site of action?

Extraction method. The choice of extraction method is profoundly affected by the chemistry of herb constituents considered responsible for therapeutic effects. For example, consider *Serenoa repens* (saw palmetto), an herb whose "active ingredients" are believed to be lipids and triterpene saponins. These groups of chemicals are minimally soluble in water but readily soluble in nonpolar solvents, such as alcohol and oils. They are also readily soluble in carbon dioxide, the basis of the technology known as supercritical CO_2 extraction. These facts lead one to the conclusion that a tea of saw palmetto berries is not the ideal form for delivery of desired constituents (not to mention that it would also taste foul). Alcohol-based extracts are a better choice in this case, as are other, newer forms of extraction based on nonpolar solvents. The ultimate decision may be based on financial rather than therapeutic concerns.

THE BASICS OF PHYTOPHARMACY

No matter what degree of technological sophistication is applied, there are two basic stages of preparation that must be taken into account when making an herbal medicine from a plant, described here. The actual procedures followed in these stages can vary, and special considerations apply to freshly harvested plants and those intended for topical delivery. In the material that follows, I will focus on different extraction methods and the ways in which extracts can be best formulated for desired medicinal effects.

Comminution

Before it can be used, the herb must be cut down to a workable size, a process known as *comminution*. The traditional tool for this process is the mortar and pestle. Today, many other devices are available for cutting or grinding unprocessed materials, such as mechanical mortars, slicing and cutting machinery, and mills of various types. For the folk herbalist, a coffee grinder provides a convenient alternative.

On a commercial scale, herbs are ground into powders with metal disk mills or hammer mills. To acquire a powder of a specific size, the processor uses sieves with a specified number of openings per square inch or centimeter. Numbers are used to indicate sizes of powders. For instance, a No. 20 powder has been passed through a sieve that has 20 parallel wires to each linear inch in either direction; such a sieve will have 400 holes per square inch.

Extraction

Extraction is the process by which soluble herb constituents are separated from inert, fibrous matter. Pharmaceutical textbooks list the following reasons for extraction:

- To make palatable, concentrated preparations, eliminating the need to use bulky or distasteful drugs
- To remove inert constituents that in some way may interfere with the action of the desired constituent(s)
- To create a product that contains only pharmacologically active constituents
- To create a product of known strength and activity that can be reliably reproduced in subsequent batches

The first step is to select a solvent capable of penetrating the tissues of the herb and dissolving the constituents. This liquid is called the *menstruum*, and the inert, fibrous, or other insoluble material that remains after the menstruum has done its work and been removed is called the *marc*. Water and alcohol are the principle solvents in common use. If the preparation must keep indefinitely, an alcohol solvent must be used.

The British Pharmacopoeia (BP) recommends four different strengths of alcohol: 45%, 60%, 70%, and 90%. The strength to be used depends on the chemical nature of the constituents to be extracted, as well as the physical density of the plant part being extracted. To ensure sterility, the solvent should contain a minimum of 20% to 25% alcohol. Other solvents may also be used for extraction, such as acetic acid, glycerol, ether, and oil.

PRINCIPAL MODES OF EXTRACTION EMPLOYED IN TRADITIONAL PHYTOPHARMACY

Well-defined classes of extraction techniques are described in the official pharmacopoeias. These may be used singly or in combination, depending on the desired outcome.

1. Maceration and expression
2. Digestion
3. Percolation
4. Infusion
5. Decoction

Maceration

Maceration is the process of softening plant material by soaking, facilitating the dissolution of the soluble constituents. It plays an important role in many official preparations, including tinctures, extracts, syrups, wines, and vinegars. Macerations differ from water-based infusions and decoctions in the following respects:

• The menstruum is usually alcohol.
• The herb remains in contact with the menstruum for a longer period of time.
• The process is conducted at ordinary temperatures.
• After straining, the liquid left in the remaining herbal material (the marc) is pressed out and mixed with the strained liquid.

The specified amount of herb, in the specified form (for example, cut or powdered), is placed with the required amount of menstruum into a vessel. The vessel is closed, to prevent the loss of alcohol, and then shaken so as to turn the contents, preferably on a daily basis. The shaking disperses the saturated layer of menstruum that surrounds the herb particles and allows fresh liquid to come into contact with the herb. Actual maceration time will depend on the specific herb, but 7 to 14 days is a good general rule of thumb.

After the prescribed amount of time, the liquid is drained from the marc. The marc is then pressed to retrieve more of the menstruum. The expressed liquid is mixed with the strained liquid, and the mixture is left to stand until it is clear, after which it is filtered.

Digestion

Digestion is a form of maceration that involves application of a gentle heat to the substance being extracted. It is used in cases in which a moderately elevated temperature will help increase the solvent powers of the menstruum. Digestion differs from decoction in that preparations made through the process of digestion are alcohol based, rather than water based.

Percolation

Percolation is a process by which a powder contained in a suitable vessel is deprived of its soluble constituents by the descent of a solvent through the material. The USP provides the following directions for percolation.

> Percolation, as directed in this Pharmacopoeia, consists in subjecting a comminuted substance or a mixture of substances, contained in a vessel called a percolator, to the solvent action of successive portions of a liquid termed the menstruum in such a manner that the liquid, as it traverses the powder in its descent to the receiver, shall extract the soluble constituents, and pass from the percolator free from insoluble matter.

The expression "until the drug is exhausted" and similar phrases used in directions for percolations indicate that the process should be continued to the point at which the valuable constituents have been as completely extracted as is possible or practical. The judgment and experience of the operator determines the point at which this has occurred.

Infusion

An *infusion* is a water-based preparation made by steeping leaves, flowers, and other nonwoody plant parts in either hot or cold water. Obviously, this method of preparation is appropriate only for herbs with water-soluble constituents.

Decoction

A *decoction* is a water-based preparation made by gently simmering the herb in boiling water. Decoction differs from infusion in that it is more appropriate for tougher plant parts, such as roots, bark, and seeds.

A COMPARISON OF OFFICIAL AND FOLK METHODS

The official sources mentioned at the beginning of this chapter provide methods and examples for all of the extraction techniques just discussed. For purposes of comparison, here we will look at some examples of officially sanctioned and modern folk techniques of herb extraction.

WATER-BASED PREPARATIONS

There are two broad ways to prepare water-based extracts: infusions and decoctions. There are some basic rules of thumb for choosing which method to use with what herb, but as with all generalizations, there are many exceptions.

- *Infusions* are appropriate for nonwoody material such as leaves, flowers, and some stems, especially herbs with a high content of volatile oils.
- *Decoctions* are necessary if the herb contains any hard or woody material, such as roots, barks, or nuts; the denser the plant or the individual cell walls, the more energy is needed to extract the cell content into the water.

Roots rich in volatile oils, such as valerian root, are an important exception to these general rules. While the woodiness might suggest that decoction is appropriate, the therapeutically important volatile oil will evaporate if the roots are simmered. With roots like this, it is better to grind the herb to a fine powder and then make an infusion.

Water extracts offer the advantage of convenience, but are limited in that some plant constituents cannot be extracted in water. Obviously, constituents that are insoluble in water will not be present in the resulting tea.

INFUSIONS

Everyone is familiar with infusions. The traditional cup of herb tea is the archetypal infusion. Of course, herb tea is not truly tea, as tea is made from the leaves of *Camellia sinensis*. However, nobody asks to be served an herb infusion!

There are many ways to make infusions, and here we shall compare official and traditional methods. As we shall see, recipes for infusions given in the USP can differ greatly from simple herbal infusions made by steeping herbs in boiling water.

Official Infusions (Infusa)

Remington's describes infusions in the following way:

These are liquid preparations made by treating herbs with either hot or cold water. The drug is not subjected to the boiling process, although it is common to pour boiling water over it; the mixture is allowed to stand in a closed vessel until cold. Cold water should be selected as the menstruum when the drug contains a valuable volatile principle, when the active agent is injured by heat, or when the desirable principles are readily soluble in water of ordinary temperature. The time required to make the infusion must also be considered, for in warm weather it is quite possible for an infusion to ferment or decompose before it is finished. Pure water should be used in making infusions, and they should not be made in large quantities unless demanded for immediate use, as, without special precautions to preserve them, they soon decompose. In making infusions the drug is usually coarsely comminuted, sliced, or bruised.

The USP gives the following general directions for a macerated infusion:

Infusions must be *freshly made from the drugs*, and, when the strength of Infusions is not otherwise directed, they are to be prepared by the following general formula:

The drug coarsely comminuted, 50 gm
Water, a sufficient quantity to make 1000 ml

Introduce the substance into a suitable vessel provided with a cover, pour upon it 1000 ml of boiling water, cover the vessel tightly, and allow it to stand for half an hour. Then strain with expression, and pass enough water through the strainer to make the infusion measure 1000 ml. If the activity of the infusion is affected by heat, cold water only should be used.

In the BP, infusions are defined this way:

Infusions are dilute solutions containing readily soluble constituents of crude drugs. They are usually prepared by diluting one volume of a concentrated infusion to ten volumes with water. For dispensing purposes, infusions should be used within 12 hours of their preparation.

On the following page are some recipes for official infusions.

Infusum Pruni Virginianae BPC 1911
(Infusion of Virginian Prune)

Virginian Prune Bark, in No 20 powder	4 g
Glycerin	5 ml
Distilled Water to	100 ml

Moisten the powdered bark with 60 ml of the water, set aside for 1 hour, pack in a percolator and percolate with more of the distilled water; collect the percolate in a vessel containing the glycerin and continue percolation until the product measures 100. Dose: 30–60 ml.

Occasionally, the older official compendia will mix methods or apply titles that might be misleading. An example is the following recipe that first infuses the ingredients in alcohol and then subjects them to a tincturing process.

Concentrated Compound Gentian Infusion BP 1980

Gentian, cut small and bruised	125 g
Dried Bitter-Orange Peel, cut small	125 g
Dried Lemon Peel, cut small	125 g
Ethanol (25%)	1200 ml

Macerate the Gentian, the dried bitter Orange peel, and the dried Lemon peel in a covered vessel for 48 hours with 1000 ml of the ethanol (25%), press out the liquid. To the pressed marc, add 200 ml of the ethanol (25%), macerate for 24 hours, press, and add the liquid to the product of the first pressing. Allow to stand for not less than 14 days; filter. Dose: 1.4–4 ml.

Folk Method of Infusion

This is perhaps the simplest method of preparing an herb. Fresh or dried herbs can be used. However, note that a larger amount of fresh herb will be needed to compensate for its higher water content. Therefore, if the instructions call for 1 part (for example, 1 teaspoon) of dried herb, the dried herb can be substituted with 3 parts (or 3 teaspoons) of fresh herb.

A Simple Hot Infusion

Gently warm a china or glass teapot and put in about 1 teaspoonful of dried herb or herb mixture for each cup of tea desired. Add 1 cup of boiling water for each teaspoonful of herb in the pot and put the lid on.

Leave to steep for 10 to 15 minutes. Infusions may be drunk hot (normally best for a medicinal tea) or cold; they may even be iced. If desired, sweeten with licorice root, honey, or brown sugar.

To make larger infusions, use a proportion of 30 g (1 oz) of herb to a half-liter (1 pint) of water. As their shelf life is not very long, infusions should be prepared when needed. Herbal tea bags may be made by filling little muslin bags with herb mixtures, but take care to remember how many teaspoonfuls you have put into each bag! These can be used in the same way as ordinary tea bags.

Infusions are appropriate for softer plant tissue such as leaves, flowers, or green stems, where the desired substances are easily accessible. If an infusion is to be made of bark, roots, seeds, or resin, it is best to powder them first to break down some of the cell walls, which will facilitate extraction. Seeds—for instance, fennel or aniseed—should be slightly bruised to release the volatile oils from the cells. All aromatic herbs should be infused in a pot with a tight-fitting lid to minimize loss of volatile oils.

Cold Infusions

Some herbs are sensitive to heat, either because they contain highly volatile oils or because their constituents break down at high temperatures. For these herbs, make a *cold infusion*. The proportion of herb to water is the same, but in this case, the infusion should be left for 6 to 12 hours in a well-scaled earthenware pot. When the liquid is ready, strain and use it.

As an alternative, cold milk can be used as a base for a cold infusion. Milk contains fats and oils that aid in the dissolution of oily constituents of plants. Milk infusions can be used for compresses and poultices, which will add the soothing action of the milk to that of the herbs. There is, however, one contraindication for the use of milk in an infusion. If there is any evidence that an individual might have a sensitivity or allergy to milk when taken internally, or if the skin becomes irritated when it is applied externally, then avoid such infusions.

Medicinal Plants Usually Prepared as Infusions

Achillea millefolium (yarrow)
Aesculus hippocastanum (horse chestnut)
Agathosma betulina (buchu)
Agrimonia eupatoria (agrimony)
Alchemilla arvensis (lady's mantle)
Althaea officinalis (marshmallow)
Anethum graveolens (dill)
Angelica archangelica (angelica)
Apium graveolens (celery)
Arctostaphylos uva-ursi (bearberry)
Artemisia absinthium (wormwood)
A. vulgaris (mugwort)
Avena sativa (oats)

Ballota nigra (black horehound)
Calendula officinalis (calendula, pot marigold)
Capsella bursa-pastoris (shepherd's purse)
Capsicum annuum (cayenne)
Carum carvi (caraway)
Cetraria islandica (Iceland moss)
Chelone glabra (balmony)
Chondrus crispus (carrageen)
Crataegus laevigata (hawthorn)
Cytisus scoparius (Scotch broom)
Daucus carota (carrot)
Drosera rotundifolia (sundew)
Elymus repens (couch grass)
Ephedra sinica (ma huang or ephedra)
Eschscholzia californica (California poppy)
Eucalyptus globulus (eucalyptus, blue gum)
Eupatorium perfoliatum (boneset)
E. purpureum (gravel root)
Euphrasia spp. (eyebright)
Filipendula ulmaria (meadowsweet)
Foeniculum vulgare (fennel)
Fucus vesiculosus (bladderwrack)
Fumaria officinalis (fumitory)
Galega officinalis (goat's rue)
Galium aparine (cleavers)
Geranium maculatum (cranesbill)
Ginkgo biloba (ginkgo)
Grindelia camporum (grindelia, gum weed)
Hieracium pilosella (mouse-ear hawkweed)
Humulus lupulus (hops)
Hypericum perforatum (St. John's wort)
Hyssopus officinalis (hyssop)
Juniperus communis (juniper)
Lactuca virosa (wild lettuce)
Lavandula officinalis (lavender)
Leonurus cardiaca (motherwort)
Linum usitatissimum (flax)
Lobelia inflata (lobelia)
Lycopus europaeus (European bugleweed)
Malva sylvestris (mallow)
Marrubium vulgare (horehound)
Matricaria recutita (chamomile)
Melissa officinalis (lemon balm)
Mentha piperita (peppermint)
M. pulegium (pennyroyal)
Mitchella repens (partridgeberry)
Nepeta cataria (catnip)
Passiflora incarnata (passionflower)
Petroselinum crispum (parsley)

Peumus boldus (boldo)
Phytolacca americana (poke)
Pimpinella anisum (anise)
Plantago major (plantain)
Polygala senega (Seneca snakeroot)
Pulsatilla vulgaris (Pasqueflower)
Rosmarinus officinalis (rosemary)
Rubus idaeus (raspberry)
R. villosus (blackberry)
Ruta graveolens (rue)
Salvia officinalis var. *rubia* (red sage)
Sambucus nigra (black elder)
Scrophularia nodosa (figwort)
Scutellaria lateriflora (skullcap)
Senna spp. (senna)
Serenoa repens (saw palmetto)
Solidago virgaurea (goldenrod)
Stellaria media (chickweed)
Symphytum officinale (comfrey)
Symplocarpus foetidus (skunk cabbage)
Tanacetum parthenium (feverfew)
Taraxacum officinale (dandelion)
Thuja occidentalis (white cedar)
Thymus spp. (thyme)
Tilia spp. (linden)
Trifolium pratense (red clover)
Tussilago farfara (coltsfoot)
Urtica dioica (nettle)
Usnea spp. (usnea)
Valeriana officinalis (valerian)
Verbascum thapsus (mullein)
Verbena officinalis (European vervain)
Vinca major (periwinkle)
Viola odorata (sweet violet)
V. tricolor (heartsease)
Zea mays (cornsilk)
Zingiber officinale (ginger)

DECOCTIONS

Pharmacopoeias once included extensive entries for decoctions. They eventually fell out of favor, as they were considered inconvenient. In fact, one of the most common mainstream criticisms of herbal medicine is that it is inconvenient. To the herbalist, however, therapeutic benefit outweighs convenience! From a different perspective, it might also be argued that the time and attention required to make a decoction provides a stress-relieving therapeutic benefit not offered by any pill.

Official Decoctions (Decocta)

Remington's describes decoctions as liquid preparations made by boiling vegetable substances with water. A general formula for decoctions can be found in the USP.

Decoctions must be freshly made, and when their strength is not otherwise directed, they are to be prepared by the following general formula:

The Drug, coarsely comminuted	50 g
Water, a sufficient quantity, to make	1000 ml

Place the drug in a suitable vessel provided with a cover, pour upon it 1000 cc. of cold water, cover and boil for fifteen minutes. Cool to about 40°C, express, strain the expressed liquid, and pass enough cold water through the strainer to make the product measure 1000 cc.

Decoctum Tussilaginis BPC 1911
(Decoction of Coltsfoot)

Coltsfoot Leaves	5 parts
Distilled Water to	100 parts

Add leaves to 120 ml of distilled water, boil for 10 minutes, strain and make up to required volume, if necessary, by passing water through the strainer. Dose: 60–120 ml or more.

Decoctum Lappae BPC 1911 (Decoction of Burdock)

Lappa	5.00 g
Distilled Water to	100.00 ml

Add the root to 150 of the distilled water and boil until the volume of the strained liquid is reduced to 100. Dose: 30–120 ml or more.

Folk Method of Decocting

Whenever the herbal material is hard and woody, making a decoction increases the likelihood that the soluble contents of the herb will actually be extracted into the water. Roots, rhizomes, wood, bark, nuts, and some seeds are hard and have strong cell walls, so to ensure an effective transfer of active constituents to the water, more heat is needed than for infusions.

A Simple Decoction

Put 1 teaspoon of dried herb (or 3 teaspoons of fresh material) for each cup of water used into a pot or saucepan. Add the appropriate amount of water to the herbs.

Bring to a boil and simmer for the time given for the mixture or specific herb, usually 10 to 15 minutes. If the herb contains volatile oils, put a lid on. Strain the tea while it is still hot.

Dried herbs should be powdered or broken into small pieces; fresh material should be cut into small pieces. When making a larger quantity of decoction, use 30 g (1 oz) of dried herb for each half-liter (1 pint) of water. The container should be glass, ceramic, or earthenware. If the container is metal, it should be enameled.

When preparing a mixture containing both soft and woody herbs, it is best to prepare an infusion (for the soft herbs) and a decoction separately, to ensure that the more delicate herbs are treated appropriately. The two can then be mixed together. However, for a woody herb rich in volatile oils, boiling will cause evaporation of important volatile constituents. For herbs like this, powder the material finely and make an infusion.

Medicinal Plants Usually Prepared as Decoctions

Angelica archangelica (angelica)
Arctium lappa (burdock)
Asclepias tuberosa (pleurisy root)
Astragalus membranaceus (astragalus)
Baptisia tinctoria (wild indigo)
Berberis vulgaris (barberry)
Betula spp. (birch)
Caulophyllum thalictroides (blue cohosh)
Chamaelirium luteum (false unicorn root)
Chionanthus virginicus (fringetree)
Cimicifuga racemosa (black cohosh)
Cola vera (kola)
Collinsonia canadensis (collinsonia, stoneroot)
Commiphora molmol (myrrh)
Dioscorea villosa (wild yam)
Echinacea spp. (echinacea, purple coneflower)
Equisetum arvense (horsetail)
Euonymus atropurpureus (wahoo)
Gentiana spp. (gentian)
Glycyrrhiza glabra (licorice)
Guaiacum officinale (guaiacum)
Hamamelis virginiana (witch hazel)
Harpagophytum procumbens (devil's claw)
Hydrangea arborescens (hydrangea)
Hydrastis canadensis (goldenseal)
Inula helenium (elecampane)
Iris versicolor (blue flag)
Juglans cinerea (butternut)
Mahonia aquifolium (Oregon grape)
Marsdenia condurango (condurango)
Menyanthes trifoliata (bogbean)
Myrica cerifera (bayberry, wax myrtle)
Panax spp. (ginseng)
Piper methysticum (kava)

Piscidia erythrina (Jamaica dogwood)
Populus tremuloides (quaking aspen)
Prunus serotina (wild cherry)
Quercus spp. (oak)
Rheum palmatum (Chinese rhubarb)
Rumex crispus (yellow dock)
Salix spp. (willow)
Sanguinaria canadensis (bloodroot)
Sassafras albidum (sassafras)
Smilax spp. (sarsaparilla)
Symphytum officinale (comfrey)
Taraxacum officinale (dandelion)
Ulmus rubra (slippery elm)
Veronicastrum virginica (culver's root)
Viburnum opulus (cramp bark)
V. prunifolium (black haw)
Vitex agnus-castus (vitex, chasteberry)
Zanthoxylum americanum (prickly ash)
Zingiber officinale (ginger)

ALCOHOL-WATER PREPARATIONS

There are three primary reasons for the widespread use of water-alcohol extracts, including tinctures. Such preparations have several advantages over purely water-based extracts:

1. Most of the constituents present, both water-soluble and alcohol-soluble, will dissolve in the extract. The only constituents that will not dissolve are the insoluble cellulose of the cell wall and any constituents bound to it.
2. Alcohol is a preservative. Infusions and decoctions are wonderful growth media for bacteria and molds and thus have a very short or nonexistent shelf life. An alcohol content of at least 20% will greatly extend the shelf life of an extract.
3. The process used to make tinctures or fluid extracts will concentrate the medicinal properties in a smaller volume of liquid.

When tinctures are prepared professionally, according to descriptions in a pharmacopoeia, specific water-to-alcohol proportions are used for each herb. Some recommendations from *The British Herbal Pharmacopoeia* can be found in chapter 26. For general use, such attention to detail is not always necessary.

Official Tincture Preparations (Tincturae)

Pharmaceutical tinctures are alcoholic solutions prepared by maceration, digestion, or percolation. The term *tincture* is also occasionally used for preparations based on glycerin or vinegar. Ethanol offers the advantage of dissolving constituents that are insoluble or sparingly soluble in water while helping to preserve them in solution. A water-alcohol menstruum can extract a larger proportion of active principles of most plants than can water alone, but at the same time contains sufficient alcohol to prevent decomposition.

The USP describes the following general procedure for the preparation of tinctures:

The proportion of drugs represented in the different kinds of tinctures is not uniform but varies according to the established standards for each. Tinctures of potent drugs represent the activity of 10 gm. of a drug of minimum U.S.P. strength, in each 100 cc. of tincture. When drugs having a higher potency than the minimum are used in preparing tinctures the finished product is assayed and adjusted to the uniform U.S.P. strength. This conforms in principle to the recommendation of the International Protocol as adopted at Brussels, and with international standards. In this group are most of the tinctures which are assayed and adjusted to standards. Most of the other tinctures represent 20 gm. of the respective drugs in each 100 cc. of tincture. Compound tinctures are made according to long established formulas, and the two official tinctures of fresh drugs are made to represent 50 gm. of the respective drugs in each 100 cc. of tincture.

There are two important variables in tinctures: the concentration of the herb and the strength of the alcohol.

Concentration of Herb

The amount of herb in a given amount of menstruum defines the concentration of the extract. Most tinctures are in concentrations of 1:4 or 1:5, but the BP also uses 1:3, 1:8, and 1:10. In the examples just given, the first number represents the weight of the herb and the second represents the volume of menstruum, so they express a ratio of weight to volume (w:v).

There are a number of ways to express concentrations. The expression *percent* may be used, according to circumstances, with one of four different meanings. In order that the meaning attached to the expression in each instance is clear, the following notations are used.

• Percent w/w (weight to weight): number of grams of active substance in 100 g of product

- Percent w/v (weight to volume): number of grams of active substance in 100 ml of product
- Percent v/v (volume to volume): number of milliliters of active substance in 100 ml of product
- Percent v/w (volume to weight): number of milliliters of active substance in 100 g of product

Strength of Alcohol

According to the BP, alcohol can be used in concentrations of 45%, 60%, 70%, and 90%. In pharmacy, the expression "70% ethanol" describes a solution made up of 70 parts of 96.4% ethanol and 30 parts of water. As an example, "Tinctura calami 1:5–70% BPC" means that this tincture of *Acorus calamus* root was made by macerating 1 part of root (in weight) in 5 parts (by volume) of a 70% ethanol solution.

The so-called mother tinctures used in homeopathy as the starting point for potentiation are usually prepared by bruising the fresh herb, expressing the juice, and adding 96% alcohol to the juice in an amount equal to one-third or one-half the volume of the fresh juice.

Folk Method of Tincturing

Alcohol is a better solvent than water for most plant constituents. A mixture of alcohol and water will dissolve nearly all of the relevant ingredients of an herb and at the same time act as a preservative. The method given here for the preparation of tinctures describes a simple and general approach. For home use, an alcohol of at least 30% concentration (60 proof) will suffice, as this is about the weakest alcohol-water mixture that still provides a long-term preservative action. Vodka is usually a good choice, although other types of alcohol can also be used.

A Simple Tincture

Put 4 ounces of finely chopped or ground dried herb into a container that can be tightly closed. (If the herb is fresh, use twice this amount.) Pour 1 pint of 30% (60 proof) vodka on the herbs and close the container tightly.

Keep the container in a warm place for two weeks and shake it well twice daily. After decanting the bulk of the liquid, pour the residue into a muslin cloth suspended in a strainer over a bowl. Wring out all the liquid. The residue (the marc) makes excellent compost. Pour the finished tincture into a dark-colored, tightly capped bottle.

Tinctures are stronger than infusions or decoctions, and thus a much smaller dosage is taken. Tinctures may be used in a variety of ways. They can be taken as is, mixed with water, or added to a cup of hot water. If added to hot water, the alcohol will largely evaporate, leaving most of the extract in the water. However, this may make the water cloudy, as resins and other constituents not soluble in water will precipitate.

Drops of tincture can be added to a bath or footbath, applied in a compress, or mixed with oil or fat to make an ointment. Suppositories and lozenges can also be made this way. Because there is no way that quantitative accuracy can be maintained when making tinctures by the folk method, it should be used only for mild herbs for which dosage is not critical.

FLUID EXTRACTS (FLUID EXTRACTA)

Another form of alcohol-based medicine is the *fluid extract*, also known as a liquid extract. In fluid extracts, which are more concentrated than tinctures, 1 part by volume of the fluid extract is equivalent to 1 part by weight of the herb. The techniques used to make these preparations are complex and involve specific skills and equipment.

The USP defines fluid extracts in the following way:

Fluid extracts are liquid preparations of vegetable drugs, containing alcohol as a solvent or as a preservative, or both, and so made that each 1 cc. contains the therapeutic constituents of 1 gm. of the standard drug which it represents.

Fluid extracts are made by percolation, and the menstruum to be used is specified in official monographs. They may be standardized if they contain constituents that can be assayed by modern methods.

Fluid extracts possess a number of advantages.

Stability is ensured by the use of an ethanol menstruum. Glycerin, which tends to retard precipitation, is used as part or all of the menstruum of some fluid extracts.

Concentration reduces the volume needed per dose.

Uniformity of dose is made possible by the precise nature of the concentration; if 1 ml of extract represents 1 g of crude herb, the dose of the fluid extract is practically the same as that of the drug.

Here are some official examples of fluid extracts.

Extractum Anthemidis Liquidum BPC 1934 (Liquid Extract of Chamomile)

Chamomile, in moderately coarse powder	1000 g
Alcohol (70%) to	1000 ml

Exhaust the Chamomile with the alcohol by percolation, reserving the first 850 ml of percolate. Evaporate the subsequent percolate to a soft extract, dissolve it in the reserved portion and add sufficient of the alcohol to produce the required volume. Dose: 2–4 ml.

Senna Liquid Extract BP 1980

Senna fruit	
Alexandrian or Tinnevelly, crushed	1000 g
Coriander oil	6 ml
Ethanol (90%)	250 ml
Purified water, freshly boiled and cooled, a sufficient quantity	

Macerate the crushed Senna fruit in 5000 ml of purified water using 2 further quantities each of 2000 ml of purified water for each maceration. Lightly press the marc, strain the expressed liquid, mix the strained liquid with the previously decanted liquid, heat the combined liquids at 80 degrees for 3 minutes in a covered vessel. Allow to stand for not less than 24 hours, filter. Evaporate the filtrate to 750 ml under reduced pressure at a temperature not exceeding 60 degrees. Separately, dissolve the Coriander oil in the ethanol (90%), add to the evaporated filtrate, and add sufficient purified water to produce 1000 ml. Allow to stand for not less than 24 hours; filter. Usual dose range: 0.5–2 ml.

SYRUPS AND ELIXIRS

Fluid medicines—whether infusions, decoctions, or tinctures—often have an unpleasant taste. Thus, it is sometimes helpful to mask the taste by adding a sweetener. One method is to use a syrup, which is the traditional way to make cough mixtures more palatable for children or to make any herbal preparation more "toothsome," as Culpeper would say.

A Simple Syrup Base

Pour 1 pint of boiling water over 2½ pounds of sugar. Place over heat and stir until the sugar dissolves and the liquid begins to boil. Remove from heat immediately.

To give this simple syrup medicinal properties, mix 1 part of tincture with 3 parts of syrup and store for future use.

To sweeten an infusion or decoction, it is simpler to add the sugar directly to the liquid. For every 1 pint of liquid, add ¾ pound of sugar. Heat gently until the sugar is dissolved. This mixture can be stored for future use in a refrigerator. Since is not advisable to consume too much sugar, syrups are best used when making gargles and cough medicines, in which the herbs tend to be rather unpalatable.

Syrupus Althaeae BPC 1911 (Syrup of Althaea)

Althaea, sliced	4.00 g
Refined sugar	90.00 g
Distilled water	56.00 ml

Macerate the Althaea in the water for 12 hours, then strain, press and filter. The filtrate should measure 45. To this add the sugar, dissolve and heat the syrup to boiling. Cool and strain through flannel. The finished product should measure about 100. Dose: 2–8 ml.

Elixirs (Elixiria)

Elixirs are another type of sweet formulation. They are defined as clear, flavored, liquid preparation containing one or more medicaments, and usually a high proportion of alcohol or sucrose. Here is one example of the 18 elixirs in the BP 1980.

Compound Fig Elixir BP 1980

Fig, cut small	320 g
Cascara Elixir	50 ml
Compound Rhubarb tincture	50 ml
Senna Liquid Extract	100 ml
Sucrose	540 g
Water	a sufficient quantity

Add the fig to 800 ml of boiling water, heat gently for one hour, strain, express, wash the pulp with sufficient warm water to produce 800 ml; evaporate the liquid to half its volume, dissolve the sucrose in the concentrated liquid, add the compound Rhubarb tincture, the Senna liquid extract, the Cascara elixir, and sufficient water to produce 1000 ml; mix.

EMULSIONS (EMULSIONES)

Emulsions are still official for both internal and external use. They are defined as dispersions of an oily liquid in an aqueous liquid, either of which may contain dissolved or suspended solids.

Emulsio Olei Amygdalae BPC 1911 (Almond Oil Emulsion)

Almond Oil	12.50 ml
Gum Acacia, in powder	3.20 g
Distilled Water to	1000 ml

Make a mucilage by triturating the gum acacia in a mortar with an equal quantity of distilled water, add the Almond oil in a slow stream, stirring lightly until the mixture appears uniform; then add gradually the remainder of the water. An alternative method of making this preparation is to triturate the Almond oil with gum acacia, add all at once twice as much distilled water as gum acacia, make a primary emulsion, and add distilled water in small quantities up to the required volume. Dose: 8–30 ml.

JUICES (SUCCI)

Juices are an excellent way of taking medicinal herbs. The effects can be dramatic and swift. The first green herbs of spring, such as cleavers (*Galium aparine*), are most useful in this form. Juices may be made at home using either a juicer or a blender.

Succus Taraxaci BPC 1911 (Juice of Dandelion)

Taraxacum juice is prepared by subjecting the bruised fresh root to pressure, adding to the expressed juice ⅓ of its volume of alcohol, allowing the mixture to stand for 7 days, and filtering. This juice is considered by many practitioners to be more effective than the liquid extract prepared from the dried root. Note: Liquor Taraxaci is prepared by adding the alcohol to the bruised fresh root before expression. Dose: 4–8 ml.

LINCTUSES (LINCTI)

The BPC 1934 defines this type of liquid preparation as follows:

Linctuses are liquid preparations of a mucilaginous, syrupy, or viscous nature containing substances which possess demulcent, expectorant, or sedative properties. They are usually administered in small doses and should be directed to be sipped and swallowed slowly without the addition of water, so that they may form a temporary protective or remedial film over the membranes of the throat.

Linctus Ipecacuanhae BPC 1923 (Linctus of Ipecacuanha)

Vinegar of Ipecacuanha	25.00 ml
Syrup of Balsam of Tolu	25.00 ml
Glycerin	25.00 ml
Mucilage of Tragacanth to	100.00 ml

Mix the liquids. Dose: 2–4 ml.

MUCILAGES

Mucilages are an interesting type of formulation that can prove quite tricky to make! The BPC 1911 has this to say about mucilages:

Mucilages are viscous preparations usually employed as emulsifying or suspending agents, or as demulcents. Mucilages which are not in constant demand should be freshly prepared as required. They deteriorate when kept, especially in warm weather, unless preservatives are added, such as solution of formaldehyde or benzoic acid. Mucilages which have been at 100 degrees for 10 minutes in small bottles and securely sealed, keep for longer periods. Such precautions are unnecessary in the case of mucilage of gum acacia or mucilage of Tragacanth if quantities limited to about a week's supply are stored in bottles of small size, as completely filled as possible. Mucilage of gum acacia, when required at short notice, can be rapidly prepared with hot water; the keeping properties of the product are inferior to mucilage prepared with cold water.

Mucilago Acaciae BPC 1911 (Mucilage of Acacia)

Gum acacia, in small pieces or coarse powder	35 g
Benzoic acid (to preserve)	0.2 g
Water to	100.00 ml

Wash the acacia quickly in distilled water, macerate with warm water (plus benzoic acid) until dissolved and make up to volume. Acacia mucilage can be sterilized by heating at 80°C for one hour.

OXYMELS

These are formulations containing acetic acid, clear honey, and enough water to give a solution with a specific gravity of 1.32, measured with a hydrometer. Usually the amount of water comes to 1 part.

Oxymel Marrubii BPC 1911 (Oxymel of Horehound)

Horehound, dried	42.50 g
Acetic acid	6.75 ml
Distilled water, boiling,	a sufficient quantity
Clarified honey to	100.00 ml

Digest the horehound with sufficient boiling water to cover it, in a water bath for one hour; then strain and press, evaporate on the water bath to 50, cool, when cold add the acetic acid and filter; make up to the required volume with the honey. Dose: 2–4 ml.

WATERS (AQUA)

Waters are traditional preparations that are still widely used as cosmetics in the form of flower waters. Aromatic waters are still official, and five are mentioned in the BP 1980.

Aqua Cinnamomi conc. BPC 1911
(Concentrated Cinnamon Water)

Oil of cinnamon	4.75 ml
Alcohol (90%)	80.00 ml
Distilled water to	100.00 ml

Dissolve the oil in the alcohol. Add the water in small amounts, shaking after each addition. One part of this solution corresponds to about 40 parts of cinnamon water.

DRY PREPARATIONS

Sometimes it is appropriate to take herbs in a dry form, and dry preparations offer certain advantages. First, they enable the patient to take the herb while avoiding the possibly unpleasant taste. Second, the patient takes the whole herb, including the fibrous material.

On the other hand, there are a number of drawbacks to dry preparations. Dry herbs are unprocessed, and thus the plant constituents are not always readily available for easy absorption. During infusion, heat and water help to break down the walls of the plant cells and dissolve the constituents, which is not always guaranteed during the digestive process in the stomach and the small intestine. When the constituents are already dissolved in liquid form, they are available to exert their actions sooner.

A more subtle drawback lies in the very fact that when herbs are taken in dry form, the patient does not taste the herb. For reasons discussed in chapter 13 and elsewhere, bitter herbs work best when tasted, as their effectiveness depends on a complex neurological reflex. When bitters are put into a capsule or a pill, their action may well be lost or diminished.

After all of these considerations have been taken into account, there are still a number of ways to use herbs in dry form. The main concern is ensuring that the herbs are powdered as finely as possible. This guarantees that the cell walls are largely broken down, and helps in the digestion and absorption of the herbs. However, the need to break down the herbs presents yet another drawback, as techniques used to grind the herbs finely will also generate much heat through friction, possibly leading to a change in chemistry.

Capsules

The easiest way to take dry powdered herbs internally is to use gelatin capsules. (Capsules not made of animal products are also available.) The size needed depends on the amount of herb prescribed per dose, the density of the plant, and the volume of the material. A size 00 capsule holds about 0.5 gram (1/6 ounce) of finely powdered herb.

Filling Capsules

Place the powdered herb in a flat dish and take the halves of the capsule apart. Move the halves of the capsules through the powder, filling them in the process. Push the halves together.

Pills

There are a number of ways to make pills, depending on the degree of technical skill you possess. The simplest way to take an unpleasant remedy is to roll the powder into a small pill with fresh bread, which works quite effectively with herbs such as goldenseal and cayenne.

Tablets

The tablet is the most commonly used oral dosage form, but is also often the most complex to make. The process of making tablets involves compressing the herb, which results in a reduction in effective surface area. The herb starts out as a very fine powder, but then is compressed into a single dosage unit. Certain tablet ingredients are included to add various physical properties to the therapeutic properties of the herb.

Common Tablet Ingredients

Drug may be poorly soluble, hydrophobic
Lubricant is usually quite hydrophobic
Granulating agents tend to help the ingredients adhere to one another
Filler may interact with the drug; it should be water-soluble
Wetting agents help water penetrate into the tablet
Disintegration agents help to break the tablet apart after ingestion

Coated tablets are used to help mask unpleasant tastes, protect tablet ingredients during storage, or simply improve the appearance of the tablet. This barrier must break down quickly, or it may hinder the drug's bioavailability. Some tablets are treated with *enteric coatings*, meaning that they are coated with a material that will dissolve in the intestine but remain intact in the stomach. Polymeric acid compounds have been used for this purpose with some success.

Lozenges (Trochisci) and Pastilles (Pastilli)

A number of formulations have been developed to pleasantly and slowly release medicinal properties in the mouth. These aromatic, medicinal forms are named after their shapes. Thus, *lozenge* is derived from the French *losange*, meaning "rhombic." *Troche*, the singular form of *trochisti*, from the Greek *trochos*, means "round." *Pastille* is from one of the French words for "food."

Trochisci Altheae BPC 1911 (Althaea Lozenges)

Althaea, in powder	6.48 g
Refined sugar, in powder	99.22 g
Gum Acacia, in powder	64.80 g
White of one egg	
Orange-flower water	a sufficient quantity

Macerate the Althaea in a sufficient quantity of orange-flower water for 12 hours, strain, add the gum acacia and sugar. Dissolve and evaporate to the consistency of honey with constant stirring; gradually add the white of an egg beaten up with more orange-flower water. Evaporate with stirring until the paste will not adhere to the hand, and divide into 100 lozenges.

EXTERNAL REMEDIES

As the body can absorb some components of herbal formulations through the skin, a wide range of methods and formulations have been developed to take advantage of this fact. Douches and suppositories, though they might appear to be internal remedies, have traditionally been categorized as external remedies.

Here are two time-honored official remedies for external application.

Peruvian Balsam NF

This balsam is made up of 60% to 64% of a volatile oil called cinnamein and 20% to 28% of resin. The higher the volatile oil content, the greater the market price of the drug. Cinnamein is a mixture of numerous compounds, of which the following have been identified: the esters benzyl benzoate, benzyl cinnamate, and cinnamyl cinnamate; the alcohol peruviol as ester; free cinnamic acid; about 0.05% of vanillin; and a trace of coumarin. It may also contain dihydrobenzoic acid, farnesol, styrol, and a phytosterol. The resin consists of the benzoic and cinnamic acid esters of the alcohol peruresinotannol, along with some free cinnamic acid.

Peruvian Balsam is a local irritant. It serves as a valuable dressing that promotes the growth of epithelial cells in the treatment of indolent ulcers, wounds, and certain skin conditions, including scabies. Ointments that contain both Peruvian Balsam and sulfur present a problem in compounding, since the resinous part of the balsam tends to separate. This difficulty may be overcome by mixing the balsam with an equal amount of castor oil before incorporating it into the base, or by mixing it with solid petroxolin.

Friar's Balsam

Friar's Balsam has been a classic herbal remedy for more than 500 years. It is an antiseptic, vulnerary, and stimulating expectorant made from the following blend of components:

Siam benzoin resin *(Styrax tonkinensis):* 47%
Storax *(Liquidambar orientalis):* 17%
Balsam of Tolu *(Myroxylon balsamum* var. *balsamum):* 17%
Balsam of Peru *(Myroxylon balsamum* var. *pereirae):* 9%
Aloe leaf latex *(Aloe vera):* 4%
Myrrh tears *(Commiphora molmol):* 4%
Angelica root *(Angelica archangelica):* 2%

The preparation is used topically as an antiseptic and to treat minor cuts and abrasions, chapped skin and lips, cracked nipples, small fissures of the skin and anus, bedsores, indolent ulcers, herpes simplex, and gingivitis. It may also be taken internally or inhaled with steam vapor as a stimulating expectorant for stubborn coughs and catarrhs, laryngitis, early stages of acute bronchitis, and chronic bronchitis. Occasionally, topical use can cause contact dermatitis.

Baths (Balneotherapy)

The use of hot water for therapeutic purposes is as ancient as humanity itself. In Europe, it has been called *balneotherapy*. The term *balneology* refers to the study of bathing, and so balneotherapy is the use of balneology in the treatment of disease. In North America, this is a field of therapeutics utilized by naturopathic physicians, and an excellent modern guide can be found in *The Textbook of Natural Medicine*. This technique has many benefits, especially when a careful selection of herbal additives is made.

Official Baths

Baths, officially known as balnea, are mentioned in the pharmacopoeias.

Balneum Sinapis BPC 1911 (Mustard Bath)

Mustard	0.25 g
Water to	100.00 ml

Rub the mustard to a smooth paste with cold water before adding it to the remainder of the water previously warmed.

Folk Method

A pleasant way of absorbing herbal compounds through the skin is by bathing in a full body bath with 1 pint of infusion or decoction added to the water. Alternatively, you can also take a foot- or hand bath, in which case the preparation would be used in undiluted form. Any herb that can be taken internally can also be used in a bath.

Another way to use herbs in baths is to simply place a handful of herbs in a muslin bag and then suspend it from the hot-water tap so that the water flows through the bag. This creates a very fresh infusion.

Bath herbs not only foster relaxation, but also can be used to give the bath an exquisite fragrance.

Fragrant, Relaxing Bath Herbs

Lavandula officinalis (lavender)
Matricaria recutita (chamomile)
Melissa officinalis (lemon balm)
Rosmarinus officinalis (rosemary)
Sambucus nigra (elder)
Tilia spp. (linden)

For a bath that will bring about a restful and healing sleep, select an infusion of one of the following to add to the bathwater. Bear in mind that although valerian is very effective, it has a strong aroma!

Sedative Bath Herbs

Lavandula spp. (lavender)
Matricaria recutita (chamomile)
Tilia spp. (linden)
Valeriana officinalis (valerian)
Viburnum opulus (cramp bark)

For children with sleep problems or babies who are teething, the gentle herbs listed here might be more appropriate than some of the strong ones mentioned above.

Bath Herbs for Children and Babies

Matricaria recutita (chamomile)
Tilia spp. (linden)
Trifolium pratense (red clover)

For feverish conditions, or to help improve circulation, stimulating and diaphoretic herbs can be used. Care should be taken to use very small amounts of the strong rubefacients, such as cayenne.

Stimulating and Diaphoretic Bath Herbs

Achillea millefolium (yarrow)
Capsicum annuum (cayenne)
Rosmarinus officinalis (rosemary)
Zingiber officinale (ginger)

These are just some of the possibilities. Ideas can be found in books on aromatherapy, a healing system based on the external application of herbs in the form of essential oils. Essential oils can also be used in baths; simply put a few drops of oil into the bathwater. Care must be taken when using these wonderful oils, as they are very concentrated, and too much of certain oils may be irritating to the skin or even toxic. For more information, refer to *Aromatherapy: A Complete Guide to the Healing Art*, by Kathi Keville and Mindy Green, one of the best books on this therapeutic modality.

Douches

Another way to use herbs externally is in a douche (the application of herbs to the vagina). This is particularly indicated for local infections.

Preparing a Douche

Prepare an infusion or decoction to be used for douching. (Be sure to prepare a fresh tea for each douche.) Allow the tea to cool to a temperature that will be comfortable for internal application. Pour the liquid into the container of a douche bag and insert applicator. Allow the liquid to rinse the inside of the vagina.

Note that because the liquid will run out of the vagina, it is easiest to douche while sitting on the toilet. It is not necessary to actively hold in the liquid. In most conditions for which douching is indicated, it is advisable to use the tea undiluted, three times daily, for a number of days, using appropriate herbal remedies internally at the same time.

If, however, a three- to seven-day course of douching (along with internal remedies) does not noticeably improve symptoms of vaginal infection, see a qualified practitioner for a diagnosis.

Enemas

Enemas and douches have both been used as official preparations. Here is an official formulation for an enema.

Enema Ulmi Fulvae BPC 1911 (Enema of Slippery Elm)

Slippery Elm in fine powder	5 g
Boiling water to	100 ml

Pour the water onto the powder, mixing thoroughly. 500 ml is about enough for one enema. The Ulmus fulva powder will almost certainly go cloudy. Just prior to the addition of the boiling water, either wet it to a thin paste with cold water or use a minimum quantity of alcohol as a wetting agent. Allow the alcohol to evaporate after the boiling water has been added.

Ointments

Ointments, or salves, are semisolid preparations that can be applied to the skin. Depending on the purpose for which they are designed, there are innumerable ways to make ointments. They can vary in texture from very greasy to a thick paste, depending on what base is used and what compounds have been mixed together. Any herb can be used for making ointments, but some that are particularly valuable in external healing mixtures are listed here.

Herbs for External Use

Achillea millefolium (yarrow)
Althaea officinalis (marshmallow)
Arnica montana (arnica)
Calendula officinalis (calendula, pot marigold)
Eucalyptus globulus (eucalyptus)
Hydrastis canadensis (goldenseal)
Plantago spp. (plantain)
Sambucus flowers (elder)
Stellaria media (chickweed)
Symphytum officinale (comfrey)
Thymus vulgaris (thyme)
Ulmus rubra (slippery elm)

Modern North American herbalism shows one of its strengths where the preparation of ointments is concerned. A cornucopia of methods and ingredients exists, and many herbalists have developed their own unique approaches. A range of materials can be used to make up the ointment base, allowing for different consistencies and different types of extraction. The reader is directed again to the books written by Rosemary Gladstar, James Green, and Christopher Hobbs, listed in Suggested Reading.

Suppositories

Suppositories are designed to enable the insertion of remedies into the orifices of the body. While they can be shaped for insertion into the nose or ears, they are most commonly used for rectal or vaginal problems. They act as carriers for any herb that is appropriate to use in this context, and there are three general categories of these:

1. Herbs that soothe mucous membranes, reduce inflammation, and aid in the healing process, such as root and leaf of *Symphytum officinale*, roots of *Althaea officinalis* and *Hydrastis canadensis*, and bark of *Ulmus rubra*
2. Astringent herbs that reduce discharge or aid in the treatment of hemorrhoids, such as *Vinca* species, *Plantago* species, *Hamamelis virginiana*, and *Rumex crispus*
3. Remedies that stimulate intestinal peristalsis and help overcome chronic constipation—in other words, laxatives

When using herbs in any of these three categories, it will often be appropriate to include an antimicrobial herb. A number of different bases may be used, but keep in mind that the base must be firm enough to be inserted into the orifice but must also melt at body temperature once inserted, to liberate the herbs it contains. The herbs should be distributed uniformly in the base; this is particularly important when using a powdered herb.

Official Suppositories

Formulas for suppositories appear in various pharmacopoeias, including the following example.

Suppositorum Ranunculus Ficaria BPC 1911 (Suppository of Lesser Celandine)

Spermaceti wax	1 g
Ranunculus ficaria ointment	3 g

Made from fresh Ranunculus digested in lard for 24 hours.

Folk Method

A simple method of making suppositories is to mix finely powdered herbs with a base, preferably cocoa butter. Mold this mixture into the desired shape, following the instructions given below. To avoid the introduction of powdered plant material into the body, however, another method must be employed: Use gelatin and vegetable glycerin as a base and add an infusion, a decoction, or a tincture in the following proportions.

Suppository

Gelatin	10 parts
Water (or infusion, decoction, tincture)	40 parts
Glycerin	15 parts

Soak the gelatin in the liquid and dissolve with the aid of gentle heating. Add glycerin and heat the whole mixture over a water bath to evaporate the water. The final consistency will depend on how much water is removed. If removed completely, a very firm consistency will be achieved.

Preparing a Mold

Shape a piece of aluminum foil to the desired dimensions. The best shape is a one-inch-long torpedo. Pour the molten base into the mold and allow to cool. Store the suppositories in their molds in the refrigerator.

Liniments

Liniments are preparations specifically formulated for easy absorption through the skin, as they are intended for use in massages that stimulate muscles and ligaments. They must be used only externally, never internally, because they usually are made with rubbing alcohol. To carry the herbal components to the muscles and ligaments, liniments are usually made of a mixture of the herb with alcohol or, occasionally, apple cider vinegar. An herb-infused or essential oil may also be added. Cayenne is a common liniment ingredient.

Linimentum Arnicae BPC 1911 (Liniment of Arnica)

Hard Soap	20.00 g
Tincture of Arnica	25.00 ml
Camphor	5.00 ml
Alcohol to	100.00 ml

Dissolve the soap in the alcohol and tincture of arnica, on a water-bath, add the camphor, dissolve, pour into suitable bottles and cool.

Jethro Kloss describes the following liniment in *Back to Eden*. It is not an official formulation, but rather an expression of the folk tradition at its best.

A Jethro Kloss Liniment

Combine:

- 2 ounces powdered myrrh
- 1 ounce powdered goldenseal
- ½ ounce cayenne pepper
- 1 quart rubbing alcohol (70%)

Mix together and let stand seven days; shake well every day, decant off, and bottle in corked bottles.

Another excellent liniment that simultaneously warms and relaxes muscles is made with equal parts *Lobelia inflata* and *Viburnum opulus* plus a pinch of *Capsicum annuum*. This can be made into a tincture or a liniment. For more examples, please refer to chapter 19.

Gargles (Gargarisma) and Mouthwashes

Mouthwashes are still official, although only one has survived to be listed in the current BP. The BP 1980 provides the following definition:

> Mouthwashes are aqueous solution of one or more medicaments. They are intended, usually after dilution with warm water, for use in contact with the mucous membranes of the oral cavity. They may contain suitable antimicrobial preservatives.

Gargarisma Myrrhea BPC 1911 (Myrrh Gargle)

Tincture of Myrrh	5.00 ml
Clarified Honey	5.00 ml
Acid Infusion of Roses to	100.00 ml

Mix the tincture of Myrrh with the clarified honey and gradually add the acid infusion of roses.

Inhalants (Vapors) and Spray Solutions (Nebulae)

These pharmacy forms represented an official use of the essential oils that have been rediscovered in the practice of aromatherapy. They facilitate the therapeutic application of the oils to the sinuses or pharynx.

Vapor Eucalapti et Mentholis Compositus BPC 1911 (Compound Eucalyptus and Menthol Inhalation)

Oil of Eucalyptus	10.00 ml
Oil of Pine	5.00 ml
Oil of Cassia	5.00 ml
Menthol	5.00 ml
Thymol	1.00 ml
Camphor	2.00 g
Tincture of Benzoin to	100.00 ml

Dissolve the oils and other ingredients in the tincture. This inhalation is an excellent basis for special medicaments. Thus, 2% of balsam of Peru may be added; 1–2% of phenol; 1–5% of cocaine; 2% of creosote; 5% of oil of tar; 1% of iodine; 5% of terebene.

Nebula Benzoini Composita BPC 1911 (Composition Benzoin Inhalation)

Oil of Pine	1.50 ml
Oil of Eucalyptus	3.00 ml
Oil of Cassia	1.50 ml
Menthol	1.00 ml
Glycerin	50.00 ml
Tincture of Benzoin to	100.00 ml

Dissolve the menthol and oils on 40 of the tincture, add the glycerin and make up to the required volume with tincture of benzoin. This preparation is suitable for use with a nebulizer.

The traditional herbal equivalents of these vapors and nebulae can be found in the medicine-making and aromatherapy books listed in Suggested Reading at the end of this chapter.

Oils

Many herbs are rich in essential oils. These include aromatic herbs like *Mentha piperita*, in which the oils are volatile. Other plants contain oils that are not particularly aromatic, such as *Hypericum perforatum*. Herbal oils can be used in two forms, depending on the mode of extraction.

1. *Pure essential oils* are extracted from the herb through a complex and careful process of distillation. These oils are best obtained from specialist suppliers who distill them for use in aromatherapy, and thus take care that they are as pure as possible.
2. *Herb-infused oils* are made through a much simpler method that resembles the technique used to make cold infusions. Instead of infusing the herb in water, put it in oil to obtain a solution of the plant's essential oils in the oil base. The best oils to use are vegetable oils, such as olive, sunflower, and almond.

A Simple Herbal Oil

Cut the herb finely, place in a clear glass container, and cover it with oil. Put the container in the sun or leave it in a warm place for 2 to 3 weeks, shaking the container daily. After that time, filter the liquid into a dark glass container for storage.

St. John's Wort Oil

Pick the flowers when they have just opened and crush them in a teaspoonful of olive oil. Place the flowers in a glass container, cover them with more oil, mix well, and put the container in the sun or a warm place for 3 to 6 weeks, at the end of which time the oil will be bright red.

Press the mixture through a cloth to filter out all the oil and leave the oil to stand. There will be some water in the liquid, which will settle on the bottom, so decant the oil from the top. Store the oil in a well-sealed, dark container.

Compresses

Compresses provide an excellent means of applying a remedy to the skin.

A Simple Compress

Soak a clean linen or cotton cloth in a hot herbal tea and apply it to the affected part of the body. Use as hot as can be tolerated. Cover the compress with a towel to hold in the heat.

When cool, replace with a fresh compress. For a cold compress, use the same method, but simply let the tea cool before application.

Poultices

This more active method of applying herbs to the outside of the body uses fresh or dried plant material, rather than a liquid.

Making a Poultice

Mash or crush fresh plant material and either heat over boiling water or mix with a small amount of boiling water to make a paste. If using dried herbs, powder them and mix with hot water to create a paste. Apply directly to the skin as hot as possible, holding the compress in place with gauze.

If using stimulating or irritating herbs such as mustard, apply them between two layers of cloth.

INCOMPATIBILITY

A problem that faces all formulators of medicines is the possibility that incompatibilities will be encountered. These fall into three broad categories.

A *therapeutic incompatibility* is defined as an undesirable pharmacological interaction between two or more ingredients that may potentiate the therapeutic effects of the ingredients, reduce the effectiveness of one or more of the ingredients, or cause toxicity in the patient.

Physical incompatibility refers to a physical or chemical interaction between two or more ingredients that leads to a visibly recognizable change. The latter may occur in the form of a precipitate, haze, or color change.

Chemical incompatibility is classified as a reaction in which an undesirable change occurs but is not visible. Since there is no visible evidence of deterioration, recognizing this type of incompatibility requires some skill.

Physical incompatibilities can often be altered or avoided. A common problem is the generation of insoluble precipitates. For example, alcohol extracts precipitate dissolved constituents when mixed with water. Such problems can often be avoided by manipulating the solvent or by adding a suspending or protective agent. The specific remedies for such problems will vary according to the substances involved.

General Methods for Overcoming Physical Incompatibilities

There are a number of simple methods that can be used to minimize or prevent physical incompatibilities.

Change the order of mixing. Combining resin-rich tinctures and water commonly causes the resin to precipitate. One possible solution is to add the tincture slowly to cold water when mixing. However, with very resin-rich tinctures, such as tincture of myrrh, it is impossible to avoid some precipitation of resin out of solution.

Change the total volume of the mixture. By simply adding more solvent, whether water or ethanol, the increased volume will provide more bulk for material to start in solution, in effect diluting the problematic constituent. The percentage of water or ethanol may be crucial, but the final outcome depends on the chemistry of the constituents in the extract.

Alter the solvents or add protective agents. Water dissolves gums, mucilage, and starch, but these are not miscible in alcohol. Alcohol dissolves most constituents. Often, the presence of alkaloids, glycosides, volatile oils, resins, or balsams in an herb necessitates the use of a higher percentage of alcohol in the extract to ensure that the constituents are extracted and will not precipitate when water is added. Glycerin can be added to replace part of the water component to decrease the chance of precipitation.

Make an emulsification or suspension with gums or syrup. For example, with acacia, do not add strong alcohol directly or the solution will "congeal." Instead, make a dilute mucilage and add alcohol slowly. This method may be used for resinous tinctures. With tragacanth, add tincture or liquid extract directly to powdered gum. Shake to mix. Water should be added in a proportion of 1 part of gum to 20 parts of water.

Chemical incompatibilities are more difficult to overcome, but rarely are an issue in phytotherapy. Chemical interactions can produce precipitation of insoluble compounds. Alkaloids form salts with metallic ions, and thus, in theory, many potential incompatibilities are possible. However, all of these can be overcome by using a solution made up of 15% to 30% alcohol.

Suggested Reading

Boyle W. *Official Herbs: Botanical Substances in the United States Pharmacopoeias, 1820–1990.* East Palestine: Buckeye Naturopathic Press, 1991.

British Herbal Pharmacopoeia. Bournemouth, UK: British Herbal Medicine Association, 1983.

British Pharmaceutical Codex 1911. London: Pharmaceutical Press, 1912.

British Pharmacopoeia. London: Constable & Co. Ltd., 1932.

Ellingwood F. *American Materia Medica, Therapeutics & Pharmacognosy, 1898,* Reprint, Sandy, OR: Eclectic Medical Publications, 1983.

Felter and Lloyd. *King's American Dispensatory,* vol. 1 & 2, Reprint, Sandy, OR: Eclectic Medical Publications, 1983.

Felter HW. *The Eclectic Materia Medica, Pharmacology & Therapeutics, 1922.* Reprint, Sandy, OR: Eclectic Medical Publications, 1983.

Gladstar R. *Family Herbal: A Guide to Living Life with Energy, Health, and Vitality.* Pownal, VT: Storey Books, 2001.

Green J. *The Herbal Medicine Maker's Handbook: A Home Manual.* Freedom, CA: Crossing Press, 2000.

Hobbs C. *Handmade Herbal Medicines: Recipes for Potions, Elixirs, and Salves.* Loveland, CO: Interweave Press, 1998.

Keville K, Green M. *Aromatherapy: A Complete Guide to the Healing Art.* Freedom, CA: Crossing Press, 1995.

Kloss J. *Back to Eden,* mass market revised edition. Twin Lakes, WI: Lotus Press, 1989.

List PH, Schmidt PC. *Phytopharmaceutical Technology.* Boca Raton, FL: CRC Press, 1989.

Osol A, ed. *Remington's Pharmaceutical Sciences,* 15th edition. Easton, PA: Mack, 1975.

Pizzorno JE, Murray MT. *The Textbook of Natural Medicine.* Edinburgh: Churchill Livingstone, 1999.

The National Formulary VI, 6th edition. Easton, PA: American Pharmaceutical Assoc., 1935.

United States Pharmacopeia, 11th edition. Easton, PA: The United States Pharmacopoeial Convention, 1936.

Wood HC, Osol A. *The Dispensatory of the United States of America,* 23rd edition. Philadelphia: JB Lippincott Co., 1943.

Part Two

TREATMENT APPROACHES
BY BODY SYSTEM

12

A MODEL OF HOLISTIC HERBAL MEDICINE

The phytotherapist must have some model to follow in formulating a prescription that addresses the needs of the whole person. The herbal component of treatment must be used in a context that also takes into account non-herbal factors, such as diet, lifestyle, and emotional, mental, and spiritual issues. In addition, all of this must take place within the framework of a particular socioeconomic situation and philosophical context. Such a model enables the practitioner to identify and address a whole range of factors, from symptoms and pathology to constitutional differences and whole body toning.

The model we will discuss here is not new, but rather is a representation of well-established and proven approaches described in holistic terms. There is little that can truly be seen as new in a field as ancient as herbalism! To choose the specific remedies that an individual needs from the vast range of possibilities nature offers can be a daunting task. However, it can be simplified if one uses a set of guidelines.

The material that follows is provided under the assumption that the prescriber has a basic grasp of human physiology and pathology. The model is based upon a five-stage process:

1. Herbal actions
2. System affinity
3. Specific remedies for the illness
4. Herbal biochemistry
5. Intuition

Herbal Actions

Herbal actions reflect the ways in which remedies affect human physiology. Plants have a direct impact on physiological activity, and knowing what body processes are involved in both disease and wellness facilitates selection of an appropriate action. Obviously, selection of actions suitable for a specific person will also depend on accurate diagnosis.

System Affinity

Some herbs show an affinity for certain organs, body systems, or even specific types of tissue. These work as tonics or nutrients for the areas involved. Many herbs can be used freely and safely as part of one's lifestyle and need not be thought of as medicines. They are at their best when used to nurture health and vitality and thus prevent the development of health problems. During illness, herbs with system affinities will enhance the general health of the particular organ or body system when combined with remedies selected for specific actions. They are especially useful when a tendency toward a certain illness has been recognized but no overt pathology is present. By using herbs in this way, one may be able to overcome a weakness that could lead to disease later in life.

Specific Remedies for Illness

The wealth of herbal knowledge that has been garnered through the generations includes the use of many plants that are traditionally *specific* for the treatment of certain diseases or symptoms. While holistic healing aims to go beyond symptomatic therapy, this knowledge deserves great respect. An understanding of specific remedies for illness can add much to a prescription based on appropriate actions and system support. However, specifics do not always exist.

Herbal Biochemistry

As discussed at length earlier in this book, increasing attention is being paid to the biochemistry of active herb constituents. Research has led to the development of many lifesaving drugs, but this is a very limited approach when it comes to using whole plants. In the hands of an experienced herbalist, knowledge of plant pharmacology can add to the healing possibilities, but not as much as is often believed.

Intuition

An intuitive rapport flowers between the experienced herbalist and the plants in their materia medica. Intuition has a special role to play in healing, and the unique relationship between plants and people augments it well. Such insightful intuition does not always flow freely, but it should be embraced when it does. Intuitive knowledge should always be checked against reference materials, if at all possible. For example, if a practitioner is not clear on the differences among bearberry, barberry, and bilberry, unfortunate misunderstandings can result!

PHYTOTHERAPEUTIC SELECTION CRITERIA

There is nothing inherent in a plant that defines the way it should be used, and considering the herbal abundance of our world, some coherent selection criteria are essential to guide phytotherapists in their healing work.

More than one-half million plants of various types present themselves as possible healing remedies. The British medical herbalist routinely uses approximately 250, while in China, the herbal practitioner can choose from about 2,000 remedies that are readily available in community pharmacies. These herbalists are obviously applying some set of guidelines in order to whittle down 500,000 possible plant remedies to a more manageable figure, but what are they? There are a number of useful ways to group the relevant criteria, but three categories are most helpful in Western herbalism:

1. Assessing the impact of herbs upon the body and mind
2. Applying nontherapeutic criteria, such as aesthetics, economics, and ecology
3. Using herbs within the context of some kind of system

Applying these three sets of criteria facilitates the formulation of treatments that are specific to the unique needs of the individual and at the same time takes into account environmental and economic considerations.

ASSESSING THE IMPACT OF HERBS ON THE INDIVIDUAL

The herbal remedies of the world vary greatly in strength, from gentle tonic or food remedies to those that are potentially lethal if taken at the wrong dosage. The holistic phytotherapist works with the underlying idea that the body is self-healing and the therapist simply supports this innate healing process. Thus, the tonic herbs are of paramount importance, as this is exactly what they do.

A characteristic of tonics is that they are all gentle remedies that have a mild yet profound effect upon the body. Of course, not all herbal remedies are tonics, as many have a powerful and immediate impact upon human physiology. These must be used with the greatest respect, and their use is best reserved for illnesses that call for strong medicine. Identifying the intensity of an herb's impact upon the body provides a useful selection criterion. Herbal remedies may be conveniently categorized as either normalizers or effectors, but bear in mind that these groupings are not absolute.

Normalizers

These are remedies that nurture and nourish the body in a way that supports its own natural processes of growth, healing, and renewal. These are the tonics, and are often used in the form of herbal foods. Nettle, cleavers, and chickweed are excellent examples of these gentle herbs.

Effectors

These are remedies that have an observable impact upon the body. They provide humanity with herbs to use for the treatment of the whole range of specific human illnesses. Effectors can in turn be divided into two groups, depending upon how they work:

Herbs with whole-plant actions. The effects of these herbs come from the impact of the whole plant on the human body. As examples, consider the immune system booster echinacea and the anti-inflammatory herb meadowsweet. It might be argued that meadowsweet works because it contains salicylates. However, as discussed in chapter 7, other actions are also at play, and the characteristic gastric inflammation caused by salicylates can even be treated with meadowsweet. This surely implies that something much broader than simple drug delivery is going on.

Herbs with specific active chemicals. These herbs exert their effects because they contain a chemical (or chemicals) with an impact so strong that whole plant effects are not usually perceived. Due to the presence of these intense chemicals, such herbs are potentially poisonous if taken at the wrong dose or in the wrong way. The cardioactive herb foxglove and the opium poppy serve as good examples.

Using Tonic Herbs

The value of tonic herbs lies in their normalizing, nurturing effects. These invaluable remedies will usually have some associated action that further indicates how they are best used. The cardiovascular tonic hawthorn is an excellent example. Hawthorn tones the whole cardiovascular system, while at the same time specifically dilates blood vessels and lowers blood pressure.

Whenever possible, the herbalist will focus on the use of such remedies, and will use stronger effectors only if absolutely necessary. In fact, chemically based effectors are used very sparingly in holistic herbalism. They are, however, the foundation of pharmacological medicine.

Tonics can play a valuable role in keeping individuals at their personal peak of health and vitality. Tonics may also be used to ward off specific known health problems or family weaknesses. There are plant remedies particularly suited for each system of the body, some of which are tonics. Selecting remedies that act as tonics for specific body systems allows the herbalist to do some impressive preventive work. When choosing, be sure to take into account the broader picture of the herb's range of actions, as this breadth of vision is needed to enable coherent choices.

For the digestive system, no one herb serves as an all-around tonic, as the system is so varied in form and function. However, bitters serve as preventive tonics. In addition, *Matricaria recutita* and *Filipendula ulmaria* are so helpful to the digestive process that they might almost be considered general tonics here.

NONTHERAPEUTIC SELECTION CRITERIA

To help further in the process of selecting among herbs with similar actions, there are a number of nontherapeutic factors to take into account. These are aesthetic, economic, and environmental.

Aesthetic Criteria

There is no reason that herbal medicines should always taste unpleasant. When possible, consider taste, aroma, and visual appeal. These factors are a matter of personal taste, but it is fine to select from a list of herbs compiled by applying both therapeutic criteria and personal aesthetic preferences. Bitter herbs constitute the only general exception. If bitterness is indicated, then the herbs must be tasted, or much of their therapeutic potential will be lost.

An example of a remedy that both works well and tastes pleasant is a cough preparation, widely used in France, that is composed of herb flowers that ease the cough reflex and help remove phlegm from the lungs. Making an herbal cough mixture that works well is straightforward enough, but effective combinations are often composed of acrid- or unpleasant-tasting plants.

Table 12.1. Tonics for Specific Body Systems

BODY SYSTEM	HERBS
Cardiovascular	*Crataegus laevigata, Allium sativum;* flavone-rich herbs, such as *Ginkgo biloba* and *Tilia platyphyllos,* help strengthen blood vessels
Respiratory	*Verbascum thapsus, Inula helenium*
Digestive	Bitter tonics, such as *Gentiana lutea, Agrimonia eupatoria,* and *Taraxacum officinale* root; *Matricaria recutita* and *Filipendula ulmaria* are generally helpful to the digestive process
Liver	Bitters, hepatics, and especially *Silybum marianum*
Urinary	*Arctostaphylos uva-ursi, Zea mays*
Reproductive	Women: *Rubus idaeus, Mitchella repens,* and other uterine tonics Men: *Serenoa repens*
Nervous	*Avena sativa, Scutellaria lateriflora, Hypericum perforatum, Verbena officinalis, Artemisia vulgaris; Eleutherococcus senticosus* and *Panax ginseng* are appropriate for those under stress
Musculoskeletal	*Apium graveolens, Menyanthes trifoliata, Urtica dioica*
Skin	*Galium aparine, Trifolium repens, Urtica dioica,* and most of the alterative remedies

The same therapeutic results are achieved with the French flower mixture, but in addition, it has a wonderful aroma, a delicate taste, and a beautiful color.

Economic Criteria

My opinions are happily out of tune with the globally rapacious capitalism of the dominant culture, but I believe that herbs (and health care) should be free of charge. Nature does not impose a financial levy on herbs, as they grow wild and free. Of course, there are environmental costs to take into account, but that is another matter. When the choice arises, use common and inexpensive herbs. Expensive does not usually equate with quality, but instead with rarity. Expensive, rare, or imported plants may not work any more effectively than common and not very glamorous nettle or cleavers. The fast-developing herb industry has a financial stake in the promotion of expensive new "wonder herbs" from exotic parts of the world.

Environmental Criteria

Understanding that ecological relationships have a bearing on the healing arts can lead to some important broad implications. While the choice of the most relevant therapy should be based on the needs of the individual, Donne's insight that "no man is an island" becomes crucial here. In a world where human impact on the environment is becoming life threatening, the broader implications of health practices must be taken into account.

Consider the Brazilian plant suma (*Pfaffia paniculata*). In recent years, it has become popular as an immune system stimulant. Quite apart from whether or not it works, one must consider the basic fact that this vine is collected from gullies in the Brazilian rain forest that are very sensitive to erosion and disturbance. Isn't it ironic that through our attempts to help people live longer and healthier lives, herbalists may be contributing to rain forest destruction, the greenhouse effect, and a potentially dramatic reduction in the life spans of our children and grandchildren? When alternatives abound, why use a remedy that carries such environmental costs?

From a green perspective, talking of chemical drugs as "unnatural" and herbal remedies as "natural" is problematic. The interactions that occur among plants and humanity on the biochemical level show us that chemistry is also natural. If a chemical exists in the body of the plant, it must be natural. If it was not natural, it could not exist without causing major trauma to life on earth. This is, of course, also the case with technological aberrations such as plutonium, but in general, how can we differentiate between what is and is not natural based simply on how it is presented to us? The real challenge is learning how to harness the chemistry of nature safely.

When the ecological effects of drug therapy and herbal therapy are compared, another vital aspect of the selection criteria is revealed. An example will clarify this point. In the treatment of gastric ulceration, a whole spectrum of options is available. A holistic approach will not only focus on treating the stomach itself, but also examine diet, lifestyle, general health, and so on. Treatment may combine dietary changes, relaxation, exercise, counseling, and other factors with the specific medicines indicated.

How should these medicines be chosen? Herbal remedies have much to offer in the treatment of digestive problems in general and ulceration in particular, and are arguably more clinically effective than drug therapy. When we compare the antiulcer drug Tagamet (cimetidine) with the herb *Althaea officinalis* (marshmallow root), we have two medications that produce equivalent symptomatic relief for the patient, but have very different environmental impacts. (See The Impact of Herbs and Drugs on the Environment: A Comparison, page 240.)

Chemical drugs used to treat gastric and duodenal ulcers lower the production of stomach acid and thereby reduce irritation of the stomach's mucosal lining. Tagamet is commonly used to inhibit gastric acid and pepsin production in the stomach by blocking histamine receptors. In the 1980s, it was one of the most widely prescribed drugs in North America.

Herbal remedies may also be selected to soothe the gastric mucosa, reduce the impact of stomach acid, and promote the healing of ulceration. Plants that are demulcent, vulnerary, and antacid are the most relevant here, and the herbalist might also include nervine herbs to reduce excessive vagal stimulation. *Symphytum officinale* (comfrey), *Althaea officinalis* (marshmallow root), *Ulmus rubra* (slippery elm), *Filipendula ulmaria* (meadowsweet), *Matricaria recutita* (chamomile), and *Calendula officinalis* (calendula) may all have a part in the treatment. When used in the context of the whole picture, herbal treatments for gastric and duodenal ulcers are extremely effective.

However, in this case we are concerned more with environmental impact than with therapeutic factors. Regardless of the relative therapeutic merits of drugs and herbs, a clear picture emerges when one compares their respective ecological costs.

The Impact of Herbs and Drugs on the Environment: A Comparison

Tagamet and the Environment

The drug Tagamet is manufactured in a process that is notoriously dirty and produces much waste. This waste must be disposed of. Even with the best intentions in the world, there will be an impact on the environment, but with less than perfect management, there will be a severe impact that causes both water and air pollution. Pollution of local rivers can lead to destruction of insect and fish populations and then, through food webs, birds. If used for irrigation, the water may have an adverse effect on the soil. The pollutants dispersed into the air not only will contribute to acid rain, but will also have a direct impact related to the specific chemicals present.

In the process of developing the drug and fulfilling government safety standards, many laboratory animals were slaughtered. The morality of this fundamental part of modern health care is dubious in the extreme. However, it is currently a necessary evil when dealing with chemical medicine, and so must be taken into account when considering the impact of chemical drugs on the environment and living beings.

Industrial production and distribution of the drug is energy intensive in a way that the resources of the planet cannot support for much longer. (The profligate use of nonrenewable energy is, of course, rampant throughout the whole industrial system, and not specifically the fault of the manufacturers of Tagamet.) The potential for political manipulation also exists, as the need for energy to manufacture drugs is cited as a justification for the development of nuclear power. The contradictions in that juxtaposition would be funny if they were not so frightening.

When using proprietary drugs, the patient and prescriber are at the same time supporting and depending on the multinational drug companies. The very existence of these vast international corporations raises political, economic, and ethical questions that go beyond the confines of this brief review. However, the patient becomes an unwitting financial supporter of these questionable organizations. Disempowerment becomes a key concept as the individual's health care needs are relegated to the experts, the physician to prescribe and the pharmacist to dispense. This is not meant as a comment on the skill or dedication of these professionals, but as a recognition that patients have relinquished personal responsibility by handing it over to experts.

Added together, these issues create a cycle of death, destruction, and exploitation perpetrated in the name of personal health. It is worth looking closer to see the hidden costs of the little tablet, as the overall cost of treatment goes far beyond the price of the pills. The cost and impact of this "simple" ulcer treatment includes environmental damage and the support of a system that may well be at the center of much planetary *dis-ease*.

Marshmallow and the Environment

The dilemma over therapeutic choice raised by these ecological, economic, and political considerations might seem daunting. However, if herbal remedies are viewed in a similar framework, a very different picture emerges.

Althaea officinalis (marshmallow), like many other herbal remedies, is produced by small-scale growers and distributed through channels that support a diversified economic system. This system provides a perfect example of how small can be beautiful. Not only does it provide the benefits of small-scale economics and ecological viability, but this also works to produce a medicine that carries the multiple advantages inherent in herb remedies.

If organic techniques were used to produce the herb, the soil was nurtured, which Welsh farmers describe as putting "heart" back into the soil. Soil structure and stability are becoming major ecological problems in much of the world, and organic farming represents a step toward remedying this situation.

In addition, a basic principle in ecology is that the more diverse a system is, the more stable it will be in the face of environmental perturbation, and organic techniques increase the diversity of soil populations. Wildcrafting plants, the practice of collecting wild plants from their natural environment, highlights the need to preserve habitats as a source of plant and seed. However, it is even more important to protect the land for the sake of Earth itself. Herbalism is part of a dawning awareness in humanity that Earth and its inhabitants do not existence solely for our use.

It is no wonder that the production of herbal medicines, and in our example marshmallow, involves no abuse of laboratory animals. The traditional use of marshmallow is ancient, and we can accept the great knowledge of its healing properties without needing to take the lives of animals. Little energy is consumed in the production of this herb, so it is an ideal medicine for a self-sufficient, low-impact economy. Even if our society does not yet function this way, we can contribute in the right way by using a sustainably produced remedy to heal any ulcers the current system generates.

The comparison between these two therapeutically equivalent medicines shows that environmental and political criteria have much to contribute when it comes to making choices. Put starkly, the choice is between being part of a cycle of death and destruction justified by personal health and being part of a life-affirming cycle that uses healing herbs for personal health. The very process of considering these perspectives is part of the healing of humanity's alienation from our world. As we think, so we become. What is it to be?

USING HERBS IN THE CONTEXT OF A THERAPEUTIC SYSTEM

Since the early history of medicine, people have been striving to make sense of the human body, the ills that assail it, and the healing remedies used to treat it. Many models or systems of medicine have been developed, most of which are found now only in texts on the history of medicine. Ways of using herbs have been repeatedly organized and reorganized into various systems that reflect the prevailing worldview held by people of different cultures and eras.

Today is no exception, as the herbal renaissance is in full bloom and the transformation of society still in mid-process. A number of systems are in current use. Some depend upon traditional knowledge, while others work within the framework of an existing philosophical system. Systems based on the folk traditions of the world vary according to the tradition used. Those that work within the framework of an existing system differ depending on the philosophy at their core.

Philosophical contexts include the profoundly holistic systems of Asia as well as the Western medical approach, which is based on what has been called the *biomedical model*. This Western model requires that herbs be used within the framework of a disease-centered approach to medicine, but nonetheless applies them in a holistic context.

Traditional Healing Systems

The traditional or folk use of herbal remedies is familiar to everyone in some form or another. This is the way in which information about herbs has been passed from generation to generation, but an unquestioning reliance on empirical evidence also gives herbalism a bad name among members of the scientific community. Their loss! Folk wisdom is of inestimable value and relevance. Generations of accrued experience and insight are not to be taken lightly.

As an example, consider the fact that these same folk remedies from around the world often point the way for pharmacologists searching for new and powerful medicines. The use of *Dioscorea* spp. (wild yam) as a source of hormone precursors and the application of *Catharanthus roseus* (Madagascar periwinkle) in anti-leukemia drugs are two good examples.

The bulk of the world's health care is still based on the traditional use of local herbal remedies. The relevance of this worldwide folk use is recognized by the World Health Organization and promoted through its Traditional Medicine Program. Every culture of the world has its own herbal tradition, which may be either a thriving aspect of modern life or a more or less moribund historical memory.

By the early 1970s, the traditional use of plant medicines appeared to be almost over in Great Britain. However, with the renewal of interest in herbs that occurred as part of a wider reawakening to the natural world, it soon became apparent that much of the tradition was alive and well. Remedies and recipes for herbal teas had been handed down from generation to generation and were still remembered. The change in social atmosphere apparently gave people "permission" to recollect these gems of knowledge.

Wales has a strong modern herbal tradition with clearly recognizable roots in the flowering of Welsh culture in the days of the old Princes of Wales (c. 1100). In rural areas are many people who know one or two herbal combinations specific for certain conditions. Often encountered are various ointments for eczema. These ointments are usually very effective, but the people using them rarely know why, and they often have no other herbal information. The recipes can usually be traced back to the medieval Physicians of Myddfai, doctors at the court of the Princes. These physicians possessed a deep and profound knowledge of herbs and the healing process, well in advance of what was available in England and the rest of non-Islamic Europe at the time.

The continuity of the tradition is paradoxically related to attempts to destroy the culture that supported the physicians. When the English invaded and conquered Wales, the royal court was destroyed. The knowledge and wisdom of the Physicians of Myddfai was in part dispersed among the people, in what would prove to be a successful attempt to preserve the traditions. It appears that certain families were given specific remedies to keep safe and pass on to future generations. These recipes and information were never shared with anyone outside the family, but the medicine was given freely to anyone who needed it. This wisdom can still be found in the hills and valleys of Wales.

However, as fundamentally valuable as traditional folk knowledge is, it has limited application within modern holistic herbal practice. An application of herbal remedies that relates specific plants to specific diseases or symptoms is little more than what we might call "organic drug therapy." Simply using remedies for symptomatic relief ignores all the insights of holistic medicine. Thus, the ancient folk traditions of the world provide a wonderful foundation upon which today's medical herbalist may build the holistic herbalism of the future.

Philosophical Systems

Phytotherapy offers the most value to holistic medicine when used within the context of a coherent philosophical system. Such systems work with intellectual, conceptual models for understanding what a human being is and what a disease process is. Each system's concept of health and human wholeness must be seen as a subset of the paradigm held by that culture as to the nature of the world itself. These paradigms are reflected in the holistic medical systems of China and India as well as in the reductionist approach taken in the biomedical model of Western medicine.

Traditional Chinese medicine, ayurveda from the Vedic tradition of Hindu India, and unani from the world of Islam represent perhaps the best-known examples of philosophical systems that are still thriving in the face of the intellectual imperialism of Western medicine. Other systems are found in such diverse cultures as Japan and Ghana and wherever herbal medicine is integrated into spirituality and transformation, as in anthroposophical medicine.

The techniques of any medical system are an expression of its ideas and theories. These, in turn, arise as specific developments in the philosophy of the culture concerned. Thus, traditional Chinese medicine (TCM) represents an application to medicine of a Confucian or Taoist worldview. Similarly, ayurveda is an expression of the profound perspectives that come from Hindu experience and spirituality.

It is important that the context within which any medical practitioner is working be clearly acknowledged and expressed. It will color all that occurs, and may either limit or facilitate the healing work undertaken. Health care does not happen in a philosophical vacuum, but instead within the context of a worldview and belief system. If this fact is not articulated overtly, it will be implied by default. The problem of cultural chauvinism often arises when comparisons are made between different health care systems of the world. In the discussion that follows, I have intended to make no value judgments. This is simply an exploration of practical considerations for both practitioners and patients in the Western world.

Western Folk Traditions and Modern Herbalism

In general, folk traditions of the Western world are vestigial or have only recently been revived by well-meaning advocates. This makes changing or developing herbal treatments problematic. Unless the herbalist is part of an active, living tradition, it is unwise to question or change information that was handed down, as the source of that knowledge no longer exists. An example may clarify this.

When in practice in West Wales, I came across a hill farmer who made an ointment for the treatment of shingles, a painful and intransigent viral infection of nerve ganglia. On two occasions, I observed that this ointment cleared trigeminal shingles in three to five days, a feat that allopathic medicine or modern herbalism would be hard pressed to duplicate. However, the farmer died childless. He never imparted the secret recipe, especially not to an upstart English herbalist from the town!

All of my attempts to identify the many herbs in the ointment failed, except for one herb out of the whole combination. This was biting stonecrop *(Sedum acre)*, an herb that is not used therapeutically today and which the seventeenth-century herbalist Culpeper insisted must not be put in any ointment. Formulation of the ointment also involved using pig urine as an extraction vehicle.

Apart from practical questions about using pig urine (such as how to collect the urine!), modern sensibilities and hygienic considerations would probably suggest using water instead. However, from a therapeutic perspective, the use of pig urine should not be discarded for hygienic reasons alone. While studying Siberian shamans in the early 20th century, researchers discovered something interesting. During visionary rituals involving the psychoactive fly agaric mushroom *(Amanita muscaria)*, the shamans would drink their own urine. This lengthened and deepened the visionary experience, because the urine contained metabolites of the alkaloid muscimole that are also psychoactive. Is it not possible that some complex interaction between herbs and pig urine produced an antiviral metabolite that could be absorbed through the skin?

While this might sound far-fetched, my observation was that the ointment worked. Unless one knows why an ingredient is included in a mixture, can it really be taken out without risking loss of the desired effect? If the recipe is changed in some way, is the formulation still the traditional one?

The ancient medical systems of the world are profoundly holistic in both diagnostic and therapeutic approaches, a direct result of the expression of their spiritually whole and integrated cultural worldviews. This is often what attracts Western herbalists to these systems but, paradoxically, it also presents the primary stumbling block. The holistic strengths of such non-reductionist systems appear to fulfill the deep need felt by Western practitioners for a meaningful, practical, and relevant holistic approach.

This confronts the Westerner with some immediate challenges. In order to harvest the therapeutic benefits inherent in these systems, the practitioner should ideally be at home with the underlying worldview of the culture that gave birth to the healing system. In TCM, the names of organs, meridians, and elements may be translated into English words, but their meaning remains different. This is due not to mistranslation, but to the fact that they represent an understanding of the human body that is very different from the Western concept. In TCM, for example, the brain is not perceived as an organ, and the focus of therapeutic work is on balancing the flow of chi (vital energy) within the body. Disease is seen as an indicator of underlying processes, rather than the focus of treatment. The Western practitioner drawn to TCM or ayurveda must embrace the implications for personal change and transformation inherent in that system.

When this occurs, the therapeutic relationship between patient and practitioner can be truly holistic, because the therapist is acting from a place of personal integration and harmony. TCM expresses ways of seeing and experiencing the world that are very different from the Western stance. When TCM techniques and protocols are used out of context, the transformative possibilities of healing are severely limited. Such attempts can become the antithesis of holistic medicine.

Recognizing the fundamental role played by cultural perspectives highlights the need for a Western context for holistic medicine. On the other hand, acceptance of the biomedical model as a useful map of the human body does not mean one must also adopt the analytical and reductionist approach that characterizes modern Western medicine. There is a dawning recognition of the possibilities that might arise if the biomedical model is used as the basis for treating the whole person, not simply the disease.

All of these issues may help to explain the frustration that plagues Western health care professionals upon initial exploration of holistic medicine. The definitive text on Western holistic medicine—a guide for the practitioner that clearly illuminates these new and exciting perspectives—has yet to be written. There is a maelstrom of activity among holistic practitioners who are exploring and applying the new ideas, but we are still in the early stages.

For some, this is just too confusing; they either abandon the endeavor or turn to one of the Asian healing systems. For others, this is a very exciting time to be involved in medicine. The lack of clarity in the situation is simply one aspect of the flowering of new ideas. There is no textbook, because the ideas have not yet reached the stage at which they can be written in stone. Instead, this is a time of flux. Many new insights are occurring, and many old ideas are being reassessed and either discarded or embraced anew. While no clear holistic context has yet been defined for Western medicine, many different approaches have made great strides in that direction.

Herbal medicine has a unique contribution to make in this time of change. As a healing modality, it is inherently holistic in that its very nature is ecological. The use of plants links both patient and practitioner to their environment in profound ways, facilitating a healing process that could be seen as therapeutic ecology. The contribution of herbs is but one part of the mosaic that will become Western holistic healing.

THE ACTIONS OF HERBS

A great deal of pharmaceutical research has gone into analyzing the active constituents of herbs to find out how and why they work. A much older approach, and one that is much more immediately useful, is to categorize herbs through an understanding of what kinds of problems they can treat.

In some cases, an herb's action may be due to a specific chemical present (for example, the antiasthma effects of ma huang). In others, actions may arise from complex, synergistic interactions among various plant constituents (the sedative valerian provides an example). However, it is best to view actions as attributes of the whole herb; any understanding of the chemistry should serve simply as an aid to prescribing. A detailed discussion of herbal actions can be found in chapter 25.

Adaptogens
Adaptogenic herbs help increase the body's resistance to stress. They improve the body's resilience by enabling it to physiologically adapt to problems before it reaches the point of collapse. An inability to cope with external pressures can have many health repercussions. Adaptogens appear to work by supporting the function of the adrenal glands.

Alteratives

Alteratives are herbs that gradually restore proper function to the body, increasing health and vitality. Some alteratives support waste elimination processes via the kidneys, liver, lungs, or skin. Others stimulate digestive function or provide antimicrobial actions, while others simply work!

Anticatarrhal Herbs

Anticatarrhal herbs help the body eliminate excess mucus, whether in the sinuses or from other parts of the body.

Anti-Inflammatory Herbs

Herbs with anti-inflammatory properties soothe inflammations or directly reduce the inflammatory response. For a detailed discussion of the many ways in which herbs may work as anti-inflammatory agents, see chapter 9.

Antimicrobial Herbs

Antimicrobials help the body destroy or resist pathogenic microorganisms. They help the body strengthen its own resistance to infective organisms and throw off the illness.

Antispasmodic Herbs

Antispasmodics ease muscle cramps. They alleviate muscular tension and, as many are also nervines, can ease psychological tension as well. Some antispasmodic herbs reduce muscle spasms throughout the body, and some work on specific organs, systems, or types of tissue.

Astringents

Astringent herbs have a binding action on mucous membranes, skin, and other tissue, which translates to an ability to shrink tissues and reduce secretions. Astringent actions are related to the presence of chemicals called tannins, so named because they are used in tanning leather. They precipitate protein molecules, reducing irritation and inflammation and creating a barrier against infection that is helpful in wounds and burns.

Bitters

Bitter-tasting herbs play a special role in preventive medicine. The bitter taste triggers a sensory response in the central nervous system, which sends a message to the gut. The gut in turn releases digestive hormones that lead to a range of effects, including stimulation of appetite and a general stimulation of the flow of digestive juices. Bitters also aid the liver in its detoxification work, increase bile flow, and stimulate gut self-repair mechanisms.

Cardiac Remedies

This is a general term for herbs that have beneficial actions on the heart and circulatory system. Some of the remedies in this group are powerful cardioactive agents, such as foxglove, while others are gentler, safer cardiotonic herbs, such as hawthorn and motherwort.

Carminatives

Plants rich in aromatic volatile oils, or carminatives, promote appropriate digestive system function, soothing the gut wall, reducing inflammation, easing griping pains, and helping the body eliminate gas from the digestive tract.

Demulcents

Herbs high in mucilage, known as demulcents, soothe and protect irritated or inflamed tissue. They reduce irritation throughout the length of the bowel, reduce sensitivity to potentially corrosive gastric acids, help prevent diarrhea, and alleviate the muscle spasms that cause colic. They also ease coughing by soothing bronchial tension and relax painful spasms of the bladder.

Diaphoretics

Diaphoretics promote perspiration, helping the body to eliminate wastes through the skin. Some produce observable sweating, while others enhance normal background perspiration. They often promote dilation of surface capillaries, thus helping to improve poor circulation. This action is especially relevant in the treatment of fever.

Diuretics

Diuretics increase the production and elimination of urine. In herbal medicine, with its ancient traditions, the term is often applied in a general way to herbs that have a beneficial action on the urinary system. They help the body eliminate waste and support the whole process of inner cleansing.

Emmenagogues

Emmenagogues stimulate menstrual flow and function. In most herbals, however, the term is used in a wider sense to indicate a remedy that normalizes and tones the female reproductive system.

Expectorants

Strictly speaking, expectorants are herbs that stimulate the removal of mucus from the lungs, but the term is also often used to refer to respiratory system tonics. There are two basic categories of expectorant herbs.

Stimulating expectorants irritate the bronchioles, causing expulsion of material.
Relaxing expectorants soothe bronchial spasms and loosen mucous secretions, helping with dry, irritating coughs.

Hepatics

Hepatics support the liver, improving function; in some cases, they also increase the flow of bile. In a broad holistic sense, hepatic herbs are of great importance because of the liver's fundamental role in health.

Hypotensives

These are plant remedies that lower abnormally elevated blood pressure.

Immunomodulators

These herbs assist with or are capable of modifying or regulating immune functions.

Laxatives

Laxatives stimulate bowel movements.

Nervines

Nervines act on the nervous system and can be subdivided into three groups.

Nervine tonics strengthen and restore nervous system function.
Nervine relaxants ease anxiety and tension by soothing both body and mind.
Nervine stimulants directly stimulate nerve activity.

Rubefacients

When applied to the skin, rubefacient herbs generate a localized increase in blood flow. They are often used to ease the pain and swelling of arthritic joints.

Tonics

Tonics nurture and enliven. Truly gifts of nature to a suffering humanity, these are whole plants that enliven whole human bodies. To ask how they work is to ask how life works!

Vulnerary Herbs

These remedies promote wound healing. While the term *vulnerary* is used mainly to describe herbs that heal skin lesions, the action is just as relevant for internal wounds, like stomach ulcers.

APPLYING THE MODEL

When selecting herbs for a given patient, many remedies present themselves as possible candidates. The problem remains: Which herbs will best address all the needs of a particular patient? The selection process can be summarized thus:

1. Through some competent diagnostic procedure, identify what physiological processes to address and in what way.
2. Select actions appropriate to address the physiological and pathophysiological processes identified through diagnosis.
3. Select relevant herbs based on their range of primary and secondary actions, thus ensuring the best fit for the needs of the patient.

The best way to approach the selection process is to follow a number of steps. This may seem a long and potentially tedious process when first starting out, but it becomes straightforward with practice.

1. List the signs and symptoms for each problem.
2. Interpret the processes behind the symptoms and the underlying pathology, and identify appropriate herbal actions to address them.
3. Using the reference lists in chapter 25, find herbs that may be helpful, based on their primary and secondary actions.
4. Identify body systems that would benefit from the use of tonic herbs and choose relevant tonics.
5. Are there any biochemical considerations? These might be positive indications for certain plants or clear contraindications.
6. Integrate the conclusions drawn in the previous steps and develop a prescription(s).
7. Identify other healing modalities and lifestyle issues that might support the actions of the herbs.

Identifying Primary and Secondary Actions

Secondary actions are additional actions that accompany the primary physiological effect of a plant. Problems may arise, however, when one tries to analyze the whole picture in a purely logical, reductionist manner. Exactly what *is* the primary action of a medicinal plant? In some cases this is obvious (for example, with an herb like senna), but in other cases, the choice is more a matter of degree. One individual may say that chamomile is primarily a relaxing nervine, while another might describe it as a carminative, anti-inflammatory herb.

When focusing on secondary actions, such decisions become even more subjective. Certain secondary effects may hover on a threshold of sorts, in that some people experience these effects fully and others not at all. This is largely why phytotherapy is as much an art as a science. We can learn the details, but it takes years of experience to become a *real* herbalist! (The only such people I've ever met were well into their 70s and wouldn't know a saponin from a satellite dish, but they were the most incredible herbal healers you can imagine.)

Identifying Relevant Tonics for Body Systems

This is where we can take advantage of the fact that some herbs show an affinity for certain organs, body systems, or even specific types of tissue. They work as tonics or nutrients for the areas involved and can be used freely.

Identifying Biochemical Considerations

Based on biochemical considerations, one might identify specific positive indications for certain plants or clear contraindications for other plants for a particular patient. This involves some degree of familiarity with phytochemistry and pharmacology. There are limits to how useful this is, as the effects of most of the herbal materia medica are not understood—either because biochemical research is lacking or because the known biochemistry does not immediately illuminate the mechanism at play.

Identifying Lifestyle Factors to Address

Human health and wholeness can rarely be adequately addressed by any one therapeutic modality, whether herbs, prescription drugs, acupuncture, or any other type of therapy. This book focuses on the herbal contribution to the therapeutic endeavor, but herbs cannot take the place of appropriate attention to a wide array of lifestyle issues.

Nutrition is often pivotal to health, but this does not mean that the individual should resort to taking dietary supplements. Instead, examine the person's normal diet to determine whether or not changes might be beneficial to healing. For example, the individual may need to alter the kinds of foods eaten, how they are cooked, or how they are eaten, among other factors.

Structural issues must also be recognized and addressed with an appropriate modality, such as osteopathy or chiropractic. Herbs cannot replace the therapeutic value of manipulation if it is indicated. On a less technical level, an assessment of exercise and movement in general is always indicated. However, this need not lead to a gym! A walk in the woods or a jog along a beach will provide not only exercise, but also the opportunity to be in nature, which is always healing.

Similarly, psychological issues should be recognized and addressed. The current vogue for pharmacological panaceas to address the emotional pain of life is very shortsighted. In my opinion, such problems require conscious and compassionate processing, not magic bullets— herbal or otherwise.

SELECTING RELEVANT HERBS

To illustrate the process to be followed in applying the model, we will look at two hypothetical case studies.

Example 1: Cystitis and Irritable Bowel Syndrome

The first step in applying the model to create a prescription for this hypothetical patient is to make a comparison of primary actions indicated for each component of the patient's condition. In this case, we will compare the primary actions indicated for cystitis with those indicated for irritable bowel syndrome. As this is a theoretical exercise, we have no other specific details on this individual's symptom picture.

Primary Actions Indicated for Cystitis

Antimicrobials appropriate for the urinary tract will help the immune system control and clear bacterial infection. Essential oil–rich diuretic plants are indicated because the oil is excreted via the kidney, thus directing it to the site of infection in the bladder

Anti-inflammatories soothe the symptom picture of pain and discomfort.

Astringents will help if there is any hematuria (blood in the urine).

Diuretics flush the urinary tract. Ideally, antimicrobial diuretics will be selected for this patient.

Antispasmodics may be necessary if there is much pain.

Primary Actions Indicated for Irritable Bowel Syndrome

Astringents will stop the diarrhea.

Bitters often normalize bowel function in such cases.

Anti-inflammatories reduce localized mucosal reactions.

Carminatives help with flatulence or colic.

Antispasmodics other than carminatives may be indicated if cramping is severe.

Nervines will help ease background stress involvement.

Actions that came up in both lists are especially relevant for this patient, and are *anti-inflammatory*, *astringent*, and *antispasmodic*. Other important actions are *antimicrobial*, *bitter*, *diuretic*, *carminative*, and *nervine*. This process of comparison gives us a basis for identifying herbs that will effectively deliver the desired primary and secondary actions.

In the herbal actions tables below, herbs that appear in more than one table are underlined to highlight the correlation. These tables summarize information provided in greater detail in chapter 25.

Table 12.2. Anti-Inflammatory Herbs and Secondary Actions

SECONDARY ACTION	HERBS
Antimicrobial	Achillea millefolium, Calendula officinalis, Hydrastis canadensis, Hypericum perforatum, Matricaria recutita, Mentha piperita, Populus tremuloides, Salvia officinalis, Solidago virgaurea
Antispasmodic	Anethum graveolens, Angelica archangelica, Apium graveolens, Asclepias tuberosa, Cimicifuga racemosa, Dioscorea villosa, Foeniculum vulgare, Glycyrrhiza glabra, Hypericum perforatum, Hyssopus officinalis, Lavandula officinalis, Matricaria recutita, Mentha piperita, Populus tremuloides, Sambucus nigra, Tilia platyphyllos, Trigonella foenum-graecum, Verbascum thapsus, Viburnum opulus, V. prunifolium
Astringent	Achillea millefolium, Aesculus hippocastanum, Agrimonia eupatoria, Calendula officinalis, Capsella bursa-pastoris, Geranium maculatum, Hydrastis canadensis, Plantago major, Populus tremuloides, Ranunculus ficaria, Salvia officinalis, Solidago virgaurea, Symphytum officinale, Tilia platyphyllos, Verbascum thapsus
Bitter	Achillea millefolium, Agrimonia eupatoria, Hydrastis canadensis, Matricaria recutita, Menyanthes trifoliata
Carminative	Achillea millefolium, Anethum graveolens, Angelica archangelica, Apium graveolens, Foeniculum vulgare, Glycyrrhiza glabra, Hyssopus officinalis, Lavandula officinalis, Matricaria recutita, Mentha piperita, Salvia officinalis, Solidago virgaurea, Tilia platyphyllos, Trigonella foenum-graecum
Diuretic	Achillea millefolium, Agrimonia eupatoria, Apium graveolens, Galium aparine, Menyanthes trifoliata, Plantago major, Sambucus nigra, Solidago virgaurea, Tilia platyphyllos, Zea mays
Nervine	Apium graveolens, Cimicifuga racemosa, Hypericum perforatum, Hyssopus officinalis, Lavandula officinalis, Matricaria recutita, Mentha piperita, Tilia platyphyllos, Viburnum prunifolium

Table 12.3. Antimicrobial Herbs and Secondary Actions

SECONDARY ACTION	HERBS
Anti-inflammatory	Artemisia absinthium, Calendula officinalis, Hypericum perforatum, Mentha piperita, Plantago major
Antispasmodic	Allium sativum, Carum carvi, Hypericum perforatum, Mentha piperita, Pimpinella anisum, Rosmarinus officinalis, Ruta graveolens, Salvia officinalis, Thymus vulgaris
Astringent	Achillea millefolium, Arctostaphylos uva-ursi, Carum carvi, Plantago major, Rosmarinus officinalis, Salvia officinalis, Thymus vulgaris
Bitter	Achillea millefolium, Artemisia absinthium, Gentiana lutea, Hydrastis canadensis, Ruta graveolens

SECONDARY ACTION	HERBS
Carminative	*Artemisia absinthium, Capsicum annuum, Carum carvi, Juniperus communis, Mentha piperita, Pimpinella anisum, Rosmarinus officinalis, Salvia officinalis, Thymus vulgaris*
Diuretic	*Achillea millefolium, <u>Arctostaphylos uva-ursi</u>, Juniperus communis, Plantago major*
Nervine	*Hypericum perforatum, Mentha piperita, Rosmarinus officinalis*

Table 12.4. Antispasmodic Herbs and Secondary Actions

SECONDARY ACTION	HERBS
Anti-inflammatory	*<u>Angelica archangelica</u>, Apium graveolens, Dioscorea villosa, Glycyrrhiza glabra, Hypericum perforatum, Hyssopus officinalis, Lavandula officinalis, <u>Matricaria recutita</u>, <u>Melissa officinalis</u>, Mentha piperita, Salvia officinalis, Sambucus nigra, Tilia platyphyllos*
Antimicrobial	*Carum carvi, Drosera rotundifolia, <u>Humulus lupulus</u>, Hypericum perforatum, Lavandula officinalis, <u>Matricaria recutita</u>, Mentha piperita, Pimpinella anisum, Pulsatilla vulgaris, Rosmarinus officinalis, Thymus vulgaris*
Astringent	*<u>Humulus lupulus</u>, Hypericum perforatum, Lycopus spp., Prunus serotina, Rosmarinus officinalis, Salvia officinalis, Tilia platyphyllos, <u>Viburnum opulus</u>, V. prunifolium*
Bitter	*Artemisia vulgaris, <u>Humulus lupulus</u>, <u>Matricaria recutita</u>*
Carminative	*<u>Angelica archangelica</u>, Anethum graveolens, Artemisia vulgaris, Carum carvi, Daucus carota, Foeniculum vulgare, <u>Humulus lupulus</u>, Hyssopus officinalis, Lavandula officinalis, Leonurus cardiaca, <u>Matricaria recutita</u>, <u>Melissa officinalis</u>, Mentha piperita, M. pulegium, Petroselinum crispum, Pimpinella anisum, Rosmarinus officinalis, Thymus vulgaris, Trigonella foenum-graecum, Valeriana officinalis, Verbena officinalis, Zingiber officinale*
Diuretic	*<u>Angelica archangelica</u>, Daucus carota, Lycopus spp., Petroselinum crispum, Sambucus nigra, Tilia platyphyllos*
Nervine	*Cimicifuga racemosa, Eschscholzia californica, <u>Humulus lupulus</u>, Hypericum perforatum, Hyssopus officinalis, Lactuca virosa, Lavandula officinalis, Leonurus cardiaca, Lobelia inflata, Lycopus spp., <u>Matricaria recutita</u>, <u>Melissa officinalis</u>, Mentha piperita, Passiflora incarnata, Piscidia erythrina, Pulsatilla vulgaris, Scutellaria lateriflora, Tilia platyphyllos, Valeriana officinalis, <u>Viburnum opulus</u>, V. prunifolium*

Table 12.5. Astringent Herbs and Secondary Actions

SECONDARY ACTIONS	HERBS
Anti-inflammatory	*<u>Agrimonia eupatoria</u>, Euphrasia officinalis, Filipendula ulmaria, Geranium maculatum, Plantago major, Polygonum bistortum, Quercus robur, Solidago virgaurea*
Antimicrobial	*Achillea millefolium, <u>Arctostaphylos uva-ursi</u>, Inula helenium, Quercus robur, Rosmarinus officinalis, Salvia officinalis, Solidago virgaurea*
Antispasmodic	*Lycopus spp., Prunus serotina, Rosmarinus officinalis, Salvia officinalis*
Bitter	*Achillea millefolium, <u>Agrimonia eupatoria</u>, Prunus serotina*
Diuretic	*Achillea millefolium, <u>Agrimonia eupatoria</u>, <u>Arctostaphylos uva-ursi</u>, Lycopus spp., Plantago major, Solidago virgaurea, Verbascum thapsus*
Nervine	*Prunus serotina, Rosmarinus officinalis*

Table 12.6. Bitter Herbs and Secondary Actions

SECONDARY ACTION	HERBS
Anti-inflammatory	*Achillea millefolium*, *Agrimonia eupatoria*, *Artemisia absinthium*, *Hydrastis canadensis*, *Matricaria recutita*
Antimicrobial	*Achillea millefolium*, *Artemisia absinthium*, *A. vulgaris*, *Hydrastis canadensis*, *Matricaria recutita*
Antispasmodic	*Marrubium vulgare*, *Matricaria recutita*, *Ruta graveolens*
Astringent	*Achillea millefolium*, *Agrimonia eupatoria*, *Hydrastis canadensis*
Carminative	*Artemisia absinthium*, *Matricaria recutita*
Diuretic	*Achillea millefolium*, *Agrimonia eupatoria*
Nervine	*Artemisia vulgaris*, *Matricaria recutita*

Table 12.7. Carminative Herbs and Secondary Actions

SECONDARY ACTION	HERBS
Anti-inflammatory	*Angelica archangelica*, *Apium graveolens*, *Artemisia absinthium*, *Matricaria recutita*, *Melissa officinalis*, *Mentha piperita*
Antimicrobial	*Allium sativum*, *Artemisia absinthium*, *Humulus lupulus*, *Juniperus communis*, *Matricaria recutita*, *Mentha piperita*, *Pimpinella anisum*, *Salvia officinalis*, *Thymus vulgaris*
Antispasmodic	*Allium sativum*, *Anethum graveolens*, *Angelica archangelica*, *Artemisia absinthium*, *Carum carvi*, *Leonurus cardiaca*, *Matricaria recutita*, *Melissa officinalis*, *Mentha piperita*, *Pimpinella anisum*, *Salvia officinalis*, *Thymus vulgaris*, *Valeriana officinalis*
Astringent	*Carum carvi*, *Humulus lupulus*, *Salvia officinalis*, *Thymus vulgaris*
Bitter	*Artemisia absinthium*, *Humulus lupulus*, *Matricaria recutita*
Diuretic	*Angelica archangelica*, *Apium graveolens*, *Juniperus communis*, *Petroselinum crispum*
Nervine	*Apium graveolens*, *Humulus lupulus*, *Leonurus cardiaca*, *Matricaria recutita*, *Melissa officinalis*, *Mentha piperita*, *Valeriana officinalis*

Table 12.8. Diuretic Herbs and Secondary Actions

SECONDARY ACTION	HERBS
Anti-inflammatory	*Agrimonia eupatoria*, *Apium graveolens*, *Eupatorium purpureum*, *Galium aparine*, *Iris versicolor*
Antimicrobial	*Achillea millefolium*, *Agathosma betulina*, *Arctostaphylos uva-ursi*, *Juniperus communis*
Astringent	*Achillea millefolium*, *Agrimonia eupatoria*, *Arctostaphylos uva-ursi*, *Cytisus scoparius*, *Galium aparine*, *Lycopus* spp.
Bitter	*Agrimonia eupatoria*, *Arctium lappa*
Nervine	*Apium graveolens*, *Lycopus* spp., *Tilia platyphyllos*

It becomes immediately apparent that there are many remedies with potential in this case. The final remedy selection for an actual patient will involve some research in primary-source herbals to clarify traditional uses of the remedies identified in this purely logical manner. Nature does not always follow human concepts of logic, so the experience of generations of herbal practitioners must be taken into account.

In the following example, I am suggesting a prescription that is designed for a person experiencing only a moderate severity of both problems.

Herbs Relevant to Cystitis and Irritable Bowel Syndrome

Agrimonia eupatoria (agrimony)
Angelica archangelica (angelica)
Arctostaphylos uva-ursi (bearberry)
Humulus lupulus (hops)
Hydrastis canadensis (goldenseal)
Matricaria recutita (chamomile)
Melissa officinalis (lemon balm)
Viburnum opulus (cramp bark)

We have the choice of adjusting the prescription to emphasize different actions, depending on individual needs, by increasing the proportions of the most relevant herbs. This process is discussed in greater detail in the next section of this chapter, Dosage and Formulation Criteria.

Stronger urinary tract effects can be obtained by increasing the proportion of diuretic antimicrobials in the mixture. We can either increase the amount of *Arctostaphylos uva-ursi* (bearberry) or add another herb, such as *Agathosma betulina* (buchu). We may also consider adding a urinary tract demulcent, such as *Zea mays* (cornsilk) or *Althaea officinalis* (marshmallow leaf).

More focus on the irritable bowel problem will result from a greater emphasis in the prescription on bitters, astringents, or carminatives. For bitter carminatives, consider *Artemisia vulgaris* (mugwort), *A. absinthium* (wormwood), or *Achillea millefolium* (yarrow). For astringents, consider *Geranium maculatum* (cranesbill) or *Filipendula ulmaria* (meadowsweet).

More attention to anxiety issues may be needed. While herbs cannot replace relaxation or appropriate lifestyle changes, stronger nervines will help. Specifics will depend upon the individual concerned, but *Valeriana officinalis* (valerian) might be helpful for this hypothetical patient.

Thus, we arrive at a possible prescription for our theoretical patient.

Prescription for Cystitis and Irritable Bowel Syndrome

Arctostaphylos uva-ursi	2 parts
Viburnum opulus	2 parts
Agrimonia eupatoria	2 parts
Angelica archangelica	1 part
Humulus lupulus	1 part
Hydrastis canadensis	1 part

Dosage: up to 5 ml of tincture three times a day

We will also recommend that the patient drink an infusion of *Matricaria recutita* (chamomile) or *Melissa officinalis* (lemon balm) often throughout the day. Table 12.9 illustrates the actions supplied by the specific herbs in this combination.

Table 12.9. Actions Supplied by Prescription for Cystitis and Irritable Bowel Syndrome

ACTION	HERBS
Diuretic	*Agrimonia eupatoria, Angelica archangelica, Arctostaphylos uva-ursi*
Antimicrobial	*Arctostaphylos uva-ursi, Humulus lupulus, Hydrastis canadensis*
Astringent	*Agrimonia eupatoria, Hydrastis canadensis, Viburnum opulus*
Bitter	*Agrimonia eupatoria, Humulus lupulus, Hydrastis canadensis, Matricaria recutita*
Anti-inflammatory	*Agrimonia eupatoria, Angelica archangelica, Hydrastis canadensis, Matricaria recutita, Melissa officinalis*
Carminative	*Angelica archangelica, Humulus lupulus, Matricaria recutita, Melissa officinalis*
Antispasmodic	*Angelica archangelica, Humulus lupulus, Matricaria recutita, Melissa officinalis, Viburnum opulus*
Nervine	*Humulus lupulus, Matricaria recutita, Melissa officinalis, Viburnum opulus*

Example 2: A Complex of Conditions

Now we will apply a similar process to a hypothetical patient with a much more complicated pathological picture. This patient has uterine fibroids, premenstrual syndrome (PMS), hypertension, and constipation. The following table illustrates the primary actions needed in order to address each part of the complex.

Table 12.10. Herbal Actions Needed for Specific Conditions

CONDITION	SIGN/SYMPTOM	ACTIONS NEEDED
Uterine fibroids	Dysmenorrhea	Anti-spasmodic, uterine tonic, hormonal normalizer
	Menorrhagia (and, possibly, anemia)	Astringent, uterine tonic, hormonal normalizer
	Abdominal congestion	Diuretic, uterine tonic, hormonal normalizer, lymphatic, circulatory stimulant, peripheral vasodilator
Premenstrual tension	Psychological symptoms (irritability, agitation, fatigue, depression, anxiety, palpitations)	Nervine relaxant, hormonal normalizer
	Neurological symptoms (headache, vertigo)	Nervine relaxant, hormonal normalizer
	Edema	Diuretic, hormonal normalizer
	Skin problems	Alterative, hormonal normalizer
Hypertension	Often	Hypotensive asymptomatic
Constipation	Difficult or infrequent passage of feces	Laxative

All of the actions mentioned above can be categorized into two groups, as illustrated in table 12.11. The choice of herbs from the first group (for symptom relief) depends upon the individual's symptom picture, which will also affect the strength of remedies chosen and their proportions in the final prescription. The herbs in the second group are, of course, more pivotal to the healing process.

Table 12.11. Actions Indicated for Complex of Conditions

PRIMARILY SYMPTOMATIC RELIEF	MORE FUNDAMENTAL HEALING ACTIONS
Antispasmodic	Uterine tonic
Astringent	Hormonal normalizer
Nervine relaxant	Alterative
Diuretic	Lymphatic
Hypotensive	Circulatory stimulant
Laxative	Peripheral vasodilator

Table 12.12. Possible Herb Choices for Hypothetical Patient

ACTION	HERBS
Antispasmodic	*Dioscorea villosa, Cimicifuga racemosa, Viburnum prunifolium*
Astringent	*Vinca major, Geranium maculatum, Achillea millefolium*
Nervine relaxant	*Scutellaria* spp., *Tilia platyphyllos, Leonurus cardiaca*
Diuretic	*Taraxacum officinale, Galium aparine, Achillea millefolium*
Hypotensive	*Crataegus* spp., *Tilia* spp., *Achillea millefolium*
Laxative	*Rumex crispus*
Uterine tonic	*Mitchella repens, Caulophyllum thalictroides*
Hormonal normalizer	*Vitex agnus-castus*
Alterative	*Cimicifuga racemosa, Galium aparine, Rumex crispus*
Lymphatic	*Galium aparine*
Circulatory stimulant	*Zanthoxylum americanum*

The most important contraindication in this case would be for anthraquinone-containing laxatives, such as senna. These are too stimulating to the musculature of the abdomen and would worsen pain related to uterine cramping. From a review of the conditions present in this hypothetical person, it should be apparent that tonic support is needed for the following body systems:

- Reproductive
- Nervous
- Cardiovascular
- Digestive

Thus, by incorporating tonics and effectors, we can develop two specific formulas for this patient, one to address the symptoms and underlying pathologies of uterine fibroids, hypertension, and constipation and one for PMS. These prescriptions can be altered in a number of ways, depending upon the therapeutic interpretation made by the practitioner.

Hypothetical Prescription for Fibroids, Hypertension, and Constipation

Vinca major	2 parts
Dioscorea villosa	2 parts
Caulophyllum thalictroides	1 part
Vitex agnus-castus	1 part
Rumex crispus	1 part
Crataegus spp.	1 part
Galium aparine	1 part
Tilia spp.	1 part
Viburnum opulus	1 part

Dosage: 5 ml of tincture three times a day

Hypothetical Prescription for PMS

Scutellaria lateriflora	2 parts
Cimicifuga racemosa	1 part

Dosage: 5 to 15 ml of tincture as needed for PMS symptoms

Table 12.13. Actions Supplied by Hypothetical Prescriptions

ACTION	HERBS
Uterine tonic	*Caulophyllum thalictroides, Cimicifuga racemosa*
Uterine astringent	*Vinca major*
Alterative	*Galium aparine, Cimicifuga racemosa, Caulophyllum thalictroides*
Antispasmodic	*Cimicifuga racemosa, Scutellaria lateriflora, Tilia* spp., *Viburnum opulus*
Lymphatic	*Galium aparine*
Nervine	*Scutellaria lateriflora, Tilia* spp., *Cimicifuga racemosa*
Antispasmodic	*Scutellaria lateriflora, Valeriana officinalis, Cimicifuga racemosa*
Diuretic	*Galium aparine, Crataegus* spp., *Tilia* spp.
Uterine tonic	*Cimicifuga racemosa, Vitex agnus-castus*
Hormonal normalizer	*Vitex agnus-castus*
Hypotensive	*Crataegus* spp., *Tilia* spp., *Viburnum opulus*

The final step in addressing the myriad issues presented by this patient is to identify other healing modalities and lifestyle changes that will support the healing actions of the herbs.

DOSAGE AND FORMULATION CRITERIA

An aspect of phytotherapy that often seems cloaked in mystery is the process of formulating prescriptions and determining dosages. What guidelines does the practitioner use in deciding upon dosages or proportions to use when combining the selected remedies? Here I shall attempt to give this process some structure. For readers who disagree, or apply a different sequence of considerations, please remember that this is only one phytotherapist's opinion.

Phytotherapy does not provide the same clear, quantitative, and logical criteria for dosage and prescribing that clinical pharmacology provides. Depending upon the perspective of the practitioner, this can be viewed either as a benefit or as a failing. For the student, it is undoubtedly problematic, but for the practitioner with some experience, it becomes evident that this relative looseness provides valuable flexibility.

As with the selection criteria we use to choose the herbs in the first place, we must integrate considerations about the plants themselves with the patient's therapeutic issues.

Physiological impact of the herb. The strongest effector herbs should usually be prescribed in smaller amounts, while gentle normalizers can be prescribed at higher dosages.

Desired therapeutic effects. This issue is theoretically difficult to quantify, as desired effects will vary with each individual and, potentially, even with each consultation. However, the following points offer a few guidelines.

- The dosage of herbs intended to have the greatest effect can often be increased.
- Tonics and mild normalizing herbs should generally be used in higher proportions.
- Additive effects, such as the cumulative effect of all astringent herbs in a prescription, must be taken into account.

Age or constitution of the patient. The younger or frailer a patient is, the lower the dosage that should be used. As discussed in more detail later, this may not be important if only normalizers are prescribed.

Convenience and simplicity. This can be important for patients who may have trouble complying with the prescribed regimen.

As long as potentially toxic herbs are avoided, it is safe to say that exact dosage is usually not too critical. The problem is often that too little is prescribed, rather than too much. From my British perspective, the dosages used in North America are absurdly low, the reason probably being (in most cases) expense rather than any therapeutic criteria. To clarify what I mean here, we can generalize about dosage by using three roughly defined categories.

Normalizers. These are herbs that can also be considered foods (such as *Urtica dioica* and *Galium aparine*), are usually used in dosages of 2 to 4 g of herb or 2 to 4 ml of tincture three times a day, so it is not critical to be exact.

Stronger herbs. These effectors are given in a dosage range of 1 to 2 g of herb or 1 to 2 ml of tincture, which means that one should take some care, but there is no need to get paranoid. An overdose may confer too much of the desired action, but no toxicity. Examples include *Chelone glabra* and *Drosera rotundifolia*.

Extremely strong herbs. These are effector herbs that are used in dosages of less than 1 ml of tincture. *This dosage range must be taken very seriously!* This category includes herbs such as *Lobelia inflata* and *Convallaria majalis*, for which accuracy is essential or the patient will suffer the consequences. Most of the medicinal plants that fall into this category are rarely used in modern phytotherapy, and most are not discussed in a therapeutic context in this book.

One of the most common arguments put forth by pharmacologists against the use of herbal medicines becomes relevant here. Pointing to the variable amounts of active constituents that occur naturally in plants, the pharmacologist will say that it is impossible to accurately prescribe or ensure a standardized dosage protocol. As phytotherapy is founded upon the use of normalizers or, at most, effectors that do not contain potent constituents, this issue is irrelevant. However, it becomes very pertinent when discussing potentially toxic plants. The inherent variability in plant constituent levels makes establishing appropriate dosage extremely problematic when using such strong plants.

The "Part" as a Unit of Measurement

European herbalists use the metric system of measurement, and so milliliters (ml) and grams (g) are the units used in dispensing herbs. The North American use of drops or dropperfuls is both confusing and quantitatively inaccurate. The size of a drop is variable, as it depends on the size of the hole in the dropper and other factors.

The prescriptions presented in this book have been developed using the concept of measurement known as the *part.* Using parts allows for great flexibility in creating formulations. One part can represent 1 ml of tincture or 1 g of dried herb. The main drawback to this easy method is that when mixing different kinds of preparations, one must still keep specific dosage considerations in mind. For example, a fluid extract is much more concentrated than a tincture, so combining tinctures with fluid extracts will necessitate some math to ensure that appropriate levels of each herb are used. In other words, if the fluid extract is twice as strong as the tincture, only half as much should be used.

Two related issues to consider are convenience for the dispensary and ease of use for the patient. It does not matter how good a prescription is; it will not work if the patient does not take it. The following points provide some guidelines on simplifying the measurement of doses.

A dosage of 5 ml is roughly equivalent to 1 teaspoonful. This makes a single dose easy to take, and can contribute greatly to patient compliance.

A dosage of 5 ml taken three times a day amounts to 105 ml a week. This can usually be rounded down to 100 ml a week, making calculating and dispensing a simple matter.

There is no need for a 5 ml single dose to consist purely of tincture. For children, or when using stronger effectors, the 5 ml dose can be made up partly with water, thus maintaining the ease of use while still lowering dosage. The prescription writer or dispenser must perform the calculation and physical measurements, as the whole point is to make the patient's experience as straightforward as possible.

In the examples that follow, we will assume that the herbs are in equivalent forms.

A Prescription for Irritable Bowel Syndrome

Myrica cerifera	2 parts
Artemisia vulgaris	1 part
Matricaria recutita	1 part
Mentha piperita	1 part
Dioscorea villosa	1 part
Valeriana officinalis	1 part

Dosage: 5 ml of tincture three times a day

In this particular case, the prescription assumes that diarrhea is a dominant component of the symptom picture and thus includes a larger proportion of *Myrica cerifera*, an effective astringent. If colic pain was a major issue, then the proportion of antispasmodic and nervine remedies might be increased.

A Prescription for Osteoarthritis

Menyanthes trifoliata	2 parts
Filipendula ulmaria	1 ½ parts
Cimicifuga racemosa	1 part
Zanthoxylum americanum	1 part
Apium graveolens	1 part
Angelica archangelica	1 part
Achillea millefolium	1 part

Dosage: 5 ml of tincture three times a day

This combination includes antirheumatic herbs with a range of relevant actions, but the emphasis is on the *Menyanthes* because it has such a good effect in osteoarthritis. *Filipendula* serves as a source of salicylates that does not irritate the stomach, and so is included in a larger proportion.

A Prescription for Psoriasis

Arctium lappa	1 part
Rumex crispus	1 part
Galium aparine	1 part
Scutellaria lateriflora	1 part

Dosage: up to 5 ml of tincture three times a day

The herbs are included in equal proportions here, as none of the limiting criteria comes into play. There are no strong effectors and no overriding therapeutic concerns.

A Prescription for Psoriasis with Anxiety and Tension

Arctium lappa	1 part
Rumex crispus	1 part
Galium aparine	1 part
Valeriana officinalis	1 part
Verbena officinalis	1 part

Dosage: up to 5 ml of tincture three times a day

In this case, the nervine component has been increased by replacing the *Scutellaria* with *Valeriana* and *Verbena*. The inclusion of *Verbena* is based upon its combination of relaxing nervine and hepatic actions. On the other hand, the percentage of *Scutellaria* could have been increased to 2 or 3 parts to achieve a similar increased nervine effect without the hepatic action.

A Prescription for Unresponsive Psoriasis

Arctium lappa	2 parts
Rumex crispus	2 parts
Smilax spp.	2 parts
Verbena officinalis	2 parts
Phytolacca americana	1 part

Dosage: 5 ml of tincture three times a day

Because a stronger alterative combination was needed, the prescription includes the effector *Phytolacca americana*. The best way to work out the parts when using strong effectors is to assign a 1-part proportion to the strongest herb and increase the proportions of the other herbs. This prescription, for example, includes 1 part of *Phytolacca* and 2 parts each of the other herbs.

A Prescription for Premenstrual Syndrome

Scutellaria lateriflora	2 parts
Valeriana officinalis	1 part
Taraxacum officinale leaf	1 part

Dosage: 5 ml of tincture as needed to alleviate symptoms

Prescription II for Premenstrual Syndrome

Vitex agnus-castus	2 parts
Cimicifuga racemosa	1 part

Dosage: 5 ml of tincture once a day throughout menstrual cycle

Notice that the dosage instructions for the first formula include the term "as needed." This is a recognition of the cyclical nature of the stress response; each person will find different times of the day more challenging than others. As this is largely symptomatic medication, the dosage may be increased until the patient experiences relief. The dosage regimen may be altered as necessary, changing the size of the dose and varying the time of day at which it is taken to suit individual needs. For example, the patient may take a large dose first thing in the morning or smaller amounts at frequent intervals throughout the day.

The patient's experience is the guiding principle here. Always treat the human being, not the theory behind the disease!

Dosage Considerations for the Elderly

As the body ages, a number of factors alter the way it utilizes substances. This can have a significant impact on determining appropriate dosages for elderly people. In the context of the selection criteria used throughout this book, such considerations are rarely an issue. The focus on tonics and gentle effector herbs allows the phytotherapist largely to avoid potential toxicity.

In the context of orthodox medicine, however, these considerations are very important when prescribing drugs with a narrow therapeutic index. They become even more significant for people who are frail or malnourished. The main concern is pharmacokinetic changes that affect how drugs are excreted from the body. The three primary factors involved here are normal physiological processes related to aging, pathophysiological changes, and iatrogenic causes.[1]

Normal Physiological Changes Related to Aging

Older people are smaller, have a higher percentage of body fat, and have less body water content.

The rate of absorption in the elderly is reduced, but not the amount of absorption. The elderly have decreased stomach acidity and intestinal blood flow. The amount of time it takes to empty the stomach also slows as a person ages. These changes decrease the rate, but not the amount, of absorption. This may delay the onset of action and peak effect of medications.

Gastric acid secretion is reduced at a rate of about 5% per decade after age 50.

Renal function declines. This is the most important age-related pharmacokinetic change. The efficiency of this vital function declines by approximately 10% per decade after age 40. A number of factors influence this:

- Reduction in glomerular filtration rate in the nephrons
- Reduction in renal blood flow
- Decrease in active tubular secretion in the nephrons

Hepatic metabolism and clearance of many drugs decline at approximately 1% per year after age 40. There is a relative reduction in Phase I metabolism, as compared with Phase II (see chapter 9 for more information).

Pathophysiological Changes

A number of disease processes can produce changes in normal functioning that have a direct impact on a whole range of pharmacokinetic factors. The specifics are complex and vary from disease to disease and drug to drug. In general, however, the most important are kidney diseases, liver and gallbladder diseases, and heart disease.

Iatrogenic Causes

Iatrogenic problems are those induced inadvertently by a physician, surgeon, medical treatment, or diagnostic procedure. Many common problems are caused by drug interactions. Other obvious examples are surgery and dialysis. Keep in mind that herbs and herbalists can also be the cause of such problems. However, if the phytotherapist follows the approach presented in this book, the risk of causing iatrogenic problems is minimal.

Dosage Adjustments for Children

Children have special needs, and special plants address these needs. As with the elderly, the herbal focus should be on tonics and gentle effectors. The healing capacity of children can be quite incredible, but attention must be paid to proper dosage. Obviously, a lower dosage will be required for children.

Appropriate dosage for children varies according to age, and a number of mathematical formulae have been developed to facilitate this. For our purposes, however, it will not be necessary to get out the calculator. Dosage proportionate to age can be adequately approximated using a method developed many years ago by Dr. Young; this is illustrated in table 12.14. There are some exceptions to this general rule, but they involve medicinal plants that the FDA has restricted.

Table 12.14. Dosage Adjustments for Children[2]

AGE	PROPORTION OF ADULT DOSE	EXAMPLES
Adult	1	1.0 g, 2.0 g, 10.0 g, 1.0 ml
12 years old	$1/2$	0.5 g, 1.0 g, 5.0 g, 0.5 ml
8 years old	$2/5$	0.4 g, 0.8 g, 4.0 g, 0.4 ml
4 years old	$1/4$	0.25 g, 0.5 g, 2.5 g, 0.25 ml
2 years old	$1/8$	0.125 g, 0.25 g, 1.25 g, 0.125 ml
1 year old	$1/16$	0.0625 g, 0.125 g, 0.625 g, 0.0625 ml

With the advent of potent modern pharmaceuticals, dosage measurements became much more critical. A number of methods have been developed to cope with the need for such accuracy. The British National Formulary provides three ways of arriving at an appropriate dosage for children.[3]

Age-Related Adjustment

This is a more refined version of Dr. Young's method.

Table 12.15. Dosage Adjustment by Age

AGE	IDEAL BODY WEIGHT (kg/lb)	HEIGHT (mm/in)	BODY SURFACE (m²)*	PERCENTAGE OF ADULT DOSE
Newborn	3.4 / 7.5	500 / 20	0.23	12.5
1 month	4.2 / 9	550 / 22	0.26	14.5
3 months	5.6 / 12	590 / 23	0.32	18
6 months	7.7 / 17	670 / 26	0.40	22
1 year	10 / 22	760 / 30	0.47	25
3 years	14 / 31	940 / 37	0.62	33
7 years	23 / 51	1200 / 47	0.88	50
12 years	37 / 81	1480 / 58	1.25	75
Adult female	56 / 123	1626 / 64	1.6	100
Adult male	68 / 150	1727 / 68	1.8	100

*m² (meters squared) is a measurement of body surface area.

Calculation by Body Weight

This method is another way to calculate an appropriate dose, but bear in mind that young children may require a higher dose per kilogram of body weight than adults because of their higher metabolic rates.

Basic Conversion Formula

$$\frac{\text{Patient's weight in kg [x] adult dose}}{70}$$

or

$$\frac{\text{Patient's weight in lb [x] adult dose}}{150}$$

Body Surface Measurements

These are a challenge to calculate, but it is amazing what you can do with a calculator. For the sake of completeness, here is the formula. I am not necessarily recommending that you try to measure the surface area of any young child of your acquaintance!

Basic Conversion Formula

$$\frac{\text{Surface area of patient (m}^2) \text{ [x] adult dose}}{1.8}$$

OUTLINE OF TREATMENT CHAPTERS

The second half of this book delves into herbal approaches to the plethora of pathologies that practitioners are called upon to treat. Each of these body system treatment chapters follows the same basic format, which is explained here. This basic format, along with the information provided in chapters 25 and 26, gives the practitioner a structure upon which to build throughout a lifelong exploration of medical herbalism.

The treatment discussions are organized as follows.

Name of the Pathology or Condition

This will reflect the terminology most commonly used in Western medicine.

Definition

The medical definitions are taken from either *The Merck Manual* or *The Merriam-Webster Medical Dictionary*.

Condition Overview

Here I provide a brief description of the condition, including relevant information for the herbalist about etiology, signs and symptoms, and prognosis. These brief introductions in no way intended to replace a comprehensive text on Western medicine that describes the pathology and its treatment in Western orthodox medicine.

Treatment of the Condition

This is a discussion of herbal selection issues to consider in developing a prescription for the condition, with an emphasis on tonic needs. Harnessing the toning and nurturing potential of herbs can be best facilitated by identifying which body systems, organs, or tissues will benefit most. This ability to tone and nurture is unique and one of the most important contributions that herbal remedies make to wellness and healing.

Actions Indicated

This provides a discussion of relevant herbal actions indicated for the processes underlying the disease entity, along with a rationale for their inclusion.

Specific Remedies

This section identifies plants that have an established tradition of use for the particular condition. I have based their selection on British usage, but as far as possible, I have included insights from the American tradition as well.

Traditional use implies demonstrable efficacy. The research scientist may consider this "mere" empirical observation and thus not scientifically valid. To the medical herbalist, on the other hand, information about traditional use provides evidence that the herb has valuable effects. These observations are based upon clinical tests performed by generations of people in the most challenging of environments: the sickroom. If certain herbs were ineffective, these practitioners would have tried something else, as they had no vested interest in proving a belief system.

However, traditional knowledge does not explain the effects produced, nor does it indicate the processes that underlie the plant's effects or any wider impact upon human physiology. This is where modern, investigative science has so much to offer—much more than can be achieved through scientific attempts to either justify or debunk the clinical use of herbs.

A Prescription for the Condition

Here I offer a suggested herbal combination that incorporates the ideas developed earlier. This is not intended as a formulaic treatment for the pathology, but rather as an example of how to build on ideas about relevant actions, tonics, biochemistry, and specific remedies to arrive at an appropriate treatment.

It is important to remember that a given prescription is in no way the "correct" or only solution. In all cases, many possible herbal choices exist. Part of the skill of the phytotherapist is the ability to engage in a therapeutic dance with the complex of variables at play. A useful exercise is to compare treatment approaches suggested by a number of herbal clinicians. When the works of herbalists within the Western tradition are compared and contrasted, it often becomes clear that the differences in herbs used are only apparent disagreements. Usually, you will find that the practitioners employed similar therapeutic criteria and that the differences simply reflect the richness of the herbal materia medica. Students (including all of us herbalists) should embrace such differences as an opportunity for developing comprehension and insight.

Actions Supplied by the Prescription

The prescription suggestion is followed by an analysis of the herbal remedies in terms of their actions. This is intended to clarify why these particular herbs were included, and, I hope, to illuminate ways in which the combination may be adjusted or altered. Except for the specifics discussed above, the herbs selected for inclusion in the prescriptions are open to challenge. However, the actions supplied are pivotal to success. By knowing which herbs supply the necessary actions, the practitioner is able to select alternative plants that still ensure the appropriate blend of herbal actions for the condition.

Broader Context of Treatment

Phytotherapy cannot be holistic unless it is used within a relevant broader context appropriate for both the individual and the condition involved. In this section, I offer suggestions concerning other therapeutic modalities, nutrition, and lifestyle issues to augment the herbal treatment.

References

1. Bennett JC, Plum F, eds. *Cecil Textbook of Medicine*, 20th edition. Philadelphia: Saunders, 1996.

2. Osol A, ed. *Remington's Pharmaceutical Sciences*, 15th ed. Easton, PA: Mack, 1975.

3. *British National Formulary*. London: Pharmaceutical Society of Great Britain, 1966.

13

THE DIGESTIVE SYSTEM

Herbal medicine is uniquely suited for the treatment of digestive system illnesses. Throughout human evolution, our food has been our medicine, ensuring that the healing properties of the herbs we consume have a direct effect on the lining of the alimentary canal. Herbs affect digestive system function not only through absorption and metabolism of the whole range of plant chemicals, but also through direct actions upon the tissue of the gut.

Much of the digestive system illness in our society is due simply to abuse. Today's average diet contains a preponderance of overly processed foods and has a high content of chemical additives. The gastrointestinal tract is subject to direct chemical irritation from alcohol, carbonated drinks, and tobacco. In this context, it is easy to see why herbal remedies can be so helpful in treating the various inflammations and reactions that plague abusers. The direct soothing action of demulcents, healing properties of astringents, and general toning of bitters have much to offer in reversing such damage.

However, as with all true healing, any potential "cure" lies beyond the range of medicines, whether herbal or synthetic. The healing process must incorporate lifestyle changes to eliminate dietary indiscretions and chemical abuses as well as reduce stress. Herbal medicine can bring about dramatic improvements in even profound digestive system problems, but the potential to maintain these benefits long term lies in the hands of the person seeking treatment.

Used within such a broad context, herbal medicine offers specific remedies for particular pathological syndromes as well as tonics and normalizers that can help prevent problems from manifesting in the first place. It is possible to treat these problems within a context of general nurturing that speeds improvement and helps reestablish health and harmony. In the hands of a skilled phytotherapist, much can be achieved therapeutically. While the array of factors will be different for each individual with, for example, a gastric ulcer, it is possible to identify some general herbal guidelines.

Of all herbal traditions, that of using herbs to aid digestion has remained the most prominent in the memory of modern Europe. Whether culinary herbs such as rosemary or medicinal liqueurs like vermouth and chartreuse, therapeutic remedies are used in large quantities. The very name *vermouth* comes from the bitter herb wormwood. Herbs maintain their foothold in official pharmacopoeias as major therapeutic agents, in the form of digestive bitters, carminatives, and laxatives of varying strengths.

The ideal is to preserve health and maintain wellness, rather than merely treat illness. Of course, there is much more to preventive medicine than consuming medicinal substances, whether medicinal plants or chemical drugs. We can help put this in perspective by recalling the World Health Organization (WHO) definition of health:

> Health is a state of complete physical, emotional, mental and social well being and not merely the absence of disease or infirmity.

This should serve to remind us that any attempt to promote wellness and prevent the development of disease must address the whole complex of factors that WHO identified. While we cannot explore this concept in depth in this book, it nonetheless can help us to identify a number of risk factors that can be minimized, as well as positive factors to be emphasized. As the focus of this book is on herbs and their safe use, we shall address the non-herbal issues only in passing. This is not meant to imply that they are less significant, but is simply a reflection of space constraints.

HERBS AND GOOD DIET

By far the most important contribution made by plants to the health of the human digestive system is in the quality of the foods we eat. Often the only real difference between a salad vegetable and a medicinal herb is that one tastes better! The body requires more than 40 nutrients for energy, growth, and tissue maintenance. All of these are found in a well-rounded diet, and many of them are found both in medicinal herbs and in plants eaten as grains, vegetables, or fruits. Of course, eating a balanced diet is a major contributing factor to a healthy lifestyle. Using medicinal herbs does not negate the importance of eating a high-quality diet.

Water

As the most plentiful component in the body, water is also crucial to survival. It is the medium for bodily fluids such as blood and lymph, in which forms it transports nutrients into cells and carries out waste products and toxins.

Carbohydrates

Carbohydrates, proteins, and fats—a group of dietary components known as macronutrients—provide fuel in the form of calories. Carbohydrates, the body's main energy source, can be divided into two types. *Simple carbohydrates* are sugars; *complex carbohydrates* include starches, such as those found in potatoes and bread.

Proteins

Proteins support tissue growth and repair and help produce antibodies, hormones, and enzymes, which are essential for all chemical reactions in the body. Dietary protein sources include meat, fish, dairy products, poultry, dried beans, nuts, and eggs.

Fats

Dietary fat protects internal organs, provides energy, insulates against cold, and helps the body absorb certain vitamins. There are three kinds of fats. *Saturated fats* are found in meat, dairy products, and coconut oil. *Monounsaturated fats* occur in olive, peanut, and canola oils; *polyunsaturated fats* are found in corn, cottonseed, safflower, soy, and sunflower oils.

A very important group of polyunsaturated fats are the essential fatty acids (EFAs) known as arachidonic acid, linoleic acid, and alpha-linolenic acid. Linoleic and arachidonic acid are the basis of the omega-6 EFAs, and alpha-linolenic acid is the basis of the omega-3 EFAs. They are essential to the human diet because they cannot be synthesized in the body from other nutrients. Essential fatty acids are necessary for the formation of healthy cell membranes, the proper development and functioning of the brain and nervous system, and the production of the eicosanoids (thromboxanes, leukotrienes, and prostaglandins).

Linoleic acid is found primarily in seeds, nuts, grains, and legumes. Alpha-linolenic acid is found in green leaves, phytoplankton and algae, and selected seeds, nuts, and legumes. Arachidonic acid is obtained from meat, and the important omega-3 EFA eicosapentaenoic acid is found in fish.

Vitamins and Minerals

The diet also supplies the important micronutrients known as vitamins and minerals. They are needed only in trace amounts, but an absence or deficiency of just one vitamin or mineral can cause major illness.

Dietary Fiber

The body also needs a supply of dietary fiber, the indigestible portion of plant foods. A high-fiber diet reduces the risks of various gastrointestinal problems and promotes cardiovascular health.

The official dietary guidelines, established jointly by the U.S. Departments of Agriculture and Health and Human Services, include seven basic recommendations.

1. Eat a variety of foods. This will help ensure that you get enough calories, protein, and fiber, as well as the vitamins, minerals, and other nutrients you need.
2. Control your weight. Keep within recommended weight limits for your age, sex, and build. Obesity is defined as being 20% above normal weight.
3. Eat a low-fat, low-cholesterol diet. Ideally, no more than 30% of daily calories should come from fat, and no more than 10% should come from saturated fat. Choose polyunsaturated fats over saturated fats when possible.
4. Eat plenty of vegetables, fruits, and grains. They are rich in nutrients, fiber, and complex carbohydrates but low in fat. More than half of one's daily calories should come from carbohydrates, and 80% of these calories should come from complex carbohydrates.
5. Eat sugar in moderation. Sugar is high in calories and promotes tooth decay.
6. Use salt in moderation. Too much salt increases the risk of developing high blood pressure. Prepared foods are often high in salt or other forms of sodium.
7. If you drink alcohol, do so in moderation. Alcohol provides calories but no nutrients, and too much is harmful.

When one eats a consistently well-balanced diet of fresh fruits, vegetables, grains, and some animal protein, nutritional supplementation is unnecessary. Multinutrient supplements may be of value when eating well poses a challenge—and can be indispensable during pregnancy and times of disease, injury, and extreme stress or physical exertion.

FIBER

Dietary fiber is largely composed of the cellulose-like components of plant cell walls. Its composition varies from plant to plant, but it always comprises a complex of constituents. This fiber is the part of fruits, vegetables, and grains that the body cannot digest. *Soluble fiber* dissolves easily in water and takes on a soft, jellylike texture in the intestines. *Insoluble fiber* passes almost unchanged through the intestines.

Both soluble and insoluble fiber helps make stools soft and easy to pass. Fiber also prevents constipation. As this natural complexity is missing from supplements, they cannot replace a diet rich in high-fiber foods. The importance of dietary fiber in human health is well established.

An abundance of research confirms the association between fiber and human health. Table 13.1 highlights a variety of conditions associated with a low-fiber diet.

Table 13.1. Diseases Associated with a Low-Fiber Diet

TYPE OF DISORDER	SPECIFIC CONDITIONS
Metabolic	Obesity, gout, diabetes, kidney stones, gallstones
Cardiovascular	Hypertension, cerebrovascular disease, ischemic heart disease, varicose veins, deep vein thrombosis, pulmonary embolism
Colon	Constipation, appendicitis, diverticulosis, diverticulitis, hemorrhoids, colon cancer, irritable bowel syndrome, ulcerative colitis, Crohn's disease
Other	Dental caries, autoimmune disorders, pernicious anemia, multiple sclerosis, thyrotoxicosis, dermatological conditions

A high-fiber diet is associated with a decreased incidence of most of the degenerative diseases of Western society. This is not related simply to fiber content. A high-fiber diet is generally high in other important nutrients as well, most of which are also deficient in the typical Western diet. The best source of dietary fiber is whole foods, although specific types of fibers have a role in the treatment of specific diseases. There is no substitute for a

Benefits of Dietary Fiber

Shortens intestinal transit time

Delays gastric emptying, resulting in reduced after-meal elevations of blood sugar

Increases satiety

Stimulates pancreatic secretions

Increases stool weight

Improves solubility of bile

Elevates numbers of beneficial intestinal microflora

Raises production of short-chain fatty acids

Lowers serum lipid levels

healthy diet—a diet composed of foods in a form as close to their original as possible. The American Dietetic Association recommends that 20 to 35 g of fiber be consumed each day. Table 13.2 illustrates the amount of fiber in many commonly eaten foods.

Table 13.2. Dietary Fiber Content of Selected Foods

FOOD	SERVING	GRAMS OF FIBER
Fruits		
Apple (with skin)	1 medium	3.5
Banana	1 medium	2.4
Cantaloupe	1/4 melon	1.0
Cherries, sweet	10	1.2
Grapefruit	1/2 medium	1.6
Orange	1 medium	2.6
Peach (with skin)	1	1.9
Pear (with skin)	1/2 large	3.1
Prunes	3	3.0
Raisins	1/4 cup	3.1
Raspberries	1/2 cup	3.1
Strawberries	1 cup	3.0

FOOD	SERVING	GRAMS OF FIBER
Vegetables, Raw		
Bean sprouts	1/2 cup	1.5
Celery, diced	1/2 cup	1.1
Cucumber	1/2 cup	0.4
Lettuce	1 cup	0.9
Mushrooms	1/2 cup	1.5
Pepper, green	1/2 cup	0.5
Spinach	1 cup	1.2
Tomato	1 medium	1.5
Vegetables, Cooked		
Asparagus, cut	1 cup	2.0
Beans, green	1 cup	3.2
Broccoli	1 cup	4.4
Brussels sprouts	1 cup	4.6
Cabbage, red	1 cup	2.8
Carrots	1 cup	4.6
Cauliflower	1 cup	2.2
Corn	1/2 cup	2.9
Kale	1 cup	2.8
Parsnip	1 cup	5.4
Potato (with skin)	1 medium	2.5
Potato (without skin)	1 medium	1.4
Spinach	1 cup	4.2
Sweet potato	1 medium	3.4
Zucchini	1 cup	3.6
Legumes		
Baked beans	1/2 cup	8.8
Dried peas, cooked	1/2 cup	4.7
Kidney beans, cooked	1/2 cup	7.3
Lima beans, cooked	1/2 cup	4.5
Lentils, cooked	1/2 cup	3.7
Navy beans, cooked	1/2 cup	6.0

FOOD	SERVING	GRAMS OF FIBER
Rice, Breads, Pasta, and Flour		
Bran muffins	1 muffin	2.5
Bread, white	1 slice	0.4
Bread, whole wheat	1 slice	1.4
Crisp bread, rye	2 crackers	2.0
Rice, brown, cooked	1/2 cup	1.0
Rice, white, cooked	1/2 cup	0.2
Spaghetti, cooked	1/2 cup	1.1
Spaghetti, whole wheat, cooked	1/2 cup	3.9
Breakfast Cereals		
All-Bran	1/3 cup	8.5
Bran Chex	2/3 cup	4.6
Corn Bran	2/3 cup	5.4
Cornflakes	1 1/4 cup	0.3
Grape-Nuts	1/4 cup	1.4
Oatmeal	3/4 cup	1.6
Raisin bran–type	2/3 cup	4.0
Shredded wheat	2/3 cup	2.6
Nuts		
Almonds	10 nuts	1.1
Filberts	10 nuts	0.8
Peanuts	10 nuts	1.4

From Michael Murray, N.D., *The Encyclopedia of Nutritional Supplements* (Roseville, Calif.: Prima Publishing, 1996).

TOBACCO

In addition to the well-known heart and lung diseases caused by tobacco, it is also responsible for changes in the digestive system. Smoking has been shown to impact all parts of the digestive system and to contribute to such common problems as heartburn and peptic ulcers. Increases in the risk of Crohn's disease and possibly even gallstones have also been observed. While most of these effects on the digestive system appear to be reversible, they send a clear message: Tobacco impairs digestive system health.

Heartburn

Heartburn occurs when acidic digestive juices splash from the stomach into the esophagus, a process known as *reflux*. Normally, a muscular valve at the lower end of the esophagus keeps the acid solution in the stomach and out of the esophagus. Smoking weakens this valve, allowing the contents of the stomach to flow backward into the esophagus. Smoking also may directly injure the esophagus, making it more prone to corrosive damage from refluxed material.

Peptic Ulcer

A peptic ulcer is an open sore in the lining of the stomach or the duodenum, the first part of the small intestine. The exact cause of ulcers is not known. A relationship between smoking cigarettes and ulcers, especially duodenal ulcers, does exist. The 1989 Surgeon General's report stated that ulcers are more likely to occur, less likely to heal, and more likely to cause death in smokers than in nonsmokers.

Liver Disease

Among a multitude of other vital functions, the liver processes drugs, alcohol, and other toxins to remove them from the body. Smoking impairs the ability of the liver to handle these substances. Some research also suggests that smoking can aggravate the course of liver disease caused by excessive alcohol intake.

Crohn's Disease

Crohn's disease causes inflammation deep in the lining of the intestine. The disease, which is associated with pain and diarrhea, usually affects the small intestine, but it can occur anywhere in the digestive tract. Both current and former smokers have a higher risk of developing Crohn's disease than do nonsmokers. Smoking is associated with higher rates of relapse, repeat surgeries, and immunosuppressive treatments.

DIGESTIVE SYSTEM DISORDERS

A number of overall processes, patterns, and symptoms are seen in conditions affecting the digestive system. By knowing herbal approaches to take in addressing general patterns, the herbalist will go a long way toward understanding treatments for specific pathologies. However, the phytotherapist's role is not merely to alleviate the discomfort caused by specific symptoms. The focus, as in all holistic approaches to health, must go beyond the treatment of symptoms.

Table 13.3. Primary Actions for the Digestive System

ACTION	HERBS
Demulcent	*Symphytum officinale, Althaea officinalis, Ulmus rubra, Glycyrrhiza glabra*
Bitter	*Artemisia absinthium, Gentiana lutea, Hydrastis canadensis*
Milder bitter	*Achillea millefolium, Matricaria recutita*
Astringent	*Agrimonia eupatoria, Geranium maculatum, Filipendula ulmaria, Myrica cerifera*
Carminative (aromatics)	*Foeniculum vulgare, Zingiber officinale, Mentha piperita, Matricaria recutita, Melissa officinalis*
Anti-inflammatory	*Matricaria recutita*
Antispasmodic	*Matricaria recutita, Valeriana officinalis, Viburnum opulus, Dioscorea villosa,* carminatives
Aperient and laxative	*Rumex crispus, Senna alexandrina, Taraxacum officinale*
Hepatic and cholagogue	*Taraxacum officinale, Chelone glabra,* bitters
Nervine	*Matricaria recutita, Valeriana officinalis, Artemisia vulgaris*
Anthelmintic	*Artemisia absinthium, Dryopteris filix-mas*
Other Actions	As needed to ensure good general health

FLATULENCE

Everyone produces gas and eliminates it by burping or passing it through the rectum. On average, most people produce 1 to 3 pints of gas a day and pass gas at least 14 times a day. Most people do not realize that passing gas 14 to 23 times a day is normal. Gas is made up primarily of odorless vapors: carbon dioxide, oxygen, nitrogen, hydrogen, and sometimes methane. The unpleasant odor of flatulence comes from bacteria in the colon that release small amounts of sulfur-containing gases.

Intestinal gas comes from two main sources: swallowed air and the breakdown of undigested foods by bacteria naturally present in the colon. Air swallowing *(aerophagia)* is a common cause of gas in the stomach. We all swallow some air when eating and drinking. However, eating or drinking rapidly, chewing gum, smoking, or wearing loose dentures may lead to the intake of more air. Burping is the usual way air leaves the stomach, but any remaining gas moves into the small intestine, where it is partially absorbed. A small amount travels into the large intestine for release through the rectum.

Certain carbohydrates are not digested and absorbed in the small intestine because the body lacks enzymes necessary to break them down. This undigested food passes into the large intestine, where bacteria may break it down, producing the gases hydrogen, carbon dioxide, and, in about one third of all people, methane. Research has not provided any answers as to why some people produce methane and others do not. In addition, foods that produce gas in one person may not cause gas in another.

Which Foods Cause Gas?

Fats and protein cause little gas, but foods containing carbohydrates may produce gas.

Sugars

The sugars that cause gas include raffinose, lactose, fructose, and sorbitol.

Raffinose is present in large amounts in beans. Smaller amounts are found in cabbage, brussels sprouts, broccoli, asparagus, certain other vegetables, and whole grains.

Lactose, the sugar in milk, is found in all milk products, including cheese and ice cream, and processed foods, such as bread, cereal, and salad dressing. Many people have low levels of the enzyme lactase, which is needed to digest lactose. As people age, levels of lactase may decrease.

Fructose is naturally present in onions, artichokes, pears, and wheat. It is also used as a sweetener in some soft drinks.

Sorbitol is a sugar found naturally in fruits, including apples, pears, peaches, and prunes.

Starches

Most starch sources, such as potatoes, corn, noodles, and wheat, produce gas as they are broken down in the large intestine. Rice is the only starch that does not cause gas.

Fiber

Soluble fiber dissolves easily in water and takes on a soft, gel-like texture in the intestines. Found in oat bran, beans, peas, and most fruits, soluble fiber is not broken down until it reaches the large intestine, where digestion causes gas. Insoluble fiber, on the other hand, passes essentially unchanged through the intestines and produces little gas. Wheat bran and some vegetables contain insoluble fiber.

CONSTIPATION

Infrequent or hard stools, or difficulty passing stools. May involve pain during the passage of a bowel movement, the inability to pass a bowel movement after straining or pushing for more than 10 minutes, or no bowel movements after more than 3 days. (*The Merriam-Webster Medical Dictionary*)

Constipation can be defined as difficult or infrequent passage of feces. It must be seen as a symptom, not a disease state in its own right. Proper diagnosis is thus vitally important. Acute constipation constitutes a definite, recognizable change for an individual, and an abrupt change in bowel habits can indicate the presence of organic disease. In chronic constipation, however, there is an ongoing problem with normal bowel movements. In such cases, the ideal is to normalize and regularize bowel movements through dietary change.

The most common cause of constipation in Western cultures is lack of dietary fiber. However, there are some important but less common causes that the practitioner should bear in mind. Examples range from irritable bowel syndrome, diverticular disease, and serious infections (for example, appendicitis) to painful anal conditions that make people afraid to open their bowels. The condition may be congenital, or may be caused by endocrine disorders, nervous system conditions, or diseases of the large intestine. Other possible causes of chronic constipation include drugs or toxins that affect bowel motility, long periods of immobility, stress, and depression. Whenever a specific cause can be determined, it should be treated.

There are many herbs that can help alleviate the discomfort of constipation. Rather than discuss all of the individual plant species, we instead can generalize about appropriate herbal actions. Laxative remedies are obviously relevant, but others must be considered. For example, bitters may be very helpful because they cause a general stimulation of the digestive process. When stress or depression is a factor, consider relaxing nervine, antispasmodic, and antidepressant herbs.

A number of different types of laxative herbs may be used. *Bulk laxatives* are fiber-rich foods and herbs that offer the only truly safe, long-term treatment possibilities. They act slowly and gently and are best used by gradually increasing the dose taken every morning and evening until a softer, bulkier stool is achieved. *Secretory laxatives* promote bowel movement through stimulation of bile production in the liver. (Hepatic herbs act as secretory laxatives.) *Stimulant laxatives* are anthraquinone-containing herbs that stimulate peristaltic movement directly via an impact on the nerve ganglia of the gut. Carminatives may be helpful in easing the pain and discomfort that is often associated with constipation.

Laxatives

Laxatives promote defecation, relieving constipation. As noted, constipation itself is not a disease, but rather a symptom that may result from any of a broad range of underlying causes. In addition to the possible causes discussed earlier, constipation may be related to a variety of subjective factors, such as stress and diet, or from a patient's impression of what constitutes "normal" bowel habits.

Normal size, frequency, and consistency of fecal output are difficult to quantify and are subject both to personal variation and to sociological patterning, of which the makers of laxatives take full advantage. There is no distinct advantage to having frequent bowel movements. While having a bowel movement once daily may be considered average, having one several times a day to once every several days may also be seen as normal. If hepatic function is normal, fear of "autointoxication" due to retention of colon contents is unfounded.

However, increased hardness of feces and reduced colonic motility, frequency, and bulk do occur, mainly due to dehydration of material that remains too long in the colon before expulsion. Bulk, softness, and hydration of feces are very dependent on the fiber and water content of the diet. Thus, sufficient intake of dietary fiber and water is a mainstay in any regimen for the treatment of constipation.

Types of Laxatives

The precise mechanisms by which laxatives work remain uncertain because of the complex factors that affect colonic function. However, there are three main ways in which laxatives work.

1. Cause retention of fluid in the contents of the colon, thereby increasing bulk and softness and facilitating transit due to their hydrophilic or osmotic properties.
2. Reduce net absorption of water and salt through both direct and indirect actions on the colonic mucosa.
3. Increase intestinal motility, decreasing the absorption of salt and water because of decreased transit

time. Indeed, abnormal colonic motility may be a contributing factor in constipation.

Bulk-Forming Agents

Bulking and swelling agents are gentle laxatives that simulate the physiologic effects of a high-fiber diet. Bulk-forming agents are widely recognized for their value in the long-term management of irritable bowel disease and chronic diverticulitis. These agents, which can be utilized as supplements to dietary fiber, are polysaccharides and celluloses derived from grains, seed husks, or kelp and include bran, psyllium, methylcellulose, and carboxymethylcellulose.

Bulking agents are normal components of food. Indigestible carbohydrates, which undergo complete or partial breakdown by the intestinal flora, physically stimulate activity through their bulking action, speeding the transit of material through the intestinal tract. Swelling agents are distinguished by their capacity to form mucilage or gels. Mucilaginous swelling agents are generally taken in some medicinal form (for example, psyllium husks) rather than as foods per se. Like bulking agents, they are composed of indigestible carbohydrates, but they undergo little or no degradation by intestinal flora. Bulk-forming laxatives have little effect on transit time through the small intestine, but they do affect colonic transit time. The heavier the stool weight, the shorter the colonic transit time.

These agents also stimulate bowel motility by modifying the intestinal flora. The colon is inhabited by more than 400 species of bacteria. The precise makeup of this intestinal flora is determined by the nature of the available substrate. Fecal bulk provides the bacteria with a substrate for proliferation, which causes an increase in bacterial mass and stool weight. Because the bacteria are specific to particular substrates, a latency period of four to six weeks is needed in order to establish a more suitable intestinal flora.

Human digestive enzymes do not affect the celluloses, hemicelluloses, lignins, and pectins contained in bulk-forming agents, so these pass unchanged through the small intestine into the colon. There, bacteria break down all or part of the bulk materials, releasing short-chain fatty acids, along with methane, carbon dioxide, and molecular hydrogen. The short-chain fatty acids promote the absorption of salts and water and provide osmotic stimuli that encourage motility. Swelling agents also soften the stool, facilitating passage through the bowel.

Gases generated in the lower bowel may cause bloating and flatulence, and constipation may initially worsen when bulking agents are introduced. Generally, this issue is resolved once a new intestinal flora is established. Starting treatment with half the normal dosage may be helpful. It is imperative that bulk-forming agents always be taken with sufficient quantities of liquid, as esophageal and intestinal obstruction can occur when fluid intake is inadequate.

A few other cautions are in order. Intestinal obstruction and impaction may occur after the administration of bulk-forming agents, especially for patients with preexisting gastrointestinal disease. People with gastrointestinal stenosis (narrowing of passages or sphincters), ulcerations, or adhesions should also avoid these agents.

Dietary Fiber

Sources of dietary fiber include whole grains, bran, vegetables, and fruits. Plant cell walls consist of varying quantities of fibrous polysaccharides (mainly cellulose), matrix polysaccharides (pectins and hemicelluloses), lignins, cutin, waxes, and some glycoproteins that are resistant to breakdown in the digestive tract. Dietary fiber acts as a laxative by several mechanisms.

Dietary fiber binds water and ions in the colonic lumen, thereby softening the feces and increasing their bulk. However, the water-binding capacity of fiber is insufficient to combat secretory diarrhea.

Dietary fiber can support the growth of colonic bacteria, thereby increasing fecal mass.

Some components may be digested by colonic bacteria to metabolites that contribute to laxative action by adding to the osmotic activity of the luminal fluid.

Colonic fermentation of water-soluble, non-cellulose polysaccharides (such as pectins and gums) can decrease stool water, apparently by producing metabolites (such as short-chain fatty acids) that directly influence colonic mechanisms of fluid and electrolyte transport.

Foods differ widely both in fiber content and in the type of fiber they contain. Grains and cereals contain a preponderance of insoluble, poorly fermentable fibers; their ingestion shortens intestinal transit time and increases stool bulk. Fruits and vegetables contain more water-soluble fibers that result in a moist stool, but have less effect on transit time. Usually, 20 to 60 g of dietary fiber is a sufficient daily intake.

Psyllium, lignin, and pectin bind bile acids, which reduces the rate of their reabsorption by the intestine and promotes excretion. The consequent enhancement of hepatic synthesis of bile acids from cholesterol may reduce plasma levels of low-density lipoprotein (LDL) cholesterol. Over time, bulk-forming agents can help relieve symptoms of irritable bowel syndrome and diverticular disease.

Osmotic Agents

Osmotic laxatives are chemicals that cause water to be retained in the bowel through osmosis, thus increasing the water content of the stool. This mechanism underlies the action of nonabsorbable sugars, such as mannose, and sugar alcohols, including mannitol and sorbitol.

Anthraquinone Laxatives

Many well-known laxative plants owe their efficacy to the presence of polyphenolic "anthranoid" compounds. These anthraquinone laxatives include 1,8-dihydroxyanthraquinone and its glycoside derivatives, which are contained in senna, cascara sagrada, and rhubarb, as well as aloe and other members of the Liliaceae family. Senna is obtained from the dried leaflets or pods of *Senna alexandrina* and other species. Cascara sagrada ("sacred bark") is obtained from the bark of the buckthorn tree, *Rhamnus purshiana.*

Anthraquinone laxatives exert their effects by damaging epithelial cells, leading to changes in absorption, secretion, and motility. Damaged epithelial cells can be found as apoptotic bodies in darker pigmented colonic mucosa, a symptom of the condition called *pseudomelanosis coli.* Pseudomelanosis coli is caused by chronic use (in other words, abuse) of anthraquinone laxatives, and has recently been associated with an increased risk of colorectal carcinoma. In vitro and animal studies show that anthraquinone laxatives have a potential role in both initiating and promoting tumorigenesis. Studies in humans have also suggested that these laxatives have tumor-promoting properties.[1]

Although clinical evaluations of the long-term toxicity of anthraquinones have yielded conflicting results, preparations that contain 1,8-dihydroxyanthraquinone itself have been withdrawn from the market, because the chemical has been associated with hepatic and intestinal tumors in laboratory animals. Whether the naturally occurring glycosides cause similar problems is not known.

Although the short-term use of these substances is generally safe, long-term use cannot be recommended. They may cause an excessive laxative effect, leading to abdominal pain and griping. Chronic use of large doses may produce nephritis. Anthraquinone-containing herbs are contraindicated for people with partial or complete bowel obstruction, as well as for women who are pregnant or nursing. Interactions with cardiac glycosides and other drugs may occur indirectly as a result of electrolyte imbalances. Most of the metabolites are excreted in the stool; however, a fraction is absorbed and appears in the urine, turning the urine a dark yellow or even red. In nursing mothers, anthraquinone metabolites can give breast milk a brownish tinge.

Castor Oil

The bean of the castor plant, *Ricinus communis*, contains two well-known noxious ingredients: an extremely toxic protein, ricin, and an oil known as castor oil. Used externally, castor oil is a bland emollient, but within the small intestine, the action of pancreatic enzymes releases ricinoleic acid. Ricinoleic acid and its salts reduce the absorption of fluid and electrolytes and stimulate intestinal peristalsis, and hence the movement of feces. Because castor oil acts in the small intestine, accumulation of fluid and evacuation take place rapidly and are relatively complete. The cathartic effect is too strong to warrant use of this agent for common constipation.

Appropriate Use of Laxatives

In otherwise healthy patients, laxatives are of secondary importance to a fiber-rich diet, adequate fluid intake, appropriate physical activity, and other non-pharmacological means of preventing and treating constipation. If such measures are inadequate, they may be supplemented with bulk-forming agents. Stimulant laxatives should be used only in unresponsive cases.

When laxatives are employed in the treatment of constipation, they should be administered in the lowest effective dosage as infrequently as possible, and be discontinued promptly and completely when no longer needed. If constipation is drug-induced, lowered dosage or use of alternative drugs should be attempted before using laxative medication.

The use of laxatives is no substitute for treatment of an underlying disease of which constipation is a symptom. Valid uses of laxative agents include maintaining soft feces, preventing straining at the stool (especially in the elderly and patients with cardiac disease or hernia), and evacuating the bowel prior to diagnostic or surgical procedures. Laxatives frequently are indicated both before and after surgery to maintain soft feces for patients with hemorrhoids and other anorectal disorders.

For these purposes, dietary fiber or bulk-forming agents are generally satisfactory and preferable. A fiber-rich diet and related laxative agents also have an established role in the management of diverticular disease of the colon and irritable bowel syndrome. In addition to perpetuating dependence on drugs, the laxative habit may set the stage for serious gastrointestinal disturbances. Irritable bowel syndrome and other functional ills have been associated with the habitual use of stimulant laxatives.

Treatment of Constipation

As with many other functional problems of the digestive system, many specific herbs have been used to treat constipation by different herbalists in different cultures. As constipation is a symptom, there are no true specific treatments. Effective, commonly used herbs include *Rumex crispus* (yellow dock) and *Plantago ovata* (psyllium seed).

A Prescription for Constipation

Rumex crispus	2 parts
Taraxacum officinale root	2 parts
Pimpinella anisum	1 part

Dosage: up to 5 ml of tincture three times a day

A stronger combination including anthraquinone-containing herbs, such as senna, may be appropriate in some cases. However, a dietary approach focusing on the rational use of fiber is the most effective. I stress the word *rational* here, because becoming an oat bran addict is not far from drug abuse!

DIARRHEA

Frequent, loose, and watery bowel movements. *(The Merck Manual)*

As with constipation, diarrhea is an important symptom that can have many causes. These range from intestinal infection and food sensitivities to colitis and anxiety, highlighting again the importance of accurate diagnosis and the dangers of simply alleviating symptoms without addressing underlying causes. Diarrhea caused by colitis, for example, should be treated differently from the traveler's diarrhea dubbed "Delhi belly" or its New World relative, "Montezuma's revenge."

Technically speaking, the term *diarrhea* refers to loose, watery stools that occur more than three times in one day. This is a common problem that usually lasts a day or two and goes away on its own without any special treatment. However, prolonged diarrhea can be a sign of other problems. It can also cause dehydration, a condition in which the body lacks adequate fluid to function properly. Dehydration is particularly dangerous in children and the elderly, and it must be treated promptly to avoid serious health problems.

Diarrhea may be a temporary or a chronic problem. A few of the more common causes of diarrhea are listed here:

Bacterial infections caused by consumption of contaminated food or water; common culprits include *Campylobacter, Salmonella, Shigella,* and *Escherichia coli*

Viral infections, including rotavirus, Norwalk virus, cytomegalovirus, herpes simplex virus, and viral hepatitis

Food intolerances, such as intolerance of lactose, the sugar found in milk

Parasites, including *Giardia, Entamoeba,* and *Cryptosporidium*

Reactions to medicines, including antibiotics, antihypertensives, and antacids containing magnesium

Intestinal diseases, such as inflammatory bowel disease

Functional bowel disorders, for example, irritable bowel syndrome, in which the intestines do not work properly

Diarrhea may be accompanied by cramping pain, bloating, nausea, or an urgent need to use the bathroom. Fever or bloody stools may also be present. Acute diarrhea lasts less than three weeks and is usually related to an infection. Chronic diarrhea lasts longer than three weeks and is often related to functional disorders, like irritable bowel syndrome, or disease, such as inflammatory bowel disease.

Diarrhea is potentially dangerous in newborns and infants, as it can lead to dehydration. General signs of dehydration include thirst, less frequent urination, dry skin, fatigue, and light-headedness. Signs in children are dry mouth and tongue, absence of tears when crying, dry diapers for three hours or more, high fever, listlessness or irritability, skin that does not flatten when pinched and released, and sunken abdomen, eyes, or cheeks.

The fluid and electrolytes (especially potassium and sodium) lost during diarrhea must be replaced, as the body cannot function properly without them. Water is essential to prevent dehydration, but it does not contain electrolytes. To maintain electrolyte levels, drink chicken or beef broth, which contains sodium, and fruit beverages, which contain potassium. For children, use a rehydration solution that contains these necessary nutrients. Such solutions are available without a prescription.

Treatment of Diarrhea

In most cases, replacing lost fluid to prevent dehydration is the only treatment necessary for diarrhea. Medicines that stop diarrhea may be helpful in some cases, but they are not recommended for people with diarrhea caused by bacteria or parasites, as stopping the diarrhea will trap the organism in the intestines and prolong the problem.

Until diarrhea subsides, avoid milk products and foods that are greasy, high in fiber, or very sweet, as they tend to aggravate diarrhea. As the condition improves, add soft, bland foods, such as bananas, plain rice, boiled potatoes, toast, crackers, cooked carrots, and baked chicken with no skin or fat. For children, pediatricians recommend what is called the BRAT diet, which stands for *bananas, rice, applesauce,* and *toast.*

Specific Remedies

Many astringent herbs have a reputation as a specific for diarrhea. Whether they are specifics or simply good examples of herbs with general astringent effects is difficult to say. *Filipendula ulmaria* (meadowsweet) may well be the best gentle overall treatment for diarrhea, as it seems to tone the lining of the small intestine. It is especially helpful for childhood diarrhea. Other excellent remedies are *Agrimonia eupatoria, Alchemilla* spp., and *Geranium maculatum.* Stronger astringents, such as *Quercus* spp. (oak bark), should be used only as a last resort.

A Prescription for Diarrhea

Agrimonia eupatoria	1 part
Geranium maculatum	1 part
Matricaria recutita	1 part

Combine dried herbs and prepare as an infusion; drink regularly throughout the day until symptoms subside.

APHTHOUS ULCERS

Acute painful ulcers on the movable oral mucosa, occurring singly or in groups. Also called "canker sores." *(The Merck Manual)*

These painful ulcers can appear singly or in clusters almost anywhere in the mouth. They are usually between 1 and 15 mm in diameter, have regular borders, and may be covered in a pseudomembrane. Aphthous ulcers generally heal within 7 to 21 days, but can be a recurrent problem for some people, a condition known as recurrent aphthous stomatitis, or RAS.

The etiology of this condition is unclear, but it is associated with lowered immune response, either locally or as a sign of a systemic problem. Stress is also strongly implicated, as are food sensitivities and nutritional deficiencies. A variety of other types of mouth ulcers often occur in people infected with human immunodeficiency virus (HIV), and may be associated with fungal, bacterial, or viral infections, or with cancer, such as non-Hodgkin's lymphoma. However, the discussion here focuses only on aphthous ulcers.

Treatment of Aphthous Ulcers

The herbal treatment guidelines given here for aphthous ulcers are best seen in the context of the general health of the mouth, stomach, and digestive tract. A stress component indicates the important role played by the nervous system.

Actions Indicated

Anti-inflammatories play a core role by reducing the localized mucosal reaction.

Antimicrobials inhibit the development of infection or prevent the spread of bacteria to the rest of the body, which can occur due to impaired buccal immune response.

Immune system support is necessary if the ulcers suggest a systemic problem.

Alteratives will help with any metabolic problems that might be present.

Demulcents help soothe and relieve symptoms.

Nervines and *adaptogens* assist the individual in coping with stress; counseling may also be indicated.

Specific Remedies

A number of specific remedies for aphthous ulcers are well known. A primary specific is *Salvia officinalis* var. *rubia* or var. *purpurea* (red sage). This is a variety of ordinary sage that contains a stronger volatile oil. While it is rarely used in cooking, it makes a perfect herb to use as a mouthwash for aphthous ulcers and other inflammatory conditions of the mouth.

A Prescription for Aphthous Ulcers

Mouthwash:

Salvia officinalis var. *rubia*	1 part
Matricaria recutita	1 part

Combine dried herbs and prepare as an infusion, to be gargled often.

Internal use:

Echinacea spp.	1 part
Galium aparine	1 part
Calendula officinalis	1 part

Dosage: up to 3 ml of tincture three times a day

Table 13.4. Actions Supplied by Aphthous Ulcer Prescription

ACTION	HERBS
Antimicrobial	*Echinacea* spp.
Alterative	*Echinacea* spp., *Galium aparine*, *Calendula officinalis*
Lymphatic	*Galium aparine*, *Calendula officinalis*
Vulnerary	*Calendula officinalis*

Broader Context of Treatment

Iron, vitamin C, vitamin B complex, and zinc supplements can be very helpful, in some cases even enough to clear the problem. Dental attention may be important, as a tooth abscess or gum disease may be the focus of the underlying problem. Similarly, a history of stomach ulceration or other gastric problems must be considered. Diet is critical, as irritants of all kinds must be avoided. These include physical irritants, such as very hot or coarse foods, as well as the chemical irritants in acid and very spicy foods, alcohol, and tobacco.

PERIODONTAL DISEASE

Pyorrhea: Inflammation or degeneration of tissues that surround and support the teeth. *(The Merck Manual)*

Gingivitis: Inflammation of the gingivae, characterized by swelling, redness, change of normal contours, watery exudate, and bleeding. *(The Merck Manual)*

Pyorrhea, a type of periodontal disease, commonly begins as gingivitis, but on rare occasions may be the presenting complaint for more serious systemic diseases, including diabetes mellitus and leukemia. Ordinarily, the major causative factor is poor dental hygiene. Gingivitis is common in puberty and pregnancy, suggesting that hormones may also play a role.

Treatment of Periodontal Disease

These very localized conditions can have a profound effect on the health of the whole body. The American Academy of Periodontology has concluded that periodontal bacteria can enter the bloodstream, travel to major organs, and begin new infections. Research suggests that this may contribute to the development of heart disease and stroke, increase a woman's risk of having a preterm, low-birth-weight baby, and pose a serious threat to people whose health is compromised by diabetes, respiratory disease, or osteoporosis.[2]

Thus, tonic support is indicated for the mouth and gums, as well as the stomach and digestion. Decaying gum tissue will be swallowed constantly and can lead to secondary digestive upsets. Pyorrhea must be treated as a whole body issue that is focused in the mouth.

Actions Indicated

Antimicrobials are essential to reduce populations of bacteria that contribute to the decay process.

Anti-inflammatories reduce any localized mucosal reaction.

Astringents lessen local bleeding and other exudations.

Circulatory stimulants promote the circulation of blood in the gums, aiding in detoxification.

Immune system support is necessary if gum disease suggests a systemic problem.

Alteratives help the body deal with any systemic problems related to the disease.

Specific Remedies

Remember that any description of specific remedies for a particular condition reflects the accrued wisdom and experience gained through generations of herbal history. However, these remedies will not replace a balanced prescription that takes into account system support in addition to all of the herbal actions indicated.

With that in mind, *Commiphora molmol* (myrrh) may be considered a specific remedy here, as it has powerful antimicrobial effects against the pathogens that cause gum disease. In addition, *Krameria triandra* (rhatany), an astringent herb from Peru, has proved uniquely effective for gum disease. Some proprietary herbal toothpastes can help support treatment by supplying the indicated herbs in that form.

A Prescription for Pyorrhea

Gum application:

Commiphora molmol	1 part
Echinacea spp.	1 part
Krameria triandra	1 part

Combine tinctures and apply to the gums three times a day using a very fine brush. An infusion of buccal anti-inflammatory herbs, such as *Salvia* and *Matricaria*, may be used as a mouthwash. Do not swallow.

Internal use:

Echinacea spp.	1 part
Galium aparine	1 part
Zanthoxylum americanum	1 part

Dosage: up to 5 ml of tincture combination three times a day

The combination of herbs for internal use supplies the following actions to support the work of the gum application.

Table 13.5. Actions Supplied by Internal Pyorrhea Prescription

ACTION	HERBS
Antimicrobial	*Echinacea* spp.
Alterative	*Echinacea* spp., *Galium aparine*, *Zanthoxylum americanum*
Lymphatic	*Echinacea* spp., *Galium aparine*, *Zanthoxylum americanum*
Circulatory stimulant	*Zanthoxylum americanum*

Broader Context of Treatment

Herbal treatment will not replace necessary dental attention. Similarly, if pyorrhea suggests deeper systemic problems, these call for skilled diagnosis. Good personal dental hygiene is essential. Avoid refined carbohydrates in the diet. Flavonoids, such as quercetin, and procyanidins have been suggested as supplements.

The following supplements may be relevant adjuncts for the long-term treatment of periodontal disease.[3]

Vitamin C: 3 to 5 g/day
Vitamin E: 400 to 800 IU/day
Vitamin A: 20,000 IU/day
Selenium: 400 mcg/day
Zinc picolinate: 30 mg/day
Folic acid: 2 mg/day

ESOPHAGITIS AND GASTROESOPHAGEAL REFLUX

> Reflux of gastric contents into the esophagus leading to localized infection. *(The Merck Manual)*

This relatively common and unpleasant problem affects the lower esophageal sphincter (LES), the muscular valve connecting the esophagus with the stomach. The condition is technically known as *gastroesophageal reflux disease* (GERD), a term in which *gastroesophageal* refers to the stomach and esophagus and *reflux* means "to flow back." Therefore, gastroesophageal reflux indicates a return of the stomach's contents back up into the esophagus. The result is heartburn or acid indigestion.

Normally, the LES valve opens to allow food to pass

into the stomach and closes to prevent food and acidic stomach juices from flowing back into the esophagus. GERD occurs when the valve is weak or relaxes inappropriately, allowing the contents of the stomach to flow up into the esophagus. The severity of GERD depends on the degree of LES dysfunction, the type and amount of fluid brought up from the stomach, and the neutralizing effect of saliva.

Dietary and lifestyle choices contribute to the development of GERD. Certain foods and drinks, including chocolate, peppermint, fried or fatty foods, coffee, and alcoholic beverages, may weaken the LES, causing reflux and heartburn. Cigarette smoking also relaxes the valve. Other causes are obesity, pregnancy, and a structural weakness of the diaphragm known as hiatus hernia.

Heartburn is the main symptom, which is experienced as a burning pain that begins behind the breastbone and moves upward to the neck and throat. The patient may feel as if food is coming back into the mouth, leaving an acid or bitter taste. This sensation might last as long as two hours, and is often worse after eating. Lying down or bending over can also result in heartburn.

Heartburn pain is sometimes mistaken for the pain associated with heart disease or a heart attack, but there are differences. Exercise may aggravate pain resulting from heart disease, while rest may relieve the pain. Heartburn pain is less likely to be associated with physical activity.

Treatment of Gastroesophageal Reflux Disease

Treatment of GERD aims at decreasing the amount of reflux or reducing damage to the lining of the esophagus from refluxed materials. Lifestyle and dietary changes are effective for most people. First, however, we shall consider relevant herbs, and then the broader context of treatment.

Actions Indicated

Demulcents soothe and coat the tissue of the esophagus, insulating the mucosal lining against acidic gastric contents.
Anti-inflammatories reduce localized mucosal reactions.
Vulneraries aid the natural healing of ulcerations and other lesions.
Astringents lessen local bleeding and other exudatations.
Alteratives help the body deal with any systemic problems related to the disease.
Carminatives may be needed if there is general disruption of digestive process.

Caution: Bitters are contraindicated in the initial stages of treatment, as they stimulate the secretion of stomach acid as well as peristaltic activity.

Specific Remedies

Any specific remedies indicated for this condition will not replace a balanced prescription that takes into account all of the herbal actions indicated and system support. Demulcent vulnerary herbs have most to offer here. Otherwise, there are no specifics as such.

A Prescription for GERD

Althaea officinalis	2 parts
Calendula officinalis	1 part
Matricaria recutita	1 part

Dosage: up to 5 ml of tincture three times a day. In addition, an infusion of the anti-inflammatory herb *Matricaria*, sipped slowly throughout the day, can be helpful. As an alternative, a cold infusion of *Althaea* root can be taken whenever needed.

Table 13.6. Actions Supplied by GERD Prescription

ACTION	HERBS
Demulcent	*Althaea officinalis*
Lymphatic	*Calendula officinalis*
Vulnerary	*Calendula officinalis*
Astringent	*Calendula officinalis*
Anti-inflammatory	*Matricaria recutita, Calendula officinalis*
Carminative	*Matricaria recutita*

Broader Context of Treatment

The following simple advice will reduce much of the symptomatic discomfort associated with GERD while treating the underlying problem.

Raise the head of the bed to reduce heartburn; raising the head of the bed allows gravity to minimize reflux of stomach contents into the esophagus.
Avoid stooping and constricting pressure on the abdomen (such as very tight clothes).
Avoid foods and beverages that weaken the LES, including chocolate, peppermint, fatty foods, coffee, and alcoholic beverages. Substances that can irritate a damaged esophageal lining, such as citrus fruits and juices, tomato products, and pepper, should also be avoided.

Decrease the size of portions at mealtime. In addition, eating meals at least two hours before bedtime may lessen reflux by allowing stomach acid to subside and the stomach to empty partially.

Lose weight. Being overweight often worsens symptoms; many overweight people find relief when they lose weight.

Avoid alcohol, as it increases the production of gastric acid, contributing to general discomfort.

Stop smoking. Cigarette smoking weakens the LES.

Overall. Deal with stress, anxiety, and any systemic health problems.

Antacids neutralize acid in the esophagus and stomach and soothe heartburn. Nonprescription antacids provide temporary relief. However, their long-term use should be avoided, as it can lead to diarrhea, altered calcium metabolism, and buildup of magnesium in the body. Too much magnesium can be a serious problem for patients with kidney disease.

GASTRITIS

Superficial, mucosal lesions of the stomach that occur very rapidly in relation to a variety of stresses. *(The Merck Manual)*

A whole range of pathologies may underlie this common complaint. Strictly speaking, the term *gastritis* means inflammation of the gastric mucosa, the tissue that lines the stomach. A number of medical subdivisions are based upon the various pathological changes that can occur in the tissue, but from an herbal perspective, these distinctions are not crucial. The approach described here may be applied in all cases, unless there is another specific problem that is more pressing than the gastritis.

Treatment of Gastritis

With gastritis, inflammation is the primary focus when selecting relevant actions and herbs. There are a number of herbs that can help reduce inflammation, but these do not replace any dietary or lifestyle changes that might also be indicated.

Actions Indicated

Demulcents soothe the lining of the stomach, by either coating the stomach or exerting anti-inflammatory actions.

Antacids have little more to offer than symptomatic relief.

Anti-inflammatories reduce localized mucosal reactions.

Astringents lessen local bleeding.

Vulneraries enhance the stomach's natural wound-healing abilities.

Nervines help ease background stress involvement.

Alteratives help the body deal with any systemic problems related to the disease.

Specific Remedies

Vulnerary and demulcent remedies such as *Symphytum* root, *Althaea* root, and *Ulmus rubra* speed healing by soothing the tissue. *Matricaria recutita* is considered a specific for gastritis in folk treatments from Europe. *Filipendula ulmaria* and *Mentha piperita* act as antacids. Remember, however, that specifics never replace a balanced prescription that takes into account all of the herbal actions indicated as well as system support.

A Prescription for Gastritis

Althaea officinalis	3 parts
Filipendula ulmaria	1 part
Matricaria recutita	1 part

Dosage: Take tincture in divided doses, to 5 ml in total, three times a day. An infusion of *Matricaria* or *Melissa* sipped slowly throughout the day will also help.

Table 13.7. Actions Supplied by Gastritis Prescription

ACTION	HERBS
Demulcent	*Althaea officinalis*
Anti-inflammatory	*Filipendula ulmaria, Matricaria recutita*
Astringent	*Filipendula ulmaria*
Vulnerary	*Matricaria recutita*
Nervine	*Matricaria recutita*

Broader Context of Treatment

Lifestyle is fundamental to both the cause and the treatment of gastritis. It is essential to eliminate food irritants, including chemicals, extreme temperatures, and fiber. Acidic foods, alcohol, tobacco, and any other factor that elicits symptoms must also be avoided. Stress will aggravate or even bring on gastritis. Work conditions, background anxiety, and related issues must all be taken into consideration. These lifestyle factors are discussed in more depth under Peptic Ulcers.

PEPTIC ULCERS

A circumscribed ulceration of the mucous membrane penetrating through the muscularis mucosa and occurring in areas exposed to acid and pepsin. *(The Merck Manual)*

Ulcerative conditions of the stomach, duodenum, and esophagus are very common in our society, and nonprescription medicines for symptom relief are major moneymakers for the pharmaceutical industry. *Gastric ulcers* occur along the lesser curvature of the stomach, while *duodenal ulcers* are found in the first few centimeters of the duodenum, or the first part of the small intestine.

Drug treatment for ulcers aims primarily to reduce the corrosive impact of stomach acid on the mucosal lining. This is accomplished with antacid chemicals or other agents that reduce acid production in the first place, either directly or indirectly. A range of plants can help here. These appear to work in a variety of ways via a multitude of mechanisms to facilitate a reversal of the condition.

Peptic ulcers result from a breakdown of the lining of the stomach and duodenum. A number of possible factors may be implicated, including increased secretion of stomach acid and pepsin and infection with the bacterium *Helicobacter pylori*. Duodenal ulcers are more common than gastric ulcers, which carry a greater risk of malignancy. Ulcers of either type may cause nausea, vomiting, loss of appetite, weight loss, and a gnawing, burning pain in the upper abdomen.

It is now believed that most peptic ulcers are caused by infection with the bacterium *Helicobacter pylori*. However, some peptic ulcers are caused by prolonged use of nonsteroidal anti-inflammatory drugs (NSAIDs), a group of pain relievers that includes aspirin, ibuprofen, and naproxen sodium. NSAIDs cause ulcers by impairing the stomach's ability to protect itself from acidic stomach juices. Normally, the stomach has three defenses against digestive juices:

1. Mucus coats the stomach lining and shields it from stomach acid.
2. The chemical bicarbonate, naturally present in the stomach, neutralizes stomach acid.
3. Blood circulation to the stomach lining aids in cell renewal and repair.

NSAIDs hinder all of these protective mechanisms. With the stomach's defenses down, digestive juices can damage the sensitive stomach lining and cause ulcers.

Peptic ulcers usually have a chronic, recurrent course with a variable symptom picture. In fact, only about half of all ulcer patients present with the characteristic symptom picture. The pain is often described as burning, gnawing or aching; there may also be a sore, empty feeling or a sensation of hunger. Antacids or milk will relieve the gastric pain. For duodenal ulcers, the typical pain is described as hunger pangs; for gastric ulcers, eating may bring on pain.

Treatment of Ulcers

Through the skilled use of plants with demulcent, antacid, astringent, and vulnerary actions, it is well within the bounds of therapeutic possibility to bring about a rapid and complete healing of any ulceration. Herbs such as *Symphytum officinale* (comfrey), *Althaea officinalis* (marshmallow), *Filipendula ulmaria* (meadowsweet), *Calendula officinalis* (calendula), *Matricaria recutita* (chamomile), and *Hydrastis canadensis* (goldenseal) are examples of remedies that may be used.

Actions Indicated

Demulcents soothe the lining of the stomach, either by coating the stomach or exerting anti-inflammatory actions.
Anti-inflammatories reduce localized mucosal reactions.
Antimicrobials are indicated for dealing with *H. pylori*. However, these herbs must be active in the stomach in order for them to be effective.
Astringents lessen local bleeding.
Vulneraries speed natural wound healing.
Carminatives will reduce any flatulence in the gastrointestinal tract.
Nervines help ease background stress involvement.
Bitters aid the healing process in the latter stages of treatment.
Alteratives help the body deal with any systemic problems related to the disease.

Caution: Emergency hospitalization is essential if the ulcer perforates or hemorrhages.

Specific Remedies

Symphytum officinale (comfrey), *Althaea officinalis* (marshmallow), *Filipendula ulmaria* (meadowsweet), *Calendula officinalis* (calendula), and *Matricaria recutita* (chamomile) can all be seen as possible specifics for the treatment of ulcers. (Please see chapter 10 for a discussion of the controversy surrounding the risks and benefits of *Symphytum officinale*.)

Based upon an understanding of their actions, the rationale for the use of these herbs to treat ulcers is very predictable. Their content of anti-inflammatory flavonoids is thought to be very important to their activity (see chapter 9). *Glycyrrhiza glabra* (licorice) is an effective remedy now used even in allopathic medicine as a treatment for ulcers. In addition to these herbs, raw cabbage juice is an effective traditional treatment. Similarly, demulcent foods such as plantain banana and even potato can help.

As mentioned, newer research suggests that the bacterium *Helicobacter pylori* is implicated in the development of many gastric and duodenal ulcers. This may help explain why *Hydrastis canadensis* (goldenseal) can be so effective against ulcers, even though digestive bitters are generally contraindicated in this condition due to the fact that they stimulate gastric secretions. *Hydrastis* is an effective antibacterial and may well be active against *Helicobacter pylori*.

The successful use of herbs to treat peptic ulceration falls into two stages. The first step is to reduce inflammation and initiate healing, and the second is to tone and complete healing. The first prescription given here focuses on reducing inflammation and beginning the healing process.

Prescription I for Peptic Ulcer

Symphytum officinale root	1 part
Althaea officinalis root	1 part
Matricaria recutita	1 part

Dosage: 5 ml of tincture combination three times a day. In addition, a cold infusion of these herbs (fresh or dried) may be drunk often to ease symptoms. *Matricaria* infusion drunk on an empty stomach will reduce inflammation and help reverse the ulcerative process.

The next prescription focuses on the second step in the healing process.

Prescription II for Peptic Ulcer

Hydrastis canadensis	1 part
Symphytum officinale	2 parts
Matricaria recutita	2 parts

Dosage: 5 ml of tincture combination three times a day

Caution: If symptoms have not subsided within a week, seek skilled diagnosis.

Table 13.8. Actions Supplied by Peptic Ulcer Prescriptions

ACTION	HERBS
Demulcent	*Symphytum officinale, Althaea officinalis*
Anti-inflammatory	*Matricaria recutita, Hydrastis canadensis*
Astringent	*Symphytum officinale, Hydrastis canadensis*
Vulnerary	*Symphytum officinale, Hydrastis canadensis, Matricaria recutita*
Nervine	*Matricaria recutita*
Carminative	*Matricaria recutita*
Bitter	*Hydrastis canadensis*

Broader Context of Treatment

Ulcer patients are vulnerable to many consequences of dietary abuse, as well as problems related to non-herbal treatments for peptic ulcer, such as antacids.

Overuse of antacids can lead to impaired absorption of certain nutrients from the diet.

Overconsumption of milk or antacids can elevate calcium levels in body tissues and urine, which can lead to kidney stones.

A bland and milky diet may contribute to obesity.

Milk can aggravate dairy sensitivity problems.

Poor appetite associated with ulcers can lead to nutritional deficiencies.

Dietary factors are fundamentally implicated in both the cause and the treatment of peptic ulceration. In some cases, ulceration may be due to a specific food allergy, but ulcers are always aggravated by sensitivity to irritants. As with other digestive system conditions, all irritant substances must be avoided, especially alcohol and tobacco. Pepper, coffee, and anything that the patient experiences as a problem should also be eliminated. Avoiding aspirin and other NSAIDs is essential.

Small meals often are tolerated better than large meals. Increasing the proportion of fiber in the diet has been shown to reduce the rate of recurrence of peptic ulceration. However, in the early stages of treatment, the patient should eat a bland diet to avoid physical irritation. Rest and reevaluation of lifestyle factors that may be causing stress are important. The creation of a stress management program uniquely suited to the needs of the patient should be a priority.

HIATUS HERNIA

Protrusion of the stomach above the diaphragm. *(The Merck Manual)*

This unpleasant yet common problem is caused when a rupture forms in the diaphragm, creating an opening in which the upper part of the stomach gets pinched (the herniation). Hiatus hernias can be caused by obesity, pregnancy, tight clothing, sudden physical exertion (such as weight lifting), straining, coughing, or abdominal injury.

Although most hiatus hernias cause no symptoms, some people experience reflux symptoms. Occasionally, reflux damages the lining of the esophagus, resulting in erosions. Postural gastric reflux, which occurs when gravity forces the stomach into the hernia, is a common presenting sign. This most frequently happens when the patient is bending over or lying down.

Treatment of Hiatus Hernia

The distressing gastric symptoms of this condition may be treated with herbal remedies, but the herniation itself can prove to be a therapeutic challenge. In severe cases, surgery may be necessary. Proper digestion and elimination are pivotal to healing, as is nervous system support. Structural issues are part of the problem, so muscular and skeletal support must be taken into account. Appropriate manipulative therapy, such as osteopathy, may be indicated.

Actions Indicated

Demulcents soothe the lining of the stomach, by either coating the mucosa or exerting anti-inflammatory actions.

Anti-inflammatories reduce localized mucosal reactions.

Vulneraries speed natural wound healing and may help strengthen the diaphragm.

Astringents lessen local bleeding.

Carminatives will help with any flatulence or colic.

Nervines help ease background stress involvement.

Specific Remedies

Symphytum officinale (comfrey), *Althaea officinalis* (marshmallow), *Filipendula ulmaria* (meadowsweet), *Calendula officinalis* (calendula), and *Matricaria recutita* (chamomile) can all be seen as possible specifics. *Symphytum* has an especially valid role because of its content of allantoin, a constituent that promotes wound healing. (See chapter 10 for a discussion of the controversy surrounding the benefits and risks of this herb.)

The main treatment goal is to reduce inflammation and facilitate natural healing through the use of demulcent and vulnerary herbs. The focus here is on easing the symptom picture.

A Prescription for Hiatus Hernia

Symphytum officinale root	1 part
Althaea officinalis root	1 part
Filipendula ulmaria	1 part

Dosage: 5 ml of tincture combination three times a day. An infusion of these herbs (fresh or dried) may be drunk often to ease symptoms. Carminative nervines may be added if stress is a major component. (*Valeriana officinalis* is a good example.)

Chamomile and the Digestive System

Chamomile tea, perhaps the best-known herbal tisane, is widely employed as a digestive remedy throughout Europe, and its therapeutic use is well documented. *Matricaria recutita* is uniquely suited for digestive problems, combining as it does carminative, antispasmodic, anti-inflammatory, antiseptic, and mild bitter actions. Analysis of its constituents reveals the presence of a volatile oil that contains, among other compounds, azulene, chamazulene, and a range of sesquiterpenes. Other constituents in chamomile provide a bitter principle, flavones, glycosides, salicylic acid, coumarin derivatives, and much more. These act together as a biologically evolved whole, each contributing specific effects to create a wonderfully rounded digestive remedy.

Through its relaxing, antispasmodic effects on smooth muscles, chamomile soothes colic, gently sedates the central nervous system, and eases the impact of stress. It exerts anti-inflammatory effects upon the lining of the gut and provides valuable antimicrobial actions. The herb also increases overall blood flow to the digestive system through local vasodilatory activity. All of these properties work together to give chamomile an invaluable role in the holistic treatment of many digestive system diseases, especially those associated with colic spasms. Various other indications for this wonderful herb are highlighted elsewhere in this book.

Table 13.9. Actions Supplied by Hiatus Hernia Prescription

ACTION	HERBS
Demulcent	*Symphytum officinale, Althaea officinalis*
Anti-inflammatory	*Filipendula ulmaria*
Vulnerary	*Symphytum officinale*
Astringent	*Symphytum officinale, Filipendula ulmaria*
Carminative	*Filipendula ulmaria*
Nervine	*Valeriana officinalis*

Broader Context of Treatment

Please refer to discussions of gastroesophageal reflux and peptic ulceration.

FUNCTIONAL DYSPEPSIA

Symptoms referred to the GI system in which a pathological condition is not present, is poorly established, or, if present, does not entirely explain the clinical state. *(The Merck Manual)*

Functional dyspepsia, often referred to as "indigestion," is a vague and variable problem that is functional in nature but usually not caused by underlying structural issues. Belching, distension, and borborygmus (rumbling sound made by the movement of gas in the bowels) often occur, along with abdominal or gastric pain. There is often an overt psychological component. While nervine remedies and addressing lifestyle issues may help, it is too easy to conclude that all indigestion is psychosomatic.

Treatment of Functional Dyspepsia

While herbal treatment centers on ensuring the health and proper functioning of the digestive system, any focus of illness in the body must also be supported with tonics. Dietary factors are often crucial. However, the symptom picture may be similar to some of the presenting signs of cardiac ischemia, peptic ulcer, or cholecystitis. Thus, differential diagnosis is essential. Any case of "'indigestion" that proves intransigent requires skilled diagnosis.

Actions Indicated

The key to correcting such functional problems is to "tune up" both metabolic and physical aspects of digestion and assimilation, while at the same time easing symptomatic discomfort with appropriate remedies.

Bitter stimulation promotes an integrated and adequate secretory response to food or hunger, as well as increased muscular tone in peristalsis.

Carminatives ease flatulence, reduce localized inflammation, decrease muscular spasms that lead to colic, and act as mild antimicrobial agents.

Antispasmodics may be indicated if carminatives do not ease abdominal cramping.

Nervines help relieve stress, anxiety, and tension; these are usually also antispasmodic.

Specific Remedies

Every herbalist in every culture has a favorite remedy for indigestion. These are often bitter carminatives or nervine carminatives. European specific remedies include *Gentiana lutea* (gentian), *Mentha piperita* (peppermint), *Matricaria recutita* (chamomile), *Melissa officinalis* (lemon balm), *Humulus lupulus* (hops), and *Valeriana officinalis* (valerian).

Often, the traditional *simple* (tea made from a single fresh remedy) is the best treatment. This should be an herb with a taste and aroma that the patient likes. Ideally, it should also be a plant he or she could easily cultivate, thus providing a steady supply of fresh leaf. The whole spectrum of an herb's actions will provide the clue as to which is the best choice for the patient. For example, of the suggested herbs (*Mentha piperita, Matricaria recutita,* and *Melissa officinalis*), *Matricaria* has nervine and mild bitter properties, while *Melissa* is also a diaphoretic. The patient's signs and symptoms will highlight the appropriate actions needed.

The simple may be augmented with a combination of bitter and carminative tinctures that aid and support the general function of the digestive system.

A Prescription for Indigestion	
Matricaria recutita	1 part
Mentha piperita	1 part
Gentiana lutea	1 part
Valeriana officinalis	1 part

Dosage: 2.5 ml of tincture combination 10 minutes before eating

Table 13.10. Actions Supplied by Indigestion Prescription

ACTION	HERBS
Carminative	*Mentha piperita, Matricaria recutita, Melissa officinalis*
Anti-inflammatory	*Mentha piperita, Matricaria recutita, Melissa officinalis*
Bitter	*Gentiana lutea, Matricaria recutita*
Nervine	*Valeriana officinalis, Matricaria recutita*

Broader Context of Treatment

Persistent problems call for skilled medical diagnosis. Because of the functional nature of this problem, just about anything that supports physiological activity or helps the person to feel at ease will be indicated. Diet is fundamental, but the problem can also be structural or psychological. Because of structural considerations, manipulative therapies, from chiropractic to rolfing, have potential value. Counseling for stress-related or deeper psychological issues may also help.

Indigestion may be disease-related, but for the most part, it results from eating too much or too quickly, eating high-fat foods, or eating during stressful situations. Smoking, alcohol, medications that irritate the stomach lining, fatigue, and ongoing stress can also aggravate or cause indigestion.

Avoiding foods and situations that seem to cause indigestion is the most successful treatment. Excess stomach acid does not cause or result from indigestion, so antacids are not an appropriate treatment, although some people report that they do help. Smokers can help relieve indigestion by quitting smoking, or at least not smoking right before eating. Exercising with a full stomach may also cause indigestion, so scheduling exercise before meals or at least an hour afterward might help.

PHYTOTHERAPY AND THE COLON

The colon, which connects the small intestine with the rectum and anus, is where water and electrolytes are absorbed from the material that enters from the small intestine. This material remains in the colon until most of the fluid and salts are absorbed into the body. The stool then passes through to the left side of the colon, where it is stored until a bowel movement occurs. The contraction of intestinal muscles and the movement of its contents are controlled by nerves, hormones, and electrical activity in the colon muscle. Movements of the colon propel the contents slowly back and forth, but mainly toward the rectum. A few times a day, strong muscle contractions push fecal material ahead. Some of these strong contractions result in a bowel movement.

A wide range of plants have a direct impact on both colon health and pathology. Astringents such as *Myrica cerifera* (bayberry), demulcents like *Althaea officinalis* (marshmallow) and *Plantago major* (plantain), and antispasmodics such as *Dioscorea villosa* (wild yam) can be very helpful in facilitating the healing of these distressing problems.

Colitis, or inflammation of the colon, appears to be caused by a number of different factors. *Mucous colitis*, also called irritable or spastic colon, is a functional disturbance in which the colon secretes an abnormally large amount of mucus that appears in the stools. The most common symptom is abdominal cramping accompanied by either constipation or diarrhea, which sometimes alternate.

Herbs offer exciting therapeutic possibilities in the treatment of mucous colitis (see Irritable Bowel Syndrome later in this chapter). Ulcerative colitis is another matter. This is a serious inflammatory disease that seems to be autoimmune in nature and poses real challenges to any therapist, whether herbalist or orthodox practitioner. However, a competent medical herbalist has much to offer in the treatment of autoimmune conditions. Inflammatory bowel diseases, including ulcerative colitis and Crohn's disease, are discussed in more detail later in this chapter.

IRRITABLE BOWEL SYNDROME

Motility disorders involving the small intestine and large bowel associated with variable degrees of abdominal pain, constipation or diarrhea, largely as a reaction to stress in a susceptible individual. *(The Merck Manual)*

Irritable bowel syndrome (IBS) is a common disorder characterized by cramping pain, gassiness, bloating, and changes in bowel habits. Symptoms can include constipation or diarrhea, or may alternate between constipation and diarrhea.

A whole panoply of symptoms can occur in IBS. These include abdominal distress, erratic frequency of bowel movements, and variability in stool consistency. Mucus may be present in stools. Often, unpleasant abdominal sensations associated with a range of generalized symptoms are present. These may vary from bloating and flatulence to headaches and anxiety.

IBS has very a diverse and sometimes obscure etiology. While stress, anxiety, and other psychological issues are often pivotal, they are but components in a multifactorial matrix. Another factor to consider is intolerance to such common foods as wheat, corn, dairy products, coffee, tea, and citrus fruit. Similarly, intolerance to the sugar lactose occurs frequently. Excessive bran consumption due to overeating of "healthy fiber" is another possible cause! Occasionally, infectious or parasitic organisms are involved (for example, *Giardia*, threadworm, *Candida*, and others). Drugs, especially antibiotics, may also be implicated.

IBS symptoms generally occur in response to some kind of trigger, which is often dietary or stress-related. While emotional conflict and stress do not *cause* IBS, they are common triggers for IBS symptoms. Stress also stimulates colonic spasms, although this process is not completely understood. Stress-reduction training or counseling and support can help relieve IBS symptoms.

Other factors are also important. In a person with IBS, the colon is more sensitive than usual and responds strongly to stimuli that would not bother most people. Eating causes contractions of the colon. Normally, this induces the urge to have a bowel movement within 30 to 60 minutes. For a person with IBS, this urge comes sooner, and is accompanied by cramps and diarrhea. The intensity is often related to the number of calories and the amount of fat in the meal. Fat, whether animal or vegetable, is a strong stimulus for colonic contractions. Many foods contain fat, especially meats of all kinds, poultry skin, whole milk, cream, cheese, butter, vegetable oil, margarine, shortening, avocados, and whipped toppings.

In some people, specific foods or medicines may act as triggers. Examples are chocolate, milk products, and alcohol. Caffeine is also likely to affect people with IBS. Even eating and distention of the colon due to gas can cause the colon to overreact. A spasm may also delay passage of stools, leading to constipation.

Two extreme varieties of IBS are commonly seen, with a spectrum of shades in between. The "spastic colon" type of IBS is characterized by alternating constipation and diarrhea, associated with and often triggered by eating. The other extreme takes the form of a painless and often uncontrollable diarrhea. This type of IBS, known as *mucous colitis*, is a functional disturbance in which the colon secretes abnormally large amounts of mucus that appears in the stools.

While normal bowel function varies from person to person, a normal movement can be described as formed but not hard, free of blood, and painless to pass. Bleeding, fever, weight loss, and persistent severe pain are not symptoms of IBS, but may indicate other problems.

Treatment of IBS

Herbs offer a wide range of therapeutic possibilities for the treatment of this condition, and often have more to offer than other therapeutic modalities. Herbal support of the digestive system and elimination is pivotal, as is help for the nervous system. However, any focus of illness in the body must also be addressed with tonics.

Actions Indicated

Astringents reverse the diarrhea and reduce any pathological mucus production.
Bitters promote appropriate digestive secretions, and often will normalize bowel function on their own.
Anti-inflammatories reduce localized mucosal reactions.
Carminatives help with any flatulence or colic.
Antispasmodics other than carminatives may be indicated if cramping is severe.
Vulneraries are indicated if there is any hint of damage to the lining of the colon.
Nervines help ease background stress.
Aperients may be indicated temporarily if constipation is present. Do not use strong herbs, however, as there may be a rapid swing back to diarrhea.

Specific Remedies

As with indigestion, many remedies can help with this functional problem, but none is a true specific. *Matricaria recutita* (chamomile) and *Mentha piperita* (peppermint) are examples of the vast range of plants that have a direct impact on IBS. With astringents such as *Myrica cerifera* (bayberry), wound-healing remedies like *Symphytum officinale* (comfrey root) and *Plantago major* (plantain), and colic-relieving antispasmodics such as *Dioscorea villosa* (wild yam), much can be done to facilitate healing.

Orthodox practitioners in the United Kingdom prescribe enteric-coated peppermint oil capsules to alleviate the symptoms of IBS. In addition, peppermint oil has been reviewed and approved by the German Commission E for safe and effective use in treating IBS. As an example of the intriguing possibilities that suggest themselves when herbs are incorporated into orthodox medicine, the instillation of peppermint oil into the colon during colonoscopy or barium enema has been reported to reduce spasm, lessening the need for intravenous spasmolytics.[4]

A Prescription for IBS

Myrica cerifera	2 parts
Artemisia vulgaris	1 part
Matricaria recutita	1 part
Mentha piperita	1 part
Dioscorea villosa	1 part
Valeriana officinalis	1 part

Dosage: 5 ml of tincture combination three times a day. In addition, a warm infusion of an appropriate carminative nervine should be drunk frequently.

Table 13.11. Actions Supplied by IBS Prescription

ACTION	HERBS
Astringent	Myrica cerifera
Bitter	Artemisia vulgaris, Matricaria recutita
Anti-inflammatory	Dioscorea villosa, Matricaria recutita
Carminative	Matricaria recutita, Mentha piperita
Antispasmodic	Dioscorea villosa, Matricaria recutita, Mentha piperita
Vulnerary	Matricaria recutita
Nervine	Matricaria recutita, Valeriana officinalis

Broader Context of Treatment

As with indigestion, because of the functional nature of IBS, just about anything that supports physiological activity or helps the individual feel at ease may be indicated. Diet is fundamental, but identifying problematic foods can be a real challenge. Structural considerations should be taken into account, as should stress and psychological issues.

Keeping a journal to record foods and situations that trigger symptoms may be the only way to identify dietary issues for a given individual. If dairy products cause symptoms to flare up, for example, the patient should cut down on these foods, or try eating yogurt instead. (Yogurt contains organisms that supply lactase, the enzyme needed to digest lactose, the sugar found in milk products.) Large meals can cause cramping and diarrhea, so symptoms may be eased if smaller meals are eaten more frequently. Similarly, eating smaller portions of foods that are low in fat and high in carbohydrates, such as pasta, rice, whole-grain breads and cereals, fruits, and vegetables, may be helpful.

In many cases, dietary fiber may help ease IBS symptoms. Whole-grain breads and cereals, beans, fruits, and vegetables are good sources of fiber. High-fiber diets keep the colon mildly distended, which may help to prevent spasms. Some forms of fiber also retain water in the stools, thereby preventing the development of hard stools that are difficult to pass. The patient should eat just enough fiber that bowel movements are painless and eas-

Herbs and IBS: A Clinical Study

A paper published in 1998 in the *Journal of the American Medical Association* details a clinical trial of traditional Chinese treatments of IBS. This is an excellent example of the use of a randomized, double-blind, placebo-controlled trial to evaluate a traditional herbal protocol. The study assessed the effectiveness of individualized treatment (a standard component of all good phytotherapeutic practice) against a placebo.[5]

Participants underwent routine IBS screening by a gastroenterologist. Chinese herbal practitioners treated the patients with confirmed diagnoses in traditional settings. Subjects were randomized into three groups: One group received individualized herbal formulations, another a standard herbal IBS formulation, and the third a placebo. The gastroenterologist evaluated the participants again at 8 weeks and at the conclusion of the 16-week treatment period.

Both groups treated with herbs responded significantly better than the placebo group. Another assessment 14 weeks after completion of treatment showed that patients who received the individualized treatment maintained improvement, while the improvement weakened somewhat in the standard formula group. It is possible that this is because the individualized treatments were effective in correcting underlying imbalances, while the standard formula addressed only symptoms.

ily passed. A high-fiber diet may initially cause gas and bloating, but within a few weeks, the body will adjust and symptoms will subside.

INFLAMMATORY BOWEL DISEASE

Inflammatory bowel disease (IBD) refers to two chronic intestinal disorders: Crohn's disease and ulcerative colitis. IBD affects 2% to 6% of Americans, or an estimated 300,000 to 500,000 people.

Crohn's disease and ulcerative colitis are serious inflammatory diseases that appear to be autoimmune in nature and pose real challenges for practitioners of all modalities. They generally present as a series of attacks of bloody diarrhea that vary in intensity and duration and alternate with symptom-free periods.

The causes of Crohn's disease and ulcerative colitis are not known, but a leading theory suggests that some agent, perhaps a virus or bacterium, alters the body's immune response, triggering an inflammatory reaction in the intestinal wall. The onset of both diseases peaks during young adulthood. Either disease may cause persistent abdominal pain, bowel sores, diarrhea, fever, intestinal bleeding, and weight loss.

The discussion that follows refers specifically to ulcerative colitis, but the herbal approach is similar for both forms of IBD.

ULCERATIVE COLITIS

A chronic, inflammatory, and ulcerative disease that arises in the colonic mucosa, characterized most often by bloody diarrhea. *(The Merck Manual)*

This disorder is a true colitis—in other words, active inflammation is a primary aspect of the condition. Ulcerative colitis usually presents as a series of attacks of bloody diarrhea varying in intensity and duration. These will alternate with periods during which the patient experiences no symptoms at all. Ulcerative colitis must be differentiated from an infectious cause. A history of recent travel or extensive antibiotic use may provide a clue.

Caution: Blood in the stools is a sign that must always be investigated by a skilled diagnostician.

Treatment of Ulcerative Colitis

Immune system issues and all they imply are crucial in ulcerative colitis (see chapter 21 for more information). Obviously, the digestive system needs a great deal of support, as do the other pathways of elimination. Because of the toll taken by stress, the nervous system may also need attention. If liver involvement is suspected, give this vital organ as much herbal support as possible with hepatic plants such as *Silybum marianum*.

Actions Indicated

Astringents may help stem blood loss.

Demulcents soothe surface irritation.

Vulneraries promote healing of ulcerations in the mucosal lining.

Anti-inflammatories aid the body in its attempt to control inappropriate inflammatory reactions.

Carminatives help relieve abdominal discomfort.

Antispasmodics help ease the muscular cramping in the bowel that causes much of the pain.

Immune system support is essential and must cover the whole range of issues involved.

Antimicrobials help combat any secondary infection that might arise.

Elimination support must be given to the other organs of elimination.

Nervines will help address the psychological components of the condition.

Specific Remedies

Allium sativum (garlic) has been advanced as a potential specific here and should be suggested as a dietary supplement. *Myrica cerifera* (bayberry) is an excellent astringent for use in this disease, but cannot be considered a specific. Because of the autoimmune basis of this deep-seated condition, one must be patient when selecting remedies, as many possible herbs will come to mind.

A Prescription for Ulcerative Colitis

Myrica cerifera	2 parts
Dioscorea villosa	2 parts
Symphytum officinale	2 parts
Valeriana officinalis	1 part
Agrimonia eupatoria	1 part
Matricaria recutita	1 part

Dosage: 5 ml of tincture combination three times a day. At least 1 clove of raw garlic should be eaten every day, and a warm infusion of an appropriate carminative nervine should be drunk often.

This prescription supplies the range of actions needed for the colon-based symptoms, but does not directly address the autoimmune problem. See chapter 21 for treatment suggestions for immune system problems. Increasing the proportions of *Myrica* or *Agrimonia* will provide greater astringency. Alternatively, add *Geranium maculatum* to the other remedies. Nervine and demulcent activity may also need to be increased, but this will vary from patient to patient.

Table 13.12. Actions Supplied by Ulcerative Colitis Prescription

ACTION	HERBS
Astringent	*Myrica cerifera, Agrimonia eupatoria, Symphytum officinale*
Demulcent	*Symphytum officinale*
Vulnerary	*Symphytum officinale, Matricaria recutita*
Anti-inflammatory	*Dioscorea villosa, Matricaria recutita*
Carminative	*Valeriana officinalis, Matricaria recutita*
Antispasmodic	*Valeriana officinalis, Matricaria recutita*
Nervine	*Valeriana officinalis, Matricaria recutita*

Broader Context of Treatment

Nutrition becomes a crucial issue in this condition, as some degree of malnutrition is likely to occur. A number of factors may contribute to nutritional deficits, each of which calls for a specific therapeutic response.

Decreased food intake may be related to therapeutic dietary restrictions or to the pain, diarrhea, nausea, and anorexia caused by the disease itself.

Malabsorption may be related to decreased absorptive surface due to disease or surgery, bile salt deficiency after surgery, bacterial flora overgrowth, or drugs, such as corticosteroids, sulfasalazine, and cholestyramine.

Increased secretion and nutrient loss can be caused by diarrhea or by the disease itself.

Increased utilization and nutrient requirements may be due to inflammation, fever, infection, or increased intestinal cell turnover.

A good multivitamin and mineral supplement will help replace lost nutrients. In *Textbook of Natural Medicine*, Drs. Pizzorno and Murray recommend vitamin supplementation at least five times the U.S. recommended daily allowance.[6] If there is loss of blood via the gut, zinc, magnesium, and iron supplementation is particularly important. If diarrhea is severe, electrolytes must be replaced.

In initial stages of treatment, avoid adding fiber to the diet, in order to minimize irritation of the inflamed mucosa. However, as symptoms are brought under control, a gradual buildup to a high-fiber diet is beneficial. Lactobacillus-rich yogurt can also be very helpful. In addition, some people respond well to diets that limit the intake of salicylate-containing foods.

DIVERTICULITIS

Inflammation of one or more diverticula, potentially leading to obstruction or perforation and to abscess and fistula formation. *(The Merck Manual)*

A *diverticulum* is a small, saclike pouch or herniation of the colonic mucosa that bulges outward through a weak spot in the colon wall; these are collectively known as *diverticula*. About half of all Americans aged 60 to 80 and almost everyone over the age of 80 has *diverticulosis*, or the condition characterized by the presence of diverticula.

When diverticula become inflamed, the disorder is called *diverticulitis*. This happens in 10% to 25% of people with diverticulosis. The characteristic signs and symptoms include pain and tenderness associated with constipation that alternates with diarrhea. Fever is often observed. Differential diagnosis is very important to rule out carcinoma of the colon.

Diverticulitis is common in industrialized countries where low-fiber diets are the norm, but rare in countries where people eat high-fiber diets rich in vegetables. Fiber, discussed in more detail earlier in this chapter, is the part of fruits, vegetables, and grains that the body cannot digest. Soluble fiber dissolves easily in water, becoming soft and jellylike in the intestines. Insoluble fiber passes almost unchanged through the intestines. Both kinds of fiber help prevent constipation and make stools soft and easy to pass.

A low-fiber diet is thought to be the primary cause of diverticulitis. The history of the condition itself provides evidence for this theory. Diverticulitis first came to the attention of American physicians in the early 1900s, a time when processed foods were becoming widely accepted and incorporated into the diet. Many processed foods are made from refined, low-fiber flour, which, unlike whole-wheat flour, contains no bran.

Straining due to constipation increases pressure in the colon, which causes weak spots to bulge out and become diverticula. Diverticulitis occurs when diverticula become infected or inflamed. An attack can develop suddenly and without warning. The most common symptom is tenderness around the left side of the lower abdomen. If infection is the cause, fever, nausea, vomiting, chills, cramping, and constipation may also be present. The severity of symptoms depends on the extent of the infection and complications.

Treatment of Diverticulitis

Problems of this nature in the large bowel will affect elimination in general, so support for the liver and kidneys is essential. In addition, the nervous system may need help. However, the problem is often associated with aging and can be linked to a whole range of health issues, from diseases to drug side effects.

Actions Indicated

Antispasmodics help relieve abdominal pain caused by cramping around diverticula.

Anti-inflammatories reduce the generalized inflammatory response within the colon.

Antimicrobials help the body deal with any infection that might be present.

Carminatives lessen discomfort due to flatulence.

Nervines ease stress, which may be either causal or a result of the condition.

Specific Remedies

Dioscorea villosa (wild yam) is a very useful specific here. It is a good antispasmodic and anti-inflammatory herb, but also has a specific impact upon this condition. Care must be taken not to induce constipation through overuse of astringent herbs.

A Prescription for Diverticulitis

Dioscorea villosa	2 parts
Valeriana officinalis	1 part
Viburnum opulus	1 part
Mentha piperita	1 part

Dosage: 5 ml of tincture combination three times a day. An infusion of *Matricaria* or *Mentha piperita* sipped slowly throughout the day will help. One clove a day of garlic *(Allium sativum)* should be eaten raw as part of the diet, or an equivalent amount taken in supplement form. The supplement should be a 600 mg oil "perle" containing 6 mg of allicin.

Table 13.13. Actions Supplied by Diverticulitis Prescription

ACTION	HERBS
Antispasmodic	*Dioscorea villosa, Viburnum opulus, Mentha piperita*
Anti-inflammatory	*Dioscorea villosa, Mentha piperita*
Antimicrobial	*Allium sativum*
Carminative	*Valeriana officinalis, Mentha piperita*
Nervine	*Valeriana officinalis, Mentha piperita*

Broader Context of Treatment

Diverticular disease appears to be associated with a low-fiber diet, and there is little doubt that most patients gain some relief from symptoms when a high-fiber diet is adopted. The underlying bowel abnormality will remain, but it will be much less likely to cause the same degree of dysfunction. However, when symptoms are acute and severe, a low-fiber diet is initially indicated to ensure that roughage does not cause physical irritation. This is especially important when the patient is not accustomed to high fiber content. As soon as the discomfort is brought under control, the proportion of fiber can be increased gradually until the patient is eating a high-fiber diet.

PHYTOTHERAPY AND LIVER DISEASE

Liver disease is particularly well suited for treatment with herbs. In the unique and often confusing language of traditional herbalism, much attention is paid to "detoxifying the liver." Liver chemistry is extraordinarily complex, and the role of the liver in human physiology is so fundamental to life that to researchers, the idea that simple plant remedies have something to offer might be laughable. This is unfortunate, because plants such as *Taraxacum officinale* (dandelion), *Silybum marianum* (milk thistle), *Chelone glabra* (balmony), and a variety of bitter tonic herbs provide a robust materia medica.

Treatment with herbs is appropriate for a range of liver conditions, from disorders requiring only gentle liver stimulation to profound liver disease. As with most claims made by the medical herbalist, pharmacological and clinical research is beginning to provide support for traditional observations and chemical insights into the mechanisms involved.

Hepatotoxin-induced liver lesions may be reversed in the early stages, but they cannot be healed simply by removing the toxins. This points to a need for effective remedies for liver diseases. Research into these plants, reviewed in chapter 9, has resulted in the isolation of a number of hepatoprotective "active principles." Well-researched herbs for the treatment of liver disorders include *Silybum marianum*, *Schisandra chinensis*, and *Glycyrrhiza glabra*.

Orthodox Western medicine does not offer many treatments for hepatitis, cirrhosis, toxic liver damage, or biliary tract disorders. In general, patients with liver disease are given supportive therapy (dietary change and removal of toxins) rather than active treatment. However, in worldwide traditional medicine systems, herbs have long been utilized for the treatment of liver disease, and a growing body of scientific evidence bears out traditional uses.

Primary Causes of Liver Disease

Viral infection

Hepatotoxic chemicals, such as:

- Ethyl alcohol
- Peroxides (particularly peroxidized edible oil)
- Toxins in food (especially aflatoxins)
- Pharmaceuticals (mainly antibiotics, chemotherapeutic agents, and CNS-active drugs)
- Environmental pollutants (xenobiotics)

Functions of the Liver

The liver is the largest solid organ in the body and has a wide range of functions:

- Metabolizes protein
- Metabolizes carbohydrates and stores glycogen
- Metabolizes lipids; synthesizes cholesterol and bile acids
- Initiates bile formation
- Biotransforms waste, toxins, and drugs
- Produces blood-clotting factors and other blood proteins
- Performs important immune functions

The liver can regenerate itself after injury or disease, but if pathology progresses beyond the capacity of the tissue to generate new cells, the body's entire metabolism will be severely impaired.

Hepatoprotection and Phytotherapy

Pharmacological investigation has resulted in the isolation of a number of antihepatotoxic (or hepatoprotective) constituents in herbs traditionally used to treat liver disease. (Please see chapter 9 for details.) The antihepatotoxic actions of herbs appear to be related to a combination of two main mechanisms:

Alteration of cell membranes, so that only small amounts of toxins can penetrate into the cell

---

Therapeutic Indications for *Silybum marianum*

Silybum marianum (milk thistle) is the primary remedy utilized to protect the liver and treat a wide range of liver disorders. Indications include:

- Toxic or metabolic liver disease (including alcohol- and drug-induced forms)
- Acute viral hepatitis
- Chronic-persistent hepatitis
- Chronic-aggressive hepatitis
- Cirrhosis of the liver
- Fatty degeneration of the liver

The best results are seen in toxic metabolic hepatitis and cirrhosis. Milk thistle arrests the course of these diseases and stimulates hepatocyte regeneration. It shortens the course of viral hepatitis, minimizes post-hepatitis complications, and strengthens the liver's defenses against trauma caused by liver surgery.

The earlier treatment commences, the better the prognosis, but effective treatment is possible at virtually every stage of these diseases. Over time, milk thistle may bring about complete restoration of the liver, with a regeneration of liver cells four times the normal rate.

The liver detoxifies many psychopharmacologic drugs and agents, and the cumulative effect of drug use on the liver can be devastating. Thus, people who want or need to take such drugs should also take milk thistle, as it has been shown to prevent the liver damage they cause.

All of this suggests that regular use of milk thistle will provide protection to either the sick or the healthy liver during the course of daily life. By stabilizing cell membranes and encouraging the regeneration of cells destroyed during the normal detoxification process, milk thistle enables the liver and the body to better cope with the deleterious effects of daily encounters with air-, water-, and food-borne toxins.

Acceleration of protein synthesis, which stimulates cell regeneration

JAUNDICE

A yellow discoloration of the skin, sclerae and other tissues due to excess circulating bilirubin. *(The Merck Manual)*

Jaundice is a symptom, not a disease in its own right. Careful differential diagnosis is required to elucidate the cause and thus the core treatment. However, a number of plants (called *cholagogues*) can have a direct effect upon the metabolism and buildup of bilirubin in the body. These can be used to ease discomfort while other remedies focus on the underlying cause.

The most common cause of jaundice is *cholestasis* (arrest or impairment of bile flow), which may itself be caused by a range of processes. This leads to a backup behind the blockage and thus to the development of jaundice. The cause of the blockage must be sought. Possible causes include swelling of inflamed tissues and blockage of ducts by gallstones, cancer, or even parasites.

Treatment of Jaundice

Herbal support of the liver, digestion, and circulation is of primary importance. However, due to the often unclear etiology of the disorder and the far-reaching effects of bilirubin, general toning is also often indicated.

Actions Indicated

Cholagogues have a direct impact on the secretion and release of bile.

Hepatics support and improve liver function and metabolism.

Bitters can serve a tonic function and also often supply actions similar to those of cholagogues and hepatics.

Eliminative support will help the whole body deal with the buildup of bilirubin and other metabolites. Laxatives, diuretics, and diaphoretics are the primary actions to consider.

Alteratives and *tonics* will support the whole body in its healing work.

Lymphatics promote tissue drainage.

Antipruritics help ease the often intense itching associated with jaundice.

Antimicrobials are critical if the jaundice has an infectious basis, and will help with surface immune support even if no infection is present.

Specific Remedies

In Europe, *Taraxacum officinale* root (dandelion) and *Verbena officinalis* (vervain) have traditionally been considered specifics. Many of the bitter hepatic and cholagogue herbs can also be seen as specifics. In addition, because *Silybum marianum* (milk thistle) can help regenerate liver cells, this herb can help ensure that bile buildup does not cause hepatotoxicity. *Chionanthus virginicus* (fringetree), *Leptandra virginica* (black root), and *Chelone glabra* (balmony) should also be considered.

A Prescription for Jaundice	
Taraxacum officinale root	2 parts
Verbena officinalis	1 part
Silybum marianum	1 part
Chionanthus virginicus	1 part
Peumus boldus	1 part

Dosage: up to 2.5 ml of tincture combination three times a day, building up to 5 ml three times a day. An infusion of *Stellaria media* or distilled witch hazel may be applied topically to relieve itching.

Table 13.14. Actions Supplied by Jaundice Prescription

ACTION	HERBS
Hepatic	*Taraxacum officinale, Verbena officinalis, Silybum marianum, Chionanthus virginicus, Peumus boldus*
Bitter	*Taraxacum officinale, Peumus boldus*
Alterative/tonic	*Taraxacum officinale, Peumus boldus*
Antipruritic	*Stellaria media*

Broader Context of Treatment

This will depend on the nature of the diagnosis.

CHRONIC HEPATITIS

An inflammatory process in the liver characterized by diffuse or patchy hepatocellular necrosis affecting all hepatocytes. *(The Merck Manual)*

The term *hepatitis* embraces a number of specific syndromes with a range of causes and prognoses. They all share a core pathology of an inflammatory response in liver cells (hepatocytes) that can lead to cellular necrosis.

An important distinction must be made between acute and chronic forms of hepatitis. In chronic hepatitis, the necrosis and inflammation lasts longer than six months to a year. Manifestations range from no symptoms at all to incapacitation due to liver failure. Such chronic inflammation may result from a range of causes, including:

- Autoimmune problems
- Viral infection
- Bacteria or other microorganisms
- Parasitic infestation
- Toxic damage due to alcohol or other drugs (recreational or therapeutic), as well as some plant toxins, such as pyrrolizidine alkaloids
- Preexisting pathology, such as Crohn's disease

Differential diagnosis is essential in order to distinguish among viral hepatitis, chronic nonviral hepatitis, and alcohol-induced liver disease. However, all forms of active hepatitis are characterized by malaise, anorexia, and fatigue. They may all begin with flulike symptoms, and are often associated with a range of specific signs and symptoms, from vomiting to jaundice.

Treatment of Hepatitis

The variety of possible etiologies necessitates a range of herbal responses. All the pathways of elimination will need support because of the extra load they will be carrying. In addition, the cardiovascular system will benefit from treatment with tonics, to deal with any complications related to portal hypertension. Other specifics will depend on the nature of the cause.

In this section, we shall first look at nonviral forms of hepatic inflammation, followed by viral hepatitis.

Actions Indicated

Hepatics help support and improve liver function and metabolism.

Antimicrobials will be critical if the hepatitis has an infectious basis, and will help with surface immune support even if no infection is present.

Bitters help with whole-system toning.

Cholagogues have a direct impact on the secretion and release of bile, and thus may be indicated if jaundice is present.

Eliminative support will help the whole body deal with the buildup of bilirubin and other metabolites. Laxatives, diuretics, and diaphoretics are the primary actions to consider.

Alteratives and *tonics* support the whole body in its healing work.

Lymphatics promote tissue drainage.

Nervines may be needed for symptomatic support.

Specific Remedies

As a whole constellation of pathologies may have a role in hepatitis, it is difficult to talk of specific herbs. Because of its regenerative potential, *Silybum marianum* (milk thistle) comes closest to being a textbook specific. The tonic hepatics are all relevant, including *Taraxacum officinale* root (dandelion), *Peumus boldus* (boldo), *Chionanthus virginicus* (fringetree), *Leptandra virginica* (black root), and *Chelone glabra* (balmony).

A Prescription for Hepatitis

Taraxacum officinale root	2 parts
Silybum marianum	2 parts
Echinacea spp.	1 part
Artemisia vulgaris	1 part
Chionanthus virginicus	1 part

Dosage: up to 2.5 ml of tincture three times a day, building up to 5 ml three times a day. *Artemisia vulgaris* is included as a bitter nervine, but this herb could be replaced with *Verbena officinalis* or another appropriate nervine.

Table 13.15. Actions Supplied by Hepatitis Prescription

ACTION	HERBS
Hepatic	*Taraxacum officinale, Silybum marianum, Chionanthus virginicus, Peumus boldus*
Antimicrobial	*Echinacea* spp.
Antihepatotoxic	*Silybum marianum*
Bitter	*Artemisia vulgaris, Taraxacum officinale, Peumus boldus*
Alterative/tonic	*Taraxacum officinale, Peumus boldus*

Broader Context of Treatment

High-dose multivitamin and mineral supplementation is recommended:[7]

Magnesium: 200 mg/day
Zinc picolinate: 50 mg/day
Vitamin A: 50,000 IU/day
Vitamin E: 200 IU/day

VIRAL HEPATITIS

Viral hepatitis consists of at least five different diseases caused by five different viruses: hepatitis A, B, C, D, and E viruses. All five viruses can lead to acute hepatitis. Hepatitis B, C, and D may also cause chronic hepatitis.

Hepatitis A

Hepatitis A virus (HAV), also known as infectious hepatitis, accounts for 32% of cases of hepatitis in the United States. HAV is spread by direct contact with an infected individual's feces or indirect fecal contamination of food, water, or food that comes from HAV-infected water sources. Symptoms of HAV may include fever, malaise, dark-colored urine, light-colored stool, and jaundice. Death is rare, but the elderly and people with immune system problems, such as AIDS, are most at risk of dying from HAV.

Hepatitis B

An estimated 5% of the world's population is infected with hepatitis B virus (HBV). In the United States, 300,000 new cases of HBV are reported yearly. Chronic liver disease develops in 5% to 10% of patients with acute HBV infection. HBV may be spread by exposure to infected body fluids and blood-clotting products, from a mother to her infant at birth or soon after, or by unprotected sex with an infected person. HBV may be asymptomatic, but if symptoms occur, they can include abdominal pain, anorexia, jaundice, malaise, nausea, and vomiting. Fever and joint pain may also develop.

Hepatitis C

Hepatitis C (formerly called non-A, non-B hepatitis) is the most commonly diagnosed hepatitis. Approximately 3 million people in the United States are chronically infected with hepatitis C virus (HCV). It is primarily spread by exposure to contaminated blood or needles; however, the mode of transmission for more than 40% of cases is unknown. HCV-infected patients rarely clear the virus from their bodies, and at least 80% of those infected become chronic disease carriers. Symptoms of HCV are similar to those of other types of hepatitis.

Hepatitis D

Hepatitis D virus (HDV) was first observed in 1977 in patients infected with chronic hepatitis B virus (HBV). When HDV occurs in a patient who already has chronic HBV, it is considered a *superinfection*; when a patient develops acute cases of both HBV and HDV at the same time, HDV is considered a *co-infection*. Among individuals with HDV superinfection, 90% develop persistent HDV infection, which eventually leads to chronic liver disease. HDV may be spread by exposure to contaminated blood products or needles and by unprotected sex with an infected person.

Hepatitis E

The hepatitis E virus (HEV) is a common cause of acute hepatitis in underdeveloped areas of the world, and travelers to these regions can acquire this form of hepatitis. Hepatitis E causes acute hepatitis that usually resolves itself. Pregnant women are prone to developing severe hepatitis due to infection with this virus. Apart from strict hygienic precautions, there are no known means of preventing or curing hepatitis E.

Treatment of Viral Hepatitis

Batchelder and Hudson have proposed the following treatment principles for viral hepatitis:[8]

- Boost immune system function
- Prevent necrosis
- Support and encourage liver regeneration
- Promote bile flow, waste elimination, and detoxification
- Address addictions (e.g., alcohol)

Actions Indicated

Table 13.16 highlights some herbs to consider, grouped by the actions they contribute.

Table 13.16. Herbs and Actions Useful in the Treatment of Viral Hepatitis

ACTION	HERBS
Adaptogen	*Eleutherococcus senticosus, Glycyrrhiza glabra, Panax ginseng, Rehmannia glutinosa, Withania somnifera*
Antidepressant	*Avena sativa, Hypericum perforatum, Verbena officinalis*
Anti-inflammatory	*Bupleurum falcatum, Matricaria recutita, Curcuma longa, Glycyrrhiza glabra, Rehmannia glutinosa*
Antioxidant	*Allium sativum, Curcuma longa, Ginkgo biloba, Silybum marianum*
Antiviral	*Astragalus membranaceus, Glycyrrhiza glabra, Hypericum perforatum, Lentinus edodes, Phyllanthus amarus, Picrorrhiza kurroa, Thuja occidentalis*

ACTION	HERBS
Detoxifying	*Schisandra chinensis, Silybum marianum, Taraxacum officinale*
Antihepatotoxic	*Curcuma longa, Cynara scolymus, Glycyrrhiza glabra, Phyllanthus amarus, Schisandra chinensis, Silybum marianum*
Immunostimulant	*Astragalus membranaceus, Echinacea* spp., *Ganoderma lucidum, Picrorrhiza kurroa*

The use of *Hypericum perforatum* in this kind of viral infection is worth exploring. The compounds hypericin and pseudohypericin are known to disrupt viral replication by damaging the integrity of the lipid envelope.[9] Viruses consist of nucleic acid enclosed in a protein coat. They lack metabolic activity and do not possess ribosomes or most of the enzymes necessary for replication. In addition, some possess a lipid envelope. Both the lipid and the protein coats protect the nucleic acid, which may be either DNA or RNA, from enzymatic degradation.

The lipid envelope of some virus types is derived from host cell membranes and modified by insertion of one or more spikelike glycoproteins. These surface spikes allow specific interactions with receptors on host cells and serve as the major antigens of the virus. Viruses with lipid envelopes include the herpes simplex viruses, hepatitis B and C, human immunodeficiency virus (HIV, or the AIDS virus), influenza A virus, Epstein-Barr virus (EBV), and others. As all of these viruses have a lipid envelope, some degree of susceptibility to *Hypericum perforatum* can be expected. The disruption caused by hypericin is a light-mediated process; however; some activity is seen in vivo.

One example of a treatment protocol for acute viral hepatitis comes from *Principles and Practice of Phytotherapy* by Simon Mills and Kerry Bone. Mills and Bone suggest the following herbal prescription.

Treatment for Acute Hepatitis[10]	
Echinacea angustifolia	35 ml
Hypericum perforatum	25 ml
Silybum marianum	20 ml
Phyllanthus amarus	20 ml
Total	100 ml

Dosage: 5 ml with water four times a day

Mills and Bone also suggest using *Picrorrhiza* at a dosage of three 500 mg tablets per day. Note that this herb can cause gastrointestinal side effects, such as cramping and diarrhea. In addition, they recommend that patients drink an infusion made from 4 g *Achillea* and 1 g dried *Zingiber* three times a day.[11]

Additional suggestions from Mills and Bone include the following:[12]

• Diaphoretics are indicated in all acute infections accompanied by fever. These include *Tilia, Sambucus,* and *Achillea,* and are best taken as an infusion.
• Diaphoretics are assisted by combination with a diffuse stimulant, such as *Zingiber.*
• Antiviral agents, which for hepatitis include *Hypericum perforatum, Phyllanthus,* and *Thuja.*
• Immune-enhancing herbs, especially *Echinacea* and *Picrorrhiza*
• Hepatoprotective agents to minimize liver damage such as *Silybum, Bupleurum, Taraxacum, Cynara* (globe artichoke), and *Picrorrhiza*

CIRRHOSIS

The disorganization of liver architecture by widespread fibrosis resulting in nodule formation. *(The Merck Manual)*

Cirrhosis is the second biggest killer of Americans between the ages of 45 and 65. Most cirrhosis is secondary to chronic alcohol abuse. Many Western sufferers are largely asymptomatic until generalized weakness, anorexia, weight loss, malaise, and loss of libido set in. In developing nations, cirrhosis often develops as a complication of viral hepatitis B.

The condition is characterized by widespread death of liver cells, accompanied by progressive fibrosis and distortion of liver architecture. This can be due to many causes, but in the United States and Europe is most commonly related to alcohol abuse.

Treatment of Cirrhosis

Primary herbal treatment is based around antihepatotoxic agents, especially *Silybum marianum* (milk thistle). Although cirrhosis is a progressive disease, the rate of progression varies and the outlook is related to many factors. In this context, herbal treatment can make a significant, positive contribution.

Actions Indicated

Hepatics support and improve liver function and metabolism.

Cholagogues have a direct upon the secretion and release of bile.

Eliminative support will help the whole body deal with the buildup of bilirubin and other metabolites. Laxatives, diuretics, and diaphoretics are the primary actions to consider.

Alteratives and *tonics* support the whole body in its healing work.

Bitters help with whole-system toning.

Lymphatics promote systemic tissue drainage.

Nervines will support any psychological work needed in alcohol withdrawal.

Antimicrobials will be helpful for surface immune support, even if no infection is present.

Specific Remedies

Because of its regenerative potential, *Silybum marianum* (milk thistle) comes closest to being a textbook specific. This wonderful remedy is essential to any treatment of cirrhosis. In addition, the tonic hepatic herbs are all relevant, and include *Taraxacum officinale* (dandelion), *Peumus boldus* (boldo), *Chionanthus virginicus* (fringetree), *Leptandra virginica* (black root), and *Chelone glabra* (balmony). *Hydrastis canadensis* (goldenseal) may be useful, as is *Cynara scolymus* (artichoke leaf).

A Prescription for Cirrhosis

Silybum marianum	2 parts
Verbena officinalis	1 part
Chelone glabra	1 part
Chionanthus virginicus	1 part

Dosage: up to 2.5 ml of tincture three times a day, building up to 5 ml three times a day

---

The alcohol base of tinctures may pose a problem. If these remedies cannot be obtained in an alcohol-free glycerite form, the medicine can be put into a small amount of hot water; the alcohol will evaporate and leave behind the herbal component. Alternatively, the patient may take *Silybum marianum* tablets or capsules, preferably standardized to 80% silymarin.

Broader Context of Treatment

Strict avoidance of any specific tissue irritants, such as alcohol, is essential. If alcohol abuse is a causative factor of the individual's cirrhosis, it must be addressed. This will include dietary advice as well as counseling support to help with alcohol cessation. In *Textbook of Natural Medicine*, Drs. Pizzorno and Murray recommend the following supplements:[13]

Vitamin A: 25,000 IU/day
Vitamin B complex: 20 times the US RDA

Vitamin C: 1 g twice a day
Vitamin E: 400 IU/day
Magnesium: 250 mg twice a day
Selenium: 200 mcg/day
Zinc: 30 mg/day
Carnitine: 500 mg twice a day
Glutamine: 1 g/day
Lactobacillus acidophilus: 1 teaspoon/day

CHOLECYSTITIS

Chronic cholecystitis: A pathologic term for a thick-walled, fibrotic, contracted gallbladder; clinically, it is used to describe chronic gallbladder disease characterized by symptoms that include recurrent biliary colic. *(The Merck Manual)*

Acute cholecystitis: Acute inflammation of the gallbladder wall, usually as a response to cystic duct obstruction by a gallstone. *(The Merck Manual)*

Cholecystitis, or gallbladder inflammation, is characterized by severe pain that becomes localized in the upper right quadrant of the abdomen, radiating to the right lower shoulder blade. Nausea and vomiting are common symptoms. Cholecystitis may be associated with gallstones, but the stones constitute a separate condition.

Treatment of Cholecystitis

Given time, cholecystitis responds well to herbal treatment, but because of the extreme pain, the patient may not be willing to wait. Diet is of fundamental importance, as consumption of any fat will precipitate pain.

Orthodox medicine tends to downplay the role of the gallbladder and bile in digestion. This may be the reason the gallbladder is so often surgically removed when gallstones are present, and why it is said that such people lead perfectly normal lives thereafter. However, even though people can tolerate the absence of the gallbladder, a healthy gallbladder helps ensure efficient digestion, which directly decreases the risks of developing arteriosclerosis, irritable bowel syndrome, hypertension, heart disease, stroke, and other major diseases.

Actions Indicated

Hepatic tonics support the work of the liver and so will have a positive metabolic effect.

Anti-inflammatories may help reduce the severity of swelling.

Antispasmodics help ease colic in the gallbladder or ducts.

Eliminative support must be provided to help the whole

body deal with the repercussions of digestive distress and systemic problems.

Alteratives and *tonics* support the whole body in its healing work.

Nervines help ease the strain from pain and general worry.

Antimicrobials will provide surface immune support even if no infection is present.

Caution: Bitters and strong cholagogues are contraindicated, because they increase the strength of peristaltic muscular contractions.

Specific Remedies

The usual hepatic tonics and antilithic (stone-dissolving) herbs will be useful here, but cannot be considered specifics per se.

A Prescription for Cholecystitis	
Dioscorea villosa	2 parts
Chionanthus virginicus	2 parts
Valeriana officinalis	2 parts
Taraxacum officinale root	1 part
Leptandra virginica	1 part

Dosage: up to 5 ml of tincture three times a day. An infusion of a carminative, antispasmodic nervine, such as *Matricaria recutita,* should be taken regularly throughout the day. In addition, the patient should take *Silybum marianum* tablets or capsules standardized to 80% silymarin. Recommended dosage is 1 capsule containing 140 mg of silymarin three times daily.

This prescription supplies antispasmodic, hepatic, nervine, and preventive antilithic actions. Many other herbs could have been used. Consider *Chelone glabra*, *Verbena officinalis*, and *Mahonia aquifolium*. The Eclectic physicians would have suggested that small amounts of *Hydrastis canadensis* and *Lobelia inflata* be added to such a mixture.

Table 13.17. Actions Supplied by Cholecystitis Prescription

ACTION	HERBS
Hepatic	*Taraxacum officinale, Chionanthus virginicus, Leptandra virginica*
Anti-inflammatory	*Taraxacum officinale*
Antispasmodic	*Dioscorea villosa, Valeriana officinalis*
Alterative/tonic	*Taraxacum officinale, Leptandra virginica*

Broader Context of Treatment

Diet and stress management are critical. Strong chemical pain relief may be indicated for severe cases.

CHOLELITHIASIS

Presence of calculi in the gallbladder (cholelithiasis) or the biliary duct (choledocholithiasis). *(The Merck Manual)*

Gallstones are pieces of solid material that form in the gallbladder. They form as hard, crystal-like particles composed of substances in the bile, primarily cholesterol and bile pigments. Stones vary in size, from as small as a grain of sand to as large as a golf ball. The gallbladder may develop a single, often large, stone or many smaller ones.

Gallstones appear to be caused by a combination of factors, including inherited body chemistry, body weight, gallbladder movement, and diet. An estimated 20 million Americans have gallstones. The following groups of people are those most likely to develop them:

- Women between 20 and 60 years of age (twice as likely as men to develop gallstones)
- Both men and women over age 60
- Pregnant women or women who have used birth control pills or estrogen replacement therapy
- Native Americans, who have the highest prevalence of gallstones in the United States (a majority of Native American men have gallstones by age 60)
- Overweight men and women
- People who go on "crash" diets or lose a lot of weight quickly

Treatment of Gallstones

Actions Indicated

Antilithics have a long tradition of use in moving or even dissolving gallstones and easing pain.

Hepatic tonics support the work of the liver and have a positive metabolic effect.

Antispasmodics relieve colic in the gallbladder or ducts.

Nervines ease the strain from pain and general worry.

Eliminative support must be provided to help the whole body deal with the repercussions of digestive distress and systemic problems.

Alteratives and *tonics* support the whole body in its healing work.

Antimicrobials will help with surface immune support, even if no infection is present.

Caution: Bitters and strong cholagogues are contraindicated, because they increase the strength of peristaltic muscular contractions.

A Prescription for Gallstones

Dioscorea villosa	2 parts
Valeriana officinalis	2 parts
Chelone glabra	1 part
Leptandra virginica	1 part
Chionanthus virginicus	1 part

Dosage: up to 5 ml of tincture three times a day. An infusion of a carminative, antispasmodic, nervine herb should be taken regularly throughout the day (for example, *Matricaria recutita*).

Table 13.18. Actions Supplied by Gallstone Prescription

ACTION	HERBS
Hepatic	*Chelone glabra, Chionanthus virginicus, Leptandra virginica*
Antilithic	*Chelone glabra, Chionanthus virginicus*
Antispasmodic	*Dioscorea villosa, Valeriana officinalis*

Broader Context of Treatment

Diet and stress management are crucial. Strong chemical pain relief may be indicated in severe cases.

HEMORRHOIDS

A mass of dilated veins in swollen tissue at the margin of the anus or nearby within the rectum; also called *piles*. (*The Merriam-Webster Medical Dictionary*)

Symptoms caused by hemorrhoids include bleeding, protrusion of tissue, and pain. Bleeding from the rectum must never be assumed to be due to hemorrhoids, but requires prompt and correct diagnosis, as it could be a sign of a serious problem.

Hemorrhoids are caused by increased pressure in the veins of the anus. The most common cause is straining during bowel movements. Constipation, prolonged sitting during bowel movements, and anal infection are contributing factors. Internal hemorrhoids occur near the beginning of the anal canal, and external hemorrhoids occur at the anal opening. Hemorrhoids may protrude outside the anus. They are very common, especially during pregnancy and after childbirth.

Treatment of Hemorrhoids

The problem is a combination of both digestive and cardiovascular system issues. Thus, the treatment should include both blood vessel tonics and lower bowel support.

Actions Indicated

Vascular tonics will help with the muscular tone and general state of well-being of the veins involved.

Astringents will reduce bleeding, if present, and tighten the tissue locally. However, if they are used internally, take care to avoid constipation.

Bitters assist digestive and eliminative processes and facilitate bowel motions.

Aperients and *laxatives* ensure easier bowel movements.

Vulneraries speed local healing of inflamed tissues.

Emollients soothe irritated tissue if applied externally.

Anti-inflammatories soothe inflamed tissues.

Specific Remedies

The materia medicas of many cultures contain herbs with a reputation for effectiveness in the treatment of this common problem. In Europe, nothing matches the action of the aptly named pilewort (*Ranunculus ficaria*)! Apart from this plant, most astringent or anti-inflammatory herbs will help if applied topically.

A Prescription for Hemorrhoids

Ginkgo biloba	1 part
Aesculus hippocastanum	1 part
Taraxacum officinale	1 part
Hydrastis canadensis	1 part
Geranium maculatum	1 part

Dosage: 5 ml of tincture three times a day

A topical application is essential to alleviate symptoms and speed healing. A number of approaches may be used to complement the internal treatment.

External Hemorrhoid Treatment

Tincture of *Aesculus hippocastanum*	10 ml
Distilled witch hazel	80 ml

Apply this combination after every bowel movement and as needed. Salves containing any of many possible herbs may also be used. Useful herbs include *Calendula officinalis, Hypericum perforatum, Matricaria recutita, Plantago* spp, and *Achillea millefolium*.

Table 13.19. Actions Supplied by Hemorrhoid Prescription

ACTION	HERBS
Vascular tonic	*Ginkgo biloba, Aesculus hippocastanum*
Astringent	*Geranium maculatum*
Bitter	*Taraxacum officinale, Hydrastis canadensis*
Aperient	*Taraxacum officinale, Hydrastis canadensis*

Broader Context of Treatment

Avoidance or elimination of constipation is often the key to alleviating hemorrhoids. Thus, in addition to direct herbal treatment of the hemorrhoids themselves, the following factors must be addressed.

Is the patient taking drugs that effect bowel motility—for example, opiates, iron supplements, some antidepressants, antacids, and laxatives?

Are any digestive conditions present, such as irritable bowel syndrome, diverticular disease, or food sensitivities?

Does the patient have a sedentary lifestyle, or have there been long periods of immobility?

Is the patient under stress or suffering from depression?

To ease bowel movements, a diet with medium- to high-fiber content is necessary. This should be introduced gradually if the patient is accustomed to low-fiber foods. During the active treatment phase, avoid the sandpaper effect that roughage can cause!

References

1. van Gorkom et al. Anthranoid laxatives and their potential carcinogenic effects. *Alimentary Pharmacology and Therapeutics* 1999 Apr; 13(4):443–52.
2. Periodontal disease as a potential risk factor for systemic diseases. *Journal of Periodontology* 1998; 69:841–50.
3. Pizzorno JE, Murray MT. *Textbook of Natural Medicine.* Edinburgh: Churchill Livingstone, 1999.
4. Kingham JGC. Commentary: Peppermint oil and colon spasm. *The Lancet* 1995 Oct 14; 346:986.
5. Bensoussan A, et al. Treatment of irritable bowel syndrome with a Chinese herbal medicine. *Journal of the American Medical Association* 1998 Nov 11; 280(18):1585–9.
6. Pizzorno JE, Murray MT. *Textbook of Natural Medicine.* Edinburgh: Churchill Livingstone, 1999.
7. Ibid.
8. Batchelder HJ, Hudson T. Therapeutic approaches to viral hepatitis. *The Protocol Journal of Botanical Medicine* 1995; 1(2):131–74.
9. Tang J, Colacino JM, Larsen SH, et al. Virucidal activity of hypericin against enveloped and non-enveloped DNA and RNA viruses. *Antiviral Research* 1990 Jun; 13(6):313–25.
10. Mills S, Bone K. *Principles and Practice of Phytotherapy: Modern Herbal Medicine.* Edinburgh: Churchill Livingstone, 1999.
11. Ibid.
12. Ibid.
13. Pizzorno JE, Murray MT. *Textbook of Natural Medicine.* Edinburgh: Churchill Livingstone, 1999.

Suggested Reading

Mills S, Bone K. *Principles and Practice of Phytotherapy: Modern Herbal Medicine.* Edinburgh: Churchill Livingstone, 1999.

Pizzorno JE, Murray MT. *Textbook of Natural Medicine.* Edinburgh: Churchill Livingstone, 1999.

14

❧

THE CARDIOVASCULAR SYSTEM

The beauty of a spring meadow in bloom, the profound sense of presence in a grove of redwood trees—the heart takes flight and the spirit is healed. However, this is not the only way in which the magnificent flora with which we share our planet brings healing to our hearts. A wide variety of herbs offer tangible, physical nourishment and healing for hearts troubled by the ills of modern society.

Consider the word *cordial*, applied to both the warming herbal drink and the human expression of heartfelt friendliness. The cordial was a medieval drink based on borage, an herb with a reputation for warming and gladdening the heart. The word derives from the Latin *cordialis*, meaning "of or for the heart," which in turn is based on the Latin *cor*, meaning "heart." The original sense of the word was medicine, food, or drink that stimulates the heart.

Herbs still maintain a central position in orthodox treatment protocols for various heart problems. Plants containing cardiac glycosides are used throughout the world to treat heart failure and certain cases of cardiac arrhythmia. In conditions like these, herbs can increase the strength and normalize the rate of the heartbeat. The real value of these herbs lies in their ability to increase the efficiency of the heart without increasing the heart muscle's need for oxygen.

However, the materia medica available to the medical herbalist embraces many more relevant possibilities than strong cardioactive remedies. Half of the annual mortality in America results from heart and blood vessel diseases. Modern cardiology is almost miraculously effective when it comes to acute emergencies, but what about maintaining good health and preventing the development of cardiovascular pathology? Can we do more for ourselves than simply minimizing risk factors, eating properly, and exercising appropriately? Emphatically, yes! Herbal tonics can contribute by offering real possibilities for the practice of preventive medicine.

Although it is resplendent with wonder drugs, the materia medica of modern medical science is sorely lacking in preventive medicines. There are also profound concerns about toxicity related to long-term use of pre-scription medications. Tonics are not mentioned in pharmacology texts, as the concept is considered illusory. Overlooking the potential of gentle toning therapies in favor of intensely active ones can be considered one of the core problems with orthodox health care. However, this need not be seen as a clash of mutually exclusive approaches. There is a place in cardiovascular medicine for gentle toning, just as there is a place for the often dramatically successful techniques of modern cardiology. In fact, used within a holistic framework, these two extremes can complement and support each other.

As discussed in chapter 9, an increasing amount of research is investigating the cardiovascular effects of plant constituents. As fascinating as this is, the benefits of such research accrue to the pharmaceutical industry, as the information is rarely about the plant from which the constituent has been extracted. It would prove almost impossible to develop herbal approaches to treatment if natural product research was the sole source of information. In the material that follows, the focus is on the traditional practitioner's approach, with newer findings referenced when relevant.

HERBS AND CARDIOVASCULAR HEALTH

The medical herbalist recognizes a broad range of relevant herbs for the cardiovascular system. As a group, they are known as *cardiac remedies*, a general term for herbs that have an action on the heart. Some of the remedies in this group are powerful *cardioactive* agents, such as *Digitalis* spp. (foxglove) and the somewhat milder *Convallaria majalis* (lily of the valley), while others are gentler and safer *cardiotonics*, such as *Crataegus* (hawthorn) and *Tilia* (linden flower).

Cardioactive herbs owe their effects on the heart to highly active substances, such as cardiac glycosides, and thus have both the strengths and the drawbacks of these powerful constituents. Cardiotonics have a beneficial action on the heart and blood vessels, but do not contain cardiac glycosides. While they do not offer the dramatic, rapid, and often life-saving benefits of many of the drugs used in modern cardiology, cardiotonics confer a definite advantage in the treatment or prevention of chronic degenerative conditions. (See chapter 9 for a more detailed discussion of the differences between cardioactive and cardiotonic agents, and chapter 10 for information on the toxicity of cardiac glycosides.)

Blood vessel or *vascular tonics* are often rich in constituents called flavonoids. These remarkable herbs include *Crataegus* spp., *Allium sativum*, *Tilia platyphyllos*, and *Ginkgo biloba*.

There are, of course, some limitations to the use of herbs to treat the heart. Perhaps the most important of these is not herbal, but human. The problem involves self-diagnosis, which can be a very hazardous pastime. In the hands of a competent clinical herbalist, medicinal plants offer a great deal in the treatment of cardiovascular conditions, but for the nonprofessional, self-diagnosis or self-selection of herbs should never replace skilled diagnosis or serve as a substitute for appropriate prescription medicines. The cardiac glycoside–containing cardioactives cannot be used safely without certain requisite medical skills, and are inappropriate for use in folk medicine. However, cardiotonic herbs can and should play a role in holistic programs designed to meet the unique needs and circumstances of each individual.

Table 14.1. Primary Actions for the Cardiovascular System

ACTION	HERBS
Cardiotonic	*Crataegus* spp., *Tilia platyphyllos*
Cardioactive	*Convallaria majalis, Cytisus scoparius, Lycopus europaeus, Scrophularia nodosa*
Circulatory stimulant	*Capsicum annuum*
Peripheral vasodilator	*Zanthoxylum americanum, Ginkgo biloba*
Hypotensive	*Tilia platyphyllos, Viscum album, Allium sativum*
Hypertensive	*Cytisus scoparius*
Diuretic	*Taraxacum officinale, Achillea millefolium,* cardioactive herbs
Vascular tonic	*Aesculus hippocastanum, Fagopyrum esculentum, Ginkgo biloba*
Nervine	*Leonurus cardiaca, Tilia platyphyllos, Valeriana officinalis*
Antispasmodic	*Viburnum opulus, Valeriana officinalis*

Tonics for the Cardiovascular System

A number of remarkable cardiovascular tonics are available to the phytotherapist. Each of the herbal traditions of the world has its own excellent tonic plants, but here we will primarily discuss cardiovascular tonics used in Western therapy.

European Cardiovascular Tonics
Crataegus spp. (hawthorn)
Allium sativum (garlic)
Tilia platyphyllos (linden)
Achillea millefolium (yarrow)
Leonurus cardiaca (motherwort)

To this list of irreplaceable European remedies, we can add others that have entered our materia medica from other parts of the world.

Cardiovascular Tonics from Other Traditions
Ginkgo biloba (ginkgo)
Selenicereus grandiflorus (night-blooming cereus)
Coleus forskohlii (coleus)
Commiphora mukul (guggul)

Crataegus laevigata (hawthorn) is one of the most useful of the cardiotonic herbs. Simply stated, hawthorn will help keep the heart healthy, preventing the development of coronary disease. It may be safely used as part of the treatment protocols for conditions such as heart failure, angina pectoris, and hypertension. While hawthorn berries are the most often used part of this shrub, the flowers and leaves may also play a role. The constituents of hawthorn highlight the importance of flavones and flavonoids in the healing impact of herbs on the cardiovascular system.

As hawthorn is one of the more aesthetic herbal remedies, a very pleasant tea may be made by infusing 1 to 2 teaspoons of the dried herb in a cup of hot water. This should be drunk regularly. Tincture is a convenient and effective way of gaining the therapeutic benefits of this special remedy. For best effects, 30 to 40 drops should be taken three times daily, then morning and evening as a long-term maintenance dose. Hawthorn may be taken over long periods of time, as there is no risk of toxicity.

Hawthorn need not be used as a medicine; it can be added to the diet as a food. For an example of how this heart tonic can be incorporated into the daily diet, try making a hawthorn conserve.

Hawthorn Berry Conserve

Soak a large handful of dried hawthorn berries in apple juice (enough to cover plus a few inches) with a cinnamon stick. Leave overnight in the refrigerator. Remove the cinnamon stick and blend the berries with a little honey. Keep refrigerated.

Ginkgo biloba, another important heart herb, is supported by an abundance of research that has revealed many important therapeutic effects. Ginkgo is recommended both for the prevention and treatment of a number of heart and blood vessel problems, especially those due to peripheral circulatory and cerebral vascular insufficiencies. Research shows that it lowers blood pressure, dilates peripheral blood vessels, and increases peripheral blood flow. In studies involving patients with peripheral arterial insufficiency, *Ginkgo* significantly improved subjects' ability to walk without pain. Other exciting applications include the treatment of circulatory disturbances related to aging and diabetes, as well as the treatment of depression, tinnitus, Alzheimer's disease, and tobacco addiction.

Another traditional European heart tonic is *Tilia platyphyllos* (linden). This herb is especially indicated when anxiety and tension are part of the spectrum of factors impacting the patient, as it is an excellent relaxing nervine. Two herbs from the ayurvedic tradition are proving to offer much in the way of tonic support of the cardiovascular system. *Coleus forskohlii* (coleus) offers a range of therapeutic possibilities that make it uniquely relevant in the treatment of cardiovascular diseases such as hypertension, congestive heart failure, and angina. *Commiphora mukul* (guggul) can be effective in lowering serum lipids. Both herbs are discussed later in this chapter.

Allium sativum (garlic) has a range of effects upon cardiovascular health. It helps reduce serum cholesterol and triglyceride levels while raising levels of high-density lipoproteins (HDL). It can also act as an effective inhibitor of platelet activating factor (PAF). Taken together, these properties provide a potential means of preventing atherosclerosis and thrombosis, hypertension, heart attacks, and stroke. Garlic's antioxidant properties help prevent the peroxidation of fats, yet another contributing factor in the development of atherosclerosis.

Other Important Cardiovascular Actions

In addition to the heart tonics, a number of other herbal actions can be helpful. Especially important are the relaxing herbs, such as *Leonurus cardiaca* (motherwort), *Scutellaria lateriflora* (skullcap), and *Valeriana officinalis* (valerian). Circulatory stimulants, such as *Capsicum annuum* (cayenne), *Zingiber officinale* (ginger), and *Zanthoxylum americanum* (prickly ash), increase blood flow, supporting oxygenation of tissue and the elimination of waste. This makes them important in circulatory problems, as well as in conditions such as rheumatism.

There are some herbs with effects on the cardiovascular system that should be avoided even though they do not contain cardiac glycosides. Examples are *Cytisus scoparius* (Scotch broom) and *Ephedra* spp. (ma huang), both of which stimulate heart activity and raise blood pressure. They are contraindicated in many conditions and should not be considered tonics.

LIFESTYLE AND RISK FACTORS

A well-rounded program for strengthening the heart and cardiovascular system must involve more than herbs. A major influence on the development of heart disease is risk factors, or habits or traits that make a person more likely to develop a disease, whose impact can be minimized. Whole forests have been turned into paper for articles about these risk factors, and anyone trying to read them all and follow the debates that rage invites a hypertensive crisis! However, some general points can be made.

The origins of heart disease are complex and can be confusing. Some of the risk factors involved are well known and provide us with clear guidelines for prevention, but simplistic statements about saturated fats, jogging, or new research can be misleading. For example, one study failed to show any association between heavy coffee consumption and long-term hypertension. However, heavy coffee drinkers also tend to be heavy smokers, which in turn may be associated with lower body weight and thus a lower blood pressure—but with an increased risk of heart attack!

Some of the risk factors for heart-related problems cannot be influenced by preventive strategies, such as genetics and age, but many others can be. Similar risk factors contribute to the development of many major pathologies that assail the cardiovascular system, so some overall preventive strategies can be applied. The major risk factors for cardiovascular disease that *can* be altered are cigarette smoking, high blood pressure, high cholesterol, obesity, and physical inactivity. Other risk factors, such as diabetes, are also potentially controllable.

Even just one risk factor raises an individual's chances of developing heart-related problems. The more risk factors a person has, the more likely he or she is to develop cardiovascular disease. From the wealth of research

Hawthorn: A Classic Cardiotonic

Hawthorn (*Crataegus* spp.) is the best known of the cardiotonic herbs, and is possibly the most valuable tonic remedy for the cardiovascular system found in the plant kingdom. There are much stronger herbs, such as foxglove, but none that provides the nourishing regeneration that hawthorn does. In addition, this invaluable heart remedy contains no cardiac glycosides.

The American Eclectic herbalist Ellingwood said of hawthorn,

. . . it is superior to any of the well known and tried remedies at present in use for the treatment of heart disease, because it seems to cure while other remedies are only palliative at best.

This was written at a time when hawthorn had just been introduced into North American medicine. It was the new wonder herb of the day, much like ginkgo or Siberian ginseng today!

Hawthorn can be considered a specific remedy for many cardiovascular diseases. A tonic in the true sense, its therapeutic benefits are realized only when a whole plant preparation is used. When the isolated constituents were tested separately in the laboratory, their individual effects were insignificant; the whole plant, however, has unique and valuable properties that have been confirmed in clinical studies. Herbal synergy again!

Indications for Hawthorn

In 1994, the German Federal Ministry of Health published a monograph officially recognizing hawthorn as a heart remedy. The monograph concluded that the herb is positively inotropic, chronotropic, and dromotropic, and that it improves coronary and myocardial circulation by dilating the coronary arteries. Perhaps most significant was the finding that hawthorn has no side effects or contraindications.

According to the ministry, the main clinical applications for hawthorn are:

- Long-term treatment of loss of cardiac function
- Any condition in which the patient notes subjective feelings of congestion and oppression in the heart region
- Mild cardiac arrhythmias
- Conditions of the aging heart that do not warrant the use of foxglove

In his book *Herbal Medicine*, German physician Rudolf Weiss suggests the following indications.[1]

- Patients with "degeneration of the cardiac muscle or coronary artery disease"

- Anginal symptoms of coronary artery disease (long-term treatment)
- Hypertension, primarily to improve cardiac function
- Weakness of the myocardium after infectious disease
- Muscular insufficiency in patients taking digitalis (hawthorn may optimize the effects of digitalis)
- Cardiac arrhythmias, mainly extrasystoles and tachycardia

In short, any degenerative condition of the cardiovascular system will benefit from the use of hawthorn. Some specific examples include myocardial problems (such as mild congestive heart failure), coronary artery disease, and associated conditions (such as hypertension). Hawthorn speeds recovery from heart attacks and lowers blood pressure in essential hypertension. Used in conjunction with other hypotensive agents, hawthorn will help keep the heart healthy and prevent the development of serious coronary disease. It will also help guard against heart weakness after infectious disease, such as pneumonia or diphtheria.

For arteriosclerosis and its complications, hawthorn is often combined with *Tilia platyphyllos* (linden flowers) or *Allium sativum* (garlic). *Viburnum opulus* (cramp bark), *Tilia,* and *Scutellaria lateriflora* (skullcap) are good complements in cases of hypertension.

In particular, hawthorn is a specific in cases in which no disease state exists but the patient is experiencing a gradual, age-related loss of cardiac function. Because of its lack of toxicity, accumulation, and habituation, it may be used long term, allowing a gradual and safe attainment of therapeutic goals, especially in the elderly.

A theoretical interaction between *Crataegus* and the cardiac glycosides should be mentioned. The theory suggests that *Crataegus* may enhance the activity of cardioactive plants (such as *Digitalis* and *Convallaria majalis*) as well as the cardiac glycoside drugs digitoxin and digoxin.[2] This could afford the clinician an opportunity to reduce the dosage of cardiac glycoside—containing substances while maintaining the desired effect—thus reducing the potential for toxicity. However, this interaction has not been confirmed.[3]

Mechanisms of Action

How does this unique herb achieve such remarkable effects? Research suggests that many of its observable effects can be explained by its ability to improve coronary circulation. It dilates the coronary arteries, relieving hypoxemia (lack of oxygen in the blood). It thus reduces the likelihood of angina attacks and relieves symptoms of angina when they occur.

The herb also directly affects the cells of the heart muscle, enhancing both activity and nutrition. It is positively inotropic, as it gently increases the force of contraction of the heart muscle. However, its activity is quite different from that of the cardiac glycoside–containing remedies. They impact the contractile fibers, while hawthorn improves the availability and utilization of energy. This facilitates a gentle but long-term, sustained effect on degenerative, age-related changes in the myocardium. Hawthorn does not produce rapid results, but the results are persistent once achieved.

Hawthorn's cardioprotective activity is generally attributed to its content of flavonoids, including flavonoglycosyls, hyperoside, rutin, and oligomeric proanthocyanidins (OPCs). Numerous flavonoid molecules have positive effects on the cardiovascular system, but the particular combination of flavonoid-based constituents in hawthorn appears to be pivotal to its beneficial cardiovascular activity.

Research suggests that OPCs in hawthorn leaves and flowers scavenge free radicals and inhibit an enzyme called human neutrophil elastase. This enzyme is released by white blood cells in greater amounts during hypoxia (lack of oxygen), and, along with free radicals, may be partly responsible for the damage to the heart that occurs under such conditions. Hawthorn extracts improve the energy dynamics of the heart muscle, exerting a protective effect on the myocardium. The well-known effects of OPCs as both free radical scavengers and inhibitors of neutrophil elastase may be the basis of this activity.

Not only do flavonoids have potent antioxidant effects, but research shows that they increase collagen cross-linking in the tissue of vascular walls, strengthening blood vessels. In addition, epidemiological studies have demonstrated an association between dietary flavonoid intake and reduced risk of heart disease, heart attacks, and stroke.[4,5,6] See chapter 9 for more information on the pharmacological effects of this important group of phytochemicals.

A Look at the Evidence

Because of its positive impact on cardiac function, hawthorn extract has been extensively studied for its effects in congestive heart failure. A commonly used classification of heart failure is that formulated by the New York Heart Association (NYHA).[7]

Table 14.2. New York Heart Association Functional Classification of Heart Failure

CLASSIFICATION	DEFINITION
Class I	No limitation of physical activity
Class II	Slight limitation of physical activity. Comfortable at rest, but ordinary physical activity results in fatigue, palpitations, dyspnea, or anginal pain
Class III	Marked limitation of physical activity. Comfortable at rest, but less than ordinary physical activity results in fatigue, palpitations, dyspnea, or anginal pain
Class IV	Unable to carry out any physical activity without discomfort

A number of placebo-controlled, double-blind clinical trials have demonstrated the value of Crataegus in NYHA class II cardiac insufficiency.[8] In fact, a recent review of the pharmacology and therapeutics of Crataegus concluded, ". . . it may be useful in the treatment of NYHA functional class II CHF."[9]

In one multicenter, double-blind study, 136 patients with class II cardiac insufficiency (according to NYHA criteria) were treated with a hawthorn extract or placebo for eight weeks. A total of 129 patients finished the trial. Throughout the eight-week trial, a statistically significant improvement in cardiac function was noted in the hawthorn group. The placebo group, however, progressively deteriorated. The patients' subjective evaluation of their main complaints (reduced exercise performance, shortness of breath, ankle edema, and nocturia) was significantly improved for subjects receiving hawthorn, compared with placebo subjects. The participants' quality of life was also improved in the hawthorn group, although not enough to be statistically significant compared with placebo.[10]

A recent study investigated the efficacy of long-term therapy with a Crataegus extract (WS 1442) as add-on therapy to preexisting diuretic treatment for patients with a more advanced stage of heart failure (NYHA class III). The data from this study confirmed that WS 1442 had a dose-dependent effect on the exercise capacity of patients with heart failure and on typical heart failure-related clinical signs and symptoms. The drug was shown to be well tolerated and safe.[11]

conducted to date, it can be concluded that the development of heart disease is definitely linked with excess dietary fat, elevated blood cholesterol levels, high blood pressure, smoking, obesity, short stature, and physical inactivity. A number of these major risk factors are discussed here.

Age and Gender

The older an individual is, the more likely he or she is to develop cardiovascular disease. Thus, the risk of heart attack is four times greater for a 50-year-old man than for a 30-year-old man. Cardiovascular problems are unusual in premenopausal women, but after menopause, the incidence of heart disease in women equals the incidence in men. Other gender-specific issues are discussed later under Socioeconomic Factors.

Oral Contraceptives

Oral contraceptives that supply high doses of estrogen increase the risk of vascular and heart disease, especially among women who smoke. However, the currently prescribed contraceptives are low-dose pills containing 35 mcg or less of estrogen. There is little additional risk of heart disease for premenopausal women who use such low-dose formulations. However, taking "the pill" does pose risks. For women taking any kind of oral contraceptive, certain guidelines are important.

Stop smoking or consider a different form of birth control. Smoking boosts the risks of serious cardiovascular problems related to oral contraceptive use (especially the risk of blood clots), particularly in women older than 35.

Use of birth control pills may increase blood pressure. If a patient is diabetic and taking oral contraceptives, her blood pressure should be monitored regularly. Oral contraceptives may not be a safe choice if the woman has had a heart attack, a stroke, problems with blood clots, or any other kind of cardiovascular disease.

Heredity

The tendency to develop certain cardiovascular diseases appears to be partially inherited. A family history of heart disease should strongly suggest the use of appropriate herbal tonics, along with dietary change and stress-reduction techniques. One inherited problem is known as *familial hyperlipidemia.* People with this condition appear to have a genetic predisposition to elevated blood lipid levels.

Tobacco

The death rate from heart disease is 300% higher in smokers than in nonsmokers in North America. Smoking by women in the United States causes one and one-half times as many deaths from heart disease as lung cancer. A smoker is two to six times more likely to suffer a heart attack than a nonsmoker, and the risk increases with the number of cigarettes smoked each day. Smoking also heightens the risk of stroke.

Of course, cardiovascular disease is not the only smoking-related health risk. Cigarette smoking is also linked with cancers of the mouth, larynx, esophagus, urinary tract, kidney, pancreas, and cervix. Smokers also are more likely to develop other kinds of lung problems, including bronchitis and emphysema. Smoking during pregnancy is linked to a number of problems, including bleeding, miscarriage, premature delivery, lower birth weight, stillbirth, and sudden infant death syndrome, or "crib death." Young children who breathe in a parent's cigarette smoke have more lung and ear infections. What more need be said?

Alcohol

Occasional consumption of small amounts of alcohol may actually benefit the circulatory system, because alcohol acts as a vasodilator. On the other hand, there is no doubt that alcohol *abuse* is a major contributing factor to heart disease. Several recent studies have reported that moderate drinkers—those who have one or two drinks per day—are less likely to develop heart disease than people who don't drink any alcohol. However, this is *not* a recommendation to start using alcohol!

Moderation is the key. More than three drinks a day can raise blood pressure, and binge drinking can lead to stroke. People who drink heavily on a regular basis have higher rates of heart disease than either moderate drinkers or nondrinkers. The government-produced "Dietary Guidelines for Americans" recommends that for overall good health, one should consume no more than one drink per day. One drink equals 12 ounces of beer, 5 ounces of wine, or 1½ ounces of 80-proof liquor.

High Blood Pressure

High blood pressure, or *hypertension*, is a major risk factor for coronary heart disease (CHD) and the most important risk factor for stroke and congestive heart failure. Research indicates that high blood pressure is the cause of three of every five cases of heart failure in women. High blood pressure also boosts the likelihood that one will develop kidney disease or blindness.

Blood pressure is the amount of force exerted by the blood against the walls of the arteries. Controlling high blood pressure is especially important for people who have active heart disease. When blood pressure is lowered, the heart does not need to work as hard. For example, a person who has experienced a heart attack is less likely to have another if high blood pressure is controlled.

Diet

The precise role of dietary factors in heart disease is unclear, but enough is known to formulate general guidelines about a possible preventive diet. These are discussed later in this chapter under Diet and Nutrition.

Cholesterol Levels

High blood cholesterol is another very important risk factor for coronary heart disease that may be amenable to change. Some cholesterol is obtained from the diet (about 25%) and the rest is manufactured by the liver. Elevated levels in serum may be a result of high dietary intake, a condition known as *exogenous hyperlipidemia*, or secondary hyperlipidemia.

Endogenous hyperlipidemia, also called primary or familial hyperlipidemia, is a disorder of cholesterol metabolism that may be caused by genetic factors. It is much less responsive to dietary and lifestyle change than the exogenous form, and is also much less common. Diseases such as diabetes mellitus, gout, hypothyroidism, obstructive jaundice, cirrhosis of the liver, and renal failure can also cause secondary hyperlipidemia.

Dietary guidelines for lowering cholesterol are provided later in this chapter under Cholesterol.

Obesity

Obese people are more likely to develop heart-related problems, even if they have no other risk factors. Excess body weight is linked with coronary heart disease, stroke, congestive heart failure, and overall mortality from heart-related causes. Obesity contributes not only to cardiovascular diseases, but also to the development of other cardiovascular risk factors, including high blood pressure, high cholesterol, and diabetes.

Results of the National Health and Nutrition Examination Survey (NHANES) of 1999 indicate that an estimated 61% of American adults are either overweight or obese, defined as having a body mass index (BMI) of 25 or more.[12] BMI, an expression of the ratio of weight to height, is a mathematical formula that represents weight levels associated with the lowest overall risk to health. It is derived by dividing body weight in kilograms by the square of the height in meters $(wt/(ht)^2)$. Individuals with a BMI of 25 to 29.9 are considered overweight; individuals with a BMI of 30 or more are considered obese.[13]

Physical Inactivity

Physical inactivity increases the risk of heart disease. It both contributes directly to heart-related problems and increases the chances of developing other risk factors, such as high blood pressure and diabetes. The Surgeon General's report and other research conclude that as little as 30 minutes of moderate activity on most, and preferably all, days of the week can help protect heart health. Examples of moderate activity are brisk walking or bicycling, raking leaves, and gardening.

Diabetes

Diabetes is a serious disorder that also raises the risk of coronary heart disease. The risk of death from heart disease is about three times higher in people with diabetes. While there is no cure for diabetes, steps can be taken to control it. In certain people, being overweight and growing older are linked with the development of the most common type of diabetes, non–insulin dependent diabetes mellitus (NIDDM). Losing excess weight and boosting physical activity may help postpone or prevent the development of this disease. See chapter 22 for more information on the management of diabetes.

Stress and Personality

Research has revealed an association between a particular type of personality and the development of heart disease. According to this model, there are two personality extremes. *Type A behavior* is characterized by a chronic sense of urgency, possibly repressed aggressiveness, and a need to strive for achievement. Type A people drive themselves to meet deadlines, many of which are self-imposed. They experience intense feelings of psychological pressure, related to both time and personal responsibility. They often try to do two or three things at once, are likely to react with hostility to obstacles, and seem temperamentally incapable of easing up.

Type B behavior is characterized by the opposite traits. These people are less preoccupied with achievement, feel less rushed, and in general are much more easygoing. They are less prone to anger, impatience, and feelings of pressure. They are also better at separating work from play, and they know how to relax.

There is much debate about the value of such personality typing, but we will not concern ourselves with these details here. The important thing is the association of behavior types with disease development. However, from a holistic standpoint, we also need to bear in mind that people cannot be simply categorized into two types! Each person is an individual, and while it may sometimes be useful to sort people into artificial categories, people cannot be identified solely in this way.

Socioeconomic Factors

Certain social and economic factors are associated with an increased risk of heart disease. However, the findings tend to vary according to the society being studied. Some studies emphasize high risk in upper socioeconomic groups, while others emphasize the opposite. Some evidence suggests that class variations disappear when the degree of physical activity is taken into account. High-risk factors include social mobility that involves a change of environment, such as moving or changing jobs.

The relatively low, though increasing, incidence of heart disease in women appears to be due to psychosocial as much as biological factors. Men are more likely to strive for dominance and to use work as a major outlet for aggression, and so are more exposed to particular stresses and conflicts. However, such behavior patterns are as damaging to women as to men.

Life Events

Particularly stressful times in an individual's life act as possible danger points for stress-related problems such as heart disease. When stressful times can be identified, it is possible to take them into account by planning ahead, making it possible to manage and lessen the impact of these stresses on health and well-being. These points of increased stress, called life events, occur in everyone's life. They are especially relevant in the development of conditions such as angina and coronary heart disease.

Goals for Decreasing Cardiovascular Risks

Quit or minimize smoking

Lower and control blood pressure

Reduce total cholesterol

Decrease LDL cholesterol

Increase HDL cholesterol

Lose weight if overweight

Increase aerobic exercise

NUTRITIONAL FACTORS FOR CARDIOVASCULAR HEALTH

The basic dietary rules for lowering cholesterol and maintaining heart health are simple: Avoid saturated fats and dietary cholesterol. Experts recommend a diet that derives not more than 30% of daily calories from fat; some say 20%. Saturated fats from animal products and tropical oils should be kept to a minimum, so avoid deep-fried foods and pay attention to nutrition labels on packaged foods. Eat more vegetables, fruits, and grains, which are cholesterol-free, virtually fat-free, and rich in fiber. Dietary recommendations are discussed in more detail later on.

Coenzyme Q_{10}

Coenzyme Q_{10} (CoQ_{10} or ubiquinone) is found in small amounts in a wide variety of foods and is synthesized in all tissues. Coenzymes are molecular cofactors upon which enzymes depend for their function. Coenzyme Q_{10} is the coenzyme for a number of mitochondrial enzymes, as well as enzymes in other parts of the cell.

Mitochondria are small, subcellular particles that exist within each cell; here is where the cell's energy production process takes place. Through a series of chemical reactions along the electron transport chains of the mitochondria, adenosine triphosphate (ATP) molecules are produced. Mitochondrial enzymes are essential for the production of ATP, and all cellular functions depend upon ATP. More than 95% of the oxygen we breathe is used solely for the purpose of making energy through this process of burning organic substances. ATP molecules in turn supply energy for the various chemical reactions necessary for life.

CoQ_{10} plays a unique role in this electron transport chain, serving as a mobile messenger link between the various enzymes in the chain. Each pair of electrons processed by the chain must first interact with CoQ_{10}, and no other substance will substitute for CoQ_{10}. Other familiar substances involved in this electron transport chain include vitamin C, riboflavin (vitamin B_2), niacinamide (vitamin B_3), and vitamin E.

CoQ_{10} is naturally present in small amounts in a wide variety of foods, but is particularly high in organ meats, such as heart, liver, and kidney, and in beef, soy oil, sardines, mackerel, and peanuts. To put dietary CoQ_{10} intake into perspective, 1 pound of sardines, 2 pounds of beef, or $2\frac{1}{2}$ pounds of peanuts provide 30 mg of CoQ_{10}. CoQ_{10} is also synthesized in all tissues, and in healthy individuals, normal levels are maintained both by CoQ_{10} intake and by synthesis in the body. It has no known toxicity or side effects. Although present in food, CoQ_{10} is not considered a vitamin, because the body is able to produce it from raw materials contained in food. Nevertheless, the body often cannot make enough for optimal function, and therefore CoQ_{10} supplements may be very helpful.

CoQ_{10} is highly concentrated in heart muscle cells, due to the high energy requirements of this type of cell. Congestive heart failure has been associated with low blood and tissue levels of CoQ_{10}. The severity of heart failure correlates with the severity of CoQ_{10} deficiency. This CoQ_{10} deficiency may well be a primary factor in some types of heart muscle dysfunction; in others, it may be a secondary phenomenon.

Whether primary, secondary, or both, deficiency of CoQ_{10} appears to be a major treatable factor in the otherwise inexorable progression of heart failure. The clinical studies that have examined the treatment of heart disease with CoQ_{10} concluded that it significantly improved heart muscle function while producing no adverse effects or drug interactions. CoQ_{10} has been used successfully for high blood pressure, congestive heart failure, angina pectoris, and cardiomyopathy, and to protect the heart from the damaging effects of the chemotherapy drug Adriamycin.

B Vitamins

Homocysteine is an amino acid found naturally in the body. High blood levels of homocysteine may increase the chances of developing heart disease, stroke, and circulation problems. Elevated levels are believed to damage arteries, predispose the blood to easy clotting, and reduce the flexibility of blood vessels.

Blood homocysteine levels are influenced by the amount of three vitamins in the diet: folic acid and vitamins B_6 and B_{12}. Ingesting less than the recommended daily amounts of these vitamins may lead to higher homocysteine levels. Daily amounts recommended by the FDA are 400 mcg of folic acid, 2 mg of B_6, and 6 mcg of B_{12}. Good sources of folic acid include citrus fruits, tomatoes, vegetables, whole grains, beans, and lentils. Foods high in B_6 include meat, poultry, fish, fruits, vegetables, and grains. Major sources of B_{12} are meat, poultry, fish, milk, and other dairy products.

Dietary Suggestions to Reduce Cardiovascular Risks

Eat more fruits and vegetables.

Eat more whole grains.

Reduce fat intake to 25% to 30% of the diet.

Reduce cholesterol intake to less than 300 mg a day.

Reduce consumption of egg yolks to three to five per week.

Minimize the use of whole milk and its products; use low-fat or nonfat milk products.

Avoid red meats; eliminate all cured meats and lunchmeats.

Eat more cold-water fish, such as sardines and salmon.

Use fresh, cold-pressed oils, such as olive and flaxseed oils, to provide essential fatty acids.

General Recommendations for Heart Health

Eat foods that you like that are low in cholesterol and saturated fats. A diet free of animal products can lower cholesterol levels and blood pressure.

Be sure to consume an adequate amount of fiber. Fiber such as that from oat bran and psyllium seeds lowers the assimilation of dietary cholesterol.

Minimize salt, avoid stimulants, and drink little or no alcohol.

Don't smoke tobacco.

Drink at least 2 pints of water a day.

Get adequate amounts of enjoyable aerobic exercise—for example, a 30-minute walk, swim, or bicycle ride several times a week, and daily if possible.

Find a relaxation program that you enjoy, and incorporate it into your daily routine.

Maintain health in general, and especially maintain normal blood pressure.

Relax—watch the grass grow!

Also, as Dr. Andrew Weil puts it, "Open your heart." That our hearts get "broken" in the emotional sense is not a coincidental use of the word. Compassion, caring, and loving respect are all heart tonics.

Recommended Supplements

In *Textbook of Natural Medicine*, Drs. Murray and Pizzorno recommend the following supplements:[14]

High-potency multiple vitamin and mineral formula

Vitamin C: 500 to 1,000 mg three times a day

Vitamin E: 400 to 800 IU/day

Inositol hexaniacinate: 550 mg three times a day with meals for two weeks, then increase dosage to 1,000 mg three times a day with meals

Vitamin B$_6$: 10 mg/day

Vitamin B$_{12}$: 2 mcg/day

Folic acid: 1,000 mcg/day

Coenzyme Q$_{10}$: 50 mg two or three times a day

WHAT IS CARDIOVASCULAR DISEASE?

Cardiovascular disease is a disorder of the heart and blood vessels of the body. Blood brings oxygen and nutrients to the heart. When blood flow to the heart is impaired, angina results. When the blood flow is critically reduced, a myocardial infarction (heart attack) may occur. Lack of blood flow to the brain or, in some cases, bleeding in the brain can cause a stroke.

Coronary heart disease (CHD) is a general term for disease of the blood vessels of the heart, known as coronary arteries. CHD causes chest pain (angina) and heart attacks. Other major cardiovascular diseases include hypertension, atherosclerosis, and various types of vascular insufficiency. A less serious but nonetheless troubling cardiovascular condition is varicose veins. In this section, we shall consider a range of such problems in the process of exploring the contribution herbs can make when used in the context of holistic medicine.

ELEVATED CHOLESTEROL

The word *cholesterol* carries very fearful implications for many executives and hamburger eaters! While elevated cholesterol is not a disease in its own right, it has been implicated as a major factor in the development of many cardiovascular diseases, especially *arteriosclerosis*, a condition discussed later in this chapter.

However, though cholesterol may contribute to the development of heart disease, it also has an important role to play in human health. Cholesterol is found in all cells of the body, primarily as a structural component of cell membranes, but it has other vital functions. Stored in the adrenal glands, testes, and ovaries, it serves as a precursor molecule for hormones (such as the sex hormones, androgens and estrogens) and adrenal corticoids (including cortisol, corticosterone, and aldosterone).

In the liver, cholesterol functions as the precursor of bile acids, which, when secreted into the intestine, aid in the digestion of food, especially fats. Cholesterol is the major sterol in the human body and is found throughout the animal kingdom. While it seldom occurs in significant amounts in higher plants, plants do contain the therapeutically important phytosterols. (See chapter 5 for more information.)

Cholesterol Levels

Blood cholesterol levels begin to increase around age of 20, but rise sharply beginning at around age 40 and continue to increase until around age 60. The higher the blood cholesterol level, the higher the risk of heart disease.

In the bloodstream, cholesterol from the diet binds with protein molecules to form various types of so-called *lipoproteins*. High-density lipoprotein (HDL) is a dense, compact microparticle that transports excess cholesterol to the liver, where it is altered and expelled in the bile. Low-density lipoprotein (LDL) is a larger, less dense particle that tends to remain in the body. Very low-density lipoproteins (VLDLs) are molecules that transport *triglycerides*, chemical compounds that store fatty acids, an essential source of energy for the body.

Normal blood levels of triglycerides range from 10 to 150 milligrams per deciliter. Elevated serum cholesterol per se is not the only indicator of atherosclerosis; triglyceride levels are used to classify primary hyperlipidemias. In certain disorders, cholesterol levels may remain fairly normal while triglyceride levels rise. It is preferable, therefore, always to measure levels of each lipoprotein fraction, especially LDL, all of which contain cholesterol.

LDL is a form of lipid often called "bad" cholesterol, because too much LDL in the blood can lead to cholesterol buildup and blockage in the arteries. HDL is a form of lipid known as "good" cholesterol, because HDL helps remove cholesterol from the blood, preventing it from piling up in the arteries.

Diets rich in saturated fats, cholesterol, and calories appear to be chiefly responsible for high blood cholesterol, and therefore are believed to promote atherosclerosis. However, the tendency of cholesterol to form plaques is influenced by the type of lipoproteins that transport it in the blood. LDL is clearly atherogenic, but HDL appears to prevent accumulation of cholesterol in the tissues.

A desirable total cholesterol level for adults without heart disease is lower than 200 mg/dl (or 200 milligrams per deciliter of blood). A level of 240 mg/dl or higher is considered high blood cholesterol. But even cholesterol levels in the "borderline high" category (200 to 239 mg/dl) increase the risk of heart disease. HDL levels are interpreted differently from total cholesterol levels. The lower the HDL level, the higher the heart disease risk. An HDL level lower than 35 is a major risk factor for heart disease. A level of 60 or higher is considered protective.

Table 14.3. Classification of Cholesterol Levels*

PARAMETER	DESIRABLE	BORDERLINE HIGH	HIGH
Total cholesterol	Lower than 200	200–239	240 and higher
LDL	Optimal 100	130–159	160 and higher
HDL	60 or higher		

*Source: National Heart, Lung, and Blood Institute. 2001. National Cholesterol Education Program. *Third report of the expert panel on detection, evaluation, and treatment of high blood cholesterol in adults (Adult Treatment Panel III)*. NIH Publication No. 01-3670.

Blood levels of these lipoproteins are partially governed by dietary factors, especially the type of vegetable lipids (phytosterols) eaten. Phytosterols are plant compounds, structurally comparable to cholesterol, that effectively block uptake of cholesterol in the liver. This highlights the value of plants as both medicine and nutrition for cardiovascular problems. Plants provide a way to balance cholesterol absorption in a way that has evolved as our bodies evolved, affecting fat metabolism and blood chemistry in an inherently integrated manner. Medical research has revealed a number of common dietary components that actively lower cholesterol levels in the blood. The processes involved are complex and not always well understood.

Plants That Lower Blood Cholesterol

Guggulipid, an herbal remedy from southern India, is gaining a reputation for reducing high blood cholesterol levels. Guggulipid is an extract from the tree *Commiphora mukul*, commonly known as guggul. The tree is a close

Garlic: Food and Medicine

The use of garlic is supported by both an ancient history and a wealth of modern research. More than 3,000 scientific papers cover its chemistry, pharmacology, and clinical uses. The therapeutic uses of garlic are extensive, but those specific to the cardiovascular system include reducing elevated cholesterol, preventing atherosclerosis and hypertension, treating poor circulation to the legs, and improving overall blood flow through antiplatelet actions.

One study involved two groups of subjects: one of 20 healthy volunteers and the other of 62 patients with coronary heart disease and elevated serum cholesterol. Both study groups ate garlic for six months. All involved experienced beneficial changes, which reached a peak at the end of eight months. The improvement in cholesterol levels persisted throughout the two months of clinical follow-up. The clinicians concluded that garlic essential oil possesses a distinct hypolipidemic (fat-reducing) action in both healthy people and patients with coronary heart disease.

Great attention is being given by Indian research workers to the value of such findings in humans. A number of clinical comparisons of the influence of garlic have been published. In one example, a group of volunteers consumed a high-fat diet for seven days. On day eight of the study, fasting blood was analyzed for content of cholesterol and other fats. The subjects then received a high-fat diet supplemented with garlic for seven days; on day fifteen, fasting blood was analyzed again. Results showed that the fat-rich diet significantly increased cholesterol levels, compared with a normal diet. However, adding garlic to the high-fat diet significantly reduced serum cholesterol levels.[15] Based on research investigating the effect of raw garlic on normal blood cholesterol levels in men, Indian research scientists advocated its daily use as a means of lowering blood cholesterol.

Garlic also possesses antiplatelet effects, or an ability to inhibit unnecessary clotting within the blood vessels. It appears to work by reducing the "stickiness" of blood platelets, decreasing platelet aggregation and inhibiting the release of clotting factors in the blood. The garlic constituent thought to be responsible for this effect is allicin, a unique thiosulfinate well known for its strong antibiotic and antifungal properties. An exciting finding indicates that garlic works selectively, inhibiting the synthesis of enzymes involved in plaque formation while sparing the vascular synthesis of important prostaglandins.[16] This finding suggest that garlic would make a safe and effective antithrombotic agent.

The traditional use of both garlic and onion in the treatment of hypertension is supported by research.[17] A recent study revealed that onion oil contains a blood pressure–lowering prostaglandin.[18] Interestingly, while garlic's antimicrobial effects are lost during cooking, its blood pressure–normalizing and cholesterol-lowering actions appear to be unaffected.

relative of myrrh (*Commiphora molmol*). Ketonic steroid compounds present in the extract, known as guggulsterones, possess cholesterol- and triglyceride-lowering actions. Guggul lowers serum triglycerides and cholesterol as well as LDL and VLDL cholesterols.[19] As antioxidants, guggulsterones keep LDL cholesterol from oxidizing, an action that protects against atherosclerosis.

Capsicum annuum (cayenne pepper) and other plants that contain the compound capsaicin may help lower blood cholesterol levels, as does the widely used spice fenugreek (*Trigonella foenum-graecum*). Caraway (*Carum carvi*) is another aromatic spice with demonstrable cholesterol-lowering properties. In addition, a whole range of Asian herbal remedies new to Western medicine are proving their value in this area, including *Phyllanthus emblica* and *Ligustrum lucidum*.

Allium sativum (garlic) and *A. cepa* (onion) have an international reputation for lowering blood pressure and generally improving the health of the cardiovascular system (see sidebar Garlic: Food and Medicine on page 301). Other herbs reputed to have cholesterol-lowering properties are *Medicago sativa* (alfalfa), *Curcuma longa* (turmeric), and *Panax ginseng* (Korean ginseng).

General Guidelines for Lowering Cholesterol and LDL

Decrease total fats in diet.

Decrease saturated fats in diet.

Decrease cholesterol in diet.

Increase essential fatty acids (polyunsaturates) in diet.

Use more monounsaturated oils, such as olive and canola.

Increase fiber (for example, by adding psyllium husks or oat bran to the diet).

Increase complex carbohydrates.

Decrease caffeine and nicotine.

Add supplemental nutrients: vitamins B_6, B_3, C, chromium, essential fatty acids.

Include garlic in the diet or take as a supplement.

Guidelines for Increasing HDL Cholesterol

Get regular aerobic exercise.

Do not smoke.

Lose weight.

Add supplemental nutrients: essential fatty acids, niacin, fiber, garlic, L-carnitine.

Dietary Fats

Cholesterol-Rich Foods

Egg yolks	Pâté
Milk fat	Liver
Other organ meats	Fatty meats
Palm oil	

Saturated Fats

Butter	Poultry
Cheese	Coconut oil
Milk	Avocado
Red meats	Margarine

Monounsaturated Fats

Olive oil	Peanuts
Olives	Cashews
Almonds	Walnuts
Pecans	Fish

Polyunsaturated Fats

Vegetable oils (sesame, safflower, sunflower, corn, soybean)

HYPERTENSION

Elevation of systolic and/or diastolic blood pressure, either primary or secondary. (*The Merck Manual*)

More than 35 million Americans have *hypertension*, or high blood pressure. For unknown reasons, the occurrence of the disorder is twice as high in African Americans as Caucasians. While hypertension is a common problem in our culture, it is rare in those that remain relatively untouched by the Western lifestyle. Lifestyle plays a major role in causing and perpetuating hypertension. Thus, dietary, psychological, and social factors must all be addressed before any real change can occur.

A distinction must be made between elevated blood pressure with no obvious medical cause, known as *primary* or *essential hypertension*, and hypertension caused by an underlying pathology, such as kidney, endocrine, or cerebral disease, which is called *secondary hypertension*. For the purposes of this discussion, we will focus on essential hypertension.

Hypertension typically causes no symptoms until complications arise, in which case symptoms can include dizziness, flushed face and skin, headache, fatigue, epistaxis (nosebleed), and nervousness. These symptoms may all be caused by other conditions as well, making it difficult to diagnose hypertension by symptoms alone.

Diagnosis must be based on a finding that both systolic and diastolic blood pressure are usually (but not always) higher than normal, and other causes of symptoms must be excluded. In general, hypertension is indicated by a blood pressure measurement higher than 140/90 mm Hg. However, "normal" blood pressure varies among individuals, and thus normal should always be viewed in terms of a range, as opposed to a specific measurement. Observable changes in retinal blood vessels are diagnostic indicators of the degree of damage caused to the body by the hypertension.

Blood pressure is the force of the blood pushing against the walls of the arteries that carry blood throughout the body. The heart beats at a rate of 60 to 70 times a minute when at rest. Each time the heart beats, it pumps blood into the arteries. Blood pressure is highest when the heart contracts to pump the blood. This is called *systolic pressure*. When the heart is at rest, in between beats, blood pressure falls. This is the *diastolic pressure*.

Blood pressure is always expressed with two numbers that represent the systolic and diastolic pressures. These numbers are measurements of millimeters (mm) of mercury (Hg). The measurement is expressed as a fraction, with the systolic number on the top and the diastolic number on the bottom. For example, a blood pressure measurement of 120/80 mm Hg is expressed verbally as "120 over 80."

Blood pressure equal to or lower than 140/90 mm Hg is considered normal, and blood pressure lower than 120/80 mm Hg is even better. Blood pressure is considered high when it stays above 140/90 mm Hg over a period of time. It was once thought that low blood pressure (for example, 105/65 mm Hg in an adult) was unhealthy. Except in rare cases, this is not true. Table 14.4, from information provided by the National High Blood Pressure Education Program, demonstrates how blood pressure levels are categorized in adults.

Blood pressure fluctuates in response to different activities. For example, when one is running, blood pressure goes up. During sleep, blood pressure goes down. Such temporary, transient changes in blood pressure are a common and normal response to the ups and downs of life. Sustained hypertension, however, is caused by greater peripheral vascular resistance. This is initiated by increased arteriolar tone and followed by the damaging structural changes of arteriosclerosis.

Table 14.4. Blood Pressure Levels for Adults[20]*

CATEGORY	BLOOD PRESSURE LEVEL (mm Hg)	
	Systolic	Diastolic
Normal	120	80
High normal	130–139	85–89
High blood pressure		
Stage 1	140–159	90–99
Stage 2	160–179	100–109
Stage 3	≥180	≥110

*People aged 18 and older who are not taking medicine for high blood pressure and not experiencing a short-term serious illness.

If left untreated, high blood pressure can lead to serious medical problems, including:

Arteriosclerosis. High blood pressure damages artery walls, causing them to become thick, stiff, and narrow; hence, the term "hardening of the arteries." Arteriosclerosis speeds the buildup of cholesterol and fats in the blood vessels, inhibiting blood flow through the body and increasing risk of heart attack or stroke.

Myocardial infarction. When the arteries that bring blood to the heart muscle become blocked, the heart cannot get enough oxygen. Reduced blood flow can cause chest pain (angina). Eventually, blood flow may be stopped completely, leading to a myocardial infarction, or heart attack.

Enlarged heart. High blood pressure makes the heart work harder. Over time, this causes the heart to thicken and stretch. Eventually, the heart fails to function normally, and fluid backs up into the lungs.

Kidney damage. The kidney acts as a filter that rids the body of wastes. Over the course of years, high blood pressure can narrow and thicken the blood vessels of the kidney so that the kidney is able to filter less fluid, and waste will build up in the blood. Eventually, the kidneys may fail altogether.

Stroke. High blood pressure contributes to arteriosclerosis, which causes arteries to narrow, so less blood can get to the brain. If a blood clot blocks one of these narrowed arteries, a stroke may occur. A stroke can also occur when very high pressure causes a weakened blood vessel in the brain (called an aneurysm) to break.

Treatment of Hypertension

The cardiovascular system needs herbal tonic support, which is supplied by the core hypotensive herbs. Other areas that need attention include the nervous system and, potentially, the lungs. Beyond this, treatment depends on the individual case. All treatment for hypertension must take place within the context of dietary and lifestyle reassessment.

Actions Indicated

Hypotensives are a broad range of remedies with the observed effect of lowering elevated blood pressure. They appear to work in a variety of ways. (See chapter 9 for a discussion of possible pharmacological mechanisms.)

Cardiotonics play a fundamental role in strengthening and toning the whole cardiovascular system when under such literal pressure. Used correctly, they facilitate beneficial changes in both the pattern and the volume of cardiac output.

Peripheral vasodilators lessen resistance within the peripheral blood vessels, thus increasing the total volume of the system and lowering pressure within it.

Diuretics help reduce the buildup of excess fluid in the body and overcome any decreased renal blood flow that might accompany the hypertension.

Vascular tonics will help nourish and tone the tissue of the arteries and veins.

Nervines address the tension and anxiety associated with any stress component in the patient's picture. Hypertension itself causes an increase in tension, which can also be eased with appropriate nervines. Most nervines are also antispasmodic.

Antispasmodics help ease peripheral resistance to blood flow by gently relaxing the muscular coat of the vessels and the muscles that the vessels pass through.

Circulatory stimulants help increase peripheral circulation.

Specific Remedies

A number of herbs have a reputation as being specific for hypertension, generally because of their impact on one or another of the processes involved in the development of the condition. The most important hypotensive plant remedy in Western medicine is hawthorn (*Crataegus* spp.), probably followed by linden (*Tilia* spp.). European mistletoe *(Viscum album)* and olive leaf *(Olea europaea)* are other well-known plants that may be considered specifics.

On the other hand, the multifactorial etiology of hypertension limits the value of the concept of specifics for this condition. Orthodox medicine has utilized *Rauvolfia serpentina* (Indian snakeroot) as a treatment for hypertension, but there are problematic side effects.

Other plants may come to mind, depending upon the individual's specific symptoms. For example, if headaches are part of the picture, then include *Stachys betonica* (wood betony) as part of the prescription. If there are associated heart palpitations, add *Leonurus cardiaca* (motherwort). A stress component would suggest increasing the nervine content, and possibly adding an adaptogen.

A Prescription for Hypertension

Crataegus spp.	2 parts
Tilia platyphyllos	1 part
Achillea millefolium	1 part
Viburnum opulus	1 part
Valeriana officinalis	1 part

Dosage: up to 5 ml of tincture three times a day. *Allium sativum* should be added to the diet or used as a dietary supplement: 1 clove of fresh garlic or 200 to 300 mg of standardized extract three times a day.

Table 14.5. Actions Supplied by Hypertension Prescription

ACTION	HERBS
Hypotensive	*Crataegus* spp., *Tilia platyphyllos, Achillea millefolium, Viburnum opulus, Valeriana officinalis*
Cardiotonic	*Crataegus* spp., *Tilia platyphyllos*
Diuretic	*Achillea millefolium, Crataegus* spp., *Tilia platyphyllos*
Antispasmodic	*Tilia platyphyllos, Viburnum opulus, Valeriana officinalis*
Vascular tonic	*Crataegus* spp., *Tilia platyphyllos, Achillea millefolium*
Nervine relaxant	*Tilia platyphyllos, Viburnum opulus, Valeriana officinalis*

Starting with a basic prescription, it is possible to fine-tune the individual's medications to address his or her unique situation. The possibilities are as endless as people are diverse. From debility and digestive problems to bronchitis and premenstrual syndrome, the phytotherapist can alter a basic formulation to readily embrace the needs of the whole patient. Note that the choice and exact proportions of herbs in the prescription will depend on the relative severity of the associated symptom picture.

A Prescription for Hypertension with a Major Stress Component

Crataegus spp.	2 parts
Tilia platyphyllos	1 part
Achillea millefolium	1 part
Eleutherococcus senticosus	1 part
Scutellaria lateriflora	1 part
Viburnum opulus	1 part
Valeriana officinalis	1 part

Dosage: up to 5 ml of tincture three times a day. *Allium sativum* should be added to the diet or used as a dietary supplement: 1 clove of fresh garlic or 200 to 300 mg of standardized extract three times a day.

A Prescription for Hypertension with Associated Headache

Crataegus spp.	2 parts
Stachys betonica	2 parts
Tilia platyphyllos	1 part
Achillea millefolium	1 part
Viburnum opulus	1 part

Dosage: up to 5 ml of tincture three times a day. *Allium sativum* should be added to the diet or used as a dietary supplement: 1 clove of fresh garlic or 200 to 300 mg of standardized extract three times a day.

A Prescription for Hypertension with Palpitations

Leonurus cardiaca	2 parts
Crataegus spp.	2 parts
Tilia platyphyllos	1 part
Achillea millefolium	1 part
Viburnum opulus	1 part

Dosage: up to 5 ml of tincture three times a day. *Allium sativum* should be added to the diet or used as a dietary supplement: 1 clove of fresh garlic or 200 to 300 mg of standardized extract three times a day.

A Prescription for Hypertension with Debility

Crataegus spp.	2 parts
Tilia platyphyllos	1 part
Achillea millefolium	1 part
Viburnum opulus	1 part
Artemisia vulgaris	1 part

Dosage: up to 5 ml of tincture three times a day. *Allium sativum* should be added to the diet or used as a dietary supplement: 1 clove of fresh garlic or 200 to 300 mg of standardized extract three times a day.

A Prescription for Hypertension with Indigestion

Crataegus spp.	2 parts
Matricaria recutita	2 parts
Tilia platyphyllos	1 part
Achillea millefolium	1 part
Viburnum opulus	1 part
Valeriana officinalis	1 part

Dosage: up to 5 ml of tincture three times a day. *Allium sativum* should be added to the diet or used as a dietary supplement: 1 clove of fresh garlic or 200 to 300 mg of standardized extract three times a day.

A Prescription for Hypertension with Bronchitis

Crataegus spp.	2 parts
Tilia platyphyllos	1 part
Achillea millefolium	1 part
Marrubium vulgare	1 part
Viburnum opulus	1 part
Verbascum thapsus	1 part

Dosage: up to 5 ml of tincture three times a day. *Allium sativum* should be added to the diet or used as a dietary supplement: 1 clove of fresh garlic or 200 to 300 mg of standardized extract three times a day.

A Prescription for Hypertension with Premenstrual Syndrome

Crataegus spp.	2 parts
Tilia platyphyllos	1 part
Achillea millefolium	1 part
Scutellaria lateriflora	1 part
Viburnum opulus	1 part
Valeriana officinalis	1 part
Vitex agnus-castus	1 part

Dosage: up to 5 ml of tincture three times a day. *Allium sativum* should be added to the diet or used as a dietary supplement: 1 clove of fresh garlic or 200 to 300 mg of standardized extract three times a day.

Broader Context of Treatment

A plethora of factors have been identified as important in the cause and treatment of essential hypertension. However, it is vital to remember that cause is always multifactorial, and statements about alcohol or calcium consumption are often too simplistic. While experts disagree about the connection between tobacco and hypertension, there is no doubt about the overall impact of smoking upon the heart, so tobacco should be avoided.

A well-known link exists between obesity and hypertension, as well as heart attack, diabetes, gallstones, osteoarthritis, and kidney disease. Weight reduction is an essential component of a treatment program for hypertension, and often lowers blood pressure more effectively than drug treatment.

Drugs represent another factor that must be considered. A number of medications raise blood pressure as an unwanted side effect. Check on all prescription drugs that the patient is using, and note that even over-the-counter nonsteroidal anti-inflammatory drugs may cause mild water retention that can elevate blood pressure. Bear in mind when taking the case history that oral contraceptives have been associated with cardiovascular and pulmonary adverse effects.

Lifestyle changes are often the key to reversing hypertension. The nature of the individual's work, relationships, worldview, and self-image may all play a role in the development of hypertension, creating a challenging job for the herbalist! Dietary changes, weight reduction, and tobacco cessation are crucial, but exercise, massage and other bodywork, relaxation techniques, and meditation can make important contributions.

Aromatherapy has much to offer when appropriate essential oils are used in the context of relaxing massage. Hypotensive oils to consider include lavender, marjoram, and ylang ylang. If the situation calls for it, relaxing oils may be also be used; consider chamomile, rose, bergamot, and neroli.

Key Therapeutic Guidelines for the Management of Hypertension

Maintain an appropriate body weight, reducing excessive weight if necessary.

Make healthy lifestyle choices:
  Avoid alcohol, caffeine, and tobacco.
  Reduce the impact of stress and incorporate stress-reduction techniques.
  Exercise regularly, but in a way that is enjoyable.

Make appropriate dietary changes:
  Eat a diet rich in fiber, complex carbohydrates, and potassium.
  Eat garlic and onions.
  Reduce or eliminate animal fats and increase intake of vegetable oils.
  Eliminate salt from the diet.

Add appropriate cardiotonic herbs.

Supplement the diet with:
  Magnesium: 800 to 1,200 mg/day
  Vitamin C: 500 to 1,000 mg three times a day
  Vitamin E: 400 to 800 IU/day
  Coenzyme Q$_{10}$: 50 mg two or three times a day
  Garlic: the equivalent of 4,000 mg a day of fresh garlic

Specific Dietary Guidelines

Salt. Average Western salt intake is about 15 times that needed by the body. Blood pressure usually falls when hypertensives cut back on salt and sodium in general. Some are more affected by sodium than others, but there is no practical way to predict this. Thus, hypertensives should eat no more than about 6 g of salt a day (approximately 1 teaspoon, or about 2,400 mg of sodium). The patient should keep track of *all* salt eaten, including the amount in processed foods.

Potassium. The relative balance between sodium and potassium is critical to many cardiovascular risk factors. Potassium levels in the diet should be raised through consumption of potassium-rich foods, such as bananas, orange juice, and potatoes. In addition, certain cooking methods are less likely to wash away this essential mineral.

Calcium and magnesium. Supplementation with these minerals can have a marked hypotensive effect.

Sugar. In some individuals, heavy sugar intake may raise blood pressure, possibly by causing sodium retention or by a direct effect on the hormonal stress response mediated by the adrenal cortex.

Alcohol. There appears to be a link between alcohol and hypertension, but not a simple one. Statistics show that people who drink a little tend to have lower blood pressure than teetotalers or those who drink a lot. Alcohol withdrawal causes a temporary increase in blood pressure, followed by a decrease. All in all, it is safe to say that individuals with a tendency to hypertension should avoid alcohol.

Caffeine. Tea, coffee, and cola drinks will aggravate hypertension because of the stimulating effect of caffeine and other alkaloids that they contain. This also goes for the caffeine-containing herbal stimulant products on the market.

Saturated fats. Apart from the impact upon blood cholesterol and other lipids, there appears to be an association between excess consumption of saturated fats and hypertension. As with all cardiovascular conditions, increasing the ratio of polyunsaturated fats to saturated fats will help in the healing process.

Vegetarian diet. A diet free of animal products lowers blood pressure and is strongly recommended for hypertensive patients. At the very least, people with hypertension should avoid red meat.

ARTERIOSCLEROSIS

Arteriosclerosis. A generic term for a number of diseases in which the arterial wall becomes thickened and loses elasticity. *(The Merck Manual)*

Atherosclerosis. A form of arteriosclerosis characterized by patchy subintimal thickening (atheromas) of medium and large arteries, which can reduce or obstruct blood flow. *(The Merck Manual)*

The term *arteriosclerosis* refers to several diseases involving arteries of various sizes and different layers of the arterial walls. From Greek words that mean "hardening of the arteries," the term originally signified the tendency of arteries to become hard and brittle through the deposition of calcium in their walls. However, this is not an important characteristic of the most familiar form of arteriosclerosis, *atherosclerosis*. This disease is characterized by fatty deposits on the intima, or inner lining, of the arteries.

Half the annual mortality in Western society results from heart and blood vessel diseases, and atherosclerosis, the most common lethal disease, is the chief cause. This is due to the impact of the disease upon the brain, heart, kidneys, and other organs of the body. Although herbs with antiarteriosclerotic properties exist, herbalism aims to prevent the disease by addressing causative factors, which include not only hypertension, but also diabetes mellitus, smoking, diet, and obesity.

Atherosclerosis is a disease of the arteries characterized by fatty deposits on the inner lining. The presence of these fatty deposits, called *arterial plaques*, leads to an important loss of arterial elasticity and a narrowing of the artery. The constriction of blood flow that results ultimately deprives vital organs of their blood supply. Clots may lodge in arteries supplying the heart, causing a heart attack, or the brain, causing stroke. Atherosclerosis may be manifested fairly rapidly in diseases in which the concentration of blood lipids is raised, such as diabetes.

Atherosclerosis is so prevalent in developed countries that many Americans assume it is a natural consequence of aging. However, overwhelming evidence links atherosclerosis closely to diet and lifestyle, suggesting that it can be prevented, slowed, or in some cases even reversed.

Depending on the location and degree of arterial damage, atherosclerosis can lead to kidney problems, high blood pressure, stroke, and other life-threatening conditions. Atherosclerosis tends to target the aorta—the body's largest artery, which leads from the heart—as well as the arteries that lead to the brain, the lower limbs, and the kidneys. Damage to the arteries that carry blood to the legs and feet can cause peripheral arterial occlusive disease, which makes walking painful. Severely restricted circulation to the limbs can also cause skin ulcers and even gangrene (tissue death).

Blockage in the coronary arteries, which feed oxygen-rich blood directly to the heart muscles, is known as *coronary artery disease* or *coronary heart disease*. Such blockage causes *ischemia*, a localized oxygen starvation affecting tissue. This disorder and its complications—angina, cardiac arrhythmias, and heart attack—are the leading causes of death in the United States and most of Europe.

Atherosclerotic deposits begin as thin, fatty streaks on an arterial wall. Such streaks may come and go in a person with a healthy lifestyle. However, if the arteries are damaged—typically from high blood pressure, stress, or smoking—the inner surface of the walls can start to deteriorate. To compensate, the artery grows new tissue that may create tiny bumps or scars. Cholesterol, white blood cells, and other deposits can begin to accumulate within these bumps, forming plaques that clog the arteries. Eventually, calcium deposits and scar tissue surround the soft plaques, making the arteries hard and inelastic. Atherosclerosis progresses over many years, which perhaps contributes to the perception that it is an affliction of aging. However, it appears that arterial deposits can begin in childhood, with significant plaque formation by the time a person is 30 years old.

People with high levels of blood cholesterol, especially LDL, are at risk for developing atherosclerosis. LDL cholesterol reacts with unstable chemical compounds called free radicals in a process that degrades both the transport mechanism for moving cholesterol through the bloodstream and the tissue lining of arterial walls. Nonetheless, most people with high cholesterol do not develop atherosclerosis, and many people with atherosclerosis have normal cholesterol levels.

A number of biochemical, physiological, and environmental risk factors increase the chance that an individual will develop atherosclerosis:

Hypertension. High blood pressure is a critical factor in the atherosclerotic process, which does not normally occur in low-pressure pulmonary arteries and veins, despite the fact that they are bathed by the same blood concentration of lipids.

Elevated serum lipid levels. The atherogenicity of cholesterol is influenced by type of lipoprotein. LDL is clearly atherogenic, but HDL appears to prevent accumulation of cholesterol in the tissues.

Obesity promotes the development of all risk factors.

Cigarette smoking increases the chances of developing this and many other diseases.

Diets rich in saturated fats, cholesterol, and calories appear to be chiefly responsible for high blood cholesterol, and such diets are therefore believed to promote atherosclerosis.

Family history of premature atherosclerotic disease appears to indicate either a propensity to higher levels of LDL or an increased susceptibility to atherosclerosis risk factors. Inborn errors in lipid metabolism also increase susceptibility.

Diabetes mellitus may lead to arteriosclerosis.

Gender. Between the ages of 35 and 44, the death rate from coronary heart disease among white men is 6.1 times that for white women. This is thought to be due to hormonal and socioeconomic influences. Overt manifestations of arteriosclerosis are rare in either sex before the age of 40, because a greater than 75% narrowing of the arteries must occur before blood flow is seriously impeded.

Aging brings about degenerative arterial changes such as dilation, tortuousness, thickening, and loss of elasticity.

Physical inactivity increases the chance that complications will develop, but the disease affects both active and sedentary individuals.

Personality type, especially type A, appears to predispose individuals to a range of cardiovascular problems.

Lifestyle factors, including diet and stress level, can contribute.

Treatment of Atherosclerosis

The cardiovascular system should be the focus of tonic attention. If any secondary problems have developed in other organs of the body because of ischemia, these must be treated. Common sites for such problems are the kidneys, eyes, and brain. The herbal guidelines must be utilized within the context of dietary and lifestyle reassessment.

Actions Indicated

Cardiotonics and *vascular tonics* help support the tissue of the cardiovascular system, possibly maintaining flexibility and tone in affected vessels.

Circulatory stimulants promote the circulation of blood, and thus oxygen availability, in the face of the increased vascular resistance characteristic of this condition.

Peripheral vasodilators have an obvious value, because they have the potential to lessen the impact of vessel blockage.

Hypotensives are indicated to help lower elevated blood pressure.

Nervines will be indicated if stress is an issue.

Antispasmodics will help relax the muscular coat of the arteries, as well as the muscles that the peripheral vessels pass through.

A Prescription for Atherosclerosis

Crataegus spp.	2 parts
Tilia platyphyllos	1 part
Achillea millefolium	1 part
Viburnum opulus	1 part
Ginkgo biloba	1 part

Dosage: up to 5 ml of tincture three times a day. *Allium sativum* should be added to the diet or used as a dietary supplement: 1 clove of fresh garlic or 200 to 300 mg of standardized extract three times a day.

It is no coincidence that this suggested prescription is similar to those given for hypertension. There is a strong correlation between the etiologies of the two conditions, and thus the specific remedies for treatment are similar.

Table 14.6. Actions Supplied by Atherosclerosis Prescription

ACTION	HERBS
Cardiotonic and vascular tonic	*Crataegus* spp., *Tilia platyphyllos*, *Achillea millefolium*, *Viburnum opulus*, *Ginkgo biloba*, *Allium sativum*
Peripheral vasodilator	*Ginkgo biloba*, *Achillea millefolium*, *Allium sativum*
Hypotensive	*Crataegus* spp., *Tilia platyphyllos*, *Achillea millefolium*, *Viburnum opulus*, *Allium sativum*
Nervine	*Tilia platyphyllos*, *Viburnum opulus*
Antispasmodic	*Crataegus* spp., *Tilia platyphyllos*, *Viburnum opulus*, *Ginkgo biloba*

Broader Context of Treatment

Atherosclerosis develops when known risk factors are compounded by genetic predisposition, so if one has a family history of atherosclerosis, the prudent course of action is to accept what cannot be changed and to change what can. In addition to the herbal medicines described, follow the general and nutritional recommendations for heart health provided earlier in this chapter.

In *Textbook of Natural Medicine*, Drs. Murray and Pizzorno recommend the following supplements:[21]

Magnesium: 800 to 1,200 mg/day

Vitamin C: 500 to 1,000 mg three times a day

Vitamin E: 400 to 800 IU/day

Flaxseed oil: 1 tablespoon/day

Coenzyme Q$_{10}$: 50 mg two or three times a day

Niacin (in the form of inositol hexaniacinate): 500 mg three times a day with meals for two weeks, then increase dosage to 1,000 mg three times a day with meals

Garlic: the equivalent of 4,000 mg a day of fresh garlic

CONGESTIVE HEART FAILURE

A common syndrome that may be caused by different etiologies whose clinical manifestations reflect a fundamental abnormality—a decrease in the myocardial contractile state such that cardiac output is inadequate for the body's needs. *(The Merck Manual)*

Congestive heart failure (CHF) is a severe condition in which the heart cannot supply the body with enough blood because it is functioning inadequately as a pump. Usually, the loss of pumping ability is a symptom of an underlying heart problem, such as coronary artery disease. The term *heart failure* suggests a sudden and complete cessation of heart activity, but in reality, the condition generally develops slowly, as the heart gradually loses its ability to pump efficiently.

Some people may experience no symptoms of congestive heart failure until years after the heart begins its decline. Most symptoms result from congestion that develops in the lungs or from backed-up blood in the veins. How critical the condition is depends on how much pumping capacity the heart has lost. The severity of the condition will determine its impact on an individual's life. Milder heart failure may have little effect, while severe heart failure can interfere with even simple activities and eventually prove fatal.

Nearly everyone's heart loses some pumping capacity with age, but a number of other factors can also lead to a potentially life-threatening loss of pumping activity. As a symptom of underlying heart disease, heart failure is closely associated with the major risk factors already discussed: smoking, high cholesterol levels, hypertension, diabetes and abnormal blood sugar levels, and obesity. Eliminating such risk factors lowers the risk of developing or aggravating heart disease and heart failure. The presence of coronary heart disease is among the greatest risks for heart failure. Muscle damage and scarring caused by a heart attack greatly increase the risk of heart failure, as does cardiac arrhythmia, or irregular heartbeat. Any disorder that causes abnormal swelling or thickening of the heart also sets the stage for heart failure.

A number of symptoms are associated with heart failure, but none is specific for the condition.

Shortness of breath is often the most prominent symptom. In heart failure, this may result from a buildup of fluid in the lungs. Breathing difficulties may occur at rest or during exercise. In some cases, congestion may be severe enough to prevent or interrupt sleep.

Fatigue or easy tiring is another symptom. As the heart's pumping capacity decreases, muscles and other tissues receive less oxygen and nutrition. Thus, the body cannot perform as much work, leading to fatigue.

Fluid retention, or edema, may cause swelling of the feet, ankles, legs, and occasionally the abdomen.

Persistent coughing is another sign, especially coughing that regularly produces mucus or pink, blood-tinged sputum. Some people develop raspy breathing or wheezing.

Because heart failure generally develops slowly, these symptoms may not appear until the condition has progressed over years. The heart hides the underlying problem by making adjustments that delay the eventual loss in pumping capacity. The heart compensates in three ways to cope with the effects of heart failure:

1. Enlargement (dilatation) allows more blood into the heart.
2. Thickening of muscle fibers (hypertrophy) strengthens the heart muscle.
3. More frequent contractions increase circulation.

By making these adjustments, or compensating, the heart can temporarily make up for losses in pumping ability, sometimes for years. However, compensation has its limits. Eventually, the heart cannot offset its lost ability to pump blood, and the signs of heart failure appear.

Treatment of Congestive Heart Failure

While herbs containing cardiac glycosides are the basis of a number of important pharmaceutical drugs for congestive heart failure, it would be inappropriate to explore the use of these cardioactive remedies in a book of this kind. As dramatically effective as they are, the key to safe and successful therapeutic application is skilled diagnosis and interpretation, as well as regular monitoring for levels of cardiac glycosides in the blood. Without this skill, these plants are extremely poisonous. However, the noncardioactive approach described here will prove effective for the treatment of mild heart failure that does not warrant the use of stronger medications, especially for elderly patients with chronic CHF.

As mild CHF is usually a result of degenerative

processes, it may be accompanied by any of the plethora of conditions that manifest in the aging process. Tonic support of the cardiovascular and respiratory systems is indicated, but beyond that, specifics will depend on the individual concerned.

Actions Indicated

Cardioactive drugs will often be the core of treatment for such problems, but are best prescribed by skilled diagnosticians who can follow the changes brought about in the heart and its functioning. Regular monitoring of cardiac glycosides in the blood is essential.

Cardiotonics will support the action of cardiac glycosides prescribed. As they theoretically may potentiate the activity of cardioactives, blood monitoring is still needed.

Peripheral vasodilators may be indicated to help with general blood circulation.

Hypotensives are often appropriate because of associated hypertension.

Diuretics ease water-retention problems. Cardioactive diuretics are often used in orthodox medicine. Replacement of flushed-out potassium is essential.

Nervines will ease stress, whether causal or a result of the heart disease.

Specific Remedies

As primary cardioactives are generally out of the range of what herbalists can use safely, we shall not use *Convallaria* or its equivalents in the prescription suggested here. Our aim is to either strengthen the heart muscle or support the work of allopathically prescribed cardiac glycosides.

Crataegus, *Tilia*, and *Allium sativum* are essential. In addition, an herb from the ayurvedic tradition is offering great hope in the treatment of a range of cardiovascular conditions. *Coleus forskohlii* and its diterpene constituent forskolin can lower blood pressure while improving the contractility of the heart.[22]

A Prescription for Mild Congestive Heart Failure

Crataegus spp.	3 parts
Ginkgo biloba	1 part
Tilia platyphyllos	1 part
Taraxacum officinale leaf	1 part
Viburnum opulus	1 part
Valeriana officinalis	1 part

Dosage: up to 5 ml of tincture three times a day. *Allium sativum* should be added to the diet or used as a dietary supplement: 1 clove of fresh garlic or 200 to 300 mg of standardized extract three times a day.

Broader Context of Treatment

The dietary and lifestyle issues already discussed all apply for congestive heart failure. Follow the general and nutritional recommendations for heart health provided earlier in this chapter.

In *Textbook of Natural Medicine*, Drs. Murray and Pizzorno recommend the following supplements:[23]

Magnesium: 200 to 400 mg three times a day
Thiamine: 200 to 250 mg/day
L-carnitine: 300 to 500 mg three times a day
Coenzyme Q_{10}: 150 to 300 mg/day

ANGINA PECTORIS

A clinical syndrome due to myocardial ischemia characterized by precordial discomfort or pressure, typically precipitated by exertion and relieved by rest or sublingual nitroglycerin. *(The Merck Manual)*

Angina pectoris, commonly known as *angina*, is a recurring pain or discomfort in the chest that indicates that the heart is not getting enough oxygen. Angina may result from blockage of the coronary arteries that supply blood to the heart or occur because the heart is overworked and thus needs more oxygen than usual.

The main underlying cause of angina is coronary artery disease, which stems from atherosclerosis of the coronary arteries. Angina may also be related to other diseases that tax the heart unduly, such as anemia, aortic valve disease, cardiac arrhythmia, and hyperthyroidism. Episodes of angina occur when the heart's need for oxygen exceeds the availability of oxygen from the blood that nourishes the heart. Physical exertion is the most common trigger for angina. Other triggers include emotional stress, extreme cold or heat, heavy meals, alcohol, and cigarette smoking.

The term *angina pectoris* literally means "choking sensation in the chest." It is usually experienced as a crushing or constricting pain that starts in the center of the chest, deep behind the breastbone, and may radiate to other parts of the body. However, the pain of angina may be felt only in peripheral locations, such as the jaw, abdomen, and arm. The pain can also be confused with indigestion, because the tight, burning sensations are similar.

An angina attack is not a heart attack! While the pain is similar, it does not last as long, usually no more than five minutes. Angina pain simply indicates that some of the heart muscle is not getting enough blood temporarily. The pain does not mean that the heart muscle is suffering irreversible, permanent damage. In addition, not all chest pain comes from the heart, and not all pain related to the heart is angina. For example, if the pain lasts for less than 30 seconds, or if it disappears during a deep breath, after drinking a glass of water, or after changing position, it almost certainly is not angina and should not cause concern. However, prolonged pain, unrelieved by rest or accompanied by other symptoms, may signal a heart attack.

Treatment of Angina Pectoris

The herbal treatment guidelines given here must be utilized within the broader context of dietary and nutritional reassessment. The herbal approach to treating angina pectoris is similar to that for hypertension and arteriosclerosis. Please refer to those sections for details.

Specific Remedies

Crataegus can be considered the closest to a specific for this condition. *Crataegus* leaves, flowers, and fruits contain a number of biologically active flavonoid substances. Studies show that *Crataegus* may inhibit the progression of atherosclerosis, increase coronary perfusion, and confer mild hypotensive effects. It may also antagonize atherogenesis and have a positive effect on the contractile ability of the heart.[24]

Salvia miltiorrhiza (dan shen) is used in traditional Chinese medicine as a circulatory stimulant, sedative, and cooling agent. It may also be valuable as an antianginal drug, because it has been shown to dilate coronary arteries in all concentrations. *S. miltiorrhiza* also appears to have a protective action against myocardial ischemia.

A Prescription for Angina

Crataegus spp.	3 parts
Leonurus cardiaca	2 parts
Achillea millefolium	1 part
Tilia platyphyllos	1 part
Viburnum opulus	1 part
Ginkgo biloba	1 part

Dosage: up to 5 ml of tincture three times a day. *Allium sativum* should be added to the diet or used as a dietary supplement: 1 clove of fresh garlic or 200 to 300 mg of standardized extract three times a day. In addition, the patient can take 5 ml of *Crataegus* tincture at the first sign of an angina attack. This will not replace the use of prescription medication.

Broader Context of Treatment

Issues similar to those covered earlier must be addressed— that is, the whole panoply of dietary and lifestyle factors that contribute to an individual's unique life experience. In addition to the herbal medicines described, follow the general and nutritional guidelines for heart health provided earlier in this chapter.

In *Textbook of Natural Medicine*, Drs. Murray and Pizzorno recommend the following supplements:[25]

Magnesium: 200 to 400 mg three times a day
Coenzyme Q_{10}: 150 to 300 mg/day
Garlic: the equivalent of 4,000 mg a day of fresh garlic

PERIPHERAL ARTERIAL OCCLUSIVE DISEASE

> Occlusion of blood supply to the extremities by atherosclerotic plaques. *(The Merck Manual)*

Peripheral arterial occlusive disease, also known as *intermittent claudication*, is a peripheral vascular disease caused by narrowing of the arteries in the legs. This restricts the flow of blood to muscles in the calves, thighs, and buttocks. While usually asymptomatic in early stages, the restricted availability of oxygen eventually causes major problems. The most striking symptoms occur upon exertion, such as walking.

Because of the limited blood supply, the muscles do not receive the oxygen they need, resulting in the buildup of lactic acid and other products of enforced anaerobic metabolism. These metabolites cause pain and cramping and interfere with the ability to walk. During rest, the pain and discomfort subside. There is a close association between the etiology of this condition and that of atherosclerosis. Please refer to that discussion for more details.

Treatment of Peripheral Arterial Occlusive Disease

In addition to the herbal suggestions given here, a complex of lifestyle issues must be addressed. The nutritional guidelines given throughout this chapter are important. Some simple behavioral pointers can help encourage blood flow back into the trunk:

Avoid crossing the legs, but if necessary, cross the legs at the ankles, not the knees.
Avoid high heels, which limit the use of the calf muscles.
Avoid restrictive clothing that limits blood flow in the groin or calf.
Avoid prolonged sitting or standing.
Take breaks to walk around to help move the blood along.
Rest and elevate the legs.

Actions Indicated

Cardiotonic. The pathology that manifests in the legs suggests that disease processes are almost certainly affecting the whole cardiovascular system.

Peripheral vasodilators facilitate blood flow to the extremities.

Hypotensives may help, as there is a close connection between hypertension and the development of this condition.

Diuretics may be appropriate if edema is present; however, edema calls for careful examination of the heart. Mild, positively inotropic remedies, such as *Crataegus*, may be adequate.

Vascular tonics are essential to tone and strengthen the blood vessels.

Nervines may be indicated, depending upon the individual's needs.

Antispasmodics may help ease the degree of muscular spasm.

Specific Remedies

Crataegus (hawthorn), *Aesculus* (horse chestnut), and *Ginkgo* may all be considered specifics for this problem. *Aesculus hippocastanum* has been the subject of numerous clinical studies on the treatment of this condition. A meta-analysis of these studies concluded that the herb was efficacious and safe.[26]

Ginkgo biloba is useful for treating peripheral vascular disease, including diabetic retinopathy and intermittent claudication. Flavonoids in *Ginkgo* reduce capillary permeability and fragility and serve as free radical scavengers. Terpene ginkgolides inhibit platelet-activating factor, decrease vascular resistance, and improve circulatory flow without appreciably affecting blood pressure. A recent meta-analysis of randomized trials of *Ginkgo* in the treatment of intermittent claudication demonstrated significant positive results.[27] Research also supports its use for treating cerebral insufficiency and secondary effects on memory and mood, as well as vertigo and tinnitus.

A Prescription for Peripheral Arterial Disease

Crataegus spp.	1 part
Aesculus hippocastanum	1 part
Ginkgo biloba	1 part
Zanthoxylum americanum	1 part
Viburnum opulus	1 part

Dosage: up to 5 ml of tincture three times a day. *Allium sativum* should be added to the diet or used as a dietary supplement: 1 clove of fresh garlic or 200 to 300 mg of standardized extract three times a day.

VARICOSE VEINS

Elongated, dilated, tortuous veins whose valves are congenitally absent or scant or have become incompetent; this condition occurs usually in the legs. *(The Merck Manual)*

Varicose veins are a common problem that affects between 10% and 20% of the population. Incidence increases with age, and it is most common in people older than 50. In addition, varicose veins are four times more common in women than in men.

The core problem is valve incompetency in the veins of the legs, which leads to dilation of the veins, loss of tissue tone, and some degree of reversal of blood flow. The abnormal swelling of veins in the legs is a symptom of generally poor blood circulation, accompanied by loss of elasticity in the walls of the veins and particularly in their valves. When they are functioning normally, these valves prevent blood from flowing back away from the heart. When their efficiency declines, some blood may stagnate in the veins, which then become swollen and tortuous (twisted), causing aching and abnormal fatigue in the legs.

Causative factors for varicose veins fit into two general groups.

1. Inadequate support of vein walls.
   Heredity. About 40% of cases have a family history of varicosity.
   Obesity. The fatty tissue that builds up in the legs provides inadequate support and results in loss of tone.
   Aging. The aging process leads to degenerative changes in supporting connective tissue, which is compounded by decreased muscular activity.
   Posture. Occupations that involve prolonged standing or sitting increase the chances that this problem will develop. This is due to a combination of the pull of gravity and lack of muscular activity in the thighs.
2. Increased resistance to the free flow of blood back into the trunk.
   Pregnancy. The growing baby may act as an obstacle to venous return.
   Thrombosis. Blockage within the vessels themselves can cause varicosities.
   Tumors. Uterine fibroids or ovarian problems, for example, can become obstructive.
   Fashion. Constriction caused by tight clothing will weaken tissue.

Treatment of Varicose Veins

The herbal treatment guidelines given here for varicose veins must be applied in the context of the lifestyle issues discussed earlier. The focus of tonic support should be the cardiovascular system, but beyond that, a range of factors may be addressed, depending upon the individual's needs. Consider musculoskeletal and connective tissue tonics if varicosity is accompanied by rheumatic problems. If the patient is pregnant, then appropriate uterine tonics are indicated.

Actions Indicated

Vascular tonics help the tissues regain tone and strength. Flavonoid-rich herbs are especially useful here, although they do not work quickly.

Circulatory stimulants assist in the process of venous return to the trunk of the body.

Astringents can support the work of the vascular tonics. The astringency is best applied externally.

Anti-inflammatories ease localized inflammation and discomfort.

Emollients and *demulcents*, used externally, lessen local discomfort.

Specific Remedies

Flavonoid-rich plants have a major role to play in toning up the muscle walls of weakened veins. Traditionally, in Europe, *Aesculus hippocastanum* (horse chestnut) has been considered an effective specific. The seeds of this plant have long been used to treat venous disorders, including varicose veins. The saponin glycoside aescin inhibits the activity of lysosomal enzymes thought to contribute to varicose veins by weakening vessel walls and increasing permeability.[28] The herb has been the subject of numerous clinical studies on the treatment of venous conditions, and a meta-analysis of some of these studies concluded that the herb was efficacious and safe.[29]

A Prescription for Varicose Veins

Crataegus spp.	1 part
Zanthoxylum americanum	1 part
Ginkgo biloba	1 part
Achillea millefolium	1 part
Aesculus hippocastanum	1 part

Dosage: up to 5 ml of tincture three times a day

Varicose Veins Lotion for External Use

Hamamelis virginiana (distilled witch hazel)	80 ml
Aesculus hippocastanum tincture	10 ml
Symphytum officinale tincture	10 ml
Total volume:	100 ml

Apply liberally as needed to ease irritation and discomfort. Rose water or another floral water may be added to make the lotion more cosmetically pleasing.

Table 14.7. Actions Supplied by Varicose Vein Prescription

ACTION	HERBS
Circulatory stimulant	*Zanthoxylum americanum, Ginkgo biloba*
Vascular tonic	*Crataegus* spp., *Aesculus hippocastanum, Achillea millefolium*
Astringent	*Achillea millefolium, Hamamelis virginiana*
Emollient and demulcent	*Symphytum officinale*
Vulnerary	*Symphytum officinale*
Anti-inflammatory	*Aesculus hippocastanum*

Broader Context of Treatment

Lifestyle factors are very important in the long-term treatment of this sometimes intransigent condition. As in other cardiovascular conditions, diet is important, and similar guidelines apply. See the general and nutritional recommendations for heart health given earlier in this chapter.

The main specific insight is that the patient should avoid postures or situations that aggravate resistance to easy venous return from the legs. In addition, anything that counteracts the effects of gravity will be helpful. Resting with the legs higher than the head for at least 10 minutes every day will help in the long term and also decrease any immediate discomfort. This may be achieved through the inverted postures of yoga, use of a slant board, or simply by lying on the floor with the legs and feet supported by a chair. The foot of the bed can be elevated 6 to 12 inches, thus facilitating drainage at night.

Gentle exercise, such as walking and stretching, is helpful. However, jogging, skipping, aerobics, and other exercises involving repeated impact can do more harm than good. Such exercise can be so uncomfortable for people with varicose veins that they are unlikely to keep it up for more than a very short time.

Aromatherapy can help improve the general tone of the veins when used in a broad, holistic context. Cypress oil, for example, has a reputation for strengthening the veins in the legs. It may be added to a bath oil or blended in a carrier oil or cream in a 3% dilution and applied very gently over the affected area. The area above the affected veins can be massaged. However, the area below the varicosity must never be massaged, as this will increase pressure in the vein.

In *Textbook of Natural Medicine*, Drs. Murray and Pizzorno recommend the following supplements:[30]

Vitamin A: 10,000 IU/day
Vitamin B complex: 10 to 100 mg/day
Vitamin C with bioflavonoids: 1 to 3 g/day
Vitamin E: 200 to 600 IU/day
Magnesium: 800 to 1,200 mg/day
Zinc: 15 to 30 mg/day

References

1. Weiss RF, Fintelmann V. *Herbal Medicine*. Stuttgart; New York: Thieme, 2000.

2. McGuffin, et al. *Botanical Safety Handbook*. Boca Raton, FL: CRC Press, 1997.

3. Brown D. Common drugs and their potential interactions with herbs or nutrients. *Review of Complementary and Integrative Medicine* 1999; 6(2):124–41.

4. Keli SO, Hertog MG, Feskens EJ, Kromhout D. Dietary flavonoids, antioxidant vitamins, and incidence of stroke: the Zutphen study. *Archives of Internal Medicine* 1996 Mar 25; 156(6):637–42.

5. Wedworth SM, Lynch S. Dietary flavonoids in atherosclerosis prevention. *Annals of Pharmacotherapy* 1995 Jun; 29(6):627–8.

6. Hertog MG, Feskens EJ, Hollman PC, et al. Dietary antioxidant flavonoids and risk of coronary heart disease: the Zutphen Elderly Study. *Lancet* 1993 Oct 23; 342(8878):1007–11.

7. *Revisions to Classification of Functional Capacity and Objective Assessment of Patients with Diseases of the Heart.* New York Heart Association (NYHA), 1994.

8. Zapfejun G. Clinical efficacy of crataegus extract WS 1442 in congestive heart failure NYHA class II. *Phytomedicine* 2001 Jul; 8(4):262–6.

9. Rigelsky JM, Sweet BV. Hawthorn: pharmacology and therapeutic uses. *American Journal of Health-System Pharmacy* 2002 Mar 1; 59(5):417–22.

10. Weikl A, Assmus KD, Neukum-Schmidt A, et al. Crataegus Special Extract WS 1442. Assessment of objective effectiveness in patients with heart failure (NYHA II). *Fortschritte der Medizin* 1996 Aug 30; 114(24):291–6.

11. Tauchert M. Efficacy and safety of crataegus extract WS 1442 in comparison with placebo in patients with chronic stable New York Heart Association class-III heart failure. *American Heart Journal* 2002 May; 143(5):910–15.

12. National Institutes of Health. *Clinical Guidelines on the Identification, Evaluation, and Treatment of Overweight and Obesity in Adults*. Bethesda, MD: Department of Health and Human Services, National Institutes of Health, National Heart, Lung, and Blood Institute, 1998.

13. Stunkard AJ, Wadden TA, eds. *Obesity: Theory and Therapy*, 2nd edition. New York: Raven Press, 1993.

14. Pizzorno JE, Murray MT. *Textbook of Natural Medicine*. Edinburgh: Churchill Livingstone, 1999.

15. Ernst E, Weihmayr T, Matrai A. Garlic and blood lipids. *British Medical Journal (Clinical Research* ed.) 1985 Jul 13; 291(6488):139.

16. Ali M. Mechanism by which garlic (Allium sativum) inhibits cyclooxygenase activity. Effect of raw versus boiled garlic extract on the synthesis of prostanoids. *Prostaglandins, Leukotrienes, and Essential Fatty Acids* 1995 Dec; 53(6):397–400.

17. Banerjee SK, Maulik SK. Effect of garlic on cardiovascular disorders: a review. *Nutrition Journal* 2002 Nov 19; 1(1):4.

18. Al-Qattan K, Khan I, Alnaqeeb MA, Ali M. Thromboxane-B2, prostaglandin-E2 and hypertension in the rat 2-kidney 1-clip model: a possible mechanism of the garlic-induced hypotension. *Prostaglandins, Leukotrienes, and Essential Fatty Acids* 2001 Jan; 64(1):5–10.

19. Satyavati G. Guggulipid: a promising hypolipidaemic agent from gum guggul (*Commiphora wightii*). In: Wagner H, Farnsworth NR, eds. *Economic and Medicinal Plant Research*, vol. 5. San Diego: Academic Press, 1991.

20. http://www.nhlbi.nih.gov/about/nhbpep/nhbp_pd.htm.

21. Pizzorno JE, Murray MT. *Textbook of Natural Medicine*. Edinburgh: Churchill Livingstone, 1999.

22. Ammon, HPT and Muller AB. Forskolin: from an ayurvedic remedy to a modern agent. *Planta Medica* (1985); 51:473–7.

23. Pizzorno JE, Murray MT. *Textbook of Natural Medicine*. Edinburgh: Churchill Livingstone, 1999.

24. Rigelsky JM, Sweet BV. Hawthorn: pharmacology and therapeutic uses. *American Journal of Health-System Pharmacy* 2002 Mar 1; 59(5):417–22.

25. Pizzorno JE, Murray MT. *Textbook of Natural Medicine.* Edinburgh: Churchill Livingstone, 1999.

26. Pittler MH, Ernst E. Horse chestnut seed extract for chronic venous insufficiency. *Cochrane Database of Systematic Reviews* 2002; (1):CD003230.

27. Pittler MH, Ernst E. Ginkgo biloba extract for the treatment of intermittent claudication: a meta-analysis of randomized trials. *The American Journal of Medicine* 2000 Mar; 108(4):276–81.

28. Kreysel H, Nissen H, Enghofer E. A possible role of lyosomal enzymes in the pathogenesis of varicosis and the reduction in their serum activity by Venostsin®. *VASA. Zeitschrift fur Gefasskrankheiten. Journal for Vascular Diseases* 1983; 12(4):377–82.

29. Pittler MH, Ernst E. Horse chestnut seed extract for chronic venous insufficiency. *Cochrane Database of Systematic Reviews* 2002; (1):CD003230.

30. Pizzorno JE, Murray MT. *Textbook of Natural Medicine.* Edinburgh: Churchill Livingstone, 1999.

15

❧

THE RESPIRATORY SYSTEM

When we draw in a breath, we share that air with all other human beings and all other life on our planet. Through respiration, our oneness with trees becomes a manifest fact, and our communion with the oceans has immediate impact. The reality of the planetary whole reveals itself, with implications for all human life, through the circulation of the gases and energy of the atmosphere. This vision underlies holistic healing as much as it does ecology. The anatomy and physiology of the respiratory system is a complex and beautiful embodiment of integration and wholeness.

Every minute, usually unconsciously, we breathe in and out between 10 and 15 times. We take a breath nearly 25,000 times a day, moving enough air to and fro to blow up several thousand balloons. This is the way in which the body extracts the oxygen it needs from the air and discharges waste carbon dioxide from the blood. The almost 10,000 liters of air inhaled each day is mostly oxygen and nitrogen. It also contains small amounts of other gases, floating bacteria, viruses, tobacco smoke, car exhaust, and other pollutants from the atmosphere.

The lungs sit within the thoracic cage, where they stretch from the *trachea* (commonly called the windpipe) to below the heart. They are textured like a finely grained sponge that can be inflated with air. About 10% of the lung is solid tissue and the rest is filled with air and blood. This unique structure facilitates gas exchange, yet is strong enough to maintain shape and function of the lungs. The lungs' main function is to rapidly exchange oxygen from inhaled air with carbon dioxide from the blood.

When we breathe, we take in air through the nose and mouth, which passes down the throat into the trachea. The air enters the lungs, where it is passes into the *bronchi*. The two main bronchi extend from the trachea into each lung, where they divide into smaller bronchi, and then a great number of smaller *bronchioles*. The bronchioles divide into a network of about 3 million alveolar ducts containing *alveoli*, commonly called air sacs.

The respiratory muscles of the thorax control the movement of the air into the lungs. These muscles, collectively called the *ventilatory apparatus*, include the diaphragm and the muscles that move the ribs. Specific nerve sites located in the brain and the neck, called *respiratory centers*, coordinate the performance of the ventilatory apparatus. The respiratory centers respond to changes in oxygen, carbon dioxide, and acid levels in the blood. Normal concentrations of these chemicals in arterial blood are maintained by changes in the breathing rate.

Gas exchange between inhaled air and blood takes place in the alveoli. A very thin membrane separates the blood from the air in the alveoli and allows oxygen and nitrogen to diffuse into the blood. This barrier is 50 times thinner than a sheet of tissue paper, but a large surface area (80 square meters, or about as large as a tennis court) is available for gas exchange. In the resting state, it takes just about a minute for the total blood volume of the body to pass through the lungs. It takes a red cell a fraction of a second to pass through the capillary network. Gas exchange occurs almost instantaneously during this short time period.

The blood carries fresh oxygen throughout the body. When the blood returns to the alveoli, carbon dioxide and other gases pass from the blood into the alveoli. These gases leave the body in the exhaled air. In a larger sense, the ebb and flow of the breath also draws life energy into the body. Thus, if respiratory disturbances inhibit gas exchange, they can lead to a lowering of the body's vitality, an increase in metabolic disorders, and degeneration of tissue.

PREVENTION OF RESPIRATORY DISEASE

We are not only what we eat, but also what we breathe. Any problem with breathing will not only affect other organs and systems, but may also cause disease in these systems. However, as the body is a whole, the reverse is also true. When the lungs need attention, we must also look at the circulatory system, so much of what was discussed in chapter 14 is also relevant to the lungs. We must also consider the condition of the digestive system and especially the organs of elimination, as the lungs share the job of eliminating waste with the bowels, kidneys, and skin.

If a problem develops in any of these systems, the body will compensate by increasing the load on the others. Many pathological tissue changes can be prevented if the environmental milieu of the cells is constantly rich in oxygen. The amount of oxygen supplied to the tissue by circulation is largely controlled by respiration.

Based on all of these considerations, it becomes apparent that two of the best preventive measures for the respiratory system are regular exercise and proper breathing. While breathing is often taken for granted, conscious and proper breathing is regarded, even in orthodox medical circles, as invaluable. The central role of the breath in many spiritual practices should perhaps provide an additional clue.

The best prophylactic is right lifestyle. Diet, exercise, and quality of life all have a profound influence on the health of the lungs. To ensure the health of the lungs, both the inner and outer environments must be in harmony. If the air we breathe is polluted, it will disrupt the ecology of the lungs just as it disrupts the ecology of the forest. We should avoid air contaminated with chemicals, particles, gases, and smoke, which brings us to the issue of tobacco.

Smoking puts a wall of tar and ash between the individual and the world and disrupts the ecology of the lungs. This disruption can lead to an impressive host of problems, from bronchitis to cancer, not to mention all the effects of diminished oxygen supply to the rest of the body. If we are to heal ourselves and our world, quitting smoking is a good place to start. The benefits of eating a whole food diet and living in the country pale a bit when combined with 20 cigarettes a day!

Other specific dangers can also be recognized and prevented. We can do our best to avoid respiratory infections, but as this is often socially impossible, we need to maintain the body's natural defenses against infection. If given the chance, the body is capable of great feats of self-defense, as long as we provide it with a balanced, vitamin-rich diet and a lifestyle that is as healthy in thought and feeling as it is in action.

In this context, it is vital to curb the misuse of antibiotics. While these drugs save lives when used at the right time and in the right way, they can also reduce the effectiveness of the body's innate defense systems to impotence. In the long run, they also contribute to the evolution of highly resistant bacteria, so that infections are becoming increasingly difficult to treat. Over the past 30 years, doctors have observed alarming developments in this direction. With correct lifestyle and the appropriate use of herbal remedies, antibiotics can often be avoided.

Air Pollutants

Air quality is the key to preventing much of the disease associated with both the upper and the lower respiratory systems. If we could avoid particulate air pollution and chemical irritants such as sulfur dioxide, many disabling conditions of the lungs would not develop. Thus, smoking (both active and passive), as well as urban and industrial pollution, is an important issue for the practitioner and the patient. Anyone concerned about lung health should become active in Friends of the Earth!

Air pollutants affect the lungs in many ways. While they may simply cause irritation and discomfort, inhaled materials can sometimes cause illness or death. The lungs have a series of built-in mechanical and biological barriers that keep harmful materials from entering the body. In addition, specific defense mechanisms inactivate some disease-causing materials. However, normal lung defenses and barriers in the lungs do not always work as well as they should.

If polluted air contains an excessive amount of dust, fumes, smoke, gases, vapors, or mists, there is an increased risk for developing a lung disease. Air pollution can irritate the eyes, throat, and lungs. Burning eyes, cough, and chest tightness are common with exposure to high levels of air pollutants. Exercise may intensify symptoms of air pollution exposure simply because it requires faster, deeper breathing. Children probably feel the effects of pollution at lower levels than adults do. They also experience more illness, such as bronchitis and earaches, in areas of high pollution than in areas with cleaner air.

For most healthy people, the symptoms of air pollution exposure resolve as soon as air quality improves. However, certain groups of people are more sensitive to the effects of air pollution than others, and responses vary greatly. Some people may notice chest tightness or cough, while others notice no effects. People with heart disease (such as angina) or lung disease (such as asthma or emphysema) may be very sensitive to air pollution and may have symptoms when others do not. During times of heavy pollution, their condition may worsen to the point that they must limit their activities or even seek additional medical care.

Air pollution is caused by the presence of gases, droplets, and particles that reduce the quality of the air. In the city, air pollution may be caused by industry and construction as well as cars, buses, and airplanes. Air pollution in the country may be caused by dust from tractors plowing fields, trucks and cars driving on dirt or gravel roads, and rock quarries, as well as by smoke from wood and crop fires. All of these particles may also be sources of airborne pesticides and herbicides.

Ground-level ozone is a major component of air pollution in most cities. Ground-level ozone is created when engine and fuel gases that have already been released into the air interact in the presence of sunlight. Ozone levels increase in cities when the air is still, the sun is bright, and the temperature is warm. Ozone irritates the respiratory tract and eyes, and exposure to high levels results in chest tightness, coughing, and wheezing. People with respiratory and heart problems are at a higher risk.

Ozone has been linked to increased hospital admissions and premature death. It also causes noticeable leaf damage in many crops, garden plants, and trees. The WHO recommends limiting exposure to 0.08 ppm to 0.1 ppm on average an hour. (Ground-level ozone should not be confused with the protective ozone that exists miles up in the atmosphere, filtering radiation.)

The Environmental Protection Agency (EPA) checks and reports on air quality in the United States. Because of its efforts, the nation's air quality has greatly improved over the past 20 years. The EPA measures the level of pollution in the air over many large cities and a number of rural areas. The Pollution Standards Index (PSI) is a scale of air quality ranging from 0 to 500 and is used in many weather reports. A PSI score higher than 100 indicates unhealthy air conditions.

Smoking and the Health Effects of Tobacco[1]

Cigarette smoking causes a variety of life-threatening diseases, including lung cancer, emphysema, chronic obstructive pulmonary disease, and heart disease. An estimated 400,000 deaths each year are directly caused by cigarette smoking. This, the single most preventable cause of death, is responsible for one in six deaths, or more deaths each year than fires, automobile crashes, alcohol, cocaine, heroin, AIDS, murders, and suicides *combined*. Passive smoking, commonly called secondhand smoke, kills some 50,000 Americans each year, making it the third leading cause of preventable death. For every eight smokers, one nonsmoker dies from the effects of secondhand smoke.

Cardiovascular Diseases

People who smoke a pack of cigarettes a day have more than twice the risk of heart attack as nonsmokers. Two or more packs a day increase the risk three times. Smoking is the principal cause of coronary heart disease, the most common cause of death in the United States. It is responsible for 21% of fatal heart disease and is an important cause of stroke, blood vessel disease, and sudden cardiac death. It also increases the risk of recurrence in people who have survived a heart attack. Smoking is also the most powerful risk factor for atherosclerosis of the arteries in the legs.

Cancers

Smoking is responsible for 32% of deaths due to cancer. Smoking causes cancer of the lung, oral cavity, pharynx, larynx, esophagus, pancreas, kidney, urinary bladder, and cervix. In addition, links may exist between smoking and cancer of the large intestine and some forms of leukemia. Smoking causes nearly 90% of all lung and throat cancers. For many years, lung cancer was the leading cause of cancer death in men, but now lung cancer has surpassed breast cancer as the leading cancer killer among women. The risk of developing cancer increases with amount and duration of smoking. Alcohol is also a risk factor for some cancers, and the combination of alcohol and smoking greatly increases cancer risk.

Respiratory Diseases

The overwhelming importance of smoking as a cause of chronic obstructive lung disease is well established. Smoking is responsible for 88% of deaths due to chronic lung disease, outweighing all other factors that cause these conditions. Smoking has an adverse effect on the body's immune system and other defense mechanisms, increasing the risk of respiratory infections, such as pneumonia and influenza. Cigarettes are a factor in up to 90% of cases of chronic bronchitis in the United States, and increase the risk of developing acute bacterial bronchitis. Air pollution also contributes to chronic bronchitis, as does working around dust or chemical fumes.

Gastrointestinal Effects

Smoking decreases the strength of the sphincter muscle between the throat and stomach, which allows stomach contents to reflux, or flow backward, into the esophagus. It may also directly injure the esophagus and impair its ability to resist further damage from refluxed material. Smoking seems to affect the liver, too, by changing the way it handles drugs and alcohol. In some people, this may influence the dose of medication necessary to treat an illness. Peptic ulcer disease is more likely to occur in smokers than in nonsmokers, and ulcers heal less readily and are more likely to recur in smokers. Current and former smokers have a higher risk of developing Crohn's disease than nonsmokers. Among people with this disease, smoking is associated with a higher rate of relapse, repeat surgery, and immunosuppressive treatment. In short, there seems to be enough evidence of harm to the digestive tract to stop smoking solely on this basis.

Effects on Teeth and Gums

Beyond oral cancer, tobacco affects oral health in a number of other ways. In a recent study of Canadians 50 years of age and older, smokers were more likely than nonsmokers to have lost all their natural teeth, to have remaining teeth with decayed and filled root surfaces, and to have significant gum disease.

Effects in Pregnancy

Smoking has a direct effect on the growth of the fetus. The more the mother smokes during pregnancy, the lower the weight of the newborn infant. Smoking increases the risk that the baby's weight at birth will be less than 2,500 grams (5½ lbs). Smoking during pregnancy may also increase the risk of miscarriage. Sudden infant death syndrome (SIDS, or crib death) occurs more frequently in infants of mothers who smoked during pregnancy. Smoking also appears to decrease the quantity and quality of breast milk, and may lead to early weaning.

Women who smoke during pregnancy incur extra risks to their own health, in addition to that of the fetus. Abnormalities of the placenta and bleeding during pregnancy are increased with smoking, and the more a pregnant woman smokes, the greater the risks.

Additional Smoking Hazards for Women

The contribution of smoking to the development of cancer of the cervix is clear. Natural menopause occurs earlier in smokers than in nonsmokers by one to two years. This may have unfavorable implications for the development of other conditions, such as coronary heart disease and osteoporosis. Smoking is also associated with an increased risk of menstrual disorders. Cigarettes and oral contraceptives are a dangerous combination that increases the risk of heart attacks, strokes, and other vascular complications.

Other Effects of Smoking

There also appears to be an association between smoking and the development of a number of other conditions:

Osteoporosis, which in turn predisposes a person to bone fractures

Decreased bone density of the lumbar spine and hip in both younger and older people

Cataracts

Graves' disease, a thyroid disorder

Decline in physical fitness

Reduction in the ability of the blood to carry oxygen

Increase in heart rate and basal metabolic rate

A decrease of blood flow in the small vessels of the skin that may damage skin components, leading to skin wrinkling and an appearance of premature aging

The Workplace

Many substances found in the workplace can cause breathing problems. Poor ventilation, closed-in working areas, and heat increase the risk.

Dusts from wood, cotton, coal, asbestos, silica, and talc, as well as from cereal grains, coffee, pesticides, drug or enzyme powders, metals, and fiberglass can all hurt the lungs.

Fumes from metals that are heated and cooled quickly result in the presence of fine, solid particles in the air. Fumes may be produced in welding, smelting, pottery making, plastics manufacture, and rubber operations.

Smoke from burning organic materials can contain a variety of dusts, gases, and vapors, depending on what is burning. Firefighters are at special risk.

Gases, such as formaldehyde, ammonia, chlorine, sulfur dioxide, ozone, and nitrogen oxides, are harmful. At greatest risk are those working around chemical reactions and in jobs involving high heat.

Vapors, such as solvents, usually irritate the nose and throat first before they affect the lungs.

Mists or sprays from paints, lacquers, hair spray, pesticides, cleaning products, acids, oils, and solvents constitute another source of pollutants.

Such substances can irritate the nose and throat, producing coldlike symptoms such as runny nose and scratchy throat. Viral infections and allergies produce similar symptoms, but a work-related illness should be suspected if nose and throat problems occur when at work. Such exposure can cause bronchitis, asthma, and emphysema.

HERBS AND THE LOWER RESPIRATORY SYSTEM

The respiratory system is the focus of gas exchange between the body and the air. The organs of the respiratory system are the nose, the pharynx, the larynx, the trachea, the bronchi and their smaller branches, and the lungs, which contain the terminal air sacs, or alveoli. Functionally, the respiratory system consists of respiratory and conducting zones. *The respiratory zone*, the actual site of gas exchange, is composed of the respiratory bronchioles, alveolar ducts, and alveoli. *The conducting zone*, sometimes called the dead air space, includes all other respiratory passageways, which serve as fairly rigid conduits to allow air to reach the gas exchange sites. The conducting zone organs also purify, humidify, and warm the incoming air. Thus, when it reaches the lungs, the air contains many fewer irritants (such as dust and bacteria) than it did when it entered the system, and it resembles the warm, damp air of the tropics.

It is convenient and therapeutically relevant to differentiate between the upper and lower respiratory systems. The lower respiratory system consists of the respiratory zone, the alveoli, and respiratory bronchioles. The air-conducting bronchi and trachea are anatomically part of this system. The upper respiratory system consists of the conducting zone, made up of the nose, sinuses, pharynx, and larynx. The system as a whole represents a major interface with the outside world and thus is a focus of much immune system activity.

Plant remedies for the respiratory system abound in pharmacopoeias, and most of the herbs still listed as official in British and American pharmacopoeias are expectorant, antitussive, or decongestant. However, the focus of orthodox medicine on effectors has led to a de-emphasis of tonic remedies. Pulmonary tonics provide the phytotherapist with the opportunity to strengthen both tissue and function, in addition to addressing symptoms of respiratory disease.

Expectorant Herbs

Phytotherapy has a great deal to offer for the treatment of respiratory disease. However, a major obstacle to correct use lies in the language herbalists use to describe respiratory herbs.

Expectorants are herbs that facilitate or accelerate the removal of bronchial secretions from the bronchi and trachea. However, in practice, this is a term that is often used somewhat loosely to refer in a general way to remedies that "do something" for the respiratory system. Chapter 25 provides a detailed discussion of the primary and secondary actions of expectorants. For the purposes of this discussion, however, we will focus briefly on two general categories of expectorant herbs: stimulating and relaxing.

Table 15.1. Actions and Herbs for the Lower Respiratory System

ACTION	HERBS
Pulmonary tonic	*Inula helenium, Tussilago farfara, Verbascum thapsus*
Stimulating expectorant	*Cephaelis ipecacuanha, Inula helenium, Marrubium vulgare, Sanguinaria canadensis*
Relaxing or demulcent expectorant	*Asclepias tuberosa, Cetraria islandica, Grindelia camporum, Lobelia inflata, Plantago* spp., *Tussilago farfara*
Antispasmodic	*Drosera rotundifolia, Euphorbia pilulifera, Lactuca virosa, Papaver* spp., *Prunus serotina*
Antimicrobial	*Allium sativum, Eucalyptus* spp., *Thymus vulgaris*
Immune support	*Echinacea* spp.
Anticatarrhal	*Hyssopus officinalis, Tussilago farfara*
Cardiotonic	*Crataegus* spp., *Leonurus cardiaca, Tilia platyphyllos*
Nervine	*Hyssopus officinalis, Lactuca virosa, Leonurus cardiaca, Lobelia inflata*

Stimulating Expectorants

Stimulating expectorants act in different ways to produce similar effects, but it is not always clear how a specific remedy works. For any given stimulating expectorant, either or both of the following mechanisms may be at play.

Irritation of the bronchioles stimulates the expulsion of any material present. This irritation initiates a reflex response that causes the body to cough.

Liquefaction of viscid sputum encourages clearing by coughing. Sputum is moved upward from the lungs by the fine hairs of the ciliated epithelium that lines the bronchiole tubes, and reduced sputum viscosity facilitates this transport.

Most stimulating expectorants contain alkaloids, saponins, or volatile oils. However, not all chemicals in these groups or plants containing these constituents have expectorant properties. The particular form of stimulation offered by this group of expectorants makes them relevant for productive coughs, in which sputum should be removed from the airways.

Relaxing Expectorants

Relaxing expectorants may also act by reflex, but here the herbs work to soothe bronchial spasm and loosen mucous secretions. This loosening occurs because relaxing expectorants facilitate the production of a less viscous mucous secretion, which helps lift up stickier material from below. This makes relaxing expectorants useful for dry, irritating coughs. You will notice that this action is similar in some respects to that of demulcents, and both actions owe a lot to their content of mucilage and occasionally volatile oils.

Tonics for the Lower Respiratory System

Herbs known as pulmonaries, or *amphoteric expectorants*, have a beneficial effect upon both lung tissue and function. Traditional remedies in this category include *Inula helenium*, *Verbascum thapsus*, and *Tussilago farfara*. Differential indications for each of these plants can be found in chapter 26, but we can generalize here that *Inula* has stimulant expectorant effects and *Verbascum* is more of a relaxing expectorant. *Tussilago* is the best of the three for children.

Tussilago farfara (coltsfoot) contains potentially liver-damaging pyrrolizidine alkaloids (PAs), especially in the roots. Animal studies that used amounts of coltsfoot hundreds of times higher than those used medicinally showed that these alkaloids can cause cancer in animals. However, this is not applicable to the size of the doses of coltsfoot usually used as medicine.[2] There has been a single case report of an infant who developed liver disease and died after the mother drank tea that supposedly contained coltsfoot during pregnancy. However, researchers found that instead of *Tussilago*, the tea contained the PA-rich plant *Adenostyles alliariae*, which has leaves similar in appearance to those of *Tussilago*.[3] To avoid any potential toxicity problems, leaf and flower formulations of *Tussilago* should not be taken for more than one consecutive month, and root products should not be used internally.

SYMPTOMS OF DISEASE

Five primary symptoms affect the lower respiratory system. While each of these symptoms may be effectively treated with herbs, they must still be seen as signposts of underlying pathology.

Dyspnea is breathlessness or shortness of breath, discussed in more detail under Types of Dyspnea below. Dyspnea is an important symptom of asthma and many other conditions.

Cough is defined as a sudden explosive expiratory maneuver that tends to clear material from the airways. Cough is caused by irritation somewhere within the respiratory tract, and is discussed in more detail later.

Chest pain is a common presenting symptom and calls for skilled differential diagnosis. Cardiovascular causes must be distinguished from the range of pulmonary problems that might be implicated.

Wheezing describes an awareness of noises associated with breathing.

Hemoptysis, or coughing up blood, calls for skilled diagnosis.

Types of Dyspnea

Dyspnea, defined as an unpleasant sensation of difficulty in breathing, has a range of clinical manifestations.

Physiological Dyspnea

This is the most common type of breathlessness and is associated with physical exertion and low-oxygen conditions. Ventilation is increased and maintained through an augmented respiratory stimulus provided by metabolic and other factors. Dyspnea is common during acute hypoxia (lack of oxygen). For example, at high altitudes, increased respiratory stimulus is due in part to the effect of arterial hypoxia on the carotid bodies. These are receptor sites in the carotid arteries that monitor the concentration of gases in the blood.

Pulmonary Dyspnea

The two major causes here are restrictive defects that impair efficient movement of the lungs or chest wall (e.g., pulmonary fibrosis) and obstructive defects that increase resistance of flow in the airways (e.g., asthma).

Cardiac Dyspnea

In the early stages of heart failure, the availability of oxygen to the tissues of the body via the blood fails to keep pace with increased metabolic needs during exercise. Respiration is increased because of tissue and cerebral acidosis, which causes hyperventilation. In later stages, the lungs become congested and edematous. The capacity of the stiff lungs is reduced and the effort needed to breathe increased.

Cardiac Asthma

This is a state of acute respiratory insufficiency; it is often very similar to other types of asthma but originates with left ventricular failure. *Orthopnea*, or breathing discomfort that occurs while a person is lying flat, is usually symptomatic of a cardiovascular basis for dyspnea.

Circulatory Dyspnea

This symptom, also known as "air hunger," is often a medical emergency that results from a lack of oxygen after hemorrhage. It may occasionally be associated with anemia.

Chemical Dyspnea

This is dyspnea related to uremia or diabetic acidosis.

Central Dyspnea

This is a symptom of cerebral lesions that affect lung function.

Psychogenic Dyspnea

Also known as "hysterical overbreathing," psychogenic dyspnea is caused by emotional or psychological factors.

COUGH

A sudden explosive expiratory maneuver that tends to clear material (sputum) from the airways. *(The Merck Manual)*

Should one soothe coughs, stimulate coughs, or suppress coughs? As with all holistic approaches, it is always preferable to focus on the underlying cause of a cough, as removing the cause will also alleviate the cough. In the sections that follow, we will discuss a number of different approaches and remedies for treating coughs.

Always select the appropriate approach for the individual's unique case. The key to treatment is achieving a correct balance among the various stimulating, demulcent, antimicrobial, and antitussive herbs available. Treat the person and his or her experience, *not* just the cough.

Coughing is a reflex response that represents an attempt by the body to clear the airways. Usually, blockages are caused by mucus secreted by membranes lining the respiratory tract. These mucous secretions help to protect the respiratory tract from all kinds of irritants by trapping and flushing out smoke particles, bacteria, and viruses. Any cough that lasts more than a few days, does not respond to treatment, or produces blood should be investigated further, as it may be a sign of serious organic disease.

In addition to the considerations just discussed, cough may be related to gastroesophageal reflux disease (GERD). In this condition, acid reflux from the stomach backs up into the throat, causing either heartburn or cough. See chapter 13 for more information about the etiology and treatment of this common condition.

Treatment of Cough

Acute inflammatory conditions of the respiratory system are primarily treated with mucilage-rich demulcents, which soothe inflamed tissue. It is difficult to explain the mechanism at play here, as the mucopolysaccharide molecules in demulcent herbs do not enter the bloodstream and thus cannot be directly active in the respiratory tissue. Instead, they are catabolized into their various components by digestive enzymes, and must exert their effects through mechanisms other than direct contact.

Stimulant, saponin-containing expectorants are best used for subacute or chronic bronchitis, for which active expectoration is indicated. However, any irritation in chronic bronchitis will indicate the need for increased demulcent action. This facilitates differentiated stages of cough therapy that can rapidly ameliorate the symptoms and shorten the duration of respiratory illness.

Traditional folk wisdom is a rich source of simple yet effective treatments for coughs. A simple cough remedy can be made with onion and honey.

A Simple Cough Elixir

Slice a large onion into rings and place them in a deep bowl. Cover the onion slices with organic honey and let stand overnight. In the morning, strain off the mixture of honey and onion juice, which makes a simple cough elixir. (Honey itself, which is often included in cough mixtures, has antimicrobial and expectorant properties.) Take a dessert spoon of this mixture four or five times a day.

A Basic Herbal Cough Tea

Tussilago farfara	2 parts
Althaea officinalis	2 parts
Hyssopus officinalis	2 parts
Glycyrrhiza glabra	1 part
Pimpinella anisum	1 part

Infuse 1 teaspoon of dried herb mixture in 1 cup of freshly boiled water; drink often until symptoms subside.

BRONCHITIS

Bronchitis is either an acute or a chronic inflammation of the mucous lining of the bronchial tubes, the main airways that carry air from the trachea to the lungs. This inflammation may be caused by viral or bacteria infection, smoking, or inhalation of chemical pollutants or dust. Types of bacteria that cause acute bronchitis include *Streptococcus pneumoniae* and *Hemophilus influenzae*.

When the cells of the bronchial lining tissue are irritated beyond a certain point, cilia that normally trap and eliminate pollutants stop functioning. The air passages become clogged by mucus, and irritation increases. In response, a heavy secretion of mucus develops, causing the characteristic cough of bronchitis.

Bronchitis makes breathing difficult and sometimes even painful. Pain may be related to the swelling of the mucous membrane in the trachea. Other common signs of bronchitis are persistent coughing, aching associated with fever, and mucus secretions. The patient will feel very fatigued due to the fact that the body is receiving less oxygen than it needs.

ACUTE BRONCHITIS

Acute inflammation of the tracheobronchial tree, generally self-limiting and with eventual complete healing and return of function. (The Merck Manual)

Acute bronchitis usually originates with a viral infection of the upper respiratory tract, such as a cold or sore throat, that can become a secondary bacterial infection and spread to the lungs. Though usually mild, it may be serious in debilitated people and those with chronic lung or heart disease.

Acute bacterial bronchitis usually lasts about a week and is accompanied by a cough that produces thick green or yellow mucus. Severe cases may also cause general malaise and chest pain. At first the cough is very dry, but as the lungs produce additional mucus in response to the infection, the cough becomes easier and less painful as the mucus lubricates the bronchi. Acute bronchitis may be accompanied by fever that lasts a few days, but persistent fever suggests the development of a pneumonia complication.

The cough of acute bronchitis may last for several weeks or even months, a reflection of the amount of time it takes for the bronchial lining to heal. However, the cough can also be a sign of other problems. For example, acute bronchitis can be confused with asthma, and pneumonia can also sometimes cause similar symptoms. Acid that comes up from the stomach and drips into the lungs during sleep may also cause bronchitis.

Acute bronchitis most commonly develops as a complication of a cold in a healthy person. It may also manifest as a flare-up in a person with chronic bronchitis. The best defense against acute bronchitis is not to smoke. Smoking damages the bronchial tree and makes it easier for viruses to cause infection. Smoking also slows healing, so it takes longer to get well.

Treatment of Acute Bronchitis

Bed rest, drinking plenty of fluids, and staying indoors in damp, cold weather are essential elements of treatment. Congestive mucus should be coughed up, so avoid the use of cough suppressants. The use of soothing, relaxing expectorants in combination with antimicrobials is often the key to successful treatment. Particularly important relaxing expectorants are *Tussilago*, *Verbascum*, *Plantago*, *Cetraria*, *Trigonella*, *Althaea*, and *Pulmonaria*.

The respiratory system will obviously need tonic and immune system support, especially if acute bronchitis is an annual event. As noted, the heart and blood vessels will benefit from tonics, such as *Crataegus* and *Allium sativum*, as there may be a deleterious impact on the tissue and its functions.

Actions Indicated

Pulmonary tonics are not crucial if the bronchitis is not a recurrent problem. However, they are clearly indicated for immunocompromised people.

Expectorants are indicated; the choice between stimulating and relaxing expectorants will depend on the individual's needs.

Demulcents augment the action of relaxing expectorants, if necessary.

Antispasmodics can help if coughing is very troublesome.

Antimicrobials are essential to deal with infection and to help the body defend against the development of secondary infection.

Anti-inflammatories may be indicated if there is extensive inflammation, and especially if the larynx or pharynx is involved.

Anticatarrhals improve the upper respiratory symptom picture.

Diaphoretics are indicated if the patient has a fever.

Cardiotonic herbs offer support if there is any history or suspicion of cardiovascular problems.

Specific Remedies

Herbal traditions from around the world offer a wealth of possible specifics. For example, osha (*Ligusticum porteri*), a plant of the American Southwest, is an excellent specific for cases of tracheobronchitis.

The specifics listed here cover a range of expectorant, antimicrobial, and antispasmodic actions. Strictly speaking, none of them is guaranteed to work in all cases, as specifics must be chosen based on the unique needs of an individual with a particular clinical picture. Please see chapter 25 for more information on the primary and secondary actions of these herbs.

Specific Remedies from Europe and North America

Allium sativum (garlic)
Althaea officinalis (marshmallow)
Asclepias tuberosa (pleurisy root)
Cephaelis ipecacuanha (ipecac)
Cetraria islandica (Iceland moss)
Chondrus crispus (Irish moss)
Drosera rotundifolia (sundew)
Glycyrrhiza glabra (licorice)
Hydrastis canadensis (goldenseal)
Hyssopus officinalis (hyssop)
Inula helenium (elecampane)
Ligusticum porteri (osha)
Lobelia inflata (lobelia)
Marrubium vulgare (white horehound)
Pimpinella anisum (anise)
Plantago spp. (plantain)
Polygala senega (Seneca snakeroot)
Populus balsamifera var. *balsamifera* (balm of Gilead)
Primula veris (cowslip)
Pulmonaria officinalis (lungwort)
Sanguinaria canadensis (bloodroot)
Symphytum officinale (comfrey)
Symplocarpus foetidus (skunk cabbage)
Thymus vulgaris (thyme)
Trigonella foenum-graecum (fenugreek)
Tussilago farfara (coltsfoot)
Verbascum thapsus (mullein)
Verbena officinalis (vervain)
Viola odorata (sweet violet)

The infusion presented here, provided by Dr. Rudolf Fritz Weiss in *Herbal Medicine*, supplies the additional benefit of increased fluid intake.[4]

A Demulcent Tea for Acute Dry Cough

Verbascum thapsus	1 part
Tussilago farfara	1 part
Althaea officinalis	1 part
Pimpinella anisum	1 part

Infuse 2 teaspoons of dry herb combination in 1 cup of boiling water for 20 minutes; drink hot three times a day

---

Table 15.2. Actions Supplied by Prescription for Acute Dry Cough

ACTION	HERBS
Pulmonary tonic	*Verbascum thapsus, Tussilago farfara*
Relaxing expectorant	*Verbascum thapsus, Tussilago farfara, Althaea officinalis, Pimpinella anisum*
Demulcent	*Verbascum thapsus, Tussilago farfara, Althaea officinalis*
Antispasmodic	*Pimpinella anisum*
Antimicrobial	*Pimpinella anisum*
Anti-inflammatory	*Verbascum thapsus, Tussilago farfara, Althaea officinalis, Pimpinella anisum*
Anticatarrhal	*Verbascum thapsus, Tussilago farfara, Althaea officinalis*

Another approach increases the stimulating expectorant component, making it more appropriate for subacute and chronic bronchitis characterized by excessive sputum production.

Prescription I to Promote Expectoration

Primula veris	1 part
Thymus vulgaris	1 part
Tussilago farfara	1 part

Infuse 2 teaspoons of dry herb combination in 1 cup of boiling water for 20 minutes; drink hot three times a day.

Table 15.3. Actions Supplied by Expectorant Prescription I

ACTION	HERBS
Pulmonary tonic	*Tussilago farfara*
Relaxing expectorant	*Tussilago farfara*
Stimulating expectorant	*Primula veris*
Demulcent	*Tussilago farfara*
Antispasmodic	*Primula veris, Thymus vulgaris*
Antimicrobial	*Thymus vulgaris*
Anti-inflammatory	*Tussilago farfara*
Anticatarrhal	*Tussilago farfara*

An alternative yet equivalent approach for acute dry cough replaces *Thymus vulgaris* with *Pimpinella anisum*. This combination also boosts the stimulating expectorant action of the prescription by increasing the proportion of saponin-rich *Primula veris*.

Prescription II to Promote Expectoration

Primula veris	2 parts
Pimpinella anisum	1 part
Tussilago farfara	1 part

Infuse 2 teaspoons of dry herb combination in 1 cup of boiling water for 20 minutes; drink hot three times a day.

A Prescription to Combat Infection in Acute Bronchitis

Inula helenium	1 part
Marrubium vulgare	1 part
Tussilago farfara	1 part
Hydrastis canadensis	1 part
Echinacea spp.	1 part

Dosage: up to 5 ml of tincture three times a day. *Allium sativum* should be eaten raw (one clove a day) or garlic oil taken as a supplement.

Table 15.4. Actions Supplied by Prescription to Combat Infection

ACTION	HERBS
Pulmonary tonic	*Inula helenium, Tussilago farfara*
Relaxing expectorant	*Tussilago farfara*
Stimulating expectorant	*Inula helenium, Marrubium vulgare*
Demulcent	*Tussilago farfara*
Antimicrobial	*Inula helenium, Hydrastis canadensis*
Immune stimulant	*Echinacea* spp.
Anti-inflammatory	*Hydrastis canadensis, Tussilago farfara*
Anticatarrhal	*Echinacea* spp., *Hydrastis canadensis, Tussilago farfara*
Bitter stimulant	*Marrubium vulgare*

Remedies for External Use

It is often possible to abort the development of a cold or even flu with a steam inhalation made from volatile oil–rich plants. When the problem is already established, inhalations help loosen the cough and clear the sinuses.

Thymus, Eucalyptus, Matricaria, and *Origanum* are good choices for steam inhalations. Pure plant essential oils may also be used. Volatile oil–rich herbs are effective decongestants and support the internal treatment by addressing some associated symptoms.

Steam Inhalation

Matricaria flowers	1 part
Thymus herb	1 part
Origanum herb	1 part

Add 1 tablespoon of dried herb combination to ½ liter (1 pint) of boiling water. Create a tent by draping a towel over the head to prevent the escape of vapors; inhale vapors rising from bowl. Inhale vapors for 5 to 10 minutes.

Aromatherapy for Acute Bronchitis

Aromatherapy treatment aims at combating infection, reducing fever, easing cough, and expelling mucus. In the first stages of acute bronchitis, when the cough is dry and painful, steam inhalation with the oils listed here may provide a great deal of relief.

Bergamot and eucalyptus oils are also effective in lowering fever, and all of these oils will help to reinforce the immune response to the infection. Dwarf pine needle oil *(Pinus pumilio)* has been the main oil used traditionally, but with the growing interest in aromatherapy, many volatile oils are now recognized as valuable remedies for inhalations. Here are some of the many possibilities.

Essential Oils for Steam Inhalation

Citrus aurantium ssp. *bergamia* (bergamot)
Eucalyptus globulus (eucalyptus)
Lavandula spp. (lavender)
Mentha arvensis var. *piperascens* (Asian mint)
M. piperita (peppermint)
Pinus pumilio (dwarf or white pine)
Santalum album (sandalwood)
Styrax benzoin (benzoin)
Thymus vulgaris (thyme)

Mentha arvensis var. *piperascens,* the source of "Chinese white flower oil," is especially rich in menthol. Menthol is anti-inflammatory, especially for the mucous membranes of the upper respiratory tract. It stimulates mucous secretions and exerts antimicrobial and mild anaesthetic actions. As with many oils, it is best used at the onset of symptoms.

Essential Oil Inhalation

Place 3 to 5 drops of essential oil in a bowl and add boiling water. Create a tent by draping a towel over the head to prevent the escape of vapors; inhale vapors rising from bowl. Inhale for 5 to 10 minutes, keeping the eyes closed to prevent irritation from vapor.

Massaging or otherwise applying oils to chest, neck, or back fosters absorption through the skin, technically called *percutaneous absorption*. Be sure to dilute the oil first in an appropriate carrier oil, such as almond oil. Essential oils absorbed through the skin are often eliminated from the body via the lungs, allowing the constituents to come in contact with the site of lung infection or inflammation. A good technique is to apply the oil and then place a clean dry cloth over the area to ensure that oils are absorbed and do not evaporate.

Post-Bronchitis Recovery

A bout of acute bronchitis is commonly followed by a period of debility. Appropriate herbs will not only speed recovery, but will also support the body in its attempt to revivify and recuperate. Emphasis should be given to respiratory tonics, bitter tonics, and support for any body system or functions indicated for the individual.

Toning remedies to consider include *Verbascum thapsus* and *Marrubium vulgare*. *Marrubium* is especially useful, for not only is it an excellent lung remedy, but it also has valuable bitter properties. If antibiotics have been used, please follow the guidelines for herbal support provided in chapter 21.

Broader Context of Treatment

Goals of treatment in the latter stages of acute bronchitis include clearing mucus from the lungs and preventing the development of complications, and any of the expectorant essential oils will be indicated. The cough may persist for some time after the fever has subsided, but applying such oils in inhalations, baths, and local massage to chest and throat will shorten the time needed for full recovery.

Expectorant Essential Oils to Aid in Recovery

Citrus aurantium ssp. *bergamia* (bergamot)
Commiphora molmol (myrrh)
Ocimum basilicum (basil)
Origanum majorana (marjoram)
Santalum album (sandalwood)
Thymus vulgaris (thyme)

The patient should be kept warm and rested, preferably in bed. It is important to avoid any factors that can aggravate the cough, such as smoke and very dry air. Given this care and treatment, most adults will recover from an attack of bronchitis fairly quickly and without complications, but the very elderly or frail, babies and young children, and people with heart conditions or a history of lung infections are at much greater risk.

CHRONIC BRONCHITIS

A condition associated with prolonged exposure to nonspecific bronchial irritants and accompanied by mucus hypersecretion and certain structural changes in the bronchi. *(The Merck Manual)*

Chronic bronchitis is a long-term condition unaccompanied by fever. It is characterized by a permanent cough with sputum that results from continual overproduction of mucus. Healthy lungs normally produce a small amount of mucus all the time, which is constantly swept up the bronchi by the cilia. This imperceptible process goes on continually, and the mucus produced is swallowed along with the saliva.

However, when infection, air pollution, smoking, or other external factors irritate the bronchi, the lungs are provoked to produce abnormally large amounts of mucus, which literally swamp the minute cilia. A deep layer of mucus covers the cilia, so they are no longer able to propel it out of the bronchi. In effect, this impairs the body's ability to expel mucus by coughing.

A series of acute bronchitis attacks, heavy smoking, or prolonged inhalation of contaminated air may result in chronic bronchitis. This implies that chronic bronchitis is preventable, as the primary causal factors are pollutants. Climate and air pollution are serious factors, especially when the two combine to produce fog, but the two most important factors are smoking and bad nutrition.

Because chronic bronchitis can be life threatening, prompt professional attention is necessary, no matter what the underlying cause. The condition is characterized by coughing up mucus nearly every day for months or years. The condition may be classified into three grades of severity.

1. *Simple chronic bronchitis* is mild but persistent with clear sputum.
2. *Mucopurulent bronchitis* is a condition in which the sputum is occasionally or always thick and often yellowish, due to the presence of pus caused by bacterial infection.

3. *Obstructive bronchitis* occurs when structural damage has been caused by continual infection, inflammation, and coughing.

In obstructive bronchitis, the bronchi become narrowed due to thickening and scarring of the membrane that lines them. The lungs lose some of their elasticity and breathing becomes more difficult, as a greater effort is needed to get a sufficient volume of air into the lungs. Damage also reduces the amount of alveolar tissue, the very thin membrane through which oxygen passes into the blood and carbon dioxide and other waste materials are extracted. Eventually, the heart may become strained in trying to maintain sufficient circulation within the lungs.

Treatment of Chronic Bronchitis

The treatment guidelines suggested here must be seen in the context of minimizing exposure to chemical and particulate air pollution, whether from tobacco smoke or industrial sources. Tonic support is vital for this chronic and debilitating condition. An inherent strength of herbal medicine reveals itself here, as the phytotherapist may select plants that not only effectively address the symptom picture, but also serve as appropriate tonics. The respiratory, cardiovascular, and immune systems all deserve special focus.

Specific Remedies

Please refer to Specific Remedies provided for acute bronchitis. In addition, the steam inhalation and aromatherapy recommendations given for acute bronchitis are also relevant to chronic bronchitis.

Actions Indicated

Pulmonary tonics are essential for supporting respiratory function and the health and general tone of the lungs.

Simulating expectorants are especially useful in cases characterized by heavy mucus production.

Relaxing expectorants are as not as important in chronic as acute bronchitis; however, they often serve as good supportive remedies.

Demulcents will soothe any associated irritation.

Diaphoretics are valuable when fever is an issue, but are not as vital here as in acute bronchitis.

Antispasmodics can help if coughing or breathlessness is severe.

Antimicrobials help the body rid itself of any accompanying infection.

Cardiotonics are essential for supporting cardiac function in the elderly, patients with cardiovascular weakness, or those with long-term chronic bronchitis.

Nervine and even *adaptogen* support may be useful in some cases.

A Prescription for Chronic Bronchitis with Debility

Inula helenium	1 part
Cetraria islandica	1 part
Tussilago farfara	1 part
Verbascum thapsus	1 part

Add 1 teaspoon of dried herb mixture to 1 cup of boiling water and infuse for 20 minutes. Drink hot three times a day.

This formulation is designed for a patient who is debilitated and weakened by chronic bronchitis. Thus, it contains a blend of stimulating and relaxing pulmonary tonics. *Cetraria* has long been used in the United Kingdom (the world capital of chronic bronchitis!) as nutritive support in such cases. To this may be added other herbs appropriate for the individual, such as *Crataegus* spp., *Eleutherococcus senticosus*, and *Galium aparine*. Please refer to chapter 26 for more information on these suggested additions.

Table 15.5. Actions Supplied by Prescription for Chronic Bronchitis with Debility

ACTION	HERBS
Pulmonary tonic	*Inula helenium, Tussilago farfara, Verbascum thapsus*
Stimulating expectorant	*Inula helenium*
Relaxing expectorant	*Cetraria islandica, Tussilago farfara, Verbascum thapsus*
Demulcent	*Cetraria islandica, Tussilago farfara, Verbascum thapsus*
Antimicrobial	*Inula helenium*
Anticatarrhal	*Inula helenium, Cetraria islandica, Tussilago farfara, Verbascum thapsus*
Diaphoretic	*Inula helenium*

A Prescription for Chronic Bronchitis with Infection

Inula helenium	1 part
Echinacea spp.	1 part
Marrubium vulgare	1 part
Verbascum thapsus	1 part

Dosage: up to 5 ml of tincture three times a day. *Allium sativum* should be eaten raw (one clove a day) or garlic oil taken as a supplement.

Table 15.6. Actions Supplied by Prescription for Chronic Bronchitis with Infection

ACTION	HERBS
Pulmonary tonic	*Inula helenium, Verbascum thapsus*
Stimulating expectorant	*Inula helenium, Marrubium vulgare*
Relaxing expectorant	*Verbascum thapsus*
Bitter	*Marrubium vulgare*
Antispasmodic	*Allium sativum*
Antimicrobial	*Inula helenium, Allium sativum*
Immune stimulant	*Echinacea* spp.
Anticatarrhal	*Inula helenium, Echinacea* spp., *Verbascum thapsus, Allium sativum*
Diaphoretic	*Inula helenium, Allium sativum*
Cardiotonic	*Allium sativum*

A Prescription for Chronic Recurrent Bronchitis with Dyspnea

Inula helenium	1 part
Dyspnea Formula (see page 332)	1 part
Marrubium vulgare	1 part
Verbascum thapsus	1 part

Dosage: up to 5 ml of tincture three times a day. *Allium sativum* should be eaten raw in the diet (one clove a day) or garlic oil taken as a supplement.

Table 15.7. Actions Supplied by Prescription for Chronic Bronchitis with Dyspnea

ACTION	HERBS
Pulmonary tonic	*Inula helenium, Verbascum thapsus*
Stimulating expectorant	*Inula helenium, Marrubium vulgare*

ACTION	HERBS
Relaxing expectorant	*Verbascum thapsus*
Antispasmodic	*Allium sativum*
Antimicrobial	*Inula helenium, Allium sativum*
Anticatarrhal	*Inula helenium, Verbascum thapsus, Allium sativum*
Diaphoretic	*Inula helenium, Allium sativum*
Cardiotonic	*Allium sativum*

Please see Asthma later in this chapter for more details about the herbs and actions added to address the dyspnea component in this prescription.

A Prescription for Chronic Recurrent Bronchitis with Severe Congestion

Inula helenium	1 part
Sanguinaria canadensis	1 part
Marrubium vulgare	1 part
Verbascum thapsus	1 part

Dosage: up to 5 ml of tincture three times a day. *Allium sativum* should be eaten raw in the diet (one clove a day) or garlic oil taken as a supplement.

Table 15.8. Actions Supplied by Prescription for Chronic Bronchitis with Severe Congestion

ACTION	HERBS
Pulmonary tonic	*Inula helenium, Verbascum thapsus*
Stimulating expectorant	*Sanguinaria canadensis, Inula helenium, Marrubium vulgare*
Relaxing expectorant	*Verbascum thapsus*
Bitter	*Marrubium vulgare*
Antispasmodic	*Sanguinaria canadensis, Allium sativum*
Antimicrobial	*Inula helenium, Sanguinaria canadensis, Allium sativum*
Anticatarrhal	*Inula helenium, Verbascum thapsus, Allium sativum*
Diaphoretic	*Inula helenium, Allium sativum*
Cardiotonic	*Allium sativum*

Broader Context of Treatment

Much of the information provided for acute bronchitis is relevant to chronic bronchitis as well. Smokers are still more likely to die from chronic bronchitis than from lung cancer, and giving up smoking is the first and most important preventive measure.

The other is improving nutrition, particularly cutting out or greatly reducing the consumption of foods that encourage the production of mucus. For most people, these are dairy products and refined starches. Dairy products appear to be the worst culprits, and cutting them right out of the diet for a time—perhaps for several weeks, or even several months if the bronchitis is long standing—will often bring about improvement. After that, dairy may be cautiously reintroduced, but only in very small amounts. For some people, it may be necessary to omit them from the diet permanently. Goat's milk may prove to promote less mucus production than cow's milk.

Starches also provoke excess mucus production, and refined starches (including white flour and all products made from it) are far worse than unrefined grains. Additives, such as chemical flavorings, colorings, and preservatives, also often trigger excess mucus production and should be avoided. The best and simplest rule is to eat foods in a state as near as possible to that in which they were grown. Avoid processed, dried, frozen, packaged, and precooked foods, and as often as possible eat foods raw or very lightly cooked.

Exercise can strengthen the muscles that facilitate breathing. Patients should exercise at least three times a week, starting with short sessions of gentle exercise and gradually building up to longer, more strenuous sessions. For example, one might begin exercising by walking slowly for 15 minutes three times a week. Next, increase the walking speed, at the same time increasing the length of time spent walking, first to 20 minutes, then to 25, and then to 30.

A special exercise program, called *pulmonary rehabilitation*, can help improve breathing; this is usually performed with the assistance of a respiratory therapist. A breathing method called *pursed-lip breathing* may also help. Take a deep breath, then breathe out slowly through the mouth while holding the lips as if about to give a kiss. Pursed-lip breathing slows the fast breathing that comes with chronic bronchitis.

PERTUSSIS

> An acute, highly communicable bacterial disease, characterized by a paroxysmal or spasmodic cough that usually ends in a prolonged, high-pitched, crowing inspiration (the whoop). *(The Merck Manual)*

Pertussis, commonly known as whooping cough, is caused by the bacterium *Bordetella pertussis*. This highly contagious infection is transmitted when the bacteria are coughed or sneezed out by an infected person and breathed in by someone else, especially during the catarrhal and early paroxysmal stages of the disease. After the third week of paroxysmal coughing, patients are no longer infectious. The incubation period averages 7 to 14 days.

B. pertussis invades the respiratory mucosa, causing increased secretion of mucus, which is initially thin. Later, the mucus becomes viscid and is not easily moved. The disease lasts about six weeks and has three well-defined stages.

1. *Catarrhal.* This stage begins slowly, with sneezing, free-flowing tears, and other signs typical of the common cold. Anorexia, listlessness, and a troublesome, hacking nocturnal cough develop next; the cough gradually becomes diurnal.
2. *Paroxysmal.* Developing after 10 to 14 days, this stage is characterized by paroxysmal coughing. Five to 15 rapidly consecutive coughs are followed by the characteristic whoop, a hurried, deep inspiration. After a few normal breaths, another paroxysm may begin. The patient may expel large quantities of thick, viscid mucus during the paroxysms. Vomiting after paroxysms is common.
3. *Convalescent.* This stage usually begins within four weeks. The frequency of paroxysms decreases, and the patient begins looking, feeling, and sounding better.

Treatment of Whooping Cough

Long-term immune system support is essential after such an infection. In addition, support for the respiratory system and potentially even the cardiovascular system may be needed.

Specific Remedies

The European herbal tradition proposes a number of herbs as possible specifics. However, these are not dramatically effective and do not replace appropriate antibiotic treatment. Instead, they support antibiotic therapy and the body's innate efforts to heal itself. Among these specifics are many antimicrobial and antispasmodic remedies.

European Specific Remedies for Pertussis

Drosera rotundifolia (sundew)

Thymus vulgaris (thyme)

Pinguicula vulgaris (butterbur)

Prunus serotina (wild cherry bark)

Eryngium planum (sea holly)

A Prescription for Pertussis and Other Paroxysmal Coughs

Thymus vulgaris	1 part
Drosera rotundifolia	1 part
Prunus serotina	1 part
Pimpinella anisum	1 part

Infuse 1 teaspoon of dried herb mixture in 1 cup of boiling water for 20 minutes. This should be drunk hot several times a day. Hot infusions are valuable in that they replace lost fluids and promote diaphoresis.

ASTHMA

A reversible obstructive lung disorder characterized by increased responsiveness of the airways. *(The Merck Manual)*

Asthma is a chronic inflammatory disorder of the airways typified by wheezing, chest tightness, coughing exacerbations, and difficult breathing.[5] An estimated 15 million Americans suffer from asthma, including 4.8 million children and adolescents.[6] Asthma can develop at any time, but is most common in young children. When it starts in childhood, asthma usually improves with age. In adult onset asthma, however, the condition often worsens with age.

A common misconception is that asthma and wheezing are the same thing. Wheezing is a sign of asthma, but many other conditions can also cause wheezing. This confusion has led to the replacement of the term *asthma* with a more descriptive name, *reactive airway disease* (RAD). People with RAD have bronchial passages that are more sensitive than normal to irritation. This hypersensitivity leads to inflammation in the tiny airways deep in the lungs. The inflammation in turn fosters the production of excess mucus and a tightening of the muscles that wind around the bronchial tubes. This combination of swelling, mucus, and tight muscles causes narrowing of the airways. Wheezing usually results, but a dry cough is sometimes the only sign.

Most asthma is characterized by one or more of the following classic symptoms.

Wheezing. This may be either a low or a loud whistle usually heard on expiration (breathing out).

Coughing. The cough of asthma is either a mild cough or a persistent hack that often occurs at night. Chest tightness, experienced as a feeling of bands strapped around the chest or a burning sensation, is another characteristic symptom.

Shortness of breath. This may be described as an inability to catch one's breath or feeling like trying to breathe through a straw. Breathing out is especially tough.

Such symptoms generally begin upon exposure to the individual's special "trigger" that sets off an attack. A sequence of events then occurs at the cellular level in the lungs.

Swelling. The bronchial tubes, often already swollen due to the chronic nature of asthma, develop the characteristic swelling of inflammation. This inflammation reduces the amount of air that can move in and out of the lungs.

Bronchoconstriction. The muscles around the bronchial tubes tighten, making breathing difficult.

Clogging. The bronchial tubes begin to produce more mucus, in turn clogging the airways. However, the tubes may be swollen and sensitive whether or not the inflammation is felt.

Asthma Triggers

Asthma attacks can be minimized by avoiding triggering factors. Several triggers can cause the airways to become more inflamed, and once exposed to a certain trigger, the airways may become more sensitive to other triggers.

Allergies

An estimated 75% of childhood asthma is allergy related, so controlling allergies may be pivotal to reducing the frequency of asthma attacks. If symptoms worsen during certain seasons, the causative factor is probably an allergy to plant pollen. When exposed to pollen, the body responds by creating antibodies that attach themselves to mast cells in the nose and airways. (Mast cells are immune system cells that detect foreign substances and initiate local inflammatory responses against them.) In turn, the mast cells produce and release a chemical called histamine, which generates the allergic response. While exposure to pollen cannot be avoided entirely, the ravages it produces in asthmatics can be minimized if some basic facts are borne in mind.

Not all pollens cause the same symptoms. Tree pollens cause problems in early spring; grass pollens strike in late spring and early summer. Weed pollens cause flare-ups in late summer.

Seasons begin at different times in different bioregions. Ragweed strikes the hardest during mid-August to late October on the East Coast and in the Midwest.

Weather and time of day also affect asthma symptoms.

Colds and Other Respiratory Infections

The most common asthma trigger is a simple cold or other respiratory infection. Colds very quickly cause the airways to become inflamed in asthmatics, even if cold symptoms remain mostly in the head.

Ingested Allergens

These may be drugs (e.g., aspirin), foods, food additives, yeasts, or molds on food.

Gastric Reflux

As much as 30% of all asthma may be caused by gastroesophageal reflux, which causes the unpleasant symptom commonly known as heartburn. Even if other specific asthma triggers have been identified, try preventing heartburn for a few weeks to see if this leads to an improvement in asthma symptoms. (See chapter 13 for more information on the treatment of gastroesophageal reflux disease.)

Exercise

Cold dry air is more aggravating than warm moist air. Simple measures, such as breathing through a scarf and taking preventive medicine before exercise, can help to minimize attacks.

Weather Changes

These include changes in barometric pressure, humidity, and temperature.

Airborne Irritants

Air pollution, dust, cigarette or wood smoke, chemical vapors, irritant gases, and even perfumes can all trigger asthma attacks.

Physical or Emotional Stress

Minimizing stress, whatever the cause, will help decrease the chance of triggering an attack.

Hormonal Changes

In some women, hormonal changes can trigger attacks at certain times in the menstrual cycle.

Childhood-Onset Asthma

Asthma that begins in childhood is closely linked with the presence of eczema, hay fever, urticaria (hives), and migraine in the patient or in close relatives. People with this kind of family history are called *atopic*. If both parents have a history of atopy, the child has a 50% chance of being affected; if only one parent is affected, the chance is 30%; and if neither parent is affected, the chance is approximately 12%. The onset of childhood asthma is often preceded for several months or even years by episodic coughing, which later develops into wheezy bronchitis and then eventually into asthma. These children often have a history of slow recovery from upper respiratory tract viral infections as well as a personal or family history of atopy.

Adult-Onset Asthma

Adult-onset asthma is more common in women than in men. There are two broad types. In the first type, no obvious reasons are apparent for asthma attacks. In the second, fairly obvious external trigger factors precipitate attacks. While the sufferer may be able to avoid these triggers, new allergens will continue to be detected, to be added to the list of external or environmental causes of the condition. Thus, a wide range of etiological factors can be involved in this all too common problem.

The two main types of adult-onset asthma are described as follows.

Extrinsic asthma is caused by allergic responses to house dust, animal fur, or various foods. This type accounts for 10% to 20% of adult-onset asthma cases.

Intrinsic asthma is caused by genetics, structural problems, infections, pollutants, and stress—both physiological and psychological. This accounts for 30% to 50% of adult-onset asthma.

Symptoms of asthma can differ greatly in frequency and degree among individuals. Some have occasional, mild, brief episodes and are otherwise symptom-free. Others experience mild coughing and wheezing much of the time, punctuated by severe exacerbations related to exposure to known allergies, viral infections, exercise, or nonspecific irritants.

Table 15.9. Stages of an Acute Asthma Attack

STAGE	SIGNS AND SYMPTOMS
Stage 1: Mild	Mild dyspnea, diffuse wheezing, adequate air exchange
Stage 2: Moderate	Respiratory distress at rest, use of accessory muscles, marked wheezing
Stage 3: Severe	Marked respiratory distress, cyanosis, use of accessory muscles, marked wheezing or absence of breath sounds
Stage 4: Respiratory failure	Severe respiratory distress, lethargy, confusion, use of accessory muscles

Treatment of Acute Asthma

Phytotherapy has much to offer for the treatment, control, and even cure of asthmatic problems, but will not replace emergency allopathic support for stages 3 and 4 of an acute attack.

Tonic support of the systems most affected by asthma is often the key to successful treatment. The respiratory system, of course, is of primary importance. In addition, attention must be paid to the cardiovascular, nervous, and digestive systems. The digestive system is implicated because the dietary sensitivities triggering asthma may also cause problems in the alimentary canal.

Actions Indicated

Pulmonary tonics are important for long-term strengthening of the lungs, but offer little short-term relief for acute attacks.

Expectorants help prevent buildup of sputum in the lungs. However, use only relaxing expectorants, as stimulant expectorants can potentially aggravate breathing difficulties.

Demulcents soothe irritation and support the action of relaxing expectorants.

Antispasmodics ease spasm responses in the muscles that facilitate respiration.

Antimicrobials help reduce the potential for secondary infection, which should be avoided at all costs.

Anticatarrhals aid the body in dealing with overproduction of sputum in lungs or sinuses.

Cardiotonics support the heart in the face of lung congestion or strain.

Nervine support is always appropriate, both because stress is a potential trigger and because asthma can cause stress, which in turn can trigger further attacks.

Specific Remedies

Ephedra sinica (ma huang) and other Asian *Ephedra* species prove exceptionally useful as bronchodilators. Although synthetic ephedrine is available, the whole herb is better tolerated and causes fewer adverse heart effects.

Ephedra stimulates the sympathetic nervous system and thus relieves the bronchospasm that underlies asthma and certain other conditions, including emphysema. Allergic reactions respond well to *Ephedra* because of its action on the sympathetic nervous system.

The ayurvedic herb *Coleus forskohlii* may be useful in asthma. The constituent forskolin raises cellular levels of cAMP, which results in relaxation of bronchial muscles and relief of asthma symptoms. Forskolin also inhibits the release of histamine and the synthesis of allergic compounds. See chapter 9 for a more detailed discussion of the possible mechanisms of action of this herb.

Herbs with Antispasmodic and Bronchodilating Effects

Ammi visnaga (khella)
Coleus forskohlii (coleus)
Drosera rotundifolia (sundew)
Ephedra spp. (ma huang or ephedra)
Euphorbia pilulifera (pill-bearing spurge)
Grindelia camporum (gumweed or grindelia)
Prunus serotina (wild cherry)

As discussed in chapter 9, the role of platelet activating factor (PAF) in bronchial asthma is receiving increased attention. *Ginkgo biloba* is an effective and safe inhibitor of PAF, making it a potentially useful herb for the control and treatment of asthma. Donald Brown, N.D., one of America's foremost naturopathic phytotherapists, advocates the use of ginkgo in the long-term management of asthma. He reports success in pediatric cases with a dosage of 80 mg/day for children 6 to 12 years old and 40 mg/day for children younger than 6 years old.[7]

Dyspnea Formula for Asthma

Grindelia camporum tincture	24 parts
Euphorbia pilulifera tincture	24 parts
Lobelia inflata tincture	12 parts
Prunus serotina tincture	12 parts
Glycyrrhiza glabra tincture	12 parts
Leonurus cardiaca tincture	12 parts
Ephedra sinica tincture	10 parts
Pimpinella anisum essential oil	1 part

Dosage: 5 ml of mixture three times a day. If *Euphorbia pilulifera* proves difficult to obtain, double the amount of *Grindelia* to make up for it.

Table 15.10. Actions Supplied by Dyspnea Formula

ACTION	HERBS
Pulmonary tonic	Lobelia inflata
Relaxing expectorant	Grindelia camporum, Euphorbia pilulifera, Lobelia inflata, Glycyrrhiza glabra
Demulcent	Glycyrrhiza glabra
Antispasmodic	Grindelia camporum, Euphorbia pilulifera, Lobelia inflata, Prunus serotina, Glycyrrhiza glabra, Pimpinella anisum, Ephedra sinica
Antimicrobial	Pimpinella anisum
Anti-inflammatory	Glycyrrhiza glabra, Pimpinella anisum
Anticatarrhal	Pimpinella anisum, Ephedra sinica
Cardiotonic	Leonurus cardiaca
Nervine	Lobelia inflata, Leonurus cardiaca

ACTION	HERBS
Anticatarrhal	Pimpinella anisum, Ephedra sinica
Cardiotonic	Leonurus cardiaca
Nervine	Lobelia inflata, Leonurus cardiaca, Trifolium pratense

A Prescription for Childhood Atopic Asthma Associated with Eczema

Dyspnea Formula (see page 332)	2 parts
Galium aparine	1 part
Trifolium pratense	1 part
Urtica dioica	1 part

Dosage: up to 5 ml of tincture three times a day

Table 15.11. Actions Supplied by Prescription for Atopic Asthma

ACTION	HERBS
Alterative	Galium aparine, Trifolium pratense, Urtica dioica
Pulmonary tonic	Lobelia inflata
Relaxing expectorant	Grindelia camporum, Euphorbia pilulifera, Lobelia inflata, Glycyrrhiza glabra
Demulcent	Glycyrrhiza glabra
Antispasmodic	Grindelia camporum, Euphorbia pilulifera, Lobelia inflata, Prunus serotina, Glycyrrhiza glabra, Pimpinella anisum, Ephedra sinica
Antimicrobial	Pimpinella anisum
Anti-inflammatory	Glycyrrhiza glabra, Pimpinella anisum

Broader Context of Treatment

Our lungs are connected to our emotions in a very obvious way—just think about what happens when we laugh or cry. If a person with asthma has difficulty expressing feelings, it is worth exploring why. Bach Flower Remedies can help here. Deep breathing exercises strengthen our connection to our feelings and, if practiced regularly, will help in the treatment of asthma. Other regular exercise, such as walking, swimming, yoga, t'ai chi, and relaxation techniques, can also aid in deepening and relaxing breathing.

Food sensitivities must be identified. It may prove beneficial to temporarily exclude eggs, wheat, dairy products, and even gluten (found in wheat, oats, barley, and rye). Lack of breast-feeding sometimes triggers early-onset asthma. Other sources of concern are alcohol (wine and beer) and preserved fruit, which often contains sulfur dioxide. Some asthmatics react to as little as 5 parts of sulfur dioxide per million.

The whole thoracic area—back and chest—should be massaged with appropriate essential oils, with particular emphasis on strokes that open the chest and shoulders. The choice of essential oils will depend on many factors, including whether or not infection is present, if the asthma is known to have an allergic component, and if emotional factors are involved. During an actual asthmatic crisis, inhalation of an antispasmodic oil is the only practical herbal help. Sniffing directly from the bottle or applying drops to a tissue is safer than using a steam inhalation, as the heat will increase inflammation of the mucous membranes and make the congestion even worse.

Essential Oils Useful in Asthma

Hyssopus officinalis (hyssop)
Lavandula spp. (lavender)
Pimpinella anisum (aniseed)
Pinus sylvestris (pine)
Rosmarinus officinalis (rosemary)

In Textbook of Natural Medicine, Drs. Pizzorno and Murray recommend the following nutritional supplements:[8]

Vitamin B$_6$: 25 mg twice a day
Vitamin B$_{12}$: 1,000 mcg a day

Vitamin C: 1 to 2g/day
Vitamin E: 400 IU/ day
Magnesium: 200 to 300 mg three times a day
Quercetin: 400 mg 20 minutes before meals
Carotene: 25,000 to 50,000 IU/day
Selenium: 250 mcg/day

EMPHYSEMA

Enlargement of the air spaces distal to terminal non-respiratory bronchioles, accompanied by destructive changes of the alveolar walls. *(The Merck Manual)*

Emphysema, which often develops as a long-term complication of chronic bronchitis, is characterized by damage to the elastic walls of the sac-like alveoli in the lungs. This damage is caused by constant coughing, the body's attempt to dislodge the bacteria and mucus blocking the swollen bronchi. In chronic bronchitis, the constant secretion of viscid mucus paralyzes the cilia that normally push out particles of dust, soot, and bacteria. Smoking and, to a lesser degree, alcohol exacerbate this condition.

Treatment of Emphysema

The herbal treatment guidelines given here offer no miracle cures, but if used consistently, they will bring about an improvement in this condition.

Actions Indicated

Pulmonary tonics are important for long-term strengthening of the lungs but offer little short-term relief for acute attacks.

Expectorants are essential to minimize the buildup of sputum in the lungs. Stimulant expectorants are necessary here because of the lessening of tone that affects the walls of the alveoli.

Demulcents soothe irritation and support the work of expectorants.

Antispasmodics ease spasm responses in the muscles that facilitate respiration.

Antimicrobials help reduce the potential for secondary infection, which should be avoided at all costs.

Anticatarrhals aid the body in dealing with overproduction of sputum in lungs or sinuses.

Cardiotonics support the heart in the face of lung congestion or strain.

Nervine support is always appropriate, as stress will exacerbate emphysema.

A Prescription for Emphysema

Dyspnea Formula (see page 332)	1 part
Sanguinaria canadensis	1 part
Inula helenium	1 part

Dosage: up to 5 ml of tincture three times a day

Table 15.12. Actions Supplied by Prescription for Emphysema

ACTION	HERBS
Pulmonary tonic	*Inula helenium, Lobelia inflata*
Stimulating expectorant	*Sanguinaria canadensis, Inula helenium, Grindelia camporum, Euphorbia pilulifera, Lobelia inflata, Glycyrrhiza glabra*
Demulcent	*Glycyrrhiza glabra*
Antispasmodic	*Inula helenium, Sanguinaria canadensis, Grindelia camporum, Euphorbia pilulifera, Lobelia inflata, Prunus serotina, Glycyrrhiza glabra, Pimpinella anisum, Ephedra sinica*
Antimicrobial	*Inula helenium, Sanguinaria canadensis, Pimpinella anisum*
Anti-inflammatory	*Glycyrrhiza glabra, Pimpinella anisum*
Anticatarrhal	*Inula helenium, Pimpinella anisum, Ephedra sinica*
Cardiotonic	*Leonurus cardiaca*
Nervine	*Lobelia inflata, Leonurus cardiaca*

Broader Context of Treatment

Great care must be taken with general health and well-being, as any health problem will aggravate emphysema. Thus, all physical and emotional factors must be addressed.

The nutritional supplements recommended for asthma are also relevant here.

Vitamin B$_6$: 25 mg twice a day
Vitamin B$_{12}$: 1,000 mcg/day
Vitamin C: 1 to 2g/day
Vitamin E: 400 IU/day
Magnesium: 200 to 300 mg three times a day
Quercetin: 400 mg 20 minutes before meals
Carotene: 25,000 to 50,000 IU/day
Selenium: 250 mcg/day

THE UPPER RESPIRATORY SYSTEM

The organs of the upper respiratory system include the nose, the pharynx, and the larynx.

Table 15.13. Actions and Herbs for the Upper Respiratory System

ACTION	HERBS
Antimicrobial	*Allium* spp., *Eucalyptus* spp., *Thymus vulgaris*, *Baptisia tinctoria*, *Commiphora molmol*, *Ligusticum porteri*
Immune stimulant	*Echinacea* spp.
Anticatarrhal	*Solidago virgaurea*, *Sambucus nigra*, *Hyssopus officinalis*, *Tussilago farfara*, *Hydrastis canadensis*, volatile oils
Astringents	*Salvia officinalis*, *Euphrasia* spp.
Diaphoretic	*Eupatorium perfoliatum*, *Tilia platyphyllos*

Tonic Support for the Upper Respiratory System

Nature abounds with herbs that have anticatarrhal effects in the upper respiratory system, but anticatarrhal herbs do not substitute for the nurturing action of tonics for this part of the body. From the European perspective, here are some appropriate tonics that also possess anticatarrhal properties.

Upper Respiratory Tract Tonics

Euphrasia spp. (eyebright)
Hydrastis canadensis (goldenseal)
Hyssopus officinalis (hyssop)
Sambucus nigra (elder)
Solidago virgaurea (goldenrod)
Urtica dioica (nettle)

Herbs and Upper Respiratory Conditions

As with many modern health problems, prevention of upper respiratory tract disease is largely a matter of avoiding pollutants and minimizing causative dietary factors. As with the lower respiratory tract, air pollution and smoking can aggravate or even cause a whole spectrum of upper respiratory problems.

Many chronic catarrhal states represent the body's response to a diet too rich in mucus-forming foods. A diet designed to minimize mucus production is essential for patients with such conditions. However, it is not always appropriate to try to dry up overproduction of normal secretions with herbs. If the body is using the mucous membranes of the sinuses as a window for removing waste through the vehicle of the catarrh, then it is best to support rather than block this activity.

The herbal approach to problems in this system is both indirect and direct. The indirect approach sees upper respiratory disease within the context of the whole person. Sometimes, the overproduction of mucus is an attempt by the body to discharge waste material that is not being properly eliminated by the bowels, kidneys, and skin. In such cases, the herbalist may prescribe bitter tonics to encourage regular bowel movements, diuretic herbs that encourage kidney elimination of retained fluids and waste materials, or diaphoretic herbs that stimulate elimination through the skin.

Patterns of Upper Respiratory Tract Disease

Treatment of many diverse pathologies becomes straightforward when one understands certain basic patterns of disease affecting the upper respiratory system.

Allergic response. The allergen must be identified and, if possible, removed from the individual's environment. This may be easy in the case of a food sensitivity, but much more problematic if the trigger is a ubiquitous environmental factor, such as pollen or house dust. (See Hay Fever for more information.)

Congestion. The production of excessive and thick mucus in the nose and other respiratory passages is a response to inflammation of the mucous membranes. This can be caused by infection, autoimmune problems, or irritants. Blockage of the sinus cavities is very common and relatively easy to treat with herbs.

Infection. Acute infections of the nose, sinuses, and throat are all too common! Occasional acute infections can be treated in a straightforward manner with antimicrobial and anticatarrhal herbs and essential oils. However, if there is a pattern of frequent, recurrent infection, attention must be focused on immune system support and other whole body issues.

Physical blockage. Any obstruction calls for skilled diagnostic investigation. Some benign problems, such as nasal polyps, may be treated with herbs, but differential diagnosis is vital to rule out more serious problems.

THE COMMON COLD

An acute, usually afebrile, viral infection of the respiratory tract, with inflammation in any or all airways, including the nose, paranasal sinuses, throat, larynx, and often the trachea and bronchi. *(The Merck Manual)*

The common cold, also known as acute rhinitis, is a viral infection of the upper respiratory tract. Many different strains of virus cause cold symptoms, and these are constantly undergoing mutation. When the mucous membranes of the nose and throat are inflamed by infection, they are far more vulnerable to attack by bacteria, and this can easily give rise to secondary infections that are more serious than the original cold, such as sinusitis, ear infections, and bronchitis. Because colds have a viral origin, antibiotic drugs that destroy bacteria are not helpful in their treatment.

Treatment of the Common Cold

There is no universally miraculous herbal cold cure. However, phytotherapy offers more than most modalities for the treatment and prevention of this all-too-common problem. With a treatment approach focusing on herbs that fit the individual's unique needs and attention to immune support, diet, and lifestyle issues, the common cold presents no real treatment challenges.

For a short-term, acute infection, there is usually no need to focus on system support. However, if the individual has frequent or recurrent colds, the use of tonic remedies will be vital. Immune system support is important, and attention must often be paid to the impact of stress in the individual's life. A tendency for colds to progress to coughs and bronchitis calls for pulmonary tonic support.

As an illustration of how other health issues may be taken into account when treating the common cold, consider this example. If the patient has a history of heart disease, cardiotonics may be used as a precautionary measure. However, *Tilia* is most appropriate, as it is diaphoretic in addition to being a heart tonic.

Actions Indicated

Antimicrobials and *immune stimulants* help the immune system combat the viral infection and help prevent secondary infection.

Anticatarrhals ease the symptomatic discomfort so characteristic of this problem. However, avoid trying to dry up mucus overproduction with herbal decongestants.

Diaphoretics help with feverishness and support the body's efforts to cope with elevated body temperature.

Expectorants help combat the development of secondary problems in the lower respiratory system.

Lymphatics are indicated if the lymph glands are swollen or there is a known history of such problems.

Specific Remedies

There are many regional and personal ideas about specific herbs for the common cold. These are often diaphoretic herbs.

To treat an infection once it has started, address the specific symptoms while at the same time supporting the body's fight against the virus. Aches and pains are common, and our materia medica offers a number of plants that will relieve these unpleasant feelings. Perhaps the best is the diaphoretic *Eupatorium perfoliatum* (boneset), especially if the patient has a fever. A hot infusion drunk often can make bearable even the worst cases of flu. Boneset's bitter taste is one of its therapeutic assets, but not one that most people relish! *Matricaria*, *Tilia*, and *Mentha piperita* tea may have similar effects, and while not as strong, they do taste much better.

Do not inhibit nasal congestion with anticatarrhal drugs, as mucus production is part of the body's normal response to infection. Herbal anticatarrhals work in a different, safer way than anticatarrhal drugs. *Matricaria*, *Mentha piperita*, or *Eupatorium perfoliatum* can help relieve much of the discomfort. Steam inhalations of eucalyptus and thyme oils will also help reduce the formation of catarrh.

Specific Remedies for the Common Cold

Achillea millefolium (yarrow)
Allium spp. (onion and garlic)
Armoracia rusticana (horseradish)
Brassica spp. (mustard)
Capsicum spp. (cayenne)
Eupatorium perfoliatum (boneset)
Matricaria recutita (chamomile)
Mentha piperita (peppermint)
Sambucus nigra (black elder)
Tilia platyphyllos (linden)

To support the immune system, use antimicrobial herbs such as echinacea and goldenseal, as well as tonics, such as cleavers and nettles. These may be combined in capsules or as tinctures. *Hydrastis canadensis* will speed recovery from infection, as will raw garlic or garlic oil capsules.

Antimicrobial Herbs

Allium spp. (onion and garlic)
Echinacea spp. (echinacea)
Eucalyptus globulus (eucalyptus)
Hydrastis canadensis (goldenseal)
Thymus vulgaris (thyme)

A Prescription for the Common Cold

Sambucus nigra	1 part
Mentha piperita	1 part
Achillea millefolium	1 part

Infuse 1 to 2 teaspoons of dried herb mixture in 1 cup of boiling water; this should be drunk hot often until symptoms pass.

Herbal Footbath for Colds

Footbaths are a traditional treatment for colds. Dissolve 1 tablespoon of mustard powder in 4 pints of hot water. Bathe the feet for 10 minutes, twice a day.

Chamomile Steam Inhalation

Place a handful of *Matricaria* flowers in a bowl and pour boiling water over them. Create a tent by draping a towel over the head to prevent the escape of vapors; inhale vapors rising from bowl for 5 to 10 minutes.

Thymus, Eucalyptus, and *Origanum* may also be used in steam inhalations, as in the following example.

Steam Inhalation Combination

Matricaria flowers	1 part
Thymus herb	1 part
Origanum herb	1 part

Add 1 tablespoon of dried herb mixture to ½ liter (1 pint) of boiling water. Follow inhalation instructions given for Chamomile Steam Inhalation.

Aromatherapy for the Common Cold

A steam inhalation of appropriate essential oils combines several beneficial effects. It clears congested nasal passages and soothes inflamed mucous membranes. At the same time, the essential oil will kill many bacteria. Some of the oils, especially *Eucalyptus* and *Melaleuca*, have an inhibitory effect on the cold virus. Use either of these two oils for inhalations in the earlier part of the day (possibly alternating with *Rosmarinus* and *Mentha piperita*), as they are mildly stimulating. At night, use inhalations of *Lavandula* or add a few drops of oil to a bath. Diffusing oil in the bedroom is helpful, especially if the patient has a cough.

Essential Oils for Steam Inhalation

Citrus aurantium ssp. *bergamia* (bergamot)
Commiphora molmol (myrrh)
Eucalyptus globulus (eucalyptus)
Lavandula spp. (lavender)
Melaleuca spp. (tea tree)
Mentha arvensis var. *piperascens* (Asian mint)
M. piperita (peppermint)
Ocimum basilicum (basil)
Origanum majorana (marjoram)
Pinus pumilio (dwarf or white pine)
Rosmarinus officinalis (rosemary)
Santalum album (sandalwood)
Styrax benzoin (benzoin)
Thymus vulgaris (thyme)

Broader Context of Treatment

Many traditional cold remedies are based on culinary ingredients, highlighting the fact that there is no real difference between medicinal and edible plants. Here is an example of a treatment that capitalizes on the value of common medicinal foods. Take this combination at the first sign of a chill or sore throat.

Kitchen Remedy to Ward Off a Cold

1 ounce fresh ginger, sliced
1 stick of cinnamon, broken
1 teaspoon coriander seeds
3 cloves
1 slice of lemon

Decoct ingredients for 15 minutes in 1 pint of water; strain. Drink a cupful hot every 2 hours. Sweeten with organic honey to taste.

For both the prevention and treatment of colds, include garlic, onions, watercress, and cayenne in the diet, and take 1 to 3 g of vitamin C daily. Diet plays a role in most cases of catarrh. Dairy products and wheat are known to promote excessive catarrh production for many people. For anyone who frequently suffers from catarrh, these foods should be excluded for a period to see if any improvement occurs. If so, the individual may need to exclude them permanently or include them in very small amounts only. Other people are sensitive to different foods, and may have to experiment to find out which foods trigger symptoms.

INFLUENZA

A specific acute viral disease characterized by fever, coryza, cough, headache, malaise, and inflamed respiratory mucous membranes. (The Merck Manual)

Influenza, commonly called the flu, is a severe form of viral respiratory tract infection with generalized bodily symptoms. New mutations of the virus arise all the time, and, unfortunately, developing immunity against one strain through previous exposure or immunization does not protect against other strains. New strains of influenza can spread extremely rapidly, and worldwide influenza epidemics are responsible for much ill health and many deaths.

Severe colds and various unidentified virus infections are often loosely referred to as flu. Some authorities would argue that this terminology is incorrect, and that true influenza is a much more severe infection that appears in the form of widespread epidemics, often at intervals of approximately 10 years. Influenza was the cause of major pandemics in the 20th century. A *pandemic* occurs over a very wide geographic area and affects an exceptionally large proportion of the population, while an *epidemic* is of a much smaller scale and tends to affect a large number of individuals within a population, community, or region at the same time.

Consider the mortality associated with some 20th century influenza pandemics:

Spanish flu (1918–1919): Caused the highest known influenza-related mortality, with approximately 500,000 deaths in the United States and 20 million worldwide
Asian flu (1957–1958): 70,000 deaths in the United States
Hong Kong flu (1968–1969): 34,000 deaths in the United States

Typical clinical features of influenza include fever (100°F to 103°F in adults and even higher in children), headache, muscle aches, extreme fatigue, and respiratory symptoms, such as cough, sore throat, and runny or stuffy nose. Although nausea, vomiting, and diarrhea can sometimes accompany influenza infection, especially in children, gastrointestinal symptoms are rarely prominent. The term *stomach flu* is actually a misnomer used to describe gastrointestinal illnesses caused by other microorganisms.

Most people recover completely in one to two weeks, but some develop serious and potentially life-threatening medical complications, such as pneumonia. Secondary bacterial infections are the greatest risk of influenza, and were responsible for most deaths in past epidemics. The use of antibiotics has dramatically reduced such deaths, although the very young and the elderly are still at risk. A really severe infection of this type may be one of the situations in which the use of antibiotics is sensible. However, if antibiotics are necessary, do not stop the herbal treatment; it can only be beneficial and will not conflict with orthodox drug treatment.

In an average year, influenza is associated with about 20,000 deaths nationwide and many more hospitalizations. Flu-related complications can occur at any age; however, the elderly and people with chronic health problems are much more likely to develop serious complications than younger, healthier people are.

Treatment of Influenza

The herbal treatment guidelines given here to use against influenza must be placed in the context of rest and recuperation, discussed later. Also consider any specific points of weakness in the individual, especially for elderly patients.

Actions Indicated

Antimicrobials support the immune system in combating viral infection and help prevent the development of secondary infection.

Diaphoretics help with symptoms of fever and support the body's efforts to cope with elevated temperature.

Anticatarrhals ease the symptomatic discomfort so characteristic of this problem. However, avoid trying to dry up mucus overproduction with herbal decongestants.

Diaphoretics help with feverishness and support the body's efforts to cope with elevated body temperature.

Expectorants help combat the development of secondary problems in the lower respiratory system.

Lymphatics are indicated if the lymph glands are swollen or there is a known history of such problems.

Bitters support the body in dealing with the debility that often follows severe viral infections.

Nervines assist the body in dealing with high fever and associated distress.

Specific Remedies

As with the common cold, there are no miracle cures here. However, certain plants can make life much more bearable during a bout of flu. These are usually diaphoretics, and my favorite is *Eupatorium perfoliatum* (boneset). This herb gets its name from its traditional use to ease the pain of what was called "break-bone fever" by European settlers in North America.

A Prescription for Influenza

Hydrastis canadensis	1 part
Echinacea spp.	1 part

Dosage: 2.5 ml of tincture every 2 hours. In addition, the patient should drink a strong hot infusion of *Eupatorium perfoliatum* every hour. If the symptom picture calls for it, follow recommendations given earlier for the common cold.

Table 15.14. Actions Supplied by Influenza Prescription

ACTION	HERBS
Antimicrobial	*Hydrastis canadensis*, *Echinacea* spp.
Diaphoretic	*Eupatorium perfoliatum*
Anticatarrhal	*Hydrastis canadensis*, *Echinacea* spp.
Lymphatic	*Echinacea* spp.
Bitter	*Hydrastis canadensis*, *Eupatorium perfoliatum*

Broader Context of Treatment

Treatment will be most effective if initiated at the *very first sign* of infection. A moderately hot bath containing a few drops of antiviral essential oil will often induce diaphoresis, followed by a deep, restful sleep. This may be enough to avert a full-blown infection, though it is a good idea to repeat this bath treatment for the next two or three days. Tea tree oil is particularly effective for this purpose. However, some people find it to be a mild skin irritant, and may not be able to tolerate more than 3 or 4 drops in a full bath.

Recovery from influenza is often slow, and the convalescing patient may feel very weak and lacking in vitality. Caffeine-containing stimulant herbs should be avoided, as the lift they confer is only temporary and will slow down recovery (see chapter 16 for more information). As pointed out above, bitter tonics will speed recovery through their metabolism-stimulating effects.

Table 15.15. Bitter Tonics for Convalescence

HERB	ACTIONS
Eupatorium perfoliatum	Bitter, diaphoretic, anticatarrhal
Gentiana spp.	Bitter, other general digestive functions
Hydrastis canadensis	Bitter, anticatarrhal, general tonic
Marrubium vulgare	Bitter, expectorant, anticatarrhal

In addition, adaptogens are often helpful, and attention to diet is essential. It may be helpful to use a multivitamin and mineral formulation until appetite and general vitality return to normal.

HAY FEVER

A symptom complex including hay fever and perennial allergic rhinitis, characterized by seasonal or perennial sneezing, rhinorrhea, nasal congestion, pruritus, and often conjunctivitis and pharyngitis. *(The Merck Manual)*

Hay fever, or *allergic rhinitis*, is a form of allergy that affects the lining of the nose and, often, the eyes and throat. As the name implies, the condition is an allergic response to the pollen of certain grasses, but the term is also used to describe similar reactions to a wide range of pollens and the spores of some fungi.

Treatment of Hay Fever

Hay fever responds well to herbal treatment, but each person is different, so a number of approaches may have to be tried until the right one is found. The immune system needs support, and stress may also be an issue. Tonic support should be provided for both the upper and lower respiratory systems.

Actions Indicated

Anticatarrhals ease the symptomatic discomfort often characteristic of this problem. Again, avoid trying to dry up mucus overproduction with herbal decongestants, as this can end up being quite painful.

Expectorants will be needed if wheezing or pulmonary congestion develops. Relaxing expectorants will usually be most relevant.

Antispasmodics are essential if there is any marked difficulty with breathing.

Bitters help tone the whole body in the face of the immune systems response.

Anti-inflammatories soothe various symptoms of inflammation as and when they arise.

Astringents often ease the symptom picture, as many anticatarrhals are also astringents.

Adaptogens and *immune support* may help long term. This overall system support should cover the liver, kidney, and any other systems that require support. See chapter 21 for more information.

Specific Remedies

Individuals may find that certain herbs suit them well, but otherwise, there is no particular specific remedy for hay fever. The well-known traditional Chinese remedy *Ephedra sinica* (ma huang) is a bronchodilator and has much to offer in the treatment of allergic reactions. Ayurveda and unani medicine use *Ammi visnaga*, a plant with a similar biochemical impact that is now being introduced to the Western world.

In addition to these alkaloid-rich plants, certain herbs might be considered specific for various types and sites of symptoms that may arise. For example, *Euphrasia* spp. ease distress that occurs in the eyes.

A Prescription for Hay Fever

Ephedra sinica	1 part
Hydrastis canadensis	1 part
Euphrasia spp.	1 part
Urtica dioica	2 parts
Solidago virgaurea	2 parts

Dosage: 5 ml of tincture three times a day. Ideally, this treatment should be started two months before hay fever season is due to commence. Start with the following dosage regimen.

Pre–Hay Fever Season Dosage Regimen

Weeks 1–2	2.5 ml once a day
Weeks 3–4	5 ml once a day
Weeks 5–6	5 ml twice a day
Weeks 7–8	5 ml three times a day

If this treatment cannot be initiated before the allergy flares up, then start with a full dose immediately, possibly increasing the dose to 5 ml four or five times a day (adults only).

Table 15.16. Actions Supplied by Hay Fever Prescription

ACTION	HERBS
Antispasmodic	*Ephedra sinica*
Anticatarrhal	*Hydrastis canadensis, Solidago virgaurea, Euphrasia* spp., *Ephedra sinica*
Anti-inflammatory	*Hydrastis canadensis, Solidago virgaurea, Euphrasia* spp., *Urtica dioica*
Antimicrobial	*Hydrastis canadensis*
Astringent	*Euphrasia* spp.
Bitter	*Hydrastis canadensis*

Broader Context of Treatment

Treating the whole person is the trick to successfully ameliorating this common problem. In addition to symptoms of the allergy, focus on general health, stress, and elimination. Dietary considerations must be based upon avoidance of specific allergens as well as general good nutrition.

Various essential oils can help with symptoms of hay fever, but the specifics vary from person to person. Oils recommended by aromatherapists include all of those listed above for the common cold, with the addition of blue chamomile, lemon balm, and lavender. If steam inhalation makes the patient feel even worse, suggest that the person put some oil on a tissue to sniff whenever needed. A massage with any of these oils can also be helpful.

SINUSITIS

An inflammatory process in the paranasal sinuses due to viral, bacterial, and fungal infections or allergic reactions.
(The Merck Manual)

The sinuses are four bony cavities positioned behind, above, and at each side of the nose and open into the nasal cavity. They act as a sound box to give resonance to the voice. Sinusitis is an inflammation of these air-containing cavities.

Like the nasal passages, the sinuses are lined with mucous membranes that react to infection by producing mucus. This represents an attempt by the body to incapacitate the infecting bacteria. Because the openings from the nose into the sinuses are very narrow, they quickly become blocked when the mucous membranes swell during a cold, hay fever, or catarrh, trapping the infection inside the sinuses.

Chronic sinusitis may occur if one or more of the drainage passages from the sinuses to the nose become blocked. This can cause headaches or a dull pain across the face and temple and around the eyes. If the maxillary sinuses above the cheeks are infected, toothache may result. Once the lining of the sinuses becomes swollen, the cilia of the nasal cavity no longer operate. The lining of the sinuses can become permanently thickened, contributing to the retention of phlegm.

Anything that blocks the sinus openings or impedes the action of the cilia can cause a sinus infection. A buildup of mucus creates an ideal environment for microorganisms to thrive.

Common Causes of Sinus Infections

Colds or upper respiratory infections
Hay fever or allergies
Air pollution and cigarette smoke
Nasal or dental procedures

Traveling at high altitudes or swimming under water

Hormone changes that occur with puberty

Pregnancy

Aging

Sinus blockages

Health conditions such as diabetes and AIDS

Treatment of Sinusitis

Success in treating this intransigent condition requires that herbal protocols be used in the context of dietary considerations. The mucous membranes, upper and lower respiratory tracts, immune system, and, possibly, the digestive system all need attention. Which systems to focus on will depend on individual indications.

Actions Indicated

Antimicrobials are pivotal in the treatment of this often entrenched condition. These herbs will help the body deal with any infection present, but also support the immune system in resisting the development of secondary infection.

Anticatarrhals ease the symptomatic discomfort characteristic of this problem and assist the body in eliminating buildup in the sinus cavities.

Astringents, often also anticatarrhals, reduce overproduction of mucus.

Anti-inflammatories are indicated, but most of the herbs with actions already listed here are also anti-inflammatory.

Diaphoretics will be indicated if feverishness is part of the symptom picture.

Analgesics may be necessary for temporary pain relief.

Lymphatics aid the drainage and immune function of this vital system.

Digestive support is indicated if overproduction of mucus causes stomach discomfort.

Adaptogens and *immune support* may help long term.

A Prescription for Sinusitis

Solidago virgaurea	2 parts
Sambucus nigra	1 part
Echinacea spp.	1 part
Baptisia tinctoria	1 part

Dosage: 5 ml of tincture three times a day

Steam inhalation is an effective technique for treating upper respiratory catarrh and sinusitis.

Steam Inhalation for Upper Respiratory Tract Catarrh and Sinusitis

Compound tincture of benzoin	30 ml
Eucalyptus essential oil	2.5 ml
Peppermint essential oil	6 drops
Lavender essential oil	5 drops
Pine essential oil	5 drops

Combine ingredients in a bottle and shake well. Put a teaspoon of the mixture in a bowl and pour on ½ liter (1 pint) boiled water. Cover the head and the bowl with a towel or cloth and inhale. **Caution:** Keep the eyes closed.

Broader Context of Treatment

Some cases of chronic mucus production are related to allergy. Sometimes, however, emotional factors like suppressed grief can result in blocked upper respiratory passages. In these cases, a good cry can help free this blocked energy and alleviate the problem.

A diet that reduces mucus production is also essential. In particular, a fruit fast for two or three days can help clear a system clogged and overburdened by toxic wastes. Hot lemon drinks reduce mucus production, as do garlic, onions, and horseradish. Suggest that the patient grate fresh horseradish root into cider vinegar or lemon juice and eat a little each day. Mustard and aromatic herbs like oregano may be added to food, and extra zinc and vitamin C can help build the body's resistance to infection.

Certain foods, especially dairy products and wheat, seem to predispose people toward sinusitis because they provoke excessive formation of mucus. During an acute attack of sinusitis, all dairy and wheat-based foods must be excluded for several days. People who have chronic or repeated attacks should be advised to exclude these foods completely for several months, and then reintroduce them in very small amounts, if at all. Goat's and sheep's milk products are sometimes better tolerated than cow's milk. Acupuncture is a very effective therapy for sinusitis and can be used alongside phytotherapy.

LARYNGITIS

Acute inflammation of the larynx. *(The Merck Manual)*

Laryngitis is an acute inflammation of the larynx, or voice box, usually associated with a common cold or overuse of the voice. It is characterized by swelling, hoarseness, pain, dryness in the throat, coughing, and inability to speak above a whisper, if at all. It is usually caused by a bacterial or viral infection, either restricted to the larynx or part of a more general infection of the upper respiratory tract. Where no clear-cut cause is found, such as infection or overuse, skilled diagnosis is required.

Treatment of Laryngitis

The lymphatic system should be the focus of tonic support, but if there is a pattern of recurrent infection, attention must also be given to strengthening the immune system.

Actions Indicated

Demulcents will soothe the mucous lining and ease discomfort.

Anti-inflammatories will reduce the immediate cause of distress.

Antimicrobials are indicated if there is a causal microorganism involved. However, they are not indicated if inflammation is due to some other cause.

Astringents are often effective as a local gargle, especially if the problem was precipitated by overuse of the vocal cords.

Bitters have a toning and stimulating effect on the mucosal lining.

Specific Remedies

The various herbal traditions of the world abound with herbs effective for conditions of the mouth, larynx, and pharynx. Osha *(Ligusticum porteri)* is an excellent specific. A small piece of the root can be chewed to ameliorate symptoms and promote the body's immune response.

In Europe, gargling with astringent herbs is the traditional approach. They should not be drunk, as they will probably also promote constipation—an unnecessary and unfortunate complication.

Astringent Herbs Relevant to Laryngitis

Achillea millefolium (yarrow)
Geranium maculatum (cranesbill)
Polygonum bistortum (bistort root)
Potentilla tormentosa (tormentil)
Quercus spp. (oak bark)
Rubus idaeus (raspberry leaf)
R. villosus (blackberry leaf)
Salvia officinalis var. *rubia* (red sage)
Sambucus nigra (black elder flower)

A Prescription for Laryngitis

Echinacea spp.	2 parts
Ligusticum porteri	2 parts
Hydrastis canadensis	1 part

Dosage: up to 1 ml of tincture every hour

A Gargle for Laryngitis

Salvia officinalis var. *rubia*	1 part
Matricaria recutita	1 part

Make a strong infusion with dried herbs. Gargle often until symptoms subside.

Gargle II for Laryngitis

Malva neglecta or *Malva sylvestris*

Infuse *Malva* flowers and leaves in lukewarm water overnight to ensure optimum extraction of mucilage. Gargle as needed.

Broader Context of Treatment

Follow the dietary advice given earlier for sinusitis. In addition, aromatherapy provides some oils that ease inflammation quite effectively, including cypress and bergamot oils. To use as a gargle, put 3 drops of essential oil in ½ cup of warm water. Gargle hourly.

TONSILLITIS

Acute inflammation of the palatine tonsils, usually due to streptococcal or, less commonly, viral infection. *(The Merck Manual)*

Tonsillitis is either an acute or a chronic inflammation of the tonsils, which are located near the back of the tongue. The adenoids, lymph glands found behind the nose, are often simultaneously inflamed. Tonsillitis usually develops suddenly as a result of a streptococcal infection, but may also be caused by a viral infection.

The condition is characterized by sore throat, fever, chills, headache, poor appetite, and weakness. The tonsils become swollen and red, and streaks of pus are often visible on their surface. Acute tonsillitis usually clears up in about a week, but antibiotics are commonly prescribed to prevent complications such as middle ear and sinus infections, formation of deep abscesses, spread of infection to other organs, and chronic tonsillitis. Chronic tonsillitis is characterized by flare-ups of acute infection. Tonsillitis is more common in children than in adults.

Tonsils are composed of the same type of tissue that makes up the lymph nodes, and they are part of the body's natural defense system. When the tonsils are infected, the lymph glands in the neck often simultaneously become enlarged and tender, signifying the body's proper reaction to the challenge of infection.

Treatment of Tonsillitis

The lymphatic system should be the focus of tonic support, but if there is a pattern of recurrent infection, attention must also be given to strengthening the immune system.

Actions Indicated

Lymphatics are of primary importance, as this is an infection of lymphatic tissue.

Antimicrobials help the immune system combat the infection, whatever the causal pathogen might be, and help prevent the development of secondary infection

Anticatarrhals are indicated if there is associated sinus congestion or middle ear involvement.

Diaphoretics help the body cope with any associated fever.

Expectorants are indicated if secondary problems develop in the lower respiratory system.

Specific Remedies

Lymphatic alteratives usually have local reputations as specifics for tonsillitis. In the United Kingdom, the most famous is *Galium aparine* (cleavers).

A Prescription for Tonsillitis

Galium aparine	2 parts
Echinacea spp.	2 parts
Baptisia tinctoria	1 part
Calendula officinalis	1 part

Dosage: up to 5 ml of tincture three times a day. Diaphoretics should be added if fever is an issue.

Broader Context of Treatment

In *Herbal Home Health Care*, Dr. Christopher recommends the following fomentation.[9] (A *fomentation* is the application of hot moist substances to the body.)

Fomentation

Verbascum thapsus	3 parts
Lobelia inflata	1 part

Make a strong infusion of dried herb mixture. Dip a cloth in the fomentation and wrap around the neck at night, repeating the procedure each night until the condition clears up.

References

1. National Center for Chronic Disease Prevention and Health Promotion. www.cdc.gov/tobacco/hlthcon.htm

2. Hirono I, Mori H, Culvenor CC. Carcinogenic activity of coltsfoot, Tussilago farfaral. *Gann* 1976 Feb; 67(1):125–29.

3. Sperl W, Stuppner H, Gassner I, et al. Reversible hepatic veno-occlusive disease in an infant after consumption of pyrrolizidine-containing herbal tea. *European Journal of Pediatrics* 1995 Feb; 154(2):112–16.

4. Weiss RF. *Herbal Medicine*. Stuttgart; New York: Thieme, 2000.

5. *Global Initiative for Asthma: Global Strategy for Asthma Management and Prevention*. NHLBI/WHO Workshop Report, March 1993. Rev edition. Washington, DC: National Institutes of Health, National Heart, Lung, and Blood Institute; January 1995. National Heart, Lung, and Blood Institute publication NIH 95–3659.

6. Centers for Disease Control. Asthma mortality and hospitalization among children and young adults—United States, 1980–1993. *Morbidity and Mortality Weekly* 1996; 45: 350–3.

7. Brown D. *Herbal Prescriptions for Better Health*. Rocklin, CA: Prima Publishing, 1996.

8. Pizzorno JE, Murray MT. *Textbook of Natural Medicine*. Edinburgh: Churchill Livingstone, 1999.

9. Christopher JR. *Herbal Home Health Care*. Springville, UT: Christopher Publications, 1976.

16

~

THE NERVOUS SYSTEM

A fascinating aspect of herbalism is the way in which plants affect human consciousness. The integration of all life revealed by the Gaia hypothesis shows us that awareness and expanded consciousness are part of the greater being we belong to. Words and names are meaningless when considering such things, but just as our Earth feeds us, heals our arthritis, and strengthens the function of our hearts, so it supports and nurtures our nervous systems.

Herbalism is a cooperative healing venture among humanity, plants, and the Earth. This experience of wholeness is spirit in action, and opens the door for change and transformation. Nature provides us with herbs that transform and enlighten as well as plants that heal and nurture the nerve tissue itself. We will consider the physical aspect of this healing here, but remember that the physical action of nervine herbs is but one side of the whole interface between plant and mind.

From one perspective, herbs are embodiments of energy and spirit, and from another they are packets of biochemicals. This dichotomy is, in fact, a microcosm of the relationship between the human brain and the mind! The complexities of the mind-body interface, so challenging to doctors concerned with psychosomatic medicine, become an aid to remedy selection for the herbalist.

All of the many herbal nervines have an impact on both somatic symptoms and the mind. A simple example is *Leonurus cardiaca* (motherwort), an herb used for treating anxiety and tension. Motherwort also has a specific affinity for the heart, easing heart palpitations and the fear that often accompanies them. This is recognized to some degree in the species name *cardiaca*, derived from the Greek word for heart.

THE NERVOUS SYSTEM AND HERBAL REMEDIES

In no other system of the body is the connection between the physical and psychological aspects of our being as apparent as in the nervous system. Clearly, the tissue of the nervous system is part of the physical makeup of the body. However, just as clearly, all psychological processes are anchored in the nervous system. Therefore, if there is *disease* on the psychological level, it will be reflected on the physiological level, and vice versa.

Orthodox medicine tends to reduce psychological problems to purely biochemical mechanisms, and assumes that appropriate drugs will sort out or at least hide the problem sufficiently to allow life to continue. Interestingly enough, some premises of complementary medicine assume or imply the other extreme: namely, that psychological factors are the cause of all disease. According to this point of view, treatment of the psyche is the only appropriate way to approach healing, and will take care of any physical problem. By bringing these two reductionist views together, we come closer to a holistic approach.

A holistic approach to healing acknowledges the interconnectedness of physiological and psychological factors, and regards the nervous system and its functions as a vital part of the treatment of the whole being. To be truly healthy, we must attend to our physical health through the right diet and lifestyle, but we are also responsible for taking care of our emotional, mental, and spiritual life. We should endeavor to live in a fulfilling, nurturing environment that supports emotional stability. Our thoughts should be creative, life enhancing, and open to the influence of intuition and imagination, rather than conceptually rigid. And we should stay open to the free flow of the higher energies of our souls, without which health is impossible.

Herbal medicine can be an ecologically and spiritually integrative tool, an ideal physical counterpart to therapeutic techniques applied on the psychological level. Herbs can benefit the nervous system in a number of ways, in addition to the rather simplistic effects of stimulation and relaxation.

Today, Western herbalism commonly recognizes three major categories of herbs that act on the nervous system, collectively called *nervines*. These are *nervine ton-*

ics, *nervine relaxants*, and *nervine stimulants*. Other important categories of nervines include hypnotics, analgesics, antispasmodics, antidepressants, and adaptogens. For more information on these actions and the primary and secondary actions of specific herbs, please see chapters 25 and 26.

Of many potential remedies that could be mentioned, table 16.1 provides a listing of the best-known nervines in European phytotherapy.

Table 16.1. Nervine Herbs Recognized in European Phytotherapy

TYPE OF NERVINE	HERBS
Tonic	Avena sativa, Hypericum perforatum, Scutellaria lateriflora
Relaxant	Cimicifuga racemosa, Eschscholzia californica, Humulus lupulus, Hypericum perforatum, Hyssopus officinalis, Lavandula spp., Leonurus cardiaca, Matricaria recutita, Melissa officinalis, Nepeta cataria, Passiflora incarnata, Piper methysticum, Piscidia erythrina, Pulsatilla vulgaris, Scutellaria lateriflora, Tilia platyphyllos, Valeriana officinalis, Viscum album
Stimulant	Cola vera, Coffea arabica, Ilex paraguayensis, Paullinia cupana, Rosmarinus officinalis
Hypnotic	Eschscholzia californica, Humulus lupulus, Lactuca virosa, Passiflora incarnata, Piper methysticum, Piscidia erythrina, Valeriana officinalis
Antispasmodic	Piper methysticum, Scutellaria lateriflora, Valeriana officinalis, Viburnum opulus, V. prunifolium
Adaptogen	Eleutherococcus senticosus, Lentinus edodes, Panax ginseng, P. quinquefolius, Shisandra chinensis, Withania somnifera
Antidepressant	Artemisia vulgaris, Avena sativa, Hypericum perforatum, Lavandula spp., Turnera diffusa
Analgesic	Dioscorea villosa, Eschscholzia californica, Gelsemium sempervirens, Piscidia erythrina, Stachys betonica, Valeriana officinalis

Table 16.2. Nervines and Body System Affinities

SYSTEM	HERB	TYPE OF NERVINE
Circulatory system	Melissa officinalis	Relaxing
	Cimicifuga racemosa	Relaxing
	Viburnum opulus	Antispasmodic
	Viscum album	Relaxing
	Lavandula spp.	Relaxing
	Tilia platyphyllos	Relaxing
	Leonurus cardiaca	Relaxing
	Valeriana officinalis	Relaxing
Respiratory system	Grindelia spp.	Antispasmodic
	Lobelia inflata	Antispasmodic
	Prunus serotina	Antispasmodic
	Lactuca virosa	Antispasmodic
Digestive system	Matricaria recutita	Relaxing
	Viburnum opulus	Antispasmodic
	Foeniculum vulgare	Antispasmodic
	Humulus lupulus	Relaxing
	Melissa officinalis	Relaxing
	Mentha piperita	Antispasmodic
	Valeriana officinalis	Relaxing
	Dioscorea villosa	Antispasmodic
Reproductive system	Viburnum prunifolium	Antispasmodic
	Viburnum opulus	Antispasmodic
	Pulsatilla vulgaris	Relaxing
	Scutellaria spp.	Relaxing
	Valeriana officinalis	Relaxing

THE ROLE OF STRESS IN HUMAN HEALTH

An examination of stress and stress management is fundamental to any discussion of nervous system health. This section provides an overview of the physiology and psychology of stress and the general adaptation syndrome, focusing on how stress relates to health and illness.

What Is Stress?

There are several ways to define *stress*. Here is perhaps the most encompassing definition: "Stress is the response of the body to any demand." Just staying alive creates demands on the body for energy to maintain life energy. Even while we are asleep, our bodies continue to function. By this definition, stress is a fundamental part of being alive and should not be avoided! The trick is to ensure that the degree of stress we experience is not overwhelming, so that life is a joy, not a drag.

From this perspective, energy usage is one characteristic of stress. Another characteristic is the lack of specificity of the stress response. Any demands made upon us in daily life bring about certain reactions in the body. These same reactions occur under a whole range of different conditions, both physical and emotional—from perceptions of hot and cold to joy and sorrow. As aware, feeling people, we generally make a big distinction between the pain caused by the loss of a loved one and the pain caused by a rapid change in temperature, but the nature of the demand is unimportant at the biological level. To the body, it is all the same, because the stress response is the same. Nerve signals travel from the brain to several glands, and these react by secreting hormones to cope with the task ahead. In short, stress is not just worry and strain. It is a keynote of life, with all its ups and downs. A new and exciting love can cause us as much stress as a cranky boss.

Stress as a Response

The most relevant way to interpret stress involves viewing it as physiological response to an adverse, or "stressful," situation. This approach is based on the work of the physiologist Hans Selye. Selye theorized that the stress response is a built-in mechanism that comes into play whenever demands are made on the individual, and is therefore a defense reaction with a protective and adaptive function. In other words, the body mounts a general physiological reaction to all forms of stress, which is usually in our own best interests. Selye called this reaction the *general adaptation syndrome* (GAS). The theory suggests a three-stage process of response:

1. An alarm reaction
2. A resistance stage, which represents a functional recovery of the body to a level superior to the pre-stress state
3. An exhaustion reaction, in which continuation of stress results in a depletion and breakdown of the recovery described in stage 2

The limitation of this inflexible, physiological model of stress is that it ignores the purely emotional or mental factors that produce wide variations in the way humans respond to potentially stressful situations.

Physiological Responses

The regulation of physiological responses to threats or stressful demands is handled mainly by the adrenal gland. Immediate response is controlled mainly, though not completely, by the adrenal gland's central medulla, while the surrounding cortex handles long-term stress responses. The initial response, or the body's preparation for what has been called the *fight-or-flight reaction*, involves a number of steps.

The first is an overall increase in nervous system activity. Next, the adrenal medulla releases adrenaline and/or noradrenaline into the bloodstream. These hormones support the nervous system through metabolic activities. The body's response to these chemicals includes an increase in heart rate and blood pressure and surface constriction of blood vessels. Surface constriction of blood vessels directs the blood away from the skin to the muscles, providing them with more sugar and oxygen. This is why we are said to "go white with shock." The release of these chemicals also mobilizes the liver's energy reserves through the release of stored glucose.

If the stressful situation is very intense or continues over a period of time, the adrenal cortex becomes increasingly involved in the stress reaction. Adrenocorticotropic hormone (ACTH), released by the anterior pituitary gland, largely controls the activity of the cortex. After information about sustained stress is processed by the central nervous system, a whole range of bodily responses occurs. These are the reactions that can adversely affect the quality of life.

Psychological Responses

In general terms, the psychological reaction to stress takes the following course:

The initial fight-or-flight reaction is accompanied by emotions such as anxiety and fear.

Individual coping strategies are activated as we attempt to find ways to deal with the harmful or unpleasant situation.

If coping strategies are successful, the fight-or-flight reaction and the anxiety state subside.

If coping strategies fail and the stress continues, a range of psychological reactions, including depression and withdrawal, may occur.

The implication is that the consequences of failing to cope can be serious. It is therefore important that we develop our own ways of adapting to and successfully dealing with stressful situations.

How Stress Causes Illness

There can be no doubt that there is a definite relationship between stress and illness. Although the exact nature of that relationship is not yet understood, a number of ideas have been suggested. Early theories tried to connect different illnesses with specific types of emotional conflict or personality and body types. According to these theories, certain body types and temperaments are more likely to develop one physical disease under stress than are others. However, there is little agreement among the experts about what correlates with what.

Selye had more to say on the subject. He maintained that the biological reactions accompanying the GAS result in both short- and long-term adverse physical changes. He called these changes *diseases of adaptation*, since they are the outcome of a system of defense responses to threatening stimuli. Selye theorized that the disease process arises as a result of a number of factors:

- The physiological effect of certain hormones from the adrenal and pituitary glands
- The impact of the inflammation process
- A general state of lowered resistance

The actual disease that manifests itself depends on a range of factors, including genetics, physical weakness, and even specific learned body responses. The GAS helps explain the effects of life changes or events on health. Life changes require adjustments that can produce physiological reactions, and sustained and unsuccessful attempts at coping with life can lower bodily resistance and promote illness. Thus, the more frequent and severe the life changes we experience, the more likely we are to become ill.

ANXIETY AS A RESPONSE TO STRESS

Stress affects our lives in many ways, and it is impossible to talk about all of the ramifications here. However, when the level of stress progresses beyond healthy stimulation and begins to adversely affect our health, it usually manifests in some form of anxiety.

Anxiety comprises various combinations of mental and physical symptoms that occur either in a persistent state or in the form of short-term panic attacks. Anxiety is often described in the following terms.

- An emotional state colored by the experienced quality of fear
- An unpleasant emotion that may be accompanied by a feeling of impending doom
- A feeling, directed toward the future, that is associated with a perceived threat of some kind
- An experience of bodily discomfort and actual bodily disturbance

In anxiety, there may be no recognizable basis for the fear or perception of threat, and the emotion provoked may be completely out of proportion to the actual stimulus. Nevertheless, the symptoms of anxiety are very real. For some people, anxiety takes the form of recurrent attacks that, although they occur unpredictably, may become associated with specific situations. These attacks begin with a sudden, intense apprehension, often combined with a feeling of impending doom and sometimes with feelings of unreality. Any of the somatic (physical) symptoms described below may occur. An anticipatory fear of loss of control often develops, so that the person may become afraid, for example, of being left alone in public places. The anticipatory fear may itself precipitate other symptoms, which escalate the attack. A whole range of reactions can be associated with anxiety.

Table 16.3. Symptoms of Anxiety

SYMPTOM	MANIFESTATIONS
Anxious mood	Worrying
	Apprehension
	Anticipation of the worst
	Irritability
Fears	The dark
	Being left alone
	Traffic
	Strangers
	Large animals
	Crowds
Cognitive symptoms	Difficulty concentrating
	Poor memory
Depressed mood	Loss of interest

SYMPTOM	MANIFESTATIONS	SYMPTOM	MANIFESTATIONS
Depression	Diurnal swing	Insomnia	Difficulty falling asleep
	Lack of pleasure in hobbies		Unsatisfying sleep
	Early awakening		Fatigue on waking
General body sensations	Tinnitus		Night terrors
	Hot and cold flushes		Broken sleep
	Prickling sensations		Dreams
	Blurred vision		Nightmares
	Feelings of weakness	General symptoms	Muscular aches and pains
Respiratory symptoms	Pressure or constriction in chest		Muscular twitching
	Tightness of breath		Muscular stiffness
	Feelings of choking		Grinding teeth
	Sighing	Cardiovascular symptoms	Tachycardia, palpitations
Genitourinary symptoms	Frequent urination		Pain in chest
	Urinary urgency		Feelings of faintness
	Suppressed menstrual periods		Throbbing of vessels
	Excessive menstrual bleeding		Skipped heartbeats
	Frigidity	Gastrointestinal symptoms	Difficulty swallowing
	Premature ejaculation		Indigestion
	Impotence		Heartburn
	Loss of erection		Looseness of bowels
Physiological aspects of behavior	Tremor of hands		Constipation
	Strained face		Flatulence
	Swallowing		Belching
	Sweating		Sensations of bloating
	Furrowed brow		Weight loss
	Facial pallor	Autonomic nervous system symptoms	Dry mouth
	Eyelid twitching		Pallor
Tension	Feelings of tension		Giddiness
	Inability to relax		Flushing
	Easily moved to tears		Tendency to sweat
	Feelings of restlessness		Raising of hair
	Fatigue		
	Startled response		
	Trembling		

Adapted from M. Hamilton, "The Assessment of Anxiety States by Rating," *British Journal of Medical Psychology* 32(1959):50–55.

MANAGING STRESS: AN OVERVIEW

There is much that can be done to ease the impact of stress and decrease the weight of the anxiety and tension we so often carry around with us. However, the very range of approaches that we have to choose from can itself become a source of stress. Where should we turn for help? Which therapy should we use? These are always difficult questions, and they are even more difficult to answer when we are not feeling our best.

The different therapies available merely represent ways to help us find the inherent peace within us. We are all, in fact, our own healers. The key is an inner attitude of taking responsibility for the quality of our own lives. We can seek aid from experts, whether medical doctors, herbalists, or practitioners of various complementary modalities, but the responsibility for healing can never be truly handed to another. Healing comes from within and is an intrinsic aspect of being alive. While healing is rarely a conscious act of harnessing inner energy, it is always an expression of our inner power.

Various tools and techniques can facilitate our healing; however, these techniques only aid in the healing process. Each of them embodies a profound truth and a great gift of healing wisdom, but humanity is very complex, and our ills are a reflection of that complexity. We need to build bridges between therapies in an effort to move toward a more holistic approach to health. In this chapter, the simple model I offer suggests ways in which we might integrate various approaches to health and wholeness to make inner peace an active part of our lives.

When people are seen as whole beings, not simply as "bodies with minds on top," it should comes as no surprise to find a deep association between psychology and physiology. This association has profound implications for all health conditions, not just stress and anxiety.

The mere fact that human beings are typically considered in terms of two separate entities—mind and body—is a demonstration of the inadequacy of our scientific approach to health. As already discussed, in reality, a human is a single whole being that cannot be separated into parts like mind and body.

Let us briefly explore the ways in which orthodox medicine views the relationship between mind and body in the development of illness. While no all-encompassing explanation for this relationship has been put forward, the medical world has considered a number of possible ideas.

Some physical illness may be psychological in origin. That is, bodily disturbances may be directly caused by psychological illnesses.

Physical illness may arise as an indirect consequence of a mental disorder. In other words, the bodily illness results from behavioral disturbances that are secondary to the psychological problem.

Physical methods of treating mental illness may cause bodily disease. Unfortunately, this is all too common with the wide use of drug therapy today.

The mental disturbance may be a manifestation of a physical illness, or an adverse effect of its treatment.

A mental or emotional problem may be a purely psychological response, either to a physical illness or to the psychological impact the illness has on the person involved.

This might all sound a bit semantic! These explanations are, however, a way to find patterns of relationship between mind and body, enabling the orthodox medical practitioner to decide which drugs to use. They help answer the question of whether the practitioner should focus on the physical problems or the mental disturbance.

From the point of view of the holistic herbalist, this is an artificial and unnecessary question. The whole must be treated as a whole in order to help both body and mind. Thus, we need not only remedies that are effective for specific symptoms, but also a management plan to help the patient cope with stress. This broader view lessens the impact of stress and creates the space for healing to take place.

EMOTIONAL AND MENTAL RESPONSES TO PHYSICAL ILLNESS

Any illness occurs within the context of our whole lives, and so will affect us psychologically and socially as well as physically. It may be useful for us to consider ways in which illness itself produces psychological problems. The difference between this type of problem and one that arises in the mind but affects the body is purely a difference of perspective.

Technically speaking, if orthodox practitioners consider the primary problem to be in the mind, they label it a *psychosomatic* problem. If they consider the root of the problem to be in the body, they label it a *somatopsychic* problem. The distinction is subtle, as shown here.

Psyche	→	(Psychosomatic)	→	Disease
Disease	→	(Somatopsychic)	→	Psyche

Relaxation Techniques

Perhaps the most important and yet the simplest tools available for lessening the impact of stress are relaxation exercises. When someone is tense and has been so for a while, the worst advice that can be given is, "Relax, take it easy." That is guaranteed to make feel anyone feel even edgier while working at trying to relax! The sad fact is that few people retain the innate skill of relaxation—a pity, but there it is. Relaxation is a skill that must be re-learned and practiced.

Many relaxation techniques exist, some based on breathing, some on muscle control, some on visualiza-tion, and some on simply listening to music. Picking the right one is matter of determining which is most suitable for the individual concerned.

Herbs and Spiritual Peace

In general, herbalists feel at home with spiritual matters. Plant remedies are potent medicines for human beings, but the plants from which they are derived are also vital for a healthy world in a number of ways. Our natural sur-roundings are important to us. Why do people fill their offices with indoor plants? They are, of course, aestheti-cally pleasing, but I suggest that aesthetic sensibilities are a part of the way in which spirituality helps us maintain our sanity. To the medieval monks, it was obvious that through the simple flowers of the field, God had given humanity a gift of healing and peace. Today, we are at last relearning this simple truth.

Gardening, Tree-Hugging, and Stress Management

If we get a bit creative, it is easy to see that the role of herbs in holistic healing need not be limited to their in-gestion. This is a perfect excuse to get into the garden, walk in the woods, and literally "smell the roses"! If one takes a very broad view of herbalism, seeing it as an ex-ploration of humanity's relationship with the plant world, some unusual healing possibilities present themselves.

In recent years, researchers from several disciplines have begun investigating the benefits of contact with plants, especially trees. In studies of the stress-reducing effects of nature, people recovered more quickly and completely from stress when exposed to plant-rich natu-ral settings, as indicated by lowered blood pressure, heart rate, muscle tension, and skin conductance. (The measur-able change in skin conductance of very small electrical charges is considered one of the best physiological mea-sures of autonomic nervous system activity and the stress response.) Direct experience of nature also facilitated psy-chological recovery, as suggested by reductions in mea-sures of fear and anger and increases in positive feelings. Physiological findings indicated that nature settings pro-duced significant recovery from stress in only four to six minutes. This rapid recovery highlights the importance for city dwellers of contact with plants, to help facilitate recuperation from various stressors, including commut-ing and work pressures.[1]

Herbal Stress Relief: Growing a Chamomile Lawn

Before the Victorians developed the grass lawn (itself a major cause of stress for some people!), lawns were made up of different varieties of herbs that could cope with being trampled. A chamomile lawn makes a wonderfully soothing place to rest, and lying upon such a lawn and breathing in its delightful aroma gently yet profoundly relaxes the body.

Growing a chamomile lawn oneself further reduces stress through the benefits of exercise and a sense of fulfillment. Specific varieties of chamomile are best for this. *Matricaria nobile* 'Treneague' is an apple-scented, nonflowering variety. This is convenient, as it saves having to re-move spent flower heads, but ordinary Roman chamomile *(Chamaemelum nobile)* can be grown from seed, which is less expensive. Prepare the soil and broadcast the seed. Cover with a thin layer of soil and keep moist but not wet. When seedlings have at least two sets of leaves, thin them to about 3 inches apart. Don't walk on them until they have started to bind together. Remove most flower heads as they appear, to ensure leaf vigor, but allow occasional flowers to remain, as they form part of the lawn's charm.

Avoid placing a chamomile lawn where it borders on a grass lawn or wild garden area, as creeping weeds will soon invade the lawn, and uprooting them will disturb the shallow-rooted chamomile plants. Surrounding the chamomile lawn with stone, brick, or paving slabs is ideal for preventing the invasion of unwanted plants as well as the spread of the chamomile.

Another study compared hospital records of gallbladder surgery patients who had window views of either a small stand of trees or a brick wall. Results showed that those with the view of trees had shorter postoperative hospital stays, required fewer potent pain drugs, and received fewer negative staff evaluations about their condition than did those with the wall view.[2]

The Role of Adaptogens

Humanity appears to have created a world of stress, pollution, lack of meaning, and lack of purpose. In the face of such cultural alienation from nature, the plethora of diseases assailing the "civilized" world should come as no surprise. To heal the ills, the causes must be addressed. Such causes are found not only within the individual, but also within our culture as a whole.

When a health problem is related to lowered resistance to disease, which in turn is caused by the increased impact of a hostile environment, the healer must also "heal" the hostile environment. In other words, even if we have found a remedy that seems to offer an increased resistance to toxic drugs, it is always preferable to remove the toxic chemical. This makes economic sense, is the right stance in Hippocratic terms, and is the right action in spiritual terms.

When attention is given to providing appropriate support for the body under stressful conditions, nature comes to our rescue. Technically, this calls for an increase in the body's nonspecific resistance to damaging man-made factors and related illnesses. A range of appropriate herbal remedies has come to light. Soviet scientists coined the term *adaptogen* to describe herbs that produce this wonderful increase in resistance and vitality. Some of the characteristics of adaptogens include:

- Nonspecific activity—in other words, an ability to increase the power of the body's resistance to physical, chemical, or biological stressors
- A normalizing influence independent of the nature of the pathological state
- An innocuous nature that does not influence normal body functions more than necessary

In these ways, adaptogens reinforce the nonspecific power of the body's resistance against stressors, increase its general capacity to withstand stressful situations, and hence guard against disease caused by overstressing the organism. The general aims of treatment with adaptogens include:

- Reduce stress reactions during the alarm phase of the stress response

- Prevent or at least delay the state of exhaustion
- Afford a certain level of protection against the effects of long-term stress

Herbs that can be described as adaptogens include *Panax ginseng* (Korean ginseng), *P. quinquefolius* (American ginseng), *Eleutherococcus senticosus* (Siberian ginseng), *Withania somnifera* (ashwaganda), *Lentinus edodes* (shiitake mushroom), and *Shisandra chinensis* (schizandra).

HERBAL REMEDIES AND STRESS MANAGEMENT

Herbs can play a fundamental role in any stress management program. When used within the context of a program that addresses a range of factors, herbs can facilitate a dramatic change in the quality of life experienced by anyone under stress. Holistic medicine reminds us to focus on an individual's unique situation, not to simply treat a diagnosed disease syndrome.

In chapter 1, I discussed the concept of *therapeutic ecology* as a model that describes the relationship of herbal medicine to other healing modalities. A well-balanced stress management program will address all of the various elements of healing discussed in that model, including physical medicine, bodywork, emotional and psychological factors, and spiritual aspects. Herbal remedies will fulfill only some needs, but they remain vital.

In addition, in the context of this therapeutic ecology, it is important to remember that the patient is *always* more important than the doctor's belief system. In other words, one person diagnosed with a stress-related problem might recuperate best when treated with dietary advice, herbs, and massage, while another may respond better to tranquilizers and psychoanalysis. The patient's needs and belief system must always be taken into account in order for meaningful change to occur.

In the treatment discussions that follow, we will focus our attention on the herbal aspects of a holistic approach to conditions affecting the nervous system, but please do not forget nutrition, relaxation, psychotherapy, spirituality, and all of the other factors that the competent practitioner must address.

A convenient way to approach stress-related problems is based on the intensity of the person's problem combined with the duration of the stressful situation, as seen in the following general list.

- Daily mild stress
- Long-standing severe stress
- Short-term severe stress

Treatment of Mild Daily Stress

If periods of stress in a person's life can be predicted, one can prepare for them ahead of time and implement herbal, dietary, and lifestyle measures that will minimize the impact. Nervine relaxants can be used regularly as gentle, soothing remedies. For some people, bitter tonics may also be important because of their metabolic toning effects.

Specific Remedies

Review the entries for specific relaxing nervines in chapter 25 to clarify their secondary actions and properties. These remedies can be drunk as teas or cold beverages, infused in massage oil, or used in relaxing baths or footbaths.

Relaxing Nervines

Artemisia vulgaris (mugwort)
Avena sativa (oats)
Lavandula spp. (lavender)
Matricaria recutita (chamomile)
Melissa officinalis (lemon balm)
Scutellaria lateriflora (skullcap)
Stachys betonica (wood betony)
Tilia platyphyllos (linden)
Valeriana officinalis (valerian)
Verbena officinalis (vervain)

A daily supplement of B-complex vitamins and vitamin C is indicated. The impact of various stressors should also be ameliorated. This is sometimes impossible, but do not automatically support the individual in putting up with something or someone, whatever the justification. People can change and change their lives. In addition to relaxation exercises, an honest reevaluation of both lifestyle and life goals is invaluable.

Treatment of Ongoing Stress

The line between chronic stress and the daily levels of stress we all put up with is fuzzy. A gentle soul with a less-than-strong constitution will cross the line into chronic stress sooner than a stronger person who copes well. Neither one of these constitutional extremes is better than the other; they merely reflect the fact that we live in a world of human diversity.

Focused attention must be given to general health. The body will often show that it is weakening through some somatic symptom. This may manifest as a long-standing complaint that gets worse, an old problem that reappears, or just an acceleration of the aging process.

Specific Remedies

The remedies suggested for daily stress relief also apply for chronic stress, but the addition of adaptogens becomes pivotal in cases of chronic stress. Important examples of adaptogens include *Eleutherococcus senticosus* (Siberian ginseng), *Panax ginseng* (Korean ginseng), and *Withania somnifera* (ashwaganda).

Treatment of Short-Term Extreme Stress

In the lives of most people, there are times when life become overwhelming and the pain of existence crescendos. Immediate herbal relief may be needed for a whole range of traumatic situations, from being involved in a car accident to personal emotional crisis. In these cases, herbs will take the edge off the trauma, but will rarely remove it.

At extremely difficult times, herbs can be seen only as an aid—one element of an approach taken to deal with the issues faced by the individual. The individual may also need to seek help from the various caring professions, go on vacation or a retreat, or even check into a hospital. However, a unique property of herbal nervines is their ability to address various associated somatic symptoms. This affords us the opportunity to focus herbal medication on the unique experience of the patient.

Specific Remedies

Many plants capable of easing intense stress are considered dangerous in our society, and because they are legally restricted substances, they will not be discussed here. However, in addition to the nervine relaxant herbs already mentioned, consider *Passiflora incarnata* (passionflower), *Valeriana officinalis* (valerian), *Piper methysticum* (kava kava) and *Lactuca virosa* (wild lettuce).

A Prescription for Acute Stress Reactions

Scutellaria lateriflora	1 part
Valeriana officinalis	1 part

Dosage: up to 5 ml of tincture as needed

Note the dosage of "up to 5 ml of tincture as needed." This represents a recognition that the stress response is cyclical, and different times of the day will be more challenging for each person. The dosage may be increased until symptoms are relieved, as this is largely symptomatic medication. The dosage regimen may also be altered as necessary, varying time of day and quantity of dose to suit individual needs. For example, the patient may wish to take a large dose first thing in the morning, or smaller amounts at frequent intervals throughout the day.

Table 16.4. Actions Supplied by Prescription for Acute Stress

ACTION	HERBS
Nervine tonic	Scutellaria lateriflora
Nervine relaxant	Scutellaria lateriflora, Valeriana officinalis
Carminative	Valeriana officinalis
Antispasmodic	Scutellaria lateriflora, Valeriana officinalis

A Prescription for Acute Stress Reaction with Indigestion and Palpitations

Scutellaria lateriflora	2 parts
Valeriana officinalis	2 parts
Leonurus cardiaca	1 part
Matricaria recutita	1 part
Artemisia vulgaris	1 part

Dosage: up to 5 ml of tincture as needed

Table 16.5. Actions Supplied by Prescription for Stress with Indigestion and Palpitations

ACTION	HERBS
Nervine tonic	Scutellaria lateriflora, Avena sativa
Nervine relaxant	Scutellaria lateriflora, Valeriana officinalis, Leonurus cardiaca
Antispasmodic	Scutellaria lateriflora, Valeriana officinalis
Bitter	Artemisia vulgaris, Matricaria recutita
Anti-inflammatory	Matricaria recutita, Valeriana officinalis
Carminative	Matricaria recutita, Valeriana officinalis, Artemisia vulgaris

Motherwort *(Leonurus cardiaca)* supports the relaxing action of the other nervines, but also has a specific calming impact upon tachycardia.

A Prescription for Acute Stress Reaction with Associated Muscle Tension

Scutellaria lateriflora	1 part
Piper methysticum	1 part

Dosage: up to 5 ml of tincture as needed

Table 16.6. Actions Supplied by Prescription for Acute Stress with Muscle Tension

ACTION	HERBS
Nervine tonic	Scutellaria lateriflora
Nervine relaxant	Scutellaria lateriflora, Piper methysticum
Antispasmodic	Scutellaria lateriflora, Piper methysticum

Muscle-Relaxant Compress

Hot chamomile compresses work well to relax painful, tense muscles. Prepare a strong infusion, using a full cup of chamomile flowers and 2 quarts of water. Cover with a lid and allow to steep for about 10 minutes; strain. Dip a towel into the infusion, wring it out, and spread it (as hot as is tolerable) on the back, shoulders, and neck. Soak another towel in the hot infusion, wring it out, and place it on top of the first towel. Now turn over both towels so that the fresh, hot compress is again in contact with the patient's skin. Remove the top towel and again soak it in the infusion. Repeat the procedure 10 to 20 times, until there is a sense of relaxation and relief of tension.

Broader Context of Treatment

Please refer to chapter 1 for a discussion of the importance of relaxation and meditation. (For more detailed information, please see my book *Successful Stress Control*, listed as suggested reading in the bibliography.) In addition, adequate intake of B vitamins is essential.

Nutritional Guidelines

A healthy diet provides optimal amounts of all known nutrients and low levels of components that are detrimental to health. It is rich in whole, unprocessed foods and especially high in plant foods—fruits, vegetables, grains, beans, seeds, and nuts. While it is impossible to come up with a detailed set of guidelines for everyone, consider the following elements of a healthy diet.

- Eat fresh, nutritious foods in season, in a form as close as possible to the original.
- Enjoy appealing and tasty foods, rotating the foods eaten for variety.
- Eat moderately and regularly.
- Balance different types of foods to ensure a nutritionally well-rounded diet.
- Eat with your senses, with full attention and with gusto

- Eat less rather than more.
- Appreciate simple foods.
- Eat vegetables, especially cruciferous vegetables.

DEPRESSION

A disorder marked especially by sadness, inactivity, difficulty with thinking and concentration, a significant increase or decrease in appetite and time spent sleeping, feelings of dejection and hopelessness, and sometimes suicidal thoughts or an attempt to commit suicide. *(The Merriam-Webster Medical Dictionary)*

Depression is a state of mind familiar to almost everyone in one form or another. In ordinary usage, the word refers to a mood state that in medicine is called *dysthymia*, in contrast with the normal state of *euthymia* and the opposite state, elation.

In psychiatric usage, disorders of mood are called *affective disorders*. Depression is either a disorder in its own right or can be a symptom of another disorder, either mental or physical. Normal human responses to some situations may include transient depression, but in medicine, these transient states are distinguished from the condition known as *clinical depression*.

Major depression occurs in 10% to 20% of the world's population in the course of a lifetime. Women are more often affected than men are, by a 2:1 ratio, and they seem to be at particular risk just before menstruation or immediately after childbirth. Relatives of people with major depression also seem to be at higher risk of developing depression, and about 2% of the population may have a chronic disorder known as depressive personality.

I was once asked to speak at a conference on the topic "Herbal Alternatives to Prozac." I spent most of the talk challenging the assumptions underlying the title! By phrasing the topic in this way, we are forced to respond to the underlying issue in terms of the efficacy of Prozac for depression, rather than by highlighting the strengths of phytotherapy when used in a holistic context.

In short, comparing the efficacy of herbs and Prozac begs the fundamental question about the underlying cause of depression. When it comes to the clinical use of herbs in major depressive illness, I want to make it clear that I do not believe there is an herbal alternative. For the majority of people with less severe depression, however, herbal alternatives will be discussed below.

I would also suggest that depression may be a rational and sane response to our society's initial manifestation of 21st century culture! As such, is a chemical "smiley face,"

whether synthetic or botanical, an ethical response? We don't suppress the inflammatory response simply because it occurs, so why suppress the emotions that accompany depression? Depression can represent an opportunity for self-exploration for the patient, and many lessons may be learned. Of course, this will entail a great challenge for both the patient and the practitioner.

Depression is defined by a standard set of symptoms described in the American Psychiatric Association's Diagnostic and Statistical Manual of Mental Disorders (DSM):

- Poor appetite and significant weight loss, or increased appetite and significant weight gain
- Insomnia or increased sleep
- Agitation or retardation of movement and thought
- Loss of interest or pleasure in usual activities; decrease in sexual drive
- Fatigue and loss of energy
- Feelings of worthlessness, self-reproach, or excessive or inappropriate guilt
- Diminished ability to think or concentrate; indecisiveness
- Recurrent thoughts of death or suicide, or suicide attempts

Not all of these characteristics will occur in each individual who becomes depressed. For purposes of psychiatric treatment, a person is considered to have experienced a major depressive episode if he or she exhibits a loss of interest or pleasure in all or almost all usual activities and shows at least four of the above symptoms nearly every day for a period of at least two weeks.

The term *depression* is often modified by words that imply either some specific factor or some chemical mechanism as the cause of the state. For example, depression that is considered a reaction to some loss of or separation from a valued person or object is called *reactive* or *exogenous depression*. In contrast, the usually more severe form of depression without apparent cause is called *endogenous depression*. *Melancholia*, a term once used to describe all depressive states, is now applied only to these most severe forms of depression.

Treatment of Depression

In terms of the herbal component of treatment protocols for depression, the nervous system must be the focus for toning, but associated symptoms may be a clue that more deep-seated issues have begun to manifest. Attention to the liver and the digestive system in general is usually a good idea.

Actions Indicated

Nervine tonics are fundamental to any long-term change in the individual's ability to cope and transform what must be changed.

Nervine relaxants may be indicated in the short term, or if the depression has an agitated or hyperactive aspect. These should not be strong herbs, which could trigger a more entrenched depression.

Nervine stimulants might help, but not predictably. If the therapist concludes that stimulation is appropriate, it is better to use bitter metabolic stimulants.

Bitters often bring about dramatic changes in patients' perceptions of themselves and of their lives. This highlights the need for a holistic perspective in such conditions.

Antispasmodics will alleviate muscular tension that might manifest as a bodily expression of psychological depression. Care should be taken not to use strong relaxants.

Adaptogens support the adrenals in coping with the stress that the whole body is experiencing.

Hepatics are indicated to support the liver's detoxification work, especially if the patient has been using prescription psychotropic drugs.

Specific Remedies

As far as this author is concerned, there are no clear-cut specifics for depression. *Hypericum perforatum* (St. John's wort) has a long tradition of use in Europe, and while it sometimes achieves remarkable results, it also sometimes does nothing. This herb requires time to work, and so must be taken for at least a month. (For more details on the actions of St. John's wort, please refer to chapter 26.)

Of numerous clinical trials performed to investigate the antidepressant effects of St. John's wort extract, a double-blind clinical trial conducted in 1993 concluded that 67% of patients experienced a positive improvement after four weeks of therapy. The study involved 105 outpatients with depressions of short duration who received either 300 mg of St. John's wort extract three times a day or placebo three times a day.[3]

A Prescription for Moderate Depression

Hypericum perforatum	2 parts
Avena sativa	1 part
Artemisia vulgaris	1 part

Dosage: up to 5 ml of tincture three times a day for at least 1 month

---

Table 16.7. Actions Supplied by Prescription for Depression

ACTION	HERBS
Nervine tonic	*Hypericum perforatum, Avena sativa*
Nervine relaxant	*Hypericum perforatum, Avena sativa, Artemisia vulgaris*
Bitter	*Artemisia vulgaris*

Broader Context of Treatment

The whole gamut of issues touched upon in this chapter must be addressed. From green salads to relaxation, spinal adjustments to changing the music one listens to—the list of factors to consider is endless. Exercise is especially important.

In *Textbook of Natural Medicine*, Drs. Pizzorno and Murray suggest the following nutritional supplements:[4]

B vitamin complex: 50 times the recommended daily dose each day
Vitamin C: 1 g three times daily
Folic acid: 400 mg/day
Vitamin B$_{12}$: 250 mcg/day
Magnesium: 500 mg/day

INSOMNIA

Difficulty in sleeping, or disturbed sleep patterns leaving the perception of insufficient sleep. *(The Merck Manual)*

The Encyclopaedia Britannica defines sleep as:

. . . normal, easily reversible, and spontaneous state of decreased and less efficient responsiveness to external stimulation. Sleep is a regularly recurring suspension of consciousness that serves recuperative and adaptive functions. Sleep usually requires the presence of flaccid or relaxed skeletal muscles and the absence of the overt, goal-directed behavior often seen in wakeful organisms. An electroencephalogram (EEG) recording the electrical activity of the human brain shows a distinctive pattern during sleep.

Let me try to translate. Sleep and rest allow the body to replenish depleted energy reserves and allow us to maintain normal physical and mental functioning. Adequate sleep is essential for good physical and mental health, as it is necessary for the body's restorative processes. These processes occur in harmony with the body's sleep cycles, which are dictated by the body's natural rhythms.

These natural rhythms, known as diurnal rhythms, are slightly more than 24 hours in length and are reset each day by light and other time cues. These rhythms dictate our need for periodic rest, so sleep is as important to our biological well-being as are food, water, warmth, and shelter.

Restful sleep in human beings consists of four patterns of brain activity, known as sleep stages. Stages 1 and 2 are considered stages of light sleep, and they typically predominate in the early part of the sleep cycle. Stages 3 and 4 are deeper, more restful sleep periods, and they tend to dominate in the latter half of the sleep cycle. All four stages come and go many times during the night. Transient awakenings usually occur during Stage 1 sleep. Most dreaming occurs during Stage 4, which is also known as REM (rapid eye movement) sleep. If this normal pattern of alternating stages is disturbed, sleep may not be fully restorative.

While sleeping approximately eight hours a night is vital to physical and mental health, dreaming is necessary for psychological health. Most theories of dream function state that dreams enable people to master their environments. In dreams, people integrate new experiences and solve conflicts from their waking lives. Another function of both sleep and dreaming is to assist in the processing and storage of memories.

The amount of sleep needed varies tremendously among individuals. There is no "normal" amount of sleep. Different people need different amounts of sleep; however, the amount of sleep that any one person needs is amazingly constant. Although one may sleep longer one night than another, depending on circumstances, the number of hours slept over a week or a month usually averages out to be very much the same. Eight hours of sleep a night is the usually cited average, although 7 to 7½ hours is more accurate for most people. Even that number is only an average, and has nothing to do with what's right or wrong. A good night's sleep can range from less than three hours to more than ten.

Causes and Consequences of Insomnia

The National Institutes of Health defines insomnia as "a disturbance or perceived disturbance of the usual sleep pattern of the individual that has troublesome consequences." In other words, insomnia is insufficient, disturbed sleep that does not fill the restorative function. This means that the individual does not get enough sleep to meet the needs of the body or to feel refreshed and energetic upon awakening and throughout the day. It is normal to wake up several times each night. Although most people don't recall these brief episodes of awakening, insomniacs typically have trouble either getting to sleep in the first place or falling back to sleep once they have awakened.

Insomnia usually has a cause, and often has multiple causes. However, the cause that initiated the problem may no longer be the one that keeps it from resolving. When trying to pinpoint the cause of insomnia, consider the following categories.

Medical Illness

Insomnia is especially related to conditions that result in pain, shortness of breath, cough, urination, nausea, diarrhea, or other bothersome symptoms that occur at night, including:

- Arthritis
- Muscles aches and pains
- Lung disease, including asthma
- Heart disease
- Diabetes
- Overactive thyroid
- Headaches
- Colitis
- Gastroesophageal reflux disease; heartburn
- Infections
- Hot flashes; menstrual pains
- Leg cramps
- Restless legs syndrome

Psychological Illness

Any psychiatric or psychological illness can interfere with sleep. Conditions associated with increased anxiety or worry often keep people from falling asleep, whereas depressive illnesses often result in early-morning awakening or trouble remaining asleep.

In addition, many prescription medications for treating psychiatric illness can compromise sleep. Antidepressants, such as Prozac, Zoloft, and Paxil, can have stimulating effects. Tranquilizers such as Valium may at first help anxious people sleep, but with prolonged use they can disturb normal sleep activity in the brain. The same is true for nicotine and alcohol use, which frequently increase during times of psychological stress.

Biological Clock Alterations

All human beings have a biological clock deep within their brains. They control regular fluctuations in body functions, such as hormone secretions, temperature regulation, and sleep-wake cycles. The clock controlling sleep-wake periods typically cycles every 25 hours; interestingly, this cycle is not synchronized with our 24-hour day. For some people, however, this normal cycle can become abnormally shortened or prolonged. One of the most common experiences of this kind of disruption is jet lag.

Medications

Prescription and over-the-counter medicines used to treat medical or psychiatric problems can also contribute to insomnia. Examples include:

- Alcohol
- Caffeine (found in coffee, tea, cola, NoDoz, and elsewhere)
- Nicotine
- Bronchodilators (asthma remedies)
- Beta-blockers (used for high blood pressure, heart disease, migraines, palpitations)
- Calcium channel blockers (used for high blood pressure, heart disease, migraines, palpitations)
- "Non-drowsy" decongestants and cold remedies
- Dilantin (diphenylhydantoin)
- Steroids (mainly prednisone and cortisone preparations)
- Thyroid hormones
- Psychotropic medications

Many people use caffeine to maintain wakefulness throughout the day. Excessive use of caffeine on a daily basis, however, can lead to withdrawal symptoms, including headache and sleeplessness at night. If caffeine is ingested too close to bedtime, its stimulating properties can also interfere with sleep. Caffeine is known to cause an increase in heart palpitations, stomach problems, diarrhea, and restless legs syndrome in certain individuals.

Negative Conditioning

Another common cause of insomnia is the way in which people respond to their inability to sleep. Not sleeping well can lead to worry, frustration, and depression, which in turn instigate additional psychological pressure to sleep. This anxiety further interferes with sleep. A cycle that may be described as "failure—worry—more failure—more worry" develops. This pattern becomes self-perpetuating. Behaviors that maintain the insomnia can aggravate the problem, as can performance anxiety.

Bad Sleep Habits

Certain behaviors, some of which are conditioned responses, commonly contribute to long-term insomnia. It is very important to recognize these causes, since in most instances they can be reduced or eliminated.

- Failing to keep to a regular sleep-wake schedule
- Depriving the body of sleep by staying up late to work or play on a frequent basis
- Trying to "catch up" on lost sleep during the weekend
- Watching late-night TV
- Excessive napping during the day
- Thinking of work-related problems while in bed
- Excessive time awareness or frequent clock watching while in bed
- Feeling "too tired" to exercise during the day
- Exercising vigorously too close to bedtime
- Drinking coffee, tea, or caffeine-containing colas too close to bedtime

Recent Stressful Events

Another common cause of insomnia, particularly in the short term, is a stressful event or crisis in a person's life. In general, the successful resolution of these problems usually leads to restoration of normal sleep.

Shift Work

Shift work is a common cause of sleep deprivation. Working the night shift on a regular basis or working different shifts on a rotating schedule produces challenges and obstacles to maintaining a normal, healthy sleep-wake pattern.

Treatment of Insomnia

There are many herbs with a reputation as an effective sleep remedy, but there are no legal plants that will put a person out. The key to successful treatment of insomnia is to find the cause and deal with it. Insomnia can push the practitioner's diagnostic skills to the limit, making the free and easy prescribing of benzodiazepine sleep aids at least understandable!

As discussed, the cause of insomnia may be anything in the realm of human life, from deep grief to constipation. Psychological issues often need attention, but so do health problems that cause pain or discomfort. Dietary indiscretions must be identified, as must an environmental factor (for example, freeway noise or a snoring spouse). In short, treatment should not depend upon substances, whether herbs or drugs.

Suggestions for Better Sleep

Sleep as much as you need to feel refreshed and healthy, but no more. Spending too much time in bed seems to be related to shallow sleep.

Get up at the same time each day, no matter when you went to bed. This will help establish a sleep-wake rhythm.

Do some sort of physical activity each day to get rid of tension and tire your body, but nothing too strenuous just before bedtime.

Do the same amount of exercise each day, preferably in late afternoon or early evening.

Make sure the bedroom is dark, cool, and quiet.

Sleep on a quality mattress and foundation.

Do not lie in bed for hours staring at the walls. If you do not fall asleep after 15 or 20 minutes, it is best to get up and do something quiet until you become drowsy.

Do not make your bed a place to watch TV, do paperwork, or eat.

Consider earplugs or eye masks if you work night shifts or live in a noisy area.

A light snack may help, but a heavy meal will not.

Unless prescribed, do not nap during the day. For most people, this can throw off the sleep schedule by confusing the body.

Natural sunlight during the day can be helpful for falling and staying asleep, so get outdoors, even for a brief walk.

Caffeine in the evening disturbs sleep, even if you don't think it does!

Alcohol causes fragmented sleep. Although it can be initially calming, liquor interferes with sleep quality.

Chronic tobacco use disturbs sleep.

Try not to rehash the day's problems or worry about tomorrow.

When you go to bed, relax your muscles, beginning with your feet and working your way up to your head.

Actions Indicated

Hypnotics are herbs with a reputation for easing a person into sleep. They are usually strong nervine relaxants, rather than "plant knockout drops"!

Nervine relaxants ease the tensions that often produce sleeplessness.

Antispasmodics address any somatic muscular tightness that might be involved.

Nervine tonics are indicated if there is any suspicion that insomnia is related to nervous exhaustion (as it often is).

Adaptogens will help in a way similar to nervine tonics, but should be used only in the morning to help deal with stress, as they might be too energizing at night.

System Support

Often the key to successful treatments lies in focusing upon a weakened or impaired body part or function. The problem must be identified and the appropriate system tonic, action, or specific herb applied. Hypnotics and nervines may be used within the context of such treatment. These should be selected according to the role they play in the system in question, and not simply upon their strength as hypnotics.

Circulatory system. Appropriate herbs include *Leonurus cardiaca*, *Tilia platyphyllos*, and *Melissa officinalis*.

Respiratory system. All of the hypnotics can be of value as antispasmodics in conditions such as asthma, if used at the right dose. *Lactuca virosa* eases irritable coughs.

Digestive system. Relaxing nervines and carminatives are important, including *Matricaria recutita*, *Verbena officinalis*, *Melissa officinalis*, *Humulus lupulus*, and *Valeriana officinalis*. Antispasmodic herbs, such as *Humulus lupulus*, *Passiflora incarnata*, *Valeriana officinalis*, and *Piscidia erythrina* will help with intestinal colic.

Urinary tract. Hypnotics are important here when used as muscle relaxants.

Reproductive system. As in the urinary tract, hypnotics may help here when used as muscle relaxants. Of particular relevance here are *Pulsatilla vulgaris* and *Piscidia erythrina*.

Musculoskeletal. All hypnotics will aid in reducing muscle tension and even the pain associated with problems in this system. They may be used internally or as lotions. Especially important are *Piscidia erythrina* and *Valeriana officinalis*.

Nervous system. All of the remedies listed here also act on the nervous system.

Skin. Matricaria recutita and *Primula veris* (cowslip) are hypnotics that also help with skin issues, but otherwise, the value of hypnotics here is to ensure that the body has a good recuperative rest each night.

Specific Remedies

Selections among the many herbal sleep aids should be made on the basis of their secondary actions or system affinities. By choosing herbs that address the specific health issues compounding the sleep difficulties, better results are obtained than if one simply chooses a strong hypnotic. For example, if a patient with insomnia also has heart palpitations, *Leonurus cardiaca* would be a good choice of nervine. This is explored in chapter 25. They may also be selected on the basis of their strength, bearing in mind the very subjective nature and individual variability in human response to these herbs. We can very roughly identify three groupings of hypnotics.

Mild Hypnotics

Matricaria recutita (chamomile)
Melissa officinalis (lemon balm)
Nepeta cataria (catnip)

Tilia platyphyllos (linden)
Trifolium pratense (red clover)

Moderate Hypnotics

Leonurus cardiaca (motherwort)
Pulsatilla vulgaris (pasqueflower)
Scutellaria lateriflora (skullcap)
Verbena officinalis (vervain)

Strong Hypnotics

Eschscholzia californica (California poppy)
Humulus lupulus (hops)
Lactuca virosa (wild lettuce)
Passiflora incarnata (passionflower)
Piper methysticum (kava kava)
Valeriana officinalis (valerian)

A Prescription for Insomnia

Passiflora incarnata	1 part
Valeriana officinalis	1 part

Dosage: 5 ml of tincture 30 minutes before bedtime

Table 16.8. Actions Supplied by Prescription for Insomnia

ACTION	HERBS
Hypnotic	*Passiflora incarnata, Valeriana officinalis*
Nervine relaxant	*Passiflora incarnata, Valeriana officinalis*
Antispasmodic	*Passiflora incarnata, Valeriana officinalis*
Carminative	*Valeriana officinalis*

A Prescription for Insomnia Associated with Menopausal Problems

Passiflora incarnata	1 part
Valeriana officinalis	1 part
Leonurus cardiaca	1 part

Dosage: 5 ml of tincture 30 minutes before bedtime, in addition to appropriate daytime treatments

---

Table 16.9. Actions Supplied by Prescription for Insomnia with Menopausal Problems

ACTION	HERBS
Hypnotic	*Passiflora incarnata, Valeriana officinalis*
Nervine relaxant	*Leonurus cardiaca, Passiflora incarnata, Valeriana officinalis*
Antispasmodic	*Leonurus cardiaca, Passiflora incarnata, Valeriana officinalis*
Carminative	*Valeriana officinalis*
Emmenagogue	*Leonurus cardiaca*

A Prescription for Insomnia Associated with Indigestion

Passiflora incarnata	1 part
Valeriana officinalis	1 part
Artemisia vulgaris	1 part
Melissa officinalis	1 part

Dosage: 7.5 ml of tincture 30 minutes before bedtime, in addition to appropriate daytime treatments. An infusion of *Matricaria, Tilia,* or *Melissa* at night may also be helpful.

Table 16.10. Actions Supplied by Prescription for Insomnia with Indigestion

ACTION	HERBS
Hypnotic	*Matricaria recutita, Passiflora incarnata, Valeriana officinalis*
Nervine relaxant	*Artemisia vulgaris, Matricaria recutita, Melissa officinalis, Passiflora incarnata, Valeriana officinalis*
Antispasmodic	*Artemisia vulgaris, Matricaria recutita, Melissa officinalis, Passiflora incarnata, Valeriana officinalis*
Carminative	*Artemisia vulgaris, Matricaria recutita, Melissa officinalis, Valeriana officinalis*
Bitter	*Artemisia vulgaris*
Anti-inflammatory	*Matricaria recutita, Melissa officinalis, Valeriana officinalis*

A Prescription for Insomnia Associated with Hypertension and Headache

Passiflora incarnata	1 part
Valeriana officinalis	1 part
Stachys betonica	1 part
Tilia platyphyllos	1 part
Viburnum opulus	1 part

Dosage: 7.5 ml of tincture 30 minutes before bedtime, in addition to appropriate daytime treatments. (Refer to chapter 14 for more information on the treatment of hypertension.) An infusion of *Tilia* or *Matricaria* at night may also be helpful.

Table 16.11. Actions Supplied by Prescription for Insomnia with Hypertension and Headache

ACTION	HERBS
Hypnotic	*Tilia platyphyllos, Passiflora incarnata, Valeriana officinalis*
Nervine relaxant	*Stachys betonica, Tilia platyphyllos, Passiflora incarnata, Valeriana officinalis, Viburnum opulus*
Antispasmodic	*Tilia platyphyllos, Passiflora incarnata, Valeriana officinalis, Viburnum opulus*
Analgesic	*Stachys betonica, Valeriana officinalis*
Hypotensive	*Tilia platyphyllos, Valeriana officinalis, Viburnum opulus*

A Prescription for Insomnia Associated with Depression

Passiflora incarnata	1 part
Valeriana officinalis	1 part
Hypericum perforatum	1 part
Artemisia vulgaris	1 part

Dosage: 7.5 ml of tincture 30 minutes before bedtime, in addition to appropriate daytime treatments. **Note:** Avoid the use of *Humulus lupulus* (hops) in depression.

Table 16.12. Actions Supplied by Prescription for Insomnia with Depression

ACTION	HERBS
Hypnotic	*Passiflora incarnata, Valeriana officinalis*
Nervine relaxant	*Artemisia vulgaris, Hypericum perforatum, Passiflora incarnata, Valeriana officinalis*

ACTION	HERBS
Antispasmodic	*Artemisia vulgaris, Hypericum perforatum, Passiflora incarnata, Valeriana officinalis*
Antidepressant	*Artemisia vulgaris, Hypericum perforatum*
Bitter	*Artemisia vulgaris*

Sleep Pillows

Pillows made with herbs, used either singly or in combination, are a long-standing remedy to facilitate a good night's sleep. Traditionally used herbs include *Matricaria recutita, Nepeta cataria, Humulus lupulus, Lavandula* spp., *Melissa officinalis, Tilia platyphyllos, Citrus aurantium* var. *amara* blossoms, and *Galium odoratum*.

Make a pillowcase lining out of linen or burlap, leaving it open at one end. Make up the herb stuffing by mixing dried herbs in the following proportions:

> 2 to 3 handfuls each of peppermint, sage, and lemon balm
> 1 to 2 handfuls of lavender, dill, lemon thyme, tarragon, woodruff, red bergamot and rosemary
> 1 to 2 tablespoons of valerian

Fill the pillow loosely with the herbs, sew closed, and put inside a soft, pretty pillowcase before use. Many other herbal combinations are possible. This is an appropriate place to experiment to find the combination and aroma that suits the individual.

Insomnia and Aromatherapy

Aromatherapy, a healing system based on the external application of herbs in the form of essential oils, has much to offer to those in search of restful sleep. A reliable and comprehensive guide to the safe use of these wonderful oils is *Aromatherapy: A Complete Guide to the Healing Art*, by Kathi Keville and Mindy Green, from which much of the following is taken.

Aromatherapy is increasingly used in hospitals in the United Kingdom, especially for sleeping difficulties. Helping an elderly patient achieve a good-quality, refreshing night's sleep is a bigger problem in hospitals than at home.[5] Lavender is the primary essential oil used to induce sleep. Placing a few drops of the oil on the pillow helps promote peaceful sleep for many patients.

A number of oils may be of service in easing the ravages of insomnia, of which the most relevant are listed below. It is very important to use essential oils in the correct way, as some oils are potentially irritating to the skin if used undiluted or may be toxic if taken internally. Here are some suggestions on how to use essential oils to treat insomnia. The dilutions given are for adults.

Massage Oils

Always dilute oils before applying them to the skin. Use a carrier oil such as sweet almond oil, grapeseed oil, jojoba oil, or any other pure, unblended vegetable oil. Do not use baby oil, as this is a mineral oil that, unlike vegetable oils, will not be absorbed by the skin. Ten to 12 drops per ounce of carrier oil (a 2% dilution) is usually appropriate.

Baths

Add up to 5 drops of pure essential oil to a bath of warm water. Float the oil on the surface and stir with your hand before relaxing in the bath for 10 to 15 minutes. For a hand or foot soak, add 2 or 3 drops of essential oil to a bowl of warm water.

Inhalation

Add 2 drops of essential oil to a bowl of hot water, cover the head and bowl with a towel to create a tent, and inhale the fragrant steam.

Essential Oils Traditionally Used for Insomnia

Bergamot
Blue chamomile
Chamomile (German or Roman)
Cypress
Frankincense
Geranium
Jasmine
Lavender
Lemon balm (Melissa)
Lemon verbena
Linden
Mandarin orange
Marjoram
Neroli
Nutmeg
Patchouli
Petitgrain
Rose
Sandalwood
Ylang ylang

Relaxing Antidepressant Essential Oil Formula

3 drops lavender oil
3 drops neroli oil
2 drops clary sage oil
2 drops marjoram oil
2 drops ylang ylang oil
1 drop German chamomile oil
1 ounce carrier oil

This can be used as either a massage or a bath oil

Fragrant Insomnia Blend (for diffuser)

25 drops lavender oil
10 drops sweet orange oil
8 drops chamomile oil
8 drops marjoram oil
6 drops ylang ylang oil

WITHDRAWAL FROM BENZODIAZEPINES

All of the commonly prescribed and abused minor tranquilizers, such as Valium and Xanax, can be safely replaced by herbal remedies when used in a broadly holistic context. The ease of replacing the drug with herbs highlights the need to avoid the development of dependence on the new herbal medicine.

Actions Indicated

Nervine tonics are fundamental to any long-term change in the individual's ability to cope with life and transform what must be changed.

Nervine relaxants will fulfill the tranquilizing role of the drug in the short term.

Nervine stimulants may be indicated in some cases, due to the long-term slowing of mind and body that results from use of these drugs in some people.

Antispasmodics alleviate muscular tension that develops in response to withdrawal.

Bitters act as safe metabolic stimulants.

Adaptogens will support the adrenals through the stressful process the body will undergo.

Hepatics may be appropriate to support the detoxification process.

System Support

Because of the stress component, both the nervous system and the adrenals will need aid. Next, focus on any body system that needs support. Body system weaknesses and ailments should be identified through the patient's medical history, current health, and observation of any temporary symptoms that might appear during the withdrawal process.

A successful transition from drugs to herbs is a gradual process. The following steps offer some guidelines for the practitioner.

1. First two to four days: Maintain regular dose of drug while adding appropriate herbs. Initially, the dosage of the herbal tincture combination described below should be 2.5 ml.
2. Reduce the dose of drug by one sixth while maintaining or increasing the dosage of herbs up to 5 ml. Maintain this regimen for four or five days.
3. Reduce the drug by one sixth every four to five days until drug use is completely discontinued, altering dosage, frequency, and strength of herbs as needed.
4. Alleviate specific somatic symptoms as indicated.

Specific Remedies

The herbal traditions of the world do not offer any ready-made specific remedies for benzodiazepine withdrawal, as these drugs are a relatively new development. However, there are an abundance of herbs that can make the withdrawal process relatively straightforward.

A few clear guidelines will assist the practitioner in the herb selection process.

Determine the strength of nervines required. One or more of the stronger relaxing nervines is usually indicated, but always remember that nature provides an abundance of nervines for a reason. An herb as mild as *Tilia* may be ideal for some individuals.

Use appropriate tonics for the nervous system and other body systems, as indicated. Nervine tonics must always be the foundation of formulations in such cases.

Identify other actions appropriate for the particular patient. For example, the liver will usually need support in its detoxification work.

Choose specifics to alleviate any symptoms that arise in the withdrawal process.

Primary Relaxing and Tonic Nervines for Withdrawal

Avena sativa (oats)
Passiflora incarnata (passionflower)
Scutellaria lateriflora (skullcap)
Valeriana officinalis (valerian)

Table 16.13. Nervines with Relevant Secondary Actions in Withdrawal

HERB	ACTIONS
Verbena officinalis	Hepatic, tonic
Artemisia vulgaris	Bitter, antidepressant
Eleutherococcus senticosus	Adaptogen
Hypericum perforatum	Antidepressant
Silybum marianum	Antihepatotoxic

Table 16.14. Herbs for Various Somatic Manifestations of Withdrawal

HERB	SOMATIC SYMPTOMS
Leonurus cardiaca	Tachycardia (palpitations)
Pulsatilla vulgaris	Menstrual problems
Lavandula spp.	Depression, digestive problems

A Prescription to Help with Benzodiazepine Withdrawal

Avena sativa	2 parts
Scutellaria lateriflora	2 parts
Valeriana officinalis	2 parts
Leonurus cardiaca	1 part
Eleutherococcus senticosus	1 part

Dosage: 2.5 ml to 5 ml of tincture three times a day

Broader Context of Treatment

As with all such treatments, many factors must be addressed when helping a patient with withdrawal. The specifics will vary according to the preferences of both practitioner and patient. The same general recommendations given for managing stress also apply here. In short, the following considerations will come into play:

- General health
- Diet and nutrition
- Lifestyle
- Belief systems, assumptions, and expectations
- Relaxation techniques

ANOREXIA NERVOSA

A disorder characterized by a disturbed sense of body image and marked anxiety about weight gain, manifested by abnormal patterns of handling food, marked weight loss, and amenorrhea in women. *(The Merck Manual)*

Anorexia nervosa is a problem typified by self-starvation. It occurs most commonly among young women, but is also observed in older women and men. For unknown reasons, anorexia nervosa has become more common in recent years, and the incidence among young women in the United States may be as high as 1% to 2% (0.1% to 0.2% in males).[6] The disorder may appear when the individual first leaves home, or may develop in connection with mental depression, peer pressure to lose weight, sexual temptation, or the discontinuation of oral contraceptives.

At the outset, the patient either stops menstruating or simply refuses to eat. In the first case, the patient later stops eating; in the second, her menstrual periods eventually cease. In either case, she may lose weight to the point of life-threatening exhaustion. In general, the patient will sleep poorly but, despite weight loss, will remain physically active, believing herself to be much fatter than she actually is. Body temperature may be low. These symptoms suggest that anorexia nervosa may be associated with a disorder of the hypothalamus, a region of the brain that regulates menstruation, eating, body temperature, and sleep.

Treatment of Anorexia Nervosa

The herbal treatment must focus on toning the nervous system, but in addition, the digestive and reproductive systems will need aid. Bitters and hepatics are especially useful in supporting the liver and digestion.

Actions Indicated

Bitters are indicated because they stimulate both appetite and general metabolism.

Nervine tonics are fundamental to any long-term change in the individual's ability to cope with life and transform what must be changed.

Nervine relaxants will alleviate associated anxiety.

Hepatics will support the detoxification process and generally benefit the body.

System tonics must be used to support any part of the body weakened by the condition or history of illness. In women, anorexia nervosa places the reproductive system under much strain.

Digestive support will be indicated if abdominal symptoms exist. Please refer to the sections on indigestion and irritable bowel syndrome in chapter 13 for more information.

Immune support may be necessary. Please refer to chapter 21 for more information.

Specific Remedies

Bitters are considered specifics here, but especially *Verbena officinalis* (vervain), a relaxing nervine with marked hepatic properties. Because it is strictly a problem of modern culture, the herbal traditions provide no information about the treatment of anorexia nervosa.

A Prescription for Anorexia Nervosa

Gentiana lutea	1 part
Avena sativa	1 part
Hypericum perforatum	1 part
Verbena officinalis	1 part

Dosage: 5 ml of tincture 10 to 15 minutes before eating, three times a day

---

Table 16.15. Actions Supplied by Prescription for Anorexia Nervosa

ACTION	HERBS
Nervine tonic	*Avena sativa, Hypericum perforatum, Verbena officinalis*
Nervine relaxant	*Hypericum perforatum, Verbena officinalis*
Bitter	*Gentiana lutea*
Hepatic	*Gentiana lutea, Verbena officinalis*

Emmenagogues might be indicated if the menstrual cycle has been disrupted. If sleep difficulties are part of the picture, please refer to Treatment of Insomnia earlier in this chapter.

Broader Context of Treatment

As with depression, the whole gamut of issues touched upon in this chapter must be addressed. As with depression, herbal therapy (or drug therapy) does not replace the fundamental need for competent and appropriate psychotherapy.

HEADACHE

> Headache (cephalalgia) is a common symptom, often associated with disability but rarely life threatening. Headache may be a primary disorder or a secondary symptom. *(The Merck Manual)*

Pain occurring over various parts of the head is one of the most common health problems affecting humanity. Several areas of the head can be afflicted, including the network of nerves that extends over the scalp and certain nerves in the face, mouth, and throat. Also sensitive to pain, because they contain delicate nerve fibers, are the muscles of the head and blood vessels found along the surface and at the base of the brain. However, the bones of the skull and the tissues of the brain itself never hurt, because they lack pain-sensitive nerve fibers.

In general, pain is a complex experience consisting of a physiological response to a painful stimulus followed by an emotional response. It is a warning mechanism that helps to protect us and is primarily associated with injury, or the threat of injury, to bodily tissues. But headache pain is different. For most headaches, even when the pain is severe, no underlying disease exists. Obviously, headache related to the presence of a brain tumor represents an exception.

The point at which a stimulus begins to cause pain is the *pain perception threshold*. Most studies have found that this point is relatively similar among disparate groups of people. However, the *pain tolerance threshold*, or the point at which pain becomes unbearable, varies significantly. Childhood experiences, cultural attitudes, genetic makeup, and gender are factors that contribute to the development of each individual's perception of and response to different types of pain. Although some people may be able to physiologically withstand pain better than others, cultural factors rather than heredity usually account for this ability.

Most headaches are caused by fatigue, emotional disorders, or allergies. Only about 2% of all headaches result from the presence of an organic disorder. These include:

- Diseases of the eye, ear, nose, throat, and sinuses
- Brain tumor
- Hypertension
- Aneurysm

Brain tissue itself is insensitive to pain, as is the bony covering of the cranium. Headache pain results from the stimulation of such pain-sensitive structures as the membranous linings of the brain (the *meninges*) and the nerves of the cranium and upper neck. This stimulation can be produced by inflammation, dilation of normal or abnormal blood vessels in the head, or muscle spasms in the neck and head.

Headaches brought on by muscle spasms are classified as *tension headaches*. Those caused by dilation of blood vessels are called *vascular headaches*. A more specialized classification, created by the International Headache Society for research purposes, further divides headaches into 14 categories.

To help the phytotherapist select appropriate remedies, headaches can be subdivided by cause into the following groupings:

Environmental. Pollutants, body posture, lighting, sound, and other factors
Stress. Physical, emotional, or mental
Dietary. Possible allergy to certain foods or additives—for example, xanthine-containing foods
Organic. Diseases such as hypertension and brain tumor

Pain may also be *referred* to the head, or felt in the head even though the site of disease is elsewhere. Referred pain may be caused by eye disorders (such as glaucoma and refractive errors), infections or tumors of the nasal sinuses, dental infections, and arthritis of the neck. In addition, headaches are one of the most common side effects of prescription and over-the-counter drugs, making it very difficult to list all potentially problematic medicines. Please refer to an appropriate reference.

Treatment of Headaches

The herbal treatment guidelines for different types of headaches must take into account a wide range of causes and issues. An important one is the abundant diversity of potential herbs that may be indicated.

Specific Remedies

Many plants might be considered specific headache herbs. Unfortunately, they do not always work for all people. A representative listing includes the following commonly available remedies.

Possible Specifics for Headache

Artemisia absinthium (wormwood)
Capsicum annuum (cayenne)
Lavandula spp. (lavender)
Matricaria recutita (chamomile)
Melissa officinalis (lemon balm)
Mentha piperita (peppermint)
Origanum marjoram (marjoram)
Piscidia erythrina (Jamaica dogwood)
Rosmarinus officinalis (rosemary)

Ruta graveolens (rue)
Sambucus nigra (elder)
Scutellaria lateriflora (skullcap)
Stachys betonica (wood betony)
Thymus vulgaris (thyme)
Valeriana officinalis (valerian)

None of these plants is a painkiller in the strict sense; that is, they do not block the experience of pain. An example of a medicinal plant that does is *Papaver somniferum* (opium poppy). The most effective plant painkillers are controlled by law, as they have the potential to lead to dependency and addiction. Because of this, it is often more effective in practice to use indirect pathways to pain relief. The herbs listed here appear to work by addressing the cause of the pain, rather than the experience of pain. These are anti-inflammatory and antispasmodic herbs that alleviate the processes underlying most muscle contractions and tension headaches.

If a clear-cut underlying pathology exists, that should be the focus of treatment. If none has been identified, herbs that will ensure good elimination, support liver function, and address any specific health needs the patient might have should be selected.

Common Headache Triggers

Almost all individuals with chronic headache have some degree of muscle irritation in the upper body—the upper back, neck, or face. The irritation is most often associated with chronic but subtle muscle tension. This applies for both tension and migraine headaches. The type of pain triggered reflects a variety of factors, including the type of headache to which the patient is prone. Over time, this tension may lead to the development of very tender muscles. It can also cause aching with normal movement, stiffness from being in one position or lying in bed for a long time, or even restrictions in the extent to which the individual can move his or her neck or jaw.

Primary headache triggers include:

Stress. Stress can be a powerful headache trigger, particularly for chronic tension headaches or migraine. A major life event such as a divorce or moving causes stress, but constant daily hassles can have an even greater effect.

Emotions. Quite ordinary emotions, such as a sense of letdown and frustration, can serve as headache triggers.

Muscle tension. Muscle irritation can produce local pain, pain at the site of muscle irritation, or referred pain in sites distant from the irritated muscle. For example, muscle irritation at the back of the neck may be felt as severe pain at the temple on the same side of the head.

Chronic muscle tension may arise from a variety of causes—poor posture, repeated muscle strain or overuse, tightening up under the effects of stress or headache itself, teeth grinding, and mannerisms such as frowning.

Change in the weather or season, altitude, or time zone.

Change in sleep patterns or meal times. Too little or too much sleep can both act as triggers.

Smoking, polluted air, or stuffy rooms. Chronic headache is one more good reason to quit smoking. Smoking in general seems to be a negative factor for people with chronic pain conditions, including headaches. Nicotine constricts the blood vessels, and inhaled carbon monoxide expands them, thus creating a condition that can trigger migraines and cluster headaches.

Blood clotting. Another cause of headaches is blood clotting, also known as platelet aggregation. Clotting creates constriction of the arteries, which results in inadequate blood supply to the brain. This is followed by rebound dilation of the blood vessels, leading to headaches.

Caffeine. Caffeine can cause headaches by increasing the body's expectation for it. When blood levels of caffeine drop, symptoms of withdrawal, including headache, may set in. That's why some heavy coffee drinkers experience "morning headache" until they have that first cup of coffee. Caffeine headaches are usually experienced as a dull, throbbing pain on both sides of the head. Once the body rids itself of caffeine, the headaches disappear on their own. Such headache sufferers, however, are often unaware that their problem is due to caffeine and will continue to drink coffee, ensuring that the problem will recur.

Foods. The following foods are known to commonly trigger headaches in sensitive people:

• Red and white wine
• Other alcohol
• Refined sugar products—for example, sodas and candy
• Dried fruit containing sulfates
• Artificial additives, colorings, and preservatives, such as aspartame (NutraSweet)
• Nuts
• Onions
• Herring
• Chocolate
• Peanut butter
• Chicken livers
• Sour cream and yogurt primarily, but potentially all dairy products
• Vinegar (except white vinegar)

- Bananas
- Anything fermented, pickled, or marinated
- Broad, lima, navy, pinto, and garbanzo beans; peas
- Foods containing large amounts of monosodium glutamate (MSG)
- Caffeine
- Citrus fruit and juices
- Fermented sausage and processed meats such as bologna, salami, pepperoni, hot dogs, and ham
- Ripened cheeses, such as Cheddar, Emmentaler, Gruyère, Stilton, Brie, and Camembert

Essential Oils for Headache

Many essential oils can be used to relieve headache. Particularly effective oils include *Lavandula* spp., *Rosmarinus officinalis*, and *Mentha piperita*, which can be used either separately or in combination. *Lavandula* may be rubbed on the temples or made into a cold compress and applied to the temples, forehead, or back of the neck. Equal parts of *Lavandula* and *Mentha piperita* may be even more effective, for *Lavandula* has the ability to enhance the action of other oils when used in blends. It is also worth noting that while *Lavandula* is a sedative, *Mentha piperita* is a stimulant, and that many commercial headache remedies combine a stimulant (usually caffeine) with one or more analgesics. This is because many painkilling drugs have a slightly sedative and sometimes even a depressant effect, and the caffeine counteracts these effects. By combining *Lavandula* and *Mentha piperita*, a similar effect is achieved without the dangers inherent in synthetic drugs.

If headache is caused by catarrh or sinus infection, inhalations with *Lavandula*, *Mentha piperita*, *Rosmarinus*, or *Eucalyptus* will usually be very effective in both relieving the headache and clearing the congestion that caused it. All of these oils are antiseptic, and will combat the nasal infection and provide immediate symptom relief.

Treatment of Tension Headaches

Because of its effectiveness in easing anxiety as a component of stress management programs, herbal medicine has most to contribute to the alleviation of tension headaches. If a period of stress can be predicted, one can be prepared ahead of time to implement appropriate herbs, diet, and lifestyle changes to minimize the impact. Nervine relaxants like those listed here can be used regularly as gentle soothing remedies, drunk as hot or cold infusions, infused in massage oil, or included in relaxing baths or footbaths.

Supportive Nervines for Tension Headaches

Artemisia vulgaris (mugwort)
Avena sativa (oats)
Matricaria recutita (chamomile)

"Natural Aspirin"

Numerous plants contain natural aspirin-type chemicals called *salicylates*, and aspirin itself was originally isolated from plant sources. In fact, the name *aspirin* comes from *Spiraea*, the old botanical genus name for meadowsweet. The word *salicylate* derives from *Salix*, the Latin name for willow.

Herbs with significant quantities of salicylates have a marked anti-inflammatory effect, without the dangers posed by aspirin itself to the stomach. In fact, meadowsweet, rich in salicylates, can be used to stanch mild stomach hemorrhage, even though synthetic salicylates cause such problems. Other plants rich in such constituents include *Salix* spp. (willow), *Gaultheria procumbens* (wintergreen), *Betula* spp. (birch), many poplars (such as *Populus tremuloides*), and *Viburnum prunifolium* (black haw). This group of herbs is most useful for inflammations of muscles, bones, and connective tissue caused by sports injuries and conditions such as osteoarthritis.

The analgesic and fever-lowering actions of these herbs are believed to be due to the ability of salicylates to interfere with the transmission of signals to parts of the hypothalamus, leading to an increase in peripheral blood flow and sweating. Salicylates are also believed to suppress the synthesis of inflammatory prostaglandins, influence arachidonic acid metabolism, increase corticoid levels, and inhibit hyaluronidase, thereby reducing inflammation.

Unlike aspirin, willow preparations do not inhibit cyclooxygenase in thrombocytes or aggregation of platelets, suggesting different mechanisms of action than those associated with salicylates. Because of this, *Salix* and other salicin-containing herbs cannot be used as substitutes for aspirin in preventive thrombolytic protocols against strokes and heart attacks.

Melissa officinalis (lemon balm)
Piper methysticum (kava kava)
Scutellaria lateriflora (skullcap)
Tilia platyphyllos (linden blossom)
Verbena officinalis (vervain)

A daily supplement of B-complex vitamins and vitamin C is also helpful. Relaxation exercises are invaluable, and the impact of various stressors should be softened. Although this may be impossible, the patient should be encouraged not to simply put up with something or someone just because it is there! It is possible for people to change themselves and to change their lives. Reevaluating choices is always valuable.

A Prescription for Tension-Related Headaches

Scutellaria lateriflora	2 parts
Valeriana officinalis	2 parts
Avena sativa	1 part

Dosage: 2.5 ml of tincture combination three times a day. If using dried herbs, infuse 2 teaspoons of the mixture in 1 cup of boiling water. This should be drunk three times a day.

A Prescription for Tension Headache with Indigestion and Palpitations

Scutellaria lateriflora	2 parts
Valeriana officinalis	2 parts
Leonurus cardiaca	1 part
Matricaria recutita	1 part
Artemisia vulgaris	1 part

Dosage: 5 ml of tincture mixture three times a day. If using dried herbs, infuse 2 teaspoons of mixture to 1 cup of boiling water. This should be drunk three times a day.

In their exceptional book *Aromatherapy: A Complete Guide to the Healing Art*, highly regarded aromatherapists Kathi Keville and Mindy Green recommend the following essential oil combination.

Essential Oil Formula for Headache Relief

3 drops lavender oil

3 drops neroli oil

2 drops marjoram oil

2 drops ylang ylang oil

1 drop German chamomile oil

1 drop clary sage oil

1 ounce carrier oil

Use as a massage or bath oil to relieve headache.

Broader Context of Treatment

The guidelines given here apply to the treatment of migraines as well as other types of headaches.

General Dietary Guidelines

• Eat smaller and more frequent meals.
• Reduce fat intake.
• Reduce caffeine (coffee, tea, cola, chocolate).
• Reduce salt.
• Increase consumption of complex carbohydrates, such as crackers, bread, rice, squash, pasta, corn, potatoes.
• Increase potassium intake with foods like milk, potatoes, asparagus, celery, apricots, grapes, carrots, broccoli, brussels sprouts, cauliflower.
• Increase magnesium intake with foods like dark green vegetables, legumes, cereal grains, milk.
• Limit alcohol intake.
• Limit sweets, and don't feed cravings.

The following supplements may also be helpful.

Magnesium: 200 to 300 mg twice daily
Fish oil: 3 to 4 g/day with meals

MIGRAINE

A paroxysmal disorder characterized by recurrent attacks of headache, with or without associated visual and gastrointestinal disturbances. *(The Merck Manual)*

Orthodox medicine considers the underlying cause of migraine to be unknown. As with most holistically oriented therapies, excellent results can be achieved with phytotherapy by focusing on factors that suggest causal links. Specific herbal remedies can prove exceptionally successful if used within a context that addresses the whole body and environment of the patient.

Common migraine may affect as many as 25% of Americans, and about 8% of all headaches treated by the average physician are migraines or some variation on migraines.[7] Attacks can occur in early childhood, but most patients first develop symptoms between the ages of 10 and 30. Many migraine patients have a family history of the problem.

The immediate cause appears to relate to spasms in the muscular walls of the blood vessels of the brain and scalp. In approximately 15% of all cases, migraine attacks are preceded by warning signs known as *auras*, such as scintillating visual effects, blind spots, zigzag flashing lights, numbness in parts of the body, and distorted visual images. These signs of an imminent attack are probably related to intracerebral vasoconstriction, and the head pain to dilation of scalp arteries.

One theory that may explain these changes suggests that the nervous system responds to a trigger by creating a spasm in the nerve-rich arteries at the base of the brain. The spasm closes down or constricts several arteries that supply blood to the brain, including the scalp artery and the carotid or neck arteries. As these arteries constrict, the flow of blood to the brain is reduced. At the same time, blood platelets clump together—a process believed to release the neurotransmitter serotonin. Serotonin is a powerful arterial constrictor and further reduces blood supply to the brain. Reduced blood flow decreases the brain's supply of oxygen. Symptoms signaling a headache, such as distorted vision and speech, may then result.

Reacting to the reduced oxygen supply, certain arteries within the brain open wider to meet the brain's energy needs, and this dilation eventually affects the neck and scalp arteries. The dilation of arteries triggers the release of pain-producing prostaglandins from various tissues and blood cells. Also released are chemicals that cause inflammation and swelling and substances that increase sensitivity to pain. The circulation of these chemicals and the dilation of the scalp arteries stimulate the pain-sensitive nociceptors. The result, according to this theory, is throbbing pain in the head.

Migraine attacks commonly take one of two forms. The most common is called *migraine without aura* (common migraine), which affects 85% of migraine sufferers. These are episodes of severe pain that affect one or both sides of the head. The pain is usually described as throbbing, but again, this is not always the case. The signature of these headaches is that they are usually, but not always, associated with feeling sick in the stomach or being sensitive to light, sound, or movement of the body.

Typically, the sufferer wishes to lie down in a dark and quiet room and wait for the storm to pass. Often, people close to the patient can predict when headache will occur because of changes in the patient's behavior, which may range from depression to exhilaration. If the headache is not relieved early by sleeping it off, it may wax and wane for days, accompanied by anorexia and nausea or vomiting, hallmarks of the so-called sick headache.

The second most common type is *migraine with aura* (classical migraine), which accounts for most of the remaining 15% of sufferers. The aura is a disturbance in the nervous system that precedes the headache. Typical disturbances involve the vision (bright flashing lights, black spots, and partial loss of vision) or the body (sensations of pins and needles moving over one limb or one side).

These disturbances usually last less than one hour for most sufferers, and almost invariably pass away, leaving no long-lasting effects.

All such symptoms may clear just before the onset of pain or merge into it. The pain may be unilateral or generalized, but tends to follow the same pattern in a particular person. Attacks may occur daily or only once every several months. Untreated attacks may last for hours or days and are often accompanied by nausea, vomiting, and photophobia. The extremities are cold and the patient will seek seclusion.

Migraine Triggers and Contributing Factors

It is critical to be aware of triggers and early signs of migraine. These signs may represent the actual onset of the headache or may be physical events that almost invariably lead to a headache. Catching the very early signs, especially before pain becomes severe, can provide important clues to controlling the migraine. These early signs may be symptoms of aura, aching muscles, cold hands, a general sense of tension, or any number of other indications.

Almost anything in one's lifestyle or environment can serve as a trigger for migraine pain. Triggers don't actually cause the pain; rather, they activate an already existing chemical mechanism in the brain. For example, if drinking red wine is usually followed by a headache within a few hours, we could call red wine a trigger.

Most migraines are triggered not by one factor, but instead by an interaction among several factors. In general, the more triggers present at any given time, the more likely that a headache will follow. In one study, migraine patients reported an average of five triggers. This has important ramifications, as it demands that triggers be observed systematically over time and that all be considered.

Factors that increase one's vulnerability to headache but do not immediately lead to one are called contributing or contextual factors. Such factors create a context in which a migraine is more likely to be set off by triggers. Some people can develop migraine not only during a period of stress but also afterward, when their vascular systems are still reacting. Migraines that wake up people in the middle of the night are also believed to result from a delayed reaction to stress.

Certain foods precipitate migraine attacks in many people. Reactions may be due to allergies or related to content of compounds known as *vasoactive amines*. These compounds can trigger migraines by causing blood vessels to expand. Many migraine sufferers have been found to have significantly lowered levels of a platelet enzyme that normally breaks down these natural dietary components. As red wine contains substances that potently inhibit this enzyme, it often triggers migraines, especially if consumed along with foods high in vasoactive amines, like cheese. Red wine and beer are among the alcoholic beverages most likely to cause problems. *Congeners*, the substances that give alcohol its distinguishing characteristics, may also be a culprit.

The naturally occurring amino acid tyramine, found in foods such as aged cheeses, Chianti wine, and pickled herring, affects several mechanisms known to be implicated in migraine. Chocolate may be another trigger. However, it is not clear if chocolate itself causes migraine or if a sudden craving for chocolate is a sign of an impending migraine. Food additives, such as sodium nitrite in hot dogs and luncheon meats and monosodium glutamate in many processed foods, may also trigger migraines for some people.

Other possible causes of migraine to consider include the range listed below. However, these will rarely all play a role for a given individual.

Foods and food sensitivities. As discussed earlier, foods containing vasoactive amines are particularly problematic. Triggers include:
- Dairy products, especially cheese
- Chocolate
- Eggs
- Wheat and wheat products
- Peanuts
- Citrus fruits
- Tomatoes
- Red meat
- Shellfish
- Alcohol (especially red wine and spirits)

Stress and fatigue. These factors will undoubtedly compound the problem and may be a clear trigger.

General toxicity. Any tendency to constipation, liver problems, or general congestion can be a marked trigger in some individuals.

Hormone levels. Occasionally, changes in levels of certain hormones may trigger an attack. This is usually related in some way to the menstrual cycle. Drugs that contain estrogen, such as birth control pills, may also serve as triggers.

Sensory irritants. These may include glaring or flickering lights and unusual odors.

Smoking, polluted air, or stuffy rooms. Smoking can cause headaches, as nicotine constricts the blood vessels while inhaled carbon monoxide expands them, thus creating a condition that can trigger migraines and cluster headaches.

Structural factors. Cranial and spinal misalignments may be involved, as may posture, even when not associated with overt skeletal problems.

Treatment of Migraine

This will depend upon the diagnosis of factors involved in any specific migraine patient. See also Broader Context of Treatment of headaches, as the recommendations given there also apply to the treatment of migraine.

Specific Remedies

It would be claiming far too much to say that herbal medicine cures migraine. However, when selected with care, certain plants have much to offer in the management of this distressing problem. By far, the most important is a European wayside plant called feverfew (*Tanacetum parthenium*). Feverfew is the only herb used in European phytotherapy known to be specific for the treatment of migraine. It is also the best example of a remedy well known to medical herbalists that has recently been accepted by allopathic medicine. (See sidebar Feverfew and Migraines on page 370.)

Feverfew is a long-term treatment, not an immediate cure for a migraine attack. Clinical experience suggests that four to six weeks of treatment is usually required before an initial response will be seen. However, average duration of use will vary among migraine patients. Success should be measured by decreased frequency, severity, and duration of migraine attacks. Don't use feverfew for patients who are pregnant or breast-feeding.

Some find that regular use of feverfew is enough to control or even prevent migraines. However, it is best to ensure that herbal support covers more factors than those addressed by feverfew. Ginkgo offers some very relevant properties, mainly related to its ability to tone the blood vessel walls and reduce the tendency for platelet aggregation. Ginkgo extract (standardized to 24% ginkgo flavone glycosides and 6% terpene lactones) at a dose of 120 mg/day in two or three divided doses is recommended.

A Prescription for the Prevention of Migraines	
Tanacetum parthenium	125 mg of dried herb taken once daily
Lavandula officinalis	Massage essential oil into temples at first sign of an attack

Feverfew and Migraines

Feverfew *(Tanacetum parthenium)* has been used throughout recorded medical history as a bitter tonic and remedy for severe headaches. Through wide media coverage, the herb has gained a reputation as a "cure" for migraine. Clinicians at the London Migraine Clinic observed that patients reported marked improvements in frequency, severity, and duration of migraine when they took the herb. Fortunately, these doctors had the inquiring and open minds of true scientists and so started their own investigations into the efficacy of feverfew. Clinical observations were soon being reported in the journals.[8]

The work of Dr. Peter Hylands and colleagues provides a good example. Seventeen patients who regularly ate fresh leaves of feverfew daily as prophylaxis against migraine were invited to participate in a double-blind, placebo-controlled trial of the herb. Of these, eight patients received capsules containing freeze-dried feverfew powder and nine a placebo. Those taking the placebo had a significant increase in the frequency and severity of headache, nausea, and vomiting during the early months of treatment. The group taking feverfew, on the other hand, continued to enjoy a reduced frequency of migraine, providing clear evidence that feverfew can prevent attacks of migraine. This led the researchers to strongly suggest the use of feverfew for migraine sufferers who have never before treated themselves with this herb. Long-term users often report beneficial side effects, such as relief from depression, nausea, and arthritic pain due to inflammation.

These findings would not at all surprise the venerable English herbalists Gerard and Culpeper! It is a pity that the patients who took placebo in this study had to experience renewed attacks of migraine to demonstrate something that the patients and herbalists already knew.

Following the clinical clues, pharmacologists began seeking the active components of the plant. The herb appears to work at least in part by inhibiting the secretion of granular contents from blood platelets and neutrophils. This may be relevant to the therapeutic value of feverfew not only in migraine, but also in other conditions, such as osteoarthritis. The five main compounds identified as having this activity were parthenolide, 3-beta-hydroxy-parthenolide, secotanapartholide A, canin, and artecanin, all of which are sesquiterpene lactones. The researchers believe it is likely that these and other sesquiterpene lactones inhibit the release of prostaglandins and histamine during the inflammatory process, thus preventing the blood vessel spasms in the head that trigger migraine attacks.

As with all such impressive research findings, do not lose sight of the importance of whole plant activity. As the dried or fresh leaf of feverfew itself is an excellent formulation, why not just suggest it to patients?

Considerable differences in parthenolide content have been observed in feverfew plants from different geographical locations. Similarly, commercial preparations of dried feverfew usually contain varying amounts of the active principle. For this reason, standardized preparations are often used. A daily dosage of 125 mg of a dried feverfew leaf preparation containing at least 0.2% parthenolide is considered appropriate for the treatment and prevention of migraines. This is approximately equivalent to 250 mcg/day of parthenolide.

A Prescription for Migraine Associated with Stress and Hypertension

Crataegus spp.	1 part
Tilia platyphyllos	1 part
Stachys betonica	1 part
Scutellaria lateriflora	1 part
Viburnum opulus	1 part

Dosage: 2.5 ml of tincture three times a day. In addition, the patient should follow instructions given in Prescription for Prevention of Migraine.

Many British phytotherapists focus upon supporting the liver during migraine treatment. As an example, consider the following mixture suggested by Mrs. Nalda Gosling, FNIMH, one of Britain's foremost herbal clinicians. Note the preponderance of hepatics and bitters in her formula.

Motherwort, vervain, dandelion root, centaury, wild carrot—each of these mixed together in equal parts and 25 g of this mixture simmered for 15 minutes in 0.5 l of water. A wineglass of this should be drunk 3 times a day.

A Cooling Compress for Migraine

1 quart ice-cold water

2 drops peppermint essential oil

1 drop ginger essential oil

1 drop marjoram essential oil

Pour the water into a 2-quart glass bowl and add the essential oils. Soak a clean cloth in the water and apply it to the head, forehead, or neck at the first sign of a migraine. Do not allow the compress to come into contact with the eyes. An ice pack applied over the compress will help keep it from getting warm.

Broader Context of Treatment

Please see Broader Context of Treatment for headache.

NEURITIS

A syndrome of sensory, motor, reflex, and vasomotor symptoms, singly or in any combination, produced by disease of a single nerve, two or more nerves in separate areas, or many nerves simultaneously. *(The Merck Manual)*

Peripheral nerve problems can be caused by a range of etiological factors, including physical trauma, collagen disease (such as rheumatoid arthritis), metabolic disease, microorganisms, toxic agents, nutritional deficiency, and malignancy. Traumatic neuritis may be induced by injury, pressure paralysis, exposure to cold, and even radiation. Appropriate treatment must be based on accurate diagnosis, which is unfortunately often problematic in this complex of conditions.

The therapeutic approach suggested here is a very basic one, ideal for traumatic neuritis, but may also be of symptomatic value in any of the conditions just mentioned.

Treatment of Neuritis

In the herbal treatment guidelines given here for neuritis, the nervous system is the focus for toning, but any associated symptoms that arise may provide a clue to deeper-seated issues.

Actions Indicated

Nervine tonics are important to nourish the traumatized nerve tissue.

Nervine relaxants ease associated pain and anxiety.

Anti-inflammatories reduce the inflammatory response.

Antispasmodics help alleviate any muscular tension developed in response to the discomfort.

Adaptogens support the body's efforts to cope with the stress of the pain and any stress-related causes.

Specific Remedies

Most of the relaxing nervines have been considered as specifics by various herbalists.

A Prescription for Neuritis

Internal use:

Hypericum perforatum	1 part
Scutellaria lateriflora	1 part
Avena sativa	1 part
Eleutherococcus senticosus	1 part

Dosage: 5 ml of tincture three times a day.

External use:

Peppermint essential oil (or any menthol-rich mint oil)

Hypericum infused oil

Colloidal oatmeal

These are three approaches to minimizing the discomfort caused by touch. Gently applying the menthol-rich oil of peppermint to sensitive skin will produce a cooling, locally anesthetic effect. Applying infused oil of *Hypericum* will reduce neurological inflammation, but must be used over a day or so. Colloidal oatmeal can act as a dry lubricant between the skin and clothing, thus minimizing irritation.

If the patient is experiencing a great deal of pain, the internal prescription may be made stronger by adding analgesic herbs, such as *Piscidia erythrina, Gelsemium sempervirens,* and possibly even *Valeriana officinalis.* However, the major drawback to these analgesics is that they can caused marked sedation at effective painkilling doses, and even then they are not necessarily as effective as the patient would like them to be! It may be appropriate to recommend prescription analgesics. Bear in mind that most of these strong drugs are derived from plants—plants that are now illegal for the herbalist to use.

Table 16.16. Actions Supplied by Prescription for Traumatic Neuritis

ACTION	HERBS
Nervine tonic	*Avena sativa, Hypericum perforatum, Scutellaria lateriflora*
Nervine relaxant	*Hypericum perforatum, Scutellaria lateriflora*
Anti-inflammatory	*Hypericum perforatum*
Antispasmodic	*Hypericum perforatum, Scutellaria lateriflora*
Adaptogen	*Eleutherococcus senticosus*

Although neuralgia, or nerve pain, is best remedied by treating the cause, essential oils do alleviate the pain, especially when used in conjunction with massage.

Essential Oils for Pain

5 drops helichrysum

3 drops chamomile

2 drops marjoram

2 drops lavender

1 ounce carrier oil

Combine ingredients and use for massage.

Broader Context of Treatment

Stress management techniques, accompanied by good quality nutrition, are essential. Vitamin B complex should be given as a supplement.

TINNITUS

The perception of sound in the absence of an acoustic stimulus. *(The Merck Manual)*

One person out of 10 has some type of hearing impairment or ear problem, and 85% of these have some associated tinnitus. While tinnitus is more common among older people, it can occur at any age, and it may not be possible to determine the cause in every patient. However, the most common causes of tinnitus are noise-induced damage and age-related hearing loss.

Because tinnitus is not a disease but a symptom, it often serves as an important marker for other conditions. Causes include concussions, cranial and cervical fractures, whiplash, and temporomandibular joint problems. In hyperthyroidism, an increased heart rate and consequent increased blood flow through the ear may cause ringing. Tinnitus is also a symptom of Ménière's disease. Transient tinnitus may follow a cold or influenza, but this generally subsides two to four months after the infection.

Whatever the underlying cause, tinnitus tends to be exacerbated by muscle spasms, stress, and tension. Substances that can accentuate tinnitus through vasoconstriction include nicotine and caffeine. Some people under stress will begin to notice ringing in their ears, often because they clench or grind their teeth. Reducing stress and relieving temporomandibular joint dysfunction generally improves tinnitus.

Damage to the fine hair cells of the inner ear may cause them to remain in a constant state of irritation. As a result, stimulation of the auditory nerve occurs randomly and spontaneously, instead of as a direct consequence of sound waves transmitted to the inner ear. These random electrical impulses are interpreted as noise, usually perceived as high-frequency ringing, because the hair cells that are most frequently damaged respond in the high-frequency range.

Unfortunately, by the time most people realize that they've suffered noise-induced tinnitus or hearing loss, hair cell damage in the inner ear is irreversible. The distress can be minimized with herbs and avoidance of aggravating factors, such as nicotine and caffeine.

Treatment of Tinnitus

The herbal treatment guidelines given here require time to work.

Specific Remedies

My training in Britain suggested the use of *Cimicifuga racemosa* (black cohosh) and *Hydrastis canadensis* (goldenseal) for tinnitus, without providing any clear reasons. However, as I worked with patients with noise-induced tinnitus from industrial South Wales, these herbs proved gratifyingly helpful. Since then, I have become aware of research investigating *Ginkgo biloba* for a range of vascular disturbances of the inner ear.

Ginkgo may help improve problems of the inner ear that result from a disturbance in blood supply. Such problems include tinnitus, vertigo, and some forms of hearing loss, including deafness due to head injury, sonic damage, and vascular problems of recent origin. Clinical research showed that many people with vertigo experienced total recovery after taking *Ginkgo* daily for several weeks. Consider the following example from the *Ginkgo* research.

The objective of a recent study in 60 patients with chronic tinnitus was to confirm the efficacy of oral treatment with a special extract of *Ginkgo*, subsequent to a 10-day treatment in which the *Ginkgo* medication was introduced directly into a vein. The primary outcome measure was the change in tinnitus volume in the more severely affected ear during treatment. The researchers concluded that *Ginkgo* was effective and safe in alleviating the symptoms associated with tinnitus.[9]

However, keep in mind that once hair cells are damaged, no medication will eliminate tinnitus completely.

A Prescription for Tinnitus

Cimicifuga racemosa	1 part
Hydrastis canadensis	1 part
Ginkgo biloba	1 part

Dosage: up to 5 ml of tincture three times a day

Broader Context of Treatment

A number of other issues should be considered in the attempt to alleviate the tinnitus. If stress is an issue, this must be addressed. This may be done with herbs, relaxation techniques, or a whole range of other approaches discussed in this chapter.

Most patients find that tinnitus is only a mild annoyance or are not aware of it most of the time. However, the constant noise can be upsetting, and for some may even lead to depression. If the depression is treated, these patients sleep better, feel better, and find the tinnitus less distracting. *Hypericum perforatum* is the main herb to consider here.

Ear protection is important, especially around potentially harmful noise. If occupational noise is a problem, the patient should try to reduce the noise level or change the working environment to avoid exposure. This is not always easy! Tinnitus can often be masked with background noise. Background music or "white noise" maybe sufficient. Patients may find this more tolerable than the internally generated tinnitus, especially elderly patients with high-frequency hearing loss.

MOTION SICKNESS

A disorder caused by repetitive angular and linear acceleration characterized primarily by nausea and vomiting. *(The Merck Manual)*

Motion sickness is a syndrome that affects some people when traveling in a vehicle, such as an automobile, airplane, or ship. Symptoms include dizziness, nausea, vomiting, drowsiness, pallor, and sweating. Why some people experience motion sickness while others do not is unknown.

The syndrome appears to arise from a disturbance in the organs of balance found in the inner ear. Psychological factors may also be involved. In the course of a long journey, the problem may disappear on its own, and in general, symptoms of motion sickness quickly resolve once travel is ended.

Treatment of Motion Sickness

Zingiber officinale (ginger) can usually be relied upon. Research published in the British medical journal *The Lancet* showed it to be more effective than Dramamine in preventing symptoms of motion sickness. Ginger may be drunk as a fresh infusion, eaten as candied ginger, or taken as capsules of the powder. For people who do not like the taste of ginger, capsules are ideal. The usual dosage for capsules is 2 to 4 as needed.

The herb *Ballota nigra* (black horehound) will also reduce this kind of nausea. One of the more effective allopathic treatments involves a dermal patch of scopalamine, a constituent of *Atropa belladonna*.

A Prescription for Motion Sickness

Ballota nigra	1 part
Mentha piperita	1 part

Dosage: 5 ml of tincture 20 minutes before travel. In addition, the patient should eat a small piece of candied ginger just before travel and as needed.

SHINGLES

An acute CNS infection involving primarily the dorsal root ganglia, characterized by vesicular eruption and neuralgic pain in the areas of the skin supplied by peripheral sensory nerves arising in the affected root ganglia. *(The Merck Manual)*

Shingles, or herpes zoster, is a viral infection of sensory nerve cells caused by the same virus (varicella zoster) that causes chicken pox. The virus remains latent in the dorsal root ganglia of the spinal cord after the initial attack of chicken pox. The disease occurs most frequently in people over the age of 50 years. It may be activated through such factors as trauma to the spinal cord resulting from surgery and X-ray therapy.

Shingles is characterized by pain along an affected nerve and its branches and the eruption of blisters over the skin areas supplied by the nerve. An attack will usually be preceded by a few days of intense pain in the affected areas. Next, many extremely painful and itchy blisters develop, which normal remain for 7 to 14 days. These eventually form crusty scabs and fall off. After such an outbreak, the pain may continue even when the blisters have disappeared, especially in the elderly. This may go on for months and can be more painful than the original infection.

Treatment of Shingles

The nervous system needs as much help as it can get! As shingles often occurs in the elderly, almost any system tonic might be appropriate. Signs and symptoms will guide the therapist.

Actions Indicated

Nervine tonics will nourish traumatized nerve tissue.
Nervine relaxants may help ease the associated pain and will definitely lessen associated anxiety or tension.

Anti-inflammatories will reduce the inflammatory response.

Antispasmodics will alleviate muscular tension developed in response to pain.

Antimicrobials may help deal with the virus infection, but it is very intransigent.

Specific Remedies

The European traditions record no specifics for shingles.

A Prescription for Shingles

Avena sativa	1 part
Hypericum perforatum	1 part
Echinacea spp.	1 part
Scutellaria lateriflora	1 part

Dosage: up to 5 ml of tincture four times a day. Topical application of *Mentha piperita* oil may reduce the pain through a mild, local numbing effect. However, this should not be attempted if the skin is extremely sensitive.

Colloidal oatmeal powder may be dusted on affected skin to act as a dry lubricant, perhaps reducing pain caused by contact with clothes.

If the patient is experiencing a great deal of pain, the internal prescription may be made stronger by adding analgesic herbs, such as *Piscidia erythrina*, *Gelsemium sempervirens*, and possibly even *Valeriana officinalis*. However, a major drawback to these analgesics is that they can cause marked sedation at effective painkilling doses, and even then they are not necessarily as effective as the patient would like them to be! It may be appropriate to recommend prescription analgesics. Bear in mind that most of these strong drugs are derived from plants—plants that are now illegal for the herbalist to use.

Table 16.17. Actions Supplied by Prescription for Shingles

ACTION	HERBS
Nervine tonic	*Avena sativa, Hypericum perforatum*
Nervine relaxant	*Hypericum perforatum, Scutellaria lateriflora, Artemisia vulgaris*
Anti-inflammatory	*Hypericum perforatum*
Antispasmodic	*Hypericum perforatum, Scutellaria lateriflora*
Antimicrobial	*Hypericum perforatum*
Immune support	*Echinacea* spp.

Broader Context of Treatment

Good nutrition and support of general health are crucial. Pain-relief medication containing acetaminophen (for example, Tylenol) may prolong the illness. Pharmacological research suggests that capsaicin, a constituent of *Capsicum annuum*, may be helpful as a pain reliever, and thus capsules of cayenne may be helpful. In addition, the following supplements are recommended.

Vitamin B complex: 100 mg three times a day with food
Vitamin C: 2 g twice a day
Lysine: 500 mg twice daily

References

1. Ulrich RS, Simons RF. Recovery from stress during exposure to everyday outdoor environments. In: Wineman J, Barnes R, Zimring C, eds. *The Costs of Not Knowing: Proceedings of the Seventeenth Annual Conference of the Environmental Design Research Association.* Washington, DC: Environmental Design Research Association, 1986.

2. Ulrich RS. View through a window may influence recovery from surgery. *Science* 1984; 224:420–21.

3. Harrer G, Sommer H. Treatment of mild/moderate depressions with Hypericum. *Phytomedicine* 1994; 1:3–8.

4. Pizzorno JE, Murray MT. *Textbook of Natural Medicine.* Edinburgh: Churchill Livingstone, 1999.

5. Price S, et al. *Aromatherapy for Health Professionals.* Edinburgh; New York: Churchill Livingstone, 1999.

6. [Information from the] National Library of Medicine Web site: www.nlm.nih.gov/medlineplus/ency/article/000362.htm

7. Bennett JC, Plum F. *Cecil Textbook of Medicine.* Philadelphia: Saunders, 1996.

8. Johnson ES, Kadam NP, Hylands DM, et al. Efficacy of feverfew as prophylactic treatment of migraine. *British Medical Journal (Clinical Research* ed.). 1985 Aug 31; 291:569–73.

9. Morgenstern C, Biermann E. The efficacy of Ginkgo special extract EGb 761 in patients with tinnitus. *International Journal of Clinical Pharmacology and Therapeutics* 2002 May; 40(5):188–97.

Suggested Reading

Hoffmann D. *Successful Stress Control: An Herbal Guide to Stress Relief.* Rochester, VT: Healing Arts Press, 1991.

17

⚜

THE URINARY SYSTEM

The importance of the urinary system cannot be overemphasized. The various physiological functions fulfilled by the kidneys and associated structures show how fundamental to bodily health and well-being they are. The maintenance of homeostasis is pivotal to any experience of wellness. With the variety of diuretics in our materia medica, the phytotherapist is uniquely endowed by nature with the means to support the complex physiology that maintains healthy kidneys and water balance in the body.

The kidneys are major organs of elimination. They work in conjunction with the liver, the lungs, the skin, and the bowels to help ensure a clean internal environment. The body disposes of excess water, toxic waste products of metabolism, and inorganic salts in the form of urine. Because of their excretory function, the kidneys are also largely responsible for maintaining the water balance of the body and the pH of the blood. The kidneys also play important roles in other body activities. For example, the kidneys release the protein erythropoietin, which stimulates the bone marrow to increase the formation of red blood cells. Because they have a role in regulating the volume of fluid in the body, they also help to control blood pressure. In addition, some drugs or their metabolites are eliminated through the kidney.

URINE PRODUCTION

The production of urine is a complex and quite wonderful process. It is far from a simple removal of water from the body. Rather, it is a process of selective filtration that removes waste and potential toxins from the blood while retaining essential molecules.

The initial site of urine production is the glomerulus of the nephrons in the kidneys. Arterial blood pressure drives a filtrate of plasma across the porous capillary walls of the glomeruli into the open space around the capillary tuft, called the Bowman's space, and is collected in the Bowman's capsule. The filtered plasma, now called glomerular filtrate, is mainly water, but also contains salts, glucose, amino acids, nitrogenous wastes such as urea, and a small amount of ammonia. Proteins, fats, and cellular elements (red blood cells, white blood cells, and platelets) are filtered out so that they remain in the general blood circulation. In normal kidneys, 100 to 140 ml of filtrate is formed each minute, a total of about 170 liters per day.

As the glomerular filtrate passes along the proximal convoluted tubule, the majority of its water content and some of its dissolved materials are reabsorbed through the walls of the tubule into the blood of the surrounding capillaries. This reabsorption process is highly selective. Water, sodium, and chloride ions, most of the bicarbonate, and all of the glucose are reabsorbed into the bloodstream, while other products, such as urea and ammonia, remain in the tubule.

During the later stage, most of the remaining filtrate is further selectively reabsorbed through Henle's loop and the distal convoluted tubule, so that only about 1% of the volume of the original filtrate is finally excreted as urine. The urine is considerably different in composition from the original filtrate.

The kidneys excrete 400 to 2,000 ml of urine or more per day. Excretion varies in volume and composition, depending on the needs of the individual. The kidneys maintain the internal fluid environment within narrow limits and are capable of adapting to a wide range of environmental situations. The cells lining the tubules are under the influence of regulating factors, such as the hormone aldosterone (from the adrenal gland), antidiuretic hormone, parathyroid hormone, and atrial natriuretic factor (from the heart).

The distal tubule regulates the overall acidity of the urine, and ultimately of the blood, by excretion of hydrogen ions. Ammonia combines with hydrogen to form ammonia ions that are secreted into the urine. Acidity is decreased by the removal of hydrogen ions.

All the blood glucose will be removed from the urine unless the blood glucose exceeds normal concentrations by a considerable amount. Other mechanisms remove most, if not all, of the other solutes, including sodium.

Much of the sodium ion in kidney filtrate is transported back to the blood, but 3 to 5 grams pass into the urine each day. As a result, most animals have strict salt requirements and must consume several grams of sodium chloride daily in order to live.

The retention of sodium is enhanced by the presence of aldosterone. This hormone is secreted into the bloodstream when the body's supply of sodium falls below normal. When there is an excess of sodium, aldosterone secretion is reduced and more sodium is excreted.

When excessive amounts of fluid are lost from the body, or the blood pressure falls below normal, the kidneys release the enzyme renin into the blood, where it promotes the formation of angiotensin. Within minutes, angiotensin causes vasoconstriction, which increases blood pressure and stimulates the secretion of aldosterone.

MAINTAINING URINARY SYSTEM HEALTH

There are not as many all-around tonics for the urinary system as there are for the cardiovascular and nervous systems. However, each herbal practitioner has favorite gentle tonics for the urinary system. These vary from bioregion to bioregion. Tonic remedies to consider for the urinary system include *Galium aparine* (cleavers), *Elymus repens* (couch grass), and *Achillea millefolium* (yarrow).

In the urinary system, the emphasis is on nourishing the tissue and helping to support the normal functioning of the various organs and tissues involved. Thus, stronger diuretics are not included in the list of possible tonics given here. The range of remedies available provides therapeutic options beyond the simple increase in diuresis so dramatically produced by *Taraxacum officinale* (dandelion leaf). The French colloquial name for dandelion, *pissé en lit* ("wet the bed"), is well deserved.

Attention to a number of straightforward factors will help maintain urinary tract health and avoid the development of illness in the whole system.

Drink adequate amounts of water, about 6 to 8 glasses a day.
Avoid too much protein in the diet, as it will tend to overload the kidneys. The kidneys deal with much of the nitrogen-rich metabolic waste these molecules produce. Under normal conditions, this is no problem. However, anyone with kidney problems should be on a low-protein diet, obtaining protein primarily from vegetable sources. Good sources of protein include peas, beans, lentils, mushrooms, and asparagus.
Practice good personal hygiene.

Avoid dietary irritants, especially foods containing oxalic acid. Do not consume coffee and tea in excess. Plant essential oils taken internally can damage the delicate tissue of the nephrons.

Table 17.1. Primary Actions for the Urinary System

ACTION	HERB
Anti-inflammatory	*Achillea millefolium, Apium graveolens, Arctostaphylos uva-ursi, Eupatorium purpureum, Galium aparine, Zea mays*
Antilithic	*Collinsonia canadensis, Eupatorium purpureum*
Antimicrobial	*Achillea millefolium, Agathosma betulina, Arctostaphylos uva-ursi, Elymus repens, Juniperus communis*
Antispasmodic	*Matricaria recutita, Valeriana officinalis, Viburnum opulus, Dioscorea villosa*, carminatives
Astringent	*Achillea millefolium, Agrimonia eupatoria, Arctostaphylos uva-ursi, Equisetum arvense, Cola vera, Cytisus scoparius*
Cardioactive	*Convallaria majalis, Cytisus scoparius, Lycopus* spp.
Demulcent	*Arctostaphylos uva-ursi, Collinsonia canadensis, Elymus repens, Zea mays*
Diaphoretic	*Achillea millefolium, Eupatorium perfoliatum, Sambucus nigra, Tilia platyphyllos*
Diuretic	All herbs listed as such in chapter 25
Hypotensive	*Achillea millefolium, Crataegus* spp., *Tilia platyphyllos*

PATTERNS OF ILLNESS IN THE URINARY SYSTEM

A number of symptoms may accompany problems in this system. Some of these symptoms are common to many health problems, but others are unique to the kidney and bladder.

Common Nonspecific Symptoms

Fever. Fever accompanies many infections and inflammatory conditions of the urinary system, although simple cystitis often involves no fever at all.
Weight loss. Marked weight loss is always an important sign, as it may indicate a number of systemic pathologies.

Malaise. A general feeling of ill health is an indicator of many disease processes.

Symptoms Unique to the Urinary System

Urinary frequency. This symptom describes increased frequency of urination without an increase in the volume of urine passed. This indication that the bladder cannot hold as much fluid as usual may be due to a range of causes.

Urinary urgency. This, a compelling need to urinate, often results from the loss of bladder tone that can accompany infection and other urinary tract problems.

Urinary tenesmus. Urinary tenesmus is experienced as a desire to urinate accompanied by an almost constant painful straining. This can continue until the cause of the irritation is removed.

Dysuria. Dysuria, or painful urination, commonly indicates possible inflammation in the bladder neck or urethra, often associated with infection. Dysuria with no infection must be carefully diagnosed.

Nocturia. The need to urinate at night can be produced by a range of factors, from drinking too much liquid before going to bed to kidney or liver disease. Such an array of minor and major causes should highlight the need for careful diagnosis.

Enuresis. Enuresis is nighttime bed-wetting.

Hesitancy, straining, and dribbling. This group of symptoms may indicate that some obstruction is inhibiting the free flow of urine from the bladder along the urethra. The most common cause is prostate problems in men.

Incontinence. Voiding of urine with little or no warning can be due to a range of factors, discussed later in this chapter.

Changes in appearance of urine. The urine might be cloudy, change color, or appear milky.

Changes in urine output. Normal urine volumes in adults range from 700 ml to 2,000 ml a day.

Pain. Pain related to kidney disease is primarily felt in the side or back, between the ribs and hips. This is caused by stretching of the capsule that covers the kidney; there are no sensory nerve endings in the organ itself. Bladder pain is usually felt above the pubic bones and referred along the urethra during urination.

Edema. Edema is swelling caused by accumulation of excess fluid in body tissues and cavities. Also called dropsy, or, preferably, hydrops, edema is symptomatic of a wide range of conditions and disorders, including heart and kidney disease. These disorders must be addressed, but diuretics can provide relief from edema by stimulating the kidneys to eliminate water from the body.

Thus, a range of signs and symptoms accompany health problems in the urinary system. In the discussion that follows, an herbal approach to these symptoms will be developed, followed by treatments for a number of specific pathologies. However, there are some conditions we shall not discuss. Serious manifestations of kidney disease, including pyelonephritis and glomerulonephritis, go beyond the range of this book. Phytotherapy can contribute much to the treatment of these conditions, but success depends upon skilled diagnosis. It is my opinion that, in this case, "a little bit of knowledge is a dangerous thing."

Thus, the focus of our discussion in this chapter will be the treatment of the more common symptoms listed above. The phytotherapist will be able to apply these treatments in a whole range of situations. I must emphasize again, however, that the ability to ameliorate a symptom is no alternative to treating underlying causes.

FREQUENCY

> Increased frequency of urination without an increase in the volume urine passed. *(The Merck Manual)*

This common symptom indicates that the bladder cannot hold as much fluid as usual. A range of processes can cause this symptom, and these causes must be identified and treated, if possible. Infection, foreign bodies, stones, and tumors can all injure the tissue of the bladder wall and cause inflammation.

Actions Indicated

Antimicrobials will help the body rid itself of any pathogens present, thus reducing inflammation and its resulting symptoms.

Anti-inflammatory herbs soothe inflamed tissue and thus reduce the irritation of local muscle spasm.

Diuretics will often help, simply because they usually will also have either antimicrobial or anti-inflammatory effects. Diuretics rich in volatile oils, such as *Juniperus communis* (juniper berry), may be contraindicated in severe cases, as it can be irritating to the nephrons.

In addition, a number of demulcent diuretic remedies work well. It is difficult to say whether they act primarily as anti-inflammatory agents to reduce inflammation or as demulcents that soothe the surface of the cells. The best examples here are *Zea mays* (cornsilk), followed by *Elymus repens* (couch grass) and *Althaea officinalis* (marshmallow leaf).

A Prescription for Urinary Frequency Associated with Infection

Zea mays	2 parts
Arctostaphylos uva-ursi	1 part

Dosage: Infuse 2 teaspoons of dry herb mixture in 1 cup of boiling water; drink 1 cup every hour until symptoms subside.

Barley Water

A traditional approach from Britain for soothing the urinary tract is barley water. This has been used in much the same way that cranberry juice has in North America. They work in different ways but achieve similar results. Barley water may be used in all cases where frequency, dysuria, or another distressing symptom occurs.

    4 oz (100 g) whole barley
    1 pint (500 ml) water
    ½ oz (15 g) lemon peel (preferably organic)

Boil the barley in a little water; strain. Pour 1 pint (500 ml) of water over the cleaned barley and add the lemon peel. Simmer until the barley is soft. Remove from heat and allow to cool until lukewarm. Strain, add a little honey, and drink several cups a day.

DYSURIA

Painful urination. *(The Merck Manual)*

A wide range of conditions can cause dysuria, so having an approach to easing this important symptom is very useful. However, successful alleviation will first depend upon accurate diagnosis, followed by appropriate treatment.

Actions Indicated

Anti-inflammatories will usually help ease the pain by reducing inflammation.

Antispasmodics soothe muscle spasms that often accompany such urinary tract problems.

Antimicrobials help the body rid itself of any pathogens, further reducing inflammation and associated symptoms.

A Prescription for Dysuria

Viburnum prunifolium	1 part
Zea mays	1 part
Arctostaphylos uva-ursi	1 part

Dosage: Infuse 2 teaspoons of dried herb mixture in 1 cup of boiling water; drink 1 cup every hour until the symptoms subside.

HEMATURIA

Blood in the urine. *(The Merck Manual)*

Hematuria can give the urine a red or brown color. If the amount of blood is small, it might not be visually apparent, but it can be detected by a number of simple tests. This symptom may be associated with a wide range of conditions, some minor and others quite severe. Competent diagnosis is crucial. The bleeding may occur at a site of physical trauma, such as where a kidney stone has cut the tissue, or from a focus of infection.

It is often possible to reduce or stop such bleeding with herbs, but this will *not* necessarily mean the trauma has been healed. The suggestions given here must be applied within the context of treatments that address the diagnosed cause.

Actions Indicated

Astringents will stanch bleeding. They may not always be powerful enough—for example, in cases of bleeding caused by large kidney stones.

Anti-inflammatories will soothe inflamed tissue, thus lessening bleeding.

Antimicrobials will help the body rid itself of any pathogens present, thus reducing inflammation and resultant bleeding.

A number of diuretic plants have an astringent effect. The most useful are *Vinca major* (periwinkle), *Equisetum arvense* (horsetail), *Alchemilla arvensis* (lady's mantle), and *Capsella bursa-pastoris* (shepherd's purse).

A Prescription for Hematuria

Vinca major	1 part
Capsella bursa-pastoris	1 part
Zea mays	1 part
Achillea millefolium	1 part

Dosage: Infuse 2 teaspoons of dried herb mixture to 1 cup of boiling water; drink 1 cup every 2 hours.

Table 17.2. Actions Supplied by Hematuria Prescription

ACTION	HERBS
Antimicrobial	*Achillea millefolium*
Astringent	*Achillea millefolium, Capsella bursa-pastoris, Vinca major*
Diuretic	*Achillea millefolium, Zea mays*
Demulcent	*Zea mays*

EDEMA

> Excessive accumulation of fluid in body tissues and cavities. *(The Merck Manual)*

Edema, or fluid retention, is an abnormal accumulation of fluid in the spaces between the cells of body tissues. This accumulation may be associated with liver or kidney disturbances, pregnancy, premenstrual syndrome, or heart failure. *Never treat water retention without addressing its causal factors.*

Here we are faced with one of the paradoxical problems associated with the current use of herbs—that is, that they work! Too often, herbs are used to address symptoms while the more fundamental healing work they can facilitate is ignored. The value of herbal diuretics in helping rid the body of excess water is a prime example of this issue. If the practitioner goes for dandelion leaf whenever edema is part of a patient's symptom picture, he or she is probably missing an opportunity for more profound healing.

Actions Indicated

Diuretics are, of course, the primary herbs to consider. The broader picture that the patient presents will suggest the appropriate treatment.

By far the most effective diuretic herb is dandelion leaf *(Taraxacum officinale)*. The diuretic effect of this herb is comparable to that of the drug furosemide. In addition to its efficacy as a diuretic, dandelion leaf provides the benefit of a rich source of potassium. One of the typical side effects of increasing diuresis by stimulating kidney function is a loss of vital potassium from the body. This can impact a range of body functions, the most critical of which is electrolyte balance in the heart muscle. If the diuretic has been prescribed to treat edema associated with congestive heart failure, any reduction in the availability of potassium will aggravate cardiac symptoms.

In dandelion leaf, however, we have one of the best natural sources of potassium. Dandelion leaf simultaneously replaces the potassium that is flushed from the body via its diuretic action. Thus, this herb provides us with an ideally balanced diuretic that may be used safely whenever this action is needed, including the treatment of edema related to heart problems.

A Prescription for Edema

Taraxacum officinale leaf

Dosage: 2.5 ml of tincture three times a day or 5 ml of tincture when needed, but not at night

---

CYSTITIS

> Acute or chronic infection of the urinary bladder. *(The Merck Manual)*

Cystitis, or inflammation of the wall and lining of the urinary bladder, may be due to bacterial infection or to mechanical abrasion from microcrystals of calcium phosphate in urine. Symptoms of cystitis include frequency, dysuria, cloudy or bloody urine, and pain and tenderness in the lower abdomen. The urine itself may be cloudy because it contains pus or blood; it may also have an unpleasant smell. These symptoms must be distinguished from those caused by vaginitis, sexually transmitted diseases, and irritations of the urethra.

Acute urinary tract infections are very common, affecting at least 15% of females at some point in their lives. Urinary tract infection is about 20 times more common in women than in men and can occur at any age. Women are more likely than men to be affected because the urethra is much shorter in women, allowing infective organisms easier access to the bladder. Such *ascending infections* are usually announced by discomfort at the urethral opening. As the condition progresses, the irritation travels upward.

These infections are usually caused by the rod-shaped bacterium called *Escherichia coli*, commonly known as *E. coli*. This is a normal bacterium found in the bowel, which, after a bowel movement, can be accidentally wiped onto the urethral opening. Less commonly, infection from the bloodstream and the kidneys descends into the bladder. These *descending infections* are usually associated with backache, headache, fatigue, and pain in the abdomen.

Many women have *bacteriuria* (bacteria in the urine) and *pyuria* (pus in the urine) in the absence of symptoms, while others may have symptoms without clinical signs. In the past, women who complained of recurrent symptoms but had no clinical signs of cystitis were diagnosed as having "urethral syndrome." Urologists now recognize a general syndrome known as interstitial cystitis, which comprises a group of urethral/bladder disorders in which the mucosa of the bladder has become eroded, resulting in ongoing symptoms in the absence of bacteriuria.

Causes of Cystitis

A variety of factors appear to increase the likelihood that an individual will develop cystitis.

Female gender. The female urethra is prone to colonization by bacteria due to its proximity to the anus, its short length (about 4 cm), and its termination inside the labia. Friction during intercourse may cause minor inflammation of the urethra, predisposing the individual to infection, or may even move pathogenic organisms into the urethra.

Pregnancy. Pregnant women may be more susceptible to infection because of hormonal changes that result in dilation and reduction in tone of the ureters of the kidney. Pressure of the uterus on the bladder and local venous congestion and pressure may also precipitate cystitis in pregnancy.

Diabetes. Diabetics and those who consume large amounts of sugar are predisposed to cystitis.

Chemical factors. Antibacterial soaps, sprays, douches, feminine deodorants, and contraceptive jellies and creams alter the vaginal environment and may cause irritation that predisposes the tissue to infection. Barrier contraceptive devices like the diaphragm may cause mechanical irritation of the urethra. Some forms of interstitial cystitis may be caused by food contaminated with pesticides.

Retention of urine. Anatomical deviations that result in retention of urine, such as a malposition of the uterus, can potentiate infection.

Oral contraceptives. Oral contraceptives may initiate infection in some individuals.

Antibiotics. Overuse of these potentially lifesaving drugs will select for resistant bacteria, often leading to cystitis.

Stress. Stress initiates the production of hormones, such as adrenocorticotropic hormone (ACTH), glucocorticoids, and aldosterone, all of which reduce circulating white blood cell counts and increase susceptibility to infection. Many who experience recurrent infection can relate stress (chemical, physical, or emotional) to the onset of symptoms.

Treatment of Cystitis

Cystitis can respond rapidly to appropriate treatment, the key being the selection of the appropriate antimicrobials. However, many well-known antimicrobial remedies (such as *Echinacea*) do not fulfill the herbalist's expectations in cystitis. It is important to use plants that are specifically active in the urinary tract. Thus, antimicrobials containing terpene essential oils are indicated. The essential oil is excreted from the body via the kidney, directing its action to the site of infection in the bladder.

Actions Indicated

Antimicrobials help the body control and then clear bacterial infection.

Anti-inflammatories soothe the pain and discomfort, but avoid overemphasizing them in the prescription. The symptomatic relief they produce must be applied in the context of removing the infection that causes the inflammation.

Astringents may be indicated if there is any hematuria.

Diuretics help flush the whole of the tract. Of course, it is best to select diuretics that possess antimicrobial and anti-inflammatory actions.

Antispasmodics may be necessary if there is much pain.

Specific Remedies

Many plants have a regional reputation for the treatment of cystitis. Often, the efficacy of these plants varies according to whether the plant is fresh or dried, what time of year it is picked, and other factors. For example, in Wales, fresh *Achillea millefolium* (yarrow), preferably harvested from sea cliffs, has a dramatic effect even in intransigent cases of cystitis. Unfortunately, tinctures or infusions made from the same plants after drying do not replicate the results achieved with fresh plant material. This is probably due to changes in the amount or relative composition of the volatile oils present.

Plants that contain antimicrobial volatile oils have most to offer. Primary examples are *Arctostaphylos uva-ursi* (bearberry) and *Agathosma betulina* (buchu).

A Prescription for Cystitis

Zea mays	2 parts
Arctostaphylos uva-ursi	2 parts
Agathosma betulina	1 part

Dosage: 5 ml of tincture three times a day. Infusion of *Achillea millefolium* (preferably fresh) should be drunk often.

Table 17.3. Actions Supplied by Prescription for Cystitis

ACTION	HERBS
Diuretic	*Arctostaphylos uva-ursi, Agathosma betulina, Zea mays*
Demulcent	*Zea mays*
Antimicrobial	*Arctostaphylos uva-ursi, Agathosma betulina*

A Prescription for Cystitis with Pain and Discomfort

Zea mays	2 parts
Arctostaphylos uva-ursi	2 parts
Viburnum prunifolium	1 part
Valeriana officinalis	1 part

Dosage: 5 ml of tincture three times a day. An infusion of *Achillea millefolium* (preferably fresh) should be drunk often.

Table 17.4. Actions Supplied by Prescription for Cystitis with Pain and Discomfort

ACTION	HERBS
Diuretic	*Arctostaphylos uva-ursi, Agathosma betulina, Zea mays*
Demulcent	*Zea mays*
Antimicrobial	*Arctostaphylos uva-ursi, Agathosma betulina*
Antispasmodic	*Valeriana officinalis, Viburnum prunifolium*

Cystitis Infusion

Hot infusions can ease symptoms dramatically. As an example, here is a combination recommended by British medical herbalist Annie McIntyre.

Althaea officinalis root	2 parts
Zea mays	2 parts
Elymus repens	2 parts
Equisetum arvense	2 parts
Arctostaphylos uva-ursi	2 parts
Agathosma betulina	1 part

Dosage: Add 1 teaspoon of this mixture to 1 cup of boiling water and infuse for 10 to 15 minutes. Drink hot four to five times a day.

Broader Context of Treatment

Cranberry juice (*Vaccinium macrocarpon*) has a strong traditional reputation for soothing symptoms of cystitis. Now, research shows that cranberry juice actually helps prevent the adherence of pathogenic bacteria to the lining of the urinary tract. Certain pathogenic *E. coli* bacteria attach themselves to the lining of the urinary tract with structures called *fimbriae*. Cranberry has been shown to inhibit the adherence of these fimbriated *E. coli* to the mucosa. It now appears that a group of flavonoids in cranberry, called proanthocyanidins, are responsible for these anti-adhesion effects.[1] Since sugar consumption is a predisposing factor for cystitis, unsweetened cranberry juice is recommended.

Here is some general advice that should be followed both during active infection and to prevent recurrent cystitis, especially for those prone to these infections.

Avoid using tampons, as they contain additives that can injure the lining of the vagina.

Discontinue use of contraceptive diaphragms, oral contraceptives, and other chemicals used in the vaginal area.

Discontinue use of deodorant soaps. These soaps are irritating to the skin and kill off normal external bacteria, which are then replaced by more virulent, less easily killed pathogens.

Increase intake of water to at least 8 to 12 glasses per day. This helps to flush out bacteria and will often reduce dysuria.

Acidify the urine. Decrease consumption of alkaline foods, such as dairy products, citrus juices, and sodas.

Eat a light diet consisting of grains, some vegetables, and specific acidifying juices.

Eliminate bladder irritants such as coffee, black tea, chocolate, and alcohol.

Discontinue intake of all high-sugar foods, including sweet vegetables and fruits, sugar, and honey.

In addition, take the following supplements.

Vitamin A: 25,000 IU/day
Vitamin C: 500 mg every 2 hours
Zinc: 30 mg/day

New studies show that ascorbic acid irritates the bladder, so vitamin C must be obtained in the form of calcium ascorbate, which is relatively buffered. Avoid vitamins containing aspartate, as it is a bladder irritant.

URINARY CALCULUS

Small hard masses somewhere in the urinary tract. *(The Merck Manual)*

An estimated 3% of all Americans will suffer from kidney stones at some time in their life, and half of these people will suffer recurrences over the next ten or more years.

While extremely painful, kidney stones rarely cause permanent loss of kidney function if properly treated, and are almost never fatal in the absence of complications.

The most important kidney stones are calcium oxalate stones, calcium phosphate stones, and uric acid stones. The vast majority of stones contain calcium in some form. Uric acid stones, which account for fewer than 10% of all stones, are an exception. In most normal people, urine is supersaturated with calcium oxalate, so all people can potentially form such stones. Normal urine is not supersaturated with respect to uric acid, cystine, or struvite. Conditions that elevate calcium oxalate supersaturation raise the risk of calcium oxalate stone formation.

Normal urine contains predictable amounts of calcium, magnesium, uric acid, and other by-products of metabolism. Normally, these substances are in solution and pass into the bladder. However, under certain conditions of high saturation, and in a complex chemical environment that is not yet completely understood, the chemicals may crystallize and form a stonelike particle in the kidney. Once formed, the particle stimulates continued crystallization. If the stone remains in the wide open spaces of the kidney, no symptoms may occur, although there may be microscopic signs of blood in the urine. However, once a piece of the stone breaks off and enters the ureter that leads to the bladder, prompt spasms occur, leading to the painful symptoms.

Two main clinical examples are hypercalciuria (excess calcium in the urine) and hyperoxaluria (excess oxalic acid in the urine). Hypercalciuria can be caused by many conditions, including hyperparathyroidism, renal tubular acidosis, sarcoidosis, vitamin D intoxication, and idiopathic factors. Hyperoxaluria may be caused by overproduction of oxalic acid and hereditary disorders of metabolism, or may be acquired through diet or intestinal disease.

Apart from overexcretion of citrates, supersaturation can be increased by abnormal interactions between urine ions. Urine citrate forms a soluble salt with calcium that normally reduces free calcium ion levels appreciably. Low urine citrate related to bowel disease, renal tubular acidosis, and, perhaps, dietary and hereditary causes can raise calcium oxalate supersaturation and promote stones. Normal women excrete more citrate and less calcium than normal men do, which may help explain why men are more likely to form stones. Low urine pH due to hereditary causes or bowel disease promotes uric acid stones. High pH related to alkali drugs or renal tubular acidosis increases calcium phosphate supersaturation.

An infection of the urinary tract can cause cellular debris to act as a focus, or "seed," on which crystals can form. Bacterial action makes the urine more alkaline, resulting in deposition of phosphates that form calcium phosphate stones. Excessive uric acid and increased excretion of calcium by the kidney, combined with an increased insolubility of calcium in the urine, can also promote stone formation. Long-term confinement to bed or even chronic lack of exercise may encourage mobilization of calcium from the bones into the blood and thus increase calcium levels in the urine. Similarly, steroids can increase blood and urine calcium levels.

Inherited tendencies and obesity can also predispose an individual to the development of kidney stones, as can several other physiological abnormalities. However, in about 20% of patients, no abnormality can be identified to explain the tendency to form calculi. Some individuals absorb excessive amounts of calcium from the intestines, overwhelming the ability of the kidney to dissolve it. Others absorb normal amounts of calcium, but the kidney allows too much to leak into the urine from the blood, and some produce urine that is too acidic, facilitating crystallization. In certain diseases that cause elevated blood calcium levels, such as hyperparathyroidism and some types of cancer, kidney stones may occur as a secondary phenomenon serving as the first clue to the underlying disease.

The pain of a kidney stone comes on suddenly. Classically, there is severe, excruciating pain in the flank on the side of the stone, coming in waves and radiating around to the lower abdomen and into the groin, scrotum, or vagina, and occasionally into the upper thigh area. The intensity of pain is as severe as most people ever experience. The patient often suffers nausea, vomiting, and profuse sweating, and there may or may not be blood in the urine. Most stones pass into the bladder, in an amount of time ranging from minutes to days or even longer, and the pain is gone. The small, usually brown or black stone may be identified in the urine, and should be kept for analysis. If fever is present, it may be due to infection that has formed behind the stone in the stagnant urine.

Indications for Surgical Treatment

In certain cases, some kind of surgery may be needed to remove a kidney stone. Surgery may be required if the stone:

- Does not pass after a reasonable period of time and causes constant pain
- Is too large to pass on its own
- Blocks the flow of urine
- Causes ongoing urinary tract infection

- Damages the kidney tissue or causes constant bleeding
- Has grown larger (as seen in follow up X-ray studies)

Treatment of Urinary Calculus

The herbal treatment guidelines given here can be quite effective, given time. Careful selection of the appropriate herbs is critical.

Actions Indicated

Antilithic remedies are the core of any treatment of renal calculus.

Anti-inflammatories are indicated to lessen the inflammation caused by the passage of hard material along the delicate tissue of this system. Such remedies will decrease the pain and discomfort to some extent.

Antispasmodics are essential to help reduce muscular spasms along the urinary tract as peristalsis moves the stone. Unfortunately, legal plant antispasmodics are not strong enough to deal with acute problems of this nature.

Demulcents will help, as they usually also act as anti-inflammatory agents in this system.

Specific Remedies

A number of plants have a long tradition of use as specifics in Europe. Important examples are *Hydrangea arborescens* (hydrangea), *Aphanes arvensis* (parsley piert), *Parietaria diffusa* (pellitory-of-the-wall), *Elymus repens* (couch grass), *Urtica dioica* (nettle), and *Solidago virgaurea* (goldenrod). To these we can add the North American plants *Eupatorium purpureum* (gravel root), *Collinsonia canadensis* (stoneroot) and *Zea mays* (corn silk).

A Prescription for Kidney Stones

Collinsonia canadensis	1 part
Eupatorium purpureum	1 part
Zea mays	1 part
Dioscorea villosa	1 part
Viburnum prunifolium	1 part

Dosage: up to 5 ml of tincture three times a day

Table 17.5. Actions Supplied by Kidney Stone Prescription

ACTION	HERBS
Diuretic	*Collinsonia canadensis, Eupatorium purpureum, Zea mays*
Demulcent	*Zea mays*
Antilithic	*Collinsonia canadensis, Eupatorium purpureum*
Antispasmodic	*Dioscorea villosa, Viburnum prunifolium, Zea mays*

Broader Context of Treatment

The treatment approach suggested here is not for the treatment of acute attacks. Rather, it is intended to help prevent subsequent attacks. Profuse sweating or low fluid intake can concentrate the urine, causing urinary salts to solidify and stones to form. The patient should avoid dehydration, especially after exercise but even on routine days, by ingesting copious amounts of fluid. Recommend that the patient drink 4 to 6 pints of fluid a day and 1 pint before going to bed—in other words, enough to ensure that 24-hour urine output is never less than 3 pints. Ideally, the patient should be drinking enough fluid for routine nighttime awakening to urinate.

When uric acid stones are the problem, the urine will be acid. To lessen the impact of these stones, the patient should eat an alkaline diet, including potatoes, vegetables, and fruits, but not citrus fruits. In addition, the patient should decrease protein intake, since protein tends to increase levels of uric acid. In particular, the patient should avoid liver, kidneys, fish roe, and sardines. Alkalinizing mineral water is a good beverage choice.

For patients with calcium oxalate stones, avoid foods that contain oxalates, such as spinach, rhubarb, beets, parsley, sorrel, and chocolate. Those who have a tendency to form oxalate stones often secrete too much calcium in their urine, which reacts with oxalic acids to form the stones. For this reason, these patients should be advised to restrict intake of dairy products, which are rich in calcium. Mineral waters rich in magnesium will increase the solubility of calcium. Both vitamin B_6 and folic acid are thought to restrict the amount of calcium formed in the body.

Calcium phosphate stones are usually formed in the presence of urinary infection. The urine is alkaline, so the patient should eat foods that acidify the urine, such as meat, fish, and eggs. However, dairy products should be avoided.

References

1. Howell AB, Vorsa N, Der Marderosian A, Foo LY. Inhibition of the adherence of P-fimbriated Esherichia coli to uroepithelial-cell surfaces by proanthocyanidin extracts from cranberries. *The New England Journal of Medicine* 1998; 339:10854 [letter].

18

THE REPRODUCTIVE SYSTEM

It should come as no surprise that nature is rich in plants that nurture the reproductive system or in some way address the process of conception and birth. However, today the phytotherapist is faced with an unfortunate 21st century dilemma. Some of the primary remedies for the female reproductive system, widely used by the Eclectic, Physiomedicalist, and Thomsonian herbalists of previous centuries, are now seriously endangered species. Currently, the most problematic of these plants are:

Chamaelirium luteum (false unicorn root)
Cypripedium spp. (lady's slipper)
Trillium erectum and *T. pendulum* (beth root)

The fact that healing plants of this importance have become endangered to the degree that they have is one of the signs of the ecological holocaust that humanity has wrought. Though these plants are still occasionally abundant locally, their ecological range has been dramatically diminished. I caution against using them unless they are from cultivated sources, which in the case of *Cypripedium* is extremely difficult. Wildcrafting this plant is an ecological crime.

REPRODUCTIVE SYSTEM HERBS AND ACTIONS

When considering the reproductive system, it is important to identify the primary tonic herbs and next determine other ways in which they impact the system (secondary actions). From the list of emmenagogues that follows, we shall select the most valuable tonics and explore their differential indications. For more details on the secondary actions of these herbs, please refer to chapters 25 and 26.

Herbal Emmenagogues

Achillea millefolium (yarrow)
Artemisia abrotanum (southernwood)
A. absinthium (wormwood)
A. vulgaris (mugwort)
Calendula officinalis (calendula)
Caulophyllum thalictroides (blue cohosh)
Cimicifuga racemosa (black cohosh)
Gentiana spp. (gentian)
Hydrastis canadensis (goldenseal)
Hyssopus officinalis (hyssop)
Lavandula spp. (lavender)
Leonurus cardiaca (motherwort)
Marrubium vulgare (horehound)
Marsdenia condurango (condurango)

Emmenagogues Demystified

The term *emmenagogue* is commonly applied to plants used to treat a range of female reproductive conditions. Strictly speaking, however, emmenagogues are remedies that stimulate menstrual flow and activity. In most modern herbals, the term is used in the wider sense to indicate a remedy that normalizes and tones the female reproductive system. Such a broad definition is almost meaningless, as it obscures the wealth of diverse actions these herbs offer. The herbs described in most herbals as emmenagogues actually provide a whole range of distinct actions that benefit the reproductive system either directly or indirectly.

Matricaria recutita (chamomile)
Mentha piperita (peppermint)
M. pulegium (pennyroyal)
Mitchella repens (partridgeberry)
Petroselinum crispum (parsley)
Pulsatilla vulgaris (pasqueflower)
Rosmarinus officinalis (rosemary)
Rubus idaeus (raspberry leaf)
Ruta graveolens (rue)
Salvia officinalis (sage)
S. officinalis var. *rubia* (red sage)
Senecio aureus (life root)
Tanacetum parthenium (feverfew)
T. vulgare (tansy)
Thymus vulgaris (thyme)
Tilia platyphyllos (linden)
Trigonella foenum-graecum (fenugreek)
Tropaeolum majus (nasturtium)
Valeriana officinalis (valerian)
Verbena officinalis (vervain)
Viburnum opulus (cramp bark)
V. prunifolium (black haw)
Vitex agnus-castus (chasteberry)
Zingiber officinale (ginger)

For further clarification, the following section discusses some of the more toning emmenagogues, presented in terms of their primary effect upon the menstrual process. Remember that all bitters will have an emmenagogue effect in the strict sense of the word—that is, they will help improve menstrual function and flow. If this is not evident, please review the information about bitters in chapter 25.

Uterine Tonics

These plants have a toning, strengthening, nourishing effect on both the tissue and the function of the female reproductive system. How and why they exert these effects is usually unknown, but this should not belittle their remarkable therapeutic contributions. Determining differential indications for these plants is one of the most confused areas in modern herbalism. Important examples of uterine tonics are *Angelica sinensis* (dong quai), *Caulophyllum thalictroides* (blue cohosh), *Cimicifuga racemosa* (black cohosh), and *Mitchella repens* (partridgeberry).

Emmenagogues

Among the many plants that can stimulate the menstrual process, some also have a tonic effect on the whole system. Of the emmenagogues listed previously, some work

through bitter stimulation and others through localized irritation. Herbs that also nourish the system to some degree include *Achillea millefolium* (yarrow), *Artemisia vulgaris* (mugwort), and *Mitchella repens* (partridgeberry).

Hormonal Normalizers

A number of plants have a direct impact upon levels of hormones in the body. Of course, there are many human hormones, and only a few impact reproductive function. Many claims can be made about plants that affect hormonal balance, but here we will limit our discussion to plants that have an observable influence. As little endocrinological research has been undertaken on these herbs, it is impossible to be specific in all cases about how they work. Thus, the herbalist tends to refer to them in terms of hormonal modulators or normalizers.

The most important of these plants in European phytotherapy is *Vitex agnus-castus* (chasteberry). It is fair to describe this plant as a normalizer, as it will tend to move the body back to normal function, regardless of which female hormone is involved and whether the problem is an excess or a deficiency of hormone. However, how it achieves this effect is a matter of conjecture. Other uterine tonics and bitters may have a similar effect because of some of their more generalized toning influences, but they are not as predictable as *Vitex*.

Uterine Astringents

An abundance of herbs reduce blood loss from the uterus, whether due to excessively heavy periods *(menorrhagia)*, bleeding between periods *(metrorrhagia)*, or organic disease, such as fibroids. The question of how they work remains unanswered, because no astringent tannin reaches the uterine tissue from the gut. Some, but not all, of these plants may influence hormonal processes. Of the many valuable astringents not on the list of emmenagogues given earlier, consider *Alchemilla vulgaris* (lady's mantle), *Capsella bursa-pastoris* (shepherd's purse), *Geranium maculatum* (cranesbill), and *Vinca major* (periwinkle).

Uterine Demulcents

Similar comments can be made about the mechanisms of action of the important reproductive system demulcent remedies. There is no way that mucopolysaccharides find their way to the uterus from the digestive process; nonetheless, there is no question that these remedies soothe inflamed tissue. The most toning is *Caulophyllum thalictroides* (blue cohosh).

Nervines and Antispasmodics

There are also a number of valuable remedies that impact the autonomic innervation of this complex system. By using the appropriate nervine or antispasmodic, much can be achieved in terms of correcting functional tone. Herbs in this category include *Viburnum opulus* (cramp bark), *V. prunifolium* (black haw), *Cimicifuga racemosa* (black cohosh), *Leonurus cardiaca* (motherwort), and *Pulsatilla vulgaris* (pasqueflower).

AMENORRHEA

> Absence of menstruation, i.e., either lack of menarche or cessation of menses. *(The Merck Manual)*

To recognize amenorrhea, one must know what constitutes normal menstruation. The duration of a menstrual period is 28 ± 3 days for 65% of women, with a range of 18 to 40 days. Once a menstrual pattern has been established, the variation does not normally exceed five days. The average duration of flow is 5 ± 2 days, with a blood loss averaging 130 ml. Flow is generally heaviest on the second day.

Amenorrhea falls into three broad categories.

Primary Amenorrhea

Women with primary amenorrhea do not begin to menstruate when expected. Because there is a wide variation in normal onset of menstruation during puberty, applying this diagnosis is problematic. In general, however, primary amenorrhea implies that menstruation has not yet started by the age of 16 years.

With the safe and effective herbs available to the phytotherapist, treatment could begin at the age of 15 if deemed necessary. However, competent diagnosis is required, as there are a number of diverse causes to consider, including imperforate hymen, ovarian dysfunction, and hormonal imbalance. Obviously, the treatment of primary amenorrhea will be dictated by the underlying cause.

Secondary Amenorrhea

Secondary amenorrhea indicates cessation of menstruation after at least one normal period. This is common, and causes include pregnancy, stress, loss or gain of weight, menopause, breast-feeding, anemia, excessive exercise, discontinuation of oral contraceptives, side effects of some drugs, ovarian cysts, and tumors.

Erratic or Irregular Menstruation

Women with erratic menstruation may have only three or four periods in a year, or three very close together followed by none for a few months. Numerous causes, similar to those for secondary amenorrhea, are possible.

Treatment of Amenorrhea

The core herbal treatment guidelines for this condition must start with tonic support for the reproductive system, but can take into account many other issues specific to the woman involved.

Actions Indicated

Emmenagogues are the classic treatment, as they can trigger the menstrual process.

Hormonal normalizers will help the body regulate levels of various hormones.

Uterine tonics will contribute their nourishing, toning power.

Other actions will be indicated by the associated symptom picture or case history. For example, if anxiety and stress are an issue, consider appropriate nervines. If severe menstrual cramps occur, use antispasmodics.

Specific Remedies

Most of the emmenagogues could be considered specifics. However, care should be taken with the stronger emmenagogues, as they may be too stimulating and cause cramping. Simple infusions can often solve this problem. Plants such as *Mentha pulegium* (pennyroyal), *Achillea millefolium* (yarrow), and *Artemisia vulgaris* (mugwort) can help initiate flow, but if they are not effective, consider the following prescription.

A Prescription for Amenorrhea Associated with Hormonal Imbalance

Caulophyllum thalictroides	2 parts
Artemisia vulgaris	2 parts
Vitex agnus-castus	1 part

Dosage: 2 ml of tincture three times a day until period starts

---

Table 18.1. Actions Supplied by Prescription for Amenorrhea with Hormonal Imbalance

ACTION	HERBS
Emmenagogue	*Artemisia vulgaris, Caulophyllum thalictroides, Vitex agnus-castus*
Hormonal normalizer	*Vitex agnus-castus*
Uterine tonic	*Caulophyllum thalictroides*

A Prescription for Amenorrhea Associated with Stress

Cimicifuga racemosa	2 parts
Verbena officinalis	2 parts
Vitex agnus-castus	1 part

Dosage: 2.5 ml of tincture three times a day until period starts

---

Table 18.2. Actions Supplied by Prescription for Amenorrhea with Stress

ACTION	HERBS
Emmenagogue	Cimicifuga racemosa, Verbena officinalis, Vitex agnus-castus
Hormonal normalizer	Vitex agnus-castus
Uterine tonic	Cimicifuga racemosa
Nervine relaxant	Cimicifuga racemosa, Verbena officinalis

Broader Context of Treatment

Considerations will depend upon the underlying cause. Thus, other therapeutic modalities, such as osteopathy and acupuncture, may be indicated.

DYSMENORRHEA

> Cyclic pain associated with menses. *(The Merck Manual)*

Dysmenorrhea, or painful menstruation, is the most common of all gynecologic complaints and the leading cause of absenteeism of women from work, school, and other activities. In addition to identifiable pathological causes, a number of constitutional factors may lower the pain threshold and thus appear to worsen dysmenorrhea. Common factors include anemia, increase in obesity, chronic illness, overwork, stress in general, diabetes, and poor nutrition. Two main forms of dysmenorrhea can be identified.

Primary Dysmenorrhea

Primary dysmenorrhea is dysmenorrhea unrelated to any definable pelvic lesion. It usually starts with the first ovulatory cycles, beginning in most cases before the age of 20 years. Primary dysmenorrhea is associated with nausea in 50% of patients, vomiting in 25% of patients, and increased stool frequency in 35% of patients. The pain is low and cramping, recurring in waves that probably correlate with uterine contractions. The pain usually begins a few hours before bleeding commences, comes to a peak intensity within a few hours, and dissipates within two days. It generally occurs over the midline of the abdomen, and is relieved by the onset of good menstrual flow.

Secondary Dysmenorrhea

Secondary dysmenorrhea is related to the presence of pelvic lesions associated with organic pelvic disease, such as endometriosis, salpingitis (also known as pelvic inflammatory disease, or PID), and postsurgical adhesions. The contraceptive intrauterine device (IUD) may cause pain problems.

Secondary dysmenorrhea begins up to a few days before menstruation and lasts several days after the onset of flow. Often it is lateralized to one side of the body, and it does not characteristically peak and diminish as clearly or quickly as primary dysmenorrhea. In general, the onset of secondary dysmenorrhea occurs later in life in women who have not had primary dysmenorrhea. However, it may also be superimposed onto a preexisting case of primary dysmenorrhea.

Treatment of Dysmenorrhea

Actions Indicated

Antispasmodics ease the muscle spasms that are the immediate cause of pain.

Nervines will help associated psychological tension or anxiety.

Diuretic remedies are indicated if dysmenorrhea is of a congestive nature, accompanied by water retention.

Uterine tonics provide the basis for any healing work in this body system.

Hormonal normalizers are indicated if the diagnosis suggests that hormonal imbalance is making a pivotal contribution.

Specific Remedies

As there are a number of possible underlying causes for this all-too-common problem, a number of remedies have been called specifics. Remedies of value in dysmenorrhea related to a whole range of different causes are *Cimicifuga racemosa* (black cohosh), *Dioscorea villosa* (wild yam), *Scutellaria lateriflora* (skullcap), *Viburnum opulus* (cramp bark), and *V. prunifolium* (black haw).

A Prescription for Dysmenorrhea

Viburnum prunifolium	1 part
Scutellaria lateriflora	1 part
Cimicifuga racemosa	1 part

Dosage: 5 ml of tincture as needed

Table 18.3. Actions Supplied by Prescription for Dysmenorrhea

ACTION	HERBS
Antispasmodic	*Viburnum prunifolium, Scutellaria lateriflora, Cimicifuga racemosa*
Nervine	*Viburnum prunifolium, Scutellaria lateriflora, Cimicifuga racemosa*
Uterine tonic	*Cimicifuga racemosa*

A Prescription for Dysmenorrhea Associated with Pelvic Lesions

Viburnum prunifolium	1 part
Dioscorea villosa	1 part
Cimicifuga racemosa	1 part

Dosage: 5 ml of tincture three times a day

Table 18.4. Actions Supplied by Prescription for Dysmenorrhea with Pelvic Lesions

ACTION	HERBS
Antispasmodic	*Viburnum prunifolium, Dioscorea villosa, Cimicifuga racemosa*
Nervine	*Viburnum prunifolium, Cimicifuga racemosa*
Uterine tonic	*Cimicifuga racemosa*

The addition of *Dioscorea villosa* will provide a more reliable antispasmodic action if a physical problem is present. This prescription will support, but *not* replace, whatever treatment is necessary for the underlying problem.

Broader Context of Treatment

Dietary and supplemental approaches are well known, but unnecessary if appropriate herbs are used. Psychological issues can be fundamental here. Low tolerance to the sensation of uterine contraction may be learned behavior.

PREMENSTRUAL SYNDROME

A condition characterized by nervousness, irritability, emotional instability, depression and possibly headaches, edema and mastalgia; it occurs during the 7 to 10 days before menstruation and disappears a few hours after onset of menstrual flow. *(The Merck Manual)*

The name *premenstrual syndrome* (PMS) describes a broad range of symptoms that occur cyclically and are severe enough to disturb a woman's life or cause her to seek help from a health practitioner. Most women experience some cyclical bodily changes during the menstrual years, corresponding to a pattern of cycling hormones. Most of these changes are normal, and many cultures observe and ritualize these subtle shifts in body response and mental and emotional focus.

Women often express a positive attitude about the conscious observance of these patterns within their own bodies. However, when the hormonal and chemical changes cause debilitating symptoms, they can disrupt the function of virtually all body systems as well as the individual's emotional life.

PMS is diagnosed on the basis of when symptoms are present. There is, by definition, a period of time for PMS sufferers during which symptoms are absent, usually just after the onset or end of menses. PMS occurs during the proliferative or luteal phase of the menstrual cycle, when levels of estrogen and progesterone are relatively high. Estrogen is a central nervous system (CNS) stimulant and progesterone is a CNS depressant. What is important is the relationship of estrogen to progesterone during the luteal phase.

A number of etiological factors have been identified for primary PMS:

Estrogen excess
Progesterone deficiency
Fluid retention
Hypoglycemia
Decreased production of prostaglandin E_1
Increased production of other prostaglandins
Magnesium deficiency
Increased prolactin levels

It is believed that many of the symptoms of PMS relate to a shift in the fluid in the water compartments of the body (intracellular, extracellular, and intravascular), with increased retention of water and water moving into the extracellular spaces. This is mediated by increased levels of ACTH and aldosterone. The cells are more receptive to insulin in the premenstrual part of the cycle, which causes relative hypoglycemia and subsequent carbohydrate cravings. Magnesium deficiency leads to decreased levels of dopamine in the brain, which leads in turn to an increase in levels of CNS stimulators (norepinephrine and serotonin). Increases in prolactin result in decreases in progesterone.

Table 18.5. The PMS Symptom Picture

SYMPTOM CATEGORY	SYMPTOM MANIFESTATIONS
Behavioral	Personality alterations may occur, in the form of nervousness, irritability, agitation, unreasonable temper, fatigue, depression. Symptoms that suggest clinical depression, such as anxiety, palpitations, tightening in the chest, and hyperventilation, are common. Violent crimes by women and suicide are often committed in the premenstrual period.
Neurological	Headache, vertigo, syncope, paresthesias of the hands or feet, and aggravation of seizure disorders have all been recorded.
Respiratory	Asthma may be intensified.
Gastrointestinal	Changes that may occur include constipation, increase or decrease in appetite, and carbohydrate cravings, particularly for sugar and chocolate.
Miscellaneous	Other symptoms include edema, weight gain, backache, enuresis, oliguria, capillary fragility, exacerbations of dermatologic disease, breast changes, and eye complaints.

Four major symptom patterns of PMS have been identified.

PMS-A. Among women with PMS, 80% have symptoms characteristic of PMS-A. Symptoms are predominantly anxiety-related, and are associated with excess estrogen as well as CNS stimulation that results in feelings of anxiety. High estrogen levels may be related to a deficiency in progesterone or, in other words, a high estrogen-to-progesterone ratio. It may also be related to the body's inability to break down estrogen, which may be due to poor liver function or vitamin B deficiency.

PMS-H. PMS-H affects about 60% of women with PMS. Here, signs and symptoms are predominantly hyperhydration (bloating and edema), increased levels of adrenocorticotropic hormone (ACTH), and increased water- and salt-saving activities in the kidneys.

PMS-C. For 40% of women with PMS, the symptom picture is dominated by carbohydrate cravings due to increased responsiveness to insulin.

PMS-D. About 5% of PMS sufferers are primarily affected by depression related to excess progesterone, which causes CNS depression.

Treatment of PMS

Note that the herbal treatment guidelines given here consist of two components, a daily prescription for working on hormonal issues and a combination to address acute PMS symptoms.

Actions Indicated

Nervines usually alleviate symptoms, but rarely clear the recurrent pattern.

Antispasmodics ease any accompanying dysmenorrhea.

Diuretics are indicated if water retention is part of the picture.

Hormonal normalizers are indicated if the diagnosis suggests that hormonal imbalance is making a pivotal contribution to PMS.

Specific Remedies

Different remedies may act as specifics for specific women, so it is difficult to generalize. From my clinical experience, I suggest that *Scutellaria lateriflora*, in the short term, is as close as possible to a specific for symptomatic relief. Longer-term specifics are likely to be hormonally focused remedies, such as *Vitex agnus-castus*.

A Prescription for Acute PMS Symptoms

Scutellaria lateriflora	2 parts
Valeriana officinalis	1 part
Taraxacum officinale leaf	1 part

Dosage: 5ml of tincture as needed to alleviate symptoms

The dosage of this symptomatic medication may be increased until the desired relief is experienced. The regimen may be altered as necessary, varying time of day and quantity of dose to suit the individual's needs. For example, she may take the entire dose first thing in the morning or smaller amounts at frequent intervals throughout the day. The woman's experience is the guiding principle here. Always treat the human being, not the theory about the condition.

A Supportive Prescription to Normalize Hormone Levels

Vitex agnus-castus	2 parts
Cimicifuga racemosa	1 part

Dosage: 5ml of tincture once a day throughout cycle. Use this prescription in combination with prescription for symptomatic relief given earlier.

Table 18.6. Actions Supplied by Two PMS Formulas

ACTION	HERBS
Nervine	*Scutellaria lateriflora, Valeriana officinalis, Cimicifuga racemosa*
Antispasmodic	*Scutellaria lateriflora, Valeriana officinalis, Cimicifuga racemosa*
Diuretic	*Taraxacum officinale* leaf
Uterine tonic	*Cimicifuga racemosa, Vitex agnus-castus*
Hormonal normalizer	*Vitex agnus-castus*

If water retention is the predominant symptom, then focus more on diuretics. Palpitations would suggest that *Leonurus cardiaca* is relevant. As an example of how this basic approach can be modified to address specific symptoms, consider the following.

A Prescription for PMS Associated with Transitory Skin Problems

Scutellaria lateriflora	2 parts
Pulsatilla vulgaris	1 part
Galium aparine	1 part
Taraxacum officinale leaf	1 part

Dosage: 5 ml of tincture as needed to alleviate symptoms. Use in combination with Prescription to Normalize Hormone Levels, given earlier.

Table 18.7. Actions Supplied by Prescriptions to Normalize Hormone Levels and for PMS with Skin Problems

ACTION	HERBS
Nervine	*Scutellaria lateriflora, Pulsatilla vulgaris, Cimicifuga racemosa*
Antispasmodic	*Scutellaria lateriflora, Pulsatilla vulgaris, Cimicifuga racemosa*
Diuretic	*Taraxacum officinale* leaf, *Galium aparine*
Alterative	*Galium aparine, Pulsatilla vulgaris*
Uterine tonic	*Cimicifuga racemosa, Vitex agnus-castus*
Hormonal normalizer	*Vitex agnus-castus*

Broader Context of Treatment

The holistic practitioner must focus on a whole gamut of relevant issues. Herbal treatment can be exceptionally effective, but the individual will also benefit from appropriate stress management techniques and possibly dietary support. A number of dietary guidelines are relevant:

Limit refined sugar, as it increases excretion of B vitamins, magnesium, and chromium and contributes to increased insulin secretion.

Limit salt to less than 3 g/day.

Limit consumption of red meat to 3 ounces a day because of its high sodium and fat content. Some evidence shows that residual hormones in red meat contribute to fibrocystic breast disease and menstrual cramps.

Limit alcohol to 1 ounce per day. Alcohol destroys B vitamins, magnesium, and chromium, and can be a potent depressant for some people.

Limit caffeine, as it intensifies anxiety and contributes to fibrocystic breast disease.

Limit dairy products. They are high in fat, interfere with magnesium absorption, and may cause constipation.

Limit fat intake to 30% of total calories.

Limit the consumption of cold foods.

Limit protein intake to 1 g/kg of body weight.

Avoid licorice. Licorice stimulates the production of aldosterone.

Minimize the consumption of oxalates, including spinach and beet greens, as they interfere with mineral absorption.

Increase complex carbohydrates to 40% of diet by adding more whole grains, leafy green vegetables, and legumes. These foods are high in fiber and B vitamins and release sugar slowly.

Increase potassium-rich foods, including sunflower seeds, dates, figs, peaches, bananas, and tomatoes. These may help prevent water retention.

Increase intake of natural diuretics, which include artichokes, asparagus, parsley, and watercress.

Researcher David Horrobin advocates the use of gamma linolenic acid (GLA). GLA is found naturally in human milk, evening primrose oil, and a few other plant oils. (See chapter 5 for more information.) Other nutrients that encourage the conversion of fatty acids to prostaglandin E_1 are magnesium, vitamin B_6, zinc, niacin, and vitamin C.

MENOPAUSE

The physiological cessation of menses as a result of decreasing ovarian function. (The Merck Manual)

Menopause is one of the major rites of human passage. In our society, however, far too many women approach menopause with dread, fearing that they will no longer be valued as women. This is a time of change in a woman's role as mother, lover, wife. However, because people have the unfortunate tendency to use their socially defined roles to create their self-images, the changes brought by menopause may be perceived in terms of loss.

On the other hand, menopause may also be viewed as a great gift in a woman's life, a liberation and an initiation. It presents an opportunity to reevaluate one's purpose in life and to change in positive ways. Women who celebrate menopause see change not as something to fear, but as an opportunity to embrace what the next stage of life will bring, to move on to greater fulfillment. It might even be said that part of the problem with the male leaders of our world is that they don't experience the gift of menopause!

Climacteric and Menopause

Menopause is the cessation of menstruation and the termination of fertility, which are not the same thing and may occur at different times. Climacteric is a transition phase that lasts for 15 to 20 years, during which time ovarian function and hormone production decline and the body readapts. Menopause is simply one event within this process.

Grasping the difference between these two natural processes is important, as it is the key to successful treatment of problems that might arise as these events unfold. Neither menopause nor climacteric is a health problem, but rather a natural part of the process of human life. Either may be accompanied by problems, and these should be addressed, but assumptions about our humanness and the role of women are as much a problem here as the biology of the process.

Advancing age brings with it inexorable changes in ovarian and menstrual function. The average length of a woman's monthly cycle gradually shortens from about 28 days at age 20 to a little longer than 26 days at age 40. At this point, the ovaries begin to lose their ability to produce mature eggs, as well as estrogen and progesterone. Thus, there is a sharp drop in fertility for women over the age of 40. The regular intervals between periods that typify menstruation for most women become interspersed with increasing numbers of cycles of shorter and longer duration. Finally, the interval between periods lengthens and menstruation ceases.

For several years before menopause, the decline in ovarian hormone production brings changes in physiology that are expressed as a variety of discomforting signs and symptoms. The years of progressive ovarian failure that lead up to menopause, a time of great emotional as well as physical adjustment, are what are referred to as the climacteric, or "change of life." In the United States, the majority of women experience menopause between the ages of 40 and 55, and the average age of menopause is 51 years.

Table 18.8 presents a comparison of menopause and climacteric, as well as other factors that affect the whole process.

Table 18.8. Differences between Menopause and Climacteric

MENOPAUSE	CLIMACTERIC
Counterpart of menarche	Counterpart of puberty
One biological event	A series of changes
Cessation of periods	Transition period in which ovarian function and hormone production decline
Termination of fertility	
Lasts 1 to 7 years	Lasts 15 to 20 years
Occurs between ages 48 and 52	Occurs between ages 40 and 60

Physical Changes after Menopause

Some atrophy of vagina, cervix, uterus, and ovaries occurs.
Vaginal wall shortens, thins, and loses muscle tone.
Labia majora become thinner, paler, less elastic.
Supporting structures lose muscle tone (sphincter muscles, bladder, rectum).
Secretion of cervical mucus is reduced.
Breast size, firmness, and shape change.
Body hair thins in most women, but increases in some.
Wrinkling and loss of skin tone occur.
Body fat is redistributed.
Bone mass is lost.
Metabolic rate slows.

Hot Flashes

The most common symptom caused by the menopausal decline in estrogen secretion is hot flashes, or flushing, described as feelings of warmth and sweating. About 85%

of women over the age of 50 are affected. The onset is sudden, and when associated with palpitations, dizziness, or faintness, they can be a frightening experience. Emotional stress, exercise, alcohol, and certain foods can bring them on for some individuals. Typically, hot flashes occur several times a day and last a few minutes at a time. *Vitex agnus-castus* is an effective remedy for this often distressing symptom.

Insomnia, Fatigue, and Depression

Menopause is often a time of emotional upheaval. Depression, insomnia, anxiety, and questions about self-worth and sexual adequacy may develop, as attention is drawn to physical ailments and declining health. The problem may be compounded by fears about what to expect from menopause. Other contributing factors may be marital discord and changes in family relationships that occur as the children mature, become more independent, and leave home.

Although some women note that their desire for sexual activity wanes after menopause, decreased estrogen secretion has no direct effect on libido. As long as vaginal symptoms are effectively treated, there is no reason why postmenopausal women should not be able to enjoy a satisfying sex life. In general, the emotional symptoms associated with menopause are caused by situational factors, not hormone deficiencies.

Genitourinary Symptoms

A variety of genital and urinary symptoms may develop during the climacteric. Falling hormone levels cause the vaginal tissues to shrink and atrophy, and there is a loss of support related to weakening of the pelvic tissues. Especially in women who have borne multiple children, the relaxation of the supporting tissues may be severe enough to allow the uterus to prolapse (drop down) into the vagina. With decreased production of natural lubricating substances, the vagina becomes dry and irritated. Itching and dyspareunia (painful sexual intercourse) may result.

Hypertension and Atherosclerosis

Heart disease and "hardening of the arteries" are less prevalent among premenstrual women than they are among men. However, in the years after menopause, these differences between the sexes gradually disappear. Similarly, women who have their ovaries surgically removed prior to natural menopause are known to have a higher incidence of heart attack and atherosclerosis.

While estrogen deficiency is believed to play a role in the development of atherosclerotic heart disease, postmenopausal estrogen replacement therapy has not yet been proved to be of benefit for this indication.

Osteoporosis

This disorder is characterized by a slow, progressive thinning and loss of calcium content of the bones. Although the process actually begins in the fourth decade in both sexes, it is accelerated in women after menopause. Thin, white, inactive female smokers are predisposed to osteoporosis. With time, their bones become brittle and more susceptible to fractures from seemingly minor injuries. When the disease is advanced, even coughing, sudden movements, or everyday activities may cause a bone to break. Wrist and hip fractures and collapse of the spinal vertebrae are especially common. The latter results in a loss of height and a forward curvature of the spine.

Estrogen deficiency plays a role in postmenopausal osteoporosis by diminishing the intestinal absorption of calcium. In addition, it increases the loss of calcium from the skeleton. Other hormonal factors are also known to be important.

Treatment of Menopausal Complaints

As discussed, while menopause and climacteric are not diseases, a series of specific symptomatic problems may arise throughout the process. In addition, other health problems may be compounded. These should be approached within the context of treating particular symptoms while supporting the menopausal changes.

In terms of tonic support, the reproductive, endocrine, nervous, and cardiovascular systems should all be taken into consideration. Of course, there is also a fundamental need for uterine tonics.

Actions Indicated

Hormonal normalizers will help the body's endocrine control mechanisms balance activity in the face of the menopausal changes.

Uterine tonics help the various organs and tissues involved move through the changes with minimal trauma.

Nervine relaxants are indicated for the anxiety and tension that often accompany menopausal changes. Of course, the nervines will ideally also be tonics.

Antidepressants will be needed if the woman experiences depression.

Bitters help in a generalized way as stimulants. These may be taken as part of the diet.

Specific Remedies

In European herbalism, *Vitex agnus-castus* and *Hypericum perforatum* have a reputation for easing the symptomatic distress that may accompany this natural process. *H. perforatum* may help lessen any depression that might occur. *Leonurus cardiaca* can help with the distressing tachycardia that often accompanies hot flashes.

In North American herbalism, *Cimicifuga racemosa* and *Senecio aureus* seem to play a similar role as potential specifics. It is worth noting that Lydia Pinkham's Compound Elixir, a women's tonic popular in the 19th century, originally contained the following herbs:

Aletris farinosa (unicorn root)
Asclepias tuberosa (pleurisy root)
Cimicifuga racemosa (black cohosh)
Senecio aureus (life root)
Trigonella foenum-graecum (fenugreek seed)

Today, there is much emphasis on isoflavone-rich herbs such as *Trifolium pratense* (red clover) and *Glycine max* (soy). Such phytoestrogen-containing herbs may have much to offer, but their use is not based on long-standing herbal experience. At best, it is based on theoretical considerations; and at worst, on marketing hype.

A Prescription for Easing Menopause Symptoms

Vitex agnus-castus	2 parts
Hypericum perforatum	1 part
Cimicifuga racemosa	1 part

Dosage: 5 ml of tincture three times a day

Table 18.9. Actions Supplied by Prescription for Menopause Symptoms

ACTION	HERBS
Hormonal normalizer	*Vitex agnus-castus*
Uterine tonic	*Cimicifuga racemosa*
Nervine relaxant and tonic	*Hypericum perforatum*
Antidepressant	*Hypericum perforatum*

A Prescription for Menopause Symptoms with Anxiety and Tachycardia

Vitex agnus-castus	2 parts
Leonurus cardiaca	2 parts
Hypericum perforatum	1 part
Cimicifuga racemosa	1 part

Dosage: up to 5 ml of tincture three times a day

Table 18.10. Actions Supplied by Prescription for Menopause Symptoms with Anxiety and Tachycardia

ACTION	HERBS
Hormonal normalizer	*Vitex agnus-castus*
Uterine tonic	*Cimicifuga racemosa*
Relaxing nervine	*Cimicifuga racemosa, Hypericum perforatum*
Antidepressant	*Hypericum perforatum*

Broader Context of Treatment

A number of excellent books explore holistic approaches to menopausal problems. Rather than try to duplicate such work, I suggest you refer to the bibliography for books I recommend as further reading.

PREGNANCY

Several herbs have been famous throughout history for preparing mothers for childbirth. Herbs can shorten labor and decrease the likelihood that complications will arise during pregnancy and in childbirth. The most widely used of these in Europe is raspberry leaf (*Rubus idaeus*). In a British medical journal, one doctor said of raspberry leaf tea,

> Somewhat shamefacedly I have encouraged expectant mothers to drink this infusion. In a great many cases labor has been free and easy from muscular spasm.[1]

Rubus idaeus leaf has a mildly soothing astringent and tonic action. The herb helps to quell nausea and is slightly sedative. Most important, it has a particular affinity for the uterus, and acts to strengthen the uterine and pelvic muscles and prevent miscarriage. In the uterus, the action of raspberry leaves is both relaxant and astringent. The relaxant properties tend to predominate and bring about tonic relaxation of the smooth muscle of the uterus, helping to reduce the pain of uterine contractions at labor. In addition, raspberry leaf tones the mucous membranes throughout the body, soothes the kidneys and urinary tract, and helps prevent hemorrhage.

Raspberry leaf has been principally used before delivery to encourage safe, easy, and speedy childbirth, and after delivery to improve milk production and speed recovery from birth.

Herbs to Avoid during Pregnancy

A literature search for plants traditionally used around the world for abortifacient or uterine stimulant actions yields a long list of plants to avoid. According to authors der Marderosian and Liberti, in *Natural Product Medicine*, 565 species from 125 families have such effects.[2] These otherwise extremely useful remedies often share chemistry that in some way irritates the placenta or causes muscular contractions in the uterus. If we limit ourselves to those plants most often encountered in Western phytotherapy, we can identify the following groupings of plants to avoid in pregnancy.

Bitters

Because bitters stimulate metabolism in general, and some bitters also act as emmenagogues to stimulate smooth muscle activity, it should be clear that bitters are contraindicated during pregnancy. All strong bitters should be excluded, particularly the following:

Aloe vera (aloe)
Artemisia abrotanum (southernwood)
A. absinthium (wormwood)
Berberis vulgaris (barberry)
Chelidonium majus (celandine)
Hydrastis canadensis (goldenseal)
Ruta graveolens (rue)
Tanacetum parthenium (feverfew)
T. vulgare (tansy)

Alkaloid-Containing Plants

Alkaloids are a diverse group of secondary plant constituents that have a wide range of pharmacological effects upon the body. The stronger representatives should be avoided during pregnancy, including the caffeine-containing social drugs coffee and tea. Some plants to avoid are:

Berberis vulgaris (barberry)
Cephaelis ipecacuanha (ipecac)
Colchicum autumnale (autumn crocus)
Cytisus scoparius (Scotch broom)
Hydrastis canadensis (goldenseal)
Lobelia inflata (lobelia)
Podophyllum peltatum (mayapple)
Sanguinaria canadensis (bloodroot)

Volatile Oil–Containing Plants

Many essential oils can have a devastating impact on the placenta and fetus if taken internally during pregnancy. Pregnant women should avoid taking all volatile oils internally. However, if used in moderation, the whole plant from which the oil was distilled will usually be fine. Important exceptions are:

Juniperus communis (juniper)
Mentha pulegium (pennyroyal)
Myristica officinalis (nutmeg, in large amounts)
Thuja occidentalis (thuja)

Strong Laxatives

The strong herbal laxatives often, but not always, owe their effects to the presence of anthraquinone constituents that stimulate peristalsis in the bowel. They may have a similar stimulating impact upon the uterus. If a laxative is needed during pregnancy, it should be either a bulk or a hepatic laxative. However, standardized senna products designed for use during pregnancy may be safe. Please refer to chapters 7 and 10 for more information on anthraquinone-containing laxatives, and 13 for more information on other types of laxatives.

Aloe vera (aloe)
Juglans cinerea (butternut)
Rhamnus cathartica (purging buckthorn)
R. frangula (buckthorn)
R. purshiana (cascara sagrada)
Rheum palmatum (Chinese rhubarb)
Senna alexandrina (senna)

Other Herbs to Avoid in Pregnancy

Other plants to be avoided do not fit into convenient categories; some are listed here. Anthelmintic remedies, for example, should be avoided because they often stimulate uterine contractions, as well as containing potentially toxic constituents. Male fern is an example of an anthelmintic remedy for the treatment of worm infestations.

Cinchona spp. (quinine)
Convallaria majalis (lily of the valley)
Dryopteris filix-mas (male fern)
Gossypium herbaceum (cotton)
Phytolacca spp. (poke)
Stillingia sylvatica (queen's delight)
Vinca spp. (periwinkle)
Viscum album (mistletoe)

Pregnancy Warnings from Botanical Safety Handbook

The following herbs are listed in the *Botanical Safety Handbook* as "not to be used during pregnancy unless otherwise directed by an expert qualified in the appropriate use of this substance."[3] Unfortunately, the authors do not adequately clarify whether inclusion in this safety category is based on actual clinical records or on theoretical extrapolation from in vitro studies on constituents. This limits the value of an otherwise excellent book.

Achillea millefolium
Achyranthes bidentata
Acorus calamus
A. gramineus
Adiantum pedatum
Agathosma betulina
A. crenulata
A. serratifolia
Albizia julibrissin
Alkanna tinctoria
Aloe ferox
A. perryi
A. vera
Andrographis paniculata
Angelica archangelica
A. atropurpurea
A. sinensis
Anthriscus cerefolium
Apium graveolens
Aralia californica
A. nudicaulis
A. racemosa
Arctostaphylos uva-ursi
Arisaema japonicum
Aristolochia clematitis
A. contorta
A. debilis
A. serpentaria
Arnica spp.
Artemisia abrotanum
A. absinthium
A. annua
A. capillaris
A. douglasiana
A. lactiflora
A. scoparia
A. vulgaris
Asarum canadense
A. europaeum
A. heteropides
A. sieboldii
Asclepias asperula
A. tuberosa
Baptisia tinctoria
Berberis vulgaris

Borago officinalis
Capsella bursa-pastoris
Carthamus tinctorius
Caulophyllum thalictroides
Cephaelis ipecacuanha
Chamaelirium luteum
Chamaemelum nobile
Changium smyrnoides
Chelidonium majus
Cimicifuga racemosa
Cinchona calisaya
C. ledgeriana
C. officinalis
C. pubescens
Cinnamomum camphora
C. cassia
C. verum
Cnicus benedictus
Coffea arabica
Cola acuminata
C. nitida
Commiphora madagascariensis
C. molmol
C. mukul
C. myrrha
Coptis chinensis
C. groenlandica
Corydalis yanhusuo
Crocus sativus
Cullen corylifolia
Cuphea balsamona
Curcuma aromatica
C. domestica
C. longa
C. zedoaria
Cyathula officinalis
Cymbopogon citratus
Daucus carota
Dryopteris filix-mas
Ephedra distachya
E. equisetina
E. gerardiana
E. intermedia
E. sinica
Equisetum hyemale
Eschscholzia californica
Eupatorium purpureum
Ferula assa-foetida
F. foetida
F. rubricaulis

Forsythia suspensa
Fouquieria splendens
Fritillaria cirrhosa
F. thunbergii
Fucus vesiculosus
Genista tinctoria
Glycyrrhiza echinata
G. glabra
G. uralensis
Gossypium herbaceum
G. hirsutum
Hedeoma pulegioides
Hepatica nobilis
Hordeum vulgare
Hydrastis canadensis
Hyssopus officinalis
Inula helenium
Iris versicolor
I. virginica
Juniperus communis
J. monosperma
J. osteosperma
J. oxycedrus
J. virginiana
Leonurus cardiaca
L. heterophyllus
L. sibiricus
Leptandra virginica
Levisticum officinale
Ligusticum chuanxiong
L. porteri
Lobelia inflata
L. siphilitica
Lomatium dissectum
Lycium barbarum
L. chinense
Lycopus americanus
L. europaeus
L. virginicus
Magnolia officinalis
Mahonia aquifolium
M. nervosa
M. repens
Marrubium vulgare
Mentha pulegium
Monarda clinopodia
M. didyma
M. fistulosa
M. pectinata
M. punctata

Myristica fragrans
Nardostachys jatamansi
Nasturtium officinale
Nepeta cataria
Paeonia suffruticosa
Panax notoginseng
Petroselinum crispum
Phellodendron amurense
P. chinense
Picrasma excelsa
Pilocarpus jaborandi
P. microphyllus
P. pennatifolius
Pimpinella anisum
Pinellia ternata
Podophyllum hexandrum
P. peltatum
Polygala senega
Portulaca oleracea
Prunus persica
Quassia amara
Rhamnus cathartica
R. frangula
R. purshiana
Rheum officinale
R. palmatum
R. tanguticum
Ricinus communis
Rosmarinus officinalis
Ruta graveolens
Salvia officinalis
Sanguinaria canadensis
Senna alexandrina
S. obtusifolia
S. tora
Symphytum officinale
Tanacetum parthenium
T. vulgare
Thuja occidentalis
Trichosanthes kirilowii
Trifolium pratense
Trigonella foenum-graecum
Trillium erectum
Tussilago farfara
Verbena hastata
V. officinalis
Vetiveria zizanoides
Vitex agnus-castus
Withania somnifera
Zanthoxylum americanum

Z. bungeanum
Z. clava-herculis
Z. schinifolium
Z. simulans
Zingiber officinale
Ziziphus spinosa

THE FIRST TRIMESTER

Counting from the first day of a woman's last menstrual period, pregnancy typically lasts 40 weeks and is often referred to in three parts, called *trimesters*. The first trimester lasts until week 12, the second spans week 13 to the end of week 27, and the third encompasses weeks 28 to 40. These divisions, however, are arbitrary. The first trimester is a time of profound changes inside the body, but the experience is very individual. For example, for one woman, the first trimester may bring increased energy and a sense of well-being, but another woman might feel increasingly tired and emotional. Still others don't notice many changes until much later in pregnancy.

Although the physical changes of early pregnancy can be uncomfortable, they almost never endanger either mother or baby's health. A number of common symptoms occur, but not all women will experience them. They include fatigue, nausea and vomiting, urinary frequency, breast tenderness, headaches, dizziness, and weight gain.

Threatened Miscarriage

For those who have suffered miscarriages in the past, herbs may prove effective in preventing repeated miscarriages. Herbs can help as long as the fetus is normal and the mother's general physical, emotional, and mental health is good. On the other hand, no herbal remedy will block appropriate miscarriage. Most cases of miscarriage are a natural rejection of a malformed fetus.

When miscarriage occurs more than once in the same woman, however, it may be related to a problem in her body, rather than the baby's. In a case like this, it is especially important to build up her general health as well as that of her partner before they attempt to conceive again. To ensure fewer complications, women should take at least 6 to 12 months between pregnancies.

When chronic poor health, inadequate diet, or trauma and stress of any kind has depleted a woman's general strength, herbs can provide extra vitality, especially to the womb, and so help avoid unnecessary miscarriage. If cramping abdominal pains or bleeding occur, medical attention is needed immediately.

Specific Remedies

A number of plants have a well-deserved reputation for preventing miscarriage. It may be significant that two of them are now endangered species; these will not be discussed. Other important plants are listed here:

Dioscorea villosa (wild yam)
Viburnum opulus (cramp bark)
V. prunifolium (black haw)

Other plants that have been widely used to prevent miscarriage are *Rosmarinus officinalis* (rosemary), *Rubus idaeus* (raspberry leaf), *Crataegus laevigata* (hawthorn), *Mitchella repens* (partridgeberry), *Leonurus cardiaca* (motherwort), *Allium sativum* (garlic), and *Trigonella foenumgraecum* (fenugreek).

A Prescription to Help Prevent Miscarriage

Viburnum prunifolium	1 part
Cimicifuga racemosa	1 part

Dosage: 2.5 ml of tincture three times a day, building up to 5 ml three times a day

---

Table 18.11. Actions Supplied by Prescription to Help Prevent Miscarriage

ACTION	HERB
Uterine tonic	*Viburnum prunifolium, Cimicifuga racemosa*
Nervine relaxant	*Viburnum prunifolium, Cimicifuga racemosa*
Antispasmodic	*Viburnum prunifolium, Cimicifuga racemosa*

Broader Context of Treatment

The woman should eat plenty of foods containing vitamins E and C. Asparagus and celery are said to be strengthening.

Morning Sickness

Morning sickness refers to the nausea and vomiting some women experience when they become pregnant. It is caused by the sudden increase in hormone levels during pregnancy. Although morning sickness is more common in the morning, it can last all day for some women. It is very common early in pregnancy, but tends to go away later, and is almost always gone by the second trimester (the fourth month). However, there is no set time for it to stop, because each woman and each pregnancy is different. Morning sickness is seen in about 50% of pregnancies, and tends to worsen with each successive pregnancy.

The exact cause of morning sickness is not known, but various theories have been proposed. One suggests that the rapid change in hormone levels in early pregnancy and the resultant high levels of progesterone may stimulate the vomit center in the brain. Progesterone relaxes smooth muscle throughout the body, including arterial smooth muscle, and this produces a drop in blood pressure, which may account for the tiredness and lethargy associated with the nausea and vomiting.

During the first 12 to 14 weeks of pregnancy, when most women experience sickness, the hormones are primarily produced in the corpus luteum in the ovaries. After this time, hormone production shifts to the placenta, which may help explain why morning sickness stops at around the same time (12 to 14 weeks). Sickness may also be related to low blood pressure; high progesterone levels may interfere with adequate circulation of blood to the brain, especially upon rising. Getting up slowly will help to relieve this.

Another theory holds that morning sickness is associated with low blood sugar, which normally occurs in early pregnancy. Elevating blood sugar levels by eating small, frequent meals may help. However, low-sugar foods should be emphasized, as sugar in the stomach can aggravate nausea.

There are no general rules for treating morning sickness, as the causes vary from one woman to another. Treatment should aim at what appears to be the underlying cause. Antiemetics are important, as they will calm the vomit reflex, no matter what the cause of morning sickness. Valuable antiemetics that are safe to use in early pregnancy are:

Ballota nigra (black horehound)
Filipendula ulmaria (meadowsweet)
Gentiana lutea (gentian)
Rosmarinus officinalis (rosemary)

In addition, many of the herbs that aid digestion will help. The carminative, antispasmodic, and relaxing nervines are especially important:

Cinnamomum aromaticum (cinnamon bark)
Dioscorea villosa (wild yam)
Foeniculum vulgare (fennel seed)
Humulus lupulus (hops)
Lavandula spp. (lavender)
Matricaria recutita (chamomile)
Melissa officinalis (lemon balm)
Mentha piperita (peppermint)
Rubus idaeus (raspberry leaf)
Syzygium aromaticum (clove)
Zingiber officinale (gingerroot)

Mucilage-rich demulcents such as *Chondrus crispus* (Iceland moss) and *Ulmus rubra* (slippery elm) help soothe the whole of the digestive tract. Both of these herbs are highly nutritious, containing many minerals and trace elements. They are also easily digested, ideal for conditions associated with weakness of the stomach.

A Prescription for Morning Sickness

Zingiber officinale	1 part
Dioscorea villosa	1 part
Ballota nigra	1 part

Dosage: 2.5 ml of tincture at night and in the morning, building up to 5 ml if needed

---

A Supplemental Infusion for Morning Sickness

Mentha piperita	1 part
Matricaria recutita	1 part

Dosage: Infuse 1 teaspoon of dried herb mixture in 1 cup of boiling water. Drink often during the day.

Broader Context of Treatment

Eat numerous small meals throughout the day, rather than three large meals.
Avoid foods and odors that bring on symptoms.
Eat small starchy snacks, such as crackers, in bed before arising.
Maintain electrolyte balance if vomiting is severe.
Vitamin B$_6$: 100 mg to 300mg/day

Constipation

High levels of progesterone relax the intestinal muscles, and thus reduce their ability to propel the contents of the bowel toward the rectum and out of the body. In addition, as pregnancy progresses, the weight of the baby and placenta increases, and the pressure they exert on the lower bowel aggravates the tendency to constipation. When the enlarged uterus impedes circulation to the bowel, the action of the intestinal muscles is also restricted. Similarly, tension and anxiety experienced by the pregnant woman also impair the action of these muscles. Other factors that can cause or exacerbate constipation during pregnancy are consumption of iron supplements and starchy meals consisting of refined flour products.

As already noted, anthraquinone-containing stimulant laxatives are not safe for use during pregnancy. Aim for gentle therapy, utilizing the following treatment considerations and the guidelines given in chapter 13.

Increase water intake to 8 glasses per day.

Increase exercise. Walking half a mile a day is an appropriate activity.

Increase intake of fresh fruits and certain dried fruits, such as prunes, raisins, and figs.

Increase fiber intake.

Use bulk laxatives, such as psyllium seeds. Take 1 tablespoon three times a day in ¼ cup of juice.

Varicose Veins

To return blood to the heart, the veins in the legs must work against gravity. This is accomplished by muscle contractions in the lower legs, which act as pumps. These muscles are toned, elastic vein walls and tiny one-way valves in the veins. The valves open as blood flows toward the heart and close to stop blood from flowing backward. Varicose veins occur when these valves malfunction, causing the blood that should be moving toward the heart to flow backward. Blood pools in the veins, and they enlarge and become varicose.

The developing fetus may become a source of physical resistance to the easy return of blood to the trunk, thus promoting the development of varicose veins. These may occur early in pregnancy but generally worsen as the pregnancy advances. Symptoms vary from painless, cosmetically problematic areas to varicosities causing mild or severe pain. Sometimes, a varicosity may occur in the labia majora. For more details on the herbal treatment of varicosities, please see chapter 14.

Fatigue and Somnolence

Some pregnant women require excessive periods of rest or sleep during the first trimester. It is normal for sleep requirements to be as great as 18 hours a day. If the woman is not working or attending school and does not have young children, she should sleep whenever possible. Ingestion of protein may help alleviate this symptom.

Some women become depressed at their inability to continue the normal pace of daily activity established before pregnancy. They should be counseled that this symptom usually completely resolves by the fourth month of gestation. Blood studies should be performed to rule out anemia. Avoid herbal stimulants, neurological or metabolic.

Anemia

Prevention of anemia is a most important aspect of antenatal care. Hemoglobin, the iron and protein compound contained in erythrocytes (red blood cells), is responsible for transporting oxygen from the lungs to all parts of the body, including the placenta and fetus. If hemoglobin levels fall, the body's ability to access oxygen falls accordingly.

During pregnancy, the blood volume increases at a faster rate than the erythrocytes multiply, so the erythrocytes are diluted by extra fluid. Hemoglobin carried by erythrocytes drops from about 11 g to approximately 1 g. Hemoglobin levels less than 1 g constitute anemia. Symptoms of anemia include lethargy, irritability, and breathlessness on slight exertion. Anemia commonly occurs during the last two months of pregnancy, when the baby utilizes a high proportion of the mother's iron. A history of menorrhagia also suggests that iron reserves might be low. Building up iron reserves before pregnancy starts is beneficial and can help the mother meet the increased iron demand without any problems.

The best approach is to increase dietary intake of iron-containing foods, as iron supplements may aggravate constipation. All iron-containing foods are better absorbed in the presence of an animal protein. Vitamin C also enhances iron absorption. Watercress, rose hips, blackberries, black currants, elderberries, parsley, spinach, dandelion leaves, and many other plant foods contain both iron and vitamin C, and natural iron never causes constipation.

Liver is a good source of iron; however, it should come from organically produced meat only. Because the liver is the detoxifying organ of mammals, it may contain chemical residues if factory reared.

Good Sources of Iron
Liver
Eggs from free-range chickens
Dairy products
Watercress
Dried apricots
Whole-wheat bread
Cocoa and carob
Cabbage
Alfalfa
Beets
Cherries
Raisins
Brown rice
Kelp
Wheat germ
Sunflower seeds
Parsley
Chicory
Lentils
Black currants, blackberries, strawberries
Spinach

Leafy herbs that can be added to salads, cooked as vegetables, and added to soups include:

Crataegus spp. (hawthorn flowers and leaves)
Rumex acetosa (sorrel)
Symphytum officinale (comfrey leaf, in moderation)
Taraxacum officinale (dandelion leaf)
Urtica dioica (nettle)

Other herbs that contain meaningful levels of iron when used as an infusion or tincture are:

Arctium lappa (burdock leaf)
Crataegus spp. (hawthorn)
Gentian lutea (gentian)
Humulus lupulus (hops)
Rubus idaeus (raspberry leaf)
Rumex crispus (yellow dock)
Scutellaria lateriflora (skullcap)
Verbena officinalis (vervain)

Dizziness

Dizziness caused by the ability of progesterone to relax the blood vessel walls is common in pregnancy. This type of dizziness, seen most frequently in early pregnancy, is a form of postural hypotension. However, hypertensive herbs such as *Cytisus scoparius* (Scotch broom) are too strong for both mother and fetus. Instead, follow these recommendations:

• Change positions slowly.
• Eat small meals throughout the day, rather than three large meals.
• Maintain blood sugar levels.

Heartburn

Heartburn, caused by reflux of gastric contents into the esophagus, is one of the most common complaints of pregnancy. Treatment approaches to this condition are discussed in chapter 13.

The relaxing effects of progesterone also reach the cardiac sphincter, the valve that guards the entrance to the stomach at the bottom of the esophagus. As the enlarging uterus pushes up against the stomach, small amounts of the stomach's contents are passed into the lower esophagus. Hydrochloric acid mixed with stomach contents irritates and burns the esophagus, resulting in an inflammatory process. In more extreme cases, parts of the stomach itself can be pushed up through the diaphragm or into the esophagus, causing some degree of hiatus hernia.

Bleeding Gums

Bleeding gums are frequently seen in pregnancy. Gingival hypertrophy, a temporary softening of the gums, is seen in 40% of pregnancies. This is a response to elevated progesterone levels in the blood. Follow the topical advice given for gingivitis in chapter 13 but *not* the internal treatment. Additional suggestions are:

• Brush gums frequently with a soft brush
• Vitamin C and bioflavonoids complex: up to 2,000 mg/day

Headache

Headache sometimes occurs in early pregnancy, but is worse between three and five months. A few cases may result from eyestrain, as pregnancy may result in a change in the amount of refractive error in the eyes. Some cases may be caused by sinusitis, and frontal headaches are seen with hypertension. Please refer to the section on headaches in chapter 16.

Hemorrhoids

Hemorrhoids may be exacerbated by or occur for the first time during pregnancy. The condition is caused by increased pressure and impairment of return of venous fluid in the veins by the pressure of the enlarging uterus. Constipation makes the problem worse. Congestion of liver function caused by intake of junk foods, refined flour, and alcohol also encourages the problem, as the hemorrhoidal veins are part of the portal drainage system. The treatment approach for this common problem of pregnancy is discussed in chapter 13.

THE SECOND AND THIRD TRIMESTERS

The second trimester consists of the period from the beginning of the 13th week until the end of the 27th week. The third trimester of pregnancy begins at the 28th week and lasts until birth. During the second trimester, the woman will usually experience decreased nausea and better sleep patterns, and have more stamina and energy than during the first trimester. The second trimester is not always trouble-free, however, as a whole new set of symptoms and sensations commonly arise. These include back pain, leg cramps, heartburn, skin changes, and constipation.

Before pregnancy, the uterus weighs about 2 ounces (56 g) and holds a volume of less than half an ounce (15 ml). At term, in addition to the weight of the baby, it weighs about 2½ pounds (a little more than 1 kg) and will have stretched to hold the baby, the placenta, and about

1 quart (approximately 1 liter) of amniotic fluid. Many of the physical symptoms of late pregnancy arise from this increase in uterine size. These may include shortness of breath, sleeping problems, varicose veins, skin changes, and hemorrhoids.

Stretch Marks

Stretch marks occur when the skin is stretched beyond its normal capacity and elasticity. In pregnancy, they are related to progesterone's softening effect on connective tissue combined with rapid weight gain. When new, stretch marks resemble purple *striae* (streaks), and after a period of time they resemble silvery scars. Genetic predisposition is the predominant factor in the development of stretch marks. The tendency to develop stretch marks can be lessened by eating appropriately and using remedies to address collagen problems in the skin.

Vitamins E, C, and B$_5$ (pantothenic acid) can help, as may zinc. These can all be obtained from the diet. In *The Herbal for Pregnancy and Childbirth*, Anne McIntyre recommends increasing consumption of the following foods:[4]

Sunflower seeds and oil
Pumpkin seeds
Wheat germ
Onions
Eggs
Lettuce
Cucumbers
Cabbage
Radishes
Horseradish
Rice bran
Asparagus
Parsnips
Brewer's yeast
Whole grains
Fish
Alfalfa
Molasses

Massaging wheat germ or vitamin E oil into the breasts, abdomen, and thighs daily will reduce the likelihood that marks will develop. *Calendula* oil mixed with wheat germ oil is especially helpful.

Backache

Elevated progesterone levels during pregnancy have a softening effect upon tendons and ligaments throughout the body, which allows them to expand as necessary to accommodate the growing baby. The spine is particularly affected, and the relaxation of the ligaments that support the spine combined with the weight of the growing abdomen often cause backache. The backward-leaning posture adopted by heavily pregnant mothers places added strain on the lower joints of the spine. Bad posture aggravates backache. Rapid weight gain in pregnancy increases strain and may exacerbate symptoms of previous damage to the back.

Yoga exercises may be helpful, and experts recommend certain asanas for pregnancy. Rest is important in preventing or relieving backache, especially in the last three months of pregnancy. Deep breathing and relaxation exercises can also help. Baths with lavender and rosemary essential oils and massage of the whole spine with a mixture of chamomile and geranium essential oils can be effective as well.

Hypertension

Gestational hypertension is characterized by a steady rise in blood pressure after the 28th week of gestation. The general rule for the upper limit of gestational hypertension is 140/90 mm Hg. Some factors that contribute to gestational hypertension are:

- Emotional and physical stress
- Obesity
- Lack of exercise
- Drugs and stimulants
- Diet (processed and heavily salted carbohydrates with inadequate protein intake)

Herbal treatment can do much to mitigate this form of secondary hypertension, but blood pressure must be monitored closely, as it can rise dangerously fast in some situations. Please refer to chapter 14 for more information on the treatment of hypertension. Other approaches that may be helpful include:

Exercise. Exercise forces blood through the vasculature. If it is healthy and flexible, the vasculature will respond by stretching and relaxing. Brisk walking or swimming is recommended. Exercise is most effective when a tendency for hypertension is first noted. It is not appropriate for very elevated blood pressure.

Practice deep relaxation or meditation techniques.

Avoid all stimulants, including caffeine, nicotine, and cocaine. All are linked to hypertension, restriction of blood flow to the placenta, and low-birth-weight babies.

Improve diet. Increase consumption of good-quality protein, vegetables, and fresh fruits.

Increase water intake.

Rest, particularly by lying on the left side.

THE POSTPARTUM PERIOD

The first six weeks of the postpartum period, or the time immediately after birth, is referred to as the *puerperium*. The first two to three days are spent bonding with the baby and waiting for the true milk to come in. True milk usually comes in at about 72 hours after the birth.

Multiparous women, or those who have had a number of children already, will have significantly more intense "after pains," or uterine contractions, to facilitate involution of the uterus to its pre-pregnant state. Early in the puerperium, there is loss of blood and later on discharge from the vagina. Fever and foul discharge indicate uterine infection.

Generally, if a woman does not nurse, she will menstruate six to eight weeks after birth. Nursing women begin to menstruate again at any time from six weeks after birth to two years after birth. However, nursing is not an adequate method of birth control, as most women ovulate before they menstruate, and a woman can become pregnant before her period returns.

After birth, estrogen and progesterone levels decrease. Postpartum depression, discussed later in this chapter, is one result of this hormonal change. Normal physiologic signs of the postpartum decrease in estrogen and progesterone include:

- Hair loss
- Return of acne
- Slowdown in nail growth
- Decrease in libido
- Thinning of the vaginal mucosa
- Increased intensity of PMS

Postpartum Depression

If the woman is lactating, she will secrete prolactin, which is actually stimulated by the sensation caused by the nursing baby. Prolactin is a mild relaxant and depressant. As prolactin levels rise, the elevated levels of estrogen and progesterone maintained throughout the pregnancy drop abruptly. This may lead to *postpartum depression*. Other factors that may contribute to such depression include:

- Emotional letdown following the excitement and fear experienced during pregnancy, labor, and delivery
- Discomforts of the puerperium
- Fatigue due to loss of sleep
- Anxiety over the ability to care for a dependent newborn
- Isolation

Postpartum depression can be treated with an approach similar to that taken for PMS in terms of herbs, diet, supplementation, and exercise. Greater emphasis can be placed on *Artemisia vulgaris* and *Hypericum perforatum*. In addition, it is important to encourage the new mother to go out and enjoy the company of other adults.

Perineal Tears or Extensive Episiotomy

The perineum (the area of skin between the vagina and the anus) may be surgically cut (an episiotomy) or may tear during birth. Usually, these will heal faster if all significant tears are stitched. A number of simple procedures can help alleviate discomfort and speed healing:

Apply ice immediately after the repair is finished to decrease swelling.

Take sitz baths with infusions of vulnerary herbs.

Apply Aloe vera *gel.*

Calendula, Symphytum, Hydrastis, and *Achillea* are all good choices of herbs for ointments or sitz baths.

Expose the area to sunlight to speed healing.

Decrease activity; severe tears heal faster with bed rest.

After Pains or Recurrent Uterine Contractions

For women who have had more than one child, after pains increase in strength with each successive pregnancy. They are helpful in that the contractions are involuting, or returning, the enlarged uterus to its previous size. Nursing will bring on or increase the intensity of these contractions. If necessary, use antispasmodic herbs and uterine tonics, such as *Cimicifuga racemosa* (black cohosh), *Dioscorea villosa* (wild yam), *Viburnum prunifolium* (black haw), and *Viburnum opulus* (cramp bark).

Stimulating Lactation

Herbal remedies called *galactogogues* encourage milk production to begin and increase total milk volume. Important examples are *Galega officinalis* (goat's rue), *Foeniculum vulgare* (fennel seed), and *Cnicus benedictus* (blessed thistle).

In addition to use of galactagogues, here are some other recommendations for increasing milk production:

- Drink plenty of fluid.
- Rest; lack of sleep produces milk shortages.
- Stimulate the nipples by allowing the baby to suck often.
- Helpful foods include apricots, asparagus, green beans, carrots, sweet potatoes, parsley, all leafy greens, and grains.

Stopping Lactation

A number of herbal approaches have been used to reduce milk flow, thus forcing the child to stop breast-feeding. There are no good reasons to stop breast-feeding at a certain time. Cultural ideas about weaning times do not provide much of a rationale, especially in light of the fact that women were discouraged from breast-feeding altogether not that long ago. *Salvia officinalis* does reduce milk flow.

Mastitis

Mastitis is inflammation of the mammary gland, usually caused by infection. Such breast infections are located in the tissue of the breast; the bacteria usually enter through cracks in the nipples. The infection then occurs in the parenchymal (fatty) tissue and causes it to swell. This swelling compresses on the milk ducts, resulting in pain and swelling of the infected breast. Such breast infections usually occur in women who are breast-feeding. The causative bacterium, *Staphylococcus aureus*, is commonly found on normal skin. Breast infections not related to breast-feeding must be differentiated from a rare form of breast cancer.

Mastitis usually occurs when the breasts become very engorged, often as a result of a missed feeding. If a baby who usually wakes up two or three times at night to nurse suddenly sleeps through the night, breast engorgement will occur. Milk that remains in the sacs becomes a breeding ground for bacteria entering through the nipple, and infection will occur. This is particularly likely if the breast has been incompletely emptied and a residual amount of milk remains over time.

In general, the following suggestions will help in the prevention and treatment of mastitis:

• Apply vulnerary and antimicrobial herbs externally, such as *Calendula*.
• Nurse in a relaxed, unhurried, thorough manner.
• Be sure the nipple area stays clean.
• Drink adequate amounts of fluid to flush the system.
• Rest.
• Maintain an adequate diet, decreasing intake of fatty and refined foods.

UTERINE FIBROIDS

Benign uterine tumors of smooth muscle origin. *(The Merck Manual)*

Fibroid tumors are benign muscle tumors that cause enlargement and distortion of the uterus in premenopausal women. They may make menstruation painful and heavy, possibly leading to anemia. Fibroids are the most common reason for hysterectomy, but unless the fibroids are causing significant problems, it is best to avoid such a drastic step. They rarely become malignant. As they depend on the presence of estrogen for their growth, they will shrink at menopause. If surgery is necessary, consider the new laser-based techniques rather than removal of the whole uterus.

Actions Indicated

Uterine tonics support the general health and vitality of the uterus.
Uterine astringents reduce blood loss.
Alteratives often help in health problems associated with benign growths. (I would love to know why!)
Antispasmodics will lessen cramping pains.
Lymphatics support the drainage of fluid from the womb.
Immune support may be appropriate. Please refer to chapter 21.

A Prescription for Uterine Fibroids

Caulophyllum thalictroides	2 parts
Vinca major	2 parts
Vitex agnus-castus	1 part
Cimicifuga racemosa	1 part
Dioscorea villosa	1 part
Galium aparine	1 part

Dosage: 2.5 ml of tincture three times a day. This formula can be made stronger by adding more antispasmodic or astringent remedies.

Table 18.12. Actions Supplied by Prescription for Uterine Fibroids

ACTION	HERBS
Uterine tonic	*Caulophyllum thalictroides, Cimicifuga racemosa*
Uterine astringent	*Vinca major*
Alterative	*Galium aparine, Cimicifuga racemosa, Caulophyllum thalictroides*
Antispasmodic	*Cimicifuga racemosa*
Lymphatic	*Galium aparine*

Broader Context of Treatment

Attention to general health and well-being is vital. Focus on a whole range of issues to ensure that the woman can be as comfortable with her body and life as possible.

Diet. Recommend a well-balanced and nutritious diet rich in fresh green vegetables.

Bodywork. Suggest approaches that will engender an experience of bodily ease and relaxation. This may be aromatherapy massage, walks by the ocean, dancing, and so on.

Peace of mind. Relaxation exercises, meditation, or counseling may be appropriate.

Lifestyle. A reevaluation of work and home environments, relationships, and personal goals will often clarify areas for positive growth and transformation.

ENDOMETRIOSIS

The presence of endometrial tissue in abnormal locations. *(The Merck Manual)*

Endometriosis is the presence of uterine tissue (endometrium) outside its usual location on the inner lining of the uterus. Approximately 5% to 20% of women of childbearing age are affected by this troublesome condition. In addition, it is discovered during as many as 20% to 50% of all gynecologic operations. Pain, abnormal menstrual bleeding, infertility, and prolonged disability may result.

Endometrial tissue may implant itself on the ovaries, fallopian tubes, pelvic ligaments, abdominal organs, old scars, and, in rare cases, the chest, lungs, spinal cord, and extremities. The site of implantation of the endometrial tissue will largely control the degree or severity of symptoms. Over time, the implants may enlarge, bleed, cause scarring, and form tough fibrous adhesions between pelvic and abdominal structures.

A number of predisposing factors have been suggested. Hormonal factors are known to be important. Implants often regress during pregnancy, and first pregnancy at a young age seems to protect against the development of endometriosis. In addition, the disease is more common in women who choose to either postpone or reject childbearing. The average age at diagnosis is 37 years, and the majority of cases occur in women between the ages of 25 and 40 years. Endometriosis is rare before the onset of menstruation and after menopause.

Although the underlying cause is still in question, there are three major theories about the etiology of endometriosis.

1. The transportation theory holds that endometrial tissue that originates in the uterus passes in a retrograde fashion through the fallopian tubes to implant on the ovaries, pelvis, and abdomen at the time of menstruation. Bloodstream and lymph vessel transport may also occur.

2. The second hypothesis suggests that endometriosis occurs at sites outside the uterus in tissues that have the potential for developing into uterine glands.

3. The induction theory combines the above two ideas to suggest that transported endometrial tissue induces the development of endometriosis through direct contact with sites on adjacent organs and structures.

Endometriosis is a notoriously difficult condition to diagnose; the conclusion is often reached only after all other problems have been excluded. Conclusive diagnosis often necessitates exploratory laparoscopy. An estimated 25% to 50% of infertile women have endometriosis. It may be largely asymptomatic, but is also often characterized by the following symptoms:

- Dysmenorrhea, especially if this begins after several years of pain-free menses
- Dyspareunia, or painful sexual intercourse
- Lower abdominal or rectal pain
- Metrorrhagia or menorrhagia

In mild or moderate cases of endometriosis, herbal medication has much to offer, but in severe cases, surgery may be indicated.

Treatment of Endometriosis

The herbal treatment of this often intransigent condition can be quite effective. However, careful selection of herbs is crucial.

Actions Indicated

Hormonal normalizers, such as *Vitex,* appear to help the body alter underlying hormonal problems.

Uterine tonics are essential for their tonic actions on endometrial tissue. In theory, this will help wherever such tissue is.

Antispasmodics ease the muscular, cramping pain that is so distressing in this condition.

Nervine relaxants help with stress and pain.

Specific Remedies

There are no traditional specifics for endometriosis, but *Dioscorea villosa* (wild yam) is almost specific for the pain, although it is not very strong. *Vitex agnus-castus* may be considered the most appropriate remedy for the underlying processes involved.

A Prescription for Endometriosis

Vitex agnus-castus	2 parts
Cimicifuga racemosa	1 part
Dioscorea villosa	1 part
Scutellaria lateriflora	1 part

Dosage: 5 ml of tincture three times a day

Table 18.13. Actions Supplied by Prescription for Endometriosis

ACTION	HERBS
Hormonal normalizer	*Vitex agnus-castus*
Uterine tonic	*Cimicifuga racemosa*
Antispasmodic	*Cimicifuga racemosa, Dioscorea villosa, Scutellaria lateriflora*
Nervine relaxant	*Scutellaria lateriflora, Cimicifuga racemosa, Dioscorea villosa*

FIBROCYSTIC BREAST DISEASE

A condition in which breast pain, cysts, and noncancerous lumpiness occur together. *(The Merck Manual)*

Fibrocystic breast disease, also known as chronic cystic mastitis, is the most common nonmalignant breast disease. It is characterized by growth of fibrous tissue that most frequently appears when a woman is in her 30s or 40s but disappears with menopause. While uncomfortable, the condition is not dangerous, and up to 20% of women develop some degree of fibrocystic breast disease during their lives. Accurate diagnosis to differentiate from breast cancer is, of course, essential and potentially life saving.

Breast cysts are largely influenced by hormonal fluctuations and become larger and more painful just prior to the onset of menstrual bleeding. The key to successful treatment lies in normalizing hormonal fluctuations, especially as the role of estrogen and progesterone in this condition is not clear.

Fibrocystic breast disease is aggravated by situations that increase the hormone shifts. The condition usually improves during pregnancy and breast-feeding and after menopause, unless hormone replacement therapy is undertaken. Women more likely to develop the condition include:

- Teenagers with slow establishment of regular periods
- Women who have children late in life
- Obese women
- Women on estrogen replacement therapy
- Women under stress

Treatment of Fibrocystic Breast Disease

The herbal treatment guidelines given here must be applied for a couple of months before results can be expected.

Actions Indicated

Hormonal normalizers help the body balance hormones and regularize swings, enabling a move toward complete alleviation of the problem.

Lymphatics assist with drainage and the general vitality of the lymphatic tissue in the breast.

Antispasmodics may help if there are excessive dragging pains.

Nervine relaxants are indicated if the problem is associated with PMS.

Diuretics help if there is associated water retention, but should not be used alone.

Specific Remedies

No true specifics are known for this condition, but *Vitex* is undoubtedly strongly indicated. Evening primrose oil may also be of great value.

A Prescription for Fibrocystic Breast Disease

Vitex agnus-castus	2 parts
Galium aparine	1 part
Scutellaria lateriflora	1 part

Dosage: 2.5 ml of tincture three times a day. In addition, the patient should take evening primrose oil *(Oenothera biennis)* at a dosage of five 500 mg capsules a day.

Table 18.14. Actions Supplied by Prescription for Fibrocystic Disease

ACTION	HERBS
Hormonal normalizer	*Vitex agnus-castus*
Lymphatic	*Galium aparine*
Diuretic	*Galium aparine*
Nervine relaxant	*Scutellaria lateriflora*
Antispasmodic	*Scutellaria lateriflora*

Broader Context of Treatment

It has been shown clearly that methylxanthines aggravate the problem. The most common dietary sources of such natural products are coffee, tea, chocolate, and soft drinks. These should be avoided totally. Other research shows that vitamin E at dosages of 400 to 800 IU daily may help. It is important to eat no meat, poultry, eggs, or dairy products from animals given hormones to promote growth.

In *Textbook of Natural Medicine*, Drs. Pizzorno and Murray recommend the following supplements:[5]

B-complex: 10 times the recommended daily dose
Choline: 500 to 1,000 mg/day
Methionine: 500 to 1,000 mg/day
Vitamin B$_6$: 25 to 50 mg three times a day
Vitamin C: 500 mg three times a day
Vitamin E: 400 to 800 IU/day (d-alpha tocopherol)
Beta-carotene: 50,000 to 300,000 IU/day
Iodine: 70 to 90 mcg/kg body weight
Zinc: 15 mg/day
Flaxseed oil: 1 tablespoon/day
Lactobacillus acidophilus: 1 teaspoon three times a day

THE MALE REPRODUCTIVE SYSTEM

Prostate diseases generally fall into three categories: infectious, malignant, and hypertrophic. Infection and malignancy are discussed in chapter 21. Our discussion here will focus on benign prostatic hypertrophy (BPH).

BENIGN PROSTATIC HYPERTROPHY

Benign adenomatous hyperplasia of the periurethral prostate gland commonly seen in men over age 50, causing variable degrees of bladder outlet obstruction. *(The Merck Manual)*

The prostate gland is present in all men from birth, and assumes importance when fertility is achieved. The prostate produces the fluid that accompanies the sperm during ejaculation. Located deep within the pelvis, it sits on top of the urethra, the tube that connects the penis to the bladder. As it achieves adult size, the prostate wraps itself around the urethra, into which its secretions empty. The gland is normally about the size of a chestnut.

Because of its location, if it becomes inflamed or enlarged, it may exert pressure on the urethra or block the outlet to the bladder, thus obstructing the flow of urine. This can cause interrupted or difficult urination (dribbling incontinence) as well as urgent or frequent urina-

tion, especially at night *(nocturia)*. *Dysuria* (painful or difficult urination) is another possible symptom. Urine trapped in the bladder may become infected, causing cystitis, and backward pressure can lead to kidney infection.

Congestion and overgrowth of the prostate gland is virtually universal in men older than 60. Why it happens is not understood, but theories suggest that it may be caused by the response of glandular cells in the prostate to age-related hormonal changes. Levels and composition of androgen and other hormones in the blood vary with age. This does not cause problems for all older men, but the ones who are not so lucky take little consolation in that fact!

Researchers believe that BPH is caused by accumulation of testosterone in the prostate. However, once in the prostate, testosterone is converted to dihydrotestosterone (DHT). DHT, a hormone more potent than testosterone, exerts effects on the prostate gland and other sexual organs. It is produced from testosterone by the enzyme 5-α reductase.

DHT is necessary for the normal growth and development of the prostate, but its presence is also necessary for the pathologic enlargement of the prostate that occurs in BPH. Thus, one therapeutic approach to treating the condition is to reduce the formation of DHT by blocking the enzyme 5-α reductase. *Serenoa repens* (saw palmetto) has this effect.

As prostate swelling progresses, flow of urine through the urethra is obstructed, and the bladder grows thicker and stronger to compensate for the increased resistance it must overcome. Eventually, the bladder is no longer able to completely overcome such forces. As it becomes increasingly difficult for the man to completely empty the bladder, urine stagnates there. If the obstruction is severe, pressure may back up urine to the kidneys, causing damage. When it becomes impossible to empty the bladder of all its contents, the occasional bacteria present in the urinary tract are able to multiply, and urinary tract infection may occur. This, in turn, may worsen the swelling already present in the prostate.

The earliest symptoms of BPH are usually urinary hesitancy, weakening of the urinary stream, and incomplete emptying of the bladder with urination. Dribbling of urine may occur. If infection sets in, burning, blood in the urine, and fever may occur. In the most severe cases, the man may experience a total inability to urinate, sometimes with massive enlargement of the bladder. A small number of enlarged or inflamed prostates may be cancerous. This fact underscores the need for a proper medical investigation.

Treatment of Benign Prostatic Hypertrophy

A Prescription for Benign Prostatic Hypertrophy (Internal)

Serenoa repens	2 parts
Hydrangea arborescens	2 parts
Smilax spp.	1 part
Zea mays	1 part
Arctostaphylos uva-ursi	1 part

Dosage: up to 5 ml of tincture three times a day

An Infusion for Benign Prostatic Hypertrophy (for Sitz Bath)

Equisetum arvense	1 part
Elymus repens	1 part
Arctostaphylos uva-ursi	1 part

Dosage: Infuse 2 oz of the mixture to each 1 pint of boiling water. Add infusion to sitz bath.

Broader Context of Treatment

If the symptoms are not markedly impairing the patient's lifestyle, and if recurrent, serious, or resistant infections or kidney damage is not present, conservative therapy may be adequate for long periods of time.

Conservative therapy consists of:

- Treatment of any infection (see chapter 21)
- Occasional massage of the gland through rectal exam, to relieve congestion
- Frequent ejaculations on the patient's part, for the same purpose as prostatic massage
- Avoidance of drugs that reduce bladder tone, include antidepressants, certain tranquilizers, and antihistamines

References

1. Bamford DS. Raspberry leaf tea: a new aspect to an old problem. *British Journal of Pharmacology* 1970 Sep; 40(1):161.

2. Der Marderosian AH, Liberti LE. *Natural Product Medicine*. Philadelphia: G. F. Stickley, 1988.

3. McGuffin, Hobbs, Upton, Goldberg, eds. *American Herbal Products Association's Botanical Safety Handbook*. Boca Raton, FL: CRC Press, 1997.

4. McIntyre A. *The Herbal for Pregnancy and Childbirth*. Shaftesbury, UK: Element Books, l992.

5. Pizzorno JE, Murray MT. *The Textbook of Natural Medicine*. Edinburgh: Churchill Livingstone, 1999.

Suggested Reading

Gladstar R. *Herbal Healing for Women*. New York: Simon & Schuster, 1993.

Green J. *Male Herbal: Health Care for Men and Boys*. Freedom, CA: Crossing Press, 1991.

Hudson T. *Women's Encyclopedia of Natural Medicine*. Los Angeles: Lowell House; Chicago: Contemporary Books, 1999.

McQuade Crawford A. *The Herbal Menopause Book*. Freedom, CA: The Crossing Press, 1996.

Nissim R. *Natural Healing in Gynecology*. San Francisco: HarperCollins, 1996.

Weed S. *Menopausal Years*. Woodstock, NY: Ash Tree, 1992.

19

THE MUSCULOSKELETAL SYSTEM

Our skeleton, connective tissue, muscles, and joints give us our form and hold us together, enabling us to stand and to move. These structures are extensively used (and misused) and are the focus of much physical wear and tear. However, the health of these structures and the tissues that compose them does not depend only upon the use to which they are put. It also depends, to a large extent, on our inner environment: the state of our metabolism, diet, and lifestyle. Of course, genetically based weaknesses can play a very important role in the health of this body system, but if these issues are recognized, much can be done to minimize problems.

Extensive skeletal misalignment can impair the function of the neurological system and other organs and disrupt the harmony of the whole body. Osteopathic or chiropractic techniques can be of great value in realigning the body, as can methods of psychophysical adjustment, such as rolfing, the Alexander technique, and Feldenkrais. However, the contribution of systemic, whole-body problems to the development of musculoskeletal ills cannot be overemphasized. The health and wholeness of this system can be maintained only as long as the inner environment and metabolism of the body remain in harmony. If our biochemical and metabolic processes are out of tune, the body will be under much strain to remove waste and toxins. If this condition persists unnoticed for years—as it often does—toxins can build up in the connective tissue of the joints. This can sow the seeds for the development of rheumatism and arthritis, particularly if there is a genetic disposition to such conditions.

HERBS AND THE MUSCULOSKELETAL SYSTEM

Among all of the problems that can affect this important body system, herbal medicine has most to offer in the treatment of chronic, degenerative ailments. As discussed in depth later in this chapter, *rheumatism* is a very general term used to describe any of various conditions characterized by inflammation or pain in muscles, joints, or connective tissue. *Arthritis*, on the other hand, specifically describes inflammation of joints, which may be due to infectious, metabolic, or constitutional causes.

Table 19.1. Primary Actions for the Musculoskeletal System

ACTION	HERBS
Antirheumatic	See Antirheumatic Herbs, page 409
Anti-inflammatory	*Angelica archangelica, Apium graveolens, Betula* spp., *Caulophyllum thalictroides, Cimicifuga racemosa, Dioscorea villosa, Gaultheria procumbens, Harpagophytum procumbens, Filipendula ulmaria, Guaiacum officinale, Menyanthes trifoliata, Populus tremuloides, Salix* spp., *Tanacetum parthenium*
Alteratives	*Arctium lappa, Cimicifuga racemosa, Guaiacum officinale, Iris versicolor, Mahonia aquifolium, Menyanthes trifoliata, Rumex crispus, Smilax* spp.
Antispasmodic	*Cimicifuga racemosa, Valeriana officinalis, Viburnum opulus*
Circulatory stimulant	*Capsicum annuum, Zanthoxylum americanum, Zingiber officinale*
Rubefacient	*Capsicum annuum, Brassica* spp., *Mentha piperita, Urtica dioica, Zanthoxylum americanum*
Analgesic	*Filipendula ulmaria, Piscidia erythrina, Salix* spp., *Valeriana officinalis*
Diuretic	*Achillea millefolium, Apium graveolens, Eupatorium perfoliatum*
Nervine	*Apium graveolens, Piscidia erythrina, Valeriana officinalis*
Other	As needed to ensure good elimination and general health—e.g., bitters, hepatics, expectorants, emmenagogues

In most cases, successful herbal treatment of musculoskeletal illness will be based on supporting the whole body, because systemic factors so often lay the foundation for degenerative musculoskeletal conditions. Thus, the primary actions of the truly healing antirheumatic herbs can usually be identified as alterative, diuretic, or some other systemically beneficial action. In general, anti-inflammatory herbs simply improve the symptom picture. As desirable as this is for the patient, it does not usually indicate a beneficial alteration in the disease process. Conditions in which active inflammation is worsening pathological change to bone tissue represent an important exception to this generalization.

Antirheumatic Actions

A vast array of herbs have a reputation for preventing, relieving, or curing rheumatic problems. The antirheumatic herbs presented here have a variety of different primary actions. They should be chosen according to the needs of the whole body, as this group includes alteratives, anti-inflammatory agents, rubefacients, diuretics, stimulants, and digestive remedies.

Antirheumatic herbs are remedies that have been observed to improve the patient's experience of rheumatic problems. However, that is not meant to imply that they have a specific effect upon disease processes or even upon the musculoskeletal tissue itself. To say that these herbs have an observable effect on symptoms is a description of outcome, rather than of process. As such, the concept has a limited application, unless the actions at play for each herb are understood (see table 19.2).

Antirheumatic Herbs

Achillea millefolium (yarrow)
Angelica archangelica (angelica)
Apium graveolens (celery seed)
Arctium lappa (burdock)
Arctostaphylos uva-ursi (bearberry)
Armoracia rusticana (horseradish)
Arnica montana (arnica)
Artemisia absinthium (wormwood)
A. vulgaris (mugwort)
Betula spp. (birch)
Brassica spp. (mustard)
Capsicum annuum (cayenne)
Caulophyllum thalictroides (blue cohosh)
Cimicifuga racemosa (black cohosh)
Dioscorea villosa (wild yam)
Eupatorium perfoliatum (boneset)
E. purpureum (gravel root)

Filipendula ulmaria (meadowsweet)
Fucus vesiculosus (bladderwrack)
Gaultheria procumbens (wintergreen)
Guaiacum officinale (guaiacum)
Harpagophytum procumbens (devil's claw)
Iris versicolor (blue flag)
Juniperus communis (juniper)
Mahonia aquifolium (Oregon grape)
Menyanthes trifoliata (bogbean)
Myrica cerifera (bayberry)
Petroselinum crispum (parsley)
Phytolacca americana (poke)
Populus tremuloides (aspen)
Rosmarinus officinalis (rosemary)
Rumex crispus (yellow dock)
Salix spp. (willow)
Smilax spp. (sarsaparilla)
Tanacetum parthenium (feverfew)
Taraxacum officinale (dandelion)
Urtica dioica (nettle)
Viburnum opulus (cramp bark)
Zanthoxylum americanum (prickly ash)
Zingiber officinale (ginger)

The activity of these herbs as antirheumatic agents can be explained as an expression of a more broadly relevant action, either the plant's main action or a more holistic synergy of a number of plant actions. For example, alteratives can work in a variety of different ways, as can anti-inflammatory herbs. Of course, the main actions that contribute to an herb's antirheumatic activity cannot always be identified.

Table 19.2. Possible Mechanism of Action of Antirheumatic Herbs

ACTION	HERBS
Anti-inflammatory	*Angelica archangelica, Apium graveolens, Betula* spp., *Dioscorea villosa, Filipendula ulmaria, Gaultheria procumbens, Guaiacum officinale, Harpagophytum procumbens, Menyanthes trifoliata, Populus tremuloides, Tanacetum parthenium*
Alterative	*Arctium lappa, Mahonia aquifolium, Fucus vesiculosus, Guaiacum officinale, Harpagophytum procumbens, Iris versicolor, Menyanthes trifoliata, Phytolacca americana, Rumex crispus, Smilax* spp., *Urtica dioica*

ACTION	HERBS
Diuretic	Achillea millefolium, Apium graveolens, Arctostaphylos uva-ursi, Eupatorium perfoliatum, E. purpureum, Juniperus communis, Petroselinum crispum, Taraxacum officinale
Circulatory stimulant	Armoracia rusticana, Brassica spp., Capsicum annuum, Myrica cerifera, Rosmarinus officinalis, Zanthoxylum americanum, Zingiber officinale
Antispasmodic	Cimicifuga racemosa, Viburnum opulus
Other action (or basis unclear)	Arnica montana, Artemisia absinthium, A. vulgaris, Caulophyllum thalictroides

Rubefacients

Rubefacients are herbs that, when applied to the skin, stimulate circulation in that area, increasing blood supply and relieving congestion and inflammation. This action makes rubefacients particularly useful in liniments for muscular rheumatism and similar conditions. Rubefacients are for topical use only. They should be used with care on sensitive skin, and not used at all when the skin is damaged.

Rubefacient Herbs

Armoracia rusticana (horseradish)
Brassica spp. (mustard)
Capsicum annuum (cayenne)
Gaultheria procumbens (wintergreen)
Mentha piperita (peppermint oil)
Rosmarinus officinalis (rosemary oil)
Senecio jacobaea (ragwort)
Zingiber officinale (ginger)

Diuretics

Diuretics support the work of the kidneys in eliminating metabolic wastes, toxins, and the products of inflammation. This action is essential in musculoskeletal conditions, as these waste products and toxins lie at the root of many problems, including arthritis and rheumatism. If any kidney problems exist, they must also be treated. For supporting the vital work of the kidneys, the following herbs are often considered specific for rheumatism.

Diuretic Herbs

Achillea millefolium (yarrow)
Apium graveolens (celery seed)
Arctostaphylos uva-ursi (bearberry)
Eupatorium perfoliatum (boneset)

Eupatorium purpureum (gravel root)
Petroselinum crispum (parsley)
Taraxacum officinale (dandelion leaf)

Circulatory Stimulants

Another way to cleanse the body of toxins is by stimulating blood circulation, which increases blood flow to muscles and joints. To accomplish this without straining the heart, we can use herbs that stimulate peripheral circulation.

Herbs That Stimulate Peripheral Circulation

Capsicum annuum (cayenne)
Phytolacca americana (poke root)
Rosmarinus officinalis (rosemary)
Zanthoxylum americanum (prickly ash)
Zingiber officinale (ginger)

Pain Relievers

While the purist never merely treats symptoms, the healer aims to relieve suffering. Thus, it may be necessary to use herbs with the intention of lessening the often severe pain of conditions like rheumatism. These, of course, should be used only as one part of an approach designed to treat the cause of disease. Anti-inflammatory herbs will relieve pain to some extent, but the only truly effective way to alleviate pain is to clear the underlying problem. Herbs listed here can be used to help relieve pain in the context of a whole body approach.

Herbal Analgesics

Guaiacum officinale (guaiacum)
Hypericum perforatum (St. John's wort)
Piscidia erythrina (Jamaica dogwood)
Valeriana officinalis (valerian)

Digestive System Tonics

The digestive system must be in good working order, as nutrients must be properly absorbed in order for the musculoskeletal system to operate at its peak. Bitter tonics may be helpful here.

Useful Bitter Tonic Herbs

Achillea millefolium (yarrow)
Artemisia absinthium (wormwood)
Gentiana lutea (gentian)
Hydrastis canadensis (goldenseal)

If the patient is troubled by constipation, laxatives may be indicated, especially those that act by stimulating the liver.

Hepatic Stimulants

Rheum palmatum (rhubarb root)
Rumex crispus (yellow dock)
Taraxacum officinale (dandelion root)

RHEUMATIC DISEASES AND ARTHRITIS

More than 100 conditions are technically classified as *rheumatic diseases*. The conditions that make up this group of health problems share many common symptoms, including pain, stiffness, and swelling of joints and the supporting structures of the body, such as muscles, tendons, ligaments, and bones. Some of these diseases may also affect other parts of the body.

Although the term *arthritis* is often used as a general descriptor for all rheumatic diseases, this is incorrect. The word *arthritis* literally means "joint inflammation," and is correctly applied to describe the swelling, redness, heat, and pain caused by tissue injury or joint disease. The many different types of arthritis comprise just a portion of the total group of rheumatic diseases.

Some rheumatic diseases are described as *connective tissue diseases* because they primarily affect the body's connective tissues—the supporting framework of the body and its internal organs. Connective tissue is found everywhere in the body and includes cartilage, bone, and the binding, supportive components of the skin. Other rheumatic conditions are classified as *autoimmune diseases* because they are associated with a systemic problem in which the immune system harms the body's own healthy tissues.

Here we will look briefly at a few examples of some of the more common rheumatic diseases. Treatment approaches are detailed later in this chapter.

Osteoarthritis

Also known as *degenerative joint disease*, osteoarthritis is the most common type of arthritis, affecting an estimated 20.7 million American adults. Osteoarthritis primarily affects cartilage, the tissue that cushions the ends of bones in the joints. The condition occurs when cartilage begins to fray, wear, and decay. In extreme cases, the cartilage may wear away entirely. Bony spurs (pointy outcroppings of bone) may form at the edges of a joint. Osteoarthritis causes joint pain, reduced joint motion, loss of function, and disability.

Rheumatoid Arthritis

Rheumatoid arthritis is an inflammatory disease of the lining of the joint that results in pain, stiffness, swelling, deformity, and loss of joint function. The inflammation most often affects joints of the hands and feet and tends to occur equally on both sides of the body. This symmetry helps distinguish rheumatoid arthritis from other types of arthritis. About 2.1 million Americans are afflicted with rheumatoid arthritis.

Although the symptoms of rheumatoid arthritis are caused by inflammation of the connective tissues, the cause is not at all clear. A characteristic sign of rheumatoid arthritis is chronic inflammation of the synovial membranes, or inner linings of the joint capsules. The synovial mass proliferates and destroys cartilage, bone, and adjacent structures. The widespread inflammation may also affect other tissues, leading to painful joints, loss of mobility, and generalized soreness and depression. Blood tests often reveal the presence of rheumatoid factors, proteins produced by the immune system in response to the rheumatic process.

Fibromyalgia

Fibromyalgia causes pain and stiffness throughout the tissues that support and move the bones and joints. Pain and localized tender points occur in the muscles and tendons, particularly those of the neck, spine, shoulders, and hips. Patients may experience widespread pain, fatigue, and sleep disturbances.

Systemic Lupus Erythematosus

Systemic lupus erythematosus (also known as lupus or SLE) is an autoimmune disease in which the immune system harms the body's tissues. In SLE, this can result in inflammation of and damage to joints, skin, kidneys, heart, lungs, blood vessels, and brain.

Ankylosing Spondylitis

This is a type of arthritis that primarily affects the spine, but it may also impact the hips, shoulders, and knees. The tendons and ligaments around the bones and joints in the spine become inflamed, resulting in pain and stiffness, especially in the lower back. Ankylosing spondylitis tends to affect people in late adolescence or early adulthood.

Gout

This form of arthritis is caused by deposits of needlelike crystals of uric acid in the connective tissue, joint spaces, or both. Uric acid is a normal breakdown product of purines, which are present in body tissues and in many foods. Normally, uric acid passes through the kidney into urine and is eliminated. However, if the concentration of uric acid in the blood rises above normal levels, sodium urate crystals may form. These needlelike crystals cause inflammation, swelling, and pain in the affected joint. The joint most commonly affected is the big toe.

Psoriatic Arthritis

This form of arthritis affects some patients with psoriasis, a common scaling skin disorder. Psoriatic arthritis often affects the joints at the ends of the fingers and is accompanied by changes in the fingernails and toenails. In some people, the spine is also involved.

Bursitis

This condition involves inflammation of the bursae, small, fluid-filled sacs that serve to reduce friction between bones and other moving structures in the joints. The inflammation may result from arthritis in the joint or from injury to or infection of the bursae. Bursitis produces pain and tenderness and may limit the movement of nearby joints.

Tendinitis

This refers to inflammation of tendons (tough cords of tissue that connect muscle to bone) caused by overuse, injury, or related rheumatic conditions. Tendinitis produces pain and tenderness and may restrict the movement of nearby joints.

ARTHRITIS AND PAIN

Pain is the body's warning system. The International Association for the Study of Pain defines *pain* as an unpleasant experience associated with actual or potential tissue damage to a person's body. Specialized cells called neurons transmit pain signals and are found throughout the skin and other body tissues. These cells respond to trauma, such as injury or tissue damage. For example, when a knife cuts the skin, chemical signals travel from neurons in the skin through nerves in the spinal cord to the brain, where they are interpreted as pain.

The pain of arthritis may be acute or chronic. Acute pain is temporary; it may last a few seconds or longer, but wanes as healing occurs. Some conditions that cause acute pain are burns, cuts, and fractures. Chronic pain, such as that caused by osteoarthritis and rheumatoid arthritis, ranges from mild to severe and can last a lifetime.

Arthritic pain may be caused by a number of processes, including muscle strain, fatigue, and inflammation of the synovial membranes of the joints, the tendons, or the ligaments. A combination of these factors contributes to the intensity of the pain. For reasons that are not clearly understood, the experience of arthritis pain varies greatly from person to person. Contributing factors include swelling within the joint, amount of heat or redness present, and damage that has occurred within the joint. In addition, pain levels are affected by different activities. Some patients note pain in their joints when they first get out of bed in the morning, while others develop pain after prolonged use of the joint. Each individual has a different threshold and tolerance for pain, which is affected by both physical and emotional factors.

Conventional Arthritis Medications

A number of over-the-counter medications can help relieve acute pain. Because osteoarthritis involves little inflammation, pain relievers like acetaminophen may prove effective. The pain of rheumatoid arthritis is generally caused by inflammation, and thus may respond better to aspirin or another nonsteroidal anti-inflammatory drug (NSAID), such as ibuprofen.

Nonsteroidal Anti-Inflammatory Drugs

Nonsteroidal anti-inflammatory drugs, or NSAIDs, are the most widely used drugs in the United States. They are used to treat pain, fever, and inflammation that occur as a result of acute injuries, rheumatoid arthritis, and osteoarthritis. They are not curative, but do help to lessen pain and inflammation.

Unfortunately, NSAIDs are not without side effects, and some of these can be life threatening. For example, gastrointestinal bleeding due to use of NSAIDs kills almost 9,000 Americans each year. In addition, all of these drugs can produce a number of similar mild, temporary side effects.

Minor Side Effects of NSAIDs

Gastrointestinal: Heartburn, dyspepsia, diarrhea, constipation, abdominal pain, nausea, stomatitis, decreased appetite, vomiting
Central nervous system: Headache, insomnia, dizziness, drowsiness, tinnitus, confusion, unusual weakness
Visual: Loss of visual acuity, blurred or double vision
Skin: Itching, rash, photosensitivity reactions, eruptions, hives
Cardiovascular: Edema, palpitations, rapid heartbeat
Genitourinary: Burning or painful urination, vaginal bleeding, blood in urine, cystitis

Unfortunately, these drugs can also produce far more serious problems. Adverse effects in the kidneys are of particular concern in the elderly, because kidney function is often already compromised by aging or complications of chronic diseases, such as diabetes and hypertension.

Serious Side Effects of NSAIDs

Gastrointestinal: Gastric and/or duodenal ulceration, gastrointestinal bleeding (advanced age is a risk factor)

Cardiovascular: Angina, cardiac arrhythmias, exacerbation of congestive heart failure

Kidney: Interstitial nephritis, acute renal failure, hyperkalemia (high serum potassium)

Skin: Exfoliative dermatitis, erythema multiforme, other unusual skin problems

Blood: Anemia, leukopenia

Liver: Jaundice, hepatitis

If NSAIDs are being used, the patient should follow a number of simple steps to lessen the impact of side effects. Take NSAIDs with food, and drink six to eight glasses of water each day to decrease gastrointestinal side effects. Also, the patient should not recline within a half hour of taking NSAIDs. If the person is at risk for ulceration, he or she should consult with a physician and pharmacist on a routine basis to decrease the chances of a life-threatening gastrointestinal ulceration. As serious ulcerations do not necessarily produce any symptoms, do not rely upon symptoms to predict ulcer development.

Risk Factors for Ulceration with NSAIDs

Advanced age

History of peptic ulcer disease or cardiovascular disease

High-dose NSAID use

Long duration of NSAID use

Heavy smoking or drinking

Kidney or liver failure

Use of certain drugs, such as Coumadin and prednisone

A number of powerful prescription drugs may be used to treat rheumatoid arthritis that does not respond to treatment with NSAIDs. These include methotrexate, hydroxychloroquine, penicillamine, and gold injections. These drugs are thought to influence and correct the immune system abnormalities responsible for diseases like rheumatoid arthritis. Use of these medications requires careful monitoring by the physician to minimize the ravages of side effects.

Corticosteroids, such as prednisone, are prescribed for a number of rheumatic conditions because they decrease inflammation and suppress the activity of the immune system. Short-term side effects of corticosteroids include swelling, increased appetite, weight gain, and emotional swings. These side effects usually disappear when the drug is discontinued. However, discontinuing corticosteroids suddenly is dangerous. Side effects that may occur after long-term use include stretch marks, excessive hair growth, osteoporosis, high blood pressure, damage to the arteries, high blood sugar, infections, and cataracts.

COMPONENTS OF A HOLISTIC TREATMENT PROGRAM FOR ARTHRITIS

One of the long-term goals of arthritis treatment is to help the patient cope with having a chronic, often disabling disease. The patient may be caught in a self-reinforcing cycle of pain, depression, and stress. Breaking out of this cycle is easier if the patient is empowered by taking on a role as an active participant, along with the health care professional, in managing the pain.

Some simple methods can alleviate pain for short periods of time. This temporary relief can make it easier for people who have arthritis to exercise.

Diet

An important part of any treatment program for arthritis is a well-balanced diet. Along with exercise, a well-balanced diet helps control weight and maintains overall good health. Weight control is particularly important here, because extra weight puts pressure on some joints and can aggravate arthritis.

One of the proposed causes of rheumatism and arthritis is accumulation of toxins or waste products in the affected tissue. A major contributing factor is inappropriate diet—consumption of foods that are either wrong for the individual's body or so devitalized and adulterated that they are detrimental for that reason alone. Dietary measures are especially essential for people with gout. These patients should avoid alcohol and foods high in purines, such as organ meats (liver, kidney), sardines, and anchovies.

As a general guideline, any foods that cause bodily reactions should be avoided, as should foods that cause digestive problems or other adverse effects, including subtle allergic reactions. Ideally, one should consume foods that are fresh and untreated, as opposed to processed foods full of additives and preservatives.

Dairy products and gluten (mainly from wheat products) often cause either overt allergic reactions or subtle ones, such as the minor digestive upsets of heartburn and flatulence. If these foods cause reactions, they should be avoided. In general, the patient should minimize consumption of meat, eggs, and dairy products, as well as very acidic foods like vinegar and pickles. The patient should also shun foods rich in oxalic acid, including rhubarb, gooseberries, black currants, and red currants. Coffee, black tea, alcohol, sugar, salt, and any food or beverage made from red grapes should also be avoided.

Instead, the patient should increase consumption of fruits and vegetables, especially green and root vegetables. Citrus fruits, which, in spite of their citric acid, appear to have an alkalinizing effect on the metabolism, are fine. The patient should drink at least 3 pints (1.5 liters) of fluid daily to help flush the body. This fluid should preferably be water with a low mineral content or water mixed with a little apple cider vinegar or apple juice. Taking at least 500 mg/day of vitamin C supplement is recommended. Fish and white meat may be eaten.

Glucosamine Sulfate

Glucosamine sulfate is a nutritional supplement that may enhance the reconstruction and healing of cartilage. Glucosamine is an amino sugar, a molecule composed of an amino acid and a simple sugar. The body uses about 20 different amino sugars as sources of energy or ingredients for the assembly of tissue components. Amino sugars are the structural basis of connective tissue and lubricating fluids.

Just as amino acids are the building blocks of proteins, amino sugars are the building blocks of very large molecules called glycosaminoglycans (GAGs), also known as mucopolysaccharides. GAGs are large, spongy, water-holding molecules that form the gel-like matrix of ground substance, or the "glue" that holds our bodies together. This substance is found in all connective tissue and mucous membranes. Glucosamine macromolecules are the basic substrate of cartilage, ligaments, tendons, and bones.

During normal use, connective tissue is constantly broken down and either replaced or restructured, creating a continuous demand for glucosamine. The normal diet is not a good source of glucosamine, so the body synthesizes it from glucose and the amino acid glutamine. Normally, the body produces enough glucosamine, but under some conditions, the production of glucosamine and its subsequent assembly into larger GAGs may be impaired. These conditions include severe stress, surgery, burns, and major injuries, as well as aging. A lack of glycoproteins or other substances based on amino sugars has been observed in many diseases, including osteoarthritis.

It appears that supplementation with glucosamine sulfate might stimulate the synthesis of the missing glycoproteins. A number of studies have compared glucosamine sulfate with ibuprofen for the treatment of osteoarthritis.[1] A recent randomized, double-blind, controlled clinical trial compared the use of glucosamine sulfate and ibuprofen in patients diagnosed with temporomandibular joint (TMJ) osteoarthritis. The researchers concluded that both glucosamine sulfate and ibuprofen reduced pain levels in these patients. However, glucosamine sulfate had a significantly greater influence in reducing pain produced during function and pain caused by daily activities.

Glucosamine sulfate is indicated for joint problems such as osteoarthritis. Onset of action is seen after two to eight weeks of treatment, as it works by stimulating the endogenous synthesis of the missing macromolecules. The suggested dose for osteoarthritis is 500 mg three times a day.

In commercial formulations, glucosamine sulfate is often combined with chondroitin sulfate. However, the evidence for the actual efficacy of chondroitin sulfate when taken by mouth is equivocal.

Heat and Cold Therapy

Heat and cold can both be used to reduce the pain and inflammation of arthritis. Studies have shown that heat and cold therapies are equally effective in alleviating pain, although they are usually avoided in acute gout. The decision to use heat or cold for arthritis pain depends on the type of arthritis.

Heat therapy increases blood flow, pain tolerance, and flexibility. Heat therapy can involve treatment with paraffin wax, microwaves, ultrasound, or moist heat. Physical therapists are needed to apply paraffin wax, microwave, or ultrasound therapy, but anyone can apply heat on his or her own. Applying moist heat, such as a warm bath or shower, or dry heat, such as a heating pad, to the painful joint for about 15 minutes often relieves pain. Deep heat is not recommended for patients with acutely inflamed joints, but deep heat is often used around the shoulder in people with osteoarthritis to relax tight tendons before stretching exercises.

Cold therapy numbs the nerves around the joint, reducing pain, relieving inflammation, and easing muscle spasms. Cold therapy can involve cold packs, ice massage, soaking in cold water, or the use of over-the-counter sprays or ointments that cool the skin and joints. Wrapping an ice pack (or a bag of frozen vegetables) in a towel and placing it on the sore area for about 15 minutes may help to reduce swelling and stop the pain. Cold therapy is often used for acutely inflamed joints; however, people with Raynaud's disease should not use this method.

Weight Reduction

Excess weight puts extra stress on joints, such as the knees and hips. A recent study found that when obese arthritis patients lost weight, they experienced significant reductions in pain and stiffness as well as an improvement in their quality of life.[2]

Devices

Splints and braces are commonly used in the treatment of arthritis pain. These help support weakened joints or allow them to rest. Some of these devices prevent the joint from moving; others allow some movement. A splint or brace should be used only with professional guidance to ensure that the device fits properly and is worn correctly. Incorrect use can cause joint damage, stiffness, and pain.

Other kinds of devices may also help ease pain. For example, using a cane when walking can take weight off an arthritic joint. A shoe insert may ease pain caused by arthritis of the foot or knee while walking.

Hydrotherapy, Mobilization Therapy, and Relaxation Therapy

Hydrotherapy involves exercising or relaxing in warm water, which helps relax tense muscles and relieve pain. This type of exercise improves muscle strength and joint movement.

Mobilization therapies include traction (gentle, steady pulling), massage, and manipulation (using the hands to restore normal movement to stiff joints). When performed by a trained professional, these methods can help control pain, increase joint motion, and improve muscle and tendon flexibility. Appropriate massage will increase blood flow and warmth to a stressed area. However, arthritis-stressed joints are very sensitive, so the therapist must be familiar with the problems of the disease.

Relaxation therapy helps reduce pain by teaching patients various ways to release muscle tension throughout the body. In one method of relaxation therapy, known as progressive relaxation, the patient tightens one muscle group at a time, then slowly releases the tension.

Exercise

Exercise can benefit patients with arthritis in many ways. It lessens joint pain and stiffness and increases flexibility, muscle strength, and endurance. It also helps with weight reduction and contributes to an improved sense of well-being. Exercise plans for patients with arthritis may include instruction about proper use of joints as well as ways to conserve energy and eliminate unnecessary motion. The amount and type of exercise for a given patient with arthritis will vary according to which joints are involved, the amount of inflammation, how stable the joints are, and whether the patient has undergone a joint replacement procedure.

In general, three types of exercise are best for people with arthritis:

Range-of-motion exercises help maintain normal joint movement, relieve stiffness, and help maintain or increase flexibility.

Strengthening exercises help maintain or increase muscle strength. Strong muscles support and protect arthritic joints.

Aerobic or endurance exercises improve cardiovascular fitness and help control weight, which is critical, as excess weight puts extra pressure on many joints.

OTHER CONSIDERATIONS FOR MUSCULOSKELETAL HEALTH

The various forms of arthritis are perhaps the most important inflammatory conditions that affect humanity, and throughout the world herbal medicines are used to treat them. About one in seven Americans exhibits some form of arthritis, which is usually characterized by inflammation in the affected tissue. The typical signs of inflammation (warmth, redness, swelling, and pain) are often present.

In some types of arthritis, inflammation is caused by autoimmune reactions. Why the body sometimes mounts an immune system reaction against its own tissue is unknown. We do know that such autoimmune reactions result in inflammation when "anti-self" antibodies react with intact connective tissue and synovial membranes. Rheumatoid arthritis is a common autoimmune form of arthritis.

Utilizing a broad holistic approach, herbal medicine works with the whole body to promote amelioration of the condition while alleviating pain and discomfort. Simply using anti-inflammatory and antirheumatic remedies is not enough. Therapy must focus on improving liver function, circulation, and elimination, as well as the quality of the patient's life and experience.

We need not look in too much depth at the differences among the various kinds of arthritis. A finely detailed differential diagnosis may not even be necessary for holistic treatment. It is necessary, however, to recognize the influence of the patient's genetic framework and the contributions of various factors, including lifestyle and diet, to the development of the condition for the particular individual. These conditions occur as a result of the body's inability to deal with pressures from wrong diet and lifestyle or other stresses. The aim of treatment is not to attack the symptoms in an effort to regain vitality, but rather to help the individual attain a state of health in which the body will be better able to take care of itself.

Arthritis and Friction

The concept of friction provides us with an important insight as to how to approach these conditions. The joint changes that occur in arthritis cause bones to rub together in a manner that causes friction, but often a long history of friction precedes these physical changes. Friction can be caused by particular physical activities—for example, when a farmer develops osteoarthritis in the shoulder on which he has carried hay bales every morning for years. It may also be related to muscle tension that binds joints too tightly together, which is usually due to a history of friction in life.

The Collins Dictionary defines *friction* in the following way:

> A resistance encountered when one body moves relative to another body with which it is in contact . . . disagreement or conflict.

When considering the roots of rheumatic and arthritic problems, this definition seems to cover it all—whether the "two bodies" involved are bones, people, or differing emotions and beliefs. Conflicts and the friction they engender may take many forms, but the experience is fundamentally an inner one. For some, conflict is a state of mind, or an attitude with which to relate to the world. Such conflict really takes place between inner aspects of the individual, as a manifestation of psychological disharmony. The inner conflict may be externalized as conflict in relationships or lifestyle, but the roots are often deep in the psyche.

When trying to create an environment conducive to healing within the body, as much attention must be paid to emotional and mental harmony as to diet and herbal medicine. An outlook on life that is tight, defensive, and lacking in vulnerability and openness will tend to feed the rheumatism. On the other hand, initiating an inner process of relaxation to reduce emotional friction, allow free interaction with other people, and open up emotions and beliefs sets the stage for the miracle of self-healing to occur. Herbs can facilitate this process.

It is possible to cleanse the whole system and to remove the source of the rheumatic or arthritic develop-ment by using appropriate herbs in combination with other techniques that support and aid the entire body. Such treatment takes time, as a degenerative process that developed over time cannot be reversed in just one month. However, when the right treatment is initiated, the practitioner may hear comments like "I already feel better within myself" long before the actual symptoms of pain or stiffness are gone.

With rheumatic and arthritic problems, perhaps more than with any other condition, it is essential to treat the whole person. Otherwise, improvement will be only slight or temporary. When one takes the individual's unique picture into account, it is possible to open the gates for a quite miraculous healing to occur. Although a general need for cleansing will be common to all patients, each must also be approached as a unique being. Does the digestive system need any kind of help? Are the kidneys working well? Is the patient under much stress? Is the endocrine system working harmoniously? How is the diet?

EXTERNAL APPLICATIONS FOR MUSCULOSKELETAL PROBLEMS

External applications of various herbs can help relieve discomfort. This plethora of prescriptions leans heavily on the wealth of traditional experience that characterizes herbalism. They may be used safely in myalgia and osteoarthritis, but those containing hot spices (such as cayenne, mustard, and ginger) should not be used by patients with rheumatoid arthritis.

These remedies may be antispasmodic, rubefacient, or anti-inflammatory in nature. There are many possible external applications of herbs, and the choice will often depend upon what plants are available and local traditions. Here is a brief list of external applications used traditionally for musculoskeletal conditions, taken from many different sources and organized by primary herbal component.

Black Mustard (*Brassica nigra*)

Mustard seeds can be applied externally to ease acute local pain, sciatica, and gout. Prepare a poultice by mixing powdered mustard seeds with warm water to form a paste. Spread onto brown paper and apply to affected area. For rheumatic pain, mustard oil, a powerful local irritant, may be incorporated into liniments for application to affected areas. This treatment should not be used in rheumatoid arthritis.

White Mustard (Brassica alba)

Poultices made with mustard flowers, bread crumbs, and vinegar are a traditional treatment for rheumatic and sciatic pains. As an alternative, mix white mustard seeds with black mustard seeds. Although mustard poultices may redden the skin, they are very stimulating and efficient.

Cayenne (Capsicum annuum)

Cayenne is an important ingredient in this traditional stimulating application, used to increase local circulation in arthritis and rheumatism.

Capsicum annuum powder	1 part
Verbascum thapsus leaf	1 part
Ulmus rubra powder	1 part
Apple cider vinegar	Enough to dampen the mixture

Mix ingredients to make a poultice. If the cayenne causes too powerful a burning sensation, cover the skin with vegetable oil before applying poultice.

Another way to use cayenne is to mix equal parts of cayenne and glycerin, shake well, and apply to painful joints. As in the above application, if cayenne causes a burning sensation, apply vegetable oil first. Cayenne powder or tincture may also be rubbed on inflamed areas for added relief.

Lavender Essential Oil (Lavandula spp.)

A small amount of essential oil of lavender, added to a fixed oil (such as almond oil) is a useful anti-inflammatory for the treatment of rheumatic complaints.

Lobelia (Lobelia inflata)

For cramps or the relief of rheumatic pain, try this traditional antispasmodic tincture.

Lobelia inflata powder (crushed seed and herb)	1 oz
Symplocarpus foetidus (root and rhizome)	1 oz
Scutellaria lateriflora (herb)	1 oz
Commiphora molmol (gum myrrh)	1 oz
Valeriana officinalis (root)	1 oz
Capsicum annuum (dried fruit)	½ oz

Infuse herbs for one week in 1 quart of brandy in a closely corked, wide-necked bottle. Shake well daily. Strain, press out clear liquid, and rub mixture on affected areas.

Mullein (Verbascum thapsus)

Mullein combines well with Cimicifuga racemosa and Lobelia inflata in liniments. For swollen joints, and to relieve the aches and pains of arthritis and rheumatism, rub mullein oil thoroughly into skin, or saturate a piece of cotton with the mullein oil, apply to skin, and cover with a dry dressing. Prepare mullein oil by infusing mullein flowers in olive oil.

For the treatment of painful and swollen joints, pour boiling vinegar over a small quantity of mullein, cover, and simmer slowly for 20 to 30 minutes. Strain; add a small amount of tinctures of cayenne and lobelia. Apply to affected areas.

Sassafras (Sassafras albidum)

Here is a recipe for a traditional North American liniment for rheumatic problems.

Sassafras albidum tincture	1 oz
Zanthoxylum americanum tincture	1 oz
Capsicum annuum tincture	1 oz
Commiphora molmol tincture	1 oz
Camphor tincture	1 oz
Distilled water	8 oz

Shake ingredients together well and apply to affected parts.

MYALGIA

A group of common nonarticular rheumatic disorders characterized by achy pain, tenderness, and stiffness of muscles, areas of tendon insertions, and adjacent soft-tissue structures. (The Merck Manual)

Myalgia, also generally called rheumatism, is a notoriously vague and misused description for aches and pains in the musculature. Since these symptoms are also common to the early stages of many infections and a range of autoimmune conditions, they may call for a more detailed differential diagnosis. A safe rule of thumb is to consider the problem more deeply if symptoms cannot be eased to some degree within two weeks.

Treatment of Myalgia

An important aspect of treatment is to support the musculoskeletal system by using appropriate tonics. Beyond that, many other parts of the body may also be involved, depending upon the individual.

Sports injuries. If myalgia is the result of long-standing sports injuries, the addition of antispasmodics can help loosen the muscles. Connective tissue must also be strengthened.

Digestive disorders. If the patient has a history of digestive problems, appropriate digestive tonics are indicated.

Cardiovascular issues. Cardiovascular tonics should be added if the patient has hypertension or overt heart disease. The balance of herbs for active treatment of both rheumatism and cardiovascular problems must be determined by the professional judgment of the herbalist.

Stress. Long-standing stress can lead to the development of tension and tightness in the muscles. This, in turn, may hold the joints too tightly, resulting in friction. Over the course of years, this can develop into "wear-and-tear" arthritis (osteoarthritis), but in the short term will cause pain and stiffness.

Actions Indicated

Antirheumatics help because of their general value for this body system.

Anti-inflammatories are especially indicated if there is much sensitivity to touch.

Alteratives are indicated if there is a suspicion of a systemic problem.

Antispasmodics ease any associated muscular tension, often the core of this problem.

Circulatory stimulants may help by increasing local circulation; however, they are usually best used in the form of rubefacients.

Rubefacients stimulate circulatory activity, thus increasing removal of tissue waste and the local supply of oxygen and nutrients.

Analgesics are of limited, symptomatic value only.

Diuretics appear to be very effective in easing vague rheumatic aches and pains.

Nervines may be indicated.

Specific Remedies

Most of the salicylate-containing anti-inflammatory herbs are considered specifics in the various folk traditions of the world. Especially important are *Filipendula ulmaria* (meadowsweet), *Gaultheria procumbens* (wintergreen), *Populus tremuloides* (aspen), and *Salix* spp. (willow bark). In addition, we can add *Angelica archangelica* (angelica), *Apium graveolens* (celery seed), and, in fact, all of the herbs in the general antirheumatic category. External applications will often help. These may be rubefacients, circulatory stimulants, salicin-containing essential oils, or even antispasmodic herbs. The choice will ultimately depend upon the patient's response to different remedies.

A Prescription for Myalgia

Salix spp.	2 parts
Angelica archangelica	1 part
Urtica dioica	1 part

Dosage: up to 5 ml of tincture three times a day

An Antispasmodic Rub

Lobelia inflata	1 part
Viburnum opulus	1 part

Rub tincture mixture into painful muscles as needed.

The internal treatment supplies a basic range of antirheumatic herbs that provide salicylate anti-inflammatory actions, along with support for the digestive process and more generalized alterative effects. Possible external treatments are so numerous that the choice is as much a matter of cultural preference as of therapeutic judgment.

Table 19.3. Actions Supplied by Myalgia Prescriptions

ACTION	HERBS
Anti-inflammatory	*Angelica archangelica, Salix* spp., *Viburnum opulus*
Antispasmodic	*Lobelia inflata, Viburnum opulus*
Alterative	*Urtica dioica*
Diuretic	*Angelica archangelica, Urtica dioica*

Broader Context of Treatment

Dietary factors must be considered. Please see suggestions given in the section on osteoarthritis. A careful review of the patient's lifestyle will help clarify issues related to posture, work conditions, stress, and other factors. Chiropractic, osteopathy, aromatherapy, massage, and attention to appropriate exercise may all prove useful.

OSTEOARTHRITIS

An arthropathy with altered hyaline cartilage and characterized by loss of articular cartilage and hypertrophy of bone, producing osteophytes. *(The Merck Manual)*

Osteoarthritis, also called degenerative joint disease, is the most common form of arthritis. It affects about one in six Americans, including 80% of people over the age of 70. By implication, more than 20 million people in the United States probably have osteoarthritis. The disease affects both men and women, but is more common in men before age 45 and more common in women after age 45.

In a healthy joint, the ends of the bones are encased in smooth cartilage. They are protected by a joint capsule, which is lined with a synovial membrane that produces synovial fluid. The capsule and fluid protect the cartilage, muscles, and connective tissues. The joint includes the following components:

Cartilage. This forms a hard but slippery coating on the end of each bone.

Joint capsule. This tough membrane sac holds all the bones and other joint parts together.

Synovial fluid. Synovial fluid lubricates the joint and keeps the cartilage smooth and healthy.

Muscles, ligaments, and tendons. Together, muscles and connective tissues keep the bones stable and allow the joint to bend and move. Ligaments are tough, cordlike connective tissues that connect one bone to another. Tendons are tough, fibrous connective tissue cords that connect muscles to bones.

Osteoarthritis primarily affects the cartilage of the joints. Healthy cartilage allows the bones to glide smoothly over one another, and also absorbs energy from the shock of physical movement, such as walking or repetitive motions. In osteoarthritis, the surface layer of this cartilage breaks down and wears away. The bones under the cartilage are then able to rub together, causing pain, swelling, and loss of motion. Over time, the joint may lose its normal shape, and bone spurs may grow on the edges of the joint. Bits of bone or cartilage can break off and float inside the joint space, causing still more pain and damage.

Unlike some other forms of arthritis, osteoarthritis affects joints only, not internal organs. Rheumatoid arthritis, for example, impacts other parts of the body in addition to the joints. Although osteoarthritis can occur in any joint, it most often affects the ends of the fingers, thumbs, neck, lower back, knees, and hips.

Body Parts Commonly Affected by Osteoarthritis

Hands. Small, bony knobs (called Heberden's nodes) appear on the end joints of the fingers. Similar knobs may appear on the middle joints of the fingers. The fingers can become enlarged and gnarled, and may ache or feel stiff and numb. The base of the thumb joint is also commonly affected.

Knees. Knees, the body's primary weight-bearing joints, are commonly affected by osteoarthritis, becoming stiff, swollen, and painful.

Hips. Osteoarthritis in the hips can cause pain, stiffness, and severe disability. The pain may be felt in the hips, groin, inner thighs, or knees. Osteoarthritis in the hip can limit the individual's ability to move and bend, making daily activities a challenge.

Spine. Osteoarthritis of the spine can cause stiffness and pain in the neck or in the lower back. Weakness or numbness of the arms or legs may also occur.

Treatment of Osteoarthritis

In addition to attention to musculoskeletal issues, the digestive system needs special care. Beyond that, treatment will depend upon the individual's specific case. Always remember the general principles of good elimination, but never resort to strenuous "purging and puking."

Actions Indicated

Antirheumatics will usually help, but selection must be based on a sound therapeutic rationale.

Anti-inflammatories are fundamental here, as their use not only eases the symptom picture but also helps arrest degenerative changes to bony tissue. Salicylate-based herbs, such as *Filipendula ulmaria*, are especially helpful.

Alteratives are the key to any attempt to transform systemic problems (if present). However, if the osteoarthritis is associated primarily with physical wear-and-tear, alteratives are not quite as fundamental. In cases like this, *Menyanthes trifoliata* is primarily indicated.

Antispasmodics lessen the impact of physical friction by relaxing the muscular envelope around the arthroses. *Cimicifuga racemosa* proves effective here.

Circulatory stimulants support the healing process by increasing blood flow through the tissue. The bark and berries of *Zanthoxylum americanum* are good choices.

Specific Remedies

Both *Menyanthes trifoliata* (bogbean) and *Harpagophytum procumbens* (devil's claw) could be considered specifics here. However, because of the multifactorial etiology of osteoarthritis, it is unlikely that there will be any one specific remedy.

Urtica dioica (nettle) is a traditional European remedy that is both taken internally and used externally as a rubefacient. This external use involves fresh, raw leaf and is not for the fainthearted! One study, performed in 1999 at Plymouth Medical School in the United Kingdom, examined the traditional reputation of nettle sting for relieving joint pain.[3] The results showed that nettle sting was markedly effective in relieving pain for many patients. The authors noted, "No observed side effects were reported, except a transient urticarial rash," which should come as no surprise to anyone familiar with this plant!

A Prescription for Osteoarthritis

Menyanthes trifoliata	2 parts
Filipendula ulmaria	1½ parts
Cimicifuga racemosa	1 part
Zanthoxylum americanum	1 part
Apium graveolens	1 part
Angelica archangelica	1 part
Achillea millefolium	1 part

Dosage: up to 5 ml of tincture three times a day. In addition, use external treatments as indicated. If the patient experiences stomach irritation related to *Menyanthes*, add *Althaea*.

Table 19.4. Actions Supplied by Prescription for Osteoarthritis

ACTION	HERBS
Alterative	Menyanthes trifoliata, Cimicifuga racemosa
Anti-inflammatory (salicylate)	Filipendula ulmaria
Anti-inflammatory (general)	Angelica archangelica, Menyanthes trifoliata, Cimicifuga racemosa
Nervine antispasmodic	Cimicifuga racemosa, Apium graveolens
Peripheral vasodilator	Zanthoxylum americanum
Diuretic	Apium graveolens, Achillea millefolium
Carminative	Angelica archangelica, Apium graveolens
Bitter tonic	Menyanthes trifoliata, Achillea millefolium

External Treatments for Osteoarthritis

External remedies may be used to ease pain and reduce inflammation, at the same time helping to eliminate toxins by stimulating circulation to the affected area. While such treatment will not lead to a fundamental change on its own, it will contribute to the healing process and ease discomfort.

A Warming, Stimulating Liniment

A very straightforward liniment can be made by mixing equal parts of glycerin and tincture of cayenne. Rub this into the affected joints or muscles. Care must be taken not to use the liniment on broken skin or on the sensitive skin of the face, as it will cause a burning sensation. This is the "heat" that relieves pain in cold, aching joints and stiff muscles.

St. John's Wort Oil

If there is pain in the muscle tissue or any nerve pain, St. John's wort oil (*Hypericum perforatum*) can be effective. Make St. John's wort oil in late summer by picking fresh blossoms and putting them into oil:

Fresh, just-opened *Hypericum perforatum* flowers	100 g (4 oz)
Olive or sunflower oil	1 pint (½ liter)

Crush the flowers in a tablespoon of the oil and place in a clear glass container. Pour the rest of the oil over the flowers and mix well. Leave the container open in a warm place for three to five days, then seal the container well and place it in sunshine or another warm place for three to six weeks. Shake daily until the oil takes on a bright red color. Next, press the mixture through a cloth and let stand for a day to allow the oil to separate from the water. Carefully pour off the oil and store in an airtight, opaque container. St. John's wort oil may be rubbed on areas of rheumatic pain, used for neuralgic or sciatic pains, or applied to minor burns.

Broader Context of Treatment

Exercise is an essential component of any treatment plan for osteoarthritis. Appropriate activity improves mood and outlook, decreases pain, increases flexibility, improves heart health and blood flow, helps reduce or maintain weight, and promotes general physical fitness. However, determining the amount and form of exercise to recommend for a patient with osteoarthritis will depend on which joints are involved, how stable they are, and whether the patient has undergone a joint replacement procedure. The specifics will vary from individual to individual, so the patient should seek advice from a doctor or physical therapist.

Strength training. Exercise bands are inexpensive devices that are useful for resistance training.

Aerobic exercise. This form of activity helps keep the lungs and circulatory system in shape.

Range of motion exercises. These activities help keep the joints limber.

Agility activities. These exercises are intended to help the patient maintain daily living skills.

When exercising and during normal daily activities, it is important for the patient to stay aware of the need to rest and protect the joints. The patient must learn to recognize the body's signals, and know when to stop or slow down in order to prevent pain. For some people, relaxation, stress reduction, and biofeedback techniques can help. Others may need to use canes or splints to take pressure off the joints. Splints provide extra support for weakened joints and can help keep the joint in the correct position. However, splints should be used for limited periods only, because joints and muscles must be exercised to prevent stiffness and weakness.

Exercise and a healthy diet facilitate weight control, another essential component of osteoarthritis treatment. Losing weight reduces stress on weight-bearing joints and limits further injury.

Nutrition is another very important factor in the successful treatment of osteoarthritis. While there is a certain degree of controversy as to which foods or supplements are most effective, it is always appropriate to focus on avoiding foods that definitely aggravate arthritic problems.

For a basic osteoarthritis exclusion diet, the patient should avoid the following foods and beverages:

Coffee, both regular and decaffeinated
Red meat of any kind
Vinegar and anything based upon vinegar (for example, pickles), with the possible exception of apple cider vinegar
Plants in the Solanaceae (nightshade) family, such as tomatoes, eggplant, peppers, potatoes, and tobacco
High-acid vegetables, such as tomatoes and rhubarb
High-acid berries, such as gooseberries, red currants, and black currants
Refined white flour products
Artificial additives, flavorings, and preservatives
Processed foods
Red wine, port, and sherry
Carbonated drinks
Shellfish
Any food or beverage that causes specific problems for the patient

Exclusion diets produce the best results in earlier, more painful stages of this long-term condition. In longstanding osteoarthritis, a balance must be struck between the adoption of good eating habits that will have a positive psychological impact on the patient and adherence to a nutritional dogma that may, in the long run, be of questionable efficacy.

Pain relief is, of course, an ongoing concern in the management of this chronic condition. As discussed earlier, there are a number of nonpharmaceutical ways to relieve the pain of osteoarthritis. Warm towels, hot packs, and warm baths represent ways to apply moist heat to the joint, relieving pain and stiffness. In some cases, a cold pack (such as a bag of ice or frozen vegetables wrapped in a towel) can relieve pain or numb the sore area. Water therapy in a heated pool may also relieve pain and stiffness.

In *Textbook of Natural Medicine*, Drs. Pizzorno and Murray suggest the following supplements:[4]

Glucosamine sulfate: 1,500 mg/day
Vitamin E: 600 IU/day
Vitamin A: 5,000 IU/day
Vitamin C: 1 to 3g/day
Vitamin B_6: 50 mg/day
Pantothenic acid: 12.5 mg/day
Methionine: 400 mg three times a day
Zinc: 45 mg/day
Copper: 1 mg/day

Numerous physical aids and supports are available for patients who have become disabled by this disease. A wealth of simple inventions, called activities of daily living (ADL) devices, can help patients manage everyday life tasks. These range from specially designed kitchen devices (such as cutlery, can openers, and faucet grips) to brushes with extended handles and adaptations to help with using the telephone. These devices can enormously improve the patient's quality and experience of life. More information can be obtained from occupational therapists and other physical therapy specialists. Other sources of information are the Arthritis Foundation and local agencies dedicated to the concerns of aging.

RHEUMATOID ARTHRITIS

A chronic syndrome characterized by nonspecific, usually symmetric inflammation of the peripheral joints, potentially resulting in progressive destruction of articular and periarticular structures; generalized manifestations may also be present. (The Merck Manual)

Rheumatoid arthritis is a chronic inflammatory condition that involves not only the joints, but other connective tissue as well. About 2.1 million Americans, or 1% of the adult population of the United States, have rheumatoid arthritis. Rheumatoid arthritis affects all races and ethnic groups. The disease most often begins in middle age and occurs with increased frequency in older people, but it may also affect children and young adults. Like some other forms of arthritis, rheumatoid arthritis occurs much more frequently in women than in men. Two to three times as many women as men develop the disease.

Rheumatoid arthritis is one of several autoimmune arthritic diseases. An important laboratory finding in this condition is the presence of rheumatoid factor (RF), a special antibody active against the normal antibodies in the bloodstream. Why RF develops is unknown, but current theories point to an exaggerated immune response to long-term stimulation by infectious agents or foreign substances. RF itself is not directly responsible for the inflammatory process, but functions solely as a marker for the disease.

The joint destruction that occurs in severe rheumatoid arthritis is caused by inflammation of the synovial membrane, the thin, smooth capsule that lines the joints. As part of the immune response to the unknown stimulus, white blood cells and antibodies infiltrate the synovial membranes, inducing them to proliferate and fold over on themselves. Persistent or recurrent inflammation results in permanent damage to the joint cartilage, bones, ligaments, and tendons. This widespread inflammatory process may also involve other tissues, including blood vessels, skin, nerves, muscles, heart, and lungs. The result is painful joints, loss of mobility, and generalized soreness and depression.

Several special features distinguish rheumatoid arthritis from other types of arthritis. For example, rheumatoid arthritis generally occurs symmetrically. That is, if one knee or hand is involved, the other will be also. The disease often affects the wrist joints and the finger joints closest to the hand. It can also impact other parts of the body, and may be associated with fatigue, occasional fever, and a general sense of malaise.

Signs and Symptoms of Rheumatoid Arthritis

Joint pain, aching, and stiffness come on gradually, followed in a few weeks by joint swelling, redness, and warmth.

Presentation is usually symmetrical. The hands, wrists, shoulders, elbows, feet, ankles and knees on both sides of the body are typically involved, but the patient may initially present with inflammation of a single joint.

Symptoms tend to be worst in the morning and diminish as the day goes on.

Rheumatoid nodules (small, firm lumps beneath the skin) appear in some patients, especially around the elbows.

Fatigue. The patient often experiences distressing fatigue in the early afternoon and has difficulty sleeping in general.

Other organs may be affected. Vasculitis, or inflammation of the blood vessels, may cause skin rashes, ulcers, and gangrene. Other manifestations include scarring of the lungs, inflammation of the membranes surrounding the heart and lungs, nerve damage, dry eyes and mouth (Sjögrens syndrome), and enlargement of the spleen and lymph nodes.

The experience of rheumatoid arthritis varies greatly from person to person. The condition may last only a few months and resolve without causing any noticeable damage. It may take the form of mild or moderate disease with periods of worsened symptoms, called flares, and periods during which the patient feels better, called remissions. The most severe form of rheumatoid arthritis is active most of the time, lasts for many years, and leads to serious joint damage and disability.

For about 5% to 10% of rheumatoid arthritis patients, the arthritis is mild or limited to one or two episodes. Another 25% have an erratic pattern of prolonged remissions and periods of relapse. In the majority, however, the clinical course is progressive with intermittent flare-ups. Most patients continue to function despite pain and discomfort, but about 10% of rheumatoid arthritis patients progress to severe permanent joint deformity, limitation of movement, or serious disability.

Treatment of Rheumatoid Arthritis

The herbal treatment guidelines given here ensure that appropriate tonics are included. Potentially, every system and organ of the body may need tonic support in this autoimmune condition that so severely affects connective tissue. The two primary foci for support are the musculoskeletal and immune systems. Nervine tonics are also indicated. If there are problems with the digestive system, emphasize tonics as well as remedies for specific symptoms.

Actions Indicated

Because of the nature of the inflammation in rheumatoid arthritis, this is where phytosterol-containing anti-inflammatory herbs, such as *Dioscorea villosa* (wild yam) and *Bupleurum*, come into their own. However, the salicylate-containing herbs are still helpful. *Filipendula ulmaria* (meadowsweet) fits perfectly. Phytosterol- and salicylate-containing herbs complement one another well.

The complex of potential causes of this autoimmune condition includes aspects of psychology. Even if a causal role cannot be proved, there can be no doubt that anxiety and depression are major aggravating factors for rheumatoid arthritis. Nervine relaxants also help as antispasmodics, and nervine tonics will ease the constant stress caused by the pain and discomfort.

Antirheumatics will help, but their selection must be based on a rationale that takes into account the individual's unique issues.

Anti-inflammatories are very important here, as much of the symptom picture is the direct result of the inflammatory process.

Alteratives play a pivotal role in any immune system work. *Menyanthes trifoliata* is essential.

Antispasmodics, such as *Cimicifuga racemosa*, will ease any associated muscular tension.

Circulatory stimulants are not as crucial in rheumatoid arthritis as they are in osteoarthritis.

Rubefacients are not as relevant here as in osteoarthritis, and, in fact, can aggravate symptoms of rheumatoid arthritis.

Analgesics will ease both the pain and the stress response to the pain.

Nervines are especially relevant, considering the acknowledged psychosomatic contribution to this problem. Tonics and antidepressants will support the patient in coping with this extremely tiring and debilitating condition. Nervine relaxants help as antispasmodics.

Hypnotics will help with sleep in the face of pain.

Specific Remedies

There are no specific remedies for rheumatoid arthritis. This is to be expected, due to the multifactorial nature of this immune-mediated condition. However, alterative-based antirheumatic herbs are of special relevance here, with an emphasis on the alterative action. These include *Menyanthes trifoliata* (bogbean), *Harpagophytum procumbens* (devil's claw), and *Arctium lappa* (burdock). *Guaiacum* and *Dioscorea villosa* (wild yam) are especially useful as anti-inflammatories. *Tanacetum parthenium* (feverfew) can be very helpful for some people.

Beyond this, appropriate treatment and herb selection are largely a reflection of the diagnostic skill of the practitioner. Much will depend on the patient's adoption of appropriate dietary and lifestyle changes and adherence to the dosage regimen.

A Prescription for Rheumatoid Arthritis

Menyanthes trifoliata	2 parts
Filipendula ulmaria	1½ parts
Dioscorea villosa	1½ parts
Guaiacum officinale	1 part
Valeriana officinalis	1 part
Cimicifuga racemosa	1 part
Apium graveolens	1 part
Angelica archangelica	1 part
Achillea millefolium	1 part
Hypericum perforatum	1 part

Dosage: up to 5 ml of tincture three times a day

A Prescription for Sleep and Pain Relief

Valeriana officinalis	1 part
Piscidia erythrina	1 part
Passiflora incarnata	1 part

Dosage: 5 to 15 ml of tincture one-half hour before retiring

The digestive system must be working well, so treat any stomach irritation as a priority. These prescriptions do not take such problems into account. As in osteoarthritis, if the patient is experiencing epigastric tenderness due to the harshness of *Menyanthes* or *Guaiacum*, add *Althaea*.

Table 19.5. Actions Supplied by Prescription for Rheumatoid Arthritis

ACTION	HERBS
Alterative	*Menyanthes trifoliata, Guaiacum officinale, Cimicifuga racemosa*
Anti-inflammatory (salicylate)	*Filipendula ulmaria*
Anti-inflammatory (saponin)	*Guaiacum officinale*
Anti-inflammatory (general)	*Angelica archangelica, Menyanthes trifoliata, Guaiacum officinale, Cimicifuga racemosa*
Nervine (antispasmodic)	*Valeriana officinalis, Cimicifuga racemosa, Apium graveolens*
Nervine (tonic and antidepressant)	*Hypericum perforatum*
Diuretic	*Apium graveolens, Achillea millefolium*
Carminative	*Angelica archangelica, Valeriana officinalis, Apium graveolens*
Bitter tonic	*Menyanthes trifoliata, Achillea millefolium*

Broader Context of Treatment

As in osteoarthritis, the patient must strike a good balance between rest and exercise, resting more when the disease is active and exercising more when it is not. Rest helps reduce active joint inflammation and pain and eases fatigue. Short rest breaks every now and then are more helpful than long ones. Exercise maintains healthy and strong muscles, preserving joint mobility and flexibility. Exercise can also help with sleep problems, reduce pain, foster a positive attitude, and facilitate weight loss.

Rheumatoid arthritis is often as much an emotional challenge as a physical one. People with this condition commonly experience fear, anger, and frustration—emotions that can greatly increase the level of stress already generated by pain and physical limitation. Although stress does not appear to cause rheumatoid arthritis, it makes coping with the disease much more difficult. A number of techniques can help patients cope with stress. Regular rest periods can be beneficial, as can relaxation, distraction, or visualization exercises. See chapter 16 for more suggestions on managing stress.

The daily living aids mentioned in the discussion on osteoarthritis can be just as helpful for patients with rheumatoid arthritis. The general dietary suggestions given for osteoarthritis are also pertinent here. However, the nutritional supplement recommendations are different. In *Textbook of Natural Medicine*, Drs. Pizzorno and Murray suggest the following supplements:[5]

DHEA: 50 to 200 mg/day
EPA: 1.8 g/day; or flaxseed oil: 1 tablespoon/day
Pantothenic acid: 500 mg four times a day
Quercetin: 250 mg three times a day, between meals
Vitamin C: 1 to 3 g/day
Vitamin E: 400 IU/day
Copper: 1 mg/day
Manganese: 15 mg/day
Selenium: 200 mcg/day
Zinc: 45 mg/day

OSTEOPOROSIS

A generalized, progressive diminution in bone tissue mass per unit volume, causing skeletal weakness, even though the ratio of mineral to organic elements is unchanged in the remaining morphologically normal bone. *(The Merck Manual)*

Osteoporosis is a disease that weakens bones to the point at which they break easily, especially those in the hip, spine, and wrist. About 25 million Americans have osteoporosis, and 80% of these people are women. One of two women and one in eight men over the age of 50 will at some point have an osteoporosis-related fracture.

Although the exact cause of osteoporosis is unknown, the process by which the bone becomes porous is understood. Normally, 6% to 12% of an adult's total skeleton is replaced each year. After skeletal mass peaks—usually around the age of 35—bones begin to lose calcium faster than they can replace it. For women, the loss of bone den-sity speeds up during the first three to seven years after menopause, and then slows down again. This post-menopausal increase in bone loss is believed to be caused by the decline in estrogen production.

Certain conditions that impair the body's ability to absorb calcium, such as kidney disease, Cushing's syndrome, and hyperthyroidism, can also lead to osteoporosis. Other factors associated with osteoporosis are surgical removal of part of the stomach or intestine and excessive use of glucocorticoids, other steroids, or anticonvulsant drugs. Prolonged immobility due to paralysis or illness can cause calcium loss, leading to eventual bone loss.

Osteoporosis is preventable. A diet rich in calcium, vitamin D, and phytoestrogens and a lifestyle that includes regular exercise are thought to be the best ways to prevent osteoporosis.

Calcium

Calcium-rich foods, such as dairy products, are the preferred source of calcium. Calcium-fortified foods and calcium supplements are other means by which optimal calcium intake can be reached in those who cannot meet this need by ingesting conventional foods.

Phosphorus-rich foods should be avoided, as they can promote bone loss. High-phosphorus foods include red meats, soft drinks, and foods containing phosphate additives. Overconsumption of alcohol and caffeine is thought to impair calcium absorption and should be avoided.

Good Food Sources of Calcium

Low-fat dairy products, such as cheese, yogurt, and milk
Canned fish with edible bones, such as salmon and sardines
Dark green leafy vegetables, such as kale, collards, and broccoli
Calcium-fortified foods, such as bread made with calcium-fortified flour and calcium-fortified orange juice

As most women get only one half to one third as much calcium as they need from the diet, calcium supplements can make up the difference. The chelated forms of calcium supplements are most effective. These include calcium citrate and calcium gluconate.

Conclusions of a panel convened by the National Institutes of Health were published in the December 28, 1994, issue of the *Journal of the American Medical Association*. The panel's recommended intake levels, presented in table 19.6, include both dietary and supplemental calcium.

Table 19.6. Optimal Calcium Intake[6]

AGE	RECOMMENDED INTAKE
Birth–6 months	400 mg/day
6–12 months	600 mg/day
1–5 years	800 mg/day
6–10 years	800–1,200 mg/day
11–24 years	1,200–1,500 mg/day
Women 25–50 years	1,000 mg/day
Pregnant or lactating women	1,200–1,500 mg/day
Postmenopausal women on estrogen replacement therapy	1,000 mg/day
Postmenopausal women not on estrogen therapy	1,500 mg/day
Men 25–65 years	1,000 mg/day
Women and men over 65	1,500 mg/day

Vitamin D and Magnesium

Adequate vitamin D is essential for optimal calcium absorption. Even a brief period of sun exposure each day provides enough vitamin D for most people. Taking vitamin D supplements (400 to 800 IU/day) may be helpful if the individual does not live in a sunny climate. Magnesium is also necessary to help the body absorb calcium. The recommended daily dose of magnesium is 250 to 350 mg.

Exercise

Exercise not only builds bone strength, but it also helps prevent bone loss. Weight-bearing exercises that put stress on bones, such as dancing, running, walking, stair climbing, and aerobics, reduce bone loss and help prevent osteoporosis. To benefit from the exercise, it must be done at least three times a week for 30 to 45 minutes.

Phytoestrogens

Plant estrogenic substances, or *phytoestrogens*, are constituents of many herbs with a historical use for conditions that are now treated with synthetic estrogens. They may be suitable alternatives to estrogens for the prevention of osteoporosis in menopausal women. Given the protective benefits of soy isoflavones against breast cancer alone, the regular consumption of soy foods is encouraged.

Herbal and Nutritional Treatments for Osteoporosis

Herbal and nutritional treatment cannot eliminate osteoporosis, but it can slow the process. The North American tradition relies on herbs such as *Equisetum arvense* (horsetail), *Avena sativa* (oat straw), and *Urtica dioica* (nettles) for the long-term treatment of osteoporosis. Some believe that they are effective because they have a high calcium content. In fact, these herbs do not contain particularly high levels of calcium, but they are often effective anyway!

Taking into account the physiological processes that underlie osteoporosis, herbal hormonal normalizers may be helpful if started early enough. Antirheumatic herbs can help with pain in the joints and muscles, and anti-inflammatory herbs will similarly reduce the discomfort associated with this problem.

A Prescription for Osteoporosis

Vitex agnus-castus	2 parts
Equisetum arvense	1 part
Avena sativa	1 part
Urtica dioica	1 part

Dosage: up to 5 ml of tincture three times a day

Broader Context of Treatment

Here are some general preventive guidelines.

Eat foods rich in calcium, such as nonfat milk, low-fat yogurt, broccoli, cauliflower, salmon, tofu, sesame seeds, almonds, and leafy green vegetables.

Eat foods that contain plant estrogens, especially tofu and other soy products.

Avoid foods that can interfere with absorption of calcium, such as red meats, soft drinks, and excessive amounts of alcohol and caffeine.

Do weight-bearing exercises for 30 to 45 minutes at least three times a week.

Do not smoke. Some studies have shown that women who smoke increase their risk of developing osteoporosis by 50%.

Avoid antacids containing aluminum, as they can prevent calcium absorption by binding with phosphorus in the intestines.

In addition, the following supplements are recommended to help prevent and treat osteoporosis:[7]

High-potency multiple vitamin and mineral formula
Calcium: 800 to 1,200 mg/day
Vitamin D: 400 IU/day

Magnesium: 400 to 800 mg/day
Boron (as sodium tetrahydraborate): 3 to 5 mg/day

GOUT

A metabolic disease marked by a painful inflammation of the joints, deposits of urates in and around the joints, and usually an excessive amount of uric acid in the blood. *(The Merriam-Webster Medical Dictionary)*

Gout is one of the most painful of the rheumatic diseases. It is caused by deposits of needlelike crystals of uric acid in the connective tissue, joint spaces, or both. The inflammatory process here is initiated by the deposition of uric acid from the bloodstream in the joint. When these crystals are ingested by white blood cells, the cells release enzymes that generate inflammation.

Gout accounts for about 5% of all cases of arthritis. *Pseudogout*, also a crystal-induced arthritis, is a condition with similar symptoms that results from deposits of calcium pyrophosphate dihydrate crystals in the joints. It may also be called calcium pyrophosphate deposition disease, crystal deposition disease, or chondrocalcinosis.

To understand gout, it is first necessary to have a basic knowledge of the chemistry of uric acid. This naturally occurring substance is a product of the chemical breakdown of the purine bases that compose the genetic material, DNA. As cells die and release DNA from their chromosomes, purines are converted into uric acid that is excreted in the urine and, to a lesser extent, through the intestinal tract. The amount of uric acid dissolved in the bloodstream is directly related to this delicate balance between uric acid production and excretion.

Normally, uric acid is dissolved in the blood and passes through the kidneys into the urine, where it is eliminated. If the body increases its production of uric acid or if the kidneys do not eliminate enough uric acid from the body, uric acid builds up, resulting in a condition called *hyperuricemia*. Hyperuricemia may also occur when a person eats too many high-purine foods, such as liver, dried beans and peas, anchovies, and gravies. Hyperuricemia by itself is not dangerous, but if hyperuricemia leads to the formation of uric acid crystals, gout may develop. However, only 1 in 20 people with hyperuricemia goes on to develop gout.

Acute attacks of gout are caused by the body's inflammatory reaction to the intermittent precipitation of uric acid crystals into the joints. The excess crystals build up in the joint spaces, causing inflammation. Deposits of uric acid, called *tophi*, can appear as lumps under the skin around the joints and at the rim of the ear. In addition, uric acid crystals can collect in the kidneys and cause kidney stones. For many people, gout first affects the joints of the big toe, a condition called *podagra*.

Risk Factors for the Development of Hyperuricemia and Gout

Genetics may play a role in determining a person's risk, since 6% to 18% of people with gout have a family history of the disease.

Obesity increases the risk of developing hyperuricemia and gout, because excessive food intake increases the body's production of uric acid.

Overconsumption of alcohol can lead to hyperuricemia, because it interferes with the elimination of uric acid from the body.

Eating too many purine-rich foods can cause or aggravate gout.

An enzyme defect that interferes with the way the body breaks down purines causes gout in a small number of people.

Exposure to lead in the environment can cause gout.

Some people are at risk for developing high uric acid levels because they have coexisting medical conditions or because they take certain medicines. The following medicines can lead to hyperuricemia because they reduce the body's ability to eliminate uric acid:

- Diuretics
- Salicylates, or medicines made from salicylic acid, such as aspirin
- The vitamin niacin, also called nicotinic acid
- Cyclosporine, a medicine used to control the body's rejection of transplanted organs
- Levodopa, a medicine used to treat Parkinson's disease

Treatment of Gout

Actions Indicated

Diuretics play a pivotal role in any attempt to go beyond mere symptom relief, as they can help flush the urates from the body.

Anti-inflammatories may help, but probably not nearly as much as the patient would like. Inflammation is an appropriate body response to the presence of crystals.

Specific Remedies

Colchicine, from *Colchicum autumnale* (autumn crocus), is a specific allopathic drug. However, use of the whole plant is very unsafe, due to its inherent toxicity.

A Prescription for Gout

Eupatorium purpureum	2 parts
Elymus repens	2 parts
Apium graveolens	2 parts
Guaiacum officinale	1 part

Dosage: up to 5ml of tincture three times a day. In addition, a strong infusion of *Urtica dioica* should be drunk often.

Broader Context of Treatment

Gout appears to be common among people who eat diets that include meat and animal fats, but is unusual in people who follow vegetarian diets. In addition, rapid weight-loss diets may increase uric acid levels in the blood.

Here are some recommendations to help predisposed people avoid gout attacks:

Drink 6 pints of fluid a day. Slightly alkaline, natural spring-water is recommended. This helps dilute the urine and promote excretion of uric acid through continued flushing of the kidneys.

Avoid purine-rich foods, such as anchovies, asparagus, crab, fish roe, herring, kidney, liver, sweetbreads, meat gravies and broth, mushrooms, mussels, peas, beans, and sardines.

Avoid all alcoholic beverages.

Eat raw fruit, vegetables, grains, seeds, and nuts. Cherries are especially recommended; the patient should consume 1/2 pound of fresh or canned cherries a day.

Exercise regularly and maintain a healthy body weight. Lose weight if overweight.

Cherries are particularly effective in lowering uric acid levels and preventing attacks of gout. Cherries, hawthorn berries, blueberries, and other dark red-blue berries are rich sources of constituents called anthocyanidins and proanthocyanidins. These compounds give those fruits their deep red-blue color, and have the ability to prevent breakdown of collagen in connective tissue.

Anthocyanidins and proanthocyanidins affect collagen metabolism in a number of ways:

- Reinforce the collagen matrix of connective tissue (ground substance, cartilage, tendons, etc.)
- Minimize free radical damage through antioxidant activity
- Inhibit the breakdown of collagen during inflammation

These effects on collagen structures make flavonoids extremely useful in the treatment of a wide variety of inflammatory conditions, including gout and rheumatoid arthritis.

There are a number of simple ways to reduce pain and inflammation during an acute gout attack. However, if the joint is too painful to touch, they can be difficult to implement. If the pain is not too severe, apply a plastic bag containing a few ice cubes or a bag of frozen vegetables to the joint to relieve painful swelling. Wrap the cold bag in a soft cloth or towel and hold it against the painful area for up to five minutes at a time, then repeat as needed. Because even the pressure of a sheet or blanket can cause pain in a gout-afflicted joint, at bedtime rest the gouty foot inside a cardboard box or a plastic laundry basket turned on its side.

BURSITIS AND TENDINITIS

Bursitis: Acute or chronic inflammation of a bursa. *(The Merck Manual)*

Tendinitis: Inflammation of a tendon (tendinitis) and the lining of the tendon sheath (tenosynovitis), usually occurring simultaneously. *(The Merck Manual)*

A bursa is a pocket of connective tissue adjacent to a joint. Lined by a smooth inner surface, the bursa facilitates the gliding movements of muscles and tendons over bony protuberances. *Bursitis* is inflammation of a bursa that results in pain, tenderness, stiffness, and, in some cases, swelling and redness. The inflammatory process may affect any bursa, but bursitis is most common in the shoulder, elbow, hip, and knee.

Bursitis that occurs in the knees is often called "housemaid's knee"; it is called "tennis elbow" when it affects that joint. The condition may be caused by a hard knock or accident or by slow, gradual change. When it is part of the gradual development of rheumatic tendencies, it should be treated as described in the section on myalgia. When acute (often due to an accident or injury), the best treatment is to use a compress or stimulating liniment on the affected area. (See External Applications for Musculoskeletal Problems earlier in this chapter.) Both will help reduce inflammation and ease pain. However, if the problem continues, an internal treatment program should be initiated. See treatment recommendations for myalgia.

Bursitis is associated with strenuous activity, particularly among manual workers and athletes. However, it can also affect otherwise sedentary people who push their bodies past reasonable limits. Warming up before strenuous exercise and cooling down afterward is the most effective way to avoid bursitis and other strains affecting the bones, muscles, and ligaments.

Tendinitis is an inflammation in or around a tendon, the fibrous tissue that connects muscle to bone. Tendons withstand bending, stretching, and twisting, but can become inflamed because of overuse, disease, or injury. The pain can be significant, and worsens if continued use of the joint furthers the damage. Most tendinitis heals in about two weeks, but chronic tendinitis can take more than six weeks to resolve, especially if the sufferer does not give the tendon adequate time to heal before using it.

Tendons can become inflamed when overstressed by any activity, but the most common cause by far is *repetitive stress*—using the same joint for the same stressful movement again and again. This happens not only in sports, but also in many types of office work and other situations.

Treatment of Bursitis and Tendinitis

While the patient may be tempted to "tough out" the pain, this is not a good idea. Left untreated, chronic bursitis can lead to the formation of calcium deposits in soft tissues, and may even cause permanent limitation of motion in the affected joint.

Actions Indicated

Antirheumatics often help; the choice will depend upon the practitioner's interpretation of the patient's total picture.

Anti-inflammatories provide the primary action needed for symptomatic relief. *Salix* is an example.

Antispasmodics, such as *Viburnum opulus*, ease local muscle tension.

Circulatory stimulants and *rubefacients* contribute by increasing local blood circulation.

Analgesics may help with pain. However, the legal herbal analgesics can do very little in such cases, so pain relief is best achieved with anti-inflammatories and antispasmodics.

A Prescription for Bursitis or Tendinitis

Salix spp.	2 parts
Viburnum opulus	2 parts
Apium graveolens	2 parts
Zanthoxylum americanum	1 part

Dosage: up to 5 ml of tincture three times a day

An Antispasmodic Rub

Lobelia inflata	1 part
Viburnum opulus	1 part

Rub tincture mixture into painful muscles as needed

Table 19.7. Actions Supplied by Prescription for Bursitis and Tendinitis

ACTION	HERBS
Anti-inflammatory (salicylate)	*Salix* spp.
Anti-inflammatory (general)	*Apium graveolens*
Antispasmodic	*Lobelia inflata, Viburnum opulus, Apium graveolens*
Circulatory stimulant	*Zanthoxylum americanum*

Broader Context of Treatment

Diathermy (deep-heat therapy) can help relieve the discomfort and inflammation of bursitis and tendinitis and also soothe tense muscles, nerves, and tendons. The goals of treatment are to restore painless movement to the joint and to maintain the strength of surrounding muscles while giving the injured tissues time to heal. Adequate rest is crucial. Returning too soon to the activity that caused the injury can lead to chronic tendinitis or torn tendons. An immediate treatment for tendinitis and bursitis is known by the acronym RICE, which stands for *rest, ice, compression,* and *elevation.*

Rest is mainly a matter of remembering not to use the joint, especially for the same action by which it was injured.

Ice can be a bag of frozen vegetables if no ice pack is handy.

Compression is best provided by wrapping the area snugly, but not painfully tight, with a sports bandage.

Elevation reduces blood pressure in the injured area. Elevate the ankle by putting it on a footstool, for example, or elevate the elbow onto a table.

RESTLESS LEGS SYNDROME

Restless legs syndrome is a puzzling neurological disorder for which a cure remains elusive. The syndrome is characterized by tingling or crawling sensations deep in the legs, associated with an overwhelming desire to move the legs to relieve the discomfort. The symptoms often worsen at night.

Restless legs syndrome is believed to be a genetic neurological condition that is activated by a chemical imbalance in the brain. Research shows that caffeine can aggravate symptoms. The syndrome has also been linked to iron or folic acid deficiency, especially in people with kidney disease.

Treatment of Restless Legs Syndrome

Herbs with strong relaxing qualities may be effective in reducing muscle tension and relieving pain. Such herbs include *Passiflora incarnata*, *Valeriana officinalis*, *Piper methysticum*, and *Cimicifuga racemosa*. *Viburnum opulus* may also help relax muscles.

To help correct nutrient deficiencies that may contribute to symptoms, the patient should take vitamin E, a multivitamin containing iron, and B complex. These should be taken in the standard RDA doses. To offset folic acid deficiency, the patient should take 400 to 1,000 mcg/day of this nutrient.

Other recommendations include:

Avoid stimulants, such as caffeine and decongestants.
Avoid stimulating activities up to three hours before bed, including exercising and consuming a heavy meal.
Keep the bedroom quiet and cool; an overly warm room appears to aggravate restless legs syndrome.
Practice relaxation techniques, such as yoga, biofeedback, and meditation, to reduce stress.
Soak the feet in cool water for relief. Never use ice water, which can cause nerve damage.

Leg Massage

1. Sit on the floor and bend one knee, keeping the foot flat. Grasp the calf in both hands and use the thumbs to find the muscle that runs along the outside of the shinbone, below the kneecap. Massage the muscle all the way down to the anklebone.
2. Place both thumbs on the inside of the leg near the anklebone. Keeping the hands around the calf for support, massage the inside of the leg vigorously with both thumbs, moving from the ankle up to the knee.
3. Finally, use the thumbs and fingers of both hands to knead the back and sides of the calf muscle. Work from the knee down to the ankle. When finished massaging one leg, repeat the entire process on the other. Alternately massage both legs several times.

References

1. Thie NM, Prasad NG, Major PW. Evaluation of glucosamine sulfate compared to ibuprofen for the treatment of temporomandibular joint osteoarthritis: a randomized double blind controlled 3 month clinical trial. *The Journal of Rheumatology* 2001 Jun; 28(6):1347–55.
2. Messier SP, Loeser RF, Mitchell MN, et al. Exercise and weight loss in obese older adults with knee osteoarthritis: a preliminary study. *Journal of the American Geriatrics Society* 2000 Sep; 48(9):1062–72.
3. Randall, et al. Nettle sting of Urtica dioica for joint pain—an exploratory study of this complementary therapy." *Complementary Therapies in Medicine* 1999 Sep; 7(3):126–31.
4. Pizzorno JE, Murray MT. *Textbook of Natural Medicine.* Edinburgh: Churchill Livingstone, 1999.
5. Ibid.
6. NIH Consensus Conference. Optimal calcium intake. NIH Consensus Development Panel on Optimal Calcium Intake. *The Journal of the American Medical Association* 1994; 272:1942–48.
7. Pizzorno JE, Murray MT. *Textbook of Natural Medicine.* Edinburgh: Churchill Livingstone, 1999.

Suggested Reading

Hoffmann D. *Healthy Bones and Joints: A Natural Approach to Treating Arthritis, Osteoporosis, Tendinitis, Myalgia, Bursitis.* Pownal, VT: Storey Books, 2000.

20

⤞

THE SKIN

The skin is the body's largest organ. It consists of a thin outer layer called the *epidermis* and a much thicker inner layer called the *dermis*. Beneath the dermis is a layer of little lobes of fat bound together by tough fibers that extend down from the dermis. Between the epidermis and dermis is the basement membrane, to which both layers are attached. This characteristic layering of cells, from the live and actively replicating cells of the stratum germinatum to the dead flakes on the surface, provides the unique setting for the skin diseases.

The skin fulfills a number of important functions. As the interface between the body's internal structures and the environment, the skin serves as a protective coat for the body against mechanical injury and attack by bacteria, fungi, viruses, and parasites. The pigment melanin protects against ultraviolet radiation. The skin is also a major organ of elimination through the functions of sweating and sloughing off dead skin cells. In addition, a number of immune responses occur in the skin.

In various ways, the skin also plays a vital role in temperature regulation. Variable amounts of heat are lost through the skin by transfer from the dermis capillaries to the cooler epidermal cells. The amounts lost vary according to constriction or dilation of the dermal blood cells. The layer of insulating fat modifies the amount of heat conducted from the depths of the body. Sweating cools the epidermis through evaporation.

The skin also serves as a primary sensory organ. The five sensations that arise from stimulation of skin nerves are touch, pain, heat, cold, and pressure. Other skin sensations, such as vibration, are composites of these basic sensations. In hairy skin, the nerve endings are simple, threadlike, naked terminals. In skin that is not hairy, there are several types of specialized nerve endings. Although they look the same, each nerve ending is capable of responding to only one of the five basic types of sensation.

Finally, the skin is the interface between our consciousness and the world, the vehicle through which we express, communicate, and perceive. Thus, psychological and spiritual aspects of the individual impact and are impacted by the skin.

This array of functions highlights the complexity of the relationships among the skin, the internal organs, and the psychology of the individual. From this awareness comes an important therapeutic insight: Effective phytotherapeutic treatment of skin disease must be mediated through internal medication, not topical application.

Treatment of skin problems must take into account the whole panoply of issues involved. Similarly, the widely held view that many skin problems are caused by "nerves" is not very helpful. There is a deep and complex relationship between the epidermis and the nervous system. Developmentally, nerve and skin cells derive from the same tissue in the human embryo. The close functional relationship between the skin and the nervous system facilitates many aspects of homeostasis, such as body temperature control.

In addition, the psychological relationship between the individual and the skin is deep and complex. An individual expresses and experiences much of his or her self-image through the skin. Thus, perception of the world and communication to the world are also vital skin functions.

To conclude that there is a simple causal relationship between the nervous system and skin disorders ignores all of the insights gained through the holistic perspective. Anyone with obvious skin problems may well become stressed, developing psychological coping mechanisms that appear to be manifestations of nervous system issues. But which comes first?

HERBS FOR THE TREATMENT OF SKIN PROBLEMS

Internal treatment of skin problems will often be relevant, but it may be appropriate to also apply herb externally for local effects.

Alteratives

As with the musculoskeletal system, the skin is often the focus for manifestations of systemic illness. For the phytotherapist, it should come as no surprise that alterative herbs are again the cornerstone of any fundamental healing transformation. The therapist is continually faced with the challenge of selecting appropriate alteratives for given individuals. Because of its focus on secondary actions and system affinities, our herb selection model often helps, but sometimes it is not the answer.

I have found the following generalization to be helpful. Bear in mind that as with all generalizations, there are many exceptions. However, it is possible to broadly group alterative herbs according to their botany and their impact on elimination.

Table 20.1. Alteratives Grouped by Plant Part and Route of Elimination

PLANT PART USED	PRIMARY ELIMINATION PATHWAY/ACTION	HERBAL EXAMPLES
Leaf	Kidney/diuretic	*Galium aparine, Trifolium pratense, Urtica dioica*
Root, rhizome, wood	Liver/hepatic	*Arctium lappa, Mahonia aquifolium, Rumex crispus*

Herbs for Topical Application

Herbs offer a range of actions that directly impact the skin, and can be applied directly by choosing the most relevant method. *Stellaria media* (chickweed), for example, is an extremely effective remedy for the relief of itching. The only itching for which it offers little relief is that due to jaundice. It is most effective in a nongreasy form, such as a bath, fomentation, poultice, lotion, or cream.

Herbal actions useful for topical application can be divided into two broad groups.

1. Actions that exert specific local effects on areas of skin to which herbs are applied include anti-inflammatory, antimicrobial, antipruritic, astringent, emollient, rubefacient, and vulnerary.
2. Actions intended primarily for internal effect but enter the body via absorption through the skin potentially include all herbal actions. However, alterative actions have been most commonly applied in this way.

Table 20.2. Herbs and Actions for Topical Use

ACTION	HERBS
Antipruritic	*Calendula officinalis, Hamamelis virginiana, Hypericum perforatum, Stellaria media*
Anti-inflammatory	*Calendula officinalis, Hypericum perforatum, Matricaria recutita, Plantago* spp., various anti-inflammatory essential oils
Emollient	*Althaea officinalis, Malva sylvestris, Symphytum officinale, Ulmus rubra*
Astringent	*Achillea millefolium, Geranium maculatum, Hamamelis virginiana*
Vulnerary	*Symphytum officinale*
Antimicrobial	*Allium sativum, Commiphora molmol, Hydrastis canadensis*; strongly antimicrobial essential oils including *Thymus vulgaris, Eucalyptus globulus, Melaleuca* spp.

Herbs for Topical Application: Pharmacy Considerations

The whole array of topical herbal formulations developed over the years deserves a special mention. See chapter 11 for more details on these various applications.

Baths

Baths, also known as *balneotherapy*, represent one of the most pleasant ways to apply medications to the skin! They are especially useful in treating widespread skin eruptions, removing crusts and scales, and relieving inflammation and itching. In short, any remedy added to a bath counts as balneotherapy. Some commonly used bath additions are:

Salts. These range from simple table or Epsom salts to the therapeutically important salt from the Dead Sea.
Oils. Essential oils can be added to supply a wide range of properties. In the bath, they act through the skin but also via the nose. Fixed oils may be added to baths too, for their lubricating and softening properties.
Herbal extracts. These can be infusions, decoctions, or tinctures.
Colloidal oatmeal. This remedy can be very antipruritic and drying for conditions such as weeping eczema and psoriasis.

Fomentations and Compresses

These methods facilitate the local application of liquid formulations. They have the advantage of convenience and relative cleanliness, as compared with poultices. Infusions, decoctions, tinctures, and oils can all be applied in this way.

Poultices

Poultices are similar to fomentations and compresses but instead incorporate the herb in some solid form, whether whole leaf, mashed cut herb, or any relevant plant part applied directly to the skin and held in place with a cloth.

Lotions

Lotions are liquid formulations for carrying the herbs. The specific effects will depend upon both herbs and vehicle. However, no matter what remedies they contain, lotions will usually have a cooling effect due to evaporation. They rarely need to be washed off, as part will be absorbed and the rest will evaporate.

Creams

Creams are suspensions of oil in water, and can be formulated to be either greasy or nongreasy. They are primarily emollient and protective. An advantage of creams is that they do not insulate the skin too much and thus will not cause a localized increase in skin temperature. Overheating can aggravate itching in many skin problems.

Ointments (Salves)

An ointment is a semisolid, lipid-based application. Because fats are used as ointment bases (for example, cocoa butter and beeswax), they extract plant constituents well. In addition, the fats soften at skin temperature and thus make the extracted material available to the skin. Like creams, ointments and salves are emollient and protective, but they remain on the skin longer. This tenacity will confer a local warming effect.

Pastes

A paste, or a mixture of powder in an ointment base, is a traditional pharmaceutical formulation that is, unfortunately, becoming rare. This is largely a matter of convenience for dispensers, because they can be very time-consuming to make. Pastes are indicated when the goal is to keep the effects of the herbs on the surface for extended periods of time. Their contents are not absorbed well, but do impact the skin surface. They are useful in conditions such as psoriasis, in which they facilitate the removal of scales.

Powders

These are dry, finely powdered herbs or minerals. Examples include colloidal oatmeal, *Lycopodium* powder, cornstarch, and various clays. Their primary benefit is that they take up moisture—for example, perspiration or exudates of eczema. They can also be antipruritic and antimicrobial.

ECZEMA AND DERMATITIS

> Superficial inflammation of the skin, characterized by vesicles (when acute), redness, edema, oozing, crusting, scaling, and usually itching. *(The Merck Manual)*

The terms *eczema* and *dermatitis* are the cause of much confusion. In keeping with the broad guidelines given in *The Merck Manual*, we shall use these terms synonymously to indicate superficial inflammation of the skin. The dermatologist subdivides dermatitis and eczema into a range of different disease entities distinguished by location and appearance. For the phytotherapist, however, the most important distinction is between cases with an internal or endogenous cause and those with a contact or exogenous cause.

In cases of dermatitis or eczema of exogenous cause, it is often possible to solve the problem simply by removing or avoiding the surface irritant, if it can be identified! Such problems, often called *contact dermatitis*, are commonly caused by:

- Industrial solvents
- Dyes
- Nickel and other metals
- Leather-tanning chemicals
- Some soaps

In such cases, eczema is the final result of a complex series of internal reactions to allergens and irritants. It is often associated with other allergic diseases, such as hay fever and asthma, but may also occur alone. The rash of eczema is very itchy, peeling, thickened, and sometimes weepy, and is typically seen in the creases of joints and around the trunk. The rash may fluctuate seasonally and can even change over the course of the day. Scratching may lead to bleeding and infection. Blood tests in individuals with eczema reveal increased levels of cells and chemicals associated with general allergic reactions.

One variation of eczema occurs on the palms of the hands and sometimes on the soles of the feet. This type may be quite frustrating to treat, because the common exposure to moisture, irritants, and injury of these areas leads to self-perpetuation of the disease. Furthermore, the thickness of the skin in these regions makes topical therapy more difficult.

A number of factors can aggravate eczema, although the specifics vary from person to person. Dietary factors are particularly important, especially in children. Milk and milk products are the most common triggers. Primary aggravating factors for eczema are:

- Stress
- Mechanical irritation
- Heat
- Dietary factors

Treatment of Eczema

Eczema requires the practitioner to be at his or her most insightful. Ideally, the nature of the underlying cause will identify what systems call for toning. However, with the exception of obvious allergies or contact irritants, this can be problematic for a skin problem like eczema.

The skin obviously needs support, but in addition the nervous system, digestive system and liver, immune system, and others may need attention. In many ways, the therapeutic conclusion will depend upon the herbalist's theoretical interpretation of eczema, rather than the patient's case history.

Actions Indicated

Alteratives are the classic remedies for the treatment of eczema. How they work is unclear, but they can often be dramatically effective.

Antipruritics, remedies that reduce the sensation of itching, are indicated, not simply to make the patient feel better, but also to reduce physical trauma caused by scratching.

Anti-inflammatories applied topically and taken internally speed the curative work of the alteratives, but do not replace them.

Lymphatic tonics, which may be considered a type of alterative, are especially helpful for eczema in children.

Nervine relaxants help with the commonly associated problem of anxiety. They also often ease itching and even inflammation in the skin because of their relaxing effect on the peripheral nerves of the autonomic nervous system.

Diuretics ensure adequate elimination through the kidneys. Diuretic alteratives are most relevant.

Hepatics will contribute support for liver function and the digestive process. Hepatic alteratives are best here.

Vulneraries support the healing of skin lesions when applied topically, but do not replace appropriate internal treatment.

Astringents, used topically, reduce any weeping or oozing of fluids.

Emollient herbs are suitable for topical applications where soothing is needed. The demarcation among emollient, anti-inflammatory, and antipruritic herbs is rather meaningless here.

Specific Remedies

For internal treatment, the leafy alteratives are often considered the closest to specifics for this often intransigent condition. These are also often diuretic and lymphatic remedies. Herbs in this group include:

Fumaria officinalis (fumitory)
Galium aparine (cleavers)
Scrophularia nodosa (figwort)
Trifolium pratense (red clover)
Urtica dioica (nettle)
Viola tricolor (heartsease)

The rooty alteratives tend to be hepatic in nature. They can often be too strong for eczema, aggravating the problem instead of healing it. For intransigent cases unresponsive to the herbs already listed, stronger remedies are indicated. For eczema, effective examples include:

Arctium lappa (burdock)
Hydrastis canadensis (goldenseal)
Mahonia aquifolium (Oregon grape)

Relevant herbs for topical use abound. However, always bear in mind that healing must be based upon internal medication, not salves. Select remedies according to the actions most appropriate for the individual's specific symptoms. The choice often will also depend on factors such as availability and aesthetics. Examples include:

Calendula officinalis (calendula)
Hydrastis canadensis (goldenseal)
Plantago spp. (plantain)
Stellaria media (chickweed)
Urtica dioica (nettle)

A Prescription for Eczema

Galium aparine	1 part
Urtica dioica	1 part
Trifolium pratense	1 part

Dosage: up to 5 ml of tincture three times a day. In addition, the patient should drink an infusion of fresh *Urtica dioica* or *Galium aparine* two or three times a day.

Table 20.3. Actions Supplied by Prescription for Eczema

ACTION	HERBS
Alterative	Galium aparine, Urtica dioica, Trifolium pratense
Lymphatic tonic	Galium aparine, Urtica dioica
Nervine relaxant	Trifolium pratense
Anti-inflammatory	Galium aparine
Diuretic	Galium aparine, Urtica dioica
Hepatic (mild)	Galium aparine, Trifolium pratense

A Prescription for Persistent Eczema Unresponsive to Mild Alteratives

Galium aparine	1 part
Arctium lappa	1 part
Scrophularia nodosa	1 part

Dosage: 2.5 ml of tincture three times a day. Build up the dosage to 5 ml three times a day. In addition, the patient should drink an infusion of fresh or dried Urtica dioica two or three times a day.

Care should be taken initially with Scrophularia nodosa, as it can produce the opposite of the desired result in some patients. If there is a flare-up of the skin eruption, cut down on the Scrophularia and try again. This is not a healing crisis!

Table 20.4. Actions Supplied by Prescription for Persistent Eczema

ACTION	HERBS
Alterative	Scrophularia nodosa, Galium aparine, Urtica dioica, Arctium lappa
Lymphatic tonic	Galium aparine, Urtica dioica
Nervine relaxant	Trifolium pratense
Anti-inflammatory	Galium aparine
Diuretic	Galium aparine, Urtica dioica, Arctium lappa
Hepatic (mild)	Galium aparine, Arctium lappa

A Prescription for Atopic Eczema Associated with Asthma

Urtica dioica	2 parts
Trifolium pratense	2 parts
Dyspnea Formula	1 part (see chapter 15, page 332)

Dosage: up to 5 ml of tincture three times a day. The relative proportion of alterative herbs to Dyspnea Formula will depend upon the patient's specific needs. In addition, the patient should drink an infusion of fresh Urtica dioica or Galium aparine two or three times a day.

Broader Context of Treatment

If dietary triggers can be identified, it is essential for the patient to avoid them completely. Often, patients may find it challenging to adhere to specific food restrictions, especially young children. The parents who must enforce the diet will need much support from the therapist (and maybe some *Scutellaria*!). Even if no obvious food triggers exist, it is always worth excluding milk and milk products. This may be particularly relevant for children who were not breast-fed or were weaned too soon. Researchers at the Hospital for Sick Children in London have shown that children often develop eczema when weaned from breast milk to cow's milk or other foods. Goat's milk, sheep's milk, and soy milk rarely trigger allergy problems.

Here are some common eczema triggers:

- Cow's milk
- Eggs
- Cheese
- Fish
- Sugar
- Food additives

Supplements suggested for inclusion in a broad therapeutic approach to the treatment of eczema by Drs. Pizzorno and Murray in *Textbook of Natural Medicine* include:[1]

Vitamin A: 50,000 IU/day
Vitamin E: 400 IU/day (mixed tocopherols)
Zinc: 50 mg/day as picolinate (decrease dosage as condition clears)
Quercetin: 200 to 400 mg three times a day (taken 5 minutes before meals)
EPA and DHA: 540 mg and 360 mg/day, or flaxseed oil: 10g daily
Evening primrose oil: 3,000 mg/day

Other authorities have recommended supplementation with vitamin C and vitamin B complex in addition to the other supplements listed.

PSORIASIS

A chronic and recurrent disease characterized by dry, well-circumscribed, silvery, scaling papules and plaques of various sizes. *(The Merck Manual)*

This is a common skin disease of unknown cause that affects up to 3% of the American population. Onset usually occurs before age 20, but all age groups may be affected. The severity of this condition can vary from the presence of one or two cosmetically annoying lesions to a physically disabling and disfiguring affliction of the entire body surface. The condition is not contagious in any way, and general health usually is not affected. However, it is no exaggeration to say that in extreme cases, psoriasis be ruinous to the individual's physical, emotional, and economic well-being. In addition, some cases are associated with a severe form of arthritis, called *psoriatic arthritis*, that affects general health in much the same way as rheumatoid arthritis does.

Psoriasis usually develops slowly, following a typical course of remission and recurrence. The characteristic *psoriatic plaques*, or lesions, are sharply demarcated, red and raised, covered with silvery scales, and bleed easily. These plaques do not usually itch, and will heal without leaving scar tissue or affecting hair growth. The nails may become pitted. Some patients have a tendency to develop psoriasis at the sites of physical trauma or irritation (called Koebner phenomena).

Common sites for psoriasis are:

- Bony protuberances (knees, elbows, sacrum)
- Scalp
- External parts of ears
- Nails, eyebrows
- Back, buttocks, and, occasionally, generalized on the trunk
- Skin folds, such as the umbilicus

Treatment of Psoriasis

To develop a therapeutic approach to this intransigent condition, it is important to understand the processes that underlie the turnover of cells in the skin. In normal skin, it takes about 28 days for an epidermal cell to go from creation to shedding or scaling. Psoriatic cells complete this process in three or four days, or almost nine times faster than usual. However, there appears to be no impairment of the normal regulatory mechanisms of cell division. Thus, the result is often enormous cell buildup, inadequate maturation, and finally plaque formation. Much of psoriasis therapy is directed toward removing these plaques in a non-traumatic fashion and to easing any attendant discomfort.

The underlying cause of the rapid epithelial cell turnover characteristic of psoriasis is not known. Theories abound and vary according to the practitioner's particular belief system. Some believe the cause is primarily nutritional. Others invoke stress and psychological factors, while those with reductionist inclinations put it down to genetics.

Undoubtedly, the immune system is involved on some level, leading some authorities to describe psoriasis as an autoimmune condition. Flare-ups commonly accompany infections, especially infections of the upper respiratory tract. Environmental factors, such as injury, stress, and cold climate, are important for some patients. About one third of patients experience spontaneous remission of disease.

In short, psoriasis represents a classic example of a condition for which a holistic perspective is essential. In designing a treatment program, the practitioner must explore as many aspects of the individual's life as is feasible.

Actions Indicated

Alteratives are important, as they are for all internally generated skin problems. In practice, the rooty hepatic alteratives often are the best choice.

Anti-inflammatories, applied topically and taken internally, will speed the curative work of the alteratives, but not replace them. They are most helpful during flare-ups and exacerbations.

Lymphatic tonics improve the health of the internal environment.

Nervine relaxants ease the anxiety that often accompanies psoriasis. They will also soothe skin discomfort, including itching and even inflammation, due to their relaxing effects on the peripheral nerves of the autonomic nervous system.

Diuretics ensure adequate elimination via the kidneys.

Hepatics support liver function and the digestive process.

Vulneraries support the healing of skin lesions when applied topically, but are not as effective here as one might hope. Remember, there is no wound to heal.

Astringents, used topically, may help in reducing redness, heat, and itching through local vasoconstrictor effects.

Emollients assist in the process of scale removal.

Antipruritics used topically may help, but itching is not a major factor in psoriasis.

Diaphoretics have been suggested as a means of increasing circulation in the skin, thus promoting elimination and, in theory, general skin health.

It is important to be aware that while they may be helpful, diaphoretics may also aggravate psoriasis in some people. They may cause local overstimulation, with an end result of increasing cell replication rates and thus desquamation. This is not a major contraindication, but keep it in mind.

Specific Remedies

Many different herbs have been described as specific for psoriasis, depending upon local botany and cultural preferences. However, there are probably no true specifics. This is to be expected in light of the multifactorial, systemic nature of psoriasis. Some people respond incredibly well to one herb, while others show no response at all. This can prove both challenging and frustrating for the practitioner, let alone the patient!

The woody, hepatic alteratives are the herbs that come closest to being specifics for psoriasis. Herbs in this group include:

Arctium lappa (burdock)
Mahonia aquifolium (Oregon grape)
Rumex crispus (yellow dock)
Smilax spp. (sarsaparilla)

Of course, any of the other alteratives may prove to be specific for a given individual. Important leafy alteratives to consider include:

Galium aparine (cleavers)
Larrea tridentata (chaparral)
Scrophularia nodosa (figwort)
Trifolium pratense (red clover)
Urtica dioica (nettle)
Viola tricolor (heartsease)

Numerous herbs are relevant for topical application. An important goal is to lift and remove psoriatic scales while reducing local inflammation. This often means that the form of the topical application is as important as any remedies it contains. Choice of topical application will be governed to some extent by the personal preferences of the patient, so experimentation may be necessary. Widely used plants include:

Calendula officinalis (calendula)
Plantago spp. (plantain)

Populus balsamifera var. *balsamifera* (balm of Gilead)
Stellaria media (chickweed)
Thuja occidentalis (thuja)

A Prescription for Psoriasis

Arctium lappa	1 part
Rumex crispus	1 part
Galium aparine	1 part
Scutellaria lateriflora	1 part

Dosage: up to 5 ml of tincture three times a day. In addition, the patient should drink an infusion of fresh *Urtica dioica* or *Galium aparine* two or three times a day.

Table 20.5. Actions Supplied by Prescription for Psoriasis

ACTION	HERBS
Alterative	Arctium lappa, Galium aparine, Rumex crispus, Urtica dioica
Lymphatic tonic	Galium aparine, Urtica dioica
Nervine relaxant	Scutellaria lateriflora
Anti-inflammatory	Galium aparine
Diuretic	Arctium lappa, Galium aparine, Urtica dioica
Hepatic	Arctium lappa, Galium aparine, Rumex crispus

A Prescription for Psoriasis with Anxiety and Tension

Arctium lappa	1 part
Rumex crispus	1 part
Galium aparine	1 part
Valeriana officinalis	1 part
Verbena officinalis	1 part

Dosage: up to 5 ml of tincture three times a day. The patient also should drink an infusion of *Matricaria recutita* as desired.

Table 20.6. Actions Supplied by Prescription for Psoriasis with Anxiety

ACTION	HERBS
Alterative	Arctium lappa, Galium aparine, Rumex crispus, Urtica dioica
Lymphatic tonic	Galium aparine, Urtica dioica
Nervine relaxant	Valeriana officinalis, Verbena officinalis

ACTION	HERBS
Anti-inflammatory	*Galium aparine*
Diuretic	*Arctium lappa, Galium aparine, Urtica dioica*
Hepatic	*Arctium lappa, Galium aparine, Rumex crispus, Verbena officinalis*

A Prescription for Intransigent, Unresponsive Psoriasis

Arctium lappa	2 parts
Rumex crispus	2 parts
Smilax spp.	2 parts
Phytolacca americana	1 part
Valeriana officinalis	1 part

Dosage: 5 ml of tincture three times a day. In addition, the patient should drink an infusion of fresh *Urtica dioica* or *Galium aparine* two or three times a day.

Care must be taken with this combination, and it is not advisable for children because of the inclusion of *Phytolacca americana* (poke root).

Table 20.7. Actions Supplied by Prescription for Unresponsive Psoriasis

ACTION	HERBS
Alterative	*Arctium lappa, Galium aparine, Phytolacca americana, Rumex crispus, Smilax* spp., *Urtica dioica*
Lymphatic tonic	*Galium aparine, Phytolacca americana, Urtica dioica*
Nervine relaxant	*Valeriana officinalis*
Anti-inflammatory	*Galium aparine*
Diuretic	*Arctium lappa, Galium aparine, Urtica dioica*
Hepatic	*Arctium lappa, Galium aparine, Rumex crispus, Smilax* spp.

A Prescription for a Patient with Psoriasis and Hypertension

Arctium lappa	2 parts
Rumex crispus	2 parts
Galium aparine	2 parts
Valeriana officinalis	1 part
Crataegus spp.	1 part
Tilia platyphyllos	1 part
Achillea millefolium	1 part

Dosage: 5 ml of tincture three times a day. The patient should also drink an infusion of *Matricaria recutita, Tilia platyphyllos,* or *Trifolium pratense* as desired. *Allium sativum* should be added to the diet or used as a dietary supplement: 1 clove of fresh garlic or 200 to 300 mg of standardized extract three times a day.

The last prescription is designed for a case in which hypertension is not the primary concern. Thus, the bulk of the dose consists of alterative herbs, rather than hypotensive remedies.

Table 20.8. Actions Supplied by Prescription for Psoriasis with Hypertension

ACTION	HERBS
Alterative	*Arctium lappa, Galium aparine, Phytolacca americana, Rumex crispus, Smilax* spp., *Urtica dioica*
Lymphatic tonic	*Galium aparine, Phytolacca americana, Urtica dioica*
Nervine relaxant	*Tilia platyphyllos, Valeriana officinalis*
Anti-inflammatory	*Galium aparine*
Diuretic	*Achillea millefolium, Arctium lappa, Crataegus* spp., *Galium aparine, Tilia platyphyllos, Urtica dioica*
Hepatic	*Allium sativum, Arctium lappa, Galium aparine, Rumex crispus, Smilax* spp.
Hypotensive	*Achillea millefolium, Allium sativum, Crataegus* spp., *Tilia platyphyllos, Valeriana officinalis*

Broader Context of Treatment

Both practitioner and patient should be aware of the many non-herbal treatment and coping options for psoriasis. Psoriasis is a condition in which patient empowerment becomes vital. Patients bear the burden of the label "psoriasis sufferer," and so they suffer. They are often told little about the range of simple nursing techniques that could make their negative skin experience easier to live with.

The skin is an interface between the person and his or her world. It senses and expresses. Psoriasis impacts the individual's experience of the world in two broad ways:

The *physical distress* makes it difficult for the patient to feel at ease.

The *psychological trauma* of feeling "disfigured" may lead to social isolation and depression.

The therapist must be prepared to help and advise in these areas as well as with the purely herbal issues. Stress management is critically important, and will ideally be part of an overall reevaluation by the patient of lifestyle, personal goals, and life vision.

For most people with psoriasis, exposure to sunlight helps alleviate and sometimes even clear the condition. Unfortunately, we have disrupted our environment so greatly that this can no longer be generally recommended, as UV light entering through the depleted ozone layer is potentially more damaging than helpful. However, the Dead Sea may be safer, because it is so far below sea level. Here occurs a quality of UV light not found anywhere else on the planet. Because the light passes through additional layers of air on its way to this area, more of the harmful spectrum may be filtered out. The salts of the Dead Sea itself are also beneficial for psoriasis. (Of course, none of this takes into account possible human dangers, such as war!)

Much of the nutritional advice available for psoriasis is contradictory. In my therapeutic experience, I have seen success with both a grapefruit fast and a no-citrus diet! Psoriasis is the epitome of a "holistic" disease, it being almost impossible to generalize about recommendations. Specifics of diet must be based upon the individual, not the pathology.

Supplements suggested for inclusion in a broad therapeutic approach to the treatment of psoriasis by Pizzorno and Murray in *Textbook of Natural Medicine* are:[2]

High-potency multiple vitamin and mineral formula
Flaxseed oil: 1 tablespoon/day
Vitamin A: 50,000 IU/day (do not use in pregnancy or for women planning to become pregnant)

Vitamin E: 400 IU/day
Chromium: 400 IU/day
Selenium: 200 mcg/day
Zinc: 30 mg/day

ACNE

A common inflammatory pilosebaceous disease characterized by comedones, papules, pustules, inflamed nodules, superficial pus-filled cysts, and, in extreme cases, canalizing and deep, inflamed, sometimes purulent, sacs. *(The Merck Manual)*

Acne is a common, potentially disfiguring skin disease. Unfortunately, it often affects those in an emotionally vulnerable stage of life—adolescents. Acne involves the sebaceous glands in the skin, which secrete lubrication (sebum) for the hair follicles (pilosebaceous follicles) and surrounding skin. These are located in greatest concentrations on the face, back, shoulders, and chest. Acne is most common in adolescents, with a peak in the late teens. Acne may, however, appear for the first time in the mid-20s or later and can persist into the 40s or 50s.
Acne lesions are commonly of three types:

Blackheads are glands plugged with excessive material that discolors on exposure to air.

Whiteheads are small collections of pus within glands.

Nodules or papules are the red and inflamed areas of more extensive infection.

A complex of causes underlies acne. Unfortunately, determining underlying causes is rarely as simple as blaming fats, chocolate, and sugar. Important predisposing factors include:

Genetic predisposition. Statistics suggest that the strongest single factor in the development of acne is family history. While the common conclusion is that the disorder has a genetic basis, it might be argued that it is related to generations of inappropriate nutrition.

Hormonal changes in adolescence. Stimulation of the sebaceous glands seems to occur with the production of androgens (the masculinizing hormone found in both sexes) at puberty. People with acne seem to produce normal amounts of androgens, but their skin may simply be unusually sensitive to its effects.

Skin flora. The bacteria normally present on the skin, or the *skin flora*, do not cause acne. However, blackheads and whiteheads are filled with trapped sebum and bacteria.

Nutrition. Although it is popularly thought that diet is a major factor in acne, there is no clear scientific evidence to support this. However, the quality of nutritional intake is fundamental to quality of life, so it makes sense to limit the intake of saturated fats and sugar, even if they do not cause acne.

One explanation for the physiological processes behind the characteristic skin eruptions of acne suggests this sequence of events:

Stimulation by androgens (male sex hormones) causes an increase in the amount and thickness of oil secretion, so more lipid is present in the follicles.

Changes in skin ecology promote bacterial growth, especially *Propionibacterium acnes.*

Sebaceous glands become obstructed by comedones (blackheads and whiteheads).

Any consequent disruption of follicular epithelium allows discharge of pus into the dermis.

Inflammatory reaction develops.

Pathological changes ensue in the following sequence:

papules → pustules → nodules → cysts

Treatment of Acne

The endocrine system must be given tonic support. This is ideal, but general endocrine toning is not a simple thing. Toning work can be focused through the use of hepatic alteratives. If there has been long-term antibiotic use, the immune system must be strengthened. See chapter 21 for more information.

Actions Indicated

Alteratives are the core of any treatment. Hepatic alteratives are especially helpful.

Hormonal normalizers are indicated because of the androgen involvement. However, impacting these hormones in an appropriate way is not always a straightforward matter.

Antimicrobials help the body deal with secondary infection. They may be used both internally and topically.

Lymphatic tonics support lymphatic drainage from the skin and underlying tissues.

Hepatics are vital, partly for the generalized benefit imparted by their liver-toning effects, but also because they have a specific role in detoxification.

Diuretics are important in ensuring adequate elimination through the kidneys.

Anti-inflammatories can be helpful when used topically within the context of daily hygiene.

Astringents, used topically, help in cleansing and avoiding secondary infection.

Specific Remedies

Traditionally, there are no definite specifics here, other than hepatic alteratives. However, tea tree oil (*Melaleuca alternifolia*) has specifically relevant properties. The primary constituent of the oil is terpinene-4-ol, which constitutes up to 60% of the oil. Australian standards set a minimum content of 30% terpinene-4-ol. Tea tree oil and terpinene-4-ol in particular have been shown to possess significant antimicrobial properties. Organisms inhibited include *Candida albicans, Escherichia coli, Staphylococcus aureus, Staphylococcus epidermidis,* and *Propionibacterium acnes.* For acne, tea tree oil applied topically in a 5% to 15% dilution three or four times daily is recommended.

Keep in mind that there is no specific herb that normalizes levels of androgens. Occasionally, however, *Vitex* can have a beneficial effect in adolescent girls.

A Prescription for Acne

Iris versicolor	1 part
Arctium lappa	1 part
Echinacea spp.	1 part
Galium aparine	1 part

Dosage: up to 5 ml of tincture three times a day. The patient should also drink an infusion of *Urtica dioica* two or three times a day. In addition, apply *Calendula officinalis* topically as a wash, in the form of an infusion mixed with distilled *Hamamelis virginiana* (witch hazel).

Broader Context of Treatment

There are a number of non-herbal issues to address, ranging from diet and hygiene to coping with a whole complex of emotions. It is often important to explain the nature of the problem to the patient, as well as the treatment you propose. Especially for adolescents, there may be a need to address unspoken feelings, such as fear and guilt. Be sure the patient understands the following issues:

Acne is not related to sexual activity. Masturbation and sex are not causes of acne. This antiquated notion harks back to the 16th century, when excess semen secretion was believed to aggravate acne. Marriage was purported to be the cure. It has no scientific validity.

Acne is not caused by dirt and cannot be washed away. It is related to an imbalance (hormonal or chemical) that causes the oil in the skin to form blackheads.

Personal hygiene is important, but an obsession with washing can aggravate the problem. It may be helpful to review some specifics with the patient:

Keep the hands away from the face, avoiding friction of the skin.

Do not squeeze pimples or blackheads, as squeezing the skin makes the acne worse. The blackhead may be pushed deeper into the skin, possibly causing the follicle to rupture.

Keep the hair off the face, and wash the hair daily, if needed.

Avoid cosmetics that contain synthetic chemicals.

Ideas about nutrition "dos and don'ts" for acne abound. Some generalizations are clear, including avoiding refined foods, red meat, and high-fat or carbohydrate-rich foods. A diet rich in green leafy vegetables and fruit is indicated.

Textbook of Natural Medicine recommends the following supplements:[3]

Vitamin A: 100,00 IU/day for three months
Vitamin E: 400 IU/day
Vitamin C: 1,000 mg/day
Zinc: 50 mg/day (as picolinate)
Selenium: 200 mcg/day
Brewer's yeast: 1 tablespoon twice a day

References

1. Pizzorno JE, Murray MT. *The Textbook of Natural Medicine*. Edinburgh: Churchill Livingstone, 1999.

2. Ibid.

3. Ibid.

21

❧

THE IMMUNE SYSTEM

In recent years, the immune system has become an increasingly critical area of focus in all branches of medicine. This is not just because of the acquired immune deficiency syndrome (AIDS) epidemic, but also because of the statistical explosion in the incidence of a whole range of autoimmune diseases. To comprehend the possible contributions that holistic approaches can make to the treatment of these conditions, it is important to have a grasp of the biological basis for immunity.

Just as important is an understanding of the role the immune system plays in human life. The new, but still incomplete, insights granted us by the field of immunology illuminate the profound complexity of human biochemical processes—and the ways in which they interact with equally complex ecological processes. However, much more than biochemistry is involved. Herbal medicine is as limited as orthodox medicine if it is used only to affect T- and B-lymphocyte function, without the benefit of a broader holistic context.

Some important insights arise when immune system function is viewed from an ecological perspective, not simply a biochemical or medical one. Human immunity is a vital component of the interface between the individual and the world. The role of the human immune system is not simply to resist the dangers present in the environment. Rather, it is part of the complex and beautiful dance of elements flowing back and forth between the human body and the rest of the world. Seen within the context of ecology, both human and environmental, immunity is about harmony.

All of this leads us to some concepts and interpretations that raise exciting possibilities for the practitioner of holistic medicine, whether phytotherapist or medical doctor.

Human immunity is ecology in action. In other words, there is a multifactorial relationship at play between individuals and their environment. There is a complex web of interactions between the inner world of the body and mind and the outer world of the environment—its people, its culture, its food, in fact, everything. The practitioner must not only identify and understand both sides of this relationship, but must also comprehend the nature of the relationship. This can prove extremely challenging, as the relationship will be in dynamic flux at all times.

Immunity represents an ecological interface between inner and outer environments. Such interfaces are critical to the health and well-being of the Earth itself. Think of the interfaces between desert and savanna, rain forest and mountains, woodland and grassland, agriculture and wilderness. These transition zones facilitate the integration and fine-tuning of biomes and biosphere health. In human ecology, the immune system is governed by a complex of processes that allow resistance and embrace at the same time. To focus on only one side of this profound interaction is to miss the point and compromise understanding of the whole.

Immunity is an expression of homeostasis. Homeostasis is an umbrella concept that describes the profound physiological processes that maintain a stable internal environment within a human being. This inner homeostasis can be seen as a reflection of planetary homeostasis. In fact, the recognition of these planet-wide processes led James Lovelock to propose the Gaia hypothesis.

Immunity is an expression of relationship. This is implicit in everything discussed so far, but also carries the implication that the very nature of *relationship* plays a role in immune system well-being. Thus, the practitioner must explore patients' relationships with the world on all levels, from the food they eat, to the people they love (or hate), to the way they relate to nature.

In short, as with all holistic healing, any approach to whole body immunity must address the following aspects of human life:

Bodily health and wholeness. We must ensure that the physical body has the appropriate nutritional and healing support to prevent or treat any ills that may affect it.

Emotional well-being. We must ensure that the patient has a nurturing, feeling experience of life, encompassing both the joy and the pain of human existence.

Mental vision and perspective. We must help create a mind-set within which the individual can find his or her own place in the world and make life choices from the center of his or her being, not from a victim's stance.
Spiritual openness and vitality. This will take the shape of whatever feels appropriate for the individual.

The new field of psychoneuroimmunology is starting to point us in directions that hold much promise for the future. The relationship between stress and immune system suppression has been well established in both animal and human research. We now know that in the presence of stress, a large and complex array of mechanical, chemical, and immune changes take place, as the body attempts to defend itself or restore homeostasis.

The term *psychoneuroimmunology* comes from our growing understanding of these mind-body connections. *Psycho* denotes thinking, emotions, and mood states; *neuro* implies involvement of the neurological and neuroendocrine systems; and *immunology* refers to cellular structures and the immune system. An increasing body of evidence indicates that the nervous system is capable of modulating the immune response. It appears that the immune system may be able to communicate with the nervous system using neuromodulators and neurohormones secreted by lymphocytes, and receptors for these substances have been found on human T-lymphocytes. Activation of these receptors can be stimulatory or inhibitory, depending on the neuroactive substance involved.

UNDERSTANDING THE HERBAL POSSIBILITIES

The various phytotherapeutic systems of the world have much to offer the holistic practitioner working with the human immune system. However, confusion and misinformation abound in this field. Much of the "phytoperplexity" comes from ill-informed attempts to blend insights from different traditions without a clear grasp of the underlying principles.

Attempts at multicultural therapeutics are to be applauded, but must proceed from a solid understanding of the systems involved. Without such a foundation, there is no real therapy, only wishful thinking. The work of herbalist Michael Tierra provides an excellent example of what can be achieved. Consider, for example, the commonly held belief in the Western herbal community that *Panax ginseng* is for men and *Angelica sinensis* (dong quai) is for women. This is simply not the case. My minimal grasp of the profundities of traditional Chinese medicine tells me that *Panax* is the strongest yang tonic, while *A. sinensis* is the most yielding yin tonic. This leads to entirely different therapeutic implications.

It is also extremely challenging to build bridges between traditional phytotherapy and the abundance of scientific data flowing from the field of immunological research. It is too easy to discard the insights of traditional approaches in favor of research published in peer-reviewed journals. This is imprudent, because important insights may be gained when one takes into account the herbal wisdom garnered through generations of experience. By the same token, we must avoid the temptation to jump to unwarranted conclusions about the results of animal research on isolated constituents, as the implications for human therapy are not always clear. See chapter 10 for a more in-depth discussion of this important issue.

On the other hand, there are many ways to use herbs to enhance the vitality of the immune system. All of the diverse herbal traditions, with their unique cultural roots and expressions, have valuable insights into treatments and specific herbs. This should come as no surprise in light of the ecological nature of immunity already discussed. Herbal medicine is ecological medicine; it is based on an ecological relationship that has evolved through geological time. By virtue of this special relationship between plants and people, there are remedies that directly address the ecological process of human immune responses.

The contribution of phytotherapy to immune system health provides a good example of the ways in which traditional knowledge is now being confirmed by modern pharmacology. In both the laboratory and the clinic, a growing number of herbal remedies have been shown to have marked effects upon the immune system. Some stimulate immune system responses, but most can best be described as *modulators*. That is, these remedies facilitate greater immune system flexibility in the body's natural response to disease. However, rather than focus on particular plants, we shall look at the whole treatment process. An overemphasis on specific plant immunostimulants is little more than "organic drug therapy," which is not the goal of the holistic herbalist.

Immunostimulation or Immunomodulation?

As pharmacologists discover the possibilities offered by the plant kingdom, they have found it necessary to coin new words to describe how plants work. In general, these terms describe normalizing, whole-plant actions—actions that are not covered by the semantics of reductionist, active-constituent research.

Immunostimulants or *immunopotentiators* lead to a nonspecific stimulation of the immunological defense system. Nonspecific immunostimulants do not affect immune system memory cells, and because their pharmacological effects fade relatively quickly, they must be administered either at intervals or continuously. The protective immunity conferred by immunostimulants happens quickly, and has been termed *paramunity*.

Immunomodulation and *immunoregulation* are terms that have been proposed to denote any effect on immune system responsiveness. For example, herbs may also stimulate T-suppressor cells and thereby reduce immune resistance. *Immunoadjuvants* are substances that enhance the production of antibodies without acting as antigens themselves. The effects of adjuvants are often thymus-dependent.

The phytotherapist is actually quite at home with these somewhat vague concepts. After all, human life is rarely governed by logic and rational thinking! From the allopathic perspective, however, the concept of immunostimulation offers a number of therapeutic possibilities. These hint at the important changes in perspective that are under way within the field of orthodox medicine.

For example, immunostimulation may prove to offer an alternative to conventional drug treatment of infections. This may be especially true for immunocompromised patients, or those with impaired immune system function. As immunostimulation is focused on boosting the body's own immune mechanisms, it may represent an opportunity to prevent opportunistic infections in high-risk patients.

In addition, immunomodulators have potential contributions to make to the therapy of malignant diseases. It is a well-known fact that stimulation of specific components of the immune system, such as macrophages and killer cells, can inhibit tumor growth. Plant-based immunostimulators may also contribute to the treatment of autoimmune diseases.

As discussed in chapter 9, immunological defense is a complicated interplay of many factors. However, the multifactorial nature of whole plant pharmacology often confounds researchers' attempts to identify the mechanisms at work. To simplify matters, it seems clear that no matter what the primary target of the immunostimulant, whether T- or B-lymphocytes or the complement system, an increase in the activity of macrophages and granulocytes plays a central role in immunomodulation.

A PHYTOTHERAPEUTIC APPROACH TO THE IMMUNE SYSTEM

It should be apparent by now that the plant kingdom can have a major impact upon the function of the human immune system—an impact that a competent holistic practitioner can use to advantage. There are many ideas about how this can be best approached. The ideas and theories I discuss in the following sections represent an attempt to bring together the perspectives of the traditional European approach, insights offered by Asian medicine, and the contributions of pharmacological research.

Because immunity must be seen in the context of homeostatic, whole-system function, we must also emphasize general detoxification and elimination. This, in turn, illuminates some of the primary ways in which herbs contribute to preventive medicine and wellness. The important insights of herbalist Christopher Hobbs in this area are an inspiration to this author and many other herbalists.

Hobbs identifies three relevant levels of herbal activity:

- Deep immune activation
- Surface immune activation
- Adaptogenic action or hormonal modulation

Deep Immune Activation

Plants that impact the immune system within the tissue that mediates its work are generating increasing interest in the herbal and research communities. These can be termed *deep immune activators*. As discussed in chapter 9, pharmacology points to saponins and complex polysaccharides as key contributors to the role of plants in this area, but please remember that herbs act as biological wholes, not just as vehicles for active ingredients.

Important Asian immunomodulators that have been incorporated into Western herbal practice include:

Astragalus membranaceus (astragalus)
Codonopsis tangshen (codonopsis)
Ganoderma lucidum (reishi mushroom)
Lentinus edodes (shiitake mushroom)
Ligustrum lucidum (privet)
Schisandra chinensis (schizandra)

An abstruse point must be made here. It may appear that the primary herbs for immunomodulation come from Asia, usually China. By extension, it may seem that Western herbalism is at a disadvantage and suffers from a lack of research on Western plants. However, this is an artifact of research funding, not an herbal reality. Until very recently, the preponderance of research on immunomodulating plants and their constituents was performed in Asia, primarily in the People's Republic of China, India, and Japan. Funding for these studies was driven by a desire to improve the lot of the people of these countries. Consequently, and quite appropriately, the research focused on the plants used medicinally in those nations.

Comparatively little attention has been paid to plant immunomodulators by American and European researchers. This should not be taken to mean that no Western plants have such properties, only that the research community lacks the funding needed to investigate them. If we examine the properties of Western herbs traditionally used to treat immune system problems, it can be argued that the traditional alteratives, tonics, and digestive bitters address deep immune issues in a similar way to better-studied Asian herbs.

Surface Immune Activation

These are the many plants known as antimicrobials, or "immune system boosters." The more attention researchers give these plants, the greater the range of mechanisms are found to explain their activity. Examples of these plants are:

Allium sativum (garlic)
Baptisia tinctoria (wild indigo)
Calendula officinalis (calendula)
Commiphora molmol (myrrh)
Echinacea spp. (echinacea)
Thuja occidentalis (thuja)
Usnea spp. (usnea)

Hormonal Modulators

Remedies in this group work though some hormonal modulation of the immune response. As is discussed in chapter 22, a number of endocrine functions can be affected by herbs. For example, adaptogens exert their effects via the adrenal glands and the general adaptation system (GAS). See chapter 16 for more information on this important coping mechanism.

Adaptogens that work via the adrenals and the general adaptation syndrome include *Eleutherococcus senticosus* (Siberian ginseng) and *Panax* spp. (Korean and American ginseng).

HERBS AND THE IMMUNE SYSTEM

The array of available information on the immune system and herbal approaches to treatment can be truly daunting! The therapeutic suggestions that follow are based upon my training and clinical experience in England and Wales. I must emphasize this point, as the approach may seem too simplistic in light of the impressive body of research on specific plants that now exists.

Remember, the approach we are taking here is based on the needs of human beings, not on the use of specific plants. Any other approach may lead to an attempt to fit a patient into the indications for a certain plant, instead of identifying the needs of the individual and what herbs might best address them.

Immune System Pathologies

The phytotherapist can choose from among a number of therapeutic options for treating the immune system. Most exciting is the ability to generally support the system in the absence of overt pathology. Nurturing wellness through preventive medicine becomes a readily achievable goal when we use immunomodulators within the context of the holistic approach. In addition, a range of immune system pathologies may be addressed with herbs.

Immune system problems can be grouped into a number of different categories.

Immunodeficiency Diseases

These pathologies are associated with malfunction of one or more of the major aspects of the immune response. This category is usually divided into two subgroups:

Primary immune deficiency disease. This type, which may be either hereditary or acquired, is disease caused by immune deficiency.
Secondary immune deficiency disease. In this kind of immune deficiency disorder, the immune deficiency is the result of another disease or diseases. An extreme example is AIDS.

Hypersensitivity Reactions

These are normal immunity processes that become damaging rather than protective. The pathological processes arise as a result of specific interactions between an antigen and components of the immune system. Four types are known.

Type I. Anaphylactic reactions are caused by release of a pharmacologically active substance, such as histamine, from IgE-sensitized mast cells and basophils after contact with specific antigens. Other examples of Type I hypersensitivity reactions are atopic diseases, such as hay fever, and allergic asthma.
Type II. In these cytotoxic reactions, binding of antibody to an antigen on the cell surface produces damage to

that cell through a variety of mechanisms. Examples are blood transfusion and Rh incompatibility reactions.

Type III. Immune complex reactions result from deposition of soluble, circulating antigen-antibody complexes in vessels or tissue. This process seems to be implicated in autoimmune conditions such as rheumatoid arthritis.

Type IV. In cell-mediated immunity, immune responses are mediated by T-cells rather than antibodies. An example is contact sensitivity to poison oak and poison ivy. Graft rejections may also be Type IV reactions.

Autoimmune Diseases

Autoimmune diseases are conditions in which lymphocytes produce antibodies that attack the body's own cells and tissues as if they were foreign substances, thus causing pathological damage. Any organ or tissue may be involved. Conditions thought to have an autoimmune basis include rheumatoid arthritis, polyarthritis, chronic active hepatitis, multiple sclerosis, and psoriasis.

Various theories have been put forth to explain the etiology of autoimmune disease. Researchers believe that the embryonic immune system contains lymphocytes that can produce self-reacting antibodies, but which are somehow inactivated as the system develops. They suggest that autoimmune diseases arise through some kind of disruption of this inactivation mechanism. A process called *immunoregulation* has been postulated to explain the complex homeostatic mechanisms that hold the "autoreactive" cells in check.

This invocation of homeostasis has interesting implications for the holistic practitioner. In fact, the fascinating complexities of biochemical and cytological immunology can be mesmerizing to both theorist and therapist. Phytotherapists often become infatuated with the research findings on interactions between plants and the immune system at the expense of a holistic perspective that perceives the person as whole, not just a reflection of blood chemistry. However, these ideas about homeostatic immunoregulation do point to a possible bridge between the reductionist science of immunology and concepts of wholeness, whether whole plant actions or the whole body perspective of holistic medicine.

Cancer

A direct relationship exists between the immune system and the development of tumors. This highlights the possibilities for prevention and treatment that may be achieved by working with immunity. The use of herbs in a broad holistic context can help the body function and heal. This is discussed in greater detail later.

Transplant Problems

Immune system rejection of transplanted organs presents a particular problem. Successful transplantation depends on the similarity between tissues of the body and those of the transplanted organ, because cytotoxic T-cells will act vigorously to destroy any foreign tissue in the body.

After surgery, the patient receives immunosuppressive therapy to inhibit the immunological rejection. This will involve one or more of the following treatments:

- Corticosteroids to suppress inflammation
- Cytotoxic drugs
- Radiation therapy
- Anti-lymphocyte globulins
- Cyclosporine

These approaches kill rapidly dividing cells, such as activated lymphocytes, and have severe side effects. However, cyclosporine greatly improves survival from organ transplants. Cyclosporines are a group of cyclic oligopeptides first discovered in *Tolypocladium inflatum*, a white mold from Norway. Interestingly, it has been determined that in its sexual state, *T. inflatum* is actually *Cordyceps subsessilis*, an extremely rare fungus that has been reported only five or six times before.[1] However, a related species, *C. sinensis*, is a well-known remedy in traditional Chinese medicine. Recent pharmacological research shows it to have a range of immunological activities.[2] In spite of all this, however, transplant issues are inappropriate for phytotherapeutic treatment.

Where does all of this leave the phytotherapist? What actions or specific herbs are indicated for these conditions? Western herbalism seems to have got itself tied in knots around the word *immune*, and both professionals and nonprofessionals are showing symptoms of conceptual overload. Appropriate remedies for immune system problems must be selected on the basis of individual need. This can be determined only through careful diagnosis, which in turn requires the practitioner to be knowledgeable about the complexities of the process. The word *immune* does not mean *Echinacea*!

The real question involves knowing when to use immunostimulant herbs and, even more important, when not to. Stimulating immune system activity may be inappropriate in some conditions and vital in others. The classic Eclectic, Physiomedicalist, and European texts on herbal therapy do not address these considerations. In an attempt to clarify the issue for myself, I have established provisional guidelines for identifying therapeutic situations in which immunostimulation is indicated and those for which it may be contraindicated.

In general, it seems safe to say that immunostimulant plants should be avoided in conditions that involve inappropriate activity of some aspect of the immune complex. In autoimmune conditions, for example, any stimulation might increase the production or pathological impact of antibodies. The same may be said for hypersensitivity reactions, even though an external antigen may be present. Transplant rejection issues also fit into this category, but are rarely encountered by the phytotherapist.

Conditions for which immunostimulants are probably contraindicated include:

- Autoimmune diseases
- Hypersensitivity reactions
- Organ transplantation

On the other hand, immunostimulant plants are fundamentally important in conditions related to inadequate or compromised immune system activity. Individuals may become *immunocompromised* for a variety of reasons, including the presence of pathogenic or parasitic organisms and inadequate immune responses to cancerous changes in the body's own cells.

Conditions for which immunostimulants are probably indicated include:

- Infections
- Cancer
- Immunodeficiency disease (for example, AIDS)

Note my use of the word *probably* in the contraindications and indications just given. The phytotherapist is completely at home with multifaceted plant effects, as well as the diversity and mutability of people. It is a mistake to view a plant simply as an "immunostimulant." A remedy that has a specific value in the treatment of rheumatoid arthritis may also demonstrate immunostimulant activity in the laboratory. However, a longstanding use of a plant based on many generations of experience has more value in practice than theoretical concerns raised by in vitro or animal studies.

GENERAL SUPPORT PROTOCOLS

A number of general treatment guidelines have particular relevance in the broader approach taken to the immune system in this chapter. Of course, these protocols have a much wider application, and will prove useful for many patients with conditions discussed elsewhere in the book. The protocols include detoxification, preventive medicine, postoperative recovery, and general guidelines for treating infection.

DETOXIFICATION

The particular herbal approach to detoxification described here is based upon the premise that the human body is self-healing and homeostatic, and that the therapist must simply support normal processes. The body has effective and astoundingly complex mechanisms for ridding the body of waste and poisons. The phytotherapist can aid the process by using basic, simple, and safe herbs. The important point is to address eliminative processes as a whole, not just to focus on the colon.

This means that whenever such a program is undertaken, the phytotherapist must ensure that all organs of elimination receive support. In addition, it is essential to provide support for whatever specific area of the body is under the most toxic pressure—for example, the lungs of a tobacco smoker or the liver of a person who has alcohol-related problems.

Details on applying the principles of detoxification for specific conditions are given in the appropriate sections, but here is a brief summary:

- Support the *whole* process of elimination
- Provide specific support for over-taxed organs
- Alleviate symptoms and address any pathology present

Herbal Actions and Elimination

The physiological impact of certain herbal actions makes them particularly valuable for supporting various pathways of elimination in the body.

Note that no particular herbs are specified here. The skill and insight of the practitioner will determine the choice of appropriate plants. The actions model presented in this book provides a relatively straightforward method for formulating a prescription that will be effective in prompting appropriate elimination work while addressing the unique needs of the individual.

Table 21.1. Appropriate Actions to Support Specific Pathways of Elimination

BODY SYSTEM	HERBAL ACTIONS
Digestive system and colon	Aperient/laxative
Urinary system and kidneys	Diuretic
Liver and blood	Hepatic, alterative
Lymphatic system	Alterative, lymphatic tonic
Skin	Diaphoretic, alterative
Respiratory system	Expectorant, pulmonary, anticatarrhal
Whole body	Tonic, bitter, alterative, adaptogen, antimicrobial

Selection of Herbs with Appropriate Actions

Selection criteria should take into account secondary actions as well as system affinity, as described in chapter 12. However, when the goal is to stimulate elimination, the phytotherapist should emphasize gentle remedies. Overly active plants can cause an intense elimination reaction. This can be unpleasant and uncomfortable, not to mention that it is of very questionable therapeutic benefit.

The phenomenon known as "purging and puking" does not represent a healing crisis, but rather the worst aspects of 19th-century medicine. In a similar vein, I can detect no valid rationale behind wellness programs based on the fatuous concept of "no pain, no gain." I would suggest that we always keep in mind the relevance of the advice given by Hippocrates: "First do no harm."

Table 21.2 provides a brief list of herbs that effectively supply the desired actions with only a mild impact on the body.

Table 21.2. Herbs to Support Eliminative Processes

ACTION	HERBS
Alterative	*Arctium lappa, Galium aparine, Urtica dioica*
Aperient/laxative	*Rumex crispus, Taraxacum officinale* root
Diaphoretic	*Achillea millefolium, Eupatorium perfoliatum, Sambucus nigra*
Diuretic	*Galium aparine, Taraxacum officinale* leaf
Expectorant, pulmonary tonic	*Marrubium vulgare, Verbascum thapsus, Tussilago farfara*
Hepatic	*Taraxacum officinale* root, *Silybum marianum*
Lymphatic tonic	*Calendula officinalis, Galium aparine, Trifolium pratense*

THE CONTRIBUTION OF HERBS TO PREVENTIVE MEDICINE

Balance and harmony are the keys to successful preventive medicine, bringing us back to the ideas proposed at the beginning of this chapter. There must be a clear and free flow of energy throughout the various aspects of the individual's life. Thus, we must address issues that go beyond the transformative effects of herbs upon metabolic and physiological processes.

Nutrition must support the body's efforts to build itself in a way that ensures health and wholeness.

Structural factors must be addressed by a skilled practitioner, if indicated, but also through appropriate exercise, dance, or any other enjoyable expression of movement.

A conscious and free-flowing emotional life is fundamental to achieving any inner harmony. This does not mean that everyone must undergo in-depth psychotherapy, but that attention be given in an appropriate form to the individual's emotional needs.

Mental factors are crucial, as we are what we think! The Bible says that without vision, people die. Without a personal vision, life becomes a slow process of degeneration and decay. The same can be said about issues affecting self-image and personal purpose.

Attention to spiritual issues is vital. Openness to spirituality can take whatever form is meaningful to the individual—whether an organized religion, appreciation of nature or art, or a simple joy in being alive.

The plant kingdom offers much to the therapist interested in preventive medicine. The key is not to focus on specific plant remedies, but instead to understand the role of herbal actions in maintaining health and correct physiological activity. Taking into account the insights about homeostasis provided by the biomedical model, it should be clear that the proper use of herbs will support the body's own attempts to maintain a stable internal environment.

The phytotherapist should consider a number of actions and herbal processes when formulating a program of preventive medicine. A review of each part of this process will demonstrate that each step is mutually supportive. Similarly, when applying the concepts of secondary actions and system affinities, it becomes apparent that there is much overlap among herbs used to support the various aspects of whole body support.

System tonics. System tonics will nourish and tone the whole system's form and function without eliciting specific physiological or biochemical responses.

Bitter tonics. This group of herbs will have a generalized toning effect in addition to specific properties.

Detoxification. Cleansing and detoxification can be gently facilitated through herbal support of the body's eliminative functions.

Table 21.3 summarizes traditionally used system tonics in European and North American phytotherapy. Note that in the case of the digestive system, no one herb serves as an all-around tonic. In this case, choose appropriate herbal actions for the digestive system to support the work of bitters.

Table 21.3. Primary System Tonics in European and North American Phytotherapy

BODY SYSTEM	TONIC HERBS
Cardiovascular	*Crataegus* spp., *Allium sativum, Ginkgo biloba*
Respiratory	*Verbascum thapsus, Inula helenium*
Digestive	*Filipendula ulmaria, Gentiana lutea, Matricaria recutita*
Liver	*Gentiana lutea, Silybum marianum, Taraxacum officinale* root
Urinary	*Arctostaphylos uva-ursi, Zea mays*
Reproductive	
Women:	*Mitchella repens, Rubus idaeus*
Men:	*Serenoa repens*
Nervous	*Avena sativa, Scutellaria lateriflora, Hypericum perforatum*
Musculoskeletal	*Apium graveolens, Urtica dioica*
Skin	*Galium aparine, Urtica dioica, Trifolium pratense*

POSTOPERATIVE RECOVERY

While herbs can in no way replace surgery, they can contribute much to the success of surgical procedures. In the suggestions given here, we shall assume that the operation contemplated is appropriate for the patient concerned, which is not always the case! As we are in no way attempting to achieve the same goals as the surgery, the first step is to clarify what goals the herbs are intended to fulfill.

Simply stated, herbs can facilitate and support postoperative healing. While the specifics will vary from person to person, a few broad generalizations prove useful. The primary contributions herbalism offers in this area are gentle, normalizing tonics. These are inherently safe, nontoxic plants that might even be considered foods. The use of these herbs should raise no objection with the physician involved, as they will cause no negative drug interactions.

The key is to use relevant tonics to support the healing process in the tissue, organs, or body systems that will experience the most trauma during the surgery. Herbs can help with two main aspects of postoperative healing. First, they will facilitate healing of the actual tissues affected by the surgery, including skin, connective, cardiovascular, and nervous system tissues. Second, they will help support the whole body in the face of the stress it will experience.

Herbal tonics contribute the following to the postoperative recovery process:

- Support the immune system
- Help the liver and nervous system deal with the effects of anesthesia
- Alleviate symptomatic discomfort where possible or appropriate
- Facilitate optimal scar formation

Support the Specific Focus of Surgery

To support the body system that is the focus of the surgical procedure, choose relevant tonic remedies according to their nurturing effects upon specific parts of the body. For example, *Crataegus* would be an appropriate choice for a patient undergoing surgery to correct cardiovascular problems.

In addition, no matter what the purpose of the operation, it will involve cutting through layers of skin, various membranes of the body, small blood vessels, and possibly nerves. The body will normally heal such wounds quite adequately on its own, but the older the person is, the more help the tissue may require. Staying with gentle remedies, consider *Urtica* for skin and membranes, *Crataegus* and *Ginkgo* for blood vessels, and *Hypericum* for nerves.

Protect the Whole Body from the Effects of Excessive Stress

The stress experienced during surgery is not simply stress associated with worry and anxiety, but also the physiological stress of the operation itself. Adaptogens are irreplaceable here. In short, they help increase the body's resistance and resilience in the face of stress. They help the body adapt around the problem and avoid the possibility of collapse. The most relevant adaptogen is *Eleutherococcus senticosus*.

Support the Immune System

There are many issues to consider before choosing the appropriate approach. Unless one is sure of the relevance and safety of immunostimulant herbs for the particular individual and operation involved, avoid strong immunostimulants and instead use a mild alterative, such as *Urtica* or *Galium*.

Protect Against the Effects of Anesthesia

The liver is the primary site for the breakdown and elimination of the metabolic waste products of the anesthesia used during the operation. Appropriate remedies will support the liver's detoxification process, facilitating the removal of the metabolites from the body and speeding the return to normal. *Silybum* is the main herb to consider, as it is best to avoid stronger liver stimulants after an operation. Very mild bitters will have a safe and gentle stimulating effect on the nervous system and support the action of *Silybum*.

Alleviate Symptomatic Discomfort

Another primary goal is to alleviate discomfort related to the surgery, whenever and however possible. This will, of course, vary from operation to operation and person to person, but much symptomatic postoperative discomfort can be eased through the use of gentle effector herbs.

Help Facilitate Optimal Scar Formation

In the process of healing the incision, the body forms scar tissue. The amount of scar tissue that forms can be limited through the use of a variety of plant medicines without compromising the viability of the wound healing. Such wound-healing herbs have been traditionally called vulneraries. Examples are *Calendula* and *Hypericum*, which are both excellent for this purpose when blended with vitamin E oil.

Gallbladder Surgery: An Example

What herbs might we use to support postoperative recovery after successful gallbladder removal surgery? Actual remedies and protocols for treating gallbladder disease are discussed in chapter 13, but here is an example of how we might apply the process just discussed to facilitate recovery from this common surgical procedure.

Table 21.4. Actions and Herbs to Facilitate Recovery from Gallbladder Surgery

DESIRED ACTION	PREOPERATIVE	POSTOPERATIVE
Operation site tonic	*Chionanthus virginicus*	*Chionanthus virginicus*
Specific tissue tonic	*Crataegus, Equisetum*	*Ginkgo, Calendula*
Nervous system tissue tonic	*Hypericum perforatum*	*Hypericum perforatum*
Adaptogenic support	*Eleutherococcus senticosus*	*Eleutherococcus senticosus*
Immune system tonic	*Urtica dioica* or *Galium aparine*	*Urtica dioica* or *Galium aparine*
Detoxification support	*Silybum marianum*	*Silybum marianum*
Symptomatic relief	Depends on individual's symptom picture	Depends on individual's symptom picture
Scar formation	*Calendula officinalis* or *Hypericum perforatum*	*Calendula officinalis* or *Hypericum perforatum*

Actions Supplied by Pre- and Postoperative Herb Choices

For the operation site, the gallbladder, any appropriate mild tonic hepatic or cholagogue will do. An alternative to *Chionanthus virginicus* might be *Chelone glabra*. In this particular case, care must be taken to avoid herbs that strongly stimulate the liver's production of bile. However, gentle remedies are indicated to help move bile in the face of stasis.

Specific tissue tonics. In this case, the preoperative goal is to strengthen skin, connective, and cardiovascular tissues, while the postoperative goal is to facilitate healing. Postoperatively, we have replaced *Crataegus* with *Ginkgo* as the cardiovascular tonic because of its ability to help increase the availability of oxygen to the brain after anesthesia. *Equisetum* was replaced by *Calendula* for the postoperative treatment to prevent possible constipation.

Nervous system tonic. Hypericum perforatum has a unique ability to promote the healing of physically damaged nerves. One of its folk names in Germany translates as "the comfrey of the nervous system."

Adaptogenic support. Adaptogens are essential to ease the body's stress response. Stress has a major effect upon physiology and healing time, and adaptogens offer direct support. Adaptogenic herbs are more appropriate than relaxing nervines for postoperative recovery, as the patient will already be under the influence of chemical sedation.

Immune system support. Some variety of help for the immune system can be very important, but it is best to be safe and use gentle, tried-and-true alteratives.

Detoxification. The liver is the primary site for the breakdown of anesthesia metabolites. The mild bitters will have a safe, stimulating effect on the nervous system.

Symptomatic relief. A possible issue here might be constipation, which can be initially treated with a mild alterative laxative, such as *Rumex crispus*. No stimulating laxatives should be used, as they may cause straining and damage to the operation scar.

Scar formation. Apply vitamin E oil with a vulnerary, such as *Calendula officinalis* or *Hypericum perforatum*, to the incision site. Antimicrobial and anti-inflammatory essential oils may also be indicated.

In addition to the herbal suggestions given here, consider the use of homeopathic arnica before the operation. This preparation may be considered a specific when it comes to the treatment of bruising. Great attention must also be paid to diet and support for the patient from family and friends.

INFECTION

Infection seems to be a concomitant aspect of living within the biosphere of planet Earth. Human beings live in constant contact and ecological dialogue with vast numbers of bacteria, viruses, and fungi. The immune system has evolved in such a way that this interaction causes a health problem only occasionally. In fact, our well-being depends on healthy and positive relationships with a range of organisms that live in and on our body. The bacterial flora of the intestines and the microorganisms on the skin provide good examples.

Infection occurs when the body is exposed to organisms that become a threat to good health. These may be nonpathogenic under normal circumstances, but can become pathogenic to the individual for any of a variety of reasons. In any case, the immune system will be involved. If the individual's immune response is compromised in some way, the ecological balance between host and microbe will be altered, allowing the microbe to thrive. Either way, herbal treatment must focus on supporting appropriate immune response.

The herbal traditions of the world abound with plants that have a reputation for antimicrobial activity. Keep in mind, however, that they do not always achieve the desired results. When used correctly, conventional antibiotic medications can save lives. Largely because of these drugs, the scourge of epidemic infectious disease has been eliminated for the most part in the Western world. This is a truly miraculous achievement.

For severe infection, phytotherapy is not always adequate, especially for people with a weakened immune response. Such infections (for example, meningitis) require antibiotic treatment. As a dedicated herbalist who recognizes the limitations of my chosen therapy, I celebrate the existence of these medicines. The role of the healer is the alleviation of suffering, not the promotion of a belief system.

All of this is not meant to imply that whole plant medicine has nothing to offer in the treatment of infection! In fact, herbal treatment has much to contribute. Various herbal remedies can:

Boost the immune response, helping the body to rid itself of pathogens by either deep or surface immune system stimulation.

Exert direct antimicrobial effects against offending organisms. To be effective, the plant constituent must reach the site of infection, which is not always easy.

Tone and strengthen tissue, organs, or whole systems affected by the infection.

Facilitate recuperation from the infection and also from the use of antibiotics.

Antimicrobial Plants

The phytopharmacology journals are full of reports of plants that have apparent antimicrobial effects. The research usually takes the form of screening large numbers of plants, often a local flora, for an antimicrobial outcome, rather than an investigation of the specific mechanism involved. In light of this vast variety, I find the current preoccupation with *Echinacea* strange, as wonderful as this plant is. The practitioner should be familiar with a range of such herbs, their strengths and their limitations. For example, the Eclectics recommended *Baptisia tinctoria* (wild indigo) in combination with *Echinacea* for acute febrile infections. Please refer to chapters 25 and

26 for more information on the wide variety of herbal antimicrobials.

General Guidelines for Treating Infection

Because the body responds with a similar immune system response no matter what the cause of infection, it is possible to make some herbal generalizations. The details will vary somewhat with the nature of the disease, the needs of the specific individual, and other medications the patient might be taking. In the guidelines given here, the herbs mentioned are meant to serve only as suggestions. Each case must be seen afresh.

Selecting Antimicrobial Herbs

The selection of appropriate antimicrobial herbs should take into account the following considerations:

Site of infection. For example, *Arctostaphylos uva-ursi* (bearberry) may be appropriate for a bladder infection, while *Commiphora molmol* (myrrh) may be a good choice for topical application to the skin.

The patient's age and general state of health. Use gentler herbs for the young, old, or debilitated. For example, choose *Nepeta cataria* (catnip) as a diaphoretic for children, reserving *Armoracia rusticana* (horseradish) for adults.

Specifics for the particular pathogen. Unfortunately, this is not always possible.

Selecting Relevant Tonics

The antimicrobial herbs selected should always be used with appropriate tonic remedies. These may be selected based on:

The site of infection. For example, *Verbascum thapsus* may be the right choice for a lung infection, while *Galium aparine* is more appropriate for lymphatic tissue infections.

Specific prevention issues for the individual. For example, use *Crataegus* if there is any concern about cardiovascular health, or *Ginkgo biloba* for an elderly patient.

Broader insights from the medical or family health history.

Symptom Support

Support the body in dealing with any fever that might accompany the infection, using diaphoretics when appropriate. In addition, if necessary, alleviate any symptomatic discomfort. Specifics will vary with each infection.

Herbal Support for Antibiotic Therapy

There is no reason why the benefits of phytotherapy should not be utilized to support a patient under treatment with antibiotics. This assumes, of course, that the antibiotics have been prescribed for appropriate reasons!

The herbal focus must be on tonics that will help the body cope with the intense biochemical battle that is under way. Selection can be based on these criteria:

Site of infection.

The need to support the digestive system and liver, as intestinal side effects are common with antibiotics.

Specific prevention issues for the individual.

Broader insights from the individual's medical or family health history.

Immune support may be appropriate, but do not try to duplicate the work of the antibiotics by overusing antimicrobial herbs! If necessary, symptomatic support may also be appropriate, and will depend on the individual's symptom picture.

Recuperation after Antibiotic Therapy

Once a course of antibiotics has been completed, herbs may be used to speed convalescence. They may also help the individual avoid any recurrence of the infection and prevent secondary problems that may result from the temporarily weakened immune response. The focus here should be on general nutrition, as well as herbal tonics.

Actions Indicated

Bitters will safely stimulate normal metabolism.

Gentle diuretics and *hepatics* will support elimination.

Specific tonics will support the tissue affected at the site of infection and the primary sites of symptomatic discomfort.

Immune support is important. This may entail both deep and surface work. Focus on deep immune support if:

- The infection is a chronic or recurrent problem
- The patient is very debilitated after the infection
- The patient is elderly
- The patient is under much stress of any kind, and thus at risk of becoming immunocompromised

MANIFESTATIONS OF INFECTION

Manifestations of infection are very diverse, varying with the pathogen involved, the site of infection, and the bodily response of the person involved. Common signs of infection include:

- Local inflammation at the site of infection
- Systemic signs including malaise, weakness, musculoskeletal aches and pains, headache, anorexia, fever, chills
- Increase of leukocytes in the blood and other blood changes seen in the lab

Infections of the Digestive System

Infections of the intestinal tract often manifest with the predominant symptom of diarrhea. The body's attempt to rid the body of the offending pathogen sets into motion processes that empty material from the gut. Treatment should incorporate the guidelines given in chapter 13 for diarrhea, along with appropriate antimicrobial herbs. Essential oil–containing herbs are especially useful here. Chronic forms of infection may manifest as some type of colitis; please refer to chapter 13 for more information on the management of this condition.

Antimicrobial Herbs for the Digestive System

Allium sativum (garlic)
Artemisia absinthium (wormwood)
Capsicum annuum (cayenne)
Carum carvi (caraway)
Coriandrum sativum (coriander)
Gentiana lutea (gentian)
Hydrastis canadensis (goldenseal)
Rosmarinus officinalis (rosemary)
Syzygium aromaticum (clove)
Thymus vulgaris (thyme)

Cardiovascular Infections

Infections affecting the heart and blood vessels can be extremely dangerous, and herbalism is not the most appropriate therapeutic modality.

Respiratory Tract Infections

The respiratory tract is one of the most common sites of infection in the human body. Fortunately, infections of the upper and lower respiratory tracts often respond well to herbal therapy. Please refer to chapter 15 for specific information on the treatment of bronchitis, sinusitis, and other infections of this system.

Antimicrobial Herbs for the Respiratory Tract

Allium sativum (garlic)
Baptisia tinctoria (wild indigo)

Commiphora molmol (myrrh)
Echinacea spp. (echinacea)
Eucalyptus spp. (eucalyptus)
Hydrastis canadensis (goldenseal)
Inula helenium (elecampane)
Ligusticum porteri (osha)
Myroxylon balsamum var. *pereirae* (balsam of Peru)
Pimpinella anisum (anise)
Populus balsamifera var. *balsamifera* (balm of Gilead)
Thymus vulgaris (thyme)
Usnea spp. (usnea)

Nervous System Infections

Infection of nervous system tissue can be extremely dangerous and difficult to treat. Conditions such as meningitis are best treated with conventional drugs, although using herbs in a supportive role, as described above, is fine. See chapter 16 for an herbal approach to the treatment of shingles, an intransigent viral infection of the nerve ganglia.

VAGINITIS

Inflammation (as from bacterial or fungal infection, allergic reaction, or hormone deficiency) of the vagina that may be marked by irritation and vaginal discharge. *(The Merriam-Webster Medical Dictionary)*

Symptoms of vaginitis include itching, burning, and a vaginal discharge that is different from normal secretions. The discharge may vary in consistency, color, and smell. The discomfort may be inside the vagina or on the vulva just outside the vagina. Discomfort during urination or sexual intercourse may also occur.

The term *vaginitis* describes a range of disorders that cause infection or inflammation of the vagina. The disorder may result from infection with organisms such as bacteria, yeast, and viruses, but may also be caused by irritation from chemicals in creams, sprays, or clothing. In some cases, vaginitis is caused by organisms that are passed between sexual partners.

Some vaginal discharge is quite common and normal for women of childbearing age. Normally, cervical glands produce a clear mucus secretion that drains downward, mixing with bacteria, discarded vaginal cells, and Bartholin's gland secretions. These substances may turn the mucus a whitish color (leukorrhea) and the discharge turns yellowish when exposed to air.

At certain times of the menstrual cycle, the cervical glands produce more mucus, depending on the amount of estrogen produced. This is normal. Sexual excitement and emotional stress are both associated with a normal vaginal discharge. This discharge is a clear, mucuslike secretion. Disease may be indicated if vaginal discharge is abnormal in color, odor, or consistency, or if the amount of discharge is significantly increased or decreased. When the abnormal discharge is caused by a sexually transmitted disease, the sexual partner(s) may require treatment as well.

Good hygiene can help prevent some of the causes of abnormal discharge, and help treat it if it occurs. A moist environment encourages the growth of yeast bacteria, so it is important to keep the area around the vulva dry. The woman should wear cotton underpants and avoid panty hose.

Treatment of Vaginitis

The material that follows, from *Family Herbal: A Guide to Living Life with Energy, Health, and Vitality* by herbalist Rosemary Gladstar, is an example of American folk herbalism at its best. Gladstar's approach epitomizes the ways in which competent herbalism can address the real needs of real people in an affordable and accessible way.

Gladstar suggests three components of effective and safe treatment:[3]

- Herbs taken internally, to address the infection
- An herbal dusting powder, to help dry excessive moisture
- Dietary measures

In the treatment suggestion given here, Gladstar recommends the use of capsules, which have a long tradition in American folk herbalism. The core herbs have been selected for their antibacterial and antifungal properties, combined with the soothing demulcency of marshmallow to minimize stomach irritation.

A Prescription for Vaginitis[4]

Black walnut hull powder

Chaparral powder

Echinacea root powder

Goldenseal root powder (organically cultivated)

Marshmallow root powder

Pau d'arco powder

Mix equal parts of the powders thoroughly and encapsulate in size 00 capsules. Take 2 capsules three times daily for 5 days, then take 2 days off. Continue this cycle for 4 weeks, or until symptoms subside.

Dusting Powder (Yoni Powder)[5]

1 cup fine white clay

½ cup cornstarch

2 tablespoons black walnut hull powder

2 tablespoons myrrh powder

1 tablespoon goldenseal root powder (organically cultivated)

A drop or two of tea tree essential oil (optional)

Combine all the ingredients and mix together using a wire whisk. Spoon some into a jar with a shaker top for easy application. Store the remainder in a glass jar with a tight-fitting lid.

Broader Context of Treatment

Attention to diet is of paramount importance. Emphasis should be placed on light, wholesome meals that are healing to the body and help restore a normal, slightly acidic pH to the vagina.

Dietary Guidelines for Vaginitis [6]

- Eat whole grains, such as brown rice, millet, and buckwheat.
- Eat nourishing soups, such as miso, chicken, and vegetable broths.
- Include steamed vegetables, especially the dark green leafy types.
- Avoid red meat.
- Eat plenty of lemons and grapefruit, but avoid sweet citrus fruits, such as oranges.
- Cranberries and unsweetened cranberry juice are highly recommended.
- Avoid alcohol and sweets during the course of a yeast infection.

Yogurt and acidophilus help replenish the normal flora of a healthy vagina and are important elements of a dietary program to combat a yeast infection. If you have allergies to dairy foods, goat yogurt and nondairy acidophilus are available. In addition, with each meal drink 1 teaspoon of apple cider vinegar mixed with 1 teaspoon of honey in ¼ cup of warm water. This old-fashioned tonic helps restore the body's acid-alkaline balance.

GENITOURINARY TRACT INFECTIONS

A range of antimicrobials are uniquely suited to treating this part of the body. They are usually herbs rich in essential oils. Please see chapter 18 for details on appropriate herbal treatments and contraindications for these herbs. As noted there, great care must be taken in patients with a history of kidney disease to completely avoid stimulating diuretics, such as *Juniperus*. In addition, consider the treatment protocol given for prostatitis, at right.

Antimicrobial Herbs for the Genitourinary Tract

Achillea millefolium (yarrow)
Agathosma betulina (buchu)
Arctostaphylos uva-ursi (bearberry)
Elymus repens (couch grass)
Juniperus communis (juniper)
Petroselinum crispum (parsley)

PROSTATITIS

Infection of the prostate gland. *(The Merck Manual)*

Prostatitis causes a number of troublesome symptoms, including aching pain and pressure in the prostate area, dysuria (painful urination), nocturia (nighttime urination), and dribbling. Hematuria (blood in the urine) may be present. The pain and pressure may make sitting down uncomfortable. Acute cases may be accompanied by fever.

Treatment of Prostatitis

Actions Indicated

Antimicrobials that work well in the urinary system are fundamental to treatment success.
Prostate tonics are indicated, as for benign prostatic hyperplasia.
Diuretics will promote voiding of urine. However, they may be contraindicated if there is marked blockage due to prostate swelling.
Demulcents that soothe the urinary system (demulcent diuretics) can help alleviate some of the symptoms.

Specific Remedies

While not specific per se, useful antimicrobials include *Arctostaphylos uva-ursi* (bearberry), *Agathosma betulina* (buchu), and *Elymus repens* (couch grass). Useful prostatic tonics include *Serenoa repens* (saw palmetto) and *Hydrangea arborescens* (hydrangea); other herbs that might fulfill such a role are *Turnera diffusa* (damiana) and *Smilax* spp. (sarsaparilla).

A Prescription for Prostatitis

Arctostaphylos uva-ursi	1 part
Agathosma betulina	1 part
Echinacea spp.	1 part
Serenoa repens	1 part
Zea mays	1 part

Dosage: up to 5 ml of tincture three times a day. In addition, the patient should drink an infusion of equal parts of dried *Zea mays* and *Achillea millefolium* throughout the day.

Table 21.5. Actions Supplied by Combination for Prostatitis

ACTION	HERBS
Antimicrobial	*Arctostaphylos uva-ursi, Agathosma betulina, Echinacea* spp., *Achillea millefolium*
Prostate tonic	*Serenoa repens*
Diuretic	*Arctostaphylos uva-ursi, Agathosma betulina, Zea mays, Achillea millefolium*
Demulcent	*Zea mays*

Broader Context of Treatment

In *Male Sexual Vitality*, Michael Murray, N.D., suggests addressing the following factors:[7]

Relax the musculature in the region. This is best achieved through stress management and relaxation techniques, but relaxing nervines may also be indicated.
Drink plenty of pure water.
Chew pumpkin seeds (Cucurbita pepo) in amounts up to $1/2$ cup a day.

Murray also recommends the following supplements:[8]

Vitamin E: 800 IU/day
Calcium-magnesium combination: 400 to 600 mg/day
Zinc picolinate: 20 to 50 mg/day

SKIN INFECTIONS

In light of the constant exposure of our massive skin surface to injury, bacteria, and various other foreign substances, it is rather incredible that the skin is not more frequently afflicted with infections. A number of factors account for this, including the skin's keratin layer, the chemicals in sebum and perspiration, and the internal defenses present in the bloodstream. Nonetheless, skin infections do occur, and vary from trivial to life threatening. Of the many different types of bacterial infection that can occur, here we shall review a treatment for boils. Please refer to chapter 24 for a discussion of impetigo in children.

BOILS

> Acute, tender, perifollicular inflammatory nodules resulting from infection by staphylococci. *(The Merck Manual)*

Boils, also known as *furuncles*, are infections that manifest as localized abscesses starting in the hair follicles. They emerge as tender, red, pus-filled lumps in the skin that often come to a "head" and subsequently drain. When deeper furuncles form and coalesce, the term *carbuncle* applies. A carbuncle may drain at several openings in the same region. The shoulders, face, scalp, buttocks, and armpits are common sites for carbuncles.

Treatment of Boils

Actions Indicated

Alteratives offer the most benefit in the treatment of boils, although I am unable to give a satisfactory explanation of how they work or why!

Antimicrobials help the body rid itself of the infection. In this case, it is difficult to say whether they work through direct bactericidal effects or indirect stimulation of the immune response.

Lymphatic tonics promote the general drainage of fluid.

Diuretics are especially important in supporting the eliminative work of the kidneys.

Hepatics are similarly helpful for the liver.

Vulnerary, anti-inflammatory, antipruritic, and *astringent herbs* may all be helpful topically.

Specific Remedies

The stronger hepatic alteratives are often considered specifics. Their strength highlights the need to take care with dosage. Important examples of hepatic alteratives are listed here. In addition, *Echinacea* is strongly indicated.

Iris versicolor (blue flag)
Larrea tridentata (chaparral)
Phytolacca americana (poke)
Pulsatilla vulgaris (pasqueflower)

A Prescription for Boils	
Echinacea spp.	3 parts
Galium aparine	2 parts
Rumex crispus	1 part
Phytolacca americana	1 part

Dosage: up to 5 ml of tincture three times a day. In addition, the patient should drink an infusion of *Urtica dioica* (preferably made from fresh herb) twice a day.

Table 21.6. Actions Supplied by Prescription for Boils

ACTION	HERBS
Alterative	*Echinacea* spp., *Galium aparine*, *Rumex crispus*, *Phytolacca americana*, *Urtica dioica*
Antimicrobial	*Echinacea* spp.
Lymphatic tonic	*Galium aparine*, *Phytolacca americana*
Diuretic	*Galium aparine*, *Urtica dioica*
Hepatic	*Rumex crispus*

FUNGAL SKIN INFECTIONS

> Superficial infections caused by dermatophytes—fungi that invade only dead tissues of the skin or its appendages. *(The Merck Manual)*

Fungal infections of the skin are very common in people of all ages. They are caused by microscopic fungal organisms that normally live on the skin surface without causing symptoms. Under the right conditions of moisture, warmth, irritation, or minor skin injury, they begin to grow more rapidly and invasively, causing a range of health problems. Certain underlying conditions may increase the likelihood that a fungal infection will occur, and should be considered when the infection is highly resistant to treatment or follows a recurrent course. They include some endocrine disorders and immune diseases.

A variety of fungal infections can affect human skin, especially in tropical environments where the heat and humidity allow the fungi to thrive. The pathogens most frequently responsible for fungal infections are known as *dermatophytes*.

Common Fungal Skin Infections

Tinea, caused by the fungus *Trichophyton*, manifests in an itchy, red, scaly patch that spreads outward as it grows. Hairs in the area may fall out or break. The skin may crack and become secondarily infected with bacteria. The fungus is spread by hairbrushes, clothes, and other personal contact.

The most common forms of tinea are:

Tinea capitis (ringworm of the scalp or neck)

Tinea barbae (ringworm of the beard area)

Tinea corporis (ringworm involving non-hairy parts of the body, such as the arms, shoulders, and face)

Tinea cruris ("jock itch")

Tinea pedis ("athlete's foot")

The discussion below of an herbal treatment for tinea pedis can be broadly applied to the other foci of fungal infections.

Treatment of Athlete's Foot

Athlete's foot, or tinea pedis, is a fungal infection of the toes and foot characterized by an itchy, scaly, malodorous rash between the toes. Cracks, irritation, redness, and bacterial infection may complicate the picture. Sports enthusiasts are not the only ones to suffer from athlete's foot. Hot weather and shoes that do not allow the feet to "breathe" are two predisposing factors. Most susceptible are people who have previously had the infection, adult men, people whose feet perspire heavily, and those with a weakened immune response. Women, children, and people who go barefoot do not often contract it. Internal treatments do little to help, unless the infection is an expression of an immune system problem.

Fungicidal essential oils and essential oil–rich plants are the most effective topical treatments. *Allium sativum* can be both dramatically effective and extremely odorous!

Effective Antifungal Herbs

Allium sativum (garlic)

Commiphora molmol (myrrh essential oil)

Melaleuca spp. (tea tree oil)

A combination of equal parts lavender and myrrh essential oils is a long-standing treatment for athlete's foot among aromatherapists in the United Kingdom. Myrrh is fungicidal and lavender is anti-inflammatory and vulnerary. For the first few days of treatment, dissolve the oils in rubbing alcohol and apply to skin until the skin no longer seems moist or weepy. Continue treatment with an ointment or cream containing 3% to 5% essential oil until the skin is completely clear. If the skin is deeply cracked and painful, calendula oil can be valuable as well.

In addition, the following hygiene pointers are important:

Clean thoroughly and repeatedly around toenails and fingernails, as the minute fungal mycelium often lodges under the nails and causes repeated infections.

Keep the feet dry, especially between the toes.

Wear open-toed shoes or sandals when you must wear shoes. Avoid vinyl uppers and athletic shoes with rubber soles. Cotton socks are better than synthetic.

Wash the feet and soak them in a vinegar and water solution (2 to 4 tablespoons of vinegar per pint of water) for 20 minutes three times daily. The use of herbal vinegars would also be appropriate.

CANCER

A proliferation of cells whose unique trait—loss of normal controls—results in unregulated growth, lack of differentiation, local tissue invasion, and metastasis. *(The Merck Manual)*

Herbal remedies have a long and honorable history in the treatment of cancer, and it may surprise some to learn that they are still at the core of modern medicine's response to this intransigent disease. For a comprehensive historical review of plants used in treating cancer, the interested reader is referred to *Plants Used Against Cancer: A Survey*, by J. L. Hartwell.[9]

Incredible resources go into cancer research, some of which are focused on plants. However, the results from all of this research attention are nowhere near as dramatic as what might be expected. This should not lead us to the conclusion that plants have little or no role in the treatment of cancer. Rather, it illuminates the basic failing of orthodox medicine's approach to degenerative disease in general and cancer in particular. For a detailed look at plants, cancer research, and the limitations of this research approach, please refer to chapter 9.

Cancer is a general term applied to a variety of malignant diseases that affect many different parts of the body. These diseases are characterized by rapid and uncontrolled formation of abnormal cells. These may mass together to form a growth or tumor, or proliferate throughout the body, initiating abnormal cell growth at other sites. If the process is not arrested, it may progress until it causes the death of the affected individual. Cancer is encountered in all higher animals, and plants also develop growths that resemble cancer.

The search for a chemical anticancer magic bullet or specific cytotoxic plant is predicated upon a rationale that might very well be flawed—that is, the idea that specific constituents represent the basis of a plant's therapeutic effect. This is not to deny that Western medicine has garnered a harvest of great benefit for a suffering humanity. Reductionist pharmacology has furnished medicine with powerful tools for the treatment of acute, life-threatening diseases and alleviation of suffering through speedy amelioration of symptoms. However, bear in mind that the major cause of death in the Western world is now degenerative disease, not acute infection. On the one hand, this change is a reflection of the successes of the allopathic approach; smallpox has been eradicated, polio no longer occurs in epidemic proportions, and tuberculosis is no longer the scourge it once was. On the other hand, these very successes highlight the inadequacy of the conventional approach to treating degenerative diseases.

Using the unfortunate militaristic imagery made popular by allopathic advocacy groups, we can say that acute infection has been "conquered." However, the vast sums and resources that have been invested toward conquering cancer have not produced the expected results. While the lobbyists for what has been called the cancer industry might conclude that more research funds are needed, holistic practitioners may come to a different conclusion. In short, the dearth of dramatic breakthroughs in cancer research might suggest that the allopathic context is not the appropriate one within which to perceive and address the complexity of factors at play in cancer. Multifactorial interactions are the strong suit of holistic medicine. This is not meant as a commentary on the effectiveness of specific holistic techniques, but merely emphasizes the need for a context that embraces more than oncogenes, tumor pathology, and carcinogens.

From the perspective of holistic medicine, any approach to cancer must be more than just an attack on a tumor. It must take into account the whole of the individual's life. A deep process of healing and reevaluation is essential. All of the issues raised at the beginning of this chapter and throughout this book must be addressed. Herbs demonstrate their relevance and efficacy in cancer only when used as a component of a treatment program constructed to address the individual in a holistic way. Such inclusive holistic approaches are, unfortunately, rare in the West. Much of so-called holistic cancer therapy is simply chemotherapy-free therapy.

A true holistic approach to cancer will involve the following factors.

A medical approach to destroying the tumor. This may take the form of improving the body's own immune response to destroying cancer cells. Herbal immunostimulants have much to offer here. Allopathic approaches may utilize cytotoxic plants, chemotherapy, surgery, and radiation.

Therapeutics geared to supporting the whole body. These take into account the patient's non-cancer issues, and may involve the use of tonics and other means of support for normal body processes, such as elimination and general homeostatic integration.

Nutritional reevaluation. This may entail identifying foods that have either an anticancer or a carcinogenic role, but, more important, should focus on ensuring that the body receives appropriate nourishment.

Bodywork appropriate for the individual. For example, massage does not cure cancer, but may play a vital role in managing stress, making it an integral part of holistic cancer treatment.

Emotional and mental support. While it may sound simple, this is a complex and formidable proposition! Stress management is essential, but so is in-depth counseling of some kind.

Counseling helps illuminate the reactions and coping mechanisms that come into play in response to cancer. However, more exciting are the potentially life-transforming insights that the patient may gain in the process. Within the context of transpersonal psychotherapy, it is possible to see illness as a gift that offers many insights and possibilities for growth and transformation. As a component of a broad, holistic treatment approach to cancer, the process can facilitate major emotional, mental, and spiritual healing even in the face of terminal bodily disease.

Integrating all of these ideas to formulate a holistic treatment program is challenging. The phytotherapist has much to offer, but without knowledge, understanding, and experience in the modalities mentioned above, herbs are not enough. Herbs can make a major contribution, but if used in isolation, they are in principle no different from chemotherapy. They may have more to offer in terms of general body health, but are less effective cytotoxic agents.

The term *anticancer herb* can foster false hopes. The National Cancer Institute defines commonly used terms in the following way:

A cytotoxic agent is toxic to tumors in laboratory cultures.
Antitumor activity occurs if cytotoxicity demonstrated in the laboratory also occurs in tumor cells in living animals.
Anticancer is a term reserved for materials that are toxic to tumor cells in clinical trials with humans.

One conclusion that can be drawn from all of this is that the holistically oriented herbalist tends to minimize the role of cytotoxic plants when developing an approach to treating cancer. While they can be life saving, they are not the core of treatment. There are a number of inherent problems with these plants, but the most important problem is how to use such potent plants safely.

An argument against the use of herbal medicines becomes relevant here. The huge variation in amounts of constituents in individual plants makes accurate prescribing or ensuring standardized protocols impossible. As phytotherapy is founded upon the use of gentle normalizers, or, at most, effectors that do not contain potent constituents, this issue is irrelevant in most cases. However, it becomes pertinent when potentially harmful cytotoxic plants are concerned.

The mere existence of cytotoxic herbs does not mean that they must be used. Similarly, the herbalist does not necessarily use the many powerful plant poisons, narcotics, and purgatives that the natural world offers. The selection of remedies for cancer must be dictated by the practitioner's interpretation of the individual's needs, which in turn is an expression of the therapeutic philosophy within which they work. The holistic practitioner will consider using such powerful remedies only within the context of a broad, holistic approach. We must act on these insights in practice or they become nothing more than hot air—and there is enough air pollution already!

In light of these dosage issues and the therapeutic ecology discussed throughout this book, I have concluded that if a practitioner decides that direct cytotoxicity is appropriate, chemotherapy may well be safer than cytotoxic plants. This statement may offend the natural medicine purist, but the needs of the patient *always* outweigh philosophical dogma.

A Holistic Approach to the Treatment of Cancer

So how are herbs most appropriately used in the treatment of cancer? By applying herbs with immunostimulant and immunomodulating properties in a holistic context, the practitioner may develop a protocol that does not depend on potentially poisonous plants. If we apply the model developed in this book, some clear guidelines become apparent.

Herbal Actions

Application of the term *anticancer* to herbal actions may be misleading. Appropriate herbal actions for cancer may include alterative, lymphatic, and tonic. Other actions will be indicated by the symptom picture and issues unique to the type of tumor involved. In addition, the needs of the individual will suggest actions necessary for system support.

System Tonics

Tonic support for the site of the tumor is essential. Tonics can also be used to address other factors revealed by a review of the patient's medical and family history.

System Support

This will take some form of immune system support, with an emphasis on deep immune stimulation, eliminative support, and stress management.

Specific Remedies

Many plants around the world have a reputation for anticancer activity. Unfortunately, they do not work as claimed! Instead, they are largely alterative, lymphatic, hepatic, or diuretic remedies, and have much to contribute to the holistic approach suggested here. However, used in isolation, they will not replace such an approach. Common examples of such remedies from the European and North American traditions are listed here.

Herbs to Support a Holistic Approach to Cancer

Arctium lappa (burdock)
Calendula officinalis (calendula)
Galium aparine (cleavers)
Hydrastis canadensis (goldenseal)
Iris versicolor (blue flag)
Larrea tridentata (chaparral)
Phytolacca americana (poke)
Rumex crispus (yellow dock)
Sanguinaria canadensis (bloodroot)
Scrophularia nodosa (figwort)
Stillingia sylvatica (queen's delight)
Thuja occidentalis (thuja)
Trifolium pratense (red clover)
Urtica dioica (nettle)
Viola odorata (sweet violet)
Viscum album (mistletoe)

Why are no prescriptions suggested or treatment protocols given in this discussion on cancer? I have two reasons, one theoretical and one personal.

If we can draw any clear conclusion from this theoretical discussion, it is that each individual must be treated as just that—a unique individual—not a tumor site. As the holistic approach proposes that we avoid cytotoxic remedies, the factors to address within the protocol will be fundamentally the same as those for immune support in general, with a possibly greater emphasis on alterative and lymphatic remedies.

However, the main reason I have not suggested any prescriptions here is a personal one. My clinical experience with treating cancer is limited, and so I have concluded that all I can ethically write is the review of theory presented here. The herbal literature is replete with treatments and cancer cures that have no basis in reality. An exception to this is *Herbal Medicine, Healing and Cancer*, by Donald Yance. Written by an experienced, knowledgeable, and realistically compassionate herbalist, the book bodes well for the future of traditional herbalism in the United States.

Table 21.7, adapted from Yance's book, briefly summarizes his three-stage approach to the treatment of cancer. Please refer to his book for more explanation and details.

Table 21.7. Three-Stage Herbal Protocol for Cancer[10]

STAGE OF TREATMENT	ACTIONS REQUIRED
Stage 1: Tonic therapy	Herbs to strengthen the individual's constitution and vitality
	Tonics, adaptogens, and herbal immune-enhancers
Stage 2: Liver and lymph detoxification	Antioxidant, liver-detoxifying, anti-inflammatory, and anti-angiogenic herbs; alteratives and lymphatics
Stage 3: Cytotoxic therapy	Gene-repairing, enzyme-inhibiting, and cytotoxic herbs
	Herbs that can alter the action of hormonal receptor-type cancers

Adapted from Donald Yance, *Herbal Medicine, Healing and Cancer*. (Los Angeles: Keats Publishing, 1999).

Isolated Constituents with Promise in Cancer

Two plant constituents that appear to have much to offer as supplementation to an individualized protocol for the treatment of cancer are artemisinin and di-indolymethane. Artemisinin is a sesquiterpene found in *Artemisia annua*, a plant known as sweet Annie in North America and qing hao in China. It was initially introduced into Western medicine as a treatment for malaria. Extensive clinical trials have demonstrated that artemisinin is effective against *Plasmodium falciparum*, the causative parasitic protozoan that is transmitted to humans via the *Anopheles* mosquito. Subsequent research showed activity against strains of *Plasmodium* that had become resistant to chloroquine.[11] In recent years, artemisinin has attracted attention as a potential anticancer drug, and appears to be effective against a wide variety of cancers, especially leukemia and colon cancer. Intermediate activities were also shown against melanoma, breast, ovarian, prostate, CNS, and renal cancer.[12]

Di-indolylmethane is a dimer of indole-3-carbinol, a glucosinolate found in cruciferous vegetables. Both of these compounds appear to have potent anticancer properties.[13] Vegetables that contain them include brussels sprouts, broccoli, and cabbages. Di-indolylmethane and indole-3-carbinol stimulate biotransformation in the liver, converting estradiol to nontoxic metabolites.[14] These glucosinolates are believed to be responsible for the lowered risk of cancer associated with the consumption of cruciferous vegetables.[15] They appear to be especially protective against breast and cervical cancer. One reason for this may be an ability to increase the breakdown of estrogens.[16] Estradiol, for example, may have carcinogenic properties when its levels become high, while the other estrogens have noncarcinogenic or perhaps even anticarcinogenic properties. As an increasing amount of estrogen-type substances are appearing in the food and water chain (probably due primarily to the wide use of pesticides and plastics), di-indolylmethane and indole-3-carbinol may be viewed as important preventive substances.

References

1. www.news.cornell.edu/releases/Sept96/cyclosporine.hrs. html.

2. Weng SC, Chou CJ, Lin LC, et al. Immunomodulatory functions of extracts from the Chinese medicinal fungus Cordyceps cicadae. *Journal of Ethnopharmacology* 2002 Nov; 83(1–2):79–85.

3. Gladstar R, *Family Herbal: A Guide to Living Life with Energy, Health, and Vitality*. Pownal, VT: Storey Books, 2001.

4. Ibid.

5. Ibid.

6. Ibid.

7. Murray MT. *Male Sexual Vitality*. Rocklin, CA: Prima, 1994.

8. Ibid.

9. Hartwell JL. *Plants Used Against Cancer: A Survey*. Lawrence, KS: Quarterman Publications, 1984.

10. Yance DR. *Herbal Medicine, Healing and Cancer*. Los Angeles: Keats Publishing, 1999.

11. Samuelsson, G. *Drugs of Natural Origin*. Stockholm: Swedish Pharmaceutical Press, 1992.

12. Efferth, et al. Antimalaria drug is also active against cancer. *International Journal of Oncology* 2001; 18; 767–73.

13. Broadbent TA, Broadbent HS. The chemistry and pharmacology of indole-3-carbinol (indole-3-methanol) and 3-(methoxymethyl)indole [part I]. *Current Medicinal Chemistry* 1998; 5:337–52.

14. Ibid., 469–91.

15. Hecht SS. Chemoprevention of cancer by isothiocyanates, modifiers of carcinogen metabolism. *Journal of Nutrition* 1999; 129:768S–74S [review].

16. Bradlow HL, Sepkovic DW, Telang NT, and Osborne MP. Multifunctional aspects of the action of indole-3-carbinol as an antitumor agent. *Annals of the New York Academy of Sciences* 1999; 889:204–13.

Suggested Reading

Boik J. *Cancer and Natural Medicine: A Textbook of Basic Science and Clinical Research*. Princeton, MN: Oregon Medical Press, 1996.

Mills S, Bone K. *Principles and Practice of Phytotherapy: Modern Herbal Medicine*. Edinburgh: Churchill Livingstone, 1999.

Yance DR. *Herbal Medicine, Healing and Cancer*. Los Angeles: Keats Publishing, 1999.

22

∾

THE ENDOCRINE SYSTEM

The herbal traditions do not provide an abundance of information about the treatment of endocrine disorders. This is not surprising, as our understanding of the functions of this important body system is a very recent development. In addition, a comprehensive review of phytotherapy for the endocrine system has yet to be written. When used skillfully within the context of an appropriate holistic approach, herbs can make a major contribution to treatment of endocrine disorders. However, the results achieved with herbs may not adequately replace drug treatment.

The endocrine system influences cellular metabolism by means of hormones. Endocrine glands, also known as ductless glands, release hormones into the blood or lymph. Hormones are chemical messengers that are transported throughout the body. The body's responses to the presence of hormones occur after a lag period of seconds or even days, but once initiated, the responses tend to be much more prolonged than those induced by the nervous system.

The endocrine glands include the pituitary, thyroid, parathyroid, adrenal, pineal, and thymus glands. Additionally, several non-endocrine organs contain areas of endocrine tissue that produce hormones. Such organs include the pancreas and the gonads. The hypothalamus, a part of the nervous system, produces and releases hormones, so is considered a *neuroendocrine* organ.

THE THYROID GLAND

The thyroid gland is a butterfly-shaped organ located at the base of the neck, just above the collarbone. The main function of this gland is the production of thyroxine, an iodine-containing hormone. Thyroxine controls the rate and intensity of most physiologic functions. The regulation of heart rate, sweating, digestive action, body temperature, calorie consumption, and many other activities depends at least in part on this hormone.

The pituitary gland, located at the base of the front of the brain, controls the thyroid itself. The pituitary releases thyroid-stimulating hormone (TSH), required by the thyroid to produce thyroxine. In turn, production of pituitary TSH depends upon the presence of thyrotropin-releasing hormone, which comes from the hypothalamus. Thus, a complex and delicate set of interactions governs the function of the thyroid, and many physical and emotional factors can also play a role.

HYPOTHYROIDISM

The characteristic clinical response to thyroid hormone deficiency in the adult. *(The Merck Manual)*

Hypothyroidism, also known as *myxedema*, is underactivity of the thyroid that results in deficiency of thyroid hormone. Although the disorder may be caused by any of a variety of diseases that affect the hypothalamus and pituitary gland, it is primarily related to disorders of the thyroid gland itself.

Inadequate secretion of thyroid hormone leads to a general slowing of all physical and mental processes. The condition is characterized by an overall depression of most cellular enzyme systems and oxidative processes. As the metabolic activity of all cells in the body slows, there is a reduction in the rate of oxygen consumption, leading to a decrease in oxidation of nutrients for energy and less body heat production.

The signs and symptoms, all of which result from this slowdown of metabolism, range from nonspecific complaints to severe symptoms that may become life threatening if unrecognized and untreated. Fatigue, lack of energy, cold intolerance, severe constipation, heavy menstrual periods, and weight gain despite a diminishing appetite may go unnoticed or be attributed to other conditions, such as stress, depression, and overwork. As symptoms worsen, they may become more obvious with time. These can include slowed pulse, muscle aches, puffiness around the eyes, hair loss, hoarseness, sluggish reflexes, and cool, dry, coarse skin. Changes in mood and personality, simulating psychiatric disturbance, may occur. The thyroid gland may become enlarged, producing a goiter in the neck. Hypothyroidism is a risk factor for a range of problems including atherosclerosis, skin problems, and constipation.

Treatment of Hypothyroidism

Orthodox therapy for hypothyroidism is based upon daily thyroid hormone replacement therapy. As no herbs adequately fulfill this action, drug therapy will often remain the basis of treatment, and the role of phytotherapy will be to help the body deal with the repercussions of the condition and its treatment. In mild cases, the use of bitters may sometimes be enough, but it will be beneficial in all cases. Other than bitters, the seaweed *Fucus vesiculosus* (bladderwrack) has been traditionally used to treat this condition. While it has much to offer, it is only truly specific when the patient has an iodine deficiency.

Herbs can support hormone replacement therapy in a number of important ways. Hypothyroidism accelerates the development of atherosclerosis, due to deposition of mucopolysaccharides in the heart muscle, placing patients at higher risk of coronary artery disease. This damage may be lessened through the use of cardiovascular tonics, such as *Crataegus* spp., *Ginkgo biloba*, and *Allium sativum*.

In addition, herbs can help ease problems related to functional and structural changes in the skin. While they may provide only symptomatic relief, this is nonetheless essential for the patient. Emollients, circulatory stimulants, and other remedies may be valuable here, but the specifics will depend upon the patient's experience. Moisturizing actions are especially important, because the skin is usually dry and scaly in this condition.

Other symptoms may also be relieved with herbs. For chronic constipation, hepatic laxatives are the best choice, as they also support liver function. Examples of herbs that may be helpful include *Rumex crispus* (yellow dock) and *Juglans cinerea* (butternut). In extreme cases, anthraquinone-containing herbs, such as *Rhamnus purshiana* (cascara sagrada) and *Senna alexandrina*, may be required. See chapters 10 and 13 for important cautions about the use of these powerful laxatives.

Nervine tonics and other nervines may be indicated, but avoid the stronger relaxing remedies, such as *Humulus lupulus* (hops) and *Valeriana officinalis* (valerian). This is because they may have too sedating an effect on body function. Antidepressant herbs like *Hypericum perforatum* (St. John's wort) and *Artemisia vulgaris* (mugwort) can be helpful.

HYPERTHYROIDISM

A clinical condition encompassing several specific diseases, characterized by hypermetabolism and elevated serum levels of free thyroid hormones. *(The Merck Manual)*

Hyperthyroidism, or overactivity of the thyroid gland, has a number of possible causes. It may be due to the presence of a growth or tumor (either benign or malignant) or a self-limited inflammation of the gland, probably due to viral infection. The most common cause is Graves' disease, an autoimmune disorder related to the production of thyroid antibodies that have a stimulating effect on the gland. This same process causes the deposition of a thick substance within the skin, behind the eyes, and elsewhere.

Clinical manifestations of hyperthyroidism, especially excessive body heat, increased neuromuscular and cardiovascular activity, and hyperactivity, are the result of heightened metabolic rate. Accelerated pulse rate can range from 90 to 160 beats per minute.

Symptoms of Hyperthyroidism

Nervousness, hyperexcitement, irritability, apprehension, sleeplessness
Difficulty sitting quietly
Rapid pulse at rest and upon exertion; heart palpitations
Low heat tolerance, profuse perspiration, flushed skin (e.g., warm, moist hands)
Fine tremor of hands, changes in bowel habits (constipation or diarrhea)
Increased appetite and progressive weight loss
Muscle fatigue and weakness
Amenorrhea
Bulging eyes *(exophthalmos)*, producing a startled expression

Treatment of Hyperthyroidism

Symptomatic amelioration of this condition is often straightforward. However, control of the underlying cause of the symptoms—excessive production of thyroid hormones—is challenging. Used as symptomatic relief, however, herbs can support the work of prescription medications.

Actions Indicated

Relaxing nervines will ease agitation and anxiety. In this case, specific relaxing nervines are indicated (*Lycopus virginicus* or *L. europaeus*, discussed under Specific Remedies).

Cardiac tonics are indicated, to help the heart function healthily in the face of the hormone-stimulated workload.

Specific Remedies

Traditional herbal treatment for hyperthyroidism provides us with one of the best examples of a condition for which a definite specific exists. This is *Lycopus virginicus* or *L. europaeus*, commonly known as bugleweed. The herb is a useful relaxing nervine, but in addition has a sometimes dramatic effect in improving the symptom picture associated with hyperthyroid conditions. I have seen no data on changes in thyroxine serum levels in patients using *Lycopus*, and thus cannot say that the improvement is related to any direct impact of the herb on hormone levels. Nonetheless, it does seem to help.

A Prescription for Hyperthyroidism

Lycopus spp.	4 parts
Leonurus cardiaca	2 parts
Scutellaria spp.	2 parts
Crataegus spp.	1 part

Dosage: up to 5 ml of tincture three times a day

A Prescription for Insomnia Associated with Hyperthyroidism

Valeriana officinalis	1 part
Passiflora incarnata	1 part

Dosage: 5 to 15 ml of tincture a half hour before retiring

Table 22.1. Actions Supplied by Combination for Hyperthyroidism

ACTION	HERBS
Nervine tonic	*Scutellaria* spp.
Nervine relaxant	*Lycopus* spp., *Leonurus cardiaca*, *Scutellaria* spp., *Valeriana officinalis*, *Passiflora incarnata*
Cardiovascular tonic	*Crataegus* spp.

DIABETES MELLITUS

A syndrome characterized by hyperglycemia resulting from absolute or relative impairment in insulin and/or insulin action. *(The Merck Manual)*

Diabetes mellitus, characterized by glycosuria (glucose in the urine) and hyperglycemia (elevated blood sugar levels), is an unfortunately common, chronic metabolic disorder involving carbohydrate, fat, and protein metabolism. Although the most widely recognized manifestation of diabetes is hyperglycemia, this is a complex and multifaceted disease that potentially affects every organ in the body.

Regulation of blood sugar, a complex homeostatic process, is dependent upon the presence of insulin, a hormone produced in specialized cells in the pancreas, called islets of Langerhans. The insulin is absorbed into the bloodstream, which carries it to the rest of the body. Insulin fulfills several important roles:

Mobilizes glucose to leave the blood and enter the cells of various body organs.
Facilitates other metabolic processes that foster the storage of energy in fat and other body substances and regulate the release of these stores into the blood.

Insufficient levels of insulin cause blood glucose levels to rise, especially after a meal. Without insulin, body organs are unable to extract glucose from the blood and begin to rely on alternate sources of energy, especially certain fats. Their metabolites, called ketones, begin to accumulate in the blood. Metabolic changes in diabetes alter the way in which the body handles fats, including cholesterol. This leads to their accumulation in the small arteries of the body, often those of the eyes, kidneys, heart, and brain. Thus, people with diabetes have an increased incidence of blindness, kidney failure, heart attack, and stroke.

There are two different forms of diabetes.

Insulin-Dependent Diabetes Mellitus (IDDM)

Insulin-dependent or Type I diabetes is often called *juvenile onset* diabetes, since it usually first presents in childhood or young adulthood. The condition is characterized by a near total lack of insulin production; this is related to a deficiency in insulin synthesis and secretion from the islets of Langerhans, clusters of cells found in the pancreas. The pathogenesis of the disease may be autoimmune in nature or related to infection with coxsackie virus B4 or mumps virus. Type I diabetes is treated with insulin and diet; there is no role for oral hypoglycemics.

Non-Insulin-Dependent Diabetes Mellitus (NIDDM)

Non-insulin-dependent or Type II diabetes usually occurs in elderly or overweight people, and is thus also called *maturity onset* diabetes. It is caused by a deficiency in or diminished effectiveness of insulin, and is much more common than Type I. Non-insulin-dependent diabetes may be secondary to other diseases, such as pancreatitis. It may also occur as a result of insulin antagonism, such as that caused by Cushing's syndrome or steroid therapy. When NIDDM occurs in young people, a genetic component appears to be involved.

Other causes of impaired glucose tolerance include pregnancy and thyrotoxicosis, a condition resulting from the presence of excess thyroid hormone, which in turn may result from either overproduction by the thyroid gland or loss of storage function and leakage from the gland. In addition, the gradual development of relative insulin deficiency is part of the normal aging process. In NIDDM, the aim of treatment is to regularize blood sugar levels through the use of hypoglycemics, glucosidase inhibitors, sugar-restricted diets, and complex carbohydrate preparations that delay the absorption of glucose from the gut. People with NIDDM retain the ability to produce some insulin, but the response to a meal is long delayed and often inadequate.

Symptoms of either type of diabetes include fatigue, increased appetite (if enough blood sugar is lost to the urine), and increased urination, as the sugar causes the kidney to produce higher volumes to dissolve the excess load. Because of the accelerated loss of body fluid, the patient experiences greater thirst. As levels of blood sugar rise and ketosis occurs, body fluids become acidic. One of the body's defenses against acidity is to decrease the amount of carbon dioxide in the blood, which leads to an increase in the rate and depth of respiration. Complications due to arterial blockage are common, including vision loss, heart problems, kidney damage, and peripheral neuropathy. Such problems usually develop over many years.

Treatment of Diabetes

The plant world offers many hypoglycemic herbs, and these have much to contribute to a comprehensive management program for NIDDM. Insulin-dependent diabetes will rarely respond well to hypoglycemic agents, as the islets of Langerhans are largely incapacitated. Herbs will not replace necessary insulin therapy.

Laboratory screenings similar to those used to identify cytotoxic plants have demonstrated that plant hypoglycemics do exist, and many hundreds have been documented. Please see chapter 9 for a discussion about this research.

Hypoglycemic Herbs from the European Tradition

Allium sativum (garlic)
Galega officinalis (goat's rue)
Morus alba (mulberry leaf)
Olea europaea (olive leaf)
Vaccinium myrtillus (bilberry)

Interestingly, goat's rue is also an effective galactagogue, hinting at a possible effect on the pituitary or hypothalamus. Remember that gentle endocrine stimulation is also one of the properties of bitters, and for some people these herbs may be dramatically effective in lowering blood sugar.

On the experimental level, many plants have been shown to have some degree of hypoglycemic activity, but their mechanisms of action are not always clear. Here are some examples cited in *Medical Botany*, by Lewis and Elvin-Lewis.[1]

Plants with Hypoglycemic Activity in Animal Studies

Anacardium occidentale (cashew)
Apium graveolens (celery)
Arctium lappa (burdock)
Avena sativa (oats)
Capsicum annuum (cayenne)
Cimicifuga racemosa (black cohosh)
Eupatorium purpureum (gravel root)
Euphorbia pilulifera (pill-bearing spurge)
Hydrastis canadensis (goldenseal)
Lophophora williamsii (peyote)
Panax ginseng (ginseng)
Spinacia oleracea (spinach)
Taraxacum officinale (dandelion)
Trigonella foenum-graecum (fenugreek)

The challenge for the herbal practitioner is the appropriate application of hypoglycemics. Such remedies can sometimes have a rapid impact on blood sugar levels, but this will vary from patient to patient. They can be used safely only as part of a comprehensive diabetes management program suitable for the particular individual. Very close observation of glucose levels in urine and blood is required. As this is beyond the scope of this discussion, no protocols for the use of hypoglycemic agents will be given here.

On the other hand, herbal preventive work to avoid long-term complications of diabetes may be undertaken quite safely, even if no attempt is made to alter insulin levels. For the reasons discussed earlier, particular attention should be given to the cardiovascular system. Heart and vascular tonics are appropriate for long-term use, especially *Crataegus* spp., *Ginkgo biloba*, and *Vaccinium myrtillus*.

THE ADRENAL GLANDS

Ideas about remedies for the adrenal glands abound. Unfortunately, they often reflect a fundamental lack of knowledge about the physiology and function of this important part of the endocrine system. The concepts couched in the vague terms used in much "alternative" literature are often valid and helpful, but the invocation of adrenal tonic effects must be based upon an understanding of actual physiology.

One adrenal gland sits astride each kidney, deep in the back part of the abdomen. Each of these glands has two parts with markedly different functions: a *cortex*, or outer part, and a *medulla*, or central portion. Therapy intended to affect these glands must be appropriate to the adrenal function the practitioner wants to address.

The Adrenal Medulla

The adrenal medulla secretes the hormones adrenaline (epinephrine) and noradrenaline (norepinephrine), which are responsible for the rapid increases in nervous system and metabolic activity involved in the general adaptation system (GAS). Please see chapter 16 for more information on this important stress response mechanism and the contribution herbs can make to support the adrenal medulla.

Functions of Adrenaline

- Acts on α- and β-receptors
- Increases contractility and excitability of heart muscle, thus increasing cardiac output
- Facilitates blood flow to muscles, brain, and viscera
- Enhances blood sugar levels by stimulating conversion of glycogen to glucose in liver
- Inhibits smooth muscle contractions

Functions of Noradrenaline

- Acts primarily on α-receptors
- Increases peripheral vascular resistance, leading to increased blood pressure

The Adrenal Cortex

The adrenal cortex is responsible for production of glucocorticoids, such as cortisol and hydrocortisone, which help regulate metabolism, the immune system, certain aspects of behavior, and many other processes. The cortex also secretes mineralocorticoids, such as aldosterone and desoxycorticosterone. Aldosterone is fundamental to the homeostatic control of sodium and potassium secretion by the kidney. These hormones are synthesized from cholesterol.

Functions of Glucocorticoids

- Enhance protein catabolism and inhibit protein synthesis
- Antagonize action of insulin
- Increase synthesis of glucose by the liver
- Influence body defense mechanism and reactions to stress
- Influence emotions

Functions of Mineralocorticoids

- Regulate reabsorption of sodium cations
- Regulate excretion of potassium cations by renal tubules

While the cortex and medulla produce different hormones in response to different stimuli, they share a complex role in certain situations—for example, the stress response. The immediate stress response is controlled mainly, although not completely, by the medulla, while long-term stress responses are handled by the surrounding cortex. Please refer to chapter 16 for a more detailed discussion of the physiological responses that constitute this reaction.

Herbs to Support the Adrenal Medulla

Adaptogens constitute the core of herbal support for conditions affecting the adrenal medulla. Saponins, such as the eleutherosides found in *Eleutherococcus senticosus* (Siberian ginseng), directly impact this part of the adrenal gland. Nervine tonic support of some kind is usually indicated as well. Although nervines will not directly affect the medulla, they will provide general systemic support to help ease the impact of tension and anxiety. Bitter tonics can be helpful as well. Examples of useful adaptogens are *Panax* spp. (ginseng), *Eleutherococcus senticosus*, and *Withania somnifera* (ashwaganda). Relevant nervine tonics include *Scutellaria lateriflora* (skullcap), *Hypericum perforatum* (St. John's wort), and *Avena sativa* (oats).

Herbs to Support the Adrenal Cortex

Herbal medicines can affect the function of the adrenal cortex in a variety of ways. Most important are the direct effects of plants rich in saponins, such as *Glycyrrhiza glabra* (licorice) and *Dioscorea villosa* (wild yam). Adaptogens will help support the cortex in its response to adrenocorticotropic hormone (ACTH).

Glycyrrhiza is in fact proving controversial because of its effects upon the adrenal cortex. Aldosterone is part of what has been called the renin-aldosterone-angiotensin axis, a hormonal homeostatic complex that regulates the volume of urine passed and electrolyte balance in the blood. When *Glycyrrhiza* is eaten or taken in great excess, its direct impact upon aldosterone can lead to potassium depletion. This is a very rare occurrence, but it is mentioned in pharmacology books as one of the dangers of herbal medicine. Such effects must be taken seriously, however, with hypertensive patients. *Glycyrrhiza* is contraindicated for these patients.

On the other hand, case reports from the United Kingdom indicate that some people with Addison's disease benefit greatly from the use of *Glycyrrhiza*. Addison's disease results from damage to the adrenal cortex, which leads to decreased production of adrenocortical hormones.

References

1. Lewis WH, Elvin-Lewis M. *Medical Botany*. New York: J. Wiley, 2003.

23

❧

PHYTOTHERAPY AND THE ELDERLY

What is aging? To some extent, the answer to this question is a subjective one, reflecting belief system as much as fact. Here we shall briefly consider some ideas about the nature of biological aging. The more extreme proponents of the current immortality movement suggest that aging is simply an artifact of bad nutrition and cramped life vision. Because these immortality advocates tout certain herbs as part of the approach to life extension, we will focus some attention on ideas of aging.

However, I must start by acknowledging my personal bias on these issues. The very expensive products and approaches proposed by some prominent exponents of "life extension" strike me as a clever moneymaking plan based on some unsavory elitist tendencies. There is a tendency in these circles to see illness as something the patient creates or attracts into his or her life. On some level, this may well be true, as illness can provide one with the profound gift of a learning opportunity. On the other hand, this insight has become an unfortunately powerful tool for browbeating and a source of guilt and judgment for the patient. In my opinion, this is nothing short of new age fascism.

Appropriate nutrition can do much to improve quality of life, health in general, and specific illness. Similarly, as should be clear at this point in the book, I have a deep respect for the role of vision and spirituality in human life. The Bible says, "Without vision, the people die." However, it does *not* say that with vision, the people will live forever. The fundamental importance of vision and spirituality is qualitative, not quantitative. By bringing these qualities into our lives, we heal and transform ourselves and the world. Having a longer chronological life span is not the point.

The material in this chapter is structured differently from that in the other treatment chapters. We will focus primarily on a range of issues germane to elder health. Discussions on most of the specific health conditions that affect elders can be found in the appropriate body system chapters by following the cross-references given here.

Genetic Theories of Aging

One group of ideas about aging is based upon the plethora of insights provided by molecular biology about DNA and RNA function and structure. Theories have been proposed that suggest that aging is related to problems with stability of DNA over time, and with the transcription of information from the chromosomal DNA to RNA. In fact, there is a different theory for each phase of the process. For those who are interested, the most relevant ideas are known as the *error theory*, the *redundant message theory*, the *transcription theory*, and the *programmed theory*.[1]

Non-Genetic Theories of Aging

A number of non-DNA-based theories of aging have also been proposed, and it is here that herbalism may be most relevant. It should be clear by now to the reader what contribution herbs may make in each of the following areas.

The immunological theory proposes that alterations in the immune system contribute to the changes associated with old age. With advancing age, the immune system is thought to become less efficient. Its capacity to deal with infection is reduced, and there is a greater likelihood of autoimmune reactions.

The connective tissue theory relates aging to changes in the collagen, elastin, and ground substance of this ubiquitous tissue. As collagen makes up 25% of body protein, any changes to this tissue will have marked effects on overall health.

The free radical theory holds that the changes of aging are caused by the combination of free radicals with essential molecules. Free radicals are chemicals whose outer orbits contain unpaired electrons, making them highly reactive.

Free radicals are a normal but short-lived aspect of metabolism. The core problem is peroxidation of fats, which damages membranes in the body. Even though the body has a range of mechanisms to cope with it, the damage caused by free radicals can be extensive. The free radical theory is the one most often cited by the longevity movement as a key insight. The question is whether free radical production is the fundamental cause of aging or simply an ancillary phenomenon that exacerbates age-related changes due to some other cause.

Spiritual and Socioeconomic Issues

In addition to biological factors, sociological, economic, and spiritual issues play a profound role in aging. Although a detailed discussion of the complex of factors at play is beyond the scope of this book, a few brief points must be made.

Age is not a disease. Death is not an evil to be avoided at all costs. Our culture has developed some distorted perceptions about old age, seeing it as the undesirable mirror image of youth. This blinkered perception ignores the incredible value of wisdom and experience. It denies our elders a voice and disregards the valuable contributions they have to offer. Our whole culture suffers as a result. We are dealing with spiritual issues here. There must be an affirmation of aging and death, and an acknowledgment of the rites of passage that these life stages represent.

Much of the illness of elders either results from or is aggravated by socioeconomic factors that are not medical at all. Issues such as isolation and poverty that manifest in cardiovascular disease will not be helped by hawthorn. If our culture is truly going to evolve into a "kinder, gentler" one, then we must pay attention to these thorny questions.

TONING AND NURTURING HEALTH IN ELDERS

As with most theories, the truth may well be some combination of all of the ideas just discussed! Where does this leave the phytotherapist? The first step is to identify any therapeutic insights that may be gained by differentiating among alterable and largely unalterable manifestations of aging. The degree and timing of such changes will vary from person to person, depending upon genetics, lifestyle, environmental conditions, and other factors.

Largely Unalterable Manifestations of Aging

Farsightedness
Fibrosis and stiffening of arteries
Graying of hair
High-tone hearing loss
Loss of skin elasticity

Fortunately, some age-related changes can be altered or avoided through various preventive approaches. In most cases, the best way to use any applicable remedy is within a broader treatment context, as indicated in the relevant body system chapters.

Table 23.1. Possibly Alterable Manifestations of Aging

MANIFESTATION	TREATMENT STRATEGIES
Agility	Stretching exercises, appropriate herbs
Arthritis	Diet, exercise, weight control, appropriate herbs
Blood pressure	Exercise, reduced salt intake, obesity, appropriate herbs
Cancer	Diet, exercise, weight control, tobacco avoidance, herbs
Cognition	Practice, appropriate herbs
Heart disease	Diet, exercise, weight control, tobacco avoidance, herbs
Heart reserve	Aerobic exercise, appropriate herbs
Isolation	Practice, socialization
Memory	Practice, appropriate herbs
Mobility	Stretching exercises, appropriate herbs
Physical fitness	Exercise, weight control, tobacco avoidance, herbs
Reaction time	Exercise, appropriate herbs

A basic premise of my philosophy is that phytotherapy can go beyond the treatment of illness to nurture health. This strength of this approach lies in the use of tonics and gentle effector remedies; stronger effectors are reserved for use only when absolutely necessary. This is also the basis of herbal treatment for elders. Thus, everything covered so far in this book has relevance to the treatment of older individuals.

Perhaps the most outstanding contribution that herbs can make to the health of elders is through system tonics. Tonics and gentle normalizer remedies not only are largely free of side effects, but also offer possibilities—unmatched by any conventional treatments—for the maintenance of wellness and the prevention of many problems associated with aging.

Prescribing Issues Unique to Elders

When considering herbal therapy for elders, it is important to acknowledge the effects of certain age-related pharmacokinetic and pharmacodynamic changes. Safe drug or herb prescribing for older patients must be based on an understanding of the alterations in absorption, distribution, and elimination mechanisms that occur as part of the aging process. Taking such issues into consideration can prevent many complications.

Although these concerns are not as important for the phytotherapist as for the physician prescribing conventional drugs, they still exist. A brief review of some of the factors involved for both plant extracts and chemical drugs is provided here; see chapter 9 for more information. Details on calculating dosages for elders are provided in chapter 12.

Drug Absorption

In order for a substance to enter the bloodstream when taken by mouth, the absorptive lining of the gastrointestinal tract must be healthy. Medicines must remain in contact with the lining for an adequate amount of time for absorption to occur. There must also be an adequate blood flow to and from the site of absorption. Normal age-related changes impact all of these factors. There is a reduction in mucosal surface area, a decrease in blood flow to the intestines, and changes in both the amount and nature of secretions.

Plasma Binding

Plant constituents are transported via the blood once they have been absorbed from the intestines. The more complex molecules are often bound with a blood protein, such as albumin. Such protein-bound drugs can compete for binding sites, which in turn may have a profound effect on availability of medications.

Distribution

With advancing age, the proportion of body water and lean body mass decreases, while body fat increases. This favors the distribution of fat-soluble over water-soluble constituents.

Elimination

The effect of a medicine ceases when it is eliminated from the body or changed into some inactive form. This involves liver metabolism, kidney function, and elimination at other sites around the body, all factors that become less efficient with age.

Paradoxical Reactions

The main concern for elders are effects known as *paradoxical reactions*. With very elderly people, it is not unusual for a medicine to have an effect that is opposite of what is expected. For example, the tranquilizer Valium (diazepam) can have a marked stimulating effect in some elders. This is an unpredictable response, so careful observation of a patient's initial response is crucial. *It is essential to be aware of potential paradoxical responses to herbal medications.*

PREVENTION AND TREATMENT OF DISEASE IN ELDERS

Elders have special needs, and plants can address these needs. Whenever possible, the focus should be on tonics and normalizers. Careful attention must be given to the dosage of stronger effectors, because of the range of pharmacological issues just discussed. A general rule of thumb is to use a lower dosage for elders than for younger adults. Such concerns do not arise if prescriptions emphasize tonics. See chapter 12 for more information on dosages for elders.

THE CARDIOVASCULAR SYSTEM

A range of cardiovascular tonic remedies are uniquely suited for treating problems of the heart and blood vessels in elders. While they do not have the dramatic, rapid, and often lifesaving effects of many currently available drugs, they confer a definite advantage for the phytotherapist addressing the chronic degenerative conditions often found in this age group.

Each cardiovascular tonic has a distinct area of application. Considering the prevalence of water retention (edema) related to the aging heart, diuretics can be especially valuable.

Appropriate Cardiovascular Tonics for Elders

Achillea millefolium (yarrow)
Aesculus hippocastanum (horse chestnut)
Allium sativum (garlic)
Crataegus spp. (hawthorn)
Ginkgo biloba (ginkgo)
Leonurus cardiaca (motherwort)
Taraxacum officinale (dandelion leaf)
Tilia spp. (linden)
Vaccinium myrtillus (bilberry)
Viburnum opulus (cramp bark)

In addition to these gentle tonics, suggested treatments outlined in chapter 14 are relevant here. The treatment outlines given for arteriosclerosis, mild congestive heart failure, angina pectoris, hypertension, and peripheral vascular disease are all relevant for elders.

An important exception may be the use of *Cytisus scoparius* (Scotch broom) in the treatment of hypotension. It may prove too strong for some elderly people, and so should be avoided. In addition, please refer to chapters 9 and 14 for discussions on the difference between cardioactive and cardiotonic remedies and the conditions for which these herbs are appropriate.

More than with any other age group, it is essential to avoid the inappropriate use of cardiac glycoside–containing herbs in elders. Because of the pharmacodynamic and pharmacokinetic changes discussed earlier, it is all too easy to build up toxic levels of these chemicals in the body. If this kind of support for heart function is needed, it is safest to use the glycosides in a standardized form to ensure that dosage is correct. This is almost impossible with *Digitalis* (foxglove), which highlights the value of pharmaceutical preparations of digitalis glycosides. These are obtainable only as prescription drugs. In short, this is a clear example of when to avoid herbal forms of strong effectors.

Fortunately, such potent treatment is not always necessary. Perhaps more important, it is not the only option. As highlighted in chapter 14, *Crataegus* spp. (hawthorn) is the best-known and possibly the most valuable tonic remedy for the cardiovascular system found in the plant kingdom. *Crataegus* facilitates a gentle but long-term, sustained effect on degenerative, age-related changes in the myocardium. The herb is of particular value for cases in which there is no overt disease, but the patient is experiencing a loss of function due to advancing age. *Crataegus* helps to maintain the heart in a healthy condition, minimizing the risk of the development of coronary disease. See chapter 14 for specific indications.

THE RESPIRATORY SYSTEM

A lifetime of exposure to air pollution and cigarette smoke (whether one's own or secondhand) will damage even the strongest lungs. The suggested treatment outlines given in chapter 15 for acute and chronic bronchitis, asthma, and emphysema are all relevant for elder patients.

A variety of remedies are appropriate for respiratory problems in elders, each with a distinct area of application.

Appropriate Respiratory Remedies for Elders

Allium sativum (garlic)
Asclepias tuberosa (pleurisy root)
Chondrus crispus (Irish moss)
Hyssopus officinalis (hyssop)
Inula helenium (elecampane)
Leonurus cardiaca (motherwort)
Marrubium vulgare (horehound)
Prunus serotina (wild cherry bark)
Thymus vulgaris (thyme)
Verbascum thapsus (mullein)

A number of stronger effectors may be found useful in more intransigent conditions, such as emphysema. However, these should be reserved for cases in which the gentler herbs have not produced the desired results.

Stronger Effectors for Respiratory Problems in Elders

Grindelia camporum (gumweed)
Lobelia inflata (lobelia)
Sanguinaria canadensis (bloodroot)

THE NERVOUS SYSTEM

A variety of remedies are appropriate for neurological problems in elders, each with a particular area of application. Treatments for nervous system problems outlined in chapter 16 are relevant here. Particularly pertinent to elders are the discussions of stress management, depression, and insomnia, as well as the treatment approaches to peripheral neuropathy and shingles.

Nervine Tonics

Avena sativa (oats)
Hypericum perforatum (St. John's wort)
Scutellaria lateriflora (skullcap)

Nervine Relaxants

Cimicifuga racemosa (black cohosh)
Hyssopus officinalis (hyssop)
Lavandula spp. (lavender)
Leonurus cardiaca (motherwort)
Matricaria recutita (chamomile)
Melissa officinalis (lemon balm)
Tilia spp. (linden)

Hypnotics

Eschscholzia californica (California poppy)
Matricaria recutita (chamomile)
Passiflora incarnata (passionflower)
Valeriana officinalis (valerian)

Antidepressants

Avena sativa (oats)
Artemisia vulgaris (mugwort)
Hypericum perforatum (St. John's wort)
Lavandula spp. (lavender)
Verbena officinalis (vervain)

A caution must be voiced about the use of *Valeriana* with elders. A very small number of people experience a paradoxical reaction to this remedy. Instead of a relaxing or hypnotic effect, these people have the opposite physiological response—that is, a caffeinelike stimulation. This is more of a possibility with the elderly. If this happens, *Valeriana* should be avoided in the future. If a paradoxical reaction does occur, *Scutellaria* will ease the unpleasant symptoms quite effectively. Note that *Humulus lupulus* was not included in the list of relevant hypnotics. This is because it has a tendency to induce depression if used consistently.

An herb of particular relevance to the elderly is *Ginkgo biloba*. While it has a popular reputation as a "memory" herb, it should be considered a cardiovascular remedy. Ginkgo leaf extract has been shown to influence arteries, veins, capillaries, blood components (erythrocytes, platelets), arterial blood flow, capillary perfusion, and venous return. Due in part to its potent antioxidant properties, its ability to enhance peripheral and cerebral circulation, and its inhibitory effects on platelet activating factor, ginkgo's primary application lies in the treatment of cerebrovascular dysfunction and peripheral vascular disorders.

Overall, studies confirm the efficacy of ginkgo extract for treating disturbances of cerebrovascular function, especially in elderly patients.[2] Well-designed studies have demonstrated therapeutic efficacy for mild to moderate forms of degenerative dementia. In Europe, ginkgo extract is administered clinically at a total daily dosage of 120 to 240 mg of standardized extract containing at least 24% ginkgo flavone glycoside and 6% terpene lactones (ginkgolides and bilobalide) for at least eight weeks. The German Commission E recommends administration for a period of not less than eight weeks for the treatment of chronic conditions.

THE DIGESTIVE SYSTEM

Please see chapter 13 for treatment approaches to a number of specific pathologies that commonly affect the elderly. These include esophagitis and gastroesophageal reflux, gastritis, peptic ulceration, hiatus hernia, indigestion, irritable bowel syndrome, constipation, diarrhea, diverticulitis, and gallbladder disease. Of course, close at-

tention must be paid to nutrition and any prescription medications the patient is taking. The advice given under Broader Context of Treatment for each of these conditions is relevant to elders as well.

An abundance of herbal remedies are appropriate for the treatment of digestive problems in elders. Some of the many possibilities are listed here. The choice will depend in part on the herbs' secondary actions.

Herbs Appropriate for Digestive Problems in Elders

Agrimonia eupatoria (agrimony)
Althaea officinalis (marshmallow)
Chondrus crispus (Irish moss)
Filipendula ulmaria (meadowsweet)
Foeniculum vulgare (fennel)
Gentiana lutea (gentian)
Matricaria recutita (chamomile)
Mentha piperita (peppermint)
Rumex crispus (yellow dock)
Silybum marianum (milk thistle)
Symphytum officinale (comfrey)
Ulmus rubra (slippery elm)

In addition to ameliorating underlying digestive tract disease, herbs have much to offer for general symptomatic relief of digestive upsets. With safe, normalizing herbal remedies, it is possible to avoid side effects and minimize paradoxical reactions or synergistic drug interactions. This is especially the case when digestive symptoms are related to side effects of essential allopathic medications.

THE URINARY SYSTEM

Treatments outlined in chapter 17 are relevant here. In addition to general approaches to the safe herbal treatment of water retention, the chapter provides treatment suggestions for conditions such as cystitis and urinary calculus.

Of all the diuretics and other urinary system herbs, the following are especially appropriate for urinary problems in elders. Their relevance reflects a combination of safety, efficacy, and appropriate secondary actions.

Appropriate Urinary Tract Remedies for Elders

Achillea millefolium (yarrow)
Arctostaphylos uva-ursi (bearberry)
Elymus repens (couch grass)
Galium aparine (cleavers)
Sambucus nigra (elder)
Taraxacum officinale (dandelion leaf)
Vaccinium macrocarpon (cranberry)

THE REPRODUCTIVE SYSTEM

Chapter 18 includes treatment discussions for post-menopausal problems and benign prostate hypertrophy.

Reproductive System Tonics for Elders

Caulophyllum thalictroides (blue cohosh)
Cimicifuga racemosa (black cohosh)
Leonurus cardiaca (motherwort)
Mitchella repens (partridgeberry)
Serenoa repens (saw palmetto)
Viburnum opulus (cramp bark)
V. prunifolium (black haw)
Vitex agnus-castus (chasteberry)

THE MUSCULOSKELETAL SYSTEM

The plethora of musculoskeletal problems so common to elders represents an area of health care that is particularly well suited to herbal treatment. Consult the treatments outlined in chapter 19 for myalgia, rheumatism, osteoarthritis, rheumatoid arthritis, and osteoporosis. Of particular importance are the suggested guidelines concerning nutrition and lifestyle.

Once again, the phytotherapist can call upon the gift of toning herbs for the treatment of these problems. There is usually no need to resort to intense treatments for musculoskeletal problems in elders, as the milder antirheumatic herbs are often effective, given time. This is not meant to imply that these herbs can completely alleviate the damage of osteoarthritis in someone who has had the condition for years. However, the patient will feel better, perhaps better than he or she has in years, within the limitations of any structural damage that may have occurred with time.

In addition, make it a priority to address any digestive symptoms present in older patients with rheumatic conditions. Any such symptoms are an indication that the processes of digestion, assimilation, and elimination are not functioning at optimal levels. This can be related to either functional or organic problems, but the body's nutritional status will suffer no matter what the cause, which in turn may aggravate arthritic conditions.

Of the many herbs that may prove useful for treating this body system, consider the following as possible tonics.

Musculoskeletal Tonics for Elders

Apium graveolens (celery seed)
Angelica archangelica (angelica)
Betula spp. (birch)
Cimicifuga racemosa (black cohosh)
Dioscorea villosa (wild yam)

Filipendula ulmaria (meadowsweet)
Menyanthes trifoliata (bogbean)
Salix spp. (willow bark)
Urtica dioica (nettle)

A number of stronger effectors may be useful for more unresponsive cases of arthritis, but these should be reserved for patients for whom gentler herbs have not produced the desired results.

Stronger Musculoskeletal Effectors

Guaiacum officinale (guaiacum)
Harpagophytum procumbens (devil's claw)
Zanthoxylum americanum (prickly ash)

THE SKIN

Treatments outlined in chapter 20 are relevant here. Skin problems are often a lifelong challenge, and may be slow to respond to treatment in the elderly. However, the suggestions for topical symptom relief can be very beneficial. The topical anti-inflammatory activity of *Calendula officinalis* and of *Hypericum perforatum* are particularly valuable.

As with all of the body systems, a range of remedies are appropriate for skin problems in elders. Again, the emphasis should be on gentle alteratives and tonics, with extra focus on general liver, digestive, and kidney function. Many essential oils are also helpful when applied topically.

Herbs for Skin Conditions in Elders

Calendula officinalis (calendula)
Galium aparine (cleavers)
Hypericum perforatum (St. John's wort)
Plantago major (plantain)
Stellaria media (chickweed)
Trifolium pratense (red clover)
Urtica dioica (nettle)
Viola tricolor (heartsease)

References

1. Bennett JC, Plum F, eds. *Cecil Textbook of Medicine.* 20th edition. Philadelphia: Saunders, 1996.
2. McKenna DJ, Jones K, Hughes K. Efficacy, safety, and use of Ginkgo biloba in clinical and preclinical applications. *Alternative Therapies in Health and Medicine* 2001 Sep–Oct; 7(5):70–86, 88–90.

Suggested Reading

Hoffmann D. *An Elder's Herbal.* Rochester, VT: Healing Arts Press, 1993.

24

PHYTOTHERAPY AND CHILDREN

With its focus on preventive medicine, holistic approaches to health can be most helpful for many common childhood problems. Conditions brought under control during childhood can often be avoided entirely during adult life. Examples are asthma and eczema, both of which can start at a very early age and become an ongoing theme throughout a person's life. If treated successfully with herbs during childhood, the condition rarely continues into adulthood.

The healing capacity of children can be quite incredible. Not to be overlooked when treating childhood ailments is the relevance of tender loving care. Children respond to love and caring in wonderful ways. So do adults, if they give themselves the chance!

A number of useful books have been written about herbs for children. I highly recommend those listed in Suggested Reading for this chapter. In different but complementary ways, these books are all sources of therapeutic and practical insights that go beyond the experience of this author. After all, Mother knows best!

This chapter is structured differently from the specific treatment chapters. Here we will discuss a variety of issues specific to children's health, including some diseases and conditions that primarily affect children. Treatment approaches for conditions that commonly affect children as well as adults can be found by following cross-references to the appropriate body system chapters.

PRESCRIBING ISSUES UNIQUE TO CHILDREN

Normal physiology in children is different from that of adults. Similarly, children respond to medications differently, which is a reflection of pharmacokinetic issues.[1] For example, in infants, delayed gastrointestinal transit time affects drug absorption and lower levels of enzymes impact drug metabolism. These differences are most significant in infants, but can be an issue up to the age of six years. While such considerations are crucial when it comes to prescription medications, in phytotherapy they can be largely avoided through an emphasis on herbal tonics.

Care must be taken with dosage for children. Because of their smaller body size, children obviously require lower dosages than adults do, but there is no clear-cut guideline for herbal formulations. Chapter 12 provides various pharmaceutical methods of deriving dosages for children based on age or body size.

Noncompliance with therapy is widespread among children. Among pediatric patients, an estimated 34% to 82% have been reported to be noncompliant with drug therapy regimens.[2] Thus, palatability is a critical factor with children, as it impacts whether or not the child will take the herbs. The taste and smell of herbal remedies can play a vital role in enhancing compliance. This is an area in which the creativity of the herbal medicine-maker can make all the difference. For example, can the child take a tablet or capsule instead?

In dispensing herbal medicines for children, it is important to educate both parents and child. The more the parents understand the disease, the treatment, and how to administer the medicine, the more likely the child is to take the remedy. It is often important to find out who is administering the medicines and where. The dosage regimen may have to be adjusted so that medications are always given at home, as opposed to at school or some other location that is not conducive to compliance.

CHILDHOOD DISEASES

The so-called childhood diseases are viral syndromes most often seen in children who lack immunity until they have recovered from the disease. The disease rarely recurs. While these diseases are usually not serious, they can cause severe fever and discomfort, and occasionally lead to serious complications. In adults, the same diseases can have different and much more severe manifestations. Some of the most common are outlined here.

MEASLES

A highly contagious acute disease characterized by fever, cough, coryza, conjunctivitis, eruptions (Koplik's spots) on the buccal and labial mucosa, and a spreading mucopapular cutaneous rash. *(The Merck Manual)*

Measles, or rubeola, is a viral infection that can be spread by physical contact or through the air via respiratory droplets. One bout usually confers immunity for life, but a few children get measles twice. The incubation period is between 7 and 14 days. The disease is most communicable two to four days before and up to five days after the rash appears.

Measles is characterized by fever, red eyes with light sensitivity, runny nose, dry and sometimes severe cough, and white spots (Koplik's spots) on the inside of the cheeks. These are seen two days before the red rash appears, which first develops near the scalp and later spreads to the upper body. After three to four days, the rash takes on a brownish, bronzy appearance, and peeling may occur. Symptoms may be severe, and children with measles are pretty sick and miserable. The rash lasts about seven days, but the child usually begins to feel better by the fourth day.

Treatment of Measles

The herbal contribution to the treatment of measles is based on alleviation of symptomatic distress. The primary areas to address are fever, itching, eye sensitivity, and coughing. Convalescent recovery will be facilitated by good nutrition and, possibly, the use of bitter tonics such as *Gentiana lutea* (gentian) and, if the cough is persistent, *Marrubium vulgare* (horehound).

Actions Indicated

Diaphoretics help ease fever; diaphoretic teas such as *Nepeta cataria*, *Achillea millefolium*, and *Tilia* spp. are especially appropriate.

Antipruritics will help relieve itching. *Stellaria media* is particularly effective.

Demulcent expectorants help with both the cough and the sore throat. Herbs to consider include *Tussilago farfara*, *Verbascum thapsus*, and *Glycyrrhiza glabra*. If a stronger remedy is indicated, use *Marrubium vulgare*.

To relieve itching, choose an aesthetic, pleasant approach if possible. Dabbing distilled *Hamamelis virginiana* (witch hazel) on itchy skin will usually provide immediate but very temporarily relief.

Eyestrain due to photosensitivity is common, so the child should rest in a darkened room. A wash made of eyebright (*Euphrasia* spp.) or a chamomile compress (*Matricaria recutita*) will ease the discomfort, but not replace the need for reduced light. Here are refreshingly clear instructions for making an eyebright eyewash from *Natural Child Care*, by Maribeth Riggs.

Eyebright Eyewash[3]

Infuse ½ oz. of dried eyebright in 1 cup of water. It is especially important to strain well to ensure that no particles remain in the infusion. When comfortably warm for the eyes, it is ready to use. This herbal wash is to be used only once.

MUMPS

An acute contagious, generalized viral disease, usually causing painful enlargement of the salivary glands, most commonly the parotids. *(The Merck Manual)*

Mumps is a virus infection of the parotid glands, two of the six salivary glands located just below and in front of the ears. This contagious condition, spread by respiratory droplets, is seen commonly between the ages of 2 and 12 years. It has an incubation period of 14 to 24 days. It can occur in adults who did not experience the disease in childhood. The condition is much more serious in adults and can lead to sterility in men.

The common symptom picture includes fever, swelling of the parotid glands, achiness, and restlessness. The swelling of the parotids can be very alarming and change the patient's appearance quite dramatically. The jaw may become stiff because of glandular swelling. The testicles are involved in up to one fifth of males, especially older patients. Mild meningitis marked by headache or stiff neck is, unfortunately, not rare. Any development of a painfully stiff neck or severe headache calls for immediate professional help.

Treatment of Mumps

In addition to the herbal treatment suggested here, symptoms may be relieved by intermittently applying ice or heat to the affected neck area. Acetaminophen may also be appropriate for pain relief; do not give aspirin to children with a viral illness because of the risk of Reye's syndrome. Warm salt-water gargles, soft foods, and extra fluids may also help relieve symptoms.

Actions Indicated

Antimicrobials are the key to successfully clearing the infection.

Lymphatic alteratives are crucial to help drain the affected glands.

Hepatics will help if there is associated constipation. These should be very mild.

Anti-inflammatories and *demulcents* may be helpful in alleviating pain and discomfort in the throat.

Specific Remedies

No specifics in the strict sense are used in Western herbalism, but lymphatic herbs might be seen as specifics. However, lymphatics for children must be chosen very carefully. *Phytolacca* is an excellent remedy here, but great care must be taken with dosage in young children. *Phytolacca* can be a powerful emetic and purgative in higher doses.

A Prescription for Mumps

Galium aparine	4 parts
Echinacea spp.	4 parts
Urtica dioica	3 parts
Phytolacca americana	1 part

Dosage: up to 5 ml of tincture three times a day. In addition, the child should drink an infusion of equal parts *Nepeta cataria* and *Trifolium pratense* often.

Table 24.1. Actions Supplied by Prescription for Mumps

ACTION	HERBS
Antimicrobial	*Echinacea* spp.
Lymphatic	*Galium aparine*, *Echinacea* spp., *Phytolacca americana*
Alterative	*Galium aparine*, *Echinacea* spp., *Urtica dioica*, *Phytolacca americana*

THE DIGESTIVE SYSTEM

Many of the treatments outlined in chapter 13 are relevant here. Most common in children are indigestion, constipation, and diarrhea. Many gentle effector herbs are appropriate for treating children's digestive problems. Carminatives are especially important, because the volatile oils they contain are often gently anti-inflammatory and antispasmodic. Thus, they can be rapidly effective at easing colic and cramping pain.

Herbs for Digestive Problems in Children

Althaea officinalis (marshmallow)
Anethum graveolens (dill)
Chondrus crispus (Irish moss)
Filipendula ulmaria (meadowsweet)
Foeniculum vulgare (fennel)
Gentiana lutea (gentian)
Matricaria recutita (chamomile)
Melissa officinalis (lemon balm)
Mentha piperita (peppermint)
Pimpinella anisum (aniseed)
Rumex crispus (yellow dock)
Ulmus rubra (slippery elm)

COLIC

> A symptom complex of early infancy that is characterized by paroxysms of crying, apparent abdominal pain, and irritability. *(The Merck Manual)*

Colic refers to painful contractions of the gastrointestinal tract. About 10% to 15% of normal, healthy babies have colic. In true, severe colic, the baby will be difficult to console, expressing discomfort with high-pitched crying and drawing up the feet into the belly. If the baby has been crying for two hours without interruption, seek professional help in order to rule out other sources of pain, such as ear infection and intestinal obstruction.

Infantile colic usually starts at one month of age and resolves by four months. The causes are not well understood, but the condition tends to occur in babies with a sensitive or vigorous temperament and a below-average need for sleep. Ideas about causes include overly rapid feeding, overeating, swallowing excessive air, lack of burping, emotional tension between parent and child, and improper feeding technique (that is, incorrect positioning). The physiological mechanism behind colic is thought to be excessive fermentation and gas production in the intestines, and may even be related to foods eaten by the nursing mother.

The parents of colicky babies will often be under great stress. The infant may be stimulated into fussy behavior by parental stress, creating a cycle of positive feedback. Parents will frequently experience feelings of frustration, anger, despair, and helplessness, and it may be appropriate to treat the parents for stress-related problems (see chapter 16 for suggestions).

Treatment of Colic

A range of herbs may help the baby directly, but they will not replace the suggestions given below. Mild, carminative, relaxing nervines are often helpful and may be made into pleasant-tasting teas or infusions to be added to a bath. Such preparations can incorporate any of the herbs listed here. Selection will be based on taste or relevant secondary actions. For example, *Trifolium pratense* also has much to offer in the treatment of childhood eczema.

Soothing Herbs for Colicky Babies

Anethum graveolens (dill)
Foeniculum vulgare (fennel*)*
Matricaria recutita (chamomile)
Melissa officinalis (lemon balm)
Mentha piperita (peppermint)
Nepeta cataria (catnip)
Tilia spp. (linden)
Trifolium pratense (red clover)

The following illustrates some non-herbal issues to consider when treating infantile colic.

Change the nursing mother's diet. Common gas-producing foods eaten by nursing mothers include dairy products, garlic, vegetables in the cabbage family, orange juice, very spicy foods, caffeine-containing foods (such as chocolate, coffee, and tea), and anything in particular that produces gas for the mother.

Recommend soothing herb teas for the mother. Relaxing nervines may help, especially those containing carminative volatile oils. Examples include *Matricaria recutita*, *Melissa officinalis*, *Tilia* spp., and *Trifolium pratense*.

Use rhythmic motions. Rhythmic movements help ease both abdominal discomfort and emotional distress for the infant. Examples include gentle rocking, car rides, walking with the baby in a front pack, baby swings, and setting the baby in an infant seat on top of a clothes dryer.

Encourage sucking. Some babies will not suck during colic attacks, and it is not a good idea to continually feed a colicky infant. However, the infant may be encouraged to suck his or her own hand or fingers, or a teething object.

Apply heat. Lay the baby over a warm hot-water bottle wrapped in a towel; while the baby is in a flexed position rhythmically pat its back. Give the baby a warm bath.

Alter feeding position. Try feeding the baby in a sitting position to help prevent ingestion of air. Burp the baby often during feeding.

Change the formula or the type of water used to make it, if the baby is bottle-fed.

Give acidophilus. This is not usually needed for breast-fed babies; however, some babies greatly benefit from the addition of acidophilus to the diet. This can be mixed with water and fed by bottle or eyedropper. *Never give honey to babies less than one year of age*, as it has been associated with infantile botulism.

CONSTIPATION

Although constipation is rarely seen in breast-fed babies, it is not abnormal for breast-fed babies to have bowel movements as infrequently as one in seven days. Treat a breast-fed infant for constipation only if the child appears to be in pain and cries during the bowel movement.

Indications for the treatment of constipation in bottle-fed babies and young children include:

Painful passage of stools. Pain during bowel movements is abnormal, and in some cases trauma to the anal canal can lead to anal fissure. Bright red blood around the anus or on toilet paper suggests the presence of an anal fissure.

Inability to pass stools. Treatment is indicated for children who feel the need to have a bowel movement and are unable to do so. The exception is infants younger than one year of age, who may grunt, push, strain, and become flushed in the face during bowel movements. This is normal behavior, as long as the episode is not accompanied by pain.

Infrequent bowel movements, occurring less often than once in four days for young children, generally indicate that treatment is needed.

If bowel movements are accompanied by much pain, abdominal bloating, or crying, it is important to seek skilled diagnosis to rule out conditions such as Hirschsprung's disease, impaction, and other potential serious disorders. It is inappropriate to use laxative remedies with children unless absolutely necessary, as children's constipation almost always responds to dietary change.

Treatment of Children's Constipation

If the suggestions given here are not adequate, see chapter 13 for suggestions on using gentle, bulking laxative remedies. The strong, stimulant anthraquinone laxatives should be avoided with children.

The National Institute of Child Health and Development provides the following guidelines for treating constipated infants and children.[4]

Infants less than 2 months old should be examined by a physician.

Infants 2 to 4 months old may be given 1 ounce of fruit juice (grape, pear, apple, cherry, or prune) per month of age twice a day.

Infants older than 4 months who have begun solid foods may be given high-fiber baby foods (e.g., peas, beans, apricots, prunes, peaches, pears, plums, and spinach) twice a day.

Children older than 1 year will benefit from the same dietary changes as adults (i.e., more fruits, vegetables, and whole-grain foods high in fiber). In addition, increase intake of fruit juices such as apple, pear, cherry, grape, and prune.

For older children, try these suggestions:

Increase intake of water.

Increase consumption of fruits and vegetables, particularly raw foods with peels, such as figs, pears, apricots, legumes, celery, cucumber, lettuce, and apples. Raisins may also be beneficial.

Increase fiber intake with whole-grain cereals or bran muffins.

Reduce intake of constipating foods, such as dairy products, white rice, bananas, cooked carrots, and white flour.

Use psyllium seed preparations in children older than 2 years of age.

Give flavored cod-liver oil.

DIARRHEA

The number and consistency of normal stools varies greatly among infants and children. Loose stools are normal in breast-fed infants. If the baby is vomiting and having frequent watery stools, however, there is a danger of dehydration and loss of electrolyte balance. If a child has nausea or vomiting, the liquids should be given in small amounts but very frequently, often every 15 minutes.

Seek medical attention immediately if there is blood in the stool, abdominal pain causing crying for more than two hours, or signs of dehydration, such as lack of turgor, depression of the anterior fontanel, and dry mucous membranes.

Infection with the bacteria *Shigella, Salmonella*, and *Campylobacter* often results in blood-flecked diarrhea. Children on antibiotics may experience diarrhea, but this is less likely if they eat yogurt with active live cultures while taking antibiotics. However, the most common cause of children's diarrhea is mild viral infection.

Treatment of Children's Diarrhea

A number of the astringent herbs are particularly suitable for children. One of the most useful is *Filipendula ulmaria* (meadowsweet). In addition, try the following remedies.

Herbs Useful for Children's Diarrhea

Achillea millefolium (yarrow)
Euphrasia spp. (eyebright)
Geranium maculatum (cranesbill)
Plantago major (plantain)
Potentilla erecta (tormentil)
Rosmarinus officinalis (rosemary)
Rubus idaeus (raspberry leaf)
Solidago virgaurea (goldenrod)
Verbascum thapsus (mullein)

INDIGESTION

Indigestion is very common in children, but is rarely a serious health problem. It may be triggered by eating too fast, overeating, eating particular foods, or drinking carbonated drinks. In addition to the information given for functional dyspepsia in chapter 13, the overriding issue that must be taken into account for children is taste! If they do not like the medicine, they will not take it, and medicinal plants work only if they are actually taken.

Treatment of Indigestion in Children

The key to success here is selecting appropriate carminative remedies that will also be palatable to the child. Carminatives will ease the movement of food or gas through the intestinal tract. Carminative oils stimulate intestinal peristalsis, the wavelike contractions that move food through the intestine and promote the expulsion of gas from the gastrointestinal tract.

The following formula from Maribeth Riggs is a good example of what can be concocted to treat children's indigestion when taste is taken into account.

An Indigestion Tea for Children[5]

1 tablespoon fennel seed
1 tablespoon dried sweet orange peel
2 cups water
Honey to taste

Decoct the fennel seed and orange peel in water. Use a covered pot. Bring to a boil and gently simmer for 20 minutes. Strain out the herbs and discard them. Any unused portion of the tea can be kept in a refrigerator and reheated for further use. Discard any remaining tea after 2 days.

Serve the tea as warm as is comfortable for the child. Sweeten it with honey to taste. Give the child 1/2 cup of tea every 2 hours whenever she experiences stomach pain from gas.

NAUSEA

Nausea, the sensation of feeling sick in the stomach without actually vomiting, is a common symptom in children. The cause must always be ascertained to ensure that no serious health problem is developing. There is a wide range of possible causes, including infection, food sensitivities, and emotional overexcitement.

Treatment of Nausea

Relief is usually easy to achieve with carminatives, as long as the child's tastes are taken into account. Nausea in children responds readily to a tea of peppermint, and even to sucking on a peppermint candy. Peppermint often prevents vomiting, although not in cases of food poisoning or when the stomach really needs to be evacuated. Ginger can be helpful, especially when the nausea is related to motion sickness. Ginger ale and candied ginger are two good ways to give a child ginger, and both are easy to carry. Sliced, crystallized ginger is sold in the Chinese food section of many grocery stores.

THE RESPIRATORY SYSTEM

Many effective and safe herbal approaches to respiratory problems in children are recognized worldwide. Whether an acute infection, such as bronchitis, influenza, the common cold, or sinusitis, or an immune system issue, such as asthma or hay fever, treatment with herbs can be beneficial. Herbal therapy makes a particularly valuable contribution in the treatment of a form of atopic asthma closely associated with eczema. Please see chapter 15 for more details on the treatment of this and many other respiratory conditions.

Remedies Appropriate for Children's Respiratory Problems

Allium sativum (garlic)
Chondrus crispus (Irish moss)
Hyssopus officinalis (hyssop)
Inula helenium (elecampane)
Leonurus cardiaca (motherwort)
Marrubium vulgare (horehound)
Prunus serotina (wild cherry bark)
Thymus vulgaris (thyme)
Tussilago farfara (coltsfoot)
Verbascum thapsus (mullein)

Here is a prescription from Maribeth Riggs for licorice lollipops. These make a particularly tasty and effective treatment for hoarseness and sore throats of any cause.

Licorice Lollipops[6]

1 five-inch-long piece licorice root
2 tablespoons honey
1 cup water

Place the licorice root, honey, and water in a covered pot; bring to a boil and simmer for 5 minutes. (Omit the honey if you use Chinese licorice.) Strain out the herb and set it aside to cool. Keep the licorice tea to drink, or discard if you wish. When the softened licorice root is cool enough to hold comfortably in the hand, give it to the child to suck on. Keep the dried licorice root in a labeled jar with a tight-fitting lid, away from children. Discard any unused root after 6 months.

Application: Give a child with a hoarse throat softened licorice root once each day in the morning or afternoon to suck on for as long as he or she wishes. Remember that licorice root is slightly stimulating and a mild laxative, so it should be eaten only in the morning or early afternoon. The hoarse throat usually disappears after 2 days.

OTITIS MEDIA

> A bacterial or viral infection in the middle ear, usually secondary to an upper respiratory infection. *(The Merck Manual)*

Otitis media, or middle ear infection, is one of the most common early childhood diseases and is often the result of problems with the eustachian tubes in the ears. Normally, the eustachian tube is closed and flat, preventing organisms from entering the middle ear from the pharyngeal cavity. The tube opens to allow drainage of secretions produced by the middle ear mucosa and to equalize pressure between the middle ear and the outside environment. If drainage is impaired, normal secretions are retained. This causes any air in the tube to be reabsorbed and produces negative pressure within the middle ear. If the tube opens, this negative pressure will draw bacteria into the middle ear, where they quickly proliferate.

As purulent fluid accumulates in the middle ear, increasing discomfort results. Infants will become irritable and indicate discomfort by holding or pulling their ears or rolling their heads from side to side. Young children will complain of pain, to put it mildly! Otitis media may be accompanied by fever of up to 104°F.

In serious otitis media, the child may not even appear ill. There may be a feeling of fullness in the ear and a popping sensation during swallowing. The child will be less responsive and may have some painless hearing loss.

Inflammation of the tympanic membrane alone is not diagnostic of middle ear infection. Just like a child's cheeks, the tympanic membrane may become flushed with increased crying, allergy, or mild physical irritation.

Treatment of Otitis Media

Unfortunately, many pediatricians prescribe antibiotics on the basis of a slightly red tympanic membrane. Not uncommonly, children receive numerous courses of medication. It is more difficult to treat children after long-term medication has failed to ameliorate the condition.

Actions Indicated

Antimicrobials are, of course, the key to successfully clearing the infection.

Anti-inflammatories may be helpful, but work best when applied topically.

Alteratives and *lymphatic tonics* can prove most effective in treating intransigent problems.

A Prescription for Otitis Media

Echinacea spp.	2 parts
Baptisia tinctoria	1 part
Galium aparine	1 part

Dosage: up to 5 ml of tincture three times a day. Warm mullein flower oil introduced into the ear can serve as an effective anti-inflammatory.

Broader Context of Treatment

In *Textbook of Natural Medicine*, Drs. Murray and Pizzorno recommend the following supplements.[7] Note that the dosage given varies with the age of the patient (see table 12.15 for dosage adjustment by age).

Beta-carotene: age 12, 20,000 IU/day (200,000 IU/day maximum)

Vitamin C: age 12, 500 mg/day

Zinc picolinate: age 12, 2.5 mg/day (15 mg/day maximum)

Bioflavonoids: age 12, 50 mg/day (250 mg/day maximum)

Evening primrose oil: age 12, 1 capsule/day

THE NERVOUS SYSTEM

Treatments outlined in chapter 16 are relevant for children, as long as remedies are selected carefully. The core selection issue is the need to avoid stronger relaxing nervines. For children, a mild nervine chosen from one of the lists provided here is usually more than adequate.

Herbs such as *Tilia* and *Trifolium* added to a bath as an infusion will have a calming effect and will prove useful before bedtime. *Trifolium* is especially relevant for problems compounded by irritating skin conditions.

Nervine Tonics for Children

Avena sativa (oats)
Hypericum perforatum (St. John's wort)
Scutellaria lateriflora (skullcap)

Nervine Relaxants for Children

Hyssopus officinalis (hyssop)
Lavandula spp. (lavender)
Leonurus cardiaca (motherwort)
Matricaria recutita (chamomile)
Melissa officinalis (lemon balm)
Nepeta cataria (catnip)
Tilia platyphyllos (linden)
Trifolium pratense (red clover)

Hypnotics for Children

Eschscholzia californica (California poppy)
Matricaria recutita (chamomile)

ATTENTION DEFICIT DISORDER

A neurobiological condition characterized by developmentally inappropriate levels of attention, concentration, activity, distractibility, and impulsivity. *(The Merriam-Webster Medical Dictionary)*

Hyperactivity or attention deficit disorder (ADD) is a thorny issue that raises a plethora of questions. There is no doubt that extreme hyperactivity occurs and can be related to dietary factors. ADD is the most commonly diagnosed behavioral disorder of childhood, affecting an estimated 3% to 5% of school-aged children. The incidence of ADD has been increasing over the last 15 years, possibly related to either better diagnosis or over-diagnosis. The disorder is 3 to 10 times more common in male than female children.

However, there seems to be an unfortunate trend to label children "hyperactive" simply because the teacher or parents do not have the time or patience for very active, perceptive, inquisitive, or creative children. *The Merck Manual* points out that "claims that a child is hyperactive often reflect the tolerance level of the annoyed person." Since when has not fitting in to the normal mold become a disease? The use of psychopharmaceuticals to control hyperactive children sounds a little bit like the Soviet psychiatrists' solution of prescribing major tranquilizers to dissidents. Rather than sedating our children so they can deal with their world, why not change the nature of school so it is more challenging and exciting?

When the child is experiencing a real problem, however, herbs may offer some help, provided that two particular areas are in some way addressed.

Psychological factors. Such factors can be of paramount importance, but these are not herbal issues.

Food irritants. There is increasing evidence that chemical irritants may play a role in hyperactivity. These may be pollutants (such as heavy metals) or artificial food additives (such as colorings and flavors).

Herbs can contribute in two areas: by calming the nervous system and by helping the liver detoxify any offending substances. Treatment suggestions for stress-related issues can be found in chapter 16. See chapter 21 for guidelines on detoxification. Other herbs to consider in support of a broad treatment plan that also addresses dietary and psychological issues are listed here. Keep in mind that the phytotherapist can also help with parental stress and exhaustion!

Supportive Herbs for Hyperactive Children

Matricaria recutita (chamomile)
Silybum marianum (milk thistle)
Tilia spp. (linden)
Trifolium pratense (red clover)

THE SKIN

There are a number of remedies appropriate for skin problems in children. Each has a distinct area of application, and some are for external use only. Please refer to chapter 20 for herbal approaches to common childhood problems such as psoriasis and eczema. Treatments for diaper rash, cradle cap, and impetigo are discussed here. The treatment outlined in chapter 15 for atopic asthma and eczema is also relevant.

The herbs listed here for skin problems in children can often be used both internally and topically. Many essential oils can also be helpful as topical applications. For details, please refer to specific plant entries in chapter 26.

Herbs for Children's Skin Problems

Calendula officinalis (calendula)
Galium aparine (cleavers)
Hypericum perforatum (St. John's wort)
Plantago major (plantain)

Stellaria media (chickweed)
Trifolium pratense (red clover)
Urtica dioica (nettle)
Viola tricolor (heartsease)

DIAPER RASH

An irritation of the skin caused by dampness, the interaction of urine (and ammonia from the urine), and feces. A rash is any skin swelling (bumps) or blotches on a baby (can be red, skin-colored, or slightly lighter or darker than skin color). *(The Merriam-Webster Medical Dictionary)*

Diaper rash is caused by a skin reaction to irritating diapers and prolonged contact with stool, urine, perspiration, soaps, detergents, or creams. Typically, the rash affects the groin area around the genitals and buttocks. It is red and scaly with tiny bumps, blisters, or cracks. When areas outside the diaper region are affected, it is important to rule out yeast infections, eczema, psoriasis, and other problems. Fever, pus, and digestive symptoms are *not* caused by simple diaper rash, and should prompt an evaluation for other problems.

Riggs suggests a well-formulated ointment for the treatment of this common condition:

Diaper Rash Ointment[8]

This ointment is made from ingredients that will help keep the surface of an infant's skin dry, nourish the skin, and fight bacteria. Comfrey root, chickweed, and marshmallow root all have one thing in common: They contain large amounts of calcium, which can help stimulate tissue growth. Comfrey root, in particular, is noted for its healing powers, sporting common folk names like knitbone and bruisewort. These three herbs combined with goldenseal powder, which serves as a topical antiseptic, are an excellent combination for combating diaper rash. Beeswax and sweet almond oil both have skin-nourishing and soothing qualities. This ointment is also good for mild abrasions, sunburns, and hives.

1 tablespoon chickweed
1 tablespoon marshmallow root
1 tablespoon comfrey root
1/8 teaspoon goldenseal root powder
1 cup sweet almond oil
1/4 cup beeswax

Combine the chickweed, marshmallow root, comfrey root, and goldenseal root powder in a cast-iron frying pan with the sweet almond oil. Gently fry the mixture for 5 to 10 minutes. Be careful not to let the herbs burn. When the mixture is hot, add the beeswax and melt it down. When the beeswax is completely melted, strain the mixture through a cheesecloth into a small, labeled jar with a tight-fitting lid. Refrigerate the ointment until it solidifies. The final ointment is an opaque tan color and smells of beeswax and comfrey root. Keep the ointment in a convenient place near the infant's changing table, away from heat. Discard any used portion after 2 months.

Application: Apply the ointment by gently rubbing it on the diaper area each time the diaper is changed. This ointment is very soothing to a rashy infant. Three or four applications are usually enough to get rid of diaper rash. If the infant's diaper rash does not respond to this treatment, or if it keeps reappearing, investigate factors such as the proper disinfection of diapers, changes in diet, and other skin disorders.

Broader Context of Treatment

Herbs will not usually be enough to clear diaper rash, unless used in the context of appropriate attention to the following issues.

Change wet diapers promptly and frequently. Switch the type of diaper used, either from disposable to cloth or vice versa.

Use a protective ointment (beeswax, zinc oxide, calendula, or Diaper Rash Ointment, page 480).

Avoid or reduce the use of occlusive rubber pants over the diaper.

Allow baby to go without a diaper, and let air and sun dry the area.

Do not use talcum powder or cornstarch. If you must powder, use a clay product.

CRADLE CAP

An inflammatory scaling disease of the scalp, face, and occasionally other areas of the body. *(The Merck Manual)*

When this rash occurs on the scalp alone, it is known as *cradle cap*. When it extends to the face, it is termed *seborrheic dermatitis*, because it occurs where the greatest number of oil-producing sebaceous glands are located. Seborrheic dermatitis is a noninfectious form of eczema that is very common in infants, usually beginning in the first weeks of life and slowly disappearing over a period of weeks or months. Unlike atopic or contact eczema, it is rarely uncomfortable or itchy. The cause is unknown. Cradle cap and other forms of seborrheic dermatitis are not infections, signs of allergy, or related to poor hygiene.

Treatment of Cradle Cap

Calendula officinalis (calendula) and *Plantago major* (plantain) are appropriate to soothe heat, soreness, and associated dry skin. The form of topical application may be crucial for most effective symptom relief, and it may be necessary to experiment to see which best suits the baby. Both of these herbs may be used in the form of ointment, cream, lotion, or wash. Oily preparations will help to loosen scales, but might cause discomfort and heat through an insulating effect.

A mucilaginous wash made from a strong decoction of *Symphytum officinale* (comfrey root) will soothe, moisturize, and serve as an effective vulnerary. Follow the wash with an ointment made from calendula, elder flower, or plantain.

Broader Context of Treatment

The scalp should be gently washed with a mild baby shampoo, which, along with soft brushing, will help remove the scales. Stronger medicated shampoos (anti-seborrhea shampoos containing sulfur and 2% salicylic acid) may loosen the scales more quickly, but can be irritating. Applying baby oil is neither helpful nor necessary, as it allows scales to build up on the scalp. Occasionally, a secondary yeast infection may occur on the affected skin, most likely in the crease areas rather than on the scalp. The area will become extremely red and itchy.

IMPETIGO

A superficial vesiculopustular skin infection. *(The Merck Manual)*

Impetigo is an infection of the skin usually caused by a streptococcal bacterium, and occasionally by *Staphylococcus aureus*. The face is most commonly affected, but other exposed areas can be involved as well. Typically, impetigo is restricted to children and is highly contagious. The characteristic appearance is one of multiple tiny pus-filled blisters that break readily, leading to a larger, more widespread eruption forming the characteristic honey-colored crusts. Itching is common, and scratching may spread the infection.

Treatment of Impetigo

Internal support of general health, elimination, and immune response is not always necessary, but is indicated if the child is generally prone to illness.

Actions Indicated for Topical Medication

Antimicrobials are, of course, the key to clearing the infection, but work best when applied topically.

Vulneraries may be helpful after the infection has cleared, to prevent discoloration or scarring of the skin.

Antipruritics may, in theory, be useful. However, because of the pathogen present on the skin, itching may not stop until the infection is cleared.

Anti-inflammatories may be helpful, but the same comments made for antipruritics are also relevant here.

Actions Indicated for Internal Treatment

Alteratives, *antimicrobials*, *lymphatic tonics*, *diuretics*, and *hepatics* may all be appropriate, for reasons similar to those discussed in chapter 20 for eczema. They will *not* replace topical treatments.

Nervines may be indicated if the child is experiencing distress. However, it is often the parents who benefit most from nervines!

Specific Remedies

I am not aware of any specifics for impetigo, but the stronger antimicrobial herbs will help. Topical applications of *Commiphora molmol* (myrrh), *Hydrastis canadensis* (goldenseal), and *Melaleuca alternifolia* (tea tree oil) have all proved useful. Ellingwood refers to successful use of *Echinacea*, both internally and externally.

A Topical Prescription for Impetigo

Commiphora molmol	1 part
Hydrastis canadensis	1 part

Gently apply this tincture combination to the affected areas, as described below.

Broader Context of Treatment

While effective, the application of tinctures high in alcohol may be too intense for the child. They may be added to a base ointment or lotion. An ointment may also be made directly from dried herbs. Apply topically, following the guidelines given here. Be careful when touching lesions and applying herbs, as the infection can spread through contact.

Remove the crusts gently with a warm wet washcloth, as the bacteria live underneath the crusts and will continue to multiply until the crusts are removed.

Apply the tincture or ointment.

Remove crusts and apply ointment several times a day. If the lesions become too large and are not controlled, the child may develop systemic complications.

Because of the highly contagious nature of impetigo, the child should be kept out of school for at least two days after the initiation of treatment. Towels, sheets, and clothing contaminated with drainage should be washed with chlorine bleach. It may be necessary to seek medical assistance under certain circumstances to avoid systemic complications. If the child has a sore throat or fever, if the impetigo is in an inaccessible area (such as the ear canal or nostril), or if significant improvement is not seen after two to three days of treatment, consult a doctor.

References

1. Kanneh A. Paediatric pharmacological principles: an update. Part 2. Pharmacokinetics: absorption and distribution. *Pediatric Nursing* 2002 Nov; 14(9):39–43.

2. Matsui DM. Drug compliance in pediatrics. *Pediatric Clinics of North America* 1997; 44:1–13.

3. Riggs M. *Natural Child Care.* New York: Harmony Books, 1989.

4. Article on the National Library of Medicine Web site: www.nlm.nih.gov/medlineplus/ency/.

5. Riggs M. *Natural Child Care.* New York: Harmony Books, 1989.

6. Ibid.

7. Pizzorno JE, Murray MT. *Textbook of Natural Medicine.* Edinburgh: Churchill Livingstone, 1999.

8. Riggs M. *Natural Child Care.* New York: Harmony Books, 1989.

Suggested Reading

Bove M. *An Encyclopedia of Natural Healing for Children and Infants.* Chicago: Keats, 2001.

Gladstar R. *Rosemary Gladstar's Herbal Remedies for Children's Health.* Pownal, VT: Storey Books, 1999.

McIntyre, A. *The Complete Woman's Herbal: A Manual of Healing Herbs and Nutrition for Personal Well-being and Family Care.* New York: H. Holt, 1995.

Riggs, M. *Natural Child Care.* New York: Harmony Books, 1989.

25

✦

HERBAL ACTIONS

The therapeutic section of this book emphasizes traditional herbal medicine. Thus, this chapter presents a more traditional perspective on herbal actions, as opposed to results of scientific research on herbs or constituents. The actions listed here reflect traditional observations of outcome. The material may or may not be in line with current scientific thinking, although scientific research bears out many of these traditional actions. The core issue is that in clinical practice, the medical herbalist will find these actions relevant and useful in the real world with real patients.

ADAPTOGEN

Soviet scientists coined the term *adaptogen* in 1964 to describe herbs that produce an increase in bodily resistance and vitality, helping the body adapt to and defend against the effects of environmental stress. Adaptogens increase the body's nonspecific resistance to damaging man-made factors and illnesses. According to a more recent definition, adaptogens must:[1]

Show a nonspecific activity—that is, increase the body's ability to resist physical, chemical, or biological noxious agents.
Have a normalizing influence independent of the nature of the pathological state.
Be innocuous and not influence normal body functions more than required.

This implies that adaptogens reinforce the nonspecific power of the body's resistance against stressors. They increase its general capacity to withstand stressful situations, and hence guard against disease caused by overstress. The general aims of treatment with adaptogens are to reduce stress reactions during the alarm phase of the stress response and to prevent or at least delay the state of exhaustion, and thus provide a certain level of protection against long-term stress. See chapter 16 for more information on the stress response and the general adaptation syndrome.

Adaptogens appear to moderate the stress response in the following ways:

Enable a more rapid but less exaggerated response. Blood glucose rises more rapidly after the onset of stress, but does not rise as high.
Allow a more sustained peak. Blood glucose is elevated (and therefore available for cell function) for a longer period of time.
Foster a more gradual decline. There is a less precipitous drop in blood glucose.

Thus, adaptogens do not block the stress response, but instead smooth out the associated highs and lows. This conserves energy in the alarm phase for use in the resistance phase. These effects may be related to adaptogens' effects on glucose metabolism:

- Stimulate the liver to convert glycogen to glucose, leading to increased blood glucose levels
- Enhance entry of glucose into cells
- Enhance utilization of glucose within cells

The specific mechanism of adaptogenic activity has not been elucidated, but some generalizations can be made. Pretreatment with adaptogens appears to alter endocrine functions of the pituitary–adrenal gland axis. Regular pretreatment with adaptogens causes a normalization of stress hormone levels and a generally decreased predisposition to stress. Other body systems also respond to the direct or indirect regulatory influences of adaptogens. For example, adaptogens have been shown to influence the pituitary gonadal system, to confer immunostimulatory actions, and to activate cognitive functions. To date, it is still unknown which cellular mechanisms are addressed during these processes.

A number of herbs can be described as adaptogens, based upon both clinical and in vitro research. It is worth noting that most of these plants are used primarily in Asian countries. This does not mean that adaptogens are found only in Asia, but rather that only Asian scientists have gotten research grants to study them!

Adaptogenic Herbs

Acanthopanax sessiliflorum (wu jia pi)

Albizzia julibrissin (silk tree)

Aralia elata (Japanese angelica tree)

A. manshurica (Manchurian aralia)

Aralia schmidtii (Sakhalin spikenard)

Cicer arietinum (chickpea)

Codonopsis pilosula (dang shen)

Echinopanax elatus (Asian devil's club)

Eleutherococcus senticosus (Siberian ginseng)

Eucommia ulmoides (hardy rubber tree)

Ganoderma lucidum (reishi mushroom)

Hoppea dichotoma

Leuzea carthamoides (maral root)

Ocimum sanctum (holy basil)

Panax ginseng (Korean ginseng)

P. quinquefolius (American ginseng)

Rhodiola rosea (roseroot stonecrop)

Schisandra chinensis (schizandra)

Tinospora cordifolia (guduchi)

Trichopus zeylanicus (arogyappacha)

Withania somnifera (ashwaganda)

ALTERATIVE

Alteratives are herbs that gradually restore proper function to the body and increase overall health and vitality. This sounds very unclear, and, indeed, their mode of action on the body is not understood. However, their value in holistic health care cannot be denied.

In broad terms, alteratives seem to alter the body's metabolic processes to improve tissues' ability to deal with a range of body functions, from nutrition to elimination. Many of the herbs with this action help the body eliminate waste through the kidneys, liver, lungs, or skin. Some work by stimulating digestive function and some are immunomodulators. Others simply work! Folk healing traditions sometimes invoke the concept of "blood cleansing," which, while hinting at much, actually says very little. If the blood truly needed cleansing, a major medical emergency would be afoot.

Immunological research on certain secondary plant products, especially saponins, has led to some interesting suggestions for the basis of alterative action, explored in more detail in chapter 6. Remember, however, that the specifics of plant activity are the result of the way the whole plant works upon the human body, not simply the effects of "active ingredients."

Alteratives can be used safely as supportive therapy in many diverse conditions, and should be considered first for cases of chronic inflammatory and degenerative diseases. These include skin diseases, various types of arthritis, and a wide range of autoimmune problems.

Primary Alterative Herbs

Allium sativum (garlic)

Arctium lappa (burdock)

Baptisia tinctoria (wild indigo)

Chionanthus virginicus (fringetree)

Cimicifuga racemosa (black cohosh)

Echinacea spp. (echinacea)

Fumaria officinalis (fumitory)

Galium aparine (cleavers)

Guaiacum officinale (guaiacum)

Hydrastis canadensis (goldenseal)

Iris versicolor (blue flag)

Larrea tridentata (chaparral)

Mahonia aquifolium (Oregon grape)

Menyanthes trifoliata (bogbean)

Phytolacca americana (poke)

Pulsatilla vulgaris (pasqueflower)

Rumex crispus (yellow dock)

Sanguinaria canadensis (bloodroot)

Scrophularia nodosa (figwort)

Smilax spp. (sarsaparilla)

Stillingia sylvatica (queen's delight)

Trifolium pratense (red clover)

Urtica dioica (nettle)

Body System Affinities

Certain alteratives are particularly well suited to specific body systems or parts. Other remedies may also have alterative actions, as has already been pointed out, but here we shall limit ourselves to the alteratives most often indicated for each body system. See specific body system chapters for more information on how each alterative should best be used.

Cardiovascular. In general, alterative activity is not specifically indicated for this system. However, by nature, alteratives will aid circulation by helping the whole body work at its peak. Alteratives to support the lymphatic aspects of circulation include *Galium aparine*, *Phytolacca americana*, and *Echinacea* spp. *Scrophularia nodosa*, useful in chronic eczema, also has positive inotropic actions. The hypocholesteremic and hypotensive actions of *Allium sativum* are well known.

Respiratory. The main alteratives that also possess beneficial properties for the lungs and respiratory system as a whole are *Allium sativum*, *Hydrastis canadensis*, *Sanguinaria canadensis*, *Baptisia tinctoria*, and *Echinacea* spp.

Digestive. All of the alteratives that work on the liver, pancreas, and other digestive system organs are of great importance in herbal medicine. Examples include *Allium sativum*, *Arctium lappa*, *Chionanthus virginicus*, *Hydrastis canadensis*, *Iris versicolor*, *Menyanthes trifoliata*, *Rumex crispus*, *Smilax* spp., and *Urtica dioica*.

Urinary. Some of the herbs described as diuretics could be characterized as urinary system alteratives. These include *Galium aparine* and *Urtica dioica*.

Reproductive. Here, the general alteratives are always of value, but specifics include *Cimicifuga racemosa* and *Hydrastis canadensis*.

Musculoskeletal. Many alteratives are important here, including *Cimicifuga racemosa*, *Menyanthes trifoliata*, and *Arctium lappa*.

Nervous. By helping the body to be healthy and whole, all alteratives aid the strained nervous system. However, *Pulsatilla vulgaris* and *Trifolium pratense* are especially helpful as alteratives with nervine actions.

Skin. The list of alteratives for the skin could include all of the herbs listed here, plus many more. This is the system for which alteratives are most often used. It is important to remember that in holistic herbalism, aiding and supporting the whole body in its return to health is always more important than applying specific remedies. Alteratives often used for the skin are *Arctium lappa*, *Mahonia aquifolium*, *Fumaria officinalis*, *Galium aparine*, *Echinacea* spp., *Scrophularia nodosa*, *Smilax* spp., *Rumex crispus*, and *Trifolium pratense*.

Table 25.1. Alteratives and Secondary Actions

SECONDARY ACTION	HERBS
Anticatarrhal	*Allium sativum*, *Baptisia tinctoria*, *Echinacea* spp., *Hydrastis canadensis*, *Phytolacca americana*, *Urtica dioica*
Anti-inflammatory	*Galium aparine*, *Guaiacum officinale*, *Hydrastis canadensis*, *Iris versicolor*, *Menyanthes trifoliata*, *Smilax* spp.
Antimicrobial	*Agathosma betulina*, *Allium sativum*, *Baptisia tinctoria*, *Echinacea* spp., *Hydrastis canadensis*, *Larrea tridentata*, *Phytolacca americana*, *Pulsatilla vulgaris*, *Sanguinaria canadensis*
Antispasmodic	*Allium sativum*, *Cimicifuga racemosa*, *Pulsatilla vulgaris*, *Sanguinaria canadensis*, *Trifolium pratense*
Astringent	*Hydrastis canadensis*, *Urtica dioica*

SECONDARY ACTION	HERBS
Bitter	*Arctium lappa*, *Hydrastis canadensis*, *Menyanthes trifoliata*
Diaphoretic	*Allium sativum*, *Guaiacum officinale*, *Stillingia sylvatica*, *Smilax* spp.
Diuretic	*Agathosma betulina*, *Arctium lappa*, *Galium aparine*, *Guaiacum officinale*, *Iris versicolor*, *Menyanthes trifoliata*, *Smilax* spp., *Urtica dioica*
Emmenagogue	*Cimicifuga racemosa*
Expectorant	*Sanguinaria canadensis*, *Trifolium pratense*, *Verbascum thapsus*
Hepatic	*Allium sativum*, *Arctium lappa*, *Chionanthus virginicus*, *Hydrastis canadensis*, *Iris versicolor*, *Mahonia aquifolium*, *Menyanthes trifoliata*, *Phytolacca americana*, *Rumex crispus*
Hypotensive	*Allium sativum*, *Cimicifuga racemosa*, *Urtica dioica*
Nervine	*Cimicifuga racemosa*, *Pulsatilla vulgaris*, *Trifolium pratense*
Vulnerary	*Galium aparine*, *Hydrastis canadensis*

Table 25.2. Relative Strengths of Alterative Herbs

STRENGTH	HERBS
Mild	*Allium sativum*, *Baptisia tinctoria*, *Chionanthus virginicus*, *Cimicifuga racemosa*, *Echinacea* spp., *Mahonia aquifolium*, *Menyanthes trifoliata*, *Pulsatilla vulgaris*
Strong	*Arctium lappa*, *Fumaria officinalis*, *Galium aparine*, *Guaiacum officinale*, *Hydrastis canadensis*, *Rumex crispus*, *Scrophularia nodosa*, *Smilax* spp., *Trifolium pratense*, *Urtica dioica*
Very strong (use with care)	*Iris versicolor*, *Larrea tridentata*, *Phytolacca americana*, *Sassafras albidum*, *Sanguinaria canadensis*, *Stillingia sylvatica*

ANTICATARRHAL

Anticatarrhal herbs help the body remove excess mucus, whether in the sinuses or in other parts of the body. They are used mainly for ear, nose, and throat infections, but also have an essential role to play in many broader-based treatment approaches.

Mucus is an essential body product. However, in response to infection or some other problem, the body may produce excess quantities in its attempt to remove the problematic organism or wastes. Some anticatarrhal remedies work by producing a less viscous mucus secretion that is easier for the body to remove. Others reduce mucus secretion directly. This is not as desirable as it sounds, as it may cause a buildup of waste that cannot be cleared from the sinuses. While the specific mode of action of anticatarrhal herbs remains uncertain, undeniable clinical experience tells us that they work!

The following constituents have been suggested as being pivotal to the action of anticatarrhal herbs.

Tannins have an astringent action and are common to many herbs in this group.

Volatile oil–rich plants can have anticatarrhal effects, in part due to their antimicrobial and anti-inflammatory actions.

Flavones and flavonoids, including commonly found compounds like quercetin, apparently contribute to the total effect.

Important Anticatarrhal Herbs

Achillea millefolium (yarrow)
Allium sativum (garlic)
Althaea officinalis (marshmallow)
Arctostaphylos uva-ursi (bearberry)
Baptisia tinctoria (wild indigo)
Capsicum annuum (cayenne)
Cetraria islandica (Iceland moss)
Chondrus crispus (Irish moss)
Echinacea spp. (echinacea)
Eupatorium perfoliatum (boneset)
Euphrasia spp. (eyebright)
Geranium maculatum (cranesbill)
Hydrastis canadensis (goldenseal)
Hyssopus officinalis (hyssop)
Inula helenium (elecampane)
Mentha piperita (peppermint)
Salvia officinalis (sage)
Sambucus nigra (elder)
Solidago virgaurea (goldenrod)
Thymus vulgaris (thyme)
Tussilago farfara (coltsfoot)
Verbascum thapsus (mullein)

Body System Affinities

Each system of the body has plants that are particularly suited to it, some of which are anticatarrhals. Here we shall see which remedies act as primary anticatarrhals for each of the following body systems.

Cardiovascular. Anticatarrhal action is not directly relevant to the cardiovascular system. However, it could be said that anticatarrhal remedies help the system by contributing to general detoxification and elimination. Such herbs include *Capsicum annuum*, *Allium sativum*, and *Achillea millefolium*.

Respiratory. All of the herbs listed as primary anticatarrhals have a beneficial effect on both the upper and lower respiratory systems.

Digestive. Anticatarrhals that have bitter, demulcent, carminative, hepatic, or astringent properties make useful therapeutic contributions to digestive problems. Important examples are *Allium sativum*, *Althaea officinalis*, *Capsicum annuum*, *Cetraria islandica*, *Chondrus crispus*, *Eupatorium perfoliatum*, *Geranium maculatum*, *Hydrastis canadensis*, *Mentha piperita*, *Salvia officinalis*, and *Thymus vulgaris*.

Urinary. In addition to their anticatarrhal properties, *Arctostaphylos uva-ursi* and *Solidago virgaurea* are important herbs for the urinary system.

Reproductive. While the herbs listed below may all play a role in the holistic treatment of an individual with reproductive system issues, none of them is a primary remedy for male or female problems. *Achillea millefolium*, *Arctostaphylos uva-ursi*, *Geranium maculatum*, and *Hydrastis canadensis* would be the first supportive remedies to consider.

Musculoskeletal. Again, none of these plants is a primary remedy for the musculoskeletal system.

Nervous. Similarly, none of these plants is a primary remedy for the nervous system.

Skin. Anticatarrhals may be indirectly indicated for the treatment of a range of skin problems because they support the body's cleansing processes. Consider *Allium sativum*, *Baptisia tinctoria*, *Echinacea* spp., *Hydrastis canadensis*, and *Sambucus nigra*.

Table 25.3. Anticatarrhal Herbs and Secondary Actions

SECONDARY ACTION	HERBS
Alterative	*Allium sativum, Baptisia tinctoria, Echinacea* spp., *Hydrastis canadensis, Verbascum thapsus*
Anti-inflammatory	*Euphrasia* spp., *Geranium maculatum, Hydrastis canadensis, Solidago virgaurea*

SECONDARY ACTION	HERBS
Antimicrobial	*Achillea millefolium, Allium sativum, Arctostaphylos uva-ursi, Baptisia tinctoria, Capsicum annuum, Echinacea* spp., *Inula helenium, Mentha piperita, Salvia officinalis, Solidago virgaurea, Thymus vulgaris*
Antispasmodic	*Allium sativum, Eupatorium perfoliatum, Hyssopus officinalis, Mentha piperita, Salvia officinalis, Thymus vulgaris*
Astringent	*Achillea millefolium, Arctostaphylos uva-ursi, Euphrasia* spp., *Geranium maculatum, Hydrastis canadensis, Salvia officinalis, Thymus vulgaris*
Bitter	*Achillea millefolium, Eupatorium perfoliatum, Hydrastis canadensis*
Carminative	*Capsicum annuum, Hyssopus officinalis, Mentha piperita, Salvia officinalis, Solidago virgaurea, Thymus vulgaris*
Demulcent	*Althaea officinalis, Arctostaphylos uva-ursi, Cetraria islandica, Chondrus crispus, Tussilago farfara, Verbascum thapsus*
Diaphoretic	*Achillea millefolium, Allium sativum, Eupatorium perfoliatum, Hyssopus officinalis, Inula helenium, Mentha piperita, Sambucus nigra, Solidago virgaurea*
Diuretic	*Achillea millefolium, Althaea officinalis, Arctostaphylos uva-ursi, Sambucus nigra, Solidago virgaurea, Tussilago farfara, Verbascum thapsus*
Emmenagogue	*Achillea millefolium, Eupatorium perfoliatum, Salvia officinalis, Thymus vulgaris*
Expectorant	*Althaea officinalis, Cetraria islandica, Chondrus crispus, Hyssopus officinalis, Sambucus nigra, Thymus vulgaris, Tussilago farfara, Verbascum thapsus*
Hepatic	*Allium sativum, Eupatorium perfoliatum, Hydrastis canadensis*
Hypotensive	*Achillea millefolium, Allium sativum*
Laxative	*Eupatorium perfoliatum, Hydrastis canadensis, Sambucus nigra*
Nervine	*Hyssopus officinalis*

SECONDARY ACTION	HERBS
Tonic	*Achillea millefolium, Capsicum annuum, Echinacea* spp., *Eupatorium perfoliatum, Hydrastis canadensis*
Vulnerary	*Althaea officinalis, Geranium maculatum, Sambucus nigra, Verbascum thapsus*

Strengths of anticatarrhal herbs are relative, because their efficacy depends upon the nature of the cause, rather than on their potency as anticatarrhals. For example, better results may be achieved with *Echinacea* than with *Solidago* if infection is the cause.

ANTI-INFLAMMATORY

Herbs that help the body combat inflammation are known as anti-inflammatory remedies. Orthodox medicine places much emphasis on chemicals that work to reduce symptoms of inflammation and ease suffering. However, symptom alleviation is not the best way to use herbal anti-inflammatories. They are safe to use for the relief of pain and discomfort, but offer most when used in combination with other remedies to address the underlying problem.

In keeping with the theme of this chapter, the groupings given here reflect traditional observations of outcome. For a pharmacological review of anti-inflammatory natural products, please refer to chapter 9. As discussed there, secondary metabolites produce anti-inflammatory actions by interacting with the inflammatory cascade in a number of different ways. While these insights are interesting, using them to reach coherent clinical conclusions is challenging, as are all extrapolations from constituent studies to whole-plant phytotherapy.

Inflammation is a normal body response to infection and other problems. Through localized biochemical and tissue changes, the inflammatory reaction often brings about the changes necessary to heal the focus of disease and restore health. Unless this response is life threatening, it is a mistake to inhibit it. For example, simply suppressing symptoms of inflammation in the stomach to relieve discomfort will not alter the underlying causes of the symptoms, and possibly could lead to the development of a stomach ulcer.

We have become conditioned to see inflammation as something to suppress and smother, rather than to work with and support. Herbal remedies offer us the possibility to work with body processes, but as in all health matters, there is a balance to achieve. Here, we need to know when to work with inflammation and when to suppress it.

Types of Anti-Inflammatory Herbs

Attempts to classify anti-inflammatory herbs by relative strength are not very helpful. It is far more useful in the therapeutic sense to group them in terms of the body system or tissue for which they are most appropriate or by their pharmacological mode of action.

Treating inflammation with herbs is usually approached in terms of what tissue or organ is the focus of inflammation. Based upon the different ways herbal anti-inflammatories are thought to work, there are four groups of anti-inflammatory herbs. I cannot overemphasize that the action of a whole plant is always more than the action of any specific constituent chemical. Keeping this holistic perspective in mind, let us look at the following groups of anti-inflammatory remedies:

Salicylate-Containing Anti-Inflammatory Herbs

A large range of plants contain salts of salicylic acid, the molecule from which aspirin was developed. Such plants are most useful for musculoskeletal inflammations, such as arthritis. Herbs containing significant quantities of salicylic acid have a marked anti-inflammatory effect, without posing the dangers to the stomach that aspirin does. In fact, *Filipendula ulmaria*, rich in salicylates, can even be used to stanch mild stomach hemorrhage. Other plants rich in such constituents include *Salix* spp., *Gaultheria procumbens*, *Betula* spp., many poplars, and *Viburnum prunifolium*.

Plants Containing Steroid Precursors

Steroids were first isolated from plant material, and some herbs contain molecules that may be metabolized by the body into inflammation-fighting steroidal molecules. Such plants will help reduce some kinds of inflammation, especially inflammation of autoimmune origin. Examples are *Glycyrrhiza glabra* and *Dioscorea villosa*, which contains diosgenin.

Essential Oil–Rich Plants

Many aromatic herbs high in essential oils have anti-inflammatory actions. One of the best of these remedies is *Matricaria recutita*, which is rich in terpenes, such as bisabolol and chamazulene. These herbs are especially useful for digestive system inflammations when taken by mouth, for respiratory problems when inhaled in some form, and for skin inflammations when used topically.

Calendula officinalis and *Hypericum perforatum* are other well-known plants containing oils that soothe and reduce inflammation.

Resin-Containing Plants

A number of resin-containing plants reduce inflammation in some areas of the body, but often cause inflammation in the stomach. This limits their usefulness, but they are irreplaceable for some arthritic conditions. Examples are *Menyanthes trifoliata*, *Harpagophytum procumbens*, and *Guaiacum officinale*.

Other Types of Anti-Inflammatory Herbs

As is common with herbal remedies, no clear-cut chemical basis can be identified to explain the anti-inflammatory actions of some plants. This in no way negates their value, because there is more to health and well-being than pharmaceutical chemistry. It might also mean that no one has yet gotten a grant to study that plant!

One of the many remedies in this group we can mention is *Cimicifuga racemosa*. Demulcent herbs often have an *apparently* anti-inflammatory effect, but this is related to their ability to soothe inflamed surfaces, not to reductions in the cellular inflammatory response.

Major Anti-Inflammatory Herbs

Achillea millefolium (yarrow)
Aesculus hippocastanum (horse chestnut)
Alchemilla arvensis (lady's mantle)
Althaea officinalis (marshmallow)
Anethum graveolens (dill)
Angelica archangelica (angelica)
Apium graveolens (celery seed)
Asclepias tuberosa (pleurisy root)
Betula spp. (birch)
Borago officinalis (borage)
Calendula officinalis (calendula)
Capsella bursa-pastoris (shepherd's purse)
Caulophyllum thalictroides (blue cohosh)
Cetraria islandica (Iceland moss)
Chondrus crispus (Irish moss)
Cimicifuga racemosa (black cohosh)
Crataegus spp. (hawthorn)
Dioscorea villosa (wild yam)
Filipendula ulmaria (meadowsweet)
Foeniculum vulgare (fennel)
Galium aparine (cleavers)
Gaultheria procumbens (wintergreen)
Geranium maculatum (cranesbill)
Glycyrrhiza glabra (licorice)

Guaiacum officinale (guaiacum)
Hamamelis virginiana (witch hazel)
Harpagophytum procumbens (devil's claw)
Hydrastis canadensis (goldenseal)
Hypericum perforatum (St. John's wort)
Hyssopus officinalis (hyssop)
Lavandula spp. (lavender)
Malva sylvestris (mallow)
Matricaria recutita (chamomile)
Mentha piperita (peppermint)
Menyanthes trifoliata (bogbean)
Plantago major (plantain)
Populus tremuloides (quaking aspen)
Salix spp. (willow)
Salvia officinalis (sage)
Sambucus nigra (elder)
Solidago virgaurea (goldenrod)
Stellaria media (chickweed)
Symphytum officinale (comfrey)
Tilia platyphyllos (linden)
Trigonella foenum-graecum (fenugreek)
Tussilago farfara (coltsfoot)
Ulmus rubra (slippery elm)
Verbascum thapsus (mullein)
Viburnum opulus (cramp bark)
V. prunifolium (black haw)
Zea mays (cornsilk)

Body System Affinities

For each system of the body, there are plants that are particularly well suited that also act as anti-inflammatory remedies. This allows the herbalist to nurture the health and vitality of a body system while at the same time lessening any inflammation.

Circulatory. A number of herbs may be used to reduce inflammations in blood vessels, including *Tilia platyphyllos*, *Crataegus* spp., *Aesculus hippocastanum*, and *Achillea millefolium*.

Respiratory. As it is a common site for inflammatory conditions, it should come as no surprise that a whole range of anti-inflammatories work well in either the upper or the lower respiratory system. For the lower respiratory system, consider *Asclepias tuberosa*, *Cetraria islandica*, *Chondrus crispus*, *Glycyrrhiza glabra*, *Hyssopus officinalis*, *Tussilago farfara*, and *Verbascum thapsus*. For the upper respiratory system, consider *Sambucus nigra* and *Solidago virgaurea*.

Digestive. As herbal remedies go directly to the digestive system, they are particularly useful in inflammatory conditions that affect it, from stomach ulcers to colitis and hemorrhoids. Such herbs include *Matricaria recutita*, *Dioscorea villosa*, *Glycyrrhiza glabra*, *Hydrastis canadensis*, *Calendula*, and *Mentha piperita*. Demulcent remedies rich in mucilage, such as *Althaea officinalis*, can have the localized effect of reducing inflammation through contact soothing.

Urinary. A number of herbs soothe the tissue of the urinary tract directly as their anti-inflammatory constituents pass through the kidneys and bladder. Plants that soothe the tissue and fight infection will also have an anti-inflammatory action. Specific urinary tract anti-inflammatory remedies include *Solidago virgaurea* and *Zea mays*.

Reproductive. Many tonics and other specific reproductive remedies will often have anti-inflammatory actions—for example, *Alchemilla arvensis* and *Caulophyllum thalictroides*.

Musculoskeletal. For hardworking and abused muscles and bones, salicylate-containing remedies come into their own. *Salix* spp., *Filipendula ulmaria*, *Populus tremuloides*, and *Betula* spp. are excellent. Others to consider are *Menyanthes trifoliata*, *Harpagophytum procumbens*, *Cimicifuga racemosa*, *Tanacetum parthenium*, and *Dioscorea villosa*. Arthritic conditions respond well to herbal therapy, but as always, herbs work best when used as part of a holistic approach to treating the person, not simply the disease.

Nervous. While the nervous system often feels as if it needs anti-inflammatories, the best remedies for the "inflamed state of mind" are the relaxing nervines. The only direct anti-inflammatory for nervous system tissue is *Hypericum perforatum*, which helps speed the recovery of damaged nerves. However, many nervines can play a supportive role, including *Avena sativa* and *Valeriana officinalis*.

Skin. Numerous remedies reduce inflammation on the skin. A selection of these gifts of the natural world includes *Calendula officinalis*, *Hypericum perforatum*, *Commiphora molmol*, *Hydrastis canadensis*, *Arnica montana*, *Stellaria media*, and *Plantago major*.

Table 25.4. Anti-Inflammatory Herbs and Secondary Actions

SECONDARY ACTION	HERBS
Anticatarrhal	*Achillea millefolium, Althaea officinalis, Cetraria islandica, Chondrus crispus, Geranium maculatum, Hydrastis canadensis, Hyssopus officinalis, Mentha piperita, Salvia officinalis, Sambucus nigra, Solidago virgaurea, Tussilago farfara, Verbascum thapsus*
Antimicrobial	*Achillea millefolium, Calendula officinalis, Hydrastis canadensis, Hypericum perforatum, Matricaria recutita, Mentha piperita, Populus tremuloides, Salvia officinalis, Solidago virgaurea*
Antispasmodic	*Anethum graveolens, Angelica archangelica, Apium graveolens, Asclepias tuberosa, Cimicifuga racemosa, Dioscorea villosa, Foeniculum vulgare, Glycyrrhiza glabra, Hypericum perforatum, Hyssopus officinalis, Lavandula* spp., *Matricaria recutita, Mentha piperita, Populus tremuloides, Salvia officinalis, Sambucus nigra, Tilia platyphyllos, Trigonella foenum-graecum, Verbascum thapsus, Viburnum opulus, V. prunifolium*
Astringent	*Achillea millefolium, Aesculus hippocastanum, Alchemilla arvensis, Calendula officinalis, Capsella bursa-pastoris, Filipendula ulmaria, Geranium maculatum, Hamamelis virginiana, Hydrastis canadensis, Plantago major, Populus tremuloides, Salvia officinalis, Solidago virgaurea, Symphytum officinale, Tilia platyphyllos, Verbascum thapsus*
Bitter	*Achillea millefolium, Hydrastis canadensis, Matricaria recutita, Menyanthes trifoliata*
Carminative	*Achillea millefolium, Anethum graveolens, Angelica archangelica, Apium graveolens, Filipendula ulmaria, Foeniculum vulgare, Glycyrrhiza glabra, Hyssopus officinalis, Lavandula* spp., *Matricaria recutita, Mentha piperita, Salvia officinalis, Solidago virgaurea, Tilia platyphyllos, Trigonella foenum-graecum*
Cholagogue	*Calendula officinalis, Dioscorea villosa, Hydrastis canadensis, Menyanthes trifoliata*
Demulcent	*Althaea officinalis, Cetraria islandica, Chondrus crispus, Glycyrrhiza glabra, Malva sylvestris, Stellaria media, Symphytum officinale, Trigonella foenum-graecum, Ulmus rubra, Verbascum thapsus, Zea mays*
Diaphoretic	*Achillea millefolium, Angelica archangelica, Asclepias tuberosa, Guaiacum officinale, Hyssopus officinalis, Mentha piperita, Sambucus nigra, Solidago virgaurea, Tilia platyphyllos*
Diuretic	*Achillea millefolium, Alchemilla arvensis, Apium graveolens, Crataegus* spp., *Galium aparine, Menyanthes trifoliata, Plantago major, Sambucus nigra, Solidago virgaurea, Tilia platyphyllos, Zea mays*
Emmenagogue	*Achillea millefolium, Alchemilla arvensis, Calendula officinalis, Caulophyllum thalictroides, Cimicifuga racemosa, Hydrastis canadensis, Hyssopus officinalis, Lavandula* spp., *Salvia officinalis, Tilia platyphyllos, Viburnum opulus, V. prunifolium*
Expectorant	*Althaea officinalis, Asclepias tuberosa, Cetraria islandica, Chondrus crispus, Glycyrrhiza glabra, Hydrastis canadensis, Hyssopus officinalis, Malva sylvestris, Plantago major, Sambucus nigra, Tussilago farfara, Verbascum thapsus*
Hepatic	*Achillea millefolium, Calendula officinalis, Dioscorea villosa, Foeniculum vulgare, Glycyrrhiza glabra, Hydrastis canadensis, Hyssopus officinalis, Menyanthes trifoliata, Trigonella foenum-graecum*
Laxative	*Hydrastis canadensis, Glycyrrhiza glabra*
Nervine	*Apium graveolens, Borago officinalis, Cimicifuga racemosa, Hypericum perforatum, Hyssopus officinalis, Lavandula* spp., *Matricaria recutita, Mentha piperita, Tilia platyphyllos, Viburnum prunifolium*
Tonic	*Achillea millefolium, Cimicifuga racemosa, Crataegus* spp., *Filipendula ulmaria, Hydrastis canadensis, Hypericum perforatum, Verbascum thapsus*
Vulnerary	*Achillea millefolium, Alchemilla arvensis, Althaea officinalis, Calendula officinalis, Filipendula ulmaria, Hamamelis virginiana, Hypericum perforatum, Hyssopus officinalis, Malva sylvestris, Matricaria recutita, Plantago major, Stellaria media, Symphytum officinale*

ANTIMICROBIAL

Antimicrobial herbs help the body destroy or resist pathogenic microorganisms in some way. The action covers the whole gamut of microorganisms, including bacteria, fungi, and viruses. However, it would be inappropriate to talk about these plants as being "antibiotic," as this term literally means "anti-life." There are times when antibiotic drugs are essential and life saving, but not as often as they are actually used. At times, supportive and preventive remedies allow the body to bypass the need for chemical intervention. But when an emergency arises, let us be thankful for the existence of antibiotics.

When using herbal remedies, we have the opportunity to help the body strengthen its own resistance to pathogens and throw off the illness. Some plant remedies contain chemicals that are antiseptic or act as specific poisons to certain organisms. In general, however, we are talking about plants that support the immune process, augmenting the integrity of the individual's own defense system.

How Antimicrobial Herbs Work

It would be a mistake to attempt an overarching generalization about mechanisms of action for herbal antimicrobials. The use of the term *antimicrobial* is a description of expected outcome, rather than a description of process. Antimicrobial effects may be related to direct interactions with pathogens or mediated via the herb's interaction with the immune response. These herbs may also work through indirect actions by stimulating immune responses. As examples of the diversity of mechanisms involved, consider the following:

Melaleuca alternifolia (tea tree) contains an oil, rich in terpinene-4-ol, that directly interferes with a pathogen's metabolism, thus killing it.[2] Other herbs rich in volatile oils also work directly to kill microorganisms. Examples include *Allium sativum*, *Thymus vulgaris*, and *Eucalyptus* spp.

Echinacea directly stimulates the body's own immune response and thus is often an effective antimicrobial agent.

Vaccinium macrocarpon (cranberry juice) blocks the adhesion of uropathogenic *E. coli* to the walls of the bladder, thus offering a useful treatment for cystitis.[3]

Important Herbal Antimicrobials

Achillea millefolium (yarrow)
Allium sativum (garlic)
Arctostaphylos uva-ursi (bearberry)
Artemisia abrotanum (southernwood)
A. absinthium (wormwood)

Baptisia tinctoria (wild indigo)
Calendula officinalis (calendula)
Capsicum annuum (cayenne)
Carum carvi (caraway)
Commiphora molmol (myrrh)
Coriandrum sativum (coriander)
Echinacea spp. (echinacea)
Eucalyptus spp. (eucalyptus)
Gentiana lutea (gentian)
Hydrastis canadensis (goldenseal)
Hypericum perforatum (St. John's wort)
Inula helenium (elecampane)
Juniperus communis (juniper)
Ligusticum porteri (osha)
Mentha piperita (peppermint)
Myroxylon balsamum var. *pereirae* (balsam of Peru)
Olea europaea (olive)
Origanum majorana (marjoram)
Pimpinella anisum (aniseed)
Plantago major (plantain)
Rosmarinus officinalis (rosemary)
Ruta graveolens (rue)
Salvia officinalis (sage)
Syzygium aromaticum (clove)
Thymus vulgaris (thyme)
Usnea spp. (usnea)

Body System Affinities

By the nature of infection and the body's immune response to it, a general systemic treatment is always appropriate, even if given in conjunction with specific local remedies. Ways in these remedies can be used are discussed in specific body system chapters.

Cardiovascular. Among antimicrobial herbs, *Allium sativum* and *Achillea millefolium* have a reputation as tonics for this system. *Allium sativum* is especially appropriate because of its broad value for the cardiovascular system in general.

Respiratory. In addition to *Echinacea* spp., *Baptisia tinctoria*, and *Commiphora molmol*, we can add *Pimpinella anisum*, *Myroxylon balsamum* var. *pereirae*, *Syzygium aromaticum*, *Inula helenium*, *Ligusticum porteri*, and *Thymus vulgaris*, which also possess different varieties of expectorant effects.

Digestive. Many volatile oil–containing herbs and some digestive bitters have an antimicrobial effect in the intestines. Some to consider are *Echinacea* spp., *Allium sativum*, *Artemisia absinthium*, *Calendula officinalis*, *Commiphora molmol*, *Gentiana lutea*, *Hydrastis canadensis*, and *Salvia officinalis*.

Urinary. Effective remedies are *Arctostaphylos uva-ursi*, *Juniperus communis*, *Eucalyptus* spp., and *Achillea millefolium*. Be aware that if there is any suggestion of kidney disease, some of the urinary antimicrobial remedies can be too strong.

Reproductive. Here, useful herbs include *Echinacea* spp., *Allium sativum*, *Artemisia abrotanum*, and *Tropaeolum majus*, as well as urinary antimicrobials.

Musculoskeletal. *Echinacea* spp. and *Baptisia tinctoria* provide a good basis for treatment.

Nervous. *Hypericum perforatum* or *Phytolacca americana*, in combination with nervines and other antimicrobial herbs, will help with the intransigent infections that can affect the nervous system.

Skin. Many antimicrobial herbs can be used on the skin. A wash of *Thymus vulgaris*, *Rosmarinus officinalis*, *Origanum majorana*, or *Allium sativum* can be most effective. *Commiphora molmol* is one of the strongest external remedies.

Table 25.5. Antimicrobial Herbs and Secondary Actions

SECONDARY ACTION	HERBS
Alterative	*Allium sativum, Baptisia tinctoria, Echinacea* spp., *Hydrastis canadensis, Inula helenium*
Anticatarrhal	*Allium sativum, Arctostaphylos uva-ursi, Baptisia tinctoria, Capsicum annuum, Echinacea* spp., *Eucalyptus* spp., *Hydrastis canadensis, Inula helenium, Mentha piperita, Myroxylon balsamum* var. *pereirae, Salvia officinalis, Thymus vulgaris*
Anti-inflammatory	*Artemisia absinthium, Calendula officinalis, Hypericum perforatum, Mentha piperita, Plantago major*
Antispasmodic	*Allium sativum, Carum carvi, Hypericum perforatum, Mentha piperita, Pimpinella anisum, Rosmarinus officinalis, Ruta graveolens, Salvia officinalis, Thymus vulgaris*
Astringent	*Achillea millefolium, Arctostaphylos uva-ursi, Carum carvi, Commiphora molmol, Plantago major, Rosmarinus officinalis, Salvia officinalis, Thymus vulgaris*
Bitter	*Achillea millefolium, Artemisia abrotanum, A. absinthium, Gentiana lutea, Hydrastis canadensis, Ruta graveolens*

SECONDARY ACTION	HERBS
Carminative	*Artemisia absinthium, Capsicum annuum, Carum carvi, Commiphora molmol, Coriandrum sativum, Juniperus communis, Mentha piperita, Pimpinella anisum, Rosmarinus officinalis, Salvia officinalis, Syzygium aromaticum, Thymus vulgaris*
Demulcent	*Arctostaphylos uva-ursi, Plantago major*
Diaphoretic	*Achillea millefolium, Allium sativum, Baptisia tinctoria, Capsicum annuum, Inula helenium, Mentha piperita, Origanum majorana*
Diuretic	*Achillea millefolium, Arctostaphylos uva-ursi, Eucalyptus* spp., *Juniperus communis, Plantago major*
Emmenagogue	*Achillea millefolium, Artemisia abrotanum, A. absinthium, Calendula officinalis, Carum carvi, Gentiana lutea, Hydrastis canadensis, Origanum majorana, Rosmarinus officinalis, Ruta graveolens, Thymus vulgaris*
Expectorant	*Carum carvi, Commiphora molmol, Eucalyptus* spp., *Inula helenium, Ligusticum porteri, Myroxylon balsamum* var. *pereirae, Origanum majorana, Pimpinella anisum, Plantago major, Ruta graveolens, Thymus vulgaris*
Hepatic	*Allium sativum, Artemisia abrotanum, Calendula officinalis, Gentiana lutea, Hydrastis canadensis, Inula helenium, Ruta graveolens*
Hypotensive	*Achillea millefolium, Allium sativum, Olea europaea*
Laxative	*Achillea millefolium, Artemisia abrotanum, A. absinthium, Gentiana lutea, Hydrastis canadensis, Ruta graveolens*
Nervine	*Hypericum perforatum, Mentha piperita, Rosmarinus officinalis*
Tonic	*Achillea millefolium, Allium sativum, Artemisia absinthium, Calendula officinalis, Capsicum annuum, Echinacea* spp., *Gentiana lutea, Hydrastis canadensis, Hypericum perforatum, Inula helenium, Ruta graveolens*
Vulnerary	*Achillea millefolium, Calendula officinalis, Commiphora molmol, Hydrastis canadensis, Hypericum perforatum, Plantago major*

Table 25.6. Relative Strengths of Antimicrobial Herbs

STRENGTH	HERBS
Mild	*Calendula officinalis, Carum carvi, Coriandrum sativum, Gentiana lutea, Olea europaea, Origanum majorana, Pimpinella anisum, Plantago major, Syzygium aromaticum*
Moderate	*Achillea millefolium, Artemisia absinthium, Capsicum annuum, Hypericum perforatum, Mentha piperita, Rosmarinus officinalis, Ruta graveolens, Salvia officinalis*
Strong	*Allium sativum, Arctostaphylos uva-ursi, Baptisia tinctoria, Commiphora molmol, Echinacea* spp., *Eucalyptus* spp., *Hydrastis canadensis, Inula helenium, Juniperus communis, Ligusticum porteri, Myroxylon balsamum* var. *pereirae, Thymus vulgaris, Usnea* spp.

ANTIRHEUMATIC

These are remedies that improve quality of life for patients with rheumatic problems. This is not meant to suggest that they have a specific effect upon the disease or even necessarily upon the musculoskeletal tissue itself. The term *antirheumatic* is a description of an expected outcome, rather than an implied mechanism. As such, it is very limited in its applicability.

The activity of these herbs can be explained as an expression of a more broadly relevant action. This may be the herb's primary action or a more holistic synergy of the plant's actions. For example, the alteratives may work in a number of different ways in rheumatic conditions, as can anti-inflammatory herbs. Of course, it is not always possible to identify the mechanism of action.

Important Antirheumatic Herbs

Achillea millefolium (yarrow)
Angelica archangelica (angelica)
Apium graveolens (celery seed)
Arctium lappa (burdock)
Arctostaphylos uva-ursi (bearberry)
Armoracia rusticana (horseradish)
Arnica montana (arnica)
Artemisia absinthium (wormwood)
Artemisia vulgaris (mugwort)
Betula spp. (birch)
Brassica spp. (mustard)
Capsicum annuum (cayenne)
Caulophyllum thalictroides (blue cohosh)
Cimicifuga racemosa (black cohosh)
Dioscorea villosa (wild yam)
Eupatorium perfoliatum (boneset)
E. purpureum (gravel root)
Filipendula ulmaria (meadowsweet)
Fucus vesiculosus (bladderwrack)
Gaultheria procumbens (wintergreen)
Guaiacum officinale (guaiacum)
Harpagophytum procumbens (devil's claw)
Iris versicolor (blue flag)
Juniperus communis (juniper)
Mahonia aquifolium (Oregon grape)
Menyanthes trifoliata (bogbean)
Myrica cerifera (bayberry)
Petroselinum crispum (parsley)
Phytolacca americana (poke)
Populus tremuloides (aspen)
Rosmarinus officinalis (rosemary)
Rumex crispus (yellow dock)
Salix spp. (willow)
Smilax spp. (sarsaparilla)
Tanacetum parthenium (feverfew)
Taraxacum officinale (dandelion)
Urtica dioica (nettle)
Viburnum opulus (cramp bark)
Zanthoxylum americanum (prickly ash)
Zingiber officinale (ginger)

Table 25.7. Possible Mechanism of Action of Antirheumatic Herbs

ACTION	HERBS
Anti-inflammatory	*Angelica archangelica, Apium graveolens, Betula* spp., *Dioscorea villosa, Filipendula ulmaria, Gaultheria procumbens, Guaiacum officinale, Harpagophytum procumbens, Menyanthes trifoliata, Populus tremuloides, Tanacetum parthenium*
Alterative	*Arctium lappa, Mahonia aquifolium, Fucus vesiculosus, Guaiacum officinale, Harpagophytum procumbens, Iris versicolor, Menyanthes trifoliata, Phytolacca americana, Rumex crispus, Smilax* spp., *Urtica dioica*
Diuretic	*Achillea millefolium, Apium graveolens, Arctostaphylos uva-ursi, Eupatorium perfoliatum, E. purpureum, Juniperus communis, Petroselinum crispum, Taraxacum officinale*

ACTION	HERBS
Circulatory stimulant	Armoracia rusticana, Brassica spp., Capsicum annuum, Myrica cerifera, Rosmarinus officinalis, Zanthoxylum americanum, Zingiber officinale
Antispasmodic	Cimicifuga racemosa, Viburnum opulus
Other action (or basis unclear)	Arnica montana, Artemisia absinthium, A. vulgaris, Caulophyllum thalictroides

Table 25.8. Relative Strengths of Antirheumatic Herbs

STRENGTH	HERBS
Mild	Achillea millefolium, Arctostaphylos uva-ursi, Arnica montana, Artemisia absinthium, A. vulgaris, Caulophyllum thalictroides, Eupatorium perfoliatum, E. purpureum, Fucus vesiculosus, Mahonia aquifolium, Rosmarinus officinalis, Rumex crispus, Taraxacum officinale
Moderate	Angelica archangelica, Apium graveolens, Arctium lappa, Armoracia rusticana, Betula spp., Brassica spp., Capsicum annuum, Cimicifuga racemosa, Dioscorea villosa, Filipendula ulmaria, Gaultheria procumbens, Harpagophytum procumbens, Menyanthes trifoliata, Myrica cerifera, Petroselinum crispum, Populus tremuloides, Salix spp., Smilax spp., Urtica dioica, Viburnum opulus, Zanthoxylum americanum, Zingiber officinale
Strong	Guaiacum officinale, Iris versicolor, Juniperus communis, Phytolacca americana, Tanacetum parthenium

ANTISPASMODIC

Antispasmodic herbs prevent or ease spasms or cramps in the muscles. They thus reduce muscular tension in the body, and, as many antispasmodics are also nervines, they will sometimes ease psychological tension as well. The term *antispasmodic* is synonymous with *spasmolytic*.

How Antispasmodics Work

Some antispasmodics work in a general way to reduce muscle spasms throughout the body, and others specifically work on certain organs or systems. Antispasmodics relax the autonomic nervous system, but not necessarily the central nervous system. For this reason, they facilitate physical relaxation of muscles without necessarily causing a sedative effect. When needed in the intestinal tract, as in colic, carminative herbs will usually suffice as antispasmodics. The relaxing expectorants have a localized antispasmodic effect in the respiratory system, but may also have a broader effect upon the body.

General Antispasmodic Herbs

Anethum graveolens (dill)
Angelica archangelica (angelica)
Apium graveolens (celery seed)
Artemisia vulgaris (mugwort)
Carum carvi (caraway)
Cimicifuga racemosa (black cohosh)
Daucus carota (wild carrot)
Dioscorea villosa (wild yam)
Drosera rotundifolia (sundew)
Elettaria cardamomum (cardamom)
Eschscholzia californica (California poppy)
Foeniculum vulgare (fennel)
Glycyrrhiza glabra (licorice)
Humulus lupulus (hops)
Hypericum perforatum (St. John's wort)
Hyssopus officinalis (hyssop)
Lactuca virosa (wild lettuce)
Lavandula spp. (lavender)
Leonurus cardiaca (motherwort)
Lobelia inflata (lobelia)
Lycopus spp. (bugleweed)
Matricaria recutita (chamomile)
Melissa officinalis (lemon balm)
Mentha piperita (peppermint)
M. pulegium (pennyroyal)
Nepeta cataria (catnip)
Passiflora incarnata (passionflower)
Petroselinum crispum (parsley)
Pimpinella anisum (aniseed)
Piper methysticum (kava kava)
Piscidia erythrina (Jamaica dogwood)
Prunus serotina (wild cherry bark)
Rosmarinus officinalis (rosemary)
Salvia officinalis var. *rubia* (red sage)
Sambucus nigra (elder)
Scutellaria lateriflora (skullcap)
Symplocarpus foetidus (skunk cabbage)
Tanacetum parthenium (feverfew)
Thymus vulgaris (thyme)
Tilia platyphyllos (linden)
Trifolium pratense (red clover)
Trigonella foenum-graecum (fenugreek)

Turnera diffusa (damiana)
Tussilago farfara (coltsfoot)
Valeriana officinalis (valerian)
Verbascum thapsus (mullein)
Verbena officinalis (vervain)
Viburnum opulus (cramp bark)
V. prunifolium (black haw)
Zingiber officinale (ginger)

Body System Affinities

Cardiovascular. *Leonurus cardiaca, Viburnum opulus, Cimicifuga racemosa, Melissa officinalis, Lavandula* spp., and *Valeriana officinalis* are important here.

Respiratory. A range of antispasmodics are useful in the respiratory system, including *Lactuca virosa, Prunus serotina, Lobelia inflata, Grindelia camporum, Euphorbia pilulifera,* and *Pimpinella anisum.*

Digestive. All of the carminative herbs tend to act as antispasmodics in the gut, and hepatics can have such an action for gallbladder conditions. Specific herbs to consider are *Matricaria recutita, Viburnum opulus, V. prunifolium, Valeriana officinalis, Humulus lupulus, Mentha piperita, Salvia officinalis, Thymus vulgaris, Anethum graveolens, Foeniculum vulgare,* and *Dioscorea villosa.*

Urinary. Think of *Viburnum opulus, V. prunifolium,* and *Daucus carota.*

Reproductive. Here, *Viburnum opulus* and *V. prunifolium* come into their own. The nervine antispasmodics, such as *Valeriana officinalis* and *Scutellaria lateriflora,* are also helpful.

Musculoskeletal. Primary muscle relaxant remedies include *Piper methysticum, Viburnum opulus, V. prunifolium, Valeriana officinalis,* and *Scutellaria lateriflora.* Externally, *Lobelia inflata* can be helpful.

Nervous. See Nervine for more information.

Skin. Antispasmodics are not directly relevant here.

Table 25.9. Antispasmodic Herbs and Secondary Actions

SECONDARY ACTION	HERBS
Alterative	Cimicifuga racemosa, Trifolium pratense
Analgesic	Cimicifuga racemosa, Dioscorea villosa, Eschscholzia californica, Hypericum perforatum, Lactuca virosa, Mentha piperita, Passiflora incarnata, Piscidia erythrina, Valeriana officinalis
Anticatarrhal	Hyssopus officinalis, Lavandula spp., Matricaria recutita, Mentha piperita, Nepeta cataria, Salvia officinalis, Sambucus nigra, Thymus vulgaris, Tilia platyphyllos, Trigonella foenum-graecum, Tussilago farfara, Verbascum thapsus, Zingiber officinale
Anti-inflammatory	Angelica archangelica, Apium graveolens, Dioscorea villosa, Glycyrrhiza glabra, Hypericum perforatum, Hyssopus officinalis, Lavandula spp., Matricaria recutita, Melissa officinalis, Mentha piperita, Salvia officinalis, Sambucus nigra, Tilia platyphyllos, Tussilago farfara
Antimicrobial	Carum carvi, Drosera rotundifolia, Humulus lupulus, Hypericum perforatum, Lavandula spp., Matricaria recutita, Mentha piperita, Pimpinella anisum, Piper methysticum, Rosmarinus officinalis, Thymus vulgaris
Astringent	Glechoma hederacea, Humulus lupulus, Hypericum perforatum, Lycopus spp., Prunus serotina, Salvia officinalis, Rosmarinus officinalis, Tilia platyphyllos, Viburnum opulus, V. prunifolium
Bitter	Artemisia vulgaris, Humulus lupulus, Matricaria recutita
Carminative	Anethum graveolens, Angelica archangelica, Artemisia vulgaris, Carum carvi, Daucus carota, Elettaria cardamomum, Foeniculum vulgare, Humulus lupulus, Hyssopus officinalis, Lavandula spp., Leonurus cardiaca, Matricaria recutita, Melissa officinalis, Mentha piperita, M. pulegium, Nepeta cataria, Petroselinum crispum, Pimpinella anisum, Salvia officinalis var. rubia, Rosmarinus officinalis, Thymus vulgaris, Trigonella foenum-graecum, Valeriana officinalis, Verbena officinalis, Zingiber officinale
Demulcent	Drosera rotundifolia, Glycyrrhiza glabra, Trigonella foenum-graecum, Tussilago farfara, Verbascum thapsus
Diaphoretic	Angelica archangelica, Cimicifuga racemosa, Hyssopus officinalis, Mentha piperita, Nepeta cataria, Rosmarinus officinalis, Sambucus nigra, Symplocarpus foetidus, Tilia platyphyllos, Verbena officinalis, Zingiber officinale

SECONDARY ACTION	HERBS
Diuretic	*Angelica archangelica, Daucus carota, Lycopus* spp., *Nepeta cataria, Petroselinum crispum, Piper methysticum, Sambucus nigra, Tilia platyphyllos, Turnera diffusa, Tussilago farfara*
Emmenagogue	*Artemisia vulgaris, Marrubium vulgare, Carum carvi, Cimicifuga racemosa, Leonurus cardiaca, Mentha pulegium*
Expectorant	*Angelica archangelica, Carum carvi, Daucus carota, Drosera rotundifolia, Foeniculum vulgare, Glycyrrhiza glabra, Lycopus* spp., *Nepeta cataria, Petroselinum crispum, Pimpinella anisum, Symplocarpus foetidus, Thymus vulgaris, Trigonella foenum-graecum, Tussilago farfara, Verbascum thapsus*
Hepatic	*Verbena officinalis*
Hypnotic	*Eschscholzia californica, Humulus lupulus, Lactuca virosa, Matricaria recutita, Passiflora incarnata, Piper methysticum, Piscidia erythrina, Tilia platyphyllos, Valeriana officinalis*
Hypotensive	*Leonurus cardiaca, Passiflora incarnata, Scutellaria lateriflora, Tilia platyphyllos, Valeriana officinalis*
Nervine relaxant	*Cimicifuga racemosa, Eschscholzia californica, Humulus lupulus, Hypericum perforatum, Hyssopus officinalis, Lactuca virosa, Lavandula* spp., *Leonurus cardiaca, Lobelia inflata, Lycopus* spp., *Matricaria recutita, Melissa officinalis, Mentha piperita, Nepeta cataria, Passiflora incarnata, Piper methysticum, Piscidia erythrina, Prunus serotina, Scutellaria lateriflora, Tilia platyphyllos, Valeriana officinalis, Viburnum opulus, V. prunifolium*
Tonic	*Artemisia vulgaris, Hypericum perforatum, Scutellaria lateriflora, Trigonella foenum-graecum, Turnera diffusa, Tussilago farfara, Verbena officinalis*
Vulnerary	*Nepeta cataria, Hypericum perforatum, Matricaria recutita, Sambucus nigra, Trigonella foenum-graecum, Verbascum thapsus*

Table 25.10. Relative Strengths of Antispasmodic Herbs

STRENGTH	HERBS
Mild	*Anethum graveolens, Angelica archangelica, Carum carvi, Daucus carota, Elettaria cardamomum, Foeniculum vulgare, Glycyrrhiza glabra, Mentha piperita, M. pulegium, Petroselinum crispum, Pimpinella anisum, Rosmarinus officinalis, Salvia officinalis, Sambucus nigra, Trigonella foenum-graecum, Verbascum thapsus*
Moderate	*Apium graveolens, Artemisia vulgaris, Hypericum perforatum, Hyssopus officinalis, Lavandula* spp., *Matricaria recutita, Melissa officinalis, Nepeta cataria, Tilia platyphyllos, Trifolium pratense, Turnera diffusa, Tussilago farfara, Zingiber officinale*
Strong	*Cimicifuga racemosa, Dioscorea villosa, Drosera rotundifolia, Eschscholzia californica, Humulus lupulus, Lactuca virosa, Leonurus cardiaca, Lobelia inflata, Lycopus europaeus, Piper methysticum, Piscidia erythrina, Prunus serotina, Pulsatilla vulgaris, Scutellaria lateriflora, Symplocarpus foetidus, Thymus vulgaris, Valeriana officinalis, Verbena officinalis, Viburnum opulus, V. prunifolium*

ASTRINGENT

If you have ever had a cup of ordinary tea, you have experienced astringency. The tightening of the tissue of the mouth demonstrates the astringent action of the tea plant, *Camellia sinensis*. Astringents are sometimes called *styptics* when applied externally to stop bleeding, or antihemorrhagics when used for internal bleeding.

How Astringents Work

Astringent action is due to a diverse group of complex chemicals, called tannins or gallotannins, that have certain chemical and physical properties in common. All members of this group have phenolic characteristics, are soluble in water, and have molecular weights ranging from 500 to 3,000. There are two groups: derivatives of flavonols called *condensed tannins* and the more important *hydrolyzable tannins*. See chapter 7 for more details on the chemistry of tannins.

The name *tannin* comes from the use of these constituents in the tanning industry. They have the effect of precipitating, or denaturing, protein molecules. They also precipitate starch, gelatin, alkaloids, and salts of heavy metals. One of the few incompatibilities found when making herbal medicines is that astringent, tannin-rich remedies will create precipitates with herbs high in alkaloids.

This alteration of protein is how animal skin is turned into leather. In other words, astringents produce a kind of temporary leather coat on the surface of tissue. Because of this activity, tannins have a number of therapeutic benefits:

Reduce irritation on the surface of tissues through a sort of numbing action.

Reduce surface inflammation.

Create a barrier against infection, which is of great help for wounds and burns.

Astringents have a role in a wide range of problems in many parts of the body, but are of great importance in wound healing and conditions affecting the digestive system. In the gut, they reduce inflammation, improve symptoms of diarrhea, and are widely used in various diseases of digestion. However, long-term use as medicine or too much tea in the diet can be deleterious to health, as this will eventually inhibit proper food absorption across the gut wall.

Herbal Astringents

Acacia catechu (black catechu)
Achillea millefolium (yarrow)
Aesculus hippocastanum (horse chestnut)
Agrimonia eupatoria (agrimony)
Arctostaphylos uva-ursi (bearberry)
Camellia sinensis (tea)
Capsella bursa-pastoris (shepherd's purse)
Cola acuminata (kola)
Equisetum arvense (horsetail)
Euphrasia spp. (eyebright)
Filipendula ulmaria (meadowsweet)
Geranium maculatum (cranesbill)
Hamamelis virginiana (witch hazel)
Inula helenium (elecampane)
Lycopus spp. (bugleweed)
Myrica cerifera (bayberry)
Plantago major (plantain)
Polygonum bistorta (bistort)
Prunus serotina (wild cherry bark)
Quercus spp. (oak)
Rheum palmatum (rhubarb)
Rosmarinus officinalis (rosemary)
Rubus idaeus (raspberry)
R. villosus (blackberry)

Salvia officinalis (sage)
Solidago virgaurea (goldenrod)
Symphytum officinale (comfrey)
Verbascum thapsus (mullein)
Vinca major (periwinkle)

Body System Affinities

As with other actions, certain astringents are particularly suited to specific body systems. Here we shall see which remedies act as astringents for each system.

Cardiovascular. Astringents are rarely needed internally for this system, although they are used externally for bruises that can be seen under the skin. However, certain cardiovascular remedies are also astringents, including *Achillea millefolium*, *Aesculus hippocastanum*, and *Cytisus scoparius*.

Respiratory. The anticatarrhal remedies often also have astringent properties. *Achillea millefolium*, *Capsella bursa-pastoris*, *Hydrastis canadensis*, *Euphrasia* spp., and *Plantago major* are examples.

Digestive. Of many possibilities, here are a few examples of astringents for this system: *Quercus* spp., *Acacia catechu*, *Polygonum bistorta*, *Potentilla erecta*, *Hamamelis virginiana*, *Geranium maculatum*, *Symphytum officinale*, *Filipendula ulmaria*, *Agrimonia eupatoria*, *Hydrastis canadensis*, *Capsella bursa-pastoris*, and *Salvia officinalis*.

Urinary. Many of the astringents already mentioned are useful here, but some specifics are *Equisetum arvense*, *Achillea millefolium*, and *Elymus repens*.

Reproductive. Here we can mention *Geranium maculatum*, *Vinca major*, *Alchemilla arvensis*, and *Hydrastis canadensis*.

Musculoskeletal. Astringency is not often directly relevant in this system.

Nervous. Astringency is also not often directly relevant here.

Skin. Of the many external astringents, or styptics, some examples are *Achillea millefolium*, *Arnica montana*, *Capsella bursa-pastoris*, *Equisetum arvense*, *Hamamelis virginiana*, *Plantago major*, *Quercus* spp., and just about all of the other astringents mentioned above.

Table 25.11. Astringent Herbs and Secondary Actions

SECONDARY ACTION	HERBS
Anticatarrhal	*Achillea millefolium, Arctostaphylos uva-ursi, Euphrasia* spp., *Geranium maculatum, Glechoma hederacea, Inula helenium, Polygonum bistorta, Salvia officinalis, Solidago virgaurea, Verbascum thapsus*
Anti-inflammatory	*Euphrasia* spp., *Filipendula ulmaria, Geranium maculatum, Hamamelis virginiana, Plantago major, Polygonum bistorta, Quercus* spp., *Solidago virgaurea*
Antimicrobial	*Achillea millefolium, Arctostaphylos uva-ursi, Acacia catechu, Inula helenium, Quercus* spp., *Rosmarinus officinalis, Salvia officinalis, Solidago virgaurea*
Antispasmodic	*Lycopus* spp., *Prunus serotina, Rosmarinus officinalis, Salvia officinalis*
Bitter	*Achillea millefolium, Agrimonia eupatoria, Prunus serotina*
Demulcent	*Arctostaphylos uva-ursi, Plantago major, Symphytum officinale, Verbascum thapsus*
Diaphoretic	*Achillea millefolium, Inula helenium, Myrica cerifera, Solidago virgaurea*
Diuretic	*Achillea millefolium, Agrimonia eupatoria, Arctostaphylos uva-ursi, Cola acuminata, Glechoma hederacea, Lycopus* spp., *Plantago major, Solidago virgaurea, Verbascum thapsus*
Emmenagogue	*Achillea millefolium, Rubus idaeus*
Expectorant	*Glechoma hederacea, Inula helenium, Plantago major, Prunus serotina, Symphytum officinale, Verbascum thapsus*
Hepatic	*Agrimonia eupatoria*
Hypotensive	*Achillea millefolium*
Nervine	*Cola acuminata, Prunus serotina, Rosmarinus officinalis*
Tonic	*Achillea millefolium, Agrimonia eupatoria, Rubus idaeus, Verbascum thapsus*
Vulnerary	*Achillea millefolium, Agrimonia eupatoria, Geranium maculatum, Symphytum officinale*

Table 25.12. Relative Strengths of Astringent Herbs

STRENGTH	HERBS
Mild or gentle	*Arctostaphylos uva-ursi, Lycopus* spp., *Plantago major, Pulmonaria officinalis, Rosmarinus officinalis, Salvia officinalis, Solidago virgaurea, Symphytum officinale, Verbascum thapsus*
Moderate	*Achillea millefolium, Aesculus hippocastanum, Capsella bursa-pastoris, Euphrasia* spp., *Filipendula ulmaria, Geranium maculatum, Glechoma hederacea, Hieracium pilosella, Inula helenium, Potentilla erecta, Prunus serotina, Ranunculus ficaria, Rheum palmatum*
Strong	*Acacia catechu, Agrimonia eupatoria, Cola acuminata, Hamamelis virginiana, Myrica cerifera, Polygonum bistorta, Quercus* spp., *Rubus villosus, Vinca major*

BITTER

The bitters are of major importance to the digestive system and to the rest of the body. Quite simply, these are remedies that have a bitter taste. Their broad effects on tone and function offer an opportunity to treat the body as a whole. These herbs can range from mildly bitter remedies, like *Achillea millefolium* and *Taraxacum officinale* leaf, to profoundly distasteful herbs, such as *Ruta graveolens* and *Artemisia absinthium*. It is, of course, the taste of rue and wormwood that has made their names symbolic in our language of extreme distress or woe. I don't think they taste quite that bad!

Bitters have a major role in holistic herbal treatment and especially preventive herbal medicine. Because of their wide effect on the body's physiology, they help enormously in treating the body as an integrated whole.

How Bitters Work

The constituents that contribute bitterness to an herb are usually described as *bitter principles*. A range of molecular structures share the bitter property; that is, they trigger a response in the bitter receptors of the back of the tongue. Examples of such constituents are monoterpenes, iridoids, sesquiterpenes, and alkaloids.

Taste is a phenomenon of chemoreception, limited to the damp area inside the mouth. About 9,000 chemoreceptors, called taste buds, occur on the tongue in groups of 50 to 100 specialized cells. They are found largely on the perimeter of the tongue in adults, but cover the whole tongue in children. Different regions of the tongue respond to the four basic tastes: sweet, salty, sour, and bitter.

Molecules that evoke taste are described as *sapid*, which comes from the Latin *sapere*, meaning "to taste." Sapidity depends upon solubility in water, which allows a molecule to penetrate the taste buds. The sensation of taste occurs when part of a molecule fits into a taste receptor in a specific taste bud. Less is known about the receptors for bitterness than for those for the other tastes.

Absinthin, found in plants of the genus *Artemisia*, such as *A. absinthium*, is so bitter it can be tasted at dilutions of 1:30,000! Great diversity and complexity is found among these bitter principles, but it appears that they all work in a similar way by triggering a sensory response in the mouth. The sensation of bitterness, and no doubt many other taste subtleties, is directed by the nerves to the central nervous system. From there, a message goes to the gut, giving rise to the release of the digestive hormone gastrin. This in turn leads to a whole range of effects, all of value to the digestive process and general bodily health. Among the many actions of bitters, they:

Stimulate appetite. This helps in convalescence and conditions associated with reduced appetite, including depression. Of course, stimulation of appetite is not always desirable!

Stimulate release of digestive juices from the pancreas, duodenum, and liver. This will help in a wide range of problems related to inefficient or allergy-impaired digestion.

Aid the liver in detoxification work and increase the flow of bile. The possibilities here are great, as many health problems have their roots in an overworked liver. This is the apparent value of bitters taken after meals, such as coffee and liqueurs like Chartreuse.

Help regulate secretion of pancreatic hormones that regulate blood sugar, insulin, and glucagon. This means that diabetics should use caution when taking bitters for any reason, as they may upset blood sugar balance. However, in the hands of a skilled practitioner, these remedies may have some relevance in the treatment of late-onset diabetes.

Help the gut wall repair damage by stimulating self-repair mechanisms.

Other effects occur in a much broader way, supporting the healthy activity of the heart and circulation in general. Herbalists have long known about the subtle psychological effects of bitter remedies. They may even have antidepressant actions in some cases, especially after viral infection. Bitters such as *Artemisia vulgaris* and *Gentiana lutea* have a generally tonic effect on consciousness.

The therapeutic ramifications of all of these actions are many. The tonic effects of these remedies go beyond specific digestive hormone activity. As digestion and assimilation of food is basic to health, bitter stimulation can often fundamentally ameliorate an underlying pathology that has nothing to do with the digestive process. In general, these benefits will not occur unless the bitter herb is tasted, so they should not be given in a capsule intended to help the patient avoid the unpleasant taste.

In practice, there appears to be much overlap between bitter and tonic remedies. The mechanism of action of bitters is not always clear, but it is evident that these herbs act to promote health and increase self-healing and resistance—yet another wonderful gift of nature.

Contraindications for Bitters

These mirror the general indications for bitters. For example, in situations for which exocrine gland stimulation is inappropriate, bitters would also be contraindicated, as they may cause inappropriate peristaltic stimulation. Do not use bitters in the following conditions:

Pregnancy
Kidney stones
Gallbladder disease
Dysmenorrhea
Gastroesophageal reflux disease
Hiatus hernia
Gastritis
Peptic ulcer

Herbal Bitters

Achillea millefolium (yarrow)
Artemisia abrotanum (southernwood)
A. absinthium (wormwood)
A. vulgaris (mugwort)
Berberis vulgaris (bearberry)
Centaurium erythraea (centaury)
Eupatorium perfoliatum (boneset)
Gentiana lutea (gentian)
Hydrastis canadensis (goldenseal)
Marrubium vulgare (horehound)
Matricaria recutita (chamomile)
Menyanthes trifoliata (bogbean)
Ruta graveolens (rue)
Tanacetum vulgare (tansy)
Taraxacum officinale (dandelion)

Body System Affinities

Bitters range from mild herbs, including *Matricaria recutita* and *Achillea millefolium*, to quite intense remedies, such as *Artemisia absinthium*, *Gentiana lutea*, and *Ruta graveolens*. Not only do we have a choice of intensity of bitterness, but we also can select bitters based on associated actions and system affinities. By nature of their bitterness, these herbs are widely applicable in a tonic sense. A fair sprinkling of bitter herbs can still be found in official pharmacopoeias.

Cardiovascular. Anything that helps digestion and eases flatulence will take pressure off the heart. Relaxing bitters, such as *Humulus lupulus* and *Valeriana officinalis*, may have a specific role in this system.

Respiratory. Certain bitters have expectorant actions, and in the case of *Marrubium vulgare*, we have an excellent remedy for all chest problems combined with the value of a potent bitter.

Digestive. A wide range of plants can be named here. The following list takes into account the liver and pancreas as organs of the digestive system: *Artemisia vulgaris*, *A. absinthium*, *Berberis vulgaris*, *Centaurium erythraea*, *Chelidonium majus*, *Chelone glabra*, *Gentiana lutea*, *Hydrastis canadensis*, *Humulus lupulus*, *Ruta graveolens*, and *Peumus boldus*.

Urinary. The bitter action is not directly relevant to this system.

Reproductive. Many bitter herbs have the ability to initiate delayed menstrual periods. They may, however, cause some cramping, and must not be used during pregnancy. The following are the most relevant: *Artemisia abrotanum*, *A. absinthium*, *A. vulgaris*, *Ruta graveolens*, and, to a lesser degree because of its mildness, *Achillea millefolium*.

Musculoskeletal. Anything that helps with digestion and assimilation of food will benefit the musculoskeletal system. A bitter that is particularly valuable for this system is *Menyanthes trifoliata*.

Nervous. By stimulating healthy body processes, bitters support the nervous system in cases of depression and general nervous debility. Any bitter can work, but those most often used are *Gentiana lutea*, *Artemisia vulgaris*, and *A. absinthium*.

Skin. Bitters herbs may benefit the skin through an alterative-like cleansing action.

Table 25.13. Bitter Herbs and Secondary Actions

SECONDARY ACTION	HERBS
Anticatarrhal	*Achillea millefolium, Centaurium erythraea, Eupatorium perfoliatum, Hydrastis canadensis, Marrubium vulgare*
Anti-inflammatory	*Achillea millefolium, Artemisia absinthium, Hydrastis canadensis, Matricaria recutita, Menyanthes trifoliata*
Antimicrobial	*Achillea millefolium, Artemisia abrotanum, A. absinthium, A. vulgaris, Hydrastis canadensis, Matricaria recutita*
Antispasmodic	*Marrubium vulgare, Matricaria recutita, Ruta graveolens*
Astringent	*Achillea millefolium, Hydrastis canadensis*
Carminative	*Artemisia abrotanum, A. absinthium, Centaurium erythraea, Matricaria recutita, Tanacetum vulgare*
Cholagogue	*Artemisia abrotanum, A. absinthium, A. vulgaris, Berberis vulgaris, Centaurium erythraea, Gentiana lutea, Hydrastis canadensis, Tanacetum vulgare*
Diaphoretic	*Achillea millefolium, Eupatorium perfoliatum*
Diuretic	*Achillea millefolium*
Emmenagogue	*Achillea millefolium, Artemisia abrotanum, A. absinthium, A. vulgaris, Centaurium erythraea, Gentiana lutea, Hydrastis canadensis, Ruta graveolens, Tanacetum vulgare*
Expectorant	*Marrubium vulgare*
Hepatic	*Achillea millefolium, Artemisia abrotanum, A. absinthium, A. vulgaris, Berberis vulgaris, Centaurium erythraea, Gentiana lutea, Hydrastis canadensis, Ruta graveolens, Tanacetum vulgare*
Laxative	*Berberis vulgaris, Centaurium erythraea, Eupatorium perfoliatum, Gentiana lutea, Hydrastis canadensis*
Nervine	*Artemisia vulgaris, Centaurium erythraea, Matricaria recutita*
Tonic	*Achillea millefolium, Artemisia absinthium, A. vulgaris, Centaurium erythraea, Hydrastis canadensis, Marrubium vulgare, Ruta graveolens*
Vulnerary	*Achillea millefolium, Hydrastis canadensis, Marrubium vulgare, Matricaria recutita*

Table 25.14. Relative Strengths of Bitter Herbs

STRENGTH	HERBS
Mild	*Achillea millefolium, Artemisia abrotanum, A. vulgaris, Matricaria recutita, Taraxacum officinale*
Strong	*Artemisia absinthium, Berberis vulgaris, Centaurium erythraea, Eupatorium perfoliatum, Gentiana lutea, Hydrastis canadensis, Marrubium vulgare, Ruta graveolens, Tanacetum vulgare*

CARDIAC REMEDIES

This is a general category for herbal remedies that have some kind of action on the heart. Some of the remedies in this group are powerful cardioactive agents, such as *Digitalis* (foxglove), while others are gentler and safer cardiotonics, like *Crataegus* (hawthorn) and *Tilia* (linden). As discussed in chapter 9, care must be taken with these terms, as they have different meanings in orthodox and herbal medicine.

Cardiotonic

These are plants that have an observably beneficial action on the heart and blood vessels but do not contain cardiac glycosides. How they work is either completely obscure or an area of pharmacological debate, but flavones appear to be major contributors to their beneficial actions. Examples of traditionally used cardiotonic herbs in Western herbalism are *Crataegus, Tilia platyphyllos, Allium sativum,* and *Leonurus cardiaca.* The diterpene forskolin is the positively inotropic constituent of *Coleus forskohlii,* a cardiotonic herb from India that is gaining increased attention. For more details on the pharmacology of some of these plants, please refer to the discussion in chapter 9.

Cardioactive

These plants owe their effects on the heart to their content of cardiac glycosides, and thus have both the benefits and the drawbacks of these constituents. The main danger is that glycosides will accumulate in the body, as their elimination rates tend to be low. Clinically trained phytotherapists prefer to use *Convallaria majalis* over *Digitalis,* as there is less chance that such problems will develop. However, without appropriate training as to the safe use of *Convallaria,* phytotherapists should avoid the use of this herb too.

Primary Cardiovascular Remedies

Achillea millefolium (yarrow)
Aesculus hippocastanum (horse chestnut)
Allium sativum (garlic)
Capsicum annuum (cayenne)
Coleus forskohlii (coleus)
Convallaria majalis (lily of the valley)
Crataegus spp. (hawthorn)
Cytisus scoparius (broom)
Ginkgo biloba (ginkgo)
Leonurus cardiaca (motherwort)
Lycopus spp. (bugleweed)
Melissa officinalis (lemon balm)
Rosmarinus officinalis (rosemary)
Scrophularia nodosa (figwort)
Tilia platyphyllos (linden)
Urginea maritima (squill)
Zanthoxylum americanum (prickly ash)
Zingiber officinale (ginger)

Body System Affinities

As cardiac remedies are very specific to the cardiovascular system, they are not usually directly relevant to conditions involving other body systems, although they do contribute greatly to general health when indicated. However, many cardiac tonics have other actions, and these are the properties that we will explore here.

Cardiovascular. Primarily cardioactive remedies include *Convallaria majalis* and *Digitalis lanata.* Other plants that mimic this cardioactive effect but do not contain cardiac glycosides include *Cytisus scoparius, Urginea maritima, Scrophularia nodosa,* and *Lycopus* spp. All must be used with caution in order to avoid toxicity problems in heart patients. The primary cardiotonic herbs to consider will be *Crataegus* spp., *Tilia platyphyllos,* and possibly *Coleus forskohlii.* Remedies that specifically benefit blood vessels include *Crataegus* spp., *Tilia platyphyllos, Aesculus hippocastanum, Allium sativum, Ginkgo biloba,* and *Achillea millefolium.*

Respiratory. Any problem with the activity of the heart might have an effect on lung congestion due to a backup of blood waiting to be pumped. Thus, cardiac tonics may benefit the lungs by helping the heart. *Allium sativum* is renowned for its antimicrobial and generally beneficial action on the lungs.

Digestive. A number of cardiac remedies support the function of this system, including *Rosmarinus officinalis, Tilia platyphyllos, Leonurus cardiaca, Achillea millefolium, Angelica archangelica, Allium sativum,* and *Melissa officinalis.*

Urinary. Most of the herbs that have a direct impact on the heart's action also increase the amount of blood that passes through the kidneys, and so act as diuretics.

Achillea millefolium is used in urinary problems, as is *Cytisus scoparius*. Any cardioactive properties must be taken into account, especially with *Cytisus scoparius*.

Reproductive. The cardiac tonics are not directly involved in the function of this system. *Achillea millefolium* may play a role as a gentle emmenagogue.

Musculoskeletal. Herbs that act as circulatory stimulants are important here because they increase peripheral blood flow. This can reduce swelling and ease stiffness. Such herbs include *Capsicum annuum*, *Zingiber officinale*, *Zanthoxylum americanum*, *Brassica* spp., and *Armoracia rusticana*.

Nervous. *Leonurus cardiaca*, *Tilia platyphyllos*, *Melissa officinalis*, and *Rosmarinus officinalis* all have a relaxing effect on the nervous system. As we shall see, many nervines help the circulatory system by relaxing the mind and body as a whole.

Skin. The only directly applicable remedy here is *Scrophularia nodosa*. However, when a skin problem is related to varicosity in veins, cardiac tonics are very important. Herbs that can help include *Crataegus* spp., *Aesculus hippocastanum*, *Achillea millefolium*, and *Tilia platyphyllos*.

CARMINATIVE

Carminatives ease discomfort caused by flatulence. The term *carminative* describes an expected outcome, rather than a specific mechanism of action. However, to a large extent, the mode of action of carminative herbs appears to be related to the complex of volatile oils they contain. These terpene oils have local anti-inflammatory and antispasmodic effects upon the mucous lining and the muscle coats of the alimentary canal. An example is farnesene, a constituent of many complex plant volatile oils with carminative actions, such as *Matricaria recutita*. Volatile oils and their activities are discussed in more depth in chapter 6.

Origanum compactum is a species of oregano used as an antispasmodic remedy for the gastrointestinal tract, especially in Morocco.[4] Belgian researchers have found that the infusion of flowers and leaves inhibits contractions triggered in guinea pig ileum by acetylcholine, histamine, serotonin, nicotine, 1,1-dimethyl-4-phenylpiperazine iodide, and even electrical stimulation. The main active components in the essential oil were identified as thymol and carvacrol. This example may help explain the well-known actions of all of the carminative remedies.

Herbal Carminatives

Allium sativum (garlic)
Anethum graveolens (dill)
Angelica archangelica (angelica)
Apium graveolens (celery seed)
Artemisia absinthium (wormwood)
Carum carvi (caraway)
Cinnamomum spp. (cinnamon)
Elettaria cardamomum (cardamom)
Eucalyptus globulus (eucalyptus)
Foeniculum vulgare (fennel)
Gaultheria procumbens (wintergreen)
Humulus lupulus (hops)
Juniperus communis (juniper)
Leonurus cardiaca (motherwort)
Matricaria recutita (chamomile)
Melissa officinalis (lemon balm)
Mentha piperita (peppermint)
M. pulegium (pennyroyal)
Petroselinum crispum (parsley)
Pimpinella anisum (aniseed)
Salvia officinalis (sage)
Thymus spp. (thyme)
Valeriana officinalis (valerian)
Zingiber officinale (ginger)

Body System Affinities

By the nature of their actions, carminatives work on the gut, and thus may have more generalized effects on other body systems. As carminative actions are due largely to volatile oil content, some of these oils have quite specific effects on other parts of the body.

Cardiovascular. Carminatives may ease apparent cardiac symptoms by eliminating the pressure of flatulence and digestive pain. While most of the carminatives have no action on this system at all, volatile oils of the following herbs do have cardiovascular effects: *Allium sativum*, *Capsicum annuum*, *Leonurus cardiaca*, *Matricaria recutita*, *Melissa officinalis*, and *Zingiber officinale*.

Respiratory. Many carminative herbs support this system through antispasmodic, antimicrobial, or anticatarrhal actions. These include *Allium sativum*, *Angelica archangelica*, *Brassica* spp., *Eucalyptus* spp., *Mentha piperita*, *Pimpinella anisum*, *Salvia officinalis*, and *Thymus vulgaris*.

Digestive. As carminatives act specifically on the digestive tract, the list of herbs appropriate for this system is extremely long. All of the herbs listed as carminatives may be relevant.

Urinary. Because of their volatile oil content, some carminatives act as diuretics and may even irritate the kidneys. Prime examples are *Juniperus communis* and *Eucalyptus* spp.

Reproductive. Again, some volatile oils have effects upon the female reproductive system. A problematic example is *Mentha pulegium*, a plant whose oil can prove damaging to the reproductive system. However, as will be discussed in chapter 26, the whole herb does not pose the same dangers as the essential oil.

Musculoskeletal. *Apium graveolens* is a carminative that is also a specific anti-inflammatory for this system. Others include *Angelica archangelica* and *Gaultheria procumbens*.

Nervous. Many volatile oil–containing remedies will soothe the nervous system. These include *Valeriana officinalis*, *Matricaria recutita*, *Humulus lupulus*, and *Melissa officinalis*.

Skin. Carminatives may be relevant to the skin in that they support digestion and metabolism in general. In some cases, a carminative herb will be good for the skin because the plant or its oils also have other effects. An example is the antimicrobial *Thymus vulgaris*, which can be useful when applied topically for its antiseptic properties.

Table 25.15. Carminative Herbs and Secondary Actions

SECONDARY ACTION	HERBS
Alterative	*Allium sativum*
Anticatarrhal	*Allium sativum, Eucalyptus* spp., *Matricaria recutita, Mentha piperita, Salvia officinalis, Thymus vulgaris*
Anti-inflammatory	*Angelica archangelica, Apium graveolens, Artemisia absinthium, Gaultheria procumbens, Matricaria recutita, Melissa officinalis, Mentha piperita*
Antimicrobial	*Allium sativum, Artemisia absinthium, Eucalyptus* spp., *Humulus lupulus, Juniperus communis, Matricaria recutita, Mentha piperita, Pimpinella anisum, Salvia officinalis, Thymus vulgaris*
Antispasmodic	*Allium sativum, Anethum graveolens, Angelica archangelica, Artemisia absinthium, Carum carvi, Eucalyptus* spp., *Leonurus cardiaca, Matricaria recutita, Melissa officinalis, Mentha piperita, Pimpinella anisum, Salvia officinalis, Thymus vulgaris, Valeriana officinalis*

SECONDARY ACTION	HERBS
Astringent	*Carum carvi, Cinnamomum* spp., *Gaultheria procumbens, Humulus lupulus, Salvia officinalis, Thymus vulgaris*
Bitter	*Artemisia absinthium, Humulus lupulus, Matricaria recutita*
Diaphoretic	*Allium sativum, Angelica archangelica, Melissa officinalis, Mentha piperita, M. pulegium, Zingiber officinale*
Diuretic	*Angelica archangelica, Apium graveolens, Brassica* spp., *Gaultheria procumbens, Juniperus communis, Petroselinum crispum*
Emmenagogue	*Carum carvi, Gaultheria procumbens, Leonurus cardiaca, Mentha pulegium, Petroselinum crispum*
Expectorant	*Angelica archangelica, Carum carvi, Eucalyptus* spp., *Petroselinum crispum, Pimpinella anisum, Thymus vulgaris*
Galactagogue	*Anethum graveolens, Carum carvi, Eucalyptus* spp., *Gaultheria procumbens*
Hypotensive	*Allium sativum, Melissa officinalis, Valeriana officinalis*
Nervine	*Apium graveolens, Humulus lupulus, Leonurus cardiaca, Matricaria recutita, Melissa officinalis, Mentha piperita, Valeriana officinalis*
Rubefacient	*Allium sativum, Brassica* spp., *Eucalyptus* spp., *Juniperus communis, Petroselinum crispum*
Tonic	*Allium sativum, Artemisia absinthium, Matricaria recutita*
Vulnerary	*Matricaria recutita*

CHOLAGOGUE

Cholagogues have the specific effect of stimulating the flow of bile from the liver. Orthodox pharmacology differentiates between direct cholagogues, which actually increase the amount of secreted bile, and indirect cholagogues, which simply increase the amount of bile being released by the gallbladder. This distinction is not very important in herbal practice, especially as we are not going to use purified ox bile (a cholagogue used in supplements that was official in the eleventh U.S. National Formulary).

By nature of the action, cholagogues are quite specific in that they act on the liver. In general, however, they function as body tonics. The secretion of bile is of great help to the whole digestive and assimilative process. After all, "we are what we digest" just much as "we are what we eat." The role of bile is partially to facilitate fat digestion, but also to act as a natural laxative and thus cleanse the system. Without exploring the vast complexities of liver function, it is worth noting that bile formation and flow are fundamental to it all. Thus, the value of these herbs goes far beyond the simple release of bile. They help ensure a strong and healthy liver and so enliven the whole being. Most bitters and hepatics are also cholagogues.

Indications for Cholagogues

Long-term maintenance of dyskinesia of the bile duct, to stimulate normal contractions to deliver bile to the small intestine.

Disorders caused by insufficient or congested bile, such as intractable biliary constipation, jaundice, and mild hepatitis.

Symptoms of indigestion, to aid in the digestion of fat-soluble substances.

To support the liver's detoxification work.

Contraindications for Cholagogues

Painful gallstones. Increased contractile activity could further constrict the bile duct, leading to incredibly intense pain.

Acute bilious colic.

Obstructive jaundice, for the same reasons as painful gallstones.

Acute cholecystitis, unless gallstones have been ruled out. Cholecystitis can be caused by infection, but the cause must be determined before a cholagogue is used.

Acute viral hepatitis.

Extremely toxic liver disorders. A cholagogue may be too stressful for a liver that is severely damaged; but this must be weighed against the potential benefit to be derived.

Herbal Cholagogues

Baptisia tinctoria (wild indigo)
Berberis vulgaris (barberry)
Chelidonium majus (celandine)
Chelone glabra (balmony)
Chionanthus virginicus (fringetree)
Cynara scolymus (artichoke)
Dioscorea villosa (wild yam)

Euonymus atropurpureus (wahoo)
Eupatorium perfoliatum (boneset)
Fumaria officinalis (fumitory)
Gentiana lutea (gentian)
Hydrastis canadensis (goldenseal)
Iris versicolor (blue flag)
Juglans cinerea (butternut)
Leptandra virginica (black root)
Mahonia aquifolium (Oregon grape)
Melissa officinalis (lemon balm)
Peumus boldus (boldo)
Rosmarinus officinalis (rosemary)
Rumex crispus (yellow dock)
Salvia officinalis (sage)
Taraxacum officinale root (dandelion)

Body System Affinities

Cardiovascular. The value of cholagogues in this system comes through general improvement of body function. However, only when a cholagogue has additional diuretic actions can any direct claims be made for this system.

Respiratory. Certain cholagogues are also antimicrobial and anticatarrhal and in this way benefit the whole system. Some are also mucous membrane tonics, including *Eupatorium perfoliatum, Hydrastis canadensis, Rosmarinus officinalis, Salvia officinalis,* and *Baptisia tinctoria.*

Digestive. Here we have a long list that includes *Cynara scolymus, Melissa officinalis, Berberis vulgaris, Leptandra virginica, Iris versicolor, Peumus boldus, Juglans cinerea, Taraxacum officinale* root, *Chionanthus virginicus* bark, *Gentiana lutea, Chelidonium majus, Euonymus atropurpureus,* and *Dioscorea villosa.*

Urinary. Cholagogues confer only indirect benefits to this system. However, *Taraxacum officinale* root is partially diuretic in action, although weaker than the leaves. *Eupatorium perfoliatum* can be an effective diuretic in feverish conditions.

Reproductive. Cholagogue remedies such as *Hydrastis canadensis* and *Berberis vulgaris* have a marked action on the muscles of the uterus, as they are strong bitters. *Rosmarinus officinalis* has a tonic and emmenagogue action, while most bitters stimulate the womb or menstrual activity.

Musculoskeletal. Cholagogues help in this system by generally supporting the body's metabolic activity.

Nervous. Because they help with assimilation, cholagogues have an enlivening "side effect" in the nervous system. These remedies may actively ease debility and depression. *Rosmarinus officinalis* is a nervine.

Skin. Taken internally, cholagogues often aid in cleansing the body and so may help clear skin problems. Examples are *Iris versicolor*, *Taraxacum officinale*, *Fumaria officinalis*, *Hydrastis canadensis*, *Mahonia aquifolium*, and *Rumex crispus*. *Hydrastis canadensis* may also be of use externally.

Table 25.16. Cholagogues and Secondary Actions

SECONDARY ACTION	HERBS
Alterative	*Baptisia tinctoria, Chionanthus virginicus, Hydrastis canadensis, Iris versicolor, Mahonia aquifolium, Rumex crispus*
Anticatarrhal	*Baptisia tinctoria, Eupatorium perfoliatum, Hydrastis canadensis*
Anti-inflammatory	*Berberis vulgaris, Dioscorea villosa, Fumaria officinalis, Hydrastis canadensis, Iris versicolor, Rosmarinus officinalis*
Antimicrobial	*Baptisia tinctoria, Berberis vulgaris, Chelidonium majus, Hydrastis canadensis, Mahonia aquifolium, Rosmarinus officinalis, Salvia officinalis*
Antispasmodic	*Dioscorea villosa, Leptandra virginica, Rosmarinus officinalis, Salvia officinalis*
Astringent	*Rosmarinus officinalis, Salvia officinalis*
Bitter	*Baptisia tinctoria, Berberis vulgaris, Chelone glabra, Cynara scolymus, Euonymus atropurpureus, Eupatorium perfoliatum, Fumaria officinalis, Gentiana lutea, Hydrastis canadensis, Juglans cinerea, Mahonia aquifolium, Peumus boldus, Taraxacum officinale root*
Diaphoretic	*Berberis vulgaris, Dioscorea villosa, Eupatorium perfoliatum, Rosmarinus officinalis*
Diuretic	*Chionanthus virginicus, Euonymus atropurpureus, Eupatorium perfoliatum, Fumaria officinalis, Iris versicolor, Peumus boldus*
Emmenagogue	*Baptisia tinctoria, Berberis vulgaris, Chelone glabra, Cynara scolymus, Euonymus atropurpureus, Eupatorium perfoliatum, Fumaria officinalis, Gentiana lutea, Hydrastis canadensis, Juglans cinerea, Mahonia aquifolium, Peumus boldus, Rosmarinus officinalis, Taraxacum officinale root*

SECONDARY ACTION	HERBS
Laxative	All cholagogues to some degree, especially *Juglans cinerea, Taraxacum officinale* root, *Rumex crispus*
Nervine	*Rosmarinus officinalis*
Tonic	*Chelone glabra, Chionanthus virginicus, Eupatorium perfoliatum, Gentiana lutea, Hydrastis canadensis, Iris versicolor, Peumus boldus, Rumex crispus, Taraxacum officinale* root
Vulnerary	*Hydrastis canadensis*

Table 25.17. Relative Strengths of Cholagogues

STRENGTH	HERBS
Mild	*Chelone glabra, Chionanthus virginicus, Cynara scolymus, Dioscorea villosa, Euonymus atropurpureus, Eupatorium perfoliatum, Fumaria officinalis, Leptandra virginica, Peumus boldus, Rosmarinus officinalis, Rumex crispus, Salvia officinalis, Taraxacum officinale* root
Strong	*Baptisia tinctoria, Berberis vulgaris, Chelidonium majus, Gentiana lutea, Hydrastis canadensis, Iris versicolor, Juglans cinerea, Mahonia aquifolium*

DEMULCENT

Demulcent herbs are rich in mucilage and can soothe and protect irritated or inflamed internal tissue. When used topically on the skin, demulcents are called emollients.

As with many other herbal actions, pharmacology does not provide an adequate explanation for how demulcents work. They are rich in carbohydrate mucilage made up of complex polysaccharide molecules. Thus, they become slimy and gummy when they come in contact with water. This physical property has a clear and direct action on the lining of the intestines, where it soothes and reduces irritation by direct contact.

However, some demulcents have similar actions far from the site of their absorption into the body—for example, the urinary tract or lungs. Clearly, these remedies do not work through a direct action, because the mucilage breaks down into its constituent parts as it is absorbed, and thus cannot soothe by direct contact with the target tissue. However, there is no doubt that some herbs do act as demulcents to the urinary tract or lungs—it is simply unclear how they do so.

In general, all mucilage-containing demulcents have the following general properties:

Reduce irritation down the whole length of the bowel.
Lessen the sensitivity of the digestive system to gastric acids and to digestive bitters.
Help prevent diarrhea.
Reduce digestive muscle spasms that cause colic.
Ease coughing by soothing bronchial tension.
Relax painful spasms in the bladder and urinary system, and sometimes even in the uterus.

Herbal Demulcents

Althaea officinalis (marshmallow)
Avena sativa (oat)
Cetraria islandica (Iceland moss)
Chondrus crispus (Irish moss)
Elymus repens (couch grass)
Glycyrrhiza glabra (licorice)
Linum usitatissimum (flax)
Malva sylvestris (mallow)
Symphytum officinale (comfrey)
Tussilago farfara (coltsfoot)
Ulmus rubra (slippery elm)
Verbascum thapsus (mullein)
Zea mays (cornsilk)

Body System Affinities

Cardiovascular. *Tilia platyphyllos* and *Aesculus hippocastanum* have a soothing action on blood vessels.

Respiratory. Many plants soothe inflammation in the chest, throat and sinuses, including *Inula helenium*, *Symphytum officinale*, *Verbascum thapsus*, *Tussilago farfara*, *Solidago virgaurea*, *Althaea officinalis* root, *Glycyrrhiza glabra*, and *Pulmonaria officinalis*.

Digestive. Numerous plants can be used here, especially *Symphytum officinale*, *Althaea officinalis*, *Cetraria islandica*, *Chondrus crispus*, *Glycyrrhiza glabra*, *Linum usitatissimum*, and *Ulmus rubra*. These remedies can be applied freely whenever a soothing demulcent is indicated.

Urinary. Excellent kidney and bladder demulcents are *Elymus repens* and *Petroselinum crispum*.

Reproductive. There are many tonic and anti-inflammatory remedies for this system, but no real demulcents.

Musculoskeletal. Vulneraries and anti-inflammatories have a more direct value in this system than demulcents as such. The undeniable value of *Symphytum officinale* here is related to its vulnerary properties.

Nervous. Demulcents are of direct value in this system only when applied to the skin, as in shingles. However, skin tonics may be thought of as "surrogate" demulcents, especially *Avena sativa*.

Skin. The emollient herbs are all demulcent, including *Symphytum officinale*, *Althaea officinalis*, *Plantago major*, *Stellaria media*, *Ulmus rubra*, and *Linum usitatissimum*.

Table 25.18. Demulcent Herbs and Secondary Actions

SECONDARY ACTION	HERBS
Anticatarrhal	*Tussilago farfara, Verbascum thapsus*
Anti-inflammatory	*Althaea officinalis, Glycyrrhiza glabra, Malva sylvestris, Symphytum officinale, Tussilago farfara, Ulmus rubra, Verbascum thapsus*
Antimicrobial	*Elymus repens*
Antispasmodic	*Tussilago farfara, Glycyrrhiza glabra, Malva sylvestris, Verbascum thapsus*
Astringent	*Althaea officinalis, Malva sylvestris, Symphytum officinale, Tussilago farfara, Ulmus rubra*
Diaphoretic	*Verbascum thapsus*
Diuretic	*Althaea officinalis, Elymus repens, Tussilago farfara, Verbascum thapsus, Zea mays*
Expectorant	*Chondrus crispus, Glycyrrhiza glabra, Malva sylvestris, Symphytum officinale, Tussilago farfara, Verbascum thapsus*
Laxative	*Glycyrrhiza glabra, Linum usitatissimum*
Tonic	*Glycyrrhiza glabra, Tussilago farfara, Verbascum thapsus, Zea mays*
Vulnerary	*Althaea officinalis, Malva sylvestris, Symphytum officinale, Tussilago farfara, Verbascum thapsus*

DIURETIC

Diuretics are agents that help the body rid itself of excess fluids by increasing the kidneys' rate of urine production. The accumulation of excess fluids in tissues, known as edema, is symptomatic of a wide range of heart, kidney, liver, and other disorders. The underlying causes of such disorders must be addressed, but diuretics may help when used in conjunction with other herbs.

Many diuretics alter the excretion of electrolytes by the kidneys. An electrolyte is a chemical that, when dissolved in a suitable solvent, forms a medium that conducts an electric current. Electrolytes, including sodium and potassium salts, are involved in many body processes, such as the regulation of blood pressure, nerve impulse transmission, and muscle contraction.

Strictly speaking, a diuretic is a remedy that increases the secretion and elimination of urine from the body. In the ancient traditions of herbal medicine, the term *diuretic* tends to be applied more broadly to herbs that have some sort of beneficial action on the urinary system. Thus, the term may be used to describe not only true diuretics, but also urinary demulcents and anti-inflammatory remedies. Needless to say, this can lead to confusion when selecting remedies for a particular individual. In general, diuretics have a vital role to play in any holistic treatment of illness, as they help the body eliminate waste and support the whole process of inner cleansing. Many diaphoretic herbs act as diuretics when taken cold.

There are number of ways to categorize diuretics, but first, an important distinction must be made between two broad groups of plant diuretics:

- Plants that act as diuretics by increasing kidney blood flow
- Plants that reduce water reabsorption in the nephrons of the kidney

The first group of herbs includes not only diuretics like *Cytisus scoparius*, but also all cardioactive and circulatory stimulant herbs. These increase blood flow to the kidney through effects on the heart or other parts of the body. Because more blood passes through the kidney, more urine is produced. Caffeine-containing herbs, such as tea and coffee, also have this effect.

The second group may work via many different means, but as is often the case with medicinal plants, a dearth of research in this area limits the value of taking an overtly pharmacological perspective.

Types of Diuretics

As mentioned, in addition to herbs that have a straightforward diuretic impact, other so-called diuretics benefit the urinary system through very different actions. We can reduce inflammation through the use of urinary demulcents and anti-inflammatories and treat infection directly with antimicrobial diuretics. Similarly, if urinary tract problems are associated with stone formation, plants known as *antilithics* can help. These are discussed in chapter 17.

True Herbal Diuretics

Achillea millefolium (yarrow)
Agathosma betulina (buchu)
Agrimonia eupatoria (agrimony)
Apium graveolens (celery seed)
Arctium lappa (burdock)
Arctostaphylos uva-ursi (bearberry)
Cola acuminata (kola)
Collinsonia canadensis (stoneroot)
Convallaria majalis (lily of the valley)
Crataegus spp. (hawthorn)
Cucurbita pepo (pumpkin)
Cytisus scoparius (Scotch broom)
Daucus carota (wild carrot)
Equisetum arvense (horsetail)
Eryngium maritimum (sea holly)
Eupatorium perfoliatum (boneset)
E. purpureum (gravel root)
Galium aparine (cleavers)
Iris versicolor (blue flag)
Juniperus communis (juniper)
Parietaria judaica (pellitory of the wall)
Petroselinum crispum (parsley)
Peumus boldus (boldo)
Sambucus nigra (elder)
Serenoa repens (saw palmetto)
Taraxacum officinale (dandelion)
Tilia platyphyllos (linden)
Zea mays (corn silk)

Table 25.19. Types of Diuretics

ACTION	HERBS
Anti-inflammatory	*Apium graveolens, Arctostaphylos uva-ursi, Eupatorium purpureum, Galium aparine, Zea mays*
Antilithic	*Collinsonia canadensis, Eupatorium purpureum*
Antimicrobial	*Achillea millefolium, Arctostaphylos uva-ursi, Agathosma betulina, Juniperus communis*
Astringent	*Achillea millefolium, Agrimonia eupatoria, Arctostaphylos uva-ursi, Equisetum arvense, Cytisus scoparius, Cola acuminata*
Demulcent	*Arctostaphylos uva-ursi, Collinsonia canadensis, Zea mays*

Body System Affinities

Cardiovascular. As already noted, cardioactive remedies have a diuretic effect because they increase blood flow through the kidneys. All diuretics that help remove water from the body can be of benefit for the cardiovascular system, including *Convallaria majalis, Cytisus scoparius, Taraxacum officinale,* and *Achillea millefolium.* Care should be taken to ensure that the right herb is used for the specific condition. For example, *Cytisus scoparius* should not be used in people with high blood pressure.

Respiratory. If chest congestion is related to heart problems, most of the diuretics will be of value. Remedies with an affinity for this system include *Eupatorium perfoliatum, Galium aparine, Sambucus nigra, Achillea millefolium,* and *Eucalyptus* spp.

Digestive. Some laxative herbs also act as diuretics. Here we can mention *Agrimonia eupatoria, Iris versicolor, Peumus boldus, Apium graveolens, Taraxacum officinale,* and *Petroselinum crispum.*

Urinary. All of the remedies listed here are applicable to this system.

Reproductive. Antiseptic diuretics often have similar effects in the reproductive system. Of special relevance is *Arctostaphylos uva-ursi. Serenoa repens* is a mild diuretic.

Musculoskeletal. Because of their cleansing actions, many diuretics help with problems of muscles and bones. *Eupatorium perfoliatum, Apium graveolens, Achillea millefolium,* and *Eupatorium purpureum* are a few examples.

Nervous. *Lycopus* spp. is the only true diuretic that benefits the nervous system directly. However, if there is much tension, a relaxing nervine may allow the passage of more urine.

Skin. All of the diuretics can potentially help the skin through inner cleansing actions. Especially important are *Galium aparine, Elymus repens,* and *Taraxacum officinale.*

Table 25.20. Diuretics and Secondary Actions

SECONDARY ACTION	HERBS
Alterative	*Arctium lappa, Galium aparine, Iris versicolor*
Anticatarrhal	*Eupatorium perfoliatum, Sambucus nigra*
Anti-inflammatory	*Apium graveolens, Eupatorium purpureum, Galium aparine, Iris versicolor*
Antimicrobial	*Achillea millefolium, Agathosma betulina, Arctostaphylos uva-ursi, Elymus repens, Juniperus communis, Serenoa repens*
Astringent	*Achillea millefolium, Agrimonia eupatoria, Arctostaphylos uva-ursi, Cola acuminata, Cytisus scoparius, Galium aparine, Lycopus* spp.
Bitter	*Agrimonia eupatoria*
Cardioactive	*Convallaria majalis, Cytisus scoparius, Lycopus* spp.
Demulcent	*Alchemilla vulgaris, Arctostaphylos uva-ursi, Collinsonia canadensis, Elymus repens, Parietaria diffusa, Zea mays*
Diaphoretic	*Achillea millefolium, Eupatorium perfoliatum, Sambucus nigra, Tilia platyphyllos*
Emmenagogue	*Achillea millefolium, Petroselinum crispum*
Expectorant	*Petroselinum crispum, Sambucus nigra*
Hepatic	*Iris versicolor, Peumus boldus*
Hypotensive	*Achillea millefolium, Crataegus* spp., *Tilia platyphyllos*
Laxative	*Iris versicolor, Eupatorium perfoliatum*
Nervine	*Apium graveolens, Cola acuminata, Lycopus* spp., *Tilia platyphyllos*
Tonic	*Agathosma betulina, Agrimonia eupatoria, Eupatorium perfoliatum, Galium aparine, Taraxacum officinale* leaf

Table 25.21. Relative Strengths of Herbal Diuretics

STRENGTH	HERBS
Mild	*Arctium lappa, Crataegus* spp., *Iris versicolor, Peumus boldus, Serenoa repens, Tilia platyphyllos*
Moderate	*Agrimonia eupatoria, Cola acuminata, Collinsonia canadensis, Convallaria majalis, Cucurbita pepo, Lycopus* spp., *Sambucus nigra, Zea mays*
Strong	*Achillea millefolium, Agathosma betulina, Alchemilla vulgaris , Apium graveolens, Arctostaphylos uva-ursi, Cytisus scoparius, Daucus carota, Elymus repens, Galium aparine, Eryngium maritimum, Eupatorium perfoliatum, E. purpureum, Juniperus communis, Parietaria diffusa, Petroselinum crispum, Taraxacum officinale*

EMMENAGOGUE

The term *emmenagogue* is widely used to describe plants that are used to treat conditions of the female reproductive system. It has come to imply, almost by default, any remedy with some kind of effect on the function or tissue of the reproductive system. Strictly speaking, however, emmenagogues are remedies that stimulate menstrual flow and activity.

Herbal Emmenagogues

Achillea millefolium (yarrow)
Artemisia abrotanum (southernwood)
A. absinthium (wormwood)
A. vulgaris (mugwort)
Calendula officinalis (calendula)
Caulophyllum thalictroides (blue cohosh)
Cimicifuga racemosa (black cohosh)
Gentiana lutea (gentian)
Hydrastis canadensis (goldenseal)
Hyssopus officinalis (hyssop)
Lavandula spp. (lavender)
Leonurus cardiaca (motherwort)
Marrubium vulgare (horehound)
Marsdenia condurango (condurango)
Matricaria recutita (chamomile)
Mentha piperita (peppermint)
M. pulegium (pennyroyal)
Mitchella repens (partridgeberry)
Petroselinum crispum (parsley)
Phytolacca americana (poke)
Pulsatilla vulgaris (pasqueflower)
Rosmarinus officinalis (rosemary)
Rubus idaeus (raspberry)
Ruta graveolens (rue)
Salvia officinalis (sage)
Tanacetum parthenium (feverfew)
T. vulgare (tansy)
Thymus vulgaris (thyme)
Tilia platyphyllos (linden)
Trigonella foenum-graecum (fenugreek)
Tropaeolum majus (nasturtium)
Valeriana officinalis (valerian)
Verbena officinalis (vervain)
Viburnum opulus (cramp bark)
V. prunifolium (black haw)
Vitex agnus-castus (chasteberry)
Zingiber officinale (ginger)

Today, most herbals use the term *emmenagogue* broadly, to denote remedies that tone and normalize the function of the female reproductive system. Such a loose definition has little meaning, as it obscures the specific benefits these herbs offer. Emmenagogues provide a whole range of distinct actions with either direct or indirect benefits for the reproductive system. To clarify this situation, the next section groups some of the more toning "emmenagogues" in terms of their main impact on the menstrual process. Remember that all bitters have an emmenagogue effect in the strict sense of the word.

Uterine Tonics

These are plants that have a toning, strengthening, nourishing effect upon both the tissue and the function of the female reproductive system. We do not have a good understanding of how and why they work, but this should not belittle their remarkable therapeutic value. Determining differential indications for these herbs is one of the most confused areas in modern herbalism.

Uterine Tonic Herbs

Caulophyllum thalictroides (blue cohosh)
Cimicifuga racemosa (black cohosh)
Mitchella repens (partridgeberry)
Rubus idaeus (raspberry leaf)

Herbs That Stimulate Menstruation

Of the many plants that stimulate the menstrual process, some also have a tonic effect. Simply triggering menstruation implies nothing more than that. Of the emmenagogues listed here, some work through bitter stimulation and others through localized irritation. These herbs will also nourish the system to some degree.

True Emmenagogues

Achillea millefolium (yarrow)
Artemisia vulgaris (mugwort)
Mitchella repens (partridgeberry)

Hormonal Normalizers

Many claims might be made about plants that affect hormonal balance, but we will limit our discussion here to those that have an observable influence. Little endocrinological research has been undertaken on these herbs, so it is impossible to be specific about their actions. Thus, the herbalist usually talks in terms of *hormonal modulator* or *hormonal normalizers*.

The most important of these herbs in the European tradition is *Vitex agnus-castus*. It is appropriate to describe this plant as a normalizer, as it seems to bring the body back to normal function no matter which female sex hormone is deficient or in excess. The uterine tonics and bitters may have some similar effects because of their general toning abilities, but none is as dependable as *Vitex agnus-castus*.

Hormonal Normalizing Herbs

Bitter tonics
Uterine tonics
Vitex agnus-castus

Uterine Astringents

A number of herbs can reduce blood loss from the uterus, whether related to menorrhagia (excessive menstrual bleeding), metrorrhagia (bleeding between periods), or organic disease, such as fibroids. How these herbs work is an important but unanswered question. No astringent tannin can reach uterine tissue from the gut. It is possible that some, but not all, of these herbs have some kind of hormonal effect. Of the many valuable remedies listed as astringents earlier in this chapter, the most toning for the uterus is *Achillea millefolium*.

Important Uterine Astringents

Achillea millefolium (yarrow)
Alchemilla arvense (lady's mantle)
Capsella bursa-pastoris (shepherd's purse)
Geranium maculatum (cranesbill)
Vinca major (periwinkle)

Uterine Demulcents

Just as with uterine astringents, it is unclear how uterine demulcents reach the uterus. There is no way that mucopolysaccharides can find their way to the uterus from the digestive system; nonetheless, there is no question that these remedies soothe inflamed tissue in the uterus. The most important of these herbs is *Caulophyllum thalictroides*.

Nervines and Antispasmodics

There are a number of valuable remedies that impact the complex autonomic innervation of the reproductive system. The appropriate nervine or antispasmodic remedy can go a long way toward correcting functional tone.

Uterine Nervines and Antispasmodic Herbs

Cimicifuga racemosa (black cohosh)
Leonurus cardiaca (motherwort)
Pulsatilla vulgaris (pasqueflower)
Viburnum opulus (cramp bark)
V. prunifolium (black haw)

Table 25.22. Emmenagogues and Secondary Actions

SECONDARY ACTION	HERBS
Anticatarrhal	*Achillea millefolium, Hydrastis canadensis, Hyssopus officinalis, Lavandula* spp., *Matricaria recutita, Mentha piperita, Rosmarinus officinalis, Thymus vulgaris*
Anti-inflammatory	*Calendula officinalis, Caulophyllum thalictroides, Lavandula* spp., *Matricaria recutita, Mentha piperita, Tanacetum parthenium, Thymus vulgaris*
Antimicrobial	*Achillea millefolium, Artemisia abrotanum, A. absinthium, Matricaria recutita, Rosmarinus officinalis, Salvia officinalis, Tanacetum vulgare, Thymus vulgaris, Tropaeolum majus*
Antispasmodic	*Calendula officinalis, Caulophyllum thalictroides, Cimicifuga racemosa, Hyssopus officinalis, Lavandula* spp., *Leonurus cardiaca, Matricaria recutita, Mentha piperita, Rosmarinus officinalis, Thymus vulgaris, Tilia platyphyllos, Valeriana officinalis, Verbena officinalis, Viburnum opulus*
Alterative	*Cimicifuga racemosa*
Astringent	*Achillea millefolium, Artemisia absinthium, Hydrastis canadensis, Mitchella repens, Rubus idaeus, Salvia officinalis, Thymus vulgaris, Tilia platyphyllos, Viburnum opulus*
Carminative	*Artemisia abrotanum, A. absinthium, A. vulgaris, Gentiana lutea, Hyssopus officinalis, Lavandula* spp., *Matricaria recutita, Mentha piperita, Petroselinum crispum, Rosmarinus officinalis, Ruta graveolens, Salvia officinalis, Tanacetum parthenium, T. vulgare, Thymus vulgaris, Tropaeolum majus, Valeriana officinalis, Zingiber officinale*
Bitter	*Achillea millefolium, Artemisia abrotanum, A. absinthium, Gentiana lutea, Hydrastis canadensis, Marrubium vulgare, Matricaria recutita, Ruta graveolens, Tanacetum parthenium, T. vulgare, Tropaeolum majus*
Demulcent	*Trigonella foenum-graecum*
Diaphoretic	*Achillea millefolium, Hyssopus officinalis, Mentha piperita, M. pulegium, Tilia platyphyllos, Zingiber officinale*
Diuretic	*Achillea millefolium, Mitchella repens, Petroselinum crispum, Tilia platyphyllos*

SECONDARY ACTION	HERBS
Expectorant	*Hyssopus officinalis, Marrubium vulgare, Petroselinum crispum, Thymus vulgaris, Trigonella foenum-graecum*
Hepatic	*Achillea millefolium, Artemisia abrotanum, A. absinthium, Calendula officinalis, Gentiana lutea, Ruta graveolens, Verbena officinalis*
Hypotensive	*Achillea millefolium, Lavandula spp., Valeriana officinalis*
Laxative	*Hydrastis canadensis*
Nervine	*Artemisia vulgaris, Cimicifuga racemosa, Hyssopus officinalis, Lavandula spp., Leonurus cardiaca, Matricaria recutita, Mentha piperita, Rosmarinus officinalis, Tilia platyphyllos, Valeriana officinalis, Verbena officinalis*
Tonic	*Achillea millefolium, Artemisia absinthium, A. vulgaris, Caulophyllum thalictroides, Gentiana lutea, Hydrastis canadensis, Leonurus cardiaca, Matricaria recutita, Mitchella repens, Rubus idaeus, Trigonella foenum-graecum, Tropaeolum majus, Verbena officinalis, Vitex agnus-castus*
Vulnerary	*Achillea millefolium, Artemisia absinthium, Calendula officinalis, Hydrastis canadensis, Matricaria recutita*

Table 25.23. Relative Strengths of True Emmenagogues

STRENGTH	HERBS
Mild	*Achillea millefolium, Calendula officinalis, Hyssopus officinalis, Lavandula spp., Leonurus cardiaca, Matricaria recutita, Mentha piperita, Petroselinum crispum, Pulsatilla vulgaris, Rosmarinus officinalis, Salvia officinalis, Thymus vulgaris, Tilia platyphyllos, Trigonella foenum-graecum, Valeriana officinalis, Verbena officinalis, Viburnum opulus, V. prunifolium*
Moderate	*Caulophyllum thalictroides, Cimicifuga racemosa, Mentha pulegium, Mitchella repens, Rubus idaeus, Senecio aureus, Vitex agnus-castus*
Strong	*Artemisia abrotanum, A. absinthium, A. vulgaris, Gentiana lutea, Hydrastis canadensis, Marrubium vulgare, Marsdenia condurango, Ruta graveolens, Tanacetum parthenium, T. vulgare, Tropaeolum majus, Zingiber officinale*

EXPECTORANT

These are herbs that facilitate or accelerate the removal of bronchial secretions from the bronchi and trachea. However, this is another carelessly used term that in practice often simply means a remedy that "does something" for the respiratory system. To further elucidate the activity and the therapeutic indications of the various remedies known as expectorants, we may categorize them as follows.

Table 25.24. Expectorant Subcategories

TYPE OF EXPECTORANT	PROPOSED MECHANISM OF ACTION
Stimulating	Alkaloid-containing
	Saponin-containing
	Volatile oil–containing
Relaxing	Demulcent
	Anti-inflammatory (often also antimicrobial)
	Antispasmodic (alkaloid-containing)
	Volatile oil–containing

Stimulating Expectorants

Stimulating expectorants act in different ways to produce the same effect. It is not always clear how specific remedies work, but current thinking suggests the following processes:

Irritate the bronchioles to stimulate expulsion of any material present.

Liquefy viscid sputum so that it can be cleared by coughing. The sputum is moved upward by the fine hairs of the ciliated epithelium lining the bronchiole tubes. Reducing viscosity facilitates this transport.

Most stimulating expectorants contain alkaloids, saponins, or volatile oils. However, not all chemicals in these groups or plants that contain these constituents have this activity.

Alkaloid-Based Action

The major component of *Cephaelis ipecacuanha* is an alkaloid called emetine. It is emetic, induces nausea, and increases gastric secretions. This stimulation has a reflex effect on the bronchial mucosa via the gastrobronchial vagus reflex, again leading to an increase in secretion. Some other expectorants also work in this way and so can cause vomiting in high doses.

Spices promote expectoration by stimulating secretory activity in the salivary and gastric glands. Examples include anise, caraway, and fenugreek. This action results in increased production and reduced viscosity of bronchial secretions, which facilitate expectoration. This helps explain why spicy foods are beneficial in easing chronic bronchitis, while bland foods tend to encourage the condition.

Saponin-Based Action

The root of *Primula veris*, an expectorant commonly used in Europe, contains 5% to 10% saponin glycosides and 0.25% volatile oil. The plant is indicated for all forms of chronic bronchitis, especially simple coughs that persist for a long time with inadequate expectoration. The action of the saponins here is not clearly understood. It may be based on reflex mechanisms induced through gastric stimulation, which is mediated via the vagus nerve. This effect is much less marked than that of the alkaloid-containing *Cephaelis ipecacuanha*.

Stimulating Expectorant Herbs

Bellis perennis (English daisy)
Cephaelis ipecacuanha (ipecac)
Hieracium pilosella (mouse ear)
Inula helenium (elecampane)
Marrubium vulgare (horehound)
Myroxylon balsamum var. *balsamum* (Tolu balsam)
Polygala senega (Seneca snakeroot)
Populus candicans (balm of Gilead)
Primula veris (cowslip)
Sanguinaria canadensis (bloodroot)
Urginea maritima (squill)
Viola odorata (sweet violet)

Relaxing Expectorants

The relaxing expectorants seem also to act by reflex, but here the reflex action works to soothe bronchial spasm and loosen mucus secretions. These remedies help to produce a thinner mucus that is easier to expel, allowing the more viscous mucus to move and thus be eliminated. This makes relaxing expectorants useful for dry, irritating coughs. This action is similar in some respects to that of demulcents, and both actions owe much to their content of mucilage and, occasionally, volatile oils.

Relaxing Expectorant Herbs

Althaea officinalis (marshmallow)
Asclepias tuberosa (pleurisy root)
Cetraria islandica (Iceland moss)
Chondrus crispus (Irish moss)
Drosera rotundifolia (sundew)
Glycyrrhiza glabra (licorice)

Grindelia camporum (gumweed)
Hydrastis canadensis (goldenseal)
Hyssopus officinalis (hyssop)
Lobelia inflata (lobelia)
Pimpinella anisum (aniseed)
Prunus serotina (wild cherry bark)
Pulmonaria officinalis (lungwort)
Symphytum officinale (comfrey)
Symplocarpus foetidus (skunk cabbage)
Thuja occidentalis (thuja)
Thymus vulgaris (thyme)
Tussilago farfara (coltsfoot)
Verbena officinalis (vervain)

Amphoteric Remedies

A third group of expectorants is especially valuable in any broader treatment for the lungs. These may work either as relaxing or as stimulating expectorants. They have been called *amphoteric remedies*, after a phenomenon in chemistry in which the same molecule can act as either an acid or an alkali.

Amphoteric Expectorant Herbs

Allium sativum (garlic)
Sambucus nigra (elder)
Verbascum thapsus (mullein)

Body System Affinities

Cardiovascular. A congestive problem in the lungs can eventually have a deleterious effect upon the heart, so, by stretching a point somewhat, we could say that respiratory remedies may help the heart.

Respiratory. Obviously, all of the expectorants are relevant here.

Digestive. All of the stimulating expectorants may act as emetics if taken in too high a dose (for example, *Cephaelis ipecacuanha*), while the relaxing expectorants may be either demulcents (*Symphytum officinale*) or carminatives (*Pimpinella anisum*).

Urinary. Some expectorants also soothe the urinary system—for example, cornsilk (*Zea mays*). Expectorants aid the excretion of waste through the lungs, and may also have some effect upon other eliminative functions.

Reproductive. Expectorant herbs that are also antispasmodic will help with menstrual cramps (for example, *Lobelia inflata*), although the alkaloid-rich or saponin-containing emetics should be avoided during pregnancy. *Hydrastis canadensis*, which can work as an expectorant while toning the mucous membranes of the respiratory system, may also be of value in the reproductive tract.

Musculoskeletal. Stimulating expectorants can be used in liniments that increase circulation to the muscles and thus ease aches and pains. Examples include *Myroxylon balsamum* var. *pereirae* and *Thymus vulgaris*. *Lobelia inflata* is a good muscle relaxant.

Nervous. *Primula veris*, *Verbena officinalis*, *Thymus vulgaris*, and *Hyssopus officinalis* can all have relaxing nervine actions.

Skin. By supporting respiration and thus the whole of a person's health, these remedies may help the skin in a broad holistic way. Expectorants that may be used internally or externally for the skin include *Populus candicans*, *Symphytum officinale*, *Sambucus nigra*, *Inula helenium*, *Allium sativum*, and *Hydrastis canadensis*.

Table 25.25. Expectorant Herbs and Secondary Actions

SECONDARY ACTION	HERBS
Alterative	*Sanguinaria canadensis*, *Thuja occidentalis*, *Verbascum thapsus*
Anticatarrhal	*Althaea officinalis*, *Cetraria islandica*, *Chondrus crispus*, *Hyssopus officinalis*, *Sambucus nigra*, *Thymus vulgaris*, *Tussilago farfara*, *Verbascum thapsus*
Anti-inflammatory	*Althaea officinalis*, *Asclepias tuberosa*, *Cetraria islandica*, *Chondrus crispus*, *Glycyrrhiza glabra*, *Hydrastis canadensis*, *Hyssopus officinalis*, *Sambucus nigra*, *Tussilago farfara*, *Verbascum thapsus*
Antimicrobial	*Allium sativum*, *Carum carvi*, *Eucalyptus* spp., *Inula helenium*, *Ligusticum porteri*, *Myroxylon balsamum* var. *balsamum*, *Origanum majorana*, *Pimpinella anisum*, *Plantago major*, *Populus candicans*, *Ruta graveolens*, *Thymus vulgaris*
Antispasmodic	*Allium sativum*, *Angelica archangelica*, *Asclepias tuberosa*, *Carum carvi*, *Daucus carota*, *Drosera rotundifolia*, *Foeniculum vulgare*, *Glycyrrhiza glabra*, *Grindelia camporum*, *Hyssopus officinalis*, *Lobelia inflata*, *Lycopus* spp., *Marrubium vulgare*, *Nepeta cataria*, *Petroselinum crispum*, *Pimpinella anisum*, *Prunus serotina*, *Sanguinaria canadensis*, *Symplocarpus foetidus*, *Thymus vulgaris*, *Trigonella foenum-graecum*, *Tussilago farfara*, *Verbascum thapsus*
Astringent	*Glechoma hederacea*, *Hydrastis canadensis*, *Inula helenium*, *Plantago major*, *Prunus serotina*, *Symphytum officinale*, *Thuja occidentalis*, *Thymus vulgaris*, *Verbascum thapsus*

SECONDARY ACTION	HERBS
Bitter	*Hydrastis canadensis*, *Marrubium vulgare*, *Prunus serotina*
Carminative	*Asclepias tuberosa*, *Hyssopus officinalis*, *Pimpinella anisum*, *Thymus vulgaris*
Demulcent	*Cetraria islandica*, *Chondrus crispus*, *Glycyrrhiza glabra*, *Symphytum officinale* root, *Tussilago farfara*, *Verbascum thapsus*
Diaphoretic	*Allium sativum*, *Asclepias tuberosa*, *Hyssopus officinalis*, *Inula helenium*, *Polygala senega*, *Sambucus nigra* flower, *Symplocarpus foetidus*
Diuretic	*Glechoma hederacea*, *Solidago virgaurea*, *Tussilago farfara*
Emmenagogue	*Hyssopus officinalis*, *Marrubium vulgare*, *Petroselinum crispum*, *Thymus vulgaris*, *Trigonella foenum-graecum*
Nervine	*Hyssopus officinalis*, *Lobelia inflata*, *Prunus serotina*, *Verbena officinalis*
Vulnerary	*Marrubium vulgare*, *Populus candicans*, *Symphytum officinale* root, *Verbascum thapsus*

HEPATIC

Hepatics are herbal remedies that aid the work of the liver in a range of ways. Traditionally, they were considered to tone, strengthen, and, in some cases, increase the flow of bile. In a broad holistic approach to health, hepatics are of great importance because of the fundamental role the liver plays in the working of the body.

There is no single or simple answer as to how hepatics work. Bitters and cholagogues all act as hepatics, but so do a whole array of other remedies that do not have those specific actions. Hepatics are the epitome of the herbal remedy that does wonders for the body without a clearly defined mechanism of action. The lack of biochemical knowledge about the way in which they work does not keep them from working.

For a more detailed look at the phytotherapeutic approach to liver disease, please see chapter 13. The fundamentally important antihepatotoxic action of some hepatic remedies, including *Silybum marianum*, is discussed in chapter 9.

Hepatic Herbs

Achillea millefolium (yarrow)
Agrimonia eupatoria (agrimony)
Aloe vera (aloe)
Apium graveolens (celery seed)
Armoracia rusticana (horseradish)
Artemisia absinthium (wormwood)
Baptisia tinctoria (wild indigo)
Berberis vulgaris (barberry)
Centaurium erythraea (centaury)
Chelone glabra (balmony)
Chionanthus virginicus (fringetree)
Curcuma longa (turmeric)
Cynara scolymus (artichoke)
Dioscorea villosa (wild yam)
Euonymus atropurpureus (wahoo)
Foeniculum vulgare (fennel)
Fumaria officinalis (fumitory)
Galium aparine (cleavers)
Gentiana lutea (gentian)
Hydrastis canadensis (goldenseal)
Hyssopus officinalis (hyssop)
Inula helenium (elecampane)
Iris versicolor (blue flag)
Leonurus cardiaca (motherwort)
Leptandra virginica (black root)
Mahonia aquifolium (Oregon grape)
Melissa officinalis (lemon balm)
Menyanthes trifoliata (bogbean)
Peumus boldus (boldo)
Rhamnus cathartica (buckthorn)
R. purshiana (cascara sagrada)
Rumex crispus (yellow dock)
Silybum marianum (milk thistle)
Taraxacum officinale (dandelion)
Zanthoxylum americanum (prickly ash)

Body System Affinities

Cardiovascular. The value of hepatics in this system comes through general improvement of body functioning. Only when a hepatic also has diuretic action can any direct claims be made.

Respiratory. Certain hepatics are also antimicrobial and anticatarrhal, which will benefit the respiratory system. Also, mucous membrane tonics help here, including herbs such as *Eupatorium perfoliatum*, *Hydrastis canadensis*, *Rosmarinus officinalis*, *Salvia officinalis*, and *Baptisia tinctoria*.

Digestive. Here we have a long list, which includes *Agrimonia eupatoria*, *Chelone glabra*, *Berberis vulgaris*, *Leptandra virginica*, *Iris versicolor*, *Peumus boldus*, *Juglans cinerea*, *Taraxacum officinale* root, *Chionanthus virginicus* bark, *Gentiana lutea*, *Euonymus atropurpureus*, and *Dioscorea villosa*.

Urinary. Hepatics confer only an indirect benefit to this system. However, *Taraxacum officinale* root is partially diuretic in action, although weaker than the leaves. *Eupatorium perfoliatum* can be a marked diuretic in feverish conditions.

Reproductive. Hepatic plants such as *Hydrastis canadensis* and *Berberis vulgaris* have a pronounced action on the muscles of the uterus. *Rosmarinus officinalis* is a tonic and emmenagogue, and most bitters will also stimulate the uterus or menstrual activity.

Musculoskeletal. Hepatics help in this system by generally supporting the body's metabolic activity.

Nervous. Because hepatics support metabolism in general, they also have an enlivening "side effect" in the nervous system. They are appropriate for use in the treatment of debility and depression.

Skin. Taken internally, hepatic remedies often aid in cleansing and so clear skin problems. Examples are *Iris versicolor*, *Taraxacum officinale*, *Fumaria officinalis*, *Hydrastis canadensis*, *Mahonia aquifolium*, and *Rumex crispus*. *Hydrastis canadensis* may also be helpful in certain conditions when used externally.

Table 25.26. Hepatic Herbs and Secondary Actions

SECONDARY ACTION	HERBS
Alterative	*Agrimonia eupatoria, Chionanthus virginicus, Fumaria officinalis, Galium aparine, Iris versicolor, Mahonia aquifolium, Rumex crispus, Taraxacum officinale, Zanthoxylum americanum*
Anticatarrhal	*Baptisia tinctoria, Hydrastis canadensis, Mahonia aquifolium*
Anti-inflammatory	*Apium graveolens, Artemisia absinthium, Dioscorea villosa, Galium aparine, Iris versicolor, Menyanthes trifoliata*
Antimicrobial	*Achillea millefolium, Baptisia tinctoria, Berberis vulgaris, Inula helenium*
Antispasmodic	*Dioscorea villosa, Foeniculum vulgare, Hyssopus officinalis, Leonurus cardiaca, Leptandra virginica, Melissa officinalis*
Astringent	*Achillea millefolium, Agrimonia eupatoria, Berberis vulgaris, Galium aparine, Hydrastis canadensis*

SECONDARY ACTION	HERBS
Bitter	Agrimonia eupatoria, Artemisia absinthium, Berberis vulgaris, Centaurium erythraea, Gentiana lutea, Hydrastis canadensis, Menyanthes trifoliata
Carminative	Apium graveolens, Armoracia rusticana, Artemisia absinthium, Foeniculum vulgare, Hyssopus officinalis, Melissa officinalis, Zanthoxylum americanum
Diaphoretic	Achillea millefolium, Baptisia tinctoria, Berberis vulgaris, Hyssopus officinalis, Inula helenium, Leptandra virginica, Melissa officinalis, Zanthoxylum americanum
Diuretic	Achillea millefolium, Agrimonia eupatoria, Armoracia rusticana, Chionanthus virginicus, Euonymus atropurpureus, Fumaria officinalis, Galium aparine, Iris versicolor, Menyanthes trifoliata, Peumus boldus
Emmenagogue	Artemisia absinthium, Berberis vulgaris, Leonurus cardiaca
Expectorant	Foeniculum vulgare, Hyssopus officinalis, Inula helenium
Hypotensive	Achillea millefolium
Laxative	Armoracia rusticana, Chelone glabra, Chionanthus virginicus, Euonymus atropurpureus, Hydrastis canadensis, Iris versicolor, Mahonia aquifolium, Rumex crispus, Taraxacum officinale
Nervine	Apium graveolens, Hyssopus officinalis, Leonurus cardiaca, Melissa officinalis
Tonic	Agrimonia eupatoria, Chelone glabra, Chionanthus virginicus, Galium aparine, Hydrastis canadensis, Mahonia aquifolium, Taraxacum officinale, Zanthoxylum americanum
Vulnerary	Agrimonia eupatoria, Hydrastis canadensis

Table 25.27. Relative Strengths of Hepatics

STRENGTH	HERBS
Mild	Achillea millefolium, Apium graveolens, Baptisia tinctoria, Dioscorea villosa, Foeniculum vulgare, Fumaria officinalis, Galium aparine, Hyssopus officinalis, Inula helenium, Leonurus cardiaca, Melissa officinalis, Zanthoxylum americanum
Moderate	Agrimonia eupatoria, Armoracia rusticana, Artemisia absinthium, Berberis vulgaris, Centaurium erythraea, Chelone glabra, Chionanthus virginicus, Cynara scolymus, Euonymus atropurpureus, Gentiana lutea, Hydrastis canadensis, Iris versicolor, Leptandra virginica, Mahonia aquifolium, Menyanthes trifoliata, Peumus boldus, Rhamnus purshiana, Rumex crispus, Silybum marianum, Taraxacum officinale

HYPNOTIC

Hypnotics are nervine remedies that help induce a deep and healing state of sleep. These herbs vary from mild, volatile oil–containing herbs that ease psychological tensions and have gentle muscle relaxant properties to powerful remedies containing strong alkaloids that work directly on the central nervous system to induce sleep.

Hypnotic herbs should always be used within the context of a holistic approach to sleep problems—that is, one that embraces relaxation techniques, nutrition, and lifestyle in general. For a detailed approach to the therapeutic use of these herbs, please see chapter 16.

Hypnotic Herbs

Artemisia vulgaris (mugwort)
Eschscholzia californica (California poppy)
Humulus lupulus (hops)
Lactuca virosa (wild lettuce)
Leonurus cardiaca (motherwort)
Matricaria recutita (chamomile)
Passiflora incarnata (passionflower)
Phytolacca americana (poke)
Piscidia erythrina (Jamaica dogwood)
Scutellaria lateriflora (skullcap)
Stachys officinalis (wood betony)
Tilia platyphyllos (linden)
Valeriana officinalis (valerian)
Verbena officinalis (vervain)

Body System Affinities

It is safe to say that all of the hypnotic remedies can help the whole body in that sleep is so vital to overall health.

Cardiovascular. Here we can mention *Leonurus cardiaca*, *Tilia platyphyllos*, and *Melissa officinalis*. Notice that these herbs are all in the "milder" category. *Viscum album* can help but must be used with care.

Respiratory. All of the hypnotics can help as antispasmodics in conditions such as asthma if used at the right dosage. *Lactuca virosa* eases irritable coughs.

Digestive. The relaxing nervines and carminatives are important, of which we can mention *Matricaria recutita, Verbena officinalis, Melissa officinalis, Humulus lupulus, and Valeriana officinalis.* Antispasmodics will help with intestinal colic—for example, *Humulus lupulus, Piscidia erythrina, Passiflora incarnata*, and *Valeriana officinalis.*

Urinary. Hypnotics are important here when used as muscle relaxants.

Reproductive. The same comment made for the urinary system holds true here.

Musculoskeletal. All hypnotics help reduce muscle tension and even the pain associated with problems in this system. They may be used internally or as lotions. Especially important are *Piscidia erythrina* and *Valeriana officinalis.*

Nervous. All these remedies work on the nervous system.

Skin. The value of hypnotics here is to ensure that the body has a good, recuperative rest each night.

Table 25.28. Relative Strengths of Hypnotic Herbs

STRENGTH	HERBS
Mild	*Artemisia vulgaris, Stachys officinalis, Leonurus cardiaca, Matricaria recutita, Tilia platyphyllos*
Moderate	*Eschscholzia californica, Pulsatilla vulgaris, Scutellaria lateriflora, Verbena officinalis*
Strong	*Humulus lupulus, Lactuca virosa, Piscidia erythrina, Passiflora incarnata, Valeriana officinalis*

HYPOTENSIVE

Hypotensive remedies reduce elevated blood pressure, tending to normalize both systolic and diastolic pressure. A number of different mechanisms may be involved; these are explored in more depth in chapter 9. Please see chapter 14 for details on the therapeutic uses of these herbs.

Hypotensive Herbs

Achillea millefolium (yarrow)
Allium cepa (onion)
A. sativum (garlic)
Caulophyllum thalictroides (blue cohosh)
Cimicifuga racemosa (black cohosh)
Crataegus spp. (hawthorn)

Eleutherococcus senticosus (Siberian ginseng)
Fagopyrum esculentum (buckwheat)
Leonurus cardiaca (motherwort)
Passiflora incarnata (passionflower)
Petroselinum crispum (parsley)
Scutellaria lateriflora (skullcap)
Tilia platyphyllos (linden)
Trigonella foenum-graecum (fenugreek)
Urtica dioica (nettles)
Valeriana officinalis (valerian)
Verbena officinalis (vervain)
Viburnum opulus (cramp bark)
V. prunifolium (black haw)
Viscum album (mistletoe)

Table 25.29. Hypotensive Herbs and Secondary Actions

SECONDARY ACTION	HERBS
Adaptogen	*Eleutherococcus senticosus*
Alterative	*Allium sativum, Cimicifuga racemosa, Urtica dioica*
Anticatarrhal	*Allium cepa, A. sativum, Trigonella foenum-graecum*
Anti-inflammatory	*Caulophyllum thalictroides, Cimicifuga racemosa, Valeriana officinalis*
Antimicrobial	*Achillea millefolium, Allium sativum, A. cepa*
Antispasmodic	*Achillea millefolium, Allium sativum*
Astringent	*Caulophyllum thalictroides, Cimicifuga racemosa, Leonurus cardiaca, Passiflora incarnata, Scutellaria lateriflora, Tilia platyphyllos, Urtica dioica, Valeriana officinalis, Verbena officinalis, Viburnum opulus, V. prunifolium*
Bitter	*Achillea millefolium*
Cardiotonic	*Allium sativum, Crataegus* spp., *Leonurus cardiaca*
Carminative	*Petroselinum crispum, Valeriana officinalis*
Cholagogue	*Allium sativum, Verbena officinalis*
Demulcent	*Trigonella foenum-graecum*
Diaphoretic	*Achillea millefolium, Allium cepa, A. sativum, Tilia platyphyllos, Verbena officinalis*
Diuretic	*Achillea millefolium, Petroselinum crispum, Tilia platyphyllos, Urtica dioica*

SECONDARY ACTION	HERBS
Emmenagogue	*Caulophyllum thalictroides, Cimicifuga racemosa, Leonurus cardiaca, Petroselinum crispum*
Expectorant	*Allium cepa, A. sativum, Petroselinum crispum, Trigonella foenum-graecum*
Galactagogue	*Trigonella foenum-graecum*
Hepatic	*Allium cepa, Verbena officinalis*
Laxative	*Verbena officinalis*
Nervine	*Cimicifuga racemosa, Leonurus cardiaca, Passiflora incarnata, Scutellaria lateriflora, Tilia platyphyllos, Valeriana officinalis, Verbena officinalis, Viburnum opulus, V. prunifolium, Viscum album*
Vulnerary	*Allium cepa, Trigonella foenum-graecum*

Table 25.30. Relative Strengths of Hypotensive Herbs

STRENGTH	HERBS
Mild	*Allium cepa, Caulophyllum thalictroides, Cimicifuga racemosa, Urtica dioica, Verbena officinalis*
Moderate	*Achillea millefolium, Eleutherococcus senticosus, Leonurus cardiaca, Passiflora incarnata, Petroselinum crispum, Scutellaria lateriflora, Valeriana officinalis, Viburnum prunifolium*
Strong	*Allium sativum, Crataegus spp., Tilia platyphyllos, Trigonella foenum-graecum, Viburnum opulus, Viscum album*

NERVINE

A nervine is a plant remedy with some kind of beneficial effect upon the nervous system. This makes the word *nervine* another catchall term, and in order to study them properly, it is helpful to sort them into a number of categories. It may be superfluous to point this out, but any successful herbal treatment of nervous system problems must involve the whole body, heart and mind, not simply the signs of agitation and worry. Of course, herbs can reduce agitation greatly, but the whole system must be strengthened in the face of the storm!

Table 25.31. Primary Nervine Categories

NERVINE ACTION	HERBAL EXAMPLES
Tonic	*Avena sativa, Hypericum perforatum, Scutellaria lateriflora*
Relaxant	*Piper methysticum, Scutellaria lateriflora, Valeriana officinalis, Verbena officinalis*
Stimulant	*Coffea arabica, Camellia sinensis, Cola acuminata, Paullinia cupana*
Hypnotic	*Humulus lupulus, Passiflora incarnata, Valeriana officinalis*
Antispasmodic	*Piper methysticum, Valeriana officinalis, Viburnum opulus*
Antidepressant	*Artemisia vulgaris, Hypericum perforatum*
Adaptogen	*Panax spp., Eleutherococcus senticosus*
Analgesic	*Piscidia erythrina, Gelsemium sempervirens*

Nervine Tonics

Perhaps the most important contribution herbs can make to the whole field of neurology lies in their ability to strengthen and nourish the nervous system. In cases of shock, stress, and nervous debility, nervine tonics strengthen and restore tissues directly. They can contribute to the healing of damaged nervous tissue, whether due to a pathological process or to physical trauma. This invaluable group of tonic remedies is best exemplified by *Avena sativa*, which has no additional relaxing or stimulating effects. Nervine tonics that also have a relaxing effect are *Scutellaria lateriflora* and *Hypericum perforatum*.

Nervine Relaxants

This group of nervines are most important in times of stress and confusion, as they can alleviate many of the accompanying symptoms. They should always be used in a broad holistic way, not simply to tranquilize. Too much tranquilizing, even with herbal medication, can in time deplete and weigh heavily on the whole nervous system.

As illustrated in table 25.32, many nervine relaxants can be selected on the basis of their secondary actions to treat additional problems. This is one of the great benefits of using herbal remedies to help with stress and anxiety problems. The physical symptoms that can so often accompany the *dis-ease* of anxiety may be treated with herbs that work on the anxiety itself.

In addition to herbs that work directly on the nervous

system, antispasmodic herbs—those that affect the peripheral nerves and the muscle tissue—may have an indirect relaxing action on the whole system. Putting the physical body at ease promotes ease in the psyche. Many nervine relaxants have this antispasmodic action. Also see Hypnotics, which at lower dosages also have a relaxing action on the mind and body.

Nervine Relaxants

Artemisia vulgaris (mugwort)

Ballota nigra (black horehound)

Borago officinalis (borage)

Chamaemelum nobile (Roman chamomile)

Cimicifuga racemosa (black cohosh)

Eschscholzia californica (California poppy)

Humulus lupulus (hops)

Hypericum perforatum (St. John's wort)

Hyssopus officinalis (hyssop)

Lactuca virosa (wild lettuce)

Lavandula spp. (lavender)

Leonurus cardiaca (motherwort)

Lobelia inflata (lobelia)

Matricaria recutita (chamomile)

Melissa officinalis (lemon balm)

Passiflora incarnata (passionflower)

Piper methysticum (kava)

Piscidia erythrina (Jamaica dogwood)

Pulsatilla vulgaris (pasqueflower)

Scutellaria lateriflora (skullcap)

Stachys betonica (wood betony)

Tilia platyphyllos (linden)

Trifolium pratense (red clover)

Turnera diffusa (damiana)

Valeriana officinalis (valerian)

Verbena officinalis (vervain)

Viburnum opulus (cramp bark)

V. prunifolium (black haw)

Body System Affinities

Cardiovascular. *Melissa officinalis, Tilia platyphyllos,* and *Leonurus cardiaca* are all mild sedatives that are helpful to the cardiovascular system. However, most remedies that lessen overactivity of the nervous system will also aid the heart and have a positive impact on circulatory conditions, such as high blood pressure.

Respiratory. Most sedatives will help with problems accompanied by chest tension, such as asthma, but specifically, we can mention *Cimicifuga racemosa, Lactuca virosa, Leonurus cardiaca, Lobelia inflata,* and *Lycopus* spp.

Digestive. All of the antispasmodic remedies may be of value here in easing spasms or colic. However, sedatives that actively aid digestion include mild herbs such as *Melissa officinalis, Matricaria recutita,* and *Lavandula* spp., plus the stronger herbs *Humulus lupulus* and *Valeriana officinalis.*

Urinary. *Serenoa repens* is a gentle sedative that also works on the urinary system.

Reproductive. *Cimicifuga racemosa, Caulophyllum thalictroides, Viburnum* spp., *Leonurus cardiaca, Serenoa repens,* and *Lactuca virosa* all have an affinity for this system.

Musculoskeletal. All sedative remedies will help ease muscular tension and pain in this complex system. Remedies to bear in mind are *Cimicifuga racemosa, Fucus vesiculosus, Viburnum prunifolium,* and *Dioscorea villosa.*

Nervous. All of the nervine remedies are relevant here.

Skin. All nervines may help the skin in an indirect way, but the following have a good reputation for skin conditions: *Trifolium pratense, Hypericum perforatum,* and *Cimicifuga racemosa.*

Table 25.32. Nervine Relaxants and Secondary Actions

SECONDARY ACTION	HERBS
Alterative	*Cimicifuga racemosa, Trifolium pratense*
Analgesic	*Hypericum perforatum, Lactuca virosa, Matricaria recutita, Passiflora incarnata, Piscidia erythrina*
Anticatarrhal	*Hyssopus officinalis, Matricaria recutita, Tilia platyphyllos*
Anti-inflammatory	*Matricaria recutita, Melissa officinalis, Tilia platyphyllos*
Antimicrobial	*Humulus lupulus, Matricaria recutita, Phytolacca americana*
Antispasmodic	*Cimicifuga racemosa, Humulus lupulus, Hypericum perforatum, Hyssopus officinalis, Lavandula* spp., *Leonurus cardiaca, Lobelia inflata, Matricaria recutita, Melissa officinalis, Passiflora incarnata, Phytolacca americana, Piper methysticum, Scutellaria lateriflora, Tilia platyphyllos, Valeriana officinalis, Viburnum opulus, V. prunifolium*
Astringent	*Ballota nigra, Humulus lupulus, Hypericum perforatum, Tilia platyphyllos, Viburnum opulus, V. prunifolium*

SECONDARY ACTION	HERBS
Bitter	*Artemisia vulgaris, Humulus lupulus, Matricaria recutita*
Carminative	*Artemisia vulgaris, Humulus lupulus, Hyssopus officinalis, Lavandula* spp., *Leonurus cardiaca, Matricaria recutita, Melissa officinalis, Valeriana officinalis*
Diaphoretic	*Cimicifuga racemosa, Hyssopus officinalis, Tilia platyphyllos, Verbena officinalis*
Diuretic	*Tilia platyphyllos*
Emmenagogue	*Artemisia vulgaris, Ballota nigra, Cimicifuga racemosa, Leonurus cardiaca*
Expectorant	*Hyssopus officinalis, Lobelia inflata, Marrubium vulgare*
Hepatic	*Verbena officinalis*
Hypnotic	*Eschscholzia californica, Humulus lupulus, Lactuca virosa, Matricaria recutita, Passiflora incarnata, Valeriana officinalis*
Hypotensive	*Leonurus cardiaca, Passiflora incarnata, Scutellaria lateriflora, Tilia platyphyllos, Valeriana officinalis*
Vulnerary	*Borago officinalis, Hypericum perforatum, Matricaria recutita*

Table 25.33. Relative Strengths of Relaxing Nervines

STRENGTH	HERBS
Mild	*Ballota nigra, Betonica officinalis, Borago officinalis, Chamaemelum nobile, Hyssopus officinalis, Lavandula* spp., *Trifolium pratense, Melissa officinalis, Viburnum opulus, V. prunifolium*
Moderate	*Artemisia vulgaris, Cimicifuga racemosa, Hypericum perforatum, Leonurus cardiaca, Lobelia inflata, Matricaria recutita, Pulsatilla vulgaris, Scutellaria lateriflora, Tilia platyphyllos, Turnera diffusa, Verbena officinalis*
Strong	*Eschscholzia californica, Humulus lupulus, Lactuca virosa, Passiflora incarnata, Piscidia erythrina, Valeriana officinalis*

Nervine Stimulants

Direct stimulation of nervous tissue is not often needed in our hyperactive modern lives. In most cases, it is more appropriate to stimulate the body's innate vitality with the help of nervine or bitter tonics. These herbs work to augment bodily harmony, and thus have a much deeper and longer-lasting effect than nervine stimulants. In the 19th century, herbalists placed much more emphasis upon stimulant herbs. It is, perhaps, a sign of our times that the world now supplies us with more than enough stimulation.

When direct nervine stimulation is indicated, the best herb to use is *Cola acuminata*, although *Paullinia cupana, Coffea arabica, Ilex paraguayensis*, and *Camellia sinensis* may also be used. One problem with these commonly used stimulants is their side effects; they are themselves implicated in the development of certain minor psychological problems, such as anxiety and tension.

Some of the volatile oil–rich herbs are also valuable stimulants. Some of the best and most common are *Rosmarinus officinalis* and *Mentha piperita*.

STIMULANT

The very word *stimulant* has different connotations, depending upon one's assumptions. In herbal medicine, the term is used to describe an action that quickens and enlivens the physiological activity of the body. All physiological process can be stimulated to some degree. Consider stimulant laxatives, circulatory stimulants, and bitters, which often act as stimulants.

On the other hand, stimulating physiological processes is not necessarily appropriate. The individual's needs and his or her unique state of health must be taken into account. Debility may be related not only to too little activity in the body, but also to too much. This is a problem of differential diagnosis that calls for skill, knowledge, and a certain amount of intuition.

In some cases, specific stimulant effects are related to the presence of alkaloids in the plant. Caffeine, perhaps the best known and most widely used of these alkaloids, is present in such herbs as *Coffea arabica, Camellia sinensis, Ilex paraguayensis*, and *Cola acuminata*, as well as in chocolate (*Theobroma cacao*). The coca tree (*Erythroxylum coca*), the source of the drug cocaine, contains other stimulating alkaloids. Whenever stimulants of this nature are used, they should be combined with nervine tonics or relaxants to balance out any overstimulation.

Herbal Stimulants

Achillea millefolium (yarrow)
Allium sativum (garlic)
Angelica archangelica (angelica)
Armoracia rusticana (horseradish)
Artemisia abrotanum (southernwood)
A. absinthium (wormwood)
A. vulgaris (mugwort)
Brassica spp. (mustard)
Capsicum annuum (cayenne)
Carum carvi (caraway)
Cephaelis ipecacuanha (ipecac)
Chelidonium majus (celandine)
Cola acuminata (kola)
Elettaria cardamomum (cardamom)
Eupatorium perfoliatum (boneset)
E. purpureum (gravel root)
Foeniculum vulgare (fennel)
Fucus vesiculosus (kelp)
Gentiana lutea (gentian)
Inula helenium (elecampane)
Juniperus communis (juniper)
Marrubium vulgare (horehound)
Marsdenia condurango (condurango)
Mentha piperita (peppermint)
Myrica cerifera (bayberry)
Panax spp. (ginseng)
Polygala senega (Seneca snakeroot)
Rhamnus cathartica (buckthorn)
R. purshiana (cascara sagrada)
Rosmarinus officinalis (rosemary)
Ruta graveolens (rue)
Sanguinaria canadensis (bloodroot)
Senna alexandrina (senna)
Tanacetum vulgare (tansy)
Zanthoxylum americanum (prickly ash)
Zingiber officinale (ginger)

Body System Affinities

Cardiovascular. Stimulant actions must be used with care in people with cardiovascular problems, but if applied with knowledge, appropriate stimulation can often aid and support an ailing heart. *Myrica cerifera, Panax* spp., *Zanthoxylum americanum, Rosmarinus officinalis, Ruta graveolens, Artemisia absinthium,* and *Achillea millefolium* may be helpful here.

Respiratory. The diaphoretic chest remedies can be considered stimulant in action. Specifics include *Angelica archangelica, Eucalyptus* spp., *Allium sativum, Armoracia rusticana, Brassica* spp., *Glechoma hederacea, Mentha piperita, Salvia officinalis, Marrubium vulgare,* and *Achillea millefolium.*

Digestive. As already discussed, bitters may be considered stimulants. Note *Chelone glabra, Myrica cerifera, Carum carvi, Elettaria cardamomum, Cinnamomum* spp., *Taraxacum officinale* root, *Alpina galanga, Allium sativum, Gentiana lutea, Armoracia rusticana, Brassica* spp., *Mentha piperita, Rosmarinus officinalis, Ruta graveolens,* and *Artemisia absinthium.*

Urinary. Relevant stimulants with diuretic properties include *Eucalyptus* spp., *Eupatorium purpureum, Juniperus communis,* and *Achillea millefolium.*

Reproductive. Stimulants for this system usually act as emmenagogues, and so should not be used during pregnancy. Important examples include *Mentha pulegium, Ruta graveolens, Rosmarinus officinalis, Artemisia abrotanum, Tanacetum vulgare,* and *Artemisia absinthium.*

Musculoskeletal. The vital role of both *Zingiber officinale* and *Capsicum annuum* are reinforced here as stimulants of peripheral circulation. We can add *Brassica* spp. and *Armoracia rusticana.* In general, rubefacient remedies are stimulants.

Nervous. Nervous system stimulants include *Cola acuminata, Paullinia cupana, Coffea arabica, Camellia sinensis,* and *Ilex paraguayensis.*

Skin. Rubefacients are stimulants, promoting local circulation to the area of skin where they are applied. Vulneraries stimulate healing, but are not stimulants as such.

Table 25.34. Stimulant Herbs and Secondary Actions

SECONDARY ACTION	HERBS
Anti-inflammatory	*Mentha piperita*
Antimicrobial	*Achillea millefolium, Allium sativum, Artemisia abrotanum, Capsicum annuum, Inula helenium, Mentha piperita, Rosmarinus officinalis, Sanguinaria canadensis*
Astringent	*Marrubium vulgare, Carum carvi*
Bitter	*Artemisia abrotanum, A. absinthium, A. vulgaris, Gentiana lutea, Marrubium vulgare, Ruta graveolens, Tanacetum vulgare*
Carminative	*Angelica archangelica, Artemisia absinthium, Capsicum annuum, Carum carvi, Elettaria cardamomum, Foeniculum vulgare, Mentha piperita, Rosmarinus officinalis, Tanacetum vulgare, Zingiber officinale*

SECONDARY ACTION	HERBS
Diaphoretic	*Achillea millefolium, Allium sativum, Angelica archangelica, Eupatorium perfoliatum, E. purpureum, Mentha piperita, Polygala senega, Tanacetum vulgare, Zingiber officinale*
Diuretic	*Achillea millefolium, Angelica archangelica, Brassica spp., Daucus carota, Eupatorium perfoliatum, E. purpureum*
Emmenagogue	*Artemisia abrotanum, A. absinthium, A. vulgaris, Carum carvi, Marrubium vulgare, Ruta graveolens, Tanacetum vulgare*
Expectorant	*Achillea millefolium, Angelica archangelica, Carum carvi, Foeniculum vulgare, Inula helenium, Marrubium vulgare, Polygala senega, Sanguinaria canadensis*
Hepatic	*Artemisia abrotanum, A. vulgaris, Gentiana lutea*
Hypotensive	*Achillea millefolium, Allium sativum*
Vulnerary	*Achillea millefolium, Capsicum annuum*

References

1. Wagner H, Norr H, Winterhoff H. Plant adaptogens. *Phytomedicine* 1994; 1:63–76.
2. Carson CF, Riley TV. The antimicrobial activity of tea tree oil. *The Medical Journal of Australia* 1994; 160:236.
3. Howell AB, Vorsa N, Der Maderosian A, Foo LY. Inhibition of the adherence of P-fimbriated *Esherichia coli* to uroepithelial-cell surfaces by proanthocyanidin extracts from cranberries. *The New England Journal of Medicine* 1998; 339:10854 [letter].

26

❧

MATERIA MEDICA

An understanding of the herbal materia medica is the basis of herbal medicine. As pointed out in chapter 1, the list of herbs that could potentially be included here is many thousands long! However, the materia medica that follows reflects my experience and training, and so emphasizes the European and North American herbs most often encountered in Western herbal medicine. The fact that most of the herbs used in ayurveda or traditional Chinese medicine are not included is in no way a rejection of their value, but simply a reflection of my focus on Western herbalism.

MATERIA MEDICA OUTLINE

Each materia medica entry follows the same general format, explained here.

Latin binomial
Common name
Taxonomic family

Other Names or **Related Species:** Many herbs have numerous regional names. Alternative common names commonly used in North American herbalism are included under this heading. If there are nomenclature issues, such as recent binomial changes, they are also noted here. Other species commonly used medicinally are listed as Related Species.

Part Used: This entry lists the part or parts of the herb used medicinally.

Constituents: The lists provided here represent a compilation of relevant phytochemical research on the particular remedy. This is not a comprehensive constituent listing, as each plant contains many hundreds of thousands of distinct chemicals, both organic and inorganic. Thus, I have listed only the most relevant chemicals, and did not include the ubiquitous primary constituents found in all plants.

The information provided here reflects current pharmacological thinking about which chemicals are the primary contributors to the plant's actions. It is important to remember, however, that fashions and insights come in and out of favor in science as much as in any other area of human endeavor. For more details on a constituent or group of constituents, please refer to the chapters on phytochemistry in part 1 of this book.

A wealth of scientific information about the whole range of different plant components is available. However, this does not necessarily tell us much about the value and benefits of the herb when used in healing. The activity of the whole plant is always more than the sum of its parts, just as a human being is more than the sum of his or her biochemistry. Knowing the chemistry of sesquiterpenes is not the same as knowing chamomile.

Actions: This section provides an overview of the physiological actions demonstrated by the herb, which are explored in depth in chapter 25 (Herbal Actions). Knowing an herb's actions is the key to using it holistically and effectively. The approach followed here is based on the practice of medical herbalism developed during the 19th and 20th centuries in North America and the United Kingdom.

Indications: Here I provide a brief overview of the clinical indications for the herb. As there is so much variability among both people and plants (the gift of diversity!), the indications provided in herbals are rarely all encompassing. Thus, the indications listed reflect my particular training and experience.

In addition, I have included quotations from some invaluable but difficult-to-find texts from the 19th-century Eclectic and Physiomedicalist traditions. These sources of therapeutic information are based upon years of clinical experience. Much of the technical language and writing style reflects the time periods in which these physicians were practicing, so it probably sounds strange to modern ears. I have not changed their words or grammar, although I could not resist occasional comments. Their Victorian terminology and spelling have been left untouched.

Texts cited include:

Priest and Priest: from Priest and Priest, *Herbal Medications*. London: L. N. Fowler and Co. Ltd., 1982.

Ellingwood: from Ellingwood, Finley. *American Materia Medica, Therapeutics and Pharmacognosy*. 1898. Reprint, Sandy, OR: Eclectic Medical Publications, 1983.

Felter: from Felter, Harvey W. *The Eclectic Materia Medica, Pharmacology and Therapeutics*. 1922. Reprint, Sandy, OR: Eclectic Medical Publications, 1983.

King's: from Felter, Harvey W. and Lloyd, John Uri. *King's American Dispensatory* vols. 1 and 2, 1892. Reprint, Sandy, OR: Eclectic Medical Publications, 1983.

Safety Considerations: If there are any concerns about the safe use of the herb, the issues are discussed under this heading, including side effects, contraindications, and drug interactions.

Preparations and Dosage: This section lists dosage ranges for various herbal preparations, taken from a number of sources. I have provided details of concentration (weight/volume ratios, expressed as "w/v") and alcohol percentages for tinctures and liquid extracts. For example, a tincture containing 1 part herb to 5 parts solvent in a menstruum composed of 45% alcohol is denoted as "1:5 in 45%." More information on these calculations may be found in chapter 11.

References: Whenever possible, at the end of the entry I have provided a reference to a more technical monograph that covers pharmacology, clinical trials, and regulatory status for that herb.

Key to Dosage Sources

Unless otherwise indicated in the text, the sources listed here are the pharmacopoeias from which I took the official medicine-making standards cited in Preparations and Dosage. They are abbreviated in the text according to the following key:

BPC: British Pharmacopoeia Codex, 4th ed. (1898)
BHP: British Herbal Pharmacopoeia (1990)
BHC: British Herbal Compendium (1992)
Comm. E: German Commission E Monographs (1998)
USP: United States Pharmacopoeia, 9th ed. (1916)

Achillea millefolium L.
Yarrow
Asteraceae

Parts Used: Aerial parts

Constituents: 0.3% to 1.4% volatile oil (α- and β-pinene, borneol, bornyl acetate, camphor, α-caryophyllene, 1,8 cineole); sesquiterpene lactones (achillicin, achillin, achillifolin, millifin, millifolide); 3% to 4% tannins; flavonoids (apigenin, luteolin, isorhamnetin, rutin); alkaloids (betonicine, stachydrine, achiceine, moschatine, trigonelline, and others); phenolic acids (caffeic, salicylic); coumarins[1]

Actions: Diaphoretic, hypotensive, astringent, antiinflammatory, antispasmodic, diuretic, antimicrobial, bitter, hepatic

Indications: *Achillea* is an important diaphoretic herb and is a standard remedy for helping the body deal with fever. It stimulates digestion and tones blood vessels. As a urinary tract antiseptic, it is indicated in infections such as cystitis, for which it is most effective if used fresh. *Achillea* is considered a specific in thrombotic conditions associated with hypertension, and is thought to lower blood pressure through dilation of peripheral vessels. Researchers believe that its anti-inflammatory and antispasmodic actions are related to its content of flavonoids.[2] Used externally, *Achillea* aids in wound healing. Antimicrobial activity against a range of bacteria has been reported for water and ether extracts of the plant.[3]

Priest and Priest described *Achillea* as a

. . . mild, slow and stimulating diaphoretic: indicated for the first stage of acute febrile reactions. For atonic and relaxed tissues where there is free discharge or passive hemorrhage of bright red blood. Cold preparations stimulate the appetite and tone the digestive organs.

Priest and Priest gave the following specific indications: acute stage of colds, influenza, and respiratory catarrhs; chronic diarrhea and dysentery; epistaxis, intestinal hemorrhage, and bleeding hemorrhoids; uterine hemorrhage, profuse protracted menstruation, and leukorrhea.

Safety Considerations: Hypersensitivity to yarrow and other plants in the Asteraceae family has been reported. Some authorities caution against using *Achillea* during pregnancy.[4] No restrictions during lactation are suggested.

Preparations and Dosage: Tincture dosage is 2 to 4 ml (1:5 in 25%) three times a day. To make an infusion, pour 1 cup of boiling water over 1 to 2 teaspoons of dried herb and infuse for 10 to 15 minutes. This should be drunk hot three times a day. When the patient is feverish, it should be drunk hourly.

Dosage recommended by the BHC is 2 to 4 g of dried herb, 2 to 4 ml of tincture, 1 to 2 ml fluid extract (1:1 in 25%), or 3 to 5 ml pressed juice from fresh herb three times a day. Commission E recommends 4.5 g dried herb, 3 teaspoons pressed juice, or 3 g fresh flowers daily.

Yarrow, in *Herbal Medicine, Expanded Commission E Monographs*

Aesculus hippocastanum L.
Horse Chestnut
Hippocastanaceae

Other Names: Do not confuse this plant with its North American relative *Aesculus glabra*, commonly known as buckeye.

Parts Used: Seeds, pericarp

Constituents: 3% to 6% triterpene saponin glycosides, a complex mixture known as aescin (escin); 0.2% to 0.3% flavonoids; coumarin derivatives (esculetin and esculin); condensed tannins; sterols (including stigmasterol, α-spinasterol, and β-sitosterol); fatty acids (such as linolenic, palmitic, and stearic acids)[5]

Actions: Astringent, anti-inflammatory, venous tonic

Indications: *Aesculus* has unique actions on the vessels of the circulatory system. The herb appears to increase the elasticity and tone of the veins while decreasing vein permeability. It may be used internally in the treatment of phlebitis, vein inflammation, varicosities, and hemorrhoids. Externally, it may be used as a lotion for the same conditions, as well as for leg ulcers.

Aescin has antiexudative actions and a tightening effect on the vasculature. *Aesculus* extract may reduce the activity of lysosomal enzymes, which is increased in chronic pathological conditions of the veins and inhibits the breakdown of mucopolysaccharides in the capillary walls. A reduction in the activity of these enzymes has the effect of decreasing vascular permeability, leading to improvement in symptoms of chronic venous insufficiency (including sensations of tiredness, heaviness, pruritus, pain, and swelling in the legs).[6]

A study of 22 patients with venous insufficiency showed that 1,200 mg of *Aesculus* extract (standardized to 50 mg aescin per capsule) lowered capillary filtration by 22% in 3 hours.[7] A review of 13 clinical studies reported that horse chestnut was superior to placebo in improving symptoms of chronic venous insufficiency. The pooled results showed that horse chestnut reduced edema, pain, fatigue, tenseness, and in some cases, pruritus in the legs.[8]

Safety Considerations: The seed contains coumarin derivatives that may theoretically interact with anticoagulant medications.

Preparations and Dosage: Tincture dosage is 1 to 4 ml three times a day (1:5 in 40%). To make an infusion, pour 1 cup of boiling water over 1 to 2 teaspoons of dried fruit and leave to infuse for 10 to 15 minutes. This should be drunk three times a day or used as a lotion.

Commercial extracts are usually standardized to 16% triterpene glycosides, calculated as aescin. Recommended doses are the equivalent of 50 mg aescin two or three times a day (300 to 900 mg of a 16% extract). Commission E recommends a total daily dose of 100 mg aescin, corresponding to 250 to 312.5 mg extract in delayed-release form.

Horsechestnut seed, in *Principles and Practice of Phytotherapy*

Agathosma betulina (Berg.) Bartl. and Wendl.
Buchu
Rutaceae

Other Names: Until recently, the binomial was *Barosma betulina*.

Part Used: Leaf

Constituents: Volatile oils, 1.0% to 3.5% (limonene, menthone, pulegone); flavonoids (rutin, diosmetin, diosmin, hesperidin, quercetin, and derivatives); miscellaneous: vitamins of the B group, tannins, mucilage[9]

Actions: Diuretic, urinary antiseptic

Indications: Buchu is useful in infections of the genitourinary system, such as cystitis, urethritis, and prostatitis. Its healing and soothing properties indicate its use in combination with other relevant remedies for many conditions affecting this system. It is especially useful when dysuria is part of the symptom picture. However, the volatile oil content may make it too irritating for people with a history of kidney disease.

Safety Considerations: Remedies high in antimicrobial oils may be contraindicated in people with kidney disease. The volatile oil of buchu contains diosmin and pulegone, which can cause irritation. However, there have been no reports of adverse effects.

Preparations and Dosage: Tincture dosage is 1 to 2 ml three times a day (1:5 in 60%). To make an infusion, pour 1 cup of boiling water over 1 to 2 teaspoonfuls of dried herb and infuse for 10 minutes. This should be drunk three times a day.

The BHC recommends 1 to 2 g in infusion of dried herb, 2 to 4 ml tincture (1:5 in 60%), or 0.5 to 1.5 ml fluid extract (1:1 in 90%) three times daily.

Buchu, in *Principles and Practice of Phytotherapy*

Agrimonia eupatoria L.
Agrimony
Rosaceae

Parts Used: Aerial parts

Constituents: Tannins (3% to 21%); coumarins; flavonoids (glycosides of luteolin, apigenin, and quercetin); polysaccharides; glycosidal bitters[10]

Actions: Astringent, tonic, bitter, diuretic, vulnerary, antispasmodic, diaphoretic, carminative, hepatic, cholagogue

Indications: The combination of astringency and bitter tonic properties in agrimony makes this herb a valuable remedy. This is especially true when astringent activity is needed in the digestive system, as agrimony also contributes a tonic action through bitter stimulation of digestive and liver secretions. Agrimony may be used to treat indigestion, and is a specific for childhood diarrhea. It is the herb of choice in early-stage appendicitis, and its properties give it a role in the treatment of mucous colitis. It may also be helpful for urinary incontinence and cystitis. Agrimony has a long tradition of use as a spring tonic. As a gargle, it helps relieve sore throats and laryngitis. Used in ointment form, it aids in the healing of wounds and bruises.

In one study, agrimony infusion was used successfully to treat cutaneous porphyria in a group of 20 patients.[11] Results demonstrated improvements in skin eruptions as well as decreases in serum iron concentrations and urinary porphyrins. Activity against *Staphylococcus aureus* and α-hemolytic streptococci has been reported.[12]

In another study, a preparation containing agrimony was used to treat 35 patients suffering from chronic gastroduodenitis.[13] After 25 days of therapy, 75% of the patients were free of pain, 95% from dyspeptic symptoms, and 76% from palpitation pains. Gastroscopy indicated that previous erosions and hemorrhagic mucous changes had healed. No side effects or signs of toxicity were observed.

Priest and Priest described agrimony as a

. . . gently stimulating tonic with a gastro-intestinal emphasis that is suitable for both infants and the elderly. It influences mucous membranes, promotes assimilation and restores debilitated conditions.

They provided the following specific indications: general alimentary weakness, hepatic weakness, enuresis, diarrhea, leukorrhea, rheumatism, and arthritis.

Safety Considerations: No side effects or drug interactions have been reported.

Preparations and Dosage: Tincture dosage is 1 to 4 ml three times a day (1:5 in 45%). For an infusion, pour 1 cup of boiling water over 1 to 2 teaspoons of the dried herb and infuse for 10 to 15 minutes. This should be drunk three times a day.

Commission E states that the average daily dosage is 3 g of herb or equivalent preparation. Ellingwood recommended 1 dram of pulverized leaves as decoction or 0.25 to 1 dram of tincture. Dosage given in the United States Dispensatory (23rd ed.) is 1 dram (4 g) or more.

Agrimony, in *Herbal Medicines: A Guide for Health-Care Professionals*

Alchemilla vulgaris L.
Lady's Mantle
Rosaceae

Parts Used: Leaf, flowering shoots

Constituents: Tannins, consisting mainly of glycosides of ellagic acid; salicylic acid (trace amounts)[14]

Actions: Astringent, diuretic, anti-inflammatory, emmenagogue, vulnerary

Indications: This and other species of *Alchemilla* have been widely used in folk medicine throughout Europe. Lady's mantle helps reduce pains associated with menstrual periods and ameliorates excessive bleeding. It also has a role to play in easing symptoms of menopause. As an emmenagogue, it can stimulate proper menstrual flow. However, in the often apparently paradoxical way of herbal remedies, the herb is also a useful uterine astringent, helpful in both menorrhagia and metrorrhagia. Its astringency makes it beneficial in the treatment of diarrhea, as a mouthwash for sores and ulcers, and as a gargle for laryngitis.

Safety Considerations: No side effects or drug interactions have been reported.

Preparations and Dosage: Tincture dosage is 2 to 4 ml three times a day (1:5 in 25%). To make an infusion, pour 1 cup of boiling water over 2 teaspoons of dried herb and infuse for 10 to 15 minutes. This should be drunk three times a day. For use in diarrhea, or as a mouthwash or lotion, make a stronger infusion by boiling the herb for a few minutes to extract all the tannin.

Dosage recommended in the BHP is 2 to 4 g dried herb or 2 to 4 ml fluid extract (1:1 in 25%).

Lady's Mantle, *The Complete German Commission E Monographs*

Allium sativum L.

Garlic

Liliaceae

Part Used: Bulb

Constituents: Organosulfur compounds (alliin, converted to allicin in the presence of the enzyme allinase); miscellaneous: enzymes including allinase, B vitamins, minerals, flavonoids[15]

Actions: Antimicrobial, diaphoretic, hypocholesteremic, cholagogue, hypotensive, antispasmodic

Indications: Used daily, garlic aids and supports the body in ways that no other herb can match. It is an effective antimicrobial, acting on bacteria, viruses, and parasites of the alimentary tract. The volatile oil is largely excreted via the lungs, making garlic useful in infections of the respiratory system, such as chronic bronchitis, respiratory catarrh, recurrent colds, and influenza. It may also be helpful in the treatment of whooping cough and as part of a broader approach to bronchial asthma. In general, garlic may be used as preventive medicine against most infectious conditions, digestive as well as respiratory. In the digestive tract, garlic is thought to support the development of the natural bacterial flora while killing pathogenic organisms.

Garlic has a range of effects upon cardiovascular health. It reduces serum cholesterol and triglyceride levels while raising levels of high-density lipoproteins (HDL). It can also act as an effective inhibitor of platelet-activating factor (PAF). Garlic's antioxidant properties help prevent the peroxidation of fats, yet another contributing factor in the development of atherosclerosis. Taken together, these properties provide a potential way to prevent atherosclerosis, thrombosis, hypertension, heart attack, and stroke.

According to epidemiological evidence, garlic may have cancer-preventive properties, especially against cancers of the gastrointestinal tract. It has been used externally for the treatment of the fungal infection ringworm and as a suppository against pinworm (*Enterobius vermicularis*). Immune potentiation and hypoglycemic actions in humans have also been reported.

Safety Considerations: At high doses, garlic may irritate the intestinal mucosa, causing nausea, diarrhea, vomiting, and burning of the mouth. However, in humans, daily administration of high doses of garlic essential oil (approximately 120 mg, equivalent to 60 g/day fresh garlic) over a period of 3 months did not cause any adverse effects.[16] Contact dermatitis from occupational exposure has been reported.

Therapeutic doses (not dietary) of garlic may potentiate the activity of anticoagulant medications and the antithrombotic actions of anti-inflammatory medications, such as aspirin. Caution is advised both before and after surgical procedures.[17,18]

Preparations and Dosage: A clove should be eaten daily for prophylaxis. During acute infections, 1 clove three times a day is indicated. Alternatively, use garlic oil capsules at a dosage of 1 capsule a day as a prophylactic or 1 capsule three times a day for infection. Recommended dosage of standardized garlic powder (6 mg allicin yield) is 600 to 900 mg/day. Enteric-coated garlic supplements can help control after-odor on breath and skin.

Commission E suggests a daily dosage of 4 g fresh garlic or equivalent preparations.

Koch HP, Lawson D, eds. *Garlic: The Science and Therapeutic Application of* Allium sativum *L. and Related Species.* Baltimore: Williams and Wilkins Publishing Co., 1996.

Althaea officinalis L.

Marshmallow

Malvaceae

Parts Used: Root, leaf

Constituents: *Root:* Mucilage (18% to 35%, consisting of a number of polysaccharides); miscellaneous: about 35% pectin, 1% to 2% asparagine, tannins

Leaf: Mucilage (including a low-molecular-weight D-glucan); flavonoids (such as kaempferol, quercetin, and diosmetin glucosides); scopoletin (a coumarin); polyphenolic acids (including syringic, caffeic, salicylic, vanillic, *p*-coumaric)[19]

Actions: Demulcent, emollient, diuretic, anti-inflammatory, expectorant

Indications: Because of the abundance of mucilage it contains, marshmallow is an excellent demulcent that is indicated whenever such an action is needed. Marshmallow root has been used primarily in the digestive system, and leaf in the urinary system and lungs. All inflammatory disorders of the gastrointestinal tract will benefit from the application of marshmallow root, including inflammations of the mouth, gastritis, peptic ulceration, and colitis. Leaf helps in cystitis, urethritis, and urinary gravel, as well as bronchitis, respiratory catarrh, and irritating coughs.

Externally, the herb is often used as an ingredient in drawing ointments for abscesses and boils and as an emollient for varicose veins and ulcers. The mucilage has demonstrated hypoglycemic activity in nondiabetic mice.[20] Antimicrobial activity against *Pseudomonas aerugi-*

nosa, Proteus vulgaris, and *Staphylococcus aureus* has been documented.[21]

Priest and Priest considered marshmallow a

> . . . soothing demulcent indicated for inflamed and irritated states of mucous membranes. Particularly suitable for the elderly with chronic inflammatory conditions affecting the gastrointestinal system or genitourinary tract.

They gave the following specific indications: acute respiratory disease, gastroenteritis, peptic ulcer, cystitis, urethritis, inflammation of the mouth and throat, inflamed hemorrhoids and wounds, burns and scalds, bedsores, abscesses, boils, and skin ulcers.

Safety Considerations: Marshmallow may delay absorption of other drugs taken at the same time.

Preparations and Dosage: Tincture dosage is 1 to 4 ml three times a day (1:5 in 25%). A cold infusion of marshmallow root may be made by infusing overnight 2 to 4 g of root in 1 cup of cold water.

Dosage recommended by the BHC is 2 to 5 g as dried herb or cold infusion or 5 to 15 ml tincture. The BPC (1949) suggests a dosage of 2 to 10 ml of syrup. Commission E recommends a daily dosage of 6 g root or 5 g leaf.

Marshmallow leaf and Marshmallow root, in *Herbal Medicine, Expanded Commission E Monographs*

Anethum graveolens L.
Dill
Apiaceae

Part Used: Seed

Constituents: Volatile oil (mainly carvone, with dihydrocarvone, limonene, α- and β-phellandrene, eugenol, anethole, myristicin, carveole, *x*-pinene); flavonoids (kaempferol); coumarins (such as scopoletin, esculetin, bergapten, umbelliferone); xanthone derivatives, such as dillanoside; miscellaneous: triterpenes, phenolic acids, protein, fixed oil[22]

Actions: Carminative, aromatic, antispasmodic, anti-inflammatory, galactagogue

Indications: Dill is an excellent remedy for flatulence and associated colic. This is the herb of choice for children's colic. It also stimulates milk flow in nursing mothers. Chewing the seeds helps clear bad breath.

Safety Considerations: Contact with juice from the fresh plant may cause photodermatitis.

Preparations and Dosage: Tincture dosage is 2 to 4 ml three times a day (1:5 in 25%). To make an infusion, pour 1 cup of boiling water over 1 to 2 teaspoons of gently crushed seeds and infuse in a covered container for 10 to 15 minutes. For the treatment of flatulence, take a cup of this infusion before meals.

According to Commission E, average daily dosage is 3 g of seed or equivalent preparations, or 0.1 to 0.3 ml essential oil. Dosage from the United States Dispensatory (23rd ed., 1948) is 15 grains to 1 dram (1 to 4 g) seed. The BPC recommends 15 to 30 ml of dill water (hydrosol) or 0.3 to 0.2 ml of essential oil. The BHP recommends 1 to 2 g dried herb or 1 to 2 ml fluid extract. Dosage listed in the BHC is 2 to 6 g of dried herb, 2 to 4 ml tincture (1:5 in 25%), or 2 to 6 ml fluid extract (1:1 in 25%).

Dill seed, in *The Complete German Commission E Monographs*

Angelica archangelica L.
Angelica
Apiaceae

Other Name: European angelica

Parts Used: Root and leaf (medicinal); stem and seed (confectionery)

Constituents: Volatile oils (0.3% to 1.0%, highest in seeds): α- and β-phellandrene, α-pinene, α-thujene, limonene, β-caryophyllene, linalool, borneol, acetaldehyde; macrocyclic lactones; phthalates (hexamethylphthalate); furanocoumarin glycosides (angelicin, umbelliferone, psoralen, bergapten, imperatoren); miscellaneous: sugars, plant acids, flavonoids, and sterols[23]

Actions: Astringent, tonic, diuretic, vulnerary, cholagogue, anti-inflammatory

Indications: Angelica is a useful expectorant for coughs, bronchitis, and pleurisy, especially when accompanied by fever, colds, or influenza. Angelica leaf may be used as a compress to treat inflammations of the chest. The content of carminative essential oil explains its use easing intestinal colic and flatulence. As a digestive agent, angelica stimulates appetite and may be helpful in anorexia nervosa. It has also been shown to help ease rheumatic inflammations. In cystitis, it acts as a urinary antiseptic. The furanocoumarin constituent bergapten has been used in the PUVA treatment of psoriasis. (PUVA is an acronym describing oral administration of psoralen and subsequent exposure to long-wavelength ultraviolet light.)

Angelica is a common flavoring for liqueurs, such as Chartreuse and Bénédictine, and is an ingredient of gin and vermouth. The leaves may be used as a garnish or in salads, and the candied stalks in cakes and pudding.

Safety Considerations: Because of its furanocoumarin

constituents, angelica may provoke photosensitivity reactions. During treatment with angelica, patients should avoid prolonged sunbathing and exposure to strong UV radiation.

In addition, some authorities state that because of the coumarin constituents, high doses of angelica may interfere with anticoagulant therapy.

Preparations and Dosage: Tincture dosage is 2 to 5 ml three times a day (1:5 in 45%). To make a decoction, place 1 teaspoon of cut root in 1 cup of water, bring to a boil, and simmer for 2 minutes. Remove from heat and let stand for 15 minutes. Decoction dosage is 1 cup three times a day.

The BHP recommends 2.5 g dried herb, 2 to 5 ml tincture (1:5 in 45%), or 2 to 5 ml liquid extract (1:1 in 25%) three times daily. Commission E recommends a daily dose of 4.5 g dried herb, 1.5 ml tincture (1:5), or 1.5 to 3.0 ml fluid extract (1:1). The total daily essential oil dosage is in the range of 10 to 20 drops.

Angelica root, in *Herbal Medicine, Expanded Commission E Monographs*

Apium graveolens L.
Celery Seed
Apiaceae

Part Used: Dried ripe seed

Constituents: Volatile oil (2% to 3%): limonene (60%), selenine (10% to 15%), α-eudesmol and β-eudesmol, santalol; phthalides (3-*n*-butylphthalide, ligustilide, sedanolide, and sedanenolide); furanocoumarins (apigravin, bergapten, celerin, isoimperatorin, isopimpinellin, umbelliferone, 8-hydroxy-5-methoxypsoralen); flavonoids (apiin, apigenin, isoquercitrin, and others)[24]

Actions: Antirheumatic, anti-inflammatory, diuretic, carminative, antispasmodic, nervine

Indications: Celery seed finds its main use in the treatment of rheumatism, arthritis, and gout. It is especially useful in rheumatoid arthritis associated with mental depression. Its value in rheumatic conditions is related primarily to its diuretic action. Celery seed is also used as a urinary antiseptic, largely because of its content of apiol, a volatile oil constituent.

In mice, phthalide constituents showed sedative and antispasmodic activities.[25] Celery seed oil has been reported to be active against *Bacillus subtilis*, *Vibrio cholerae*, *Staphylococcus aureus*, *S. albus*, *Shigella dysenteriae*, *Corynebacterium diphtheriae*, *Salmonella typhi*, *Streptococcus faecalis*, *S. pyogenes*, *Pacillus pumilus*, and *Pseudomonas solanacearum*.[26]

No activity against *Escherichia coli*, *Sarcina lutea*, or *Pseudomonas aeruginosa* was observed.

Safety Considerations: While no problems have been documented for celery seed, photosensitivity reactions resulting from external contact with celery stems have been reported.[27] This has been attributed to their content of furanocoumarins, which are known photosensitizing agents.[28]

Preparations and Dosage: Tincture dosage is 1 to 4 ml three times a day (1:5 in 60%). To make an infusion, pour 1 cup of boiling water over 1 to 2 teaspoons of freshly crushed seeds; infuse in a covered container for 10 to 15 minutes. This should be drunk three times a day.

Dosage from the BHC is 0.5 to 3 g dried seed (or infusion), 2 to 8 ml tincture (1:5 in 90%), or 0.5 to 2 ml fluid extract (1:1 in 90%) three times a day.

Apii fructus, in *Herbal Drugs and Phytopharmaceuticals*

Arctium lappa L.
Burdock
Asteraceae

Parts Used: Root, rhizome, leaf

Constituents: Lignans (arctigenin, arctiin, and matairesinol); polyacetylenes; carbohydrates: inulin (45% to 50%), mucilage, pectin, sugars; miscellaneous: organic acids, fatty acids, and phenolic acids[29]

Actions: Alterative, diuretic, bitter

Indications: Burdock is a valuable remedy for the treatment of skin conditions that result in dry and scaly patches. It may be most effective for psoriasis if used over a long period of time. It has value when used as part of a wider treatment program for rheumatic complaints, especially when associated with psoriasis.

Part of burdock's action is related to bitter stimulation of digestive juice secretion, especially bile secretion. Thus, it helps with digestion and appetite, and has been used in anorexia nervosa and similar conditions. It has also been used to support kidney function and to treat cystitis. In general, burdock will move the body to a state of integration and health, improving indicators of systemic imbalance, such as skin problems and dandruff. Externally, burdock may be applied as a compress or poultice to speed healing of wounds and ulcers. Eczema and psoriasis may also be treated this way, but it is important to remember that such skin problems can be healed only from within, with the help of internal remedies.

Animal studies using roots and leaves of burdock plants that had not yet flowered demonstrated diuretic, hypoglycemic, and antifurunculous properties.[30] The antimicrobial activity documented for burdock has been attributed to its polyacetylene constituents, although only traces of these compounds are found in dried commercial herb.[31] Other studies have suggested that burdock may afford protection against mutagenicity.[32,33] Burdock has also shown antitumor activity.[34] In an animal study, the addition of dietary fiber (5%) from burdock roots to the diet of rats provided protection against toxicity from various artificial food colorings.[35]

Priest and Priest considered burdock a

> . . . general alterative: influences skin, kidneys, mucous and serous membranes, to remove accumulated waste products. It is specific for eruptions on the head, face and neck, and for acute irritable and inflammatory conditions.

They gave the following specific indications: eczema, psoriasis, dermatitis; boils, carbuncles, sties, sores, rheumatism, gout, and sciatica.

Safety Considerations: Potentially, burdock may cause allergic reactions in people sensitive to plants in the Asteraceae family.

Preparations and Dosage: Tincture dosage is 2 to 4 ml three times a day (1:5 in 40%). To make a decoction, put 1 teaspoon of root into 1 cup of water, bring to a boil, and simmer for 10 to 15 minutes. This should be drunk three times a day.

The BHC recommends 2 to 6 g of dried root by decoction, 8 to 12 ml tincture (1:5 in 25%), or 2 to 6 ml fluid extract (1:1 in 25%) three times a day.

Burdock root, in *The Complete German Commission E Monographs*

Arctostaphylos uva-ursi (L.) K. Spreng.
Bearberry
Ericaceae

Other Names: Uva-ursi, kinnikinnick

Part Used: Leaf

Constituents: Hydroquinones (arbutin, methylarbutin); iridoids (monotropein); flavonoids (quercitrin, isoquercitrin, myricacitrin, and others); miscellaneous: tannins; volatile oil; ursolic, malic and gallic acids[36]

Actions: Diuretic, astringent, antimicrobial, demulcent

Indications. Bearberry has a specific antiseptic and astringent effect on the membranes of the urinary system. It generally soothes, tones, and strengthens these tissues. It is specifically used for conditions in which there is gravel or ulceration in the kidney or bladder. It may be applied in the treatment of acute urinary tract infections, such as pyelitis and cystitis, or used as part of a holistic approach to chronic kidney problems. It has proved effective for some cases of bed-wetting. As a douche, it may be helpful in the treatment of vaginal ulceration and infection.

Ellingwood provided the following specific indications for bearberry:

> Its direct influence is upon relaxed conditions of the bladder walls, to which it imparts tone and induces normal contraction. It restrains excessive mucous discharges.

He recommended the herb for ulceration of the bladder, cystitis, pyelitis, pyelonephritis, and gonorrhea.

Safety Considerations: Urinary acidifiers inhibit the conversion of arbutin to active hydroquinone, rendering bearberry less effective.

Preparations and Dosage: Tincture dosage is 2 to 4 ml three times a day (1:5 in 25%). To make an infusion, pour 1 cup of boiling water over 1 to 2 teaspoons of dried leaves; infuse in a covered container for 10 to 15 minutes. This should be drunk three times a day.

Commission E recommends 10 to 12 g (equivalent to 400 to 840 mg of arbutin) in 150 ml water as infusion or cold macerate. Dosage from BHC is 1.5 to 2.5 g dried leaf infusion or cold aqueous extract, 2 to 4 ml tincture (1:5 in 25%), or 1.5 to 2.5 ml fluid extract (1:1 in 25%).

Bearberry, in *Principles and Practice of Phytotherapy*

Arnica montana L.
Arnica
Asteraceae

Part Used: Flower head

Constituents: Sesquiterpene lactones (arnifolin, arnicolides, helenalin); flavonoids (such as eupafolin, patuletin, and spinacetin); volatile oil, containing thymol and various ethers of thymol; miscellaneous: phenolic acids, coumarins, resins, bitters (arnicin), tannins, carotenes[37]

Actions: Anti-inflammatory, vulnerary

Indications: This herb should not be taken internally, as it is potentially toxic. However, arnica provides us with one of the best external remedies for local healing, and may be considered a specific when it comes to the treatment of bruises and sprains. The homeopathic preparation is entirely safe to take internally, especially when used according to homeopathic directions. The herb itself, used externally, will help relieve pain and inflammation of phlebitis, rheumatism, and similar conditions. In fact, it may be used on the skin in all cases of pain or inflammation, as long as the skin is not broken.

Arnica has been shown to be an immunostimulant, as both the sesquiterpene lactone helenalin and the polysaccharide fraction stimulate phagocytosis. Sesquiterpene lactones are known to have anti-inflammatory activity, and their biological effects appear to be mediated through immunological processes. The fact that helenalin is an anti-inflammatory sesquiterpene lactone might help account for the value of arnica for pain and inflammation.

Safety Considerations: Due to the toxicity of the sesquiterpene lactones it contains, oral use of arnica must be avoided altogether. Topical applications of arnica may cause an allergy in the form of painful, itchy, inflammatory changes to the skin in some people.

Preparations and Dosage: For topical use, a simple folk tincture will suffice. Pour $1/2$ liter (1 pint) of 70% alcohol over 50 g (2 ounces) of freshly picked flowers in a clear glass container. Seal and let stand for at least a week in the sun or a warm place. Filter and store in a sealed container; keep out of direct sunlight. Use as needed.

Arnica flowers, in *Principles and Practice of Phytotherapy*

Artemisia absinthium L.
Wormwood
Asteraceae

Parts Used: Leaf, flowering top

Constituents: Volatile oil, including α- and β-thujone (35%); sesquiterpene lactones (absinthin, artemetin, matricin, isoabsinthin, artemolin); acetylenes; flavonoids; phenolic acids; lignans (diayangambin and epiyangambin)[38]

Actions: Bitter, carminative, antimicrobial, anthelmintic, antidepressant

Indications: Traditionally, wormwood has been used in a wide range of conditions, from indigestion to depression, many of which have been validated by scientific analysis. The herb is primarily used as a bitter to stimulate and invigorate the whole digestive process. It is helpful in indigestion, especially when due to a deficient quantity or quality of gastric juices. As the name implies, wormwood is a powerful remedy against worm infestations, especially roundworm and pinworm. The herb may also be used to help the body deal with fever and infections. It has a long history of use as an antidepressant.

Safety Considerations: Adverse effects are likely only with overdose, and are due primarily to the effects of thujone, which is toxic. Taken in high doses, wormwood

preparations may cause intoxication with vomiting, severe diarrhea, retention of urine, stupor, and convulsions. Aqueous extracts contain relatively little thujone. Wormwood is contraindicated for patients with stomach hyperacidity and intestinal ulcers. Avoid during pregnancy.

Concerns about the safety of wormwood are related largely to the presence of the monoterpene constituent thujone in the essential oil (see chapter 6 for more information). Concerns about the toxicity of wormwood essential oil are well founded; however, the amount of essential oil in the dried herb is low, minimizing danger.

Thujone is also a component of certain other essential oils, including white cedar oil (from the leaves of *Thuja occidentalis*) and tansy oil (from the leaves and tops of *Tanacetum vulgare*). It is also found in the leaves of the culinary sage *(Salvia officinalis)* and of rosemary *(Rosmarinus officinalis)*. For purposes of comparison, the thujone content of selected plants is listed here.

Salvia officinalis (sage leaf): 1,453 to 12,636 ppm
Artemisia absinthium (wormwood leaf): 3,500 ppm
Rosmarinus officinalis (rosemary plant): 84 to 399 ppm

Antifertility studies were conducted in rats using dry extract of wormwood (probably containing some essential oil). Oral administration of this extract at a dosage of 200 mg/kg for 7 days caused a significant anti-implantation effect.[39] Daily oral administration of thujone to rats at 10 mg/kg produced convulsions on day 38 of the study (after intake of a total of 380 mg of thujone) in 5% of the rats. The oral LD_{50} of mixed α- and β-thujones has been determined to be 192 mg/kg in rats, 230 mg/kg in mice, and 395 mg/kg in guinea pigs; however, α-thujone is more toxic than β-thujone.[40] Overdose of wormwood in humans may cause major CNS disturbances, including convulsions and paralysis leading to unconsciousness and death. Very high doses of wormwood tincture have been reported to induce abortion.

Dilute aqueous extracts of dried wormwood contain only trace amounts of essential oil. Thujone-free wormwood extracts can be prepared with extraction procedures using either water, 30% ethanol, or supercritical carbon dioxide extraction technology.

Preparations and Dosage: Tincture dosage is 1 to 4 ml three times a day (1:1 in 25%). To make an infusion, pour 1 cup of boiling water over 1 to 2 teaspoons of the dried herb; infuse for 10 to 15 minutes. This should be drunk three times a day. To avoid the extremely bitter taste when using wormwood as an anthelmintic, powdered wormwood may be taken in pill form to eliminate worms.

Commission E lists a daily dosage of 2 to 3 g of herb as a water infusion. BPC recommends 3 to 10 ml of tincture daily. Dosage from the BHP is 1 to 2 g of dried herb or 1 to 2 ml of fluid extract (1:1 in 25%) three times a day.

Artemisiae herba, in *Herbal Drugs and Phytopharmaceuticals*

Artemisia vulgaris L.
Mugwort
Asteraceae

Parts Used: Leaf, root

Constituents: Volatile oil (linalool, l,8-cineole, β-thujone, borneol, α- and β-pinene); sesquiterpene lactones (vulgarin); flavonoids; coumarin derivatives; triterpenes[41]

Actions: Bitter tonic, stimulant, nervine tonic, emmenagogue

Indications: As a bitter, mugwort may be used whenever digestive stimulation is indicated. However, the herb supports digestion not only through bitter stimulation, but also through carminative actions conferred by the volatile oils it contains. In addition, it has a mild nervine action, which also appears to be related to volatile oil content, that may help ease depression and tension. Thus, it is essential that the volatile oil is not lost in preparation. Mugwort may also be used as an emmenagogue to promote normal menstrual flow.

Safety Considerations: Mugwort is potentially allergenic to people sensitive to plants in the Asteraceae family.

Preparations and Dosage: Tincture dosage is 1 to 4 ml three times a day (1:5 in 25%). To make an infusion, pour 1 cup of boiling water over 1 to 2 teaspoons of dried herb and infuse for 10 to 15 minutes in a covered container. This should be drunk three times a day.

Dosage from the BHP is 0.5 to 2 g of dried herb or 0.5 to 2 ml of fluid extract (1:1 in 25%) three times a day.

Mugwort, in *The Complete German Commission E Monographs*

Asclepias tuberosa L.
Pleurisy Root
Asclepiadaceae

Part Used: Rhizome

Constituents: Cardenolides (including asclepiadin); flavonoids (rutin, kaempferol, quercetin, and isorhamnetin); miscellaneous: friedalin, α- and β-amyrin, lupeol, viburnitol, choline sugars[42]

Actions: Diaphoretic, expectorant, antispasmodic, carminative, anti-inflammatory

Indications: Pleurisy root is effective against respiratory infections, reducing inflammation and promoting expectoration. It can be used in the treatment of bronchitis, influenza, and other respiratory conditions. The fact that it also has diaphoretic and antispasmodic powers explains why it is so highly valued for treating pleurisy and pneumonia. In the laboratory, low doses of extracts of *Asclepias* species stimulated uterine contractions and exhibited estrogenic effects.[43]

Priest and Priest gave the following specific indications: catarrhal complaints from cold and damp, hard dry cough, bronchitis, pleurisy, peritonitis, pneumonia, influenza, intercostal rheumatism, and other intercostal diseases. According to *King's:*

It was one of the most common medicines employed by the Eclectic fathers. The drug has fallen into unmerited neglect, and could profitably be employed at the present day for purposes for which much more powerful, and sometimes dangerous, drugs are used. It has an extensive range of usefulness, being possessed of diaphoretic, diuretic, laxative, tonic, carminative, expectorant, and probably anti-spasmodic properties.

Pleurisy root is one of the best diaphoretics of the Eclectic materia medica. It is not stimulating, and may be used to promote diaphoresis, no matter how high the degree of fever. Pleurisy root has a deservedly good reputation in respiratory diseases. It acts upon the mucous membrane of the pulmonary tract, augmenting the secretions and favoring easy expectoration. . . . As its popular name indicates, pleurisy root is of much value in treating pleurisy. Not only is its action on serous membranes marked, but it is very effectual in intercostal neuralgia and rheumatism, as well as in pericardial pains.

In pneumonia, as well as in bronchitis, it is best adapted to the acute stage, where the lesion seems to be extensive, taking in a large area of lung parenchyma and mucous tissues. In the convalescing stage of pneumonia, and other respiratory lesions, when suppression of the expectoration and dyspnoea threaten, small doses at frequent intervals will correct the trouble. It, as well as *Euphrasia* and *Matricaria*, is among our best drugs for snuffles, or acute nasal catarrh of infants.

It is an excellent remedy for ordinary colds. It is, in fact one of our best drugs for catarrhal conditions, whether of the pulmonary or gastrointestinal tract, especially when produced by recent colds. Stomach troubles, particularly those of children, are often markedly benefited by small doses.

Safety Considerations: *Asclepias* increases the risk of cardiac glycoside toxicity if taken with drugs or herbs that contain such constituents.

Preparations and Dosage: Tincture dosage is 1 to 2 ml three times a day (1:5 in 45%). To make an infusion, pour 1 cup of boiling water over ½ to 1 teaspoon of the herb and infuse for 10 to 15 minutes. This should be drunk three times a day.

Pleurisy root, in *Herbal Medicines: A Guide for Health-Care Professionals*

Astragalus membranaceus (Fisch.) Bunge
Astragalus
Fabaceae

Part Used: Root

Constituents: Triterpenoid saponin glycosides (astragalosides I-VII); flavonoid glycosides and aglycones; high-molecular-weight polysaccharides[44]

Action: Immunomodulator

Indications: Astragalus has been used since ancient times in traditional Chinese medicine. When research illuminated its effects upon the immune system, it was adopted as an important remedy in the West. Studies indicate that the polysaccharides in astragalus intensify phagocytosis in reticuloendothelial systems, stimulate pituitary-adrenal cortical activity, and restore depleted red blood cell formation in bone marrow. Astragalus is also one of the herbs known to stimulate the body's natural production of interferon.[45]

Astragalus has been used in combination with drug therapies to reduce their toxicity and ameliorate side effects. The herb has been employed to treat chronic leukopenia (low white blood cell count) related to treatment with steroids, anticancer drugs, and other therapies.[46] In an in vitro study, researchers were able to use a lower dose of interleukin 2 (IL 2), a common cancer treatment, by combining the drug with astragalus. High doses of IL 2 are associated with significant side effects.[47] The addition of astragalus potentiated IL 2 activity tenfold, thus potentially facilitating a lower dose of IL 2 for the same therapeutic outcome. In a laboratory study, astragalus prevented liver damage induced by the common anticancer drug stilbenemide.[48]

Astragalus appears to strengthen both nonspecific and specific immunity. The conclusion drawn by most Western herbalists is that astragalus is an ideal remedy for anyone who might be immunocompromised. It strengthens many functions of the immune system, helps protect the liver from damage, and may have valuable anticancer effects.

Safety Considerations: Astragalus potentiates the effects of interleukin 2 and acyclovir, but may be incompatible with immunosuppressive drugs (e.g., cyclosporine, azathioprine, and methotrexate).[49]

Preparations and Dosage: Tincture dosage is 4 to 8 ml three times a day (1:5 in 40%). To make a decoction, put 2 to 4 teaspoons of root into 1 cup of water, bring to a boil, and simmer for 10 to 15 minutes. This should be drunk three times a day. In traditional Chinese medicine, pieces of root are boiled in soups and removed prior to serving.

Astragalus, in *Principles and Practice of Phytotherapy*

Avena sativa L.
Oats
Poaceae

Other name: Oatstraw

Parts Used: Seed, whole plant

Constituents: Proteins (prolamines known as avenins); *C*-glycosyl flavones; avenacosides (spirostanol glycosides); fixed oil; vitamin E; starch[50]

Actions: Nervine tonic, antidepressant, nutritive, demulcent, vulnerary

Indications: Oats is one of the best remedies for "feeding" the nervous system, especially when the patient is under stress. It is considered a specific in cases of nervous debility and exhaustion associated with depression. Oats may be used in combination with most of the other nervines, both relaxant and stimulant, to strengthen the whole nervous system. It is also used to treat general debility.

Safety Considerations: No side effects or drug interactions have been reported.

Preparations and Dosage: Tincture dosage is 3 to 5 ml three times a day (1:5 in 25%). To make an oatstraw infusion, pour 1 cup of boiling water over 1 to 3 teaspoons of dried straw and leave to infuse 10 to 15 minutes. This should be drunk three times a day.

A soothing bath for use in treating neuralgia and irritated skin conditions can be made by boiling 1 pound of shredded oatstraw in 2 quarts of water for one-half hour. Strain the liquid and add to the bath. Alternately, put cooked rolled oats into a muslin bag and soak it in the bathwater.

Dosage recommended by the BHP is 1 to 5 ml tincture (1:5 in 45%) or 0.6 to 2 ml fluid extract (1:1 in 25%) three times daily. Commission E suggests using 100 g dried herb for one full bath.

Avenae herba, in *Herbal Drugs and Phytopharmaceuticals*

Ballota nigra L.
Black Horehound
Lamiaceae

Constituents: Diterpenes (marrubiin, ballonigrin, ballotinone)[51]

Actions: Antiemetic, nervine, astringent, emmenagogue, expectorant

Indications: Black horehound—not to be confused with white horehound (*Marrubium vulgare*)—is an excellent remedy for calming nausea and vomiting when the cause lies within the nervous system, rather than in the stomach. It may be safely used for motion sickness, for example, in which nausea is triggered through the inner ear and the central nervous system. This herb is also of value in treating nausea and vomiting caused by pregnancy or nervousness. Black horehound has a reputation as a normalizer of menstrual function and as a mild expectorant.

Safety Considerations: No side effects or drug interactions have been reported.

Preparations and Dosage: Tincture dosage is 1 to 2 ml three times a day (1:5 in 25%). To make an infusion, pour 1 cup of boiling water over 1 to 2 teaspoons of dried herb and infuse for 10 to 15 minutes. This should be drunk three times a day, or as needed.

Horehound, Black, in *Herbal Medicines: A Guide for Health-Care Professionals*

Baptisia tinctoria (L.) Venten.
Wild Indigo
Fabaceae

Part Used: Root

Constituents: Isoflavones (genistein, biochanin A); flavonoids; alkaloids (such as cytisine); coumarins; polysaccharides[52]

Actions: Antimicrobial, anticatarrhal

Indications: Wild indigo is especially valuable for the treatment of infections and catarrh of the ear, nose, and throat. It may be used for laryngitis, tonsillitis, pharyngitis, and catarrhal infections of the nose and sinuses. Taken both internally and as a mouthwash, it heals mouth ulcers and gingivitis and helps control pyorrhea. Systemically, it may be useful in the treatment of enlarged and inflamed lymph glands (lymphadenitis) and to reduce fevers. A douche of wild indigo decoction will improve leukorrhea.

Ellingwood had much to say about this neglected remedy:

The agent has been widely used for many years by our practitioners in the treatment of typhoid conditions, and has established its position as an important remedy. In scarlet fever, with its specific indications, it is a useful remedy. Large doses are not necessary, but it should be employed early and the use persisted in. In the treatment of low fevers this agent is said to exercise marked sedative power over the fever.

It is advised in all diseases of the glandular system, and in hepatic derangements especially, with symptoms of the character. In the various forms of stomatitis, putrid sore throat and scarlatina; in inflammation of the bowels, where there is a tendency to typhoid conditions, especially ulcerative inflammation of any of the internal organs; in dyspepsia, with great irritability and offensive decomposition of food; in scrofula and in cutaneous infections, the agent should be long continued. In the long protracted and sluggish forms of fevers, with great depression of the vital forces; in ulceration of the nipples or mammary glands, or of the cervix uteri, it is spoken highly of.

Safety Considerations: No side effects or drug interactions have been reported.

Preparations and Dosage: Tincture dosage is 1 ml three times a day (1:5 in 60%). To make a decoction, put 1/2 to 1 teaspoon of dried root in 1 cup of water, bring to a boil, and simmer for 10 to 15 minutes. This should be drunk three times a day.

Berberis vulgaris L.
Barberry
Berberidaceae

Part Used: Bark of root or stem

Constituents: Isoquinoline alkaloids (berberine, berbamine); miscellaneous: chelidonic acid, resin, tannins[53]

Actions: Cholagogue, hepatic, antiemetic, bitter, laxative

Indications: Barberry is a traditional remedy for correcting liver function and promoting the flow of bile. It is indicated when gallstones or gallbladder inflammation is present and when jaundice occurs due to a congested state of the liver. As a bitter tonic with mild laxative effects, it helps strengthen and cleanse the system in weak or debilitated people. Barberry has the interesting ability to reduce the size of an enlarged spleen. It has antimalarial actions and is effective against infections caused by the protozoan *Leishmania* spp.

Priest and Priest described barberry as follows:

. . . stimulating tonic hepatic: influences the mucosa generally, removing mucoid accumulations and controlling excess secretion. Improves appetite, digestion and assimilation. Indicated for "gouty" constitutions.

They provided the following specific indications: biliary catarrh with constipation and jaundice, gastritis, biliousness, debility during convalescence, ulcerative stomatitis, and eczema of the hands.

Safety Considerations: Avoid during pregnancy.

Preparations and Dosage: Tincture dosage is 1 to 2 ml three times a day (1:5 in 60%). To make a decoction, put 1 teaspoon of herb into 1 cup of cold water and bring to a boil. Simmer for 10 to 15 minutes. This should be drunk three times a day.

The BPC suggests a dosage of 1 to 3.5 ml fluid extract three times a day. Recommended dosage from the BHP is 1 to 2 g of dried herb, 2 to 4 ml tincture (1:10 in 60%), or 2 to 3 ml fluid extract (1:1 in 25%) three times a day.

Barberry, in *The Complete German Commission E Monographs*

Betula alba L.
Birch
Betulaceae

Parts Used: Young leaf, twig

Constituents: Flavonoids (mainly hyperoside, with luteolin and quercetin glycosides)[54]

Actions: Diuretic, anti-inflammatory, antiseptic, tonic

Indications: Birch leaf is an effective remedy for cystitis and other infections of the urinary system and helps eliminate excess water from the body. Perhaps because of this cleansing, diuretic activity, the plant has been used to treat gout, rheumatism, and mild arthritic pain. Birch bark helps ease muscle pain if applied externally, with the fresh, wet, internal side of the bark placed against the skin.

Safety Considerations: No side effects or drug interactions have been reported.

Preparations and Dosage: Tincture dosage is 1 to 2 ml three times a day (1:5 in 25%). To make an infusion, pour 1 cup of boiling water over 1 to 2 teaspoons of dried leaf and infuse for 10 minutes. This should be drunk three times a day.

Commission E suggests a dosage of 2 to 3 g dried herb several times a day.

Betulae folium, in *Herbal Drugs and Phytopharmaceuticals*

Brassica nigra (L.) W.D.J. Koch
Black Mustard
Brassicaceae

Other Names and Related Species: Formerly *Sinapsis nigra*. White mustard (*Brassica alba* Rabenh., non L., syn. *Sinapsis alba* L.) may be used interchangeably.

Part Used: Seed

Constituents: Glucosinolates (black mustard contains sinigrin, white mustard sinalbin); miscellaneous: sinapine, sinapic acid, fixed oil, protein, mucilage[55]

Actions: Rubefacient, irritant, stimulant, diuretic, emetic

Indications: This well-known spice finds its main use in medicine as a stimulating external application. The rubefacient action causes mild irritation to the skin, which stimulates the circulation in that area and relieves muscular and skeletal pain. This also gives it a role in the treatment of chilblains. Because of its stimulating, diaphoretic action, mustard can be applied in the same ways that cayenne and ginger are. For feverishness, colds, and influenza, mustard seed may be taken as a tea or ground and sprinkled into a bath. An infusion or poultice of mustard is useful in the treatment of bronchitis.

Safety Considerations: No side effects or drug interactions have been reported. May cause skin irritation when applied externally, especially in fair-skinned people.

Preparations and Dosage: Mustard is most commonly used as a poultice, which can be made by mixing 100 g (4 oz) of freshly ground mustard seeds with enough warm water (at about 45°C or 110°F) to form a thick paste. Spread this mixture onto a piece of cloth the size of the body area to be covered. To prevent the paste from sticking to the skin, first lay a piece of dampened gauze on the skin. Apply the cloth spread with mustard and remove after 1 minute. The skin may be reddened by this treatment, but may be soothed by the application of olive oil afterward.

To make an infusion, pour 1 cup of boiling water over 1 teaspoon of mustard flour (powder) and infuse for 5 minutes. This may be drunk three times a day. For a footbath, make an infusion using 1 tablespoon of bruised seeds to l liter (2 pints) of boiling water.

Calendula officinalis L.
Calendula
Asteraceae

Other Names: Marigold, pot marigold

Parts Used: Petals, flower head

Constituents: Triterpenes (calendulosides A-D); flavonoids (including narcissin, rutin); volatile oil; chlorogenic acid[56]

Actions: Anti-inflammatory, antispasmodic, lymphatic, astringent, vulnerary, emmenagogue, cholagogue, antifungal

Indications: Calendula may be used safely whenever there is inflammation on the skin, whether due to infection or physical damage. It may be applied for any external bleeding or wound, bruising, or strains. The herb is also of benefit for slow-healing wounds and skin ulcers, and ideal for first-aid treatment of minor burns and scalds. Calendula may be applied locally as a lotion, poultice, or compress, depending on which is most appropriate. Calendula has long been used throughout Europe for wound healing and treatment of both skin and gastric ulcers. Its healing power appears to be based at least in part on its terpene content.

When taken internally, calendula has anti-inflammatory actions in the digestive system, and thus may be used in the treatment of gastric and duodenal ulcers. As a cholagogue, it helps relieve gallbladder problems and many of the vague digestive complaints known as "indigestion."

Calendula demonstrates marked antifungal activity and may be used both internally and externally to combat fungal infections. As an emmenagogue, it has a reputation for helping with delayed menstruation and easing painful periods. In general, it is considered a normalizer of the menstrual process.

In the laboratory, calendula has demonstrated anti-inflammatory, antibacterial, and antiviral activities.[57] A combination of allantoin and calendula extract applied to surgically induced skin wounds in rats was reported to stimulate physiological regeneration and granulation. Allantoin alone exerted a much weaker action.[58]

Safety Considerations: Calendula is a possible allergen for those with known sensitivity to members of the Asteraceae family.

Calendula was shown to be nontoxic when administered chronically to mice in the form of aqueous extract.[59] No symptoms of toxicity were observed after administration of a calendula flower extract at a dosage of 0.15 g/kg to hamsters older than 18 months and rats older than 21 months.[60]

Preparations and Dosage: Tincture dosage is 1 to 4 ml three times a day (1:5 in 60%). To make an infusion, pour 1 cup of boiling water over 1 to 2 teaspoons of flowers and infuse for 10 to 15 minutes. This should be drunk three times a day. Calendula may be applied externally as a lotion or ointment for cuts, bruises, diaper rash, sore nipples, burns, and scalds.

Dosage recommended in the BHP is 1 to 4 g dried herb, 0.3 to 1.2 ml tincture, or 0.5 to 1 ml liquid extract three times daily. Commission E suggests 1 to 2 g dried herb per cup of water (150 ml) or 2 to 4 ml tincture daily.

Calendula flower, in *Herbal Medicine, Expanded Commission E Monographs*

Capsella bursa-pastoris (L.) Medikus
Shepherd's Purse
Brassicaceae

Parts Used: Aerial parts

Constituents: Flavonoids (luteolin-7-rutinoside, quercetin-3-rutinoside); plant acids (fumaric and bursic acids)[61]

Actions: Astringent, diuretic, anti-inflammatory

Indications: Shepherd's purse may be used whenever a gentle diuretic is indicated—for instance, to alleviate water retention due to kidney problems. As an astringent, the herb proves effective in the treatment of diarrhea, wounds, nosebleeds, and other conditions. It traditionally was used to stimulate the menstrual process, but is also of value in reducing excess menstrual flow.

Ellingwood recommended shepherd's purse for hematuria, passive hemorrhage, chronic menorrhagia, intestinal hemorrhage, gastric hemorrhage, atonic dyspepsia, diarrhea, and dysentery, and externally for bruised or strained muscles, bleeding piles, and rheumatic joints.

Safety Considerations: Because of its oxalic acid content, patients with kidney stones should avoid shepherd's purse.

Preparations and Dosage: Tincture dosage is 1 to 2 ml three times a day (1:5 in 25%). To make an infusion, pour 1 cup of boiling water over 1 to 2 teaspoons of dried herb and infuse for 10 to 15 minutes. For menstrual conditions, a cup should be drunk every 2 to 3 hours just before and during the period. Otherwise, it should be drunk three times a day.

Dosage listed in the BHP is 1 to 4 g dried herb or 1 to 4 ml liquid extract (1:1 in 25%) three times a day. Commission E recommends 10 to 15 g of herb or equivalent preparations daily.

Shepherd's Purse, in *Herbal Medicine, Expanded Commission E Monographs*

Capsicum annuum L.

Cayenne

Solanaceae

Part Used: Fruit

Constituents: Capsaicinoids (up to 1.5%): capsaicin, dihydrocapsaicin, others; carotenoids (capsanthin, capsorubin, carotene); steroidal saponins, known as capsicidins, in seed and root[62]

Actions: Stimulant, carminative, anticatarrhal, sialagogue, rubefacient, antimicrobial

Indications: Cayenne is the most useful of the systemic stimulants. It stimulates blood flow, strengthening the heart, arteries, capillaries, and nerves. A general tonic, it is especially useful for toning both the circulatory and digestive systems. Cayenne may be helpful in cases of flatulent dyspepsia and colic. It may also be used in conditions marked by insufficient peripheral circulation leading to cold hands and feet and, possibly, chilblains. It is also valuable for debility and for warding off colds.

Externally, cayenne is applied as a rubefacient for problems such as lumbago and rheumatic pains. As an ointment, it can help with unbroken chilblains, as long as it is used in moderation. As a gargle for laryngitis, it combines well with myrrh. This combination also makes a good antiseptic wash.

Research has shown that capsaicin blocks the transmission of pain and itching by nerve fibers in the skin. Capsaicin applied in the form of a topical cream helps relieve pain by depleting local supplies of a neurotransmitter called substance P, which transmits pain and itching signals from the nerves in the skin to the spinal cord. A link exists between many painful disorders and unusually high levels of substance P in nerve fibers. Unlike other local anesthetics, cayenne does not block impulses to all of the nerve fibers, only type C fibers, which are strictly related to pain. Thus, it does not interfere with perception of touch, temperature, and pressure.

In numerous clinical studies, a topical cream containing 0.025% or 0.075% capsaicin has proved helpful in treating painful and itchy skin disorders, including psoriasis, shingles, diabetic neuropathy, and postmastectomy pain.[63,64] Capsaicin cream may also be effective in relieving the severe, stabbing pain associated with trigeminal neuralgia, a disorder that affects the largest nerve in the face. Improvement was generally apparent after several days of applying the cream three times daily. Capsaicin cream also shows promise in reducing the pain of arthritis.[65]

King's described cayenne thus:

Capsicum is a pure, energetic, permanent stimulant, producing in large doses vomiting, purging, pains in the stomach and bowels, heat and inflammation of the stomach, giddiness, a species of intoxication and an enfeebled condition of the nervous power. The infusion is much used in colds, catarrh, hoarseness, etc. In atonic dyspepsia and catarrhal gastritis it stimulates the nerves of the stomach, promotes the secretion of the digestive juices, and assists peristaltic motion . . . Capsicum meets the debility of young and old, but is particularly useful in the elderly, when the body-heat is low, vitality depressed and reaction sluggish. Tired, painful muscles, stiffened joints and relaxation of any part are common conditions in the elderly that are, in a measure, rectified by Capsicum. Flatulence in dyspeptic states may be dispelled by capsicum.

Externally, the infusion and tincture have been found valuable as a stimulating gargle in the ulcerated throat of scarlatina. If used early in tonsillitis, with relaxation, it may abort the trouble, but if it does not, its use should be discontinued until the active inflammation has subsided. Hoarseness, from atony of the vocal cords, is relieved by it, and it is a remedy for relaxed uvula. It enters into various tinctures and liniments. The concentrated tincture of capsicum has been highly recommended in the treatment of chilblains and toothache. In the former, a piece of sponge of flannel must be saturated with it, and rubbed well over the seat of the chilblain, until a strong tingling and electrical feeling is produced. This application should be continued daily, until the disease is removed; relief will be experienced on the very first application and frequently there will be a total removal of the disease after the second or third application. This, however, will depend upon the severity of the case.

Safety Considerations: No side effects or drug interactions have been reported.

Preparations and Dosage: Tincture dosage is 0.25 to 1 ml three times a day (1:5 in 25%). To make an infusion, pour 1 cup of boiling water over 1/2 to 1 teaspoon of cayenne and infuse for 10 minutes. Mix a tablespoon of this infusion with hot water and drink when needed.

Dosage recommended in the BPC is 0.06 g of dried herb or 0.3 to 0.9 ml tincture three times daily. The BHP recommends 30 to 120 mg of dried herb or 0.3 to 1 ml of tincture three times daily.

Cayenne pepper, in *Herbal Medicine, Expanded Commission E Monographs*

Carum carvi L.
Caraway
Apiaceae

Part Used: Seed

Constituents: Volatile oil, consisting of carvone (40% to 60%) and limonene, with other constituents; flavonoids (mainly quercetin derivatives); miscellaneous: polysaccharide, protein, fixed oil, calcium oxalate[66]

Actions: Carminative, antispasmodic, expectorant, emmenagogue, galactagogue, astringent, antimicrobial

Indications: Caraway is used as a calming herb to ease flatulent dyspepsia and intestinal colic, especially in children. It also helps stimulate appetite. Its astringency makes it useful in the treatment of diarrhea and, when applied as a gargle, in laryngitis. It may be employed for bronchitis and bronchial asthma, and its antispasmodic actions help relieve menstrual pains. Caraway has been used to increase milk flow in nursing mothers.

Safety Considerations: No side effects or drug interactions have been reported.

Preparations and Dosage: Tincture dosage is 1 to 4 ml three times a day (1:5 in 40%). To make an infusion, pour 1 cup of boiling water over 1 teaspoon of freshly crushed seeds and infuse in a covered container for 10 to 15 minutes. This should be drunk three times a day.

Carvi fructus, in *Herbal Drugs and Phytopharmaceuticals*

Centaurium erythraea Rafn.
Centaury
Gentianaceae

Parts Used: Dried aerial parts

Constituents: Secoiridoids: gentiopicroside (gentiopicrin), swertiamarin; alkaloids (gentianine, gentianidine, gentioflavine); xanthone derivatives; phenolic acids; triterpenes (β-sitosterol, campesterol, brassicasterol, stigmasterol, α- and β-amyrin, erythrodiol)[67]

Actions: Bitter, hepatic

Indications: Centaury may be used whenever a digestive and gastric stimulant is needed. It is indicated primarily for appetite loss (anorexia) associated with liver weakness. Centaury is helpful in dyspepsia and any other condition involving sluggish digestion.

Safety Considerations: No side effects or drug interactions have been reported.

Preparations and Dosage: Tincture dosage is 1 to 2 ml three times a day (1:5 in 25%). To make an infusion, pour

1 cup of boiling water over 1 teaspoon of dried herb and infuse for 5 to 10 minutes. Drink 1 cup one half hour before meals.

Commission E recommends an average daily dosage of 6 g dried herb or equivalent preparations, or 1 to 2 ml extract daily.

Centaurii herba, in *Herbal Drugs and Phytopharmaceuticals*

Cephaelis ipecacuanha (Brot.) A. Rich.
Ipecacuanha
Rubiaceae

Other Name: Ipecac

Parts Used: Root, rhizome

Constituents: Isoquinoline alkaloids (2% to 3%): mainly emetine, cephaeline, psychotrine; tannins: ipecacuanhin and ipecacuanhic acid[68]

Actions: Expectorant, emetic, sialagogue, antiprotozoal

Indications: Ipecac is used mainly as an expectorant for conditions such as bronchitis and whooping cough. At higher doses, it is a powerful emetic, and as such is used to treat poisoning. Care must be taken when using this herb. After administration of an effective emetic dose, the patient should drink large amounts of water. In the same way that ipecac promotes expectoration through stimulation and subsequent elimination of mucus, it fosters the production of saliva. It has been found effective against amoebic dysentery.

Safety Considerations: Because it is an emetic, ipecac will prevent the absorption of drugs.

Preparations and Dosage: Ipecac is a very powerful herb, so only a small amount should be used. Use 0.01 to 0.25 g of herb for an infusion. Pour 1 cup of boiling water over a pea-sized amount of herb and infuse for 5 minutes. This may be drunk three times a day.

Ipecacuanhae radix, in *Herbal Drugs and Phytopharmaceuticals*

Cetraria islandica
Iceland Moss
Parmeliaceae

Part Used: Whole plant (a lichen)

Constituents: Lichen acids (fumarprotocetraric, protocetraric, cetraric, usnic); polysaccharides (about 50%): mainly lichenin and isolichenin; miscellaneous: furan derivatives, fatty acid, lactones, terpenes[69]

Actions: Demulcent, anti-inflammatory, antiemetic, expectorant

Indications: As a soothing demulcent with a high mucilage content, Iceland moss is valuable in gastritis, vomiting, and dyspepsia. It is also often used in respiratory catarrh and bronchitis to soothe mucous membranes. Its nourishing qualities give it a role in the treatment of cachexia, a state of malnourishment and debility.

King's described Iceland moss as

. . . demulcent, tonic and nutritious. Excessive doses may induce nausea and looseness of the bowels, while ordinary doses improve the appetite, digestion and general nutrition. Constipation is not produced by it, and the circulation is unaffected. Its nutritive qualities are undoubtedly due to its starch. The bitterness of cetrarin may be detected in the nursing mother's milk. Used as a demulcent in chronic catarrhs, chronic dysentery and diarrhea, and as a tonic in dyspepsia, convalescence and exhausting diseases. Boiled with milk, it forms an excellent nutritive and tonic in phthisis and general debility. It relieves the cough of chronic bronchitis.

Safety Considerations: Because of its high mucilage content, Iceland moss may impair absorption of drugs.

Preparations and Dosage: Tincture dosage is 1 to 2 ml three times a day (1:5 in 25%). To make a decoction, put 1 teaspoon of shredded moss in 1 cup of cold water. Boil for 3 minutes and let stand for 10 minutes. A cup should be drunk morning and evening.

Commission E recommends 4 to 6 g of herb or equivalent preparations daily.

Iceland moss, in *Herbal Medicine, Expanded Commission E Monographs*

Chelone glabra L.
Balmony
Scrophulariaceae

Parts Used: Dried aerial parts

Constituents: Very little research has been conducted on this plant. Only resins and bitters have been reported.

Actions: Cholagogue, hepatic, bitter, antiemetic, stimulant, laxative

Indications: Balmony is an excellent agent for liver problems and acts as a tonic for the whole digestive system. The herb stimulates the secretion of digestive juices, and in this way produces its laxative actions. Balmony is used to treat gallstones, inflammation of the gallbladder, and jaundice. It is considered a specific for gallstones that lead to congestive jaundice. The herb stimulates appetite; eases colic, dyspepsia, and biliousness; and is beneficial in

debility. Externally, it has been used to treat inflamed breasts, painful ulcers, and piles.

Priest and Priest said that balmony is a

. . . mild relaxing hepatic influencing the mucous membranes, stimulating appetite and toning the stomach. It is suitable for children and the elderly. Indicated for gastrointestinal disturbances after prolonged illness.

They gave the following specific indications: atonic conditions, malaise and debility, dyspepsia, malabsorption, roundworms and threadworms, colitis from hepatic dysfunction, and chronic jaundice.

Safety Considerations: No side effects or drug interactions have been reported.

Preparations and Dosage: Tincture dosage is 1 to 2 ml three times a day (1:10 in 40%). To make an infusion, pour 1 cup of boiling water over 2 teaspoons of dried herb and infuse for 10 to 15 minutes. This should be drunk three times a day.

Chionanthus virginicus L.
Fringetree
Oleaceae

Part Used: Bark

Constituents: Phyllyrin (a lignin glycoside); chionanthin[70]

Actions: Hepatic, cholagogue, alterative, diuretic, tonic, antiemetic, laxative

Indications: This valuable herb may be safely used for many liver problems, especially when jaundice is part of the picture. It is a specific for the treatment of gallbladder inflammation and a valuable component of treatment for gallstones. Fringetree aids the liver in general, and as such is often used as a tonic as part of a wider treatment to support the whole body. Because it stimulates the release of bile, it also acts as a gentle and effective laxative.

Ellingwood considered fringetree specific for

. . . the liver. It is a remedy for hepatic engorgement; jaundice more or less pronounced; pain over the region of the gall-bladder; pain in the epigastrium; pain radiating from the navel over the abdomen; soreness in the region of the liver, extending to the umbilicus; enlargement of the of the liver, determined by percussion; nausea; occasional vomiting; constipation with dry feces, temperature slightly above normal; skin usually yellow.

In addition, he recommended it for acute congestion of the liver, catarrh of the common bile duct, acute jaundice, jaundice of childhood, bilious headaches, malarial conditions, diabetes mellitus, sugar in the urine, and typhoid fever.

Safety Considerations: No side effects or drug interactions have been reported.

Preparations and Dosage: Tincture dosage is 1 to 2 ml three times a day (1:5 in 40%). To make an infusion, pour 1 cup of boiling water over 1 to 2 teaspoons of herb and infuse for 10 to 15 minutes. This should be drunk three times a day.

Chondrus crispus (L.) Stackh.
Irish Moss
Gigartinacea

Part Used: Dried thallus (*Note:* This is a seaweed, not a moss.)

Constituents: Polysaccharides; the extract, also known as carrageenan, consists of sulfated, straight-chain galactans. (There are a variety of grades of carrageenan of different molecular weights, including a food grade with a molecular weight of about 100,000 to 500,000.)[71]

Actions: Expectorant, demulcent, anti-inflammatory

Indications: With modern attention on dramatically effective "miracle drugs," it is refreshing to remember the nourishing and strengthening food medicines, such as Irish moss. The safety of this seaweed allows it to make some unique contributions to health care. Its main traditional use was for respiratory illness, where it often served as the core of prescriptions used to treat irritating coughs, bronchitis, and many other lung problems.

Irish moss may be freely used in digestive conditions for which a demulcent is indicated, such as gastritis and ulceration of the stomach and duodenum. Its soothing activity makes it helpful for inflammations of the urinary system, and it was once used extensively in the same way cornsilk is used today. It has also been used as a food as part of maintenance diets for people with diabetes. However, in the past, its primary role was in speeding recuperation from debilitating illness, which once received a greater focus of attention than it does today. Herbs such as Irish moss and other tonic, nutritive remedies have much to offer in facilitating proper recovery of health after major disease.

King's suggested the use of Irish moss as

. . . a demulcent in chronic affections of the air passages, chronic diarrhea and dysentery, scrofula, rickets, enlarged mesenteric glands, irritation of the bladder and kidneys, etc. As a culinary article, it may be employed in the preparation of jellies, white soup, blanc mange, etc.

Safety Considerations: Irish moss may impair absorption of drugs.

Preparations and Dosage: To use fresh, wash the seaweed well, add 1 cup to 3 cups of milk or water, and flavor to taste. Simmer slowly until most of the seaweed has dissolved. Remove any undissolved fragments and pour it into a mold to set.

The dried seaweed is best made into a decoction. Steep 1 oz of dried Irish moss in cold water for 15 minutes, boil for 10 to 15 minutes in 3 pints of water (or milk), and strain. It may be combined with licorice, lemon, ginger, or cinnamon and sweetened to taste.

Cimicifuga racemosa (L.) Nutt.
Black Cohosh
Ranunculaceae

Parts Used: Dried root and rhizome (not fresh)

Constituents: Triterpene glycosides (actein, cimicifugoside, cimifugine, racemoside, cimiracemosides); isoferulic acid; salicylic acid; miscellaneous: volatile oil, tannins[72]

Actions: Emmenagogue, antispasmodic, anti-inflammatory, antirheumatic, alterative, nervine, hypotensive

Indications: Black cohosh is a valuable relaxant and normalizer of the female reproductive system. It may be used to good effect to treat painful or delayed menstruation, and relieves cramping pain in the womb and cramping associated with ovulation. Modern interest in this herb has focused on its gynecological uses. While it is of undoubted value in this area, its contribution to the treatment of arthritic disorders should not be overlooked. It is very effective against rheumatic pain, including that of rheumatoid arthritis, osteoarthritis, and muscle problems, and is helpful for neurological pain, including sciatica and neuralgia. As a relaxing nervine, it may be used in many situations where such an agent is needed. It has also been found beneficial for tinnitus.

Black cohosh helps to ease the physical and mental changes associated with perimenopause and menopause, as well as hormonal deficits resulting from ovariectomy or hysterectomy in younger women. Clinical studies support the primary application of black cohosh for the treatment of menopausal symptoms such as hot flashes, headache, vertigo, heart palpitations, ringing in the ears, and a range of associated psychological symptoms, including irritability, sleep disturbances, and depressive moods. Black cohosh extract has also been used successfully in women younger than 40 years for treatment of hormonal deficits resulting from ovariectomy or hysterectomy. At least 8 weeks of treatment are required to alleviate symptoms. A review of clinical studies showed that trials have ranged in length from 8 weeks to as long as 6 months.[73]

Because of the wealth of accrued experience presented in *King's American Dispensatory*, I have included a passage from its extensive monograph on black cohosh:

> This is a very active, powerful, and useful remedy, and appears to fulfil a great number of indications. It possesses an undoubted influence over the nervous system. In small doses the appetite and digestion are improved, and larger amounts augment the secretions of the gastrointestinal tract. The heart-beat is slowed and given increased power by it, while arterial tension is elevated.
>
> Upon the reproductive organs it exerts a specific influence, promoting the menstrual discharge, and by its power of increasing contractility of the unstriped fibres of the uterus, it acts as an efficient parturient. . . . Few of our remedies have acquired as great a reputation in the treatment of rheumatism and neuralgia. Indeed, few cases of rheumatism, or conditions depending upon a rheumatic basis, will present, which will not be influenced for the better by *Cimicifuga*. . . .
>
> Muscular pain of a rheumatoid character, when not amounting to a true rheumatic attack, and other rheumatoid pains when acute and not of spinal origin such as gastralgia, enteralgia, tenesmic vesical pains, pleurodynia, pain in the mediastina orbits or ears, are relieved by *Cimicifuga*.
>
> By its special affinity for the female reproductive organs, it is an efficient agent for the restoration of suppressed menses. In dysmenorrhoea it is surpassed by no other drug, being of greatest utility in irritative and congestive conditions of the uterus and appendages, characterized by tensive, dragging pains, resembling the pains of rheumatism. If the patient be despondent and chilly, combine *Cimicifuga* with *Pulsatilla*, especially in anemic subjects. . . .
>
> *Cimicifuga* has proved a better agent in obstetrical practice than ergot. It produces natural intermittent uterine contractions, whereas ergot produces constant contractions, thereby endangering the life of the child, or rupture of the uterus. Where the pains are inefficient, feeble, or irregular, *Cimicifuga* will stimulate to normal action. It is an excellent "partus praeparator" if given for several weeks before confinement. It is a diagnostic agent to differentiate between spurious and true labor pains, the latter being increased, while the former are dissipated under its use. It is the best and safest agent known for the relief of after-pains, and is effectual in allaying the general excitement of the nervous system after labor. . . . Preparations of *Cimicifuga*, to be of any medicinal value, must be prepared from recently dried roots.

Safety Considerations: When used at the recommended dosage, no adverse effects are to be expected. The herb should not be used during pregnancy, except to assist birth.

Preparations and Dosage: Tincture dosage is 2 to 4 ml three times a day (1:5 in 60%). To make a decoction, pour 1 cup of water over ½ to 1 teaspoon of dried root, bring to a boil, and simmer for 10 to 15 minutes. This should be drunk three times a day.

Dosage listed in the BPC is 1.8 to 3.6 ml tincture (1:10 in 60%) or 0.3 to 1.8 ml fluid extract (1:1 in 90%). Commission E suggests a daily dosage of 40% to 60% ethanol extract corresponding to 40 mg of drug. The USP recommends 1 g dried herb or 1 ml liquid extract.

Black Cohosh, in *Principles and Practice of Phytotherapy*

Cola acuminata Schumann
Cola
Sterculiaceae

Other Names: *Cola vera*; kola

Part Used: Seed kernel (the kernel freed from the testa)

Constituents: Caffeine, with traces of theobromine; tannins and other phenolics; miscellaneous: phlobaphene (an anthocyanin pigment known as kola red), betaine[74]

Actions: Central nervous system stimulant, antidepressant, astringent, diuretic

Indications: Cola has a marked stimulating effect on human consciousness. It can be used whenever there is a need for direct stimulation, which is less often than some may believe! If the health and function of the nervous system is improved, it will usually not need such stimulation. In the short term, however, cola may be used in nervous debility, states of atony, and weakness.

Cola can be viewed as specific in cases of depression associated with weakness and debility, and may act as a specific in nervous diarrhea. It will help in general depression and, in some people, may even give rise to euphoric states. It may also be beneficial for some types of migraine. Because of its stimulant properties, it can be a valuable part of treatment for anorexia.

Safety Considerations: Because it contains caffeine, cola may cause all of the reactions and potential drug interactions associated with this constituent. In addition, it may cause cumulative caffeine effects when used in combination with coffee, black or green tea, guarana, or maté.

Preparations and Dosage: Tincture dosage is 1 to 2 ml three times a day (1:5 in 40%). To make a decoction, put 1 to 2 teaspoons of powdered cola nuts in a cup of water, bring to a boil, and simmer gently for 10 to 15 minutes. This should be drunk when needed.

Dosage recommended in the BHC is 1 to 3 g powdered cotyledons, 1 to 4 ml tincture (1:5 in 60%), or 0.6 to 1.2 ml fluid extract (1:1 in 60%) three times a day. Commission E lists a daily dosage of 2 to 6 g dried herb, 10 to 30 g tincture, or 2.5 to 7.5 g fluid extract.

Cola nut, in *Herbal Medicine, Expanded Commission E Monographs*

Collinsonia canadensis L.
Stoneroot
Lamiaceae

Parts Used: Root, rhizome

Constituents: Essential oil; tannins; saponins; alkaloids; resins; organic acid[75]

Actions: Antilithic, diuretic, diaphoretic

Indications: As its name suggests, stoneroot finds its main use in the treatment and prevention of stone and gravel in the urinary system and gallbladder. It may be used as a prophylactic, but is also an excellent remedy when the body needs assistance in passing stones or gravel. It is a strong diuretic.

In his extensive monograph, *Ellingwood* gave the following indications for stoneroot:

Hemorrhoids, catarrhal gastritis, pain in the rectum, heart tonic, rheumatic inflammation, laryngitis, pharyngitis, clergyman's sore throat, dysentery, ulcers, fistula, inflammation of the middle ear, acute cystitis, vaginismus.

Safety Considerations: No side effects or drug interactions have been reported.

Preparations and Dosage: Tincture dosage is 1 to 2 ml three times a day (1:5 in 40%). To make a decoction, put 1 to 2 teaspoons of dried root in 1 cup of water, bring to a boil, and simmer for 10 to 15 minutes. This should be drunk three times a day.

The BHP recommends 1 to 4 g dried herb, 2 to 8 ml tincture (1:5 in 40%), or 1 to 4 ml liquid extract (1:1 in 25%) three times a day.

Stone Root, in *Herbal Medicines: A Guide for Health-Care Professionals*

Commiphora molmol (Nees) Engl.
Myrrh
Burseraceae

Part Used: Gum resin

Constituents: Volatile oil (1.5% to 17%); gum (up to 60%); resins (up to 40%, average 20%); sterols[76]

Actions: Antimicrobial, astringent, carminative, anti-catarrhal, expectorant, vulnerary

Indications: Myrrh is an effective antimicrobial agent that has been shown to work in two complementary ways. Its primary action is to stimulate the production of white blood corpuscles, which have antipathogenic actions. Secondarily, it has a direct antimicrobial effect.

Myrrh may be used in a wide range of conditions appropriate for treatment with an antimicrobial agent. It finds specific use in the treatment of infections of the mouth, such as mouth ulcers, gingivitis, and pyorrhea, as well as catarrhal problems, such as pharyngitis and sinusitis. Myrrh is often employed as part of an approach to the treatment of the common cold, and may be of benefit for laryngitis and respiratory complaints. Systemically, it is useful in the treatment of boils and similar conditions, glandular fever, and brucellosis. Applied externally, it is healing and antiseptic for wounds and abrasions.

Anti-inflammatory and antipyretic actions have been documented in mice.[77] Hypoglycemic activity in both normal and diabetic rats has been reported.[78] The proposed mode of action involved a decrease in gluconeogenesis and an increase in peripheral utilization of glucose in diabetic rats.

Safety Considerations: Use of undiluted tincture of myrrh in the mouth may give rise to a transient burning sensation and irritation of the palate. Theoretically, myrrh may interfere with existing antidiabetic therapy, as hypoglycemic properties have been documented.

Preparations and Dosage: The resin dissolves much more easily in alcohol than in water, so tincture is preferred and is easily obtainable. Dosage is 1 to 4 ml three times a day (1:1 in 90%). As the resin is difficult to dissolve in water, it should be powdered well for an infusion. Pour 1 cup of boiling water over 1 to 2 teaspoons of myrrh powder and infuse for 10 to 15 minutes. This should be drunk three times a day.

For external use, Commission E recommends dabbing the skin two to three times daily with undiluted tincture. As a rinse or gargle, add 5 to 10 drops of tincture to a glass of water. Dental powders should contain 10% powdered resin.

Myrrh, in *Herbal Medicine, Expanded Commission E Monographs*

Crataegus laevigata (Poir.) DC.
Hawthorn
Rosaceae

Parts Used: Traditionally, berry; modern products often use flower and leaf

Constituents: Flavonoids (leaf and flower, up to 1.78%): vitexin, quercetin, hyperoside, rutin; oligomeric procyanidins (leaf and flower, 1.0% to 2.4%); triterpene acids (leaf and flower, up to 0.6%): ursolic, oleanolic, crataegolic acids; phenolic acids (caffeic, chlorogenic, and related phenolcarboxylic acids)[79]

Actions: Cardiotonic, diuretic, astringent, hypotensive

Indications: A tonic in the true sense, *Crataegus* can be considered a specific remedy for most cardiovascular disease. A whole plant preparation should be used, as the individual effects of isolated constituents proved insignificant when tested in the laboratory. The whole plant, on the other hand, has unique and valuable properties. After a four-year study commissioned by the German Federal Ministry of Health, *Crataegus* gained recognition as a heart remedy in Europe. Please see chapter 14 for a more detailed discussion of these research results and the possible mechanisms of action of this important herb.

Hawthorn's primary attribute appears to be an ability to improve coronary circulation. It dilates the coronary arteries, relieving cardiac hypoxemia. Consequently, it reduces the likelihood of angina attacks and relieves symptoms of angina when they occur. The herb thus directly affects the cells of the cardiac muscle, enhancing both activity and nutrition.

Crataegus is also positively inotropic; that is, it increases the contractility of cardiac muscle. However, it is quite different in activity from the cardiac glycoside-containing remedies. They impact the contractile fibers, while *Crataegus* assists with the availability and utilization of energy, facilitating a gentle but sustained reversal of degenerative, age-related changes.

Used in conjunction with other cardiac herbs, *Crataegus* helps keep the heart in healthy condition, minimizing the risk of the development of coronary disease. It is indicated for cardiovascular degenerative disease, coronary artery disease, and associated conditions, including angina pectoris, mild congestive heart failure, essential hypertension, and recovery after myocardial infarction. It is especially beneficial for loss of function due to old age that has not yet resulted in overt pathology. It causes no toxicity, accumulation, or habituation, and is safe for long-term use in the elderly.

Safety Considerations: Hawthorn enhances the activity of cardioactive drugs, such as *Digitalis* spp., *Convallaria majalis*, strophanthin, and the cardiac glycosides digitoxin and digoxin. However, because of its coronary vasodilating and antiarrhythmic effects, it also potentially reduces the toxicity of these cardiac glycosides by reducing the dosage needed to achieve the desired effect.

Hawthorn procyanidins have reportedly potentiated coronary artery dilation caused by theophylline, caffeine, papaverine, sodium nitrate, adenosine, and epinephrine. However, the European Scientific Cooperative on Phytotherapy (ESCOP) monograph does not list any interactions, so some authorities apparently do not consider these interactions significant.

Preparations and Dosage: Tincture dosage is 2.5 ml three times daily, then 2.5 ml morning and evening as a maintenance dose (1:5 in 40%). For the treatment of acute or severe conditions, use up to 5 ml three times a day. In the elderly, treatment should be continued over many months. To make an infusion, infuse 2 teaspoons of dried herb in 1 cup of boiling water; this should be drunk three times a day.

Dosage suggested in the BHP is 0.3 to 1 g dried herb, 1 to 2 ml tincture (1:5 in 45%), or 1 to 2 ml liquid extract (1:1 in 25%) three times a day. Commission E recommends 160 to 900 mg water-ethanol extract (corresponding to 30 to 168.7 mg procyanidins, calculated as epicatechin, and 3.5 to 19.8 mg flavonoids, calculated as hyperoside).

Hawthorn, in *Principles and Practice of Phytotherapy*

Daucus carota L.
Wild Carrot
Apiaceae

Parts Used: Dried aerial parts, seed

Constituents: Flavonoids; daucine (an alkaloid); volatile oil; petroselinic acid; tannins[80]

Actions: Diuretic, antilithic, carminative, antispasmodic, antirheumatic

Indications: The volatile oil present in wild carrot is an active urinary antiseptic, which helps explain its application in such conditions as cystitis and prostatitis. It has been considered a specific for the treatment of kidney stones. For the treatment of gout and rheumatism, it is used as a diuretic in combination with other remedies. The seeds may be used as a settling carminative agent for the relief of flatulence and colic.

Safety Considerations: Juice of the fresh plant may cause photosensitivity.

Preparations and Dosage: Tincture dosage is 1 to 2 ml three times a day (1:5 in 25%). To make an infusion of aerial parts, pour 1 cup of boiling water over 1 teaspoon of dried herb and infuse for 10 to 15 minutes. This should be drunk three times a day. To prepare an infusion of seeds, use $1/3$ to 1 teaspoon per cup of water. This should be drunk three times a day.

Wild Carrot, in *Herbal Medicines: A Guide for Health-Care Professionals*

Dioscorea villosa L.
Wild Yam
Dioscoreaceae

Parts Used: Dried underground parts

Constituents: Steroidal saponins, based on diosgenin: dioscin, dioscorin, and others[81]

Actions: Antispasmodic, anti-inflammatory, anti-rheumatic, hepatic, cholagogue, diaphoretic

Indications: This valuable herb was at one time the sole source of the chemicals used as raw material for the manufacture of contraceptive hormones. However, this should not be taken to mean that the herb is a source of so-called natural progesterone. The human body is incapable of converting the sapogenins to sex hormones.

In herbal medicine, wild yam is a remedy that can be used to relieve intestinal colic, soothe diverticulitis, ease dysmenorrhea, and relieve ovarian and uterine pains. It is of great use in the treatment of rheumatoid arthritis, especially the acute phase, in which there is intense inflammation.

Priest and Priest described wild yam and its indications in the following way:

> . . . autonomic nerve relaxant, especially for gastrointestinal conditions, vegetative neuroses and hyperaesthesiae. Rheumatic syndromes arising from hepatic and intestinal dysfunction.

They offered the following specific indications: bilious colic, flatulence, gastrointestinal irritation, neuralgic conditions, dysmenorrhea, uterine pains, nervousness, restlessness, and pains of pregnancy.

Ellingwood considered it specific for

> . . . sudden spasmodic griping pain in the stomach and bowels. It is specific in bilious colic, in the pain of the passing of gallstones, in mild cases, and is valuable in spasmodic colic of any kind.

In addition, *Ellingwood* recommended it for neuralgic dysmenorrhea, ovarian neuralgia, and cramplike pains.

King's provides the following monograph:

> It is a specific in bilious colic, having proved almost invariably successful in doses of $1/2$ pint of the decoction, repeated every half hour or hour. No other medicine is required, as it gives prompt and permanent relief in the most severe cases. In fact it is not only of value in bilious colic, but in all forms of colic and other painful abdominal neuroses and all forms of gastro-intestinal irritation. If it does not relieve in one hour, the medicine should be discontinued. It has allayed the pain incident to the passage of biliary calculi when given with full doses of gelsemium.
>
> It will likewise allay nausea, also spasms of the bowels and combined with equal parts of *Cornus sericea* in decoction, is eminently beneficial in the nausea and vomiting of pregnancy. This root appears to exert an action especially upon enfeebled and irritable mucous tissues that become painful from spasmodic contractions of their muscular fibers; hence its value in bilious colic, in painful dysenteric tenesmus, in dysmenorrhoea (the result of spasmodic irritation of the mucous membrane), of the cervix uteri and in spasmodic irritations of the gastric mucous membrane attended with pain, nausea and vomiting. It is reputed useful in indigestion with hepatic derangement, in chronic hepatic congestion and in the chronic gastritis of drunkards. It is also useful in after-pains.

Safety Considerations: No side effects or drug interactions have been reported.

Preparations and Dosage: Tincture dosage is 2 to 4 ml three times a day (1:5 in 40%). To make a decoction, put 1 to 2 teaspoons of herb in 1 cup of water, bring to a boil, and simmer gently for 10 to 15 minutes. This should be drunk three times a day.

The BHP recommends 2 to 4 g dried herb, 2 to 10 ml tincture (1:5 in 45%), or 2 to 4 ml fluid extract (1:1 in 45%) three times daily.

Drosera rotundifolia L.
Sundew
Droseraceae

Parts Used: Whole plant

Constituents: Naphthoquinones, including plumbagin; flavonoids (kaempferol, myricetin, quercetin, hyperoside); miscellaneous: carotenoids, plant acids, resin, tannins, ascorbic acid[82]

Actions: Antispasmodic, antitussive, expectorant

Indications: Sundew may be used to great benefit in bronchitis and whooping cough. The presence of plumbagin helps to explain its actions here, as the constituent has been shown to be active against *Streptococcus*, *Staphylococcus*, and *Pneumococcus* bacteria. Sundew is also effective against infections in other parts of the respiratory tract, and its relaxing effect upon involuntary muscles makes it useful in relieving asthma. In addition to pulmonary conditions, sundew has a long history of use for treating stomach ulcers.

Drosera prevents acetylcholine- or histamine-induced bronchospasm and has antitussive properties. These antispasmodic actions have been attributed to its naphthoquinone constituents. Antimicrobial properties have been documented for the naphthoquinones. In vivo, plumbagin demonstrated a broad spectrum of activity against various gram-positive and gram-negative bacteria, influenza viruses, pathogenic fungi, and parasitic protozoans. Successful treatment of *Microsporum* infections in guinea pigs by local applications of 0.25% to 0.5% solutions of plumbagin (in 40% alcohol) or 1% emulsions has been reported. However, plumbagin was ineffective against *Lamblia muris* and tuberculosis infection when administered orally to mice for 5 days.[83]

Safety Considerations: No side effects or toxicity has been documented. Plumbagin has a LD_{50} of 15 mg/kg body weight (i.p.) in mice.

Preparations and Dosage: Tincture dosage is 1 to 2 ml three times a day (1:5 in 60%). To make an infusion, pour 1 cup of boiling water over 1 teaspoon of dried herb and infuse for 10 to 15 minutes. This should be drunk three times a day. Commission E recommends a dosage of 3 g herb daily.

Droserae longifoliae herba, in *Herbal Drugs and Phytopharmaceuticals*

Echinacea spp.
Echinacea
Asteraceae

Other Name: Purple coneflower. The main *Echinacea* species available in commerce are *E. purpurea*, *E. angustifolia*, and *E. pallida*.

Part Used: Root

Constituents: Caffeic acid esters (0.6% to 2.1%) including echinacoside (in *E. angustifolia* but not *E. purpurea*) and cichoric acid (*E. purpurea* only); alkylamides, mostly unsaturated isobutyl amides (including dodeca-2,4,8,10-tetraenoic acid); polysaccharides (including echinacin B); polyacetylenes; essential oil[84]

Actions: Antimicrobial, immunomodulator, anti-inflammatory, anticatarrhal, vulnerary, alterative

Indications: Echinacea is one of the primary remedies for helping the body rid itself of microbial infections. It is often effective against both bacterial and viral attacks. It may be used for conditions such as boils, septicemia, and similar infections, and, in conjunction with other herbs, it may be used for any infection anywhere in the body. For example, in combination with yarrow or bearberry, it is effective against cystitis.

Echinacea is especially useful for infections of the upper respiratory tract, including laryngitis, tonsillitis, the common cold, and other catarrhal conditions of the nose and sinus. In general, it may be used widely and safely. Tincture or decoction of echinacea may be used as a mouthwash for gingivitis or pyorrhea. The herb may be applied externally as a lotion to treat septic sores and cuts.

Much research has focused upon this plant, providing important insights into its activity and potential uses. Constituents from the roots have demonstrated mild activity against *Streptococcus* and *Staphylococcus aureus*. The caffeic acid derivative echinacoside was the most active; about 6 mg were reported to be equivalent to 1 unit of penicillin.[85] Treatment with tincture reduced both the rate of growth and the rate of reproduction of *Trichomonas vaginalis*, and was deemed effective in halting recurrence of *Candida albicans* infection.[86]

In other studies, echinacea appeared to prevent infection and repair tissue damaged by infection, partially by inhibiting the activity of the enzyme hyaluronidase.[87] The hyaluronidase system is a primary defense mechanism in which connective "ground substance," composed largely of hyaluronic acid, acts as a barrier against pathogenic organisms. Some pathogens activate an enzyme, hyaluronidase, which destroys the integrity of the ground substance. The barrier then becomes leaky, allowing pathogens to invade, attach themselves to exposed cells, penetrate the membranes, and kill the cells. The result is an inflammatory infection.

Echinacea inhibits the action of hyaluronidase by bonding with it in some way, causing a temporary increase in the integrity of the barrier and impairing the ability of pathogens to stimulate the destruction of the ground substance. A range of constituents mediates this process, especially a complex polysaccharide called echinacin B. This anti-hyaluronidase action also supports the regeneration of connective tissue destroyed during infection and the elimination of pathogenic organisms that create infection.

Purified polysaccharides from echinacea strongly activate the body's macrophage-mediated defense system. Macrophages initiate the destruction of pathogens and cancer cells. Echinacea activates macrophages on its own, independent of any effect on T cells. A tumor-inhibiting principle—an oncolytic lipid-soluble hydrocarbon from the essential oil—has also been identified. The echinacoside glycosides appear to be the primary "antibiotics" in echinacea, but they probably function synergistically with many other active substances present in the plant. The polysaccharides possess the best immune-stimulating properties and are also antiviral. Other constituents have been shown to possess good antitumor, bacteriostatic, and anesthetic properties.[88]

Clinical data support the use of echinacea in a variety of situations.[89] It is indicated primarily for the prevention and treatment of acute infections, particularly colds, influenza, and other acute upper respiratory tract infections, in which it reduces both the duration and severity of symptoms. This all points to a conclusion that echinacea's actions are related on some level to immune system function, as it helps the body deal with infections and stimulates immune response. The herb activates the macrophages that destroy cancer cells and pathogens and increases phagocytosis by raising levels of white blood cells, such as neutrophils, monocytes, eosinophils, and B-lymphocytes. It also affects properidin levels, suggesting activation of the complement system.[90]

Safety Considerations: Echinacea may cause allergic reactions in people sensitive to plants in the Asteraceae family. Theoretically, it may interfere with immunosuppressant therapy.

Preparations and Dosage: *Echinacea* is often inappropriately used as "daily immune support." It is more appropriately used to treat active infection or at the first sign of an acute infection.

Tincture dosage is 1 to 4 ml three times a day (1:5 in 40%). To make a decoction, put 1 to 2 teaspoons of root in 1 cup of water and bring slowly to a boil. Let simmer for 10 to 15 minutes. This should be drunk three times a day.

The BHC recommends 1 g dried root, 2 to 5 ml tincture (1:5 in 45%), or 0.5 to 1 ml of fluid extract (1:1 in 45%) of *Echinacea angustifolia* three times daily. Commission E suggests *E. pallida* tincture (1:5 in 50%, from dry extract) corresponding to 900 mg herb or 6 to 9 ml expressed juice of *E. purpurea* daily.

Echinacea, in *Principles and Practice of Phytotherapy*

Eleutherococcus senticosus (Rupr. and Maxim.) Maxim.
Siberian Ginseng
Araliaceae

Other Names: *Acanthopanax senticosus;* eleuthero

Part Used: Root

Constituents: Eleutherosides A-E; glycosides of a range of aglycones, including sterols, lignans, and phenolics; polysaccharides[91]

Action: Adaptogen

Indications: Siberian ginseng is one of the primary adaptogens in use today. As discussed in more detail in chapter 25, an adaptogen is a substance that acts to enhance the body's nonspecific resistance to various internal and external stressors. Because of this nonspecific action, Siberian ginseng can be recommended as a general tonic with a very wide range of clinical indications.

Siberian ginseng improves the body's resistance to environmental stressors and enhances physical and mental performance. It stimulates many aspects of the immune response, is antihepatotoxic, and increases resistance to oxygen deprivation of the heart.[92] The herb is especially useful for conditions influenced by the stress response, including angina, hypertension, hypotension, various types of neuroses, chronic bronchitis, and cancer. It is beneficial against the effects of prolonged stress or overwork such as exhaustion, irritability, insomnia, and mild depression.

Siberian ginseng may also be employed to support recovery from acute or chronic diseases, trauma, surgery, and other stressful events, and can help counter the debilitating effects of treatments such as chemotherapy and radiation. It may be taken on a long-term basis to minimize the incidence of acute infections and to generally improve well-being.

Safety Considerations: Siberian ginseng may interfere with cardiac medications (including hypo- and hypertensive drugs) and hypoglycemic agents. It may also enhance some drug effects. In a clinical study, the herb appeared to increase the efficacy of the antibiotics monomycin and kanamycin, used to treat *Shigella* dysentery and *Proteus* enterocolitis.[93]

Preparations and Dosage: Based upon clinical studies, standard tincture dosage is 50 to 100 drops three times a day. An equivalent dosage for a solid extract concentrated at a ratio of 20:1 would be 100 to 200 mg. The recommended regimen is usually for a 6-week course of treatment followed by a 2-week break.

Dosage recommended in the BHC is 2 to 3 g dried root and rhizome or equivalent preparations three times daily. Commission E suggests 2 to 3 g of root daily.

Siberian Ginseng, in Principles and Practice of Phytotherapy

Elymus repens (L.) Beauvois
Couch Grass
Poaceae

Other Name: Formerly *Agropyron repens*

Part Used: Rhizome

Constituents: Carbohydrates (10%): triticin, inositol, mannitol, and mucilage; volatile oil (0.05%), mainly agropyrene; flavonoids (tricin)[94]

Actions: Diuretic, demulcent, antimicrobial

Indications: Couch grass may be used in urinary tract infections such as cystitis, urethritis, and prostatitis. Its demulcent properties soothe irritation and inflammation. The herb is of value in the treatment of benign prostatic hypertrophy (BPH, or enlarged prostate), and may also be used for kidney stones and gravel. As a tonic diuretic, couch grass has been used in combination with other herbs for rheumatism. Research has demonstrated broad antibiotic activity for the terpene constituent agropyrene and its oxidation product.

Safety Considerations: There is a theoretical risk of potassium depletion when couch grass is used in combination with potassium-depleting diuretics.

Preparations and Dosage: Tincture dosage is 2 to 4 ml three times a day (1:5 in 40%). To make a decoction, put 2 teaspoons of cut rhizome in 1 cup of water, bring to a boil, and simmer for 10 minutes. This should be drunk three times a day.

Dosage recommendations from the BHP are 4 to 8 g dried herb, 5 to 15 ml tincture (1:5 in 40%), or 4 to 8 ml fluid extract (1:1 in 25%) three times a day. The BPC lists a fluid extract dosage of 3.5 ml to 20 ml three times a day. Commission E recommends 6 to 9 g dried herb daily.

Couch Grass, in The Complete German Commission E Monographs

Ephedra sinica Stapf
Ephedra
Ephedraceae

Other Name: Ma huang

Part Used: Stem

Constituents: Alkaloids (L-ephedrine, with D-ephedrine, pseudoephedrine, norephedrine, *N*-methylephedrine, benzylmethylamine); flavonoid glycosides; glycans; proanthocyanidins[95]

Actions: Vasodilator, hypertensive, circulatory stimulant, antiallergic

Indications: Ephedra has been used in China for at least 5,000 years to treat a range of health problems. This ancient medicinal plant was also mentioned in the Hindu Vedas. With the discovery of the alkaloids in ephedra, this time-honored, traditional herbal wisdom was verified, providing modern medicine with important healing tools.

Ephedra contains a range of therapeutically active alkaloids, which sometimes amount to up to 2% of the dried herb. Various Asian *Ephedra* species provide the source material for the widely used alkaloids ephedrine and pseudoephedrine, mainly *E. sinica* and *E. equisetina* from China and *E. gerardiana* from India. The alkaloids present in ephedra have apparently opposite effects on the body. The whole plant, as used in traditional herbal medicine, has an overall beneficial, balancing action.

A brief review of the pharmacology of these alkaloids may prove illuminating. Ephedrine was the first ephedra alkaloid to find wide use in Western medicine, being hailed as a "cure for asthma" because of its ability to relax airways in the lungs. Unfortunately, as is often the way with miracle cures, it soon became clear that this isolated ephedra constituent had unacceptable side effects that dramatically limited its use. The adverse effects were related to the way in which ephedrine stimulates the autonomic nervous system, which has the effect of elevating blood pressure, among others. Studies on the whole plant, however, demonstrated only a slight blood pressure elevation. This led researchers to the discovery that pseudoephedrine, another ephedra alkaloid, slightly reduces heart rate and lowers blood pressure, thus avoiding the side effects of ephedrine.[96]

Pseudoephedrine is also an effective bronchodilator, equivalent in strength to ephedrine. However, it has the advantage of causing less stimulation of the nervous system, and thus less vasoconstriction, tachycardia, and other cardiovascular symptoms. Clinical studies have shown that pseudoephedrine has insignificant side effects. The efficacy and safety of pseudoephedrine are recognized by the Food and Drug Administration, which approved it as an over-the-counter nasal decongestant.

All of these findings confirm the traditional applications of *Ephedra sinica* as an effective treatment for nasal congestion and sinus pressure, whether due to the common cold, allergies, or sinusitis. The herb is used with great success in the treatment of asthma, bronchial asthma, bronchitis, and associated conditions, because of its power to relieve spasms in the bronchial tubes. It eases allergic reactions, giving it a role in the treatment of hay fever and other allergies. It may also be employed to treat low blood pressure and circulatory insufficiency.

Safety Considerations: Combined with cardiac glycosides or halothane, ephedra can produce cardiac arrhythmias. Guanethidine enhances the sympathomimetic effect of ephedra. Combining ephedra with monoamine oxidase inhibitors can significantly increase the sympathomimetic action of the alkaloid ephedrine in the herb, possibly causing fatal hypertension. Used in combination with secale alkaloid derivatives (e.g., ergotamine) or oxytocin can produce hypertension.[97,98]

Ephedra is contraindicated for people with certain health problems. It should not be used in the presence of cardiovascular conditions, thyroid disease, or diabetes, or by men experiencing difficulty urinating due to prostate enlargement.

Preparations and Dosage: Tincture dosage is 1 to 4 ml three times a day (1:4 in 45%). To make a decoction, put 1 to 2 teaspoons of the dried herb in 1 cup of water, bring to a boil, and simmer for 10 to 15 minutes. This should be drunk three times a day.

Commission E recommends a single daily dose corresponding to 15 to 30 mg total alkaloid.

Ephedra, in *Herbal Medicine, Expanded Commission E Monographs*

Equisetum arvense L.
Horsetail
Equisetaceae

Part Used: Dried stem

Constituents: Alkaloids (including nicotine, palustrine, and palustrinine); flavonoids (such as isoquercitrin and equicetrin); sterols (including cholesterol, isofucosterol, campesterol); silicic acid; miscellaneous: a saponin (equisitonin), dimethylsulphone, thiaminase, aconitic acid[99]

Actions: Astringent, diuretic, vulnerary

Indications: Horsetail is an excellent astringent for the genitourinary system, reducing hemorrhage. While it acts as a mild diuretic, its toning and astringent actions make it invaluable in the treatment of incontinence and bedwetting in children. It is considered a specific for cases of inflammation or benign enlargement of the prostate gland. Applied externally, it is a vulnerary that helps heal skin wounds. In some cases, it has been found to ease the pain of rheumatism and stimulate the healing of chilblains.

Safety Considerations: No side effects or drug interactions have been reported.

Preparations and Dosage: Tincture dosage is 2 to 4 ml three times a day (1:5 in 25%). To make an infusion, pour 1 cup of boiling water over 2 teaspoons of dried plant and infuse for 15 to 20 minutes. This should be drunk three times a day.

Horsetail may be used to make a bath to help with rheumatic pain and chilblains. Steep 100 g (3½ ounces) of herb in hot water for 1 hour and add to the bath.

The BHC recommends 1 to 4 g dried herb, 2 to 6 ml tincture (1:5 in 25%), or 1 to 4 ml fluid extract three times a day. Commission E suggests 6 g of herb or equivalent preparations daily.

Horsetail, in *Herbal Medicine, Expanded Commission E Monographs*

Eschscholzia californica Cham.
California Poppy
Papaveraceae

Parts Used: Dried aerial parts

Constituents: Alkaloids; flavone glycosides[100]

Actions: Nervine, hypnotic, antispasmodic, anodyne

Indications: California poppy has been used as a sedative and hypnotic for children, especially in cases of overexcitement and sleeplessness. It can be used wherever an antispasmodic remedy is indicated—for example, for colic pain. It may also be useful to treat gallbladder colic.

Safety Considerations: California poppy has additive effects when used with other sedatives.

Preparations and Dosage: Tincture (1:5 in 25%) dosage is 1 to 4 ml at night for sleeplessness in children. For antispasmodic indications, use 0.5 to 2 ml three times daily. To make an infusion, pour 1 cup of boiling water over 1 to 2 teaspoons of dried herb and infuse for 10 minutes. A cup drunk at night will promote restful sleep.

Eucalyptus globulus Labill.
Eucalyptus
Myrtaceae

Other Name: Blue gum

Parts Used: Leaf, essential oil distilled from leaf

Constituents: Volatile oil (0.5% to 3.5%): 1,8-cineole (= eucalyptol, 70% to 85%); α-pinene, p-pinene, d-limonene, α-phellandrene; polyphenolic acids (caffeic, ferulic, gallic, protocatechuic, and others); flavonoids (including eucalyptin, hyperosides, rutin)[101]

Actions: Antimicrobial, antispasmodic, expectorant, stimulant, febrifuge

Indications: Eucalyptus leaf is used topically as an antimicrobial and internally as a decongestant and expectorant. The essential oil is used in aromatherapy.

King's American Dispensatory described the way this plant was used by the Eclectic physicians. Here are some relevant excerpts:

> *Eucalyptus globulus* has for a long time been known as a remedy for intermittent fever among the natives of the countries of its origin. Aside from its alleged utility in intermittents, this agent has had other virtues attributed to it, as follows: The leaves and their preparations have been successfully used as a tonic and gently stimulating stomachic, in atonic dyspepsia, and in catarrh of the stomach and typhoid fever; also advised in mucous catarrhal affections generally; in pseudo-membranous laryngitis, in asthma, with profuse secretion, and in chronic bronchitis, with or without emphysema, and in whooping-cough; it has likewise proved efficient in chronic catarrh of the bladder, where the urine is high-colored, contains an abnormal amount of mucus, or, perhaps, some purulent matter, and micturation is attended with much pain. More recently it has been recommended as a diuretic in the treatment of dropsy. Both the leaves and the oil are excitants and deodorizers, and, as such, have been successfully employed as local applications in bronchial affections with fetid expectoration, in ozena, in fetid or profuse mucous discharges, in vaginal leucorrhoea, offensive lochial discharges, gonorrhoeal discharges, indolent, fetid wounds or ulcers, cancerous ulcerations, in septicemia, and in gangrene. The leaves may, in some cases, be applied alone, directly to the part, in form of cataplasm; or they may be combined with other articles to form a poultice. The oil may be applied of full strength, or diluted with some other agent. In throat and pulmonary maladies, a tincture diluted, or a medicated water, may be inhaled in the form of spray; if the oil be employed, it may be dropped on some cotton placed in a small tube, from which the vapor may be inhaled. As a deodorizer, the tincture or the oil may be sprinkled or sprayed upon the offensive body, or the atmosphere of an apartment may be frequently sprayed with the same. Externally applied, the oil gives relief in some forms of neuralgic and rheumatic pains. The leaves of *Eucalyptus*, made up into cigars or cigarettes, and smoked, have been advised to afford relief in bronchial catarrh, asthma, and other affections of the respiratory organs. . . . *Eucalyptus* honey, gathered by bees from *Eucalyptus* flowers, is quite active, and has been rec-

ommended for parasitic and putrescent conditions, gonorrhoea, fevers, and catarrhal diseases.

A plant preparation containing a mixture of various herbal tinctures, including eucalyptus, has been used successfully to treat chronic suppurative otitis. The efficacy of the preparation was attributed to the antibacterial and anti-inflammatory actions of the herbs.[102]

Safety Considerations: No side effects or drug interactions have been reported.

Preparations and Dosage: Tincture dosage is 1 ml three times a day (1:5 in 25%). Make an infusion with 1 to 2 teaspoons of the leaves to 1 cup of boiling water. Infuse in a covered container for 10 to 15 minutes. This should be drunk three times a day.

Commission E recommends a daily dose of 4 to 6 g leaf or 3 to 9 g tincture.

Eucalyptus leaf and oil, in *Herbal Medicine, Expanded Commission E Monographs*

Euonymus atropurpureus Jacq.
Wahoo
Celastraceae

Other Name: Spindle tree

Part Used: Root

Constituents: Cardenolides based on digitoxigenin; alkaloids, such as asparagine and atropurpurine; sterols (euonysterol, atropurpurol, homoeuonysterol)[103]

Actions: Cholagogue, hepatic, laxative, diuretic, circulatory stimulant

Indications: Wahoo is one of the primary liver herbs. It alleviates congestion in the liver, facilitating the free flow of bile and thus supporting the digestive process. It may be used to treat jaundice and gallbladder problems, such as inflammation and pain or congestion due to stones. It will relieve constipation due to liver or gallbladder problems. Because of its normalizing action upon the liver, it may be beneficial for a range of skin problems in which the liver may play a role.

Ellingwood considered wahoo specific for

> . . . indigestion with biliousness, constipation, chronic intermittents with cachexia, pulmonary phthisis with night sweats and great weakness; dropsical affections following acute disease; in convalescence from severe intermittent fever; enlargement of the liver; chronic bronchitis.

In addition, he recommended it for malarial cachexia, as a nutritive tonic, as a hepatic stimulant, and for chronic pulmonary complaints.

Safety Considerations: Wahoo is contraindicated for people taking cardiac glycosides or other cardioactive agents.

Preparations and Dosage: Tincture dosage is 1 to 2 ml three times a day (1:5 in 40%). To make a decoction, pour 1 cup of water over ½ to 1 teaspoon of herb, bring to a boil, and simmer for 10 to 15 minutes. This should be drunk three times a day.

The BHC lists a dosage of 0.3 to 1 g dried bark, 5 to 15 ml expressed juice, 0.6 to 2.6 ml tincture (1:5 in 45%), or 0.3 to 1 ml fluid extract (1:1 in 45%) three times a day.

Euonymus Bark, in *British Herbal Compendium*, vol. 1

Eupatorium perfoliatum L.
Boneset
Asteraceae

Parts Used: Dried aerial parts

Constituents: Sesquiterpene lactones (eupafolin, euperfolitin, eufoliatin, eufoliatorin, euperfolide, eucannabinolide, and helenalin); immunostimulatory polysaccharides; flavonoids (quercetin, kaempferol, hyperoside, astragalin, rutin, eupatorin, and others); miscellaneous: diterpenes (dendroidinic acid, hebenolide); sterols; volatile oil[104]

Actions: Diaphoretic, bitter, laxative, tonic, antispasmodic, carminative, astringent

Indications: Boneset is one of the best remedies for the relief of symptoms that accompany influenza. It will speedily relieve aches and pains and help the body deal with any fever present. Boneset may also be used to help clear the upper respiratory tract of mucus congestion. Its mild aperient activity eases constipation. Overall, it is a safe choice for any fever and for use as a general cleansing agent. It may also provide symptomatic relief as part of treatment for muscular rheumatism.

High dilutions of various sesquiterpene lactones isolated from *E. perfoliatum* demonstrated immunostimulant activity.[105] In addition, polysaccharide fractions from *E. perfoliatum* showed immumostimulant actions in granulocyte, macrophage, and carbon clearance tests.[106]

King's American Dispensatory included an extensive monograph on boneset, an excerpt of which is included here:

> As a tonic, it is useful in remittent, intermittent, and typhoid fevers, dyspepsia, and general debility. In intermittent fever, a strong infusion, as hot as can be comfortably swallowed, is administered for the purpose of vomiting freely. This is also attended with profuse diaphoresis, and sooner or later by an evacuation of the bowels. During the

intermission, the cold infusion or extract is given every hour as a tonic and antiperiodic. The chill and succeeding fever is slight, the skin dry, and not, as a rule, followed by perspiration; there are pains in the bones, praecordial oppression, and great thirst. If, however, the case is one in which the fever lasts all day, a slight sweating may follow at night. Another indication in ague is vomiting, especially of much bile. *Eupatorium* given as above, or sometimes in small doses, may relieve headache of intermittent character when the intermissions are irregular. In epidemic influenza the warm infusion is valuable as an emetic and diaphoretic, likewise in febrile diseases, catarrh, colds, with hoarseness and pleuritic pains, and wherever such effects are indicated. In influenza it relieves the pain in the limbs and back. Its popular name "boneset" is derived from its well-known property of relieving the deep seated pains in the limbs which accompany this disorder, and colds and rheumatism. Often this pain is periosteal, and if neuralgic in character, or due to a febrile condition, *Eupatorium* will relieve it. But it is not a remedy for periosteal pain due to inflammation or to organic changes in the periosteum. On the other hand, when given until the patient sweats, and then continued in 5-drop doses of specific eupatorium it has relieved the severe nocturnal muscular and "bone pains" of syphilis. It is a remedy for the cough of the aged, that cough in which there is an abundance of secretion, but lack of power to expectorate. The cough of measles, common colds, of asthma, and hoarseness are also relieved by it. Unless given in excess it acts as a good tonic to the gastric functions, increasing the appetite and power of digestion.

Safety Considerations: Boneset may cause allergic reactions in people sensitive to plants in the Asteraceae family.

Preparations and Dosage: Tincture dosage is 2 to 4 ml three times a day (1:5 in 45%). To make an infusion, pour 1 cup of boiling water over 1 to 2 teaspoons of dried herb and infuse for 10 to 15 minutes. This should be drunk as hot as possible. For fevers or flu, it should be drunk every half hour; otherwise, drink three times a day.

Boneset, in *Herbal Medicines: A Guide for Health-Care Professionals*

Eupatorium purpureum L.
Gravel Root
Asteraceae

Other Name: Also commonly known as Joe pye. Do not confuse with boneset (*Eupatorium perfoliatum*).

Parts Used: Rhizome, root

Constituents: Volatile oil, of unknown composition; flavonoids (including euparin); resin[107]

Actions: Diuretic, antilithic, antirheumatic

Indications: Gravel root is used primarily to treat kidney stones or gravel. It may also be of benefit in urinary tract infections, such as cystitis or urethritis, and can also play a useful role in a systemic treatment of rheumatism and gout.

Ellingwood considered it to have the following indications:

Irritation of the bladder in women from displacement and chronic inflammation of the uterus; and suppression of urine, partial or complete, during or after pregnancy.

He recommended it for dropsy, strangury, gravel, hematuria, diseases of the kidney and bladder due to an excess of uric acid, chronic endometriosis, leukorrhea, chronic uterine disease, threatened abortion, ovarian and uterine atony, dysmenorrhea, dysuria, constant desire to urinate, intermittent fever, and severe bone pains.

Safety Considerations: Gravel root may cause allergic reaction in people sensitive to plants in the Asteraceae family.

Preparations and Dosage: Tincture dosage is 2 ml three times a day (1:5 in 40%). To make a decoction, put 1 teaspoon of herb in 1 cup of water, bring to a boil, and simmer for 10 minutes. This should be drunk three times a day.

Gravel Root, in *Herbal Medicines: A Guide for Health-Care Professionals*

Euphrasia officinalis L.
Eyebright
Scrophulariaceae

Parts Used: Dried aerial parts

Constituents: Iridoid glycosides, including aucubin (0.5%); tannins (about 12%, both condensed and hydrolyzable gallic acid types); phenolic acids (including caffeic and ferulic); volatile oil (about 0.2%); flavonoids[108]

Actions: Anticatarrhal, astringent, anti-inflammatory

Indications: Eyebright is an excellent remedy for mucous membrane problems. Its combination of anti-inflammatory and astringent properties makes it relevant for many conditions. Used internally, eyebright is a powerful anticatarrhal, and thus may be used to treat nasal catarrh, sinusitis, and other congestive states. However, the herb is best known for its use in eye conditions, including acute or chronic inflammations, stinging and weeping eyes, and oversensitivity to light. It may be applied as a compress in conjunction with internal use for conjunctivitis and blepharitis.

Priest and Priest described it as a

. . . mild stimulating astringent. Vaso-constrictor to vessels of nasal and conjunctival membranes. Specific for congestive conditions of the eyes with profuse lachrymation.

They gave these specific indications: catarrhal blepharitis, rhinitis, sinusitis, conjunctivitis, hay fever, acute coryza, irritable sneezing, and lachrymation.

Safety Considerations: No side effects or drug interactions have been reported.

Preparations and Dosage: Tincture dosage is 1 to 4 ml three times a day (1:5 in 45%). To make an infusion, pour 1 cup of boiling water over 1 teaspoon of dried herb and infuse for 5 to 10 minutes. This should be drunk three times a day.

For a compress, place 1 teaspoon of 1 dried herb in ½ liter (1 pint) of water. Boil for 10 minutes and let cool slightly. Moisten a cloth in the lukewarm liquid, wring out slightly, and place over the eyes. Leave the compress in place for 15 minutes. Repeat several times a day.

Eyebright, in *Principles and Practice of Phytotherapy*

Filipendula ulmaria (L.) Maxim.
Meadowsweet
Rosaceae

Parts Used: Aerial parts

Constituents: Volatile oil; salicylaldehyde (up to 70%), ethylsalicylate, methylsalicylate, phenolic glycosides (spiraein, monotropin, gaultherin); flavonoids (flavonols, flavones, flavanones, and chalcone derivatives); polyphenolics and other tannins, mainly hydrolyzable (1% in alcohol extract, 12.5% in aqueous extract); miscellaneous: phenylcarboxylic acids, coumarin, vitamin C[109]

Actions: Antirheumatic, anti-inflammatory, carminative, antacid, antiemetic, astringent

Indications: Meadowsweet is one of the best digestive remedies available. As such, it will be indicated in many conditions, if they are approached holistically. The herb protects and soothes the mucous membranes of the digestive tract, reducing excess acidity and easing nausea. It is used in the treatment of heartburn, hyperacidity, gastritis, and peptic ulceration. Its gentle astringency is especially helpful in children's diarrhea. The presence of aspirin-like chemicals (salicylates) explains meadowsweet's ability to reduce fever and relieve the pain of rheumatism in muscles and joints.

Safety Considerations: Meadowsweet should be avoided by people with salicylate sensitivity.

Preparations and Dosage: Tincture dosage is 2 to 4 ml three times a day (1:5 in 45%). To make an infusion, pour 1 cup of boiling water over 1 to 2 teaspoons of dried herb and infuse in a covered container for 10 to 15 minutes. This should be drunk three times a day or as needed.

The BHC recommends 2 to 6 g dried herb, 2 to 4 ml tincture (1:5 in 45%), or 2 to 6 ml fluid extract (1:1 in 25%) three times daily. Commission E suggests 2.5 to 3.5 g flower or 4 to 5 g herb or equivalent preparations daily.

Meadowsweet, in *Principles and Practice of Phytotherapy*

Foeniculum vulgare Mill.
Fennel
Apiaceae

Part Used: Seed

Constituents: Volatile oil (8%): anethole (60% to 80%), fenchone (10% to 30%); flavonoids (mainly rutin, quercetin, and kaempferol glycosides); coumarins (bergapten, imperatorin, xanthotoxin, and marmesin); miscellaneous: sterols, fixed oils, sugars[110]

Actions: Carminative, aromatic, antispasmodic, anti-inflammatory, galactagogue, hepatic

Indications: Fennel is an excellent stomach and intestinal remedy that relieves flatulence and colic while stimulating digestion and appetite. It is similar to aniseed in its calming effect in bronchitis and other coughs, and is a good choice for flavoring cough remedies. Fennel may increase milk flow in nursing mothers. Used externally, the essential oil eases muscular and rheumatic pains. Fennel infusion may be used as a compress to treat conjunctivitis and blepharitis (inflammation of the eyelids).

Safety Considerations: No side effects or drug interactions have been reported.

Preparations and Dosage: Tincture dosage is 1 to 2 ml three times a day (1:5 in 40%). For an infusion, pour 1 cup of boiling water over 1 to 2 teaspoons of slightly crushed seeds and infuse in a covered container for 10 minutes. This should be drunk three times a day. To ease flatulence, take a cup ½ hour before meals.

Recommended dosage from the BHP is 0.3 to 0.6 g herb or 0.8 to 2 ml liquid extract (1:1 in 70%) three times daily. The USP suggests 1 g herb, 15 ml fennel water (hydrosol), or 0.2 ml essential oil. The BPC suggests a three times daily dose of 25 to 30 ml fennel water or 0.3 ml oil three times daily. Daily dosage recommended by Commission E is 5 to 7 g herb, 10 to 20 g syrup or honey, 5 to 7.5 ml compound fennel tincture, or equivalent preparations.

Fennel fruit, in *Principles and Practice of Phytotherapy*

Fucus vesiculosus L.
Kelp
Fucaceae

Other Name: Bladderwrack

Part Used: Whole plant (a seaweed)

Constituents: Phenolic compounds (phloroglucinol, fucols); mucopolysaccharides (algin); sulphuryl-, sulphonyl-, and phosphonyl-glycosyl ester diglycerides; polar lipids; trace metals (particularly iodine)[111]

Actions: Antihypothyroid, antirheumatic

Indications: Bladderwrack has proved useful in the treatment of underactive thyroid and goiter. By regulating thyroid function, the seaweed helps bring about improvement in all related symptoms. For cases in which obesity is associated with thyroid trouble, this herb may aid in weight loss. It has a reputation for helping to relieve symptoms of rheumatism and rheumatoid arthritis, when both taken internally and applied externally to inflamed joints.

Safety Considerations: Kelp's iodine content may cause hyper- or hypothyroidism, and it may interfere with existing treatment for abnormal thyroid function.[112] In general, brown seaweeds are known to concentrate various heavy metals and other toxic elements. Elevated urinary arsenic concentrations have been traced to ingestion of kelp tablets. Prolonged ingestion of kelp may reduce gastrointestinal iron absorption (due to the binding properties of fucoidan), resulting in a slow reduction in hemoglobin, packed cell volume, and serum iron concentrations. Prolonged ingestion may also affect absorption of sodium and potassium ions (alginic acid) and cause diarrhea.[113]

Preparations and Dosage: Kelp may be taken in tablet form as a dietary supplement or as an infusion. For an infusion, pour 1 cup of boiling water over 2 to 3 teaspoons of dried herb and steep for 10 minutes. This should be drunk three times a day.

The BHC recommends 0.8 to 2 g dried thallus, 2 to 6 ml tincture (1:5 in 25%), or 0.5 to 2 ml fluid extract (1:1 in 25%) three times daily.

Fucus, in *Herbal Drugs and Phytopharmaceuticals*

Fumaria officinalis DC.
Fumitory
Fumariaceae

Parts Used: Aerial parts

Constituents: Isoquinoline alkaloids[114]

Actions: Diuretic, laxative, alterative, hepatic

Indications: Fumitory has a long history of use for the treatment of skin problems, such as eczema and acne. Its action is probably related to general cleansing mediated via the kidneys and liver. Fumitory may also be used as an eyewash to soothe conjunctivitis.

Safety Considerations: No side effects or drug interactions have been reported.

Preparations and Dosage: Tincture dosage is 1 to 2 ml three times a day (1:5 in 25%). For an infusion, pour 1 cup of boiling water over 1 to 2 teaspoons of dried herb and infuse for 10 to 15 minutes. This may be drunk freely, but for skin problems, it should be drunk at least three times a day.

The BHC lists a dosage of 2 to 4 g dried herb or 2 to 4 ml fluid extract (1:1 in 25%) three times a day. Commission E recommends a daily dosage of 6 g dried herb.

Fumariae herba, in *Herbal Drugs and Phytopharmaceuticals*

Galega officinalis L.
Goat's Rue
Fabaceae

Parts Used: Dried aerial parts

Constituents: Amines (galegine, 4-hydroxygalegine, peganine); flavonoids; saponins[115]

Actions: Hypoglycemic, galactagogue, diuretic, diaphoretic

Indications: Goat's rue is one of many herbal remedies with the ability to reduce blood sugar levels. It is thus potentially indicated in diabetes mellitus. It cannot replace insulin therapy, however, and should be used only under professional supervision.

Goat's rue is also an effective galactagogue. It stimulates both the production and flow of breast milk, and has been shown to increase milk output by up to 50% in some cases. It may also stimulate the development of the mammary glands.

Safety Considerations: Goat's rue may potentiate the action of hypoglycemic drugs.

Preparations and Dosage: Tincture dosage is 1 to 2 ml three times a day (1:10 in 45%). For an infusion, pour 1 cup of boiling water over 1 teaspoon of dried herb and infuse for 10 to 15 minutes. This should be drunk twice a day.

Galegae herba, in *Herbal Drugs and Phytopharmaceuticals*

Galium aparine L.
Cleavers
Rubiaceae

Parts Used: Aerial parts

Constituents: Plant acids (caffeic, *p*-coumaric, gallic, *p*-hydroxybenzoic, salicylic, citric); coumarins; iridoids (asperuloside, rubichloric acid); tannins[116]

Actions: Diuretic, alterative, anti-inflammatory, tonic, astringent

Indications: Cleavers is a very valuable plant, being perhaps the best tonic available for the lymphatic system. As a lymphatic tonic with alterative and diuretic actions, it may be used safely for a wide range of problems involving the lymphatic system. These include swollen glands (lymphadenitis) anywhere in the body, especially tonsillitis and adenoid trouble.

Cleavers is helpful in skin conditions, especially the dry types, such as psoriasis. It makes a useful contribution to the treatment of cystitis and other urinary tract conditions associated with pain, and may be combined with urinary demulcents for this. There is a long tradition of using cleavers to treat ulcers and tumors. Cleavers also makes an excellent vegetable.

Priest and Priest described cleavers as a

> . . . soothing, relaxing and diffusive diuretic: increases aqueous excretion, corrects inability to pass normal catabolic wastes and relieves irritation. Preferred diuretic for exanthemas.

They gave these specific indications: dropsy, renal obstructions, bladder stone, gravel, calculi, scalding micturation, dysuria, irritable bladder, cystitis, enuresis in children, eczema, and psoriasis.

Safety Considerations: No side effects or drug interactions have been reported.

Preparation and Dosage: Tincture dosage is 4 to 8 ml three times a day (1:5 in 25%). To make an infusion, pour 1 cup of boiling water over 2 to 3 teaspoons of dried herb and infuse for 10 to 15 minutes. This should be drunk three times a day. A pleasant and effective way of using fresh cleavers is to juice or simply puree in a blender. The resulting deep green liquid must be used right away or it will ferment. However, it may be frozen immediately for future use. An ice cube-sized piece makes an ideal dose.

Dosage listed in the BHC is 2 to 4 g dried herb, 5 to 15 ml expressed juice, 4 to 10 ml tincture (1:5 in 25%), or 2 to 4 ml fluid extract (1:1 in 25%) three times a day.

Clivers, in *Herbal Medicines: A Guide for Health-Care Professionals*

Gentiana lutea L.
Gentian
Gentianaceae

Parts Used: Dried rhizome and root

Constituents: Iridoids: marogentin, gentiopicroside (= gentiopicrin), swertiamarin; xanthones (gentisein, gentisin, isogentisin); alkaloids: mainly gentianine (0.6% to 0.8%) and gentialutine; phenolic acids (including gentisic, caffeic, protocatechuic, syringic, sinapic acids); miscellaneous: sugars (such as gentianose and gentiobiose), traces of volatile oil[117]

Actions: Bitter, sialagogue, hepatic, cholagogue, antimicrobial, anthelmintic, emmenagogue

Indications: Gentian is an excellent bitter that, like all bitters, stimulates the appetite and digestion via general stimulation of digestive juices. Thus, it promotes the production of saliva, gastric juices, and bile. Because of this stimulation, it has a generally fortifying effect. It also accelerates the emptying of the stomach. It is indicated for most cases involving lack of appetite and digestive sluggishness, as well as dyspepsia and flatulence.

Priest and Priest considered it an

... intense, bitter, stimulating tonic: influences digestive organs, mucous membranes and the portal circulation. Indicated for atonic and sub-acid states: slowly promotes peristalsis and facilitates assimilation.

They offered the following specific indications: languid conditions and general debility, anorexia, alimentary insufficiency; portal congestion, biliousness, and jaundice.

Safety Considerations: In predisposed persons, gentian may cause headaches. Gentian is contraindicated during pregnancy and for those with gastric or duodenal ulcers.

Preparations and Dosage: Tincture dosage is 1 to 2 ml three times a day (1:5 in 40%), 15 to 30 minutes before meals, or any time acute stomach pains are associated with a feeling of fullness. To make a decoction, put 1/2 teaspoon of shredded root in 1 cup of water and boil for 5 minutes. This should be drunk warm about 15 to 30 minutes before meals, or according to the guidelines given for tincture.

Commission E recommends a daily dosage of 2 to 4 g root, 1 to 3 ml tincture, or 2 to 4 ml fluid extract. The USP (23th ed., 1943) suggests 1 to 2 g as decoction three times daily; the BHP recommends 0.6 to 2 g by infusion or decoction or 1 to 4 ml tincture (1:5 in 45%) three times daily.

Gentian root, in Herbal Medicine, Expanded Commission E Monographs

Geranium maculatum L.
Cranesbill
Geraniaceae

Part Used: Rhizome

Constituents: Tannins, including gallic acid (levels are highest just before flowering)[118]

Actions: Astringent, antihemorrhagic, anti-inflammatory, vulnerary

Indications: American cranesbill is an effective astringent used for diarrhea, dysentery, and hemorrhoids. When duodenal or gastric ulceration is associated with bleeding, this remedy may be used in combination with other relevant herbs. Cranesbill will help when blood is lost in the feces, although careful diagnosis is vital. It is also indicated for the treatment of menorrhagia (excessive blood loss during menstruation) or metrorrhagia (uterine hemorrhage). As a douche, it may be used to treat leukorrhea.

Safety Considerations: No side effects or drug interactions have been reported.

Preparations and Dosage: Tincture dosage is 2 to 4 ml three times a day (1:5 in 40%). For a decoction, put 1 to 2 teaspoons of rhizome in 1 cup of cold water, bring to a boil, and simmer for 10 to 15 minutes. This should be drunk three times a day.

The BHP recommends 1 to 2 g by decoction, 2 to 4 ml tincture (1:5 in 45%), or 1 to 2 ml liquid extract (1:1 in 45%) three times a day.

Ginkgo biloba L.
Ginkgo
Ginkgoaceae

Parts Used: Leaf; seed kernel is used extensively in traditional Chinese medicine

Constituents: Diterpene lactones (ginkgolides A, B, C, and J); sesquiterpene lactone (bilobalide); flavonol glycosides (mainly flavone glycosides, including ginkgetin, quercetin, and kaempferol derivatives)[119]

Actions: Anti-inflammatory, vasodilator, relaxant, digestive bitter, uterine stimulant

Indications: The modern use of ginkgo is not derived from traditional Chinese medicine, although ginkgo fruit has a long history of use in that system. Extracts of *Ginkgo biloba* leaf were introduced into Western medical practice in 1965 in Germany. Most pharmacologic studies on ginkgo leaf for the treatment of peripheral vascular disease and cerebral insufficiency have utilized the proprietary extract EGb 761 and, more recently, Ll 1370, not the crude leaf or simple extracts.[120]

Ginkgo's primary actions are to increase blood supply, antagonize platelet activating factor (PAF), and protect and enhance brain function (an action known as *cerebroprotection*). Its ability to improve circulation and thus blood supply appears to be due to both its vasodilating properties and its ability to reduce total blood viscosity.

Various mechanisms may underlie the vasodilating activity—for example, effects on prostaglandin metabolism that increase the synthesis of the vasodilator prostacyclin. Ginkgo's antioxidant, radical-scavenging properties may also play a role. Its ability to lower pathologically elevated total blood viscosity seems to be due to its PAF antagonism, which results in a reduction in erythrocyte aggregation.

The ginkgolides and bilobalide appear to be responsible for the herb's cerebroprotective properties.[121] Among other factors, researchers have studied ginkgo's ability to increase tolerance to hypoxia, protect against ischemia, improve energy metabolism, and reduce edema in order to demonstrate the protective actions of ginkgo extracts on experimentally damaged brain.

Other ginkgo actions are based on its radical-scavenging effects and PAF antagonism. The constituents of ginkgo extract with PAF-antagonistic activity are the ginkgolides. In particular, ginkgolide B has been found to be a very active PAF antagonist. As discussed elsewhere, PAF binding to PAF receptors on target cells leads to the release of mediators and to various physiologic reactions, such as vasodilation and platelet aggregation. These actions are responsible for asthma, inflammation, and anaphylaxis. PAF antagonists block the PAF receptors of target cells. This inhibition of platelet aggregation appears to be one of the most relevant actions associated with ginkgo use.

Ginkgo's main clinical indication is for the treatment of cerebral insufficiency, a common problem in the elderly.[122] Among the symptoms typical of cerebral insufficiency are difficulties with concentration and memory, absentmindedness, confusion, lack of energy, tiredness, decreased physical performance, depressed mood, and anxiety. Headache, vertigo, and tinnitus are other common complaints. These symptoms are associated with impaired cerebral circulation, and are sometimes thought to be early indications of dementia, either the degenerative or the multiple infarct type. However, in some cases, no explanation for the symptoms can be found.

Many experimental and clinical studies support the efficacy of ginkgo extract in the treatment of peripheral blood flow disorders. Vertigo, hearing disorders, and tinnitus have many and varied causes, but are often associated with insufficient perfusion of the brain or inner ear.

Vertigo is regarded as one of the pathologic conditions that respond best to ginkgo extract. Ginkgo can also contribute, as part of a broader treatment, to the control of peripheral arterial occlusive disease (intermittent claudication).

Safety Considerations: Ginkgo may have an additive effect when used with other antiplatelet agents. One patient taking 40 mg of a 50:1 concentrated extract twice daily in combination with long-term aspirin therapy experienced bleeding from the iris.[123] However, it is important to note that ginkgo has demonstrated a very low incidence of side effects and a relative lack of reported drug interactions, evidenced by the fact that many elderly patients taking ginkgo are taking multiple other medications simultaneously.

Ginkgo may potentiate the effects of papaverine used to treat male impotence.[124] Raw ginkgo fruits are reportedly toxic. Ginkgo extracts, however, are derived from the leaves.

Preparations and Dosage: Dosage of standardized extract is 120 to 240 mg/day in divided doses, 50:1 standardized leaf extract containing 22% to 27% ginkgo flavone glycosides and 5% to 7% terpene lactones (ginkgolides A, B, C, and bilobalides). For optimal results, 4 to 8 weeks of daily use are required.

Commission E recommends 120 to 240 mg dry extract in two or three doses to treat disturbances of performance related to organic brain syndromes. For other cardiovascular indications, it recommends 120 to 160 mg in two or three doses.

Ginkgo, in *Principles and Practice of Phytotherapy*

Glycyrrhiza glabra L.
Licorice
Fabaceae

Part Used: Dried root

Constituents: Oleanane triterpenes (glycyrrhizin, glycyrrhetinic acid, and phytosterols); flavanones; isoflavonoids; chalcones; polysaccharides (mainly glucans); volatile oil (containing fenchone, linalool, furfuryl alcohol, benzaldehyde); miscellaneous: starch, sugars, amino acid[125]

Actions: Expectorant, demulcent, anti-inflammatory, antihepatotoxic, antispasmodic, mild laxative

Indications: Licorice is a traditional herbal remedy with an ancient history and worldwide usage. Modern research has demonstrated that the herb has effects upon the endocrine system and the liver, among other organs. The triterpenes of *Glycyrrhiza* are metabolized in the body to molecules with a structure similar to that of the adrenal cortex hormones. This may be the basis of the herb's anti-inflammatory action.

As an antihepatotoxic, licorice can be effective in the treatment of chronic hepatitis and cirrhosis, for which it is widely used in Japan. Much of the liver-oriented research has focused upon the triterpene glycyrrhizin. Studies show that this constituent inhibits hepatocyte injury caused by carbon tetrachloride, benzene hexachloride, and polychlorinated biphenyl (PCB).[126] It inhibits the growth of several DNA and RNA viruses and irreversibly inactivates herpes simplex virus particles.[127]

Licorice has a wide range of applications for bronchial problems, including catarrh, bronchitis, and coughs in general. The herb is used in orthodox medicine as a treatment for peptic ulcers, and is similarly used in herbal medicine for gastritis and ulcers. It may also be effective in relieving abdominal colic.

King's described it thus:

> Liquorice root is emollient, demulcent and nutritive. It acts upon mucous surfaces, lessening irritation and is consequently useful in coughs, catarrhs, irritation of the urinary organs and pain of the intestines in diarrhoea. It is commonly administered in decoction, sometimes alone, at other times with the addition of other agents and which is the preferable mode of using it. As a general rule, the acrid principle should be removed previous to forming a decoction. When boiled for some time the water becomes impregnated with its acrid resin; hence, in preparing a decoction for the purpose of sweetening diet drinks or covering the taste of nauseous drugs, it should not be boiled over 5 minutes. The efficiency of the root in old bronchial affections may be due to this acrid resin. The powdered root is also employed to give the proper solidity to pills and to prevent their adhesion; the extract for imparting the proper viscidity to them. The extract, in the form of lozenge, held in the mouth until it has dissolved, is a very popular and efficient remedy in coughs and pectoral affections. The bitterness of quinine, quassia, aloes and the acrid taste of senega, guaiacum are masked by Liquorice.

Safety Considerations: Side effects are minimal if daily intake is less than 10 mg of glycyrrhizin. Chronic use may cause hypokalemia, headache, spastic numbness, hypertension, weak limbs, dizziness, and edema. Glycyrrhizin and glycyrrhetinic acid have antidiuretic, mineralocorticoid-type actions, but these constituents are removed from most commercial extracts. The resulting extracts are denoted as "deglycyrrhizinated."

Prolonged use in conjunction with thiazide and loop diuretics and cardiac glycosides is contraindicated, and licorice should not be administered in combination with spironolactone or amiloride.[128] This herb is not recommended for patients taking cardiac glycosides, hypotensive agents, corticoids, diuretic drugs, or monoamine oxidase inhibitors.

Preparations and Dosage: Tincture dosage is 1 to 3 ml three times a day (1:5 in 40%). To make a decoction, put $^1/_2$ to 1 teaspoon of root in 1 cup of water, bring to a boil, and simmer for 10 to 15 minutes. This should be drunk three times a day.

Commission E recommends an average daily dosage of 5 to 15 g root, equivalent to 200 to 600 mg of glycyrrhizin. Dosage according to the BHP is 1 to 5 g (by infusion or decoction) or 2 to 5 ml liquid extract three times a day.

Licorice, in *Principles and Practice of Phytotherapy*

Grindelia squarrosa (Pursh) Dunal
Gumweed

Asteraceae

Related Species: *Grindelia camporum*

Parts Used: Dried aerial parts

Constituents: Diterpenes (grindelic acid and others); flavonoids (including acacetin, kumatakenin, quercetin); resins[129]

Actions: Antispasmodic, expectorant, hypotensive

Indications: Gumweed acts to relax smooth muscles and heart muscles. This helps to explain its use in the treatment of asthmatic and bronchial conditions, especially when these are associated with rapid heartbeat and nervous response. The herb may be used for asthma, bronchitis, whooping cough, and upper respiratory catarrh. Because of its relaxing effect on the heart and pulse rate, it may reduce blood pressure. Externally, it can be applied in a lotion to treat poison ivy dermatitis.

King's discussed in detail the indications for two species:

> The grindelias leave in the mouth a bitter, acrid sensation, which persists for some time and is accompanied or followed by an increased flow of saliva. On account of their irritant effects upon the kidneys, they act as diuretics. The brain and cord are first stimulated by them, followed by motor impairment of the lower extremities and a desire to sleep. The number of respirations are reduced by them. *Grindelia robusta* has been found especially efficient in asthma giving prompt relief. Occasionally, however, as is, indeed, the case with all the therapeutical agents, it has

failed but the circumstances attending these failures have not yet been determined. It has likewise been found efficient in bronchial affections, in pertussis, and in some renal maladies. Prof. Scudder was partial to this remedy as a local application in chronic diseases of the skin with feeble circulation, particularly old chronic and indolent ulcers. *Grindelia squarrosa* has been highly eulogized as an efficient remedy in intermittent fever and in other malarial affections, also to remove the splenic enlargement which frequently follows those disorders. Why two plants so closely allied as the *G. robusta* and the *G. squarrosa*, and possessing nearly identical constituents, should give such discordant therapeutical results, is certainly enigmatical. The fact is, that many physicians have a great proneness to run after new remedies, especially when introduced under some pretentious name, and to place a marvelous credulity in the statements of interested parties, who are incapable of determining accurate conclusions as to the value of a remedy. [*Author's note:* This is as relevant today as it was 100 years ago!] As a local application, the fluid extract is stated to be of value in the painful eczematous inflammation and vesicular eruption resulting from contact with the poison vine or the poison oak.

Safety Considerations: Gumweed may theoretically cause allergic reactions in people sensitive to plants in the Asteraceae family.

Preparations and Dosage: Tincture dosage is 1 to 2 ml three times a day (1:5 in 60%). For an infusion, pour 1 cup of boiling water over 1 teaspoon of dried herb and infuse for 10 to 15 minutes. This should be drunk three times a day.

The BHC recommends 0.3 to 1 g resin or 1 to 4 ml tincture (1:5 in 90%) up to three times daily. According to Commission E, total daily dosage is 4 to 6 g of drug or equivalent preparations or 1.5 to 3 ml tincture (1:10 or 1:5, 60% to 80%).

Gumweed herb, in *The Complete German Commission E Monographs*

Guaiacum officinale L.
Guaiacum
Zygophyllaceae

Other Name: Guaiac

Part Used: Heartwood

Constituents: Lignans (furoguaiacidin, guaiacin, furoguaiacin, furoguaiaoxidin); resins (15% to 20%), including guaiaretic, hydroguaiaretic, guaiacic, and α- and β-guaiaconic acids; miscellaneous: vanillin, terpenoids (including guaiagutin, guaiasaponin)[130]

Actions: Antirheumatic, anti-inflammatory, laxative, diaphoretic, diuretic

Indications: Guaiacum is a specific for rheumatic complaints. It is especially useful in cases involving much inflammation and pain, and is thus valuable for chronic rheumatism and rheumatoid arthritis. It helps in the treatment of gout and may be used to prevent recurrence of this disease.

Safety Considerations: Due to the high content of resins in this valuable herb, care must be taken with patients with gastritis or peptic ulceration, who may be more likely to experience stomach upset.

Preparations and Dosage: Tincture dosage is 1 to 2 ml three times a day (1:5 in 90%). Commission E recommends 4.5 g of herb or equivalent preparations daily.

Guaiac wood, in *The Complete German Commission E Monographs*

Hamamelis virginiana L.
Witch Hazel
Hamamelidaceae

Parts Used: Twig, leaf

Constituents: Tannins (hamamelitannins); flavonoids (quercetin, kaempferol, astragalin, myricitrin); volatile oil; saponins; resin[131]

Actions: Astringent, anti-inflammatory

Indications: This herb can be found in most households in the form of distilled witch hazel. It is one of the easiest-to-use astringents for external use. As with all astringents, witch hazel may be applied in all cases of bleeding, internal and external. It is especially valuable for easing symptoms of hemorrhoids, and has a well-deserved reputation for the treatment of bruises, inflamed swellings, and varicose veins. Witch hazel helps control diarrhea and is useful in dysentery.

Ellingwood considered it specific for

> . . . soreness of muscles, muscular aching, a bruised sensation, soreness from violent muscular exertion, soreness from bruises and strains, soreness and muscular aching from cold and exposure, relaxed mucous membranes, dark blue membranes from venous stasis, veins dilated, relaxed, enlarged, and full varicoses.

In addition, he recommended it for sore throat, tonsillitis, diphtheria, acute catarrh, diarrhea, hemorrhoids, prolapse of the bowel, leukorrhea, and sore breasts.

Safety Considerations: No side effects or drug interactions have been reported.

Preparations and Dosage: Tincture dosage is 1 to 2 ml three times a day (1:5 in 40%). For an infusion, pour 1 cup of boiling water over 1 teaspoon of dried herb and infuse for 10 to 15 minutes. This should be drunk three times a day. Witch hazel can be made into an excellent ointment and many other topical formulations.

Witchhazel, in *Principles and Practice of Phytotherapy*

Harpagophytum procumbens DC. ex Meisn.
Devil's Claw
Pedaliaceae

Part Used: Rhizome

Constituents: Iridoid glycosides (harpagide, harpagoside, procumbide); flavonoids (kaempferol and luteolin glycosides); phenolic acids (chlorogenic and cinnamic acid); a quinone (harpagoquinone); miscellaneous: triterpenes, oleanolic and ursolic acid derivatives, esters, sugars[132]

Actions: Anti-inflammatory, antirheumatic, anodyne, hepatic

Indications: This valuable plant has proved effective in some cases of arthritis. This appears to be due to the presence of a glycoside called harpagoside, which reduces inflammation in the joints. Unfortunately, devil's claw is not always effective, but it is well worth considering for arthritis associated with inflammation and pain. The plant also helps with liver and gallbladder complaints.

Safety Considerations: No drug interactions have been reported. Pharmacological research suggests a potential protective action against arrhythmia, which has led to the speculation that it may interact with antiarrhythmic agents.[133]

Preparations and Dosage: Tincture dosage is 1 to 2 ml three times a day (1:5 in 40%). For a decoction, put $^{1}/_{2}$ to 1 teaspoon of rhizome into 1 cup of water, bring to a boil, and simmer for 10 to 15 minutes. This should be drunk three times a day. The regimen should be continued for at least 1 month.

Commission E recommends 1.5 g daily for loss of appetite, otherwise 4.5 g daily.

Devil's claw, in *Principles and Practice of Phytotherapy*

Humulus lupulus L.
Hops
Cannabaceae

Part Used: Inflorescence (strobile)

Constituents: Volatile oil (humulene, β-caryophyllene, myrcene, farnesene); flavonoids (mainly glycosides of kaempferol and quercetin); oleoresin (3% to 12%): humulone, lupulene; estrogenic substances of undetermined structure; miscellaneous: tannins, lipids, xanthohumol (a chalcone)[134]

Actions: Sedative, hypnotic, antimicrobial, antispasmodic, astringent

Indications: Hops has a marked relaxing effect upon the central nervous system, and is used extensively for the treatment of insomnia. It eases tension and anxiety, and is appropriate for cases in which tension leads to restlessness, headache, and indigestion. As it is also astringent, it may be valuable for conditions such as mucous colitis. However, patients experiencing significant depression should avoid hops, as it may accentuate this mood state. Externally, its antiseptic action is applied to treat skin ulcers.

Clinical studies generally refer to hops given in combination with one or more additional herbs. Hops in combination with valerian has been reported to improve sleep disturbances.[135] A combination of hops, chicory, and peppermint was shown to relieve pain in patients with chronic cholecystitis (calculus and non-calculus).[136]

Ellingwood considered hops specific for "marked cases of nerve irritation and wakefulness where anxiety and worry are the cause." He recommended it for hysteria, insomnia, acute local inflammations, facial neuralgia, delirium tremens, and excessive sexual excitement.

Safety Considerations: Do not use hops in patients with marked depression, as the sedative effect may accentuate symptoms. The sedative action may also potentiate the effects of alcohol or of existing sedative therapy.

Preparations and Dosage: Tincture dosage is 1 to 4 ml three times a day (1:5 in 40%). For an infusion, pour 1 cup of boiling water over 1 teaspoon of dried herb and infuse in a covered container for 10 to 15 minutes. A cup should be drunk at night to induce sleep. This dose may be strengthened if needed.

The BHC suggests 0.5 to 1 g dried strobiles, 1 to 2 ml tincture (1:5 in 60%), or 0.5 to 1 ml fluid extract (1:1 in 45%) three times daily and before going to bed. According to Commission E, dosage is 0.5 g dried herb as a single dose.

Hops, in *Herbal Medicine, Expanded Commission E Monographs*

Hydrangea arborescens L.
Hydrangea
Hydrangeaceae

Parts Used: Dried root and rhizome

Constituents: Flavonoids (kaempferol and quercetin); coumarin (hydrangin); saponin; volatile oil[137]

Actions: Diuretic, antilithic

Indications: Hydrangea's primary use is for the treatment of inflamed or enlarged prostate. It may also be effective against urinary stones and gravel associated with infections, such as cystitis.

Ellingwood gave the following specific symptomatology for this underutilized remedy:

> . . . frequent urination with heat, burning, accompanied with quick, sharp, acute pains in the urethra; partial suppression of urine with general irritation and aching or pain in the back, pain from the passage of renal sand, are direct indications for this agent. I am convinced after a lifetime of experience that it is more universally a sedative to pain and distress in kidneys and urinary bladder than any other one remedy.

Ellingwood also recommended hydrangea for acute nephritis, urinary gravel, backache due to urinary tract problems, and urinary irritation.

Safety Considerations: No side effects or drug interactions have been reported.

Preparations and Dosage: Tincture dosage is 2 to 4 ml three times a day (1:5 in 40%). To make a decoction, put 2 teaspoons of root in 1 cup of water, bring to a boil, and simmer for 10 to 15 minutes. This should be drunk three times a day.

Hydrangea, in *Herbal Medicines: A Guide for Health-Care Professionals*

Hydrastis canadensis L.
Goldenseal
Ranunculaceae

Parts Used: Root, rhizome

Constituents: Isoquinoline alkaloids (2.5% to 6.0%): hydrastine (1.5% to 4.0%), berberine (0.5% to6.0%); fatty acids; resin; phenylpropanoids (meconin, chlorogenic acid); phytosterins; a small amount of volatile oil[138]

Actions: Bitter, hepatic, alterative, anticatarrhal, antimicrobial, anti-inflammatory, laxative, emmenagogue, oxytocic

Indications: Goldenseal is one of our most useful remedies, and owes much of its value to its tonic effects on mucous membranes. This probably accounts for its effectiveness in digestive problems, from peptic ulcers to colitis. The alkaloids it contains stimulate bile production and secretion, and this bitter stimulant activity makes it useful for loss of appetite.

Goldenseal is effective in catarrhal conditions, especially sinus disorders. The herb's pharmacological activity, including its antimicrobial properties, is usually attributed to the isoquinoline alkaloid constituents, primarily hydrastine and berberine. Berberine has immunostimulant, antispasmodic, sedative, hypotensive, uterotonic, cholerectic, and carminative actions. It also has marked antimicrobial activity, and while not in the same league as pharmaceutical antibiotics, it has a broad spectrum of antibiotic activity. Activity has been demonstrated against a number of bacteria, protozoans, and fungi in vitro.[139]

Traditionally, *Hydrastis canadensis* was used during labor to help contractions, but for this very reason, it should not be taken during pregnancy. Applied externally, it can help with eczema, ringworm, itching, earache, and conjunctivitis.

Ellingwood recommended it for numerous conditions:

> . . . functional disorders of the stomach, catarrhal gastritis, atonic dyspepsia, chronic constipation, hepatic congestion, chronic alcoholism, hepatic congestion, general debility, protracted fevers, cerebral engorgements, prostrating night sweats, menorrhagia or metrorrhagia due to uterine subinvolution, postpartum haemorrhage, tumors, catarrhal conditions, aphthous ulcers, indolent ulcers, nasal catarrh, diphtheria, tonsillitis, inflammation of the eyes, leucorrhoea, anal fissure, eczema, gall stones, cholecystitis, congestive jaundice, goitre, non-malignant mammary tumors.

Safety Considerations: Goldenseal is contraindicated for individuals with elevated blood pressure. Prolonged use of goldenseal may decrease vitamin B absorption. Like all berberine-containing plants and strong bitters, *Hydrastis* is not recommended for use during pregnancy. Uterine stimulant properties have been reported for berberine, canadine, hydrastine, and hydrastinine.[140] Goldenseal should not be taken during lactation.

Preparations and Dosage: Tincture dosage is 1 ml three times a day (1:5 in 60%). To make an infusion, pour 1 cup of boiling water over $^1/_2$ to 1 teaspoon of powdered root and infuse for 10 to 15 minutes. This should be drunk three times a day. Decoct unpowdered root in the usual way, by simmering.

Dosage from the BPC is 2 to 4 ml tincture or 0.3 to 0.9 ml liquid extract three times a day. Dosage provided in the BHC is 0.5 to 1 g dried rhizome and root, 4 to 10 ml tincture (1:10 in 60%), or 0.3 to 1 ml fluid extract (1:1 in 60%) three times daily.

Berberis bark and Hydrastis root, in *Principles and Practice of Phytotherapy*

Hypericum perforatum L.
St. John's Wort
Clusiaceae

Parts Used: Aerial parts

Constituents: Volatile oil (caryophyllene, methyl-2-octane, *n*-nonane, *n*-octanal, *n*-decanal, α- and β-pinene); naphthodianthones (hypericin, pseudohypericin); phloroglucinols (hyperforin); catechins; proanthocyanidins; flavonoids (hyperoside, rutin)[141]

Actions: Anti-inflammatory, astringent, vulnerary, nervine, antimicrobial

Indications: Taken internally, St. John's wort has sedative and pain-relieving effects, giving it a place in the treatment of neuralgia, anxiety, tension, and similar problems. It is considered especially appropriate for use when menopausal changes trigger irritability and anxiety. St. John's wort is increasingly recommended to treat depression, an indication that is supported by numerous clinical trials in both Europe and the United States.[142] However, in my opinion these claims are overblown.

St. John's wort is helpful for neuralgic pain and will ease fibrositis, sciatica, and rheumatic pain. Externally, it is a valuable healing and anti-inflammatory remedy. Applied in lotion form, it speeds the healing of wounds and bruises, varicose veins, and mild burns. An infused oil is especially useful for the healing of sunburn.

The mechanism of action for the purported antidepressant activity of *Hypericum perforatum* is not understood. One study tested the herb in several biochemical models relevant to the mechanism of action of antidepressant drugs—for example, monoamine oxidase (MAO) inhibition. It was found to have weak MAO-A and MAO-B inhibition activity in vitro, but the study authors concluded that MAO inhibition does not explain the herb's antidepressant activity.[143] While hypericin is considered an MAO inhibitor, newer studies indicate that the constituent hyperforin is also active. Thus, based on currently available information, the whole extract must be considered the "active ingredient," as the single constituents responsible for this activity remain unknown. Consequently, dosage should be based on the quantity of total extract, not on hypericin content.

Priest and Priest described St. John's wort as a

. . . sedative nervine for muscular twitching and choreiform movements—especially indicated for nerve injuries to the extremities and teeth/gums. Promotes elimination of catabolic waste products.

They provided the following specific indications:

painful injuries to sacral spine and coccyx, traumatic shock, hemorrhoids with pain and bleeding, facial neuralgia after dental extractions and toothache, neurasthenia, chorea, and depression.

Safety Considerations: No adverse reactions have been confirmed at dose levels up to 1 mg of total hypericin.[144] Photosensitization at high doses has been reported during experimental antiviral treatment with synthetic hypericin (35 mg intravenously) in HIV-positive patients.[145] While a few instances of photosensitization have been documented, this appears to be very rare. A recent study utilizing human keratinocyte cell cultures demonstrated that usual therapeutic doses of *Hypericum* extracts are about 30 to 50 times below the phototoxic level.[146]

There have been reports of elevated serotonin levels in patients taking selective serotonin reuptake inhibitors (e.g., sertraline) in combination with St. John's wort.[147] Evidence suggests that St. John's wort affects the hepatic cytochrome P_{450} system, increasing the activity of its most abundant isozyme, CYP_3A_4. Thus, theoretically, the herb could reduce the activity of simultaneously administered drugs that are known substrates for this isozyme, including nonsedating antihistamines, oral contraceptives, certain antiretroviral agents, antiepileptic medications, calcium channel-blockers, cyclosporine, some chemotherapeutic drugs, macrolide antibiotics, and selected antifungals.

Preparations and Dosage: Tincture dosage is 2 to 4 ml three times a day (1:5 in 40%). To make an infusion, pour 1 cup of boiling water over 1 to 2 teaspoons of dried herb and infuse for 10 to 15 minutes. This should be drunk three times a day. See chapter 11 or 19 for instructions on making St. John's wort–infused oil for external application.

Based on clinical studies, dosage of standardized extract is 300 mg three times a day of extract standardized to 3% to 5% hyperforin. Dosage recommended in the BHP is 2 to 4 g dried herb, 2 to 4 ml tincture (1:10 in 45%), or 2 to 4 ml (1:1 in 25%) three times a day. Commission E suggest 2 to 4 g of herb or 0.2 to 1 mg total hypericin in other forms of application.

St John's wort, in *Principles and Practice of Phytotherapy*

Hyssopus officinalis L.
Hyssop
Lamiaceae

Parts Used: Dried aerial parts

Constituents: Diterpenes (marrubiin); triterpenoid saponins (oleanolic and ursolic acids); volatile oil (camphor, pinocaphone, thujone, and many others); flavonoids (including diosmin and hesperidin); miscellaneous: hyssopin (a glucoside), tannins (5% to 8%), resin[148]

Actions: Antispasmodic, expectorant, diaphoretic, nervine, anti-inflammatory, carminative

Indications: Hyssop has an interesting range of uses, largely attributed to the antispasmodic action of its volatile oil. The herb is used for coughs, bronchitis, and chronic catarrh. Its diaphoretic properties explain its use for the common cold. As a nervine, it may be taken for anxiety states and petit mal seizures.

King's Dispensatory considered hyssop a

... stimulant, aromatic, carminative and tonic. Principally used in quinsy and other sore throats, as a gargle, combined with sage and alum, in infusion sweetened with honey. Also recommended in asthma, coughs, and other affections of the chest, as an expectorant. The leaves applied to bruises, speedily relieve the pain, and disperse every spot or mark from the affected parts.

Safety Considerations: No side effects or drug interactions have been reported.

Preparations and Dosage: Tincture dosage is 1 to 4 ml three times a day (1:5 in 45%). For an infusion, pour 1 cup of boiling water over 1 to 2 teaspoons of dried herb and infuse in a covered container for 10 to 15 minutes. This should be drunk three times a day.

Hyssop, in *The Complete German Commission E Monographs*

Inula helenium L.
Elecampane
Asteraceae

Part Used: Rhizome

Constituents: Sesquiterpene lactones, including alantolactone (= helenalin), isoalantolactone; polysaccharides, mainly inulin (up to 44%); miscellaneous: sterols, resin[149]

Actions: Expectorant, antitussive, diaphoretic, hepatic, antimicrobial

Indications: Elecampane is a specific for irritating bronchial coughs, especially in children. It may be used whenever copious catarrh is present—for example, in bronchitis or emphysema. It can be helpful in asthma and bronchial asthma, and has been applied for the treatment of tuberculosis.

This remedy provides a good illustration of the complex and integrated ways in which herbs work. The mucilage has a relaxing effect, while the essential oils bring about stimulation, so the herb both soothes irritation and promotes expectoration. These actions are combined with

an overall antibacterial effect. Its bitter principle stimulates digestion and appetite.

Priest and Priest considered elecampane a

... gently stimulating tonic expectorant for chronic catarrhal conditions: warming, strengthening and cleansing to pulmonary mucous membranes. Indicated for chronic pectoral states with excessive catarrhal expectoration and/or a tubercular diathesis.

They suggested it for the following specific indications: bronchial and gastric catarrh, chronic bronchitis, tuberculosis, pneumoconiosis, silicosis, pertussis, emphysematous conditions, and chronic cough in the elderly.

Safety Considerations: Elecampane may cause allergic reactions in people sensitive to plants in the Asteraceae family.

Preparations and Dosage: Tincture dosage is 1 to 2 ml three times a day (1:5 in 40%). To make an infusion, pour 1 cup of cold water over 1 teaspoon of shredded root. Let stand for 8 to 10 hours. Heat and take very hot three times a day.

Helenii rhizoma, in *Herbal Drugs and Phytopharmaceuticals*

Iris versicolor L.
Blue Flag
Iridaceae

Part Used: Rhizome

Constituents: Volatile oil, containing furfural; iridin (also known as irisin, a glycoside); acids (including salicylic and isophthalic); miscellaneous: a monocyclic C_{31} triterpenoid, gum, resin, sterols[150]

Actions: Cholagogue, hepatic, alterative, laxative, diuretic, anti-inflammatory

Indications: Blue flag is used in the treatment of skin diseases, and apparently works in this area through effects on the liver, the main detoxifying organ of the body. It is valuable as part of a wider treatment for eczema and psoriasis.

Priest and Priest described blue flag as a

... positive alterative for chronic, torpid conditions: influences glandular system, lymphatics, liver and gall ducts, and intestinal glands. Specific for hepatic congestion due to venous or lymphatic stasis.

They recommended it for chronic hepatitis, rheumatic conditions, toxic sciatica, scrophulous skin conditions, eczema, psoriasis, herpes, enlarged thyroid gland, and uterine fibroids.

Safety Considerations: No side effects or drug interactions have been reported.

Preparations and Dosage: Tincture dosage is 1 ml three times a day (1:5 in 40%). To make a decoction, put 1 teaspoon of dried herb into 1 cup of water, bring to a boil, and simmer for 10 to 15 minutes. This should be drunk three times a day.

According to the BHC, dosage is 0.6 to 2 g dried rhizome (or by decoction), 3 to 10 ml tincture (1:5 in 45%), or 0.6 to 2 ml fluid extract (1:1 in 45%) three times daily.

Blue Flag, in *Herbal Medicines: A Guide for Health-Care Professionals*

Juniperus communis L.
Juniper
Cupressaceae

Part Used: Dried fruit (berry)

Constituents: Volatile oil (0.2% to 3.42%): myrcene, sabinene, α- and β-pinene, 4-cineole, camphene, limonene; condensed tannins; diterpenes; flavonoids (amentoflavone, quercetin, isoquercitrin, apigenin); miscellaneous: sugars, resin, vitamin C[151]

Actions: Diuretic, antimicrobial, carminative, antirheumatic

Indications: The actions documented for juniper are primarily associated with its volatile oil components. Juniper berries make an excellent antiseptic for urinary tract conditions such as cystitis. Their essential oil is quite stimulating to the kidney nephrons, however, so people with kidney disease should avoid this herb.

Juniper's bitter action aids digestion and eases flatulent colic. The herb is taken internally for rheumatism and arthritis, and, used externally, helps relieve pain in the joints or muscles. In the laboratory, a juniper extract demonstrated potent inhibition of herpes simplex virus type I in human cell culture.[152]

Safety Considerations: With prolonged use or overdose, juniper may cause renal damage, evidenced by renal pain with an increased urge to urinate, pain during urination, and hematuria and albuminuria (the presence of blood and protein, respectively, in the urine). People with kidney disease should not take juniper berries. They should also be avoided in pregnancy.

Preparations and Dosage: Tincture dosage is 0.5 to 1 ml three times a day (1:5 in 40%). To make an infusion, pour 1 cup of boiling water over 1 teaspoon of lightly crushed berries and infuse in a covered container for 20 minutes. This should be drunk three times a day.

Commission E recommends a total daily dosage of 2 g to a maximum of 10 g of dried juniper fruit, corresponding to 20 to 100 mg of essential oil.

Juniper berry, in *Herbal Medicine, Expanded Commission E Monographs*

Lactuca virosa L.
Wild Lettuce
Asteraceae

Part Used: Dried leaf

Constituents: Lactucin (a sesquiterpene lactone); flavonoids (mainly based on quercetin); coumarins (cichoriin and aesculin); N-methyl-β-phenethylamine[153]

Actions: Nervine, anodyne, hypnotic, antispasmodic

Indications: The latex of wild lettuce was at one time sold as "lettuce opium," or "lactucarium," as it was called in the official pharmacopoeias of the day. Wild lettuce is a valuable remedy for insomnia and restlessness. As an antispasmodic, it can be applied as part of a holistic treatment for whooping cough and dry irritated coughs in general. It relieves colic pains in the intestines and uterus, and so may be used in dysmenorrhea. It also eases muscular pains related to rheumatism. The herb has been used as an anaphrodisiac.

Safety Considerations: Wild lettuce may cause allergic reactions in people sensitive to plants in the Asteraceae family.

Preparations and Dosage: Tincture dosage is 1 to 2 ml three times a day (1:5 in 40%). To make an infusion, pour 1 cup of boiling water over 1 to 2 teaspoons of herb and infuse for 10 to 15 minutes. This should be drunk three times a day.

Dosage recommended in the BHC is 0.5 to 4 g dried herb or 0.5 to 4 ml fluid extract (1:1 in 25%) three times daily. The USP gives a dosage of 2 ml lactucarium tincture three times a day.

Wild Lettuce, in *Herbal Medicines: A Guide for Health-Care Professionals*

Lavandula angustifolia Miller
Lavender
Lamiaceae

Part Used: Flower

Constituents: Volatile oil (linalyl acetate, linalol, lavandulyl acetate, borneol, limonene, caryophyllene); coumarins (umbelliferone, herniarin, coumarin); miscellaneous: triterpenes (e.g., ursolic acid), flavonoids (e.g., luteolin)[154]

Actions: Carminative, antispasmodic, relaxing nervine, antidepressant, rubefacient, emmenagogue, hypotensive

Indications: This beautiful herb has many uses, culinary, cosmetic, and medicinal. It can help relieve headaches, particularly when they are stress-related. Lavender may be quite effective in clearing depression, especially if used in conjunction with other remedies, and can also be used to promote natural sleep. As a gentle, strengthening nervous system tonic, it may be used to treat states of nervous debility and exhaustion. The essential oil may be applied externally as a stimulating liniment to help ease aches and pains of rheumatism. The general safety and efficacy of the essential of lavender make it widely applicable in topical formulations.

Safety Considerations: No side effects or drug interactions have been reported.

Preparations and Dosage: To make an infusion to take internally, pour 1 cup of boiling water over 1 teaspoon of dried herb and infuse in a covered container for 10 minutes. This can be drunk three times a day. Lavender essential oil should not be taken internally, but can be inhaled, rubbed on the skin, or added to baths.

Commission E recommends 1 to 2 teaspoons of herb per cup of water or 1 to 4 drops (approximately 20 to 80 mg) of lavender essential oil.

Lavender flower, in *Herbal Medicine, Expanded Commission E Monographs*

Leonurus cardiaca L.
Motherwort
Lamiaceae

Parts Used: Aerial parts

Constituents: Iridoids (leonuride and others); labdane diterpenes (including leocardin); flavonoids (apigenin, kaempferol, and quercetin glucosides); caffeic acid; alkaloids (0.35%): tachydrine, betonicine, turicin, leonurine; tannins (2% to 8%); volatile oil (0.05%)[155]

Actions: Nervine, emmenagogue, antispasmodic, hepatic, cardiotonic, hypotensive

Indications: The binomial of this plant illustrates the range of uses to which it has been put. "Motherwort" indicates its relevance for menstrual and uterine conditions, while "*cardiaca*" suggests that it is beneficial in cardiovascular and circulatory system treatments.

The herb is valuable for stimulating delayed or suppressed menstruation, especially when anxiety or tension is involved, and may be used to ease false labor pains. It is a useful relaxing tonic for menopausal changes.

Motherwort is also an excellent heart tonic, strengthening without straining. It is considered a specific for tachycardia (heart palpitations), especially when brought on by anxiety or other such causes. It may be used in all heart conditions associated with anxiety and tension.

Motherwort has demonstrated cardioactivity in vitro. An alcoholic extract was found to have a direct inhibitory effect on myocardial cells: It exerted an antagonistic action against calcium chloride and stimulated both α- and β-adrenoceptors.[156]

According to *Priest and Priest*, motherwort is

. . . diffuse, stimulating and relaxing, an antispasmodic nervine: indicated for reflex conditions affecting cardiac function, and as a simple cardiac tonic. It also influences pre-menstrual nerve tension and muscular rigidity.

They provided the following specific indications: anemic nervousness and insomnia, palpitations, cardiac weakness after infections, neurosis, hyperthyroid cardiac reactions, premenstrual syndrome, congestive amenorrhea, and dysmenorrhea.

Safety Considerations: Excessive use of motherwort may interfere with other cardiovascular treatments.

Preparations and Dosage: Tincture dosage is 1 to 4 ml three times a day (1:5 in 40%). For an infusion, pour 1 cup of boiling water over 1 to 2 teaspoons of dried herb and infuse for 10 to 15 minutes. This should be drunk three times a day.

According to the BHC, dosage is 2 to 4 g dried herb, 4 to 10 ml tincture (1:5 in 45%), or 2 to 4 ml fluid extract (1:1 in 25%) three times daily. Commission E recommends 4.5 g herb or equivalent preparations.

Motherwort herb, in *The Complete German Commission E Monographs*

Leptandra virginica (L.) Nutt.
Black Root
Scrophulariaceae

Other Name: *Veronicastrum virginicum* (L.) Farw.

Parts Used: Rhizome, root

Constituents: Volatile oil (cinnamic acid, methoxycinnamic acid, dimethoxycinnamic acid); saponins; mannitol; dextrose; tannins[157]

Actions: Cholagogue, hepatic, laxative, diaphoretic, antispasmodic

Indications: Black root is used to relieve liver congestion and to treat inflamed gallbladder (cholecystitis). Black root is also appropriate for use in jaundice caused by liver congestion; in fact, it will help whenever there is any sign of liver dysfunction. For example, because chronic constipation is often related to liver problems, this herb is an ideal remedy for that condition.

Priest and Priest described black root as a

> . . . mild relaxing hepatic for torpid and congestive conditions, influencing the liver assisting the secretion of bile. It also cleanses the alimentary tract of viscid mucus and stimulates peristalsis.

They provided the following specific indications: hepatitis, cholecystitis, chronic hepatic torpor, nonobstructive jaundice, to clear the bowels in febrile states, hemorrhoids, and skin eruptions.

Safety Considerations: No side effects or drug interactions have been reported.

Preparations and Dosage: Tincture dosage is 1 to 2 ml three times a day (1:5 in 60%). To make a decoction, put 1 to 2 teaspoons of dried herb in 1 cup of cold water, bring to a boil, and simmer for 10 minutes. Take 1 cup three times a day.

Lobelia inflata L.
Lobelia
Campanulaceae

Parts Used: Aerial parts

Constituents: Piperidine alkaloids (0.48%): lobeline, lobelanidine, lobelanine; chelidonic acid; miscellaneous: resins, gums, fats[158]

Actions: Antiasthmatic, antispasmodic, expectorant, emetic, nervine

Indications: Lobelia has a general depressant action on the central and autonomic nervous systems and on neuromuscular activity. It may be used for many conditions in combination with other herbs, to further their effectiveness when relaxation is needed. Its primary specific use is for bronchial asthma and bronchitis.

Much of the pharmacological activity of lobelia is attributed to its alkaloid constituents, principally lobeline. Analysis of its action reveals apparently paradoxical effects. Lobeline has peripheral and central effects similar to those of nicotine, but is less potent. Hence, lobeline initially causes CNS stimulation, followed by respiratory depression.

Ellingwood considered lobelia specific for

> . . . irritable, spasmodic and oppressed breathing, and in respiratory problems from exalted nerve force and nerve irritation. It is contra-indicated in general relaxation and

in dyspnoea from enlarged or fatty heart, or from hydropericardium, or enfeebled heart, with valvular incompetence. It is specific in threatened spasm with exalted nerve action—a high degree of nerve tension with great restlessness and excitability, flushed face and contracted pupils. It is a prompt emetic in full doses.

The high regard that the Eclectics had for *Lobelia* is reflected in *Ellingwood's* recommendation for the following pathologies: spasmodic asthma, whooping cough, spasmodic croup, membranous croup, infantile convulsions, puerperal eclampsia, epilepsy, tetanus, hysterical paroxysms, hysterical convulsions, rigid os uteri, diphtheria, tonsillitis, and pneumonia.

Safety Considerations: The side effects of lobeline and lobelia are similar to those of nicotine and tobacco, and include nausea and vomiting, diarrhea, coughing, tremors, and dizziness. Symptoms of overdose include profuse diaphoresis, tachycardia, convulsions, hypothermia, hypotension, and coma. Lobelia should not be used during pregnancy or lactation.

Preparations and Dosage: Tincture dosage is 0.5 to 1 ml three times a day (1:5 in 40%). To make an infusion, pour 1 cup of boiling water over 1/4 teaspoon of dried herb and infuse for 10 to 15 minutes. This should be drunk three times a day.

Dosage listed in the BHC is 50 to 200 mg dried herb or 0.4 to 1.6 ml tincture (1:8 in 60%) up to three times daily.

Lobelia, in *Herbal Medicines: A Guide for Health-Care Professionals.* For more information on the Eclectic physicians' use of this important plant, see pages 235–242 of Ellingwood's *American Materia Medica, Therapeutics and Pharmacognosy* and pages 1199–1205 of *King's American Dispensatory.*

Lycopus virginicus L.
Bugleweed
Lamiaceae

Other Names: Sweet bugle, water bugle, gypsywort. Related species include *L. europaeus* and *L. americanus.*

Parts Used: Aerial parts

Constituents: Phenolic acid derivatives (caffeic, rosmarinic, chlorogenic, and ellagic acids); pimaric acid methyl ester[159]

Actions: Diuretic, peripheral vasoconstrictor, astringent, nervine, antitussive

Indications: Bugleweed is a specific for overactive thyroid, especially when symptoms include shortness of breath, palpitations, and shaking. It may also be safely used in cases of heart palpitations of nervous origin. Bugleweed will support a weak heart associated with an accumulation of water in the body. As a sedative cough reliever, it helps ease irritating coughs, especially those of nervous origin.

Ellingwood described the specific symptomatology of bugleweed thus:

> In diseases of the heart, either functional or organic, marked by irritability and irregularity of the organ, dyspnoea, feeling of oppression in the cardiac region, its administration is followed by gratifying results. Hypertrophy and dilatation have been known to undergo marked diminution in consequence of its administration.

As for its therapeutic uses, he said:

> It possesses tonic, sedative, astringent and narcotic properties and has been successfully used in incipient phthisis, hemoptysis, etc. It acts like digitalis in reducing the velocity of the pulse, but has no cumulative effects. In pericarditis and endocarditis its sedative action lessens the frequency of the pulse, irritability and its attendant inflammation, in a manner equaled by no other remedy. Exopthalmic goiter. In diseases of the respiratory apparatus lycopus has been found to be very useful. Hemoptysis, associated with rapid and tumultuous heart's action, yields readily to its influence, as does hemorrhage from any part.

Safety Considerations: Bugleweed may interfere with the action of thyroid hormones because it blocks conversion of thyroxin to T3 in the liver. In vitro, it has also been shown to interfere with thyroxin production by inhibiting thyroid-stimulating hormone.

Preparations and Dosage: Tincture dosage is 1 to 2 ml three times a day (1:5 in 40%). For an infusion, pour 1 cup of boiling water over 1 teaspoon of dried herb and infuse for 10 to 15 minutes. This should be drunk three times a day.

Commission E suggests a daily dosage of 1 to 2 g dried herb for infusion or extract equivalent to 20 mg of herb.

Bugleweed, in *The Complete German Commission E Monographs*

Mahonia aquifolium (Pursh) Nutt.
Oregon Grape
Berberidaceae

Other Names: Mountain grape, holly mahonia. Formerly *Berberis aquifolium.*

Parts Used: Rhizome, root

Constituents: Alkaloids of the isoquinoline type (berberine, berbamine, hydrastine, oxycanthine)[160]

Actions: Alterative, cholagogue, laxative, antiemetic, anticatarrhal, tonic

Indications: Oregon grape finds its main use for the treatment of chronic and scaly skin conditions, such as psoriasis and eczema. As skin problems of this nature generally have systemic causes, the tonic activity of Oregon grape on the liver and gallbladder may explain its effectiveness. It may be helpful for stomach and gallbladder conditions, especially when there is associated nausea and vomiting. As a laxative, it may be safely used to treat chronic constipation.

Ellingwood considered Oregon grape specific for:

> . . . scaly, pustular and other skin disease due to the disordered conditions of the blood. It is the most reliable alterative when the influences of the dyscrasia is apparent in the skin. It is given freely during the treatment of skin diseases where an alterative is considered an essential part of the treatment.

In addition, he recommended it for pimples, roughness, eczema capitis, eczema genitalis, pruritis, scaly eczema, psoriasis, pityriasis, chronic dermatosis, glandular indurations, ulcerations, and syphilis.

Safety Considerations: No side effects or drug interactions have been reported.

Preparations and Dosage: Tincture dosage is 1 to 4 ml three times a day (1:5 in 40%). To make a decoction, put 1 to 2 teaspoons of root in 1 cup of water, bring to a boil, and simmer for 10 to 15 minutes. This should be drunk three times a day.

The BHP recommends 1 to 2 g dried herb or 1 to 2 ml liquid extract (1:1 in 25%) three times a day.

Marrubium vulgare L.
Horehound
Lamiaceae

Other Name: White horehound

Parts Used: Dried leaf, flowering top

Constituents: Diterpene lactones: marrubiin (0.3% to 1.0%), with premarrubiin; diterpene alcohols (marruciol, marrubenol, sclareol, peregrinin, dihydroperegrinin); volatile oil (containing α-pinene, sabinene, limonene, camphene, *p*-cymol, α-terpinolene); flavonoids (apigenin, luteolin, quercetin, and their glycosides); alkaloids (traces of the pyrrolidine betonicine and its isomer turicine); miscellaneous: choline, alkanes, phytosterols, tannins[161]

Actions: Expectorant, antispasmodic, bitter, vulnerary, emmenagogue

Indications: Horehound is a valuable plant for the treatment of bronchitis, especially when the patient has a nonproductive cough. It relaxes the smooth muscles of the bronchus while promoting mucus production and thus expectoration. It is beneficial in the treatment of whooping cough. Its bitter action stimulates the flow and secretion of bile from the gallbladder, aiding digestion. Horehound is also used externally to promote wound healing.

King's described this valuable remedy in the following terms:

> Horehound is a stimulant tonic, expectorant, and diuretic. Its stimulant action upon the laryngeal and bronchial mucous membranes is pronounced and it, undoubtedly, also influences the respiratory function. It is used in the form of a syrup, in coughs, colds, chronic catarrh, asthma and all pulmonary affections. The warm infusion will produce diaphoresis, and sometimes diuresis, and has been used with benefit in jaundice, asthma, hoarseness, and amenorrhoea; the cold infusion is an excellent tonic in some forms of dyspepsia, acts as a vermifuge.

Safety Considerations: No side effects or drug interactions have been reported.

Preparations and Dosage: Tincture dosage is 1 to 2 ml three times a day (1:5 in 40%). For an infusion, pour 1 cup of boiling water over ½ to 1 teaspoon of dried herb and infuse for 10 to 15 minutes. This should be drunk three times a day.

Commission E recommends a daily dose of 4.5 g dried herb or 2 to 6 tablespoons pressed juice.

Horehound herb, in *Herbal Medicine, Expanded Commission E Monographs*

Marsdenia reichenbachii Triana
Condurango
Asclepiadaceae

Other Name: *Marsdenia condurango* Reichb. F.

Part Used: Dried bark

Constituents: Glycosides (based on condurangogenins, known as condurangoglycosides); miscellaneous: essential oil, phytosterols, sugars, starch, fat[162]

Actions: Bitter, emmenagogue

Indications: Condurango is a bitter that may be used to treat a whole range of digestive and stomach problems. It is best known for its ability to stimulate appetite, an action common to all bitters. However, in addition, this herb relaxes the nerves of the stomach, making it useful for settling indigestion associated with nervous tension and anxiety.

Ellingwood had this to say about condurango:

> The influence of the agent is exercised directly upon the stomach as a tonic and corrective of perverted action. It is of service in gastric ulcer and in the early stages of cancer of the stomach, for which it was originally lauded as a cure. It is depended upon by some enthusiastic users to retard progress of some cases of this disease and to relieve distress and urgent symptoms when fully developed. It cannot be curative. It will be found of service, probably, in catarrhal gastritis with extreme atonicity and threatened ulceration. In these cases its virtues as a tonic and restorative will find exercise to the full extent of their influence. It deserves thorough investigation and faithful trial. It may be given in the form of a warm decoction with excellent advantage. A wine of Condurango is prepared which has good influence upon the stomach. Half an ounce may be taken with the meals.

Safety Considerations: No side effects or drug interactions have been reported.

Preparations and Dosage: Tincture dosage is 1 to 2 ml three times a day (1:5 in 60%). To make an infusion, pour 1 cup of boiling water over 1 to 2 teaspoons of powdered herb and infuse for 10 to 15 minutes. This should be drunk three times a day.

Commission E suggests a daily dosage of 2 to 4 g dried bark, 2 to 5 ml tincture, or 2 to 4 ml fluid extract.

Condurango cortex, in *Herbal Drugs and Phytopharmaceuticals*

Matricaria recutita L.
German Chamomile
Asteraceae

Other Names: Do not confuse with *Chamaemelum nobile* (= *Anthemis nobilis*), commonly known as Roman chamomile.

Part Used: Flower head

Constituents: Sesquiterpenes (chamazulene, α-bisabolol, bisabolol oxide); sesquiterpene lactones (matricin, matricarin); flavonoid glycosides (6% to 8%): apigenin, luteolin, quercetin, isorhamnetin[163]

Actions: Nervine, antispasmodic, carminative, antiinflammatory, antimicrobial, bitter, vulnerary

Indications: A comprehensive list of medicinal uses for chamomile would be very long. Included would be insomnia, anxiety, menopausal depression, loss of appetite, dyspepsia, gastric ulcers, diarrhea, colic, aches and pains of flu, migraine, neuralgia, teething, vertigo, motion sickness, conjunctivitis, inflamed skin, urticaria, and many others! This may seem too good to be true, but it simply reflects the wide range of chamomile's actions in the body.

Chamomile, probably the most widely used relaxing nervine herb in the Western world, is safe for use in all types of anxiety and stress-related disorders. It relaxes and tones the nervous system, and is especially valuable when anxiety and tension produce digestive symptoms, such as gas, colic pains, and even ulcers. This ability to ease physical symptoms as well as underlying psychological tension is one of the great benefits of herbal remedies in stress and anxiety. Chamomile makes a wonderful late-night tea to ensure restful sleep. It is helpful for anxious children or teething infants when added to bathwater.

As an antispasmodic herb, chamomile works on peripheral nerves and muscles, and thus indirectly relaxes the whole body. When the physical body is at ease, the mind and heart follow. The herb prevents and eases muscle cramps, whether in the legs or in the abdomen. When added to a bath after a hard day, chamomile infusion or essential oil relaxes the body and eases the cares and weight of a troubled heart and mind.

Because chamomile is rich in essential oil, it acts on the digestive system, promoting proper function. This usually involves soothing the walls of the intestines, easing griping pains, and facilitating the elimination of gas. A cup of hot chamomile tea is a simple, effective way to relieve indigestion. It calms inflammations, such as gastritis, and helps prevent ulcers.

Used internally, it is an effective anti-inflammatory remedy for the digestive and respiratory system; it has a similar action on the skin when applied externally. A steam inhalation of chamomile essential oil puts its valuable constituents in contact with inflamed mucous membranes in the sinuses and lungs. Chamomile is also a mild antimicrobial that helps the body destroy or resist pathogenic microorganisms. As an anticatarrhal, it assists in the elimination of excess mucus buildup in the sinus area. It may be used to treat head colds and allergies, such as hay fever.

Safety Considerations: Chamomile may cause allergic reactions in people sensitive to plants in the Asteraceae family. However, such reactions are extremely rare.

Preparations and Dosage: Chamomile may be used in any of the ways plants are prepared as medicines. It may be used fresh or dried in infusions, and tincture is an excellent dosage form to ensure that all constituents are extracted and available. Chamomile essential oil is valued in aromatherapy.

For an infusion, infuse 2 to 3 teaspoons of herb in 1 cup of boiling water for 10 minutes in a covered container. This should be drunk three or four times a day. Tincture dosage is 1 to 4 ml three times a day (1:5 in 40%).

Commission E recommends a daily dosage of 3 g herb as an infusion and 3% to 10% infusion for poultice. The BHC suggests 2 to 4 g herb as infusion, 3 to 10 ml tincture (1:5 in 45%), or 1 to 4 ml liquid extract (1:1 in 45%) three times a day.

Chamomile, German, in *Principles and Practice of Phytotherapy*

Melaleuca alternifolia L.
Tea Tree
Myrtaceae

Other Name: Ti tree

Part Used: Essential oil

Constituents: Volatile oil, containing a range of terpenes and sesquiterpenes[164]

Action: Antimicrobial

Indications: Tea tree essential oil is an important antibacterial and antifungal agent. While it is undoubtedly useful, it seems to have attracted the modern equivalent of the old purveyors of "snake oil." Some of the claims made have a kernel of truth to them; however, many are exaggerated for promotional reasons.

A list of conditions for which *Melaleuca* oil has been suggested includes sinusitis, the common cold, sinus blockage, laryngitis, coughs, aphthous ulcers, boils, cuts, bites, sunburn, miliaria, parasites, head lice, herpes infection, impetigo, psoriasis, infected seborrheic dermatitis, tinea infection (including ringworm of the scalp and athlete's foot), fungal infections of the nails, thrush, and trichomonal vaginitis. All of the fungal or parasitic problems should respond well to treatment with tea tree oil.

Safety Considerations: No side effects or drug interactions have been reported.

Preparations and Dosage: Tea tree essential oil is for external use, and people with sensitive skin should dilute it first with a fixed carrier oil, such as almond oil. Currently, a wide range of products containing tea tree oil are available, including toothpaste, soap, and shampoo.

Melissa officinalis L.
Lemon Balm
Lamiaceae

Parts Used: Dried or fresh aerial parts

Constituents: Volatile oil (0.1% to 0.2%): neral and geranial, caryophyllene oxide, and a whole range of terpenes; flavonoids in low concentrations (luteolin-7-glucoside and rhamnazin); polyphenolics (including protocatechuic acid, caffeic acid, rosmarinic acid, and tannins); triterpenic acids, such as ursolic and pomolic acids[165]

Actions: Carminative, nervine, antispasmodic, antidepressant, diaphoretic, antimicrobial, hepatic

Indications: Lemon balm, an excellent carminative herb, relieves spasms in the digestive tract and is useful in flatulent dyspepsia. Because of its mild antidepressant properties, it is primarily indicated when dyspepsia is associated with anxiety or depression, as the gently sedative oils relieve tension and stress reactions. The volatile oil appears to act on the interface between the digestive tract and the nervous system. The herb has been described by some herbalists as a *trophorestorative* for the nervous system, similar in some ways to oats.

Lemon balm is appropriate for neuralgia, anxiety-induced palpitations, insomnia, and migraine associated with tension. Lemon balm has a tonic effect on the heart and circulatory system and causes mild vasodilation of peripheral vessels, thus lowering blood pressure. It may be used for feverish conditions, such as influenza.

Hot-water extracts have antiviral properties, possibly due in part to the presence of rosmarinic acid and other polyphenolics. A lotion-based extract may be applied to herpes simplex skin lesions, the antiviral activity having been confirmed in both laboratory and clinical trials.

Lemon balm's hormone-regulating effects have also been well documented in the laboratory. Freeze-dried aqueous extracts have been shown to inhibit many of the effects of thyroid-stimulating hormone (TSH) on the thyroid gland. In laboratory studies, it interfered with the binding of TSH to plasma membranes and inhibited the enzyme iodothyronine deiodinase in vitro. It also inhibits the receptor-binding and other biological activity of immunoglobulins in the blood of patients with Graves' disease, a condition that causes hyperthyroidism.

Safety Considerations: Lemon balm may interfere with the action of thyroid hormones.

Preparations and Dosage: Tincture dosage is 2 to 6 ml three times a day (1:5 in 40%). For an infusion, pour 1 cup of boiling water over 2 to 3 teaspoons of dried herb or 4 to 6 g of fresh herb and infuse in a covered container for 10 to 15 minutes. A cup of this tea should be taken morning and evening or when needed.

Commission E recommends 1.5 to 4.5 g dried herb as an infusion, taken several times a day. Dosage listed in the BHC is 2 to 4 g as infusion, 2 to 6 ml tincture (1:5 in 45%), or 2 to 4 ml liquid extract (1:1 in 45%).

Melissae folium, in *Herbal Drugs and Phytopharmaceuticals*

Mentha pulegium L.
Pennyroyal
Lamiaceae

Parts Used: Aerial parts

Constituents: Volatile oil (1% to 2%): pulegone, isopulegone, menthol, isomenthone, limonene, piperitone; miscellaneous: bitters, tannins[166]

Actions: Carminative, diaphoretic, stimulant, emmenagogue

Indications: With its richly aromatic volatile oil, pennyroyal is helpful for flatulence and related abdominal colic. It relieves spasmodic pain and eases anxiety. However, its main application is as an emmenagogue, used to stimulate the menstrual process and to strengthen uterine contractions. Pennyroyal essential oil is toxic and should be avoided completely.

Safety Considerations: Human fatalities related to ingestion of pennyroyal essential oil as an abortifacient have been reported. The dose required for an abortifacient effect is close to the toxic dose, and fatalities have been related to both nephrotoxicity and hepatotoxicity. Doses of 1 ounce have proved fatal.[167]

Preparations and Dosage: Tincture dosage is 1 to 2 ml three times a day (1:5 in 40%). To make an infusion, pour 1 cup of boiling water over 1 to 2 teaspoons of dried herb and infuse in a covered container for 10 to 15 minutes. This should be drunk three times a day.

Dosage recommended in the BHP is 1 to 4 g dried herb or 1 to 4 ml liquid extract (1:1 in 45%).

Pennyroyal, in *Herbal Medicines: A Guide for Health-Care Professionals*

Mentha x piperita L.
Peppermint
Lamiaceae

Parts Used: Aerial parts

Constituents: Phenolic acids (caffeic, chlorogenic, and rosmarinic acid); essential oil (up to 1.5%), the major components of which are menthol, menthone, and menthyl acetate; flavonoids (glycosides of apigenin, diosmetin, and luteolin); tannins[168]

Actions: Carminative, anti-inflammatory, antispasmodic, aromatic, diaphoretic, antiemetic, nervine, antimicrobial, analgesic

Indications: Peppermint is an excellent carminative with relaxing effects on the muscles of the digestive system. It combats flatulence, flatulent dyspepsia, intestinal colic, and associated conditions, and stimulates the flow of bile and digestive juices. The volatile oil acts as a mild anaesthetic to the stomach wall, allaying feelings of nausea and the desire to vomit. It also help relieve the nausea and vomiting of pregnancy and of motion sickness.

Peppermint can play a role in the treatment of ulcerative conditions of the bowels. It is a traditional treatment for fevers, colds, and influenza. As an inhalant, peppermint provides temporary relief of nasal catarrh. It may help with headaches associated with indigestion, and its nervine actions ease anxiety and tension. Used for dysmenorrhea, it relieves pain and eases associated tension. Externally, peppermint is applied to soothe itching and inflammation of the skin.

Ellingwood considered peppermint specific for

. . . flatulent colic, gastrodynia, nausea, vomiting, spasmodic pain in the bowels, hiccough, palpitation from indigestion, griping, irritability of the stomach, diarrhoea with abdominal pain, nervous headache, painful gonorrhoea.

In addition, he recommended it for fevers associated with nausea and vomiting, local pain relief in rheumatism (essential oil), symptomatic relief of asthma and chronic bronchitis, toothache, acute indigestion, and pruritis ani.

Safety Considerations: No side effects or drug interactions have been reported.

Preparations and Dosage: Tincture dosage is 1 to 2 ml three times a day (1:5 in 40%). To make an infusion, pour 1 cup of boiling water over a heaping teaspoon of dried herb and infuse in a covered container for 10 minutes. This may be drunk as often as desired.

According to Commission E, daily dosage is 3 to 6 g herb, 5 to 15 g tincture, or equivalent preparations. For essential oil, it suggests a daily dosage internally of 6 to 12 drops, or 3 to 4 drops in hot water as an inhalation. For irritable colon, it recommends a single dose of 0.2 ml, or an average daily dose of 0.6 ml essential oil in enteric-coated capsules. (Enteric-coated capsules are designed to dissolve after they pass the stomach, thus facilitating activity in the intestines.) The BHC suggests 2 to 3 g herb by infusion or 2 to 4 ml tincture (1:5 in 45%) three times a day.

Menthae piperitae folium, in *Herbal Drugs and Phytopharmaceuticals*

Menyanthes trifoliata L.
Bogbean
Menyanthaceae

Other Name: Buckbean

Part Used: Leaf

Constituents: Anthraquinones (including emodin, aloe-emodin, chrysophanol, and rhein glycosides); flavonoid glycosides (hyperin, kaempferol, quercetin, rutin, trifolioside); alkaloids (gentianin and gentianidine); coumarins (scopoletin); iridoids[169]

Actions: Bitter, diuretic, cholagogue, antirheumatic

Indications: Bogbean is a most useful herb for rheumatism, osteoarthritis, and rheumatoid arthritis. However, because of its stimulating effects in the digestive system, it should not be used for rheumatism accompanied by colitis or diarrhea. It acts as an aperient by stimulating the walls of the colon, and markedly promotes secretion of digestive juices and bile flow. It is thus useful for debilitated states related to sluggish digestion, indigestion, and disorders of the liver and gallbladder.

Safety Considerations: Excessive doses of bogbean may irritate the gastrointestinal tract, causing diarrhea, griping pains, nausea, and vomiting.[170]

Preparations and Dosage: Tincture dosage is 1 to 4 ml three times a day (1:5 in 40%). For an infusion, pour 1 cup of boiling water over 1 to 2 teaspoons of dried herb and infuse for 10 to 15 minutes. This should be drunk three times a day.

According to the BHC, dosage is 0.5 to 2 g dried leaf, 4 to 10 ml tincture (1:5 in 25%), or 1 to 2 ml fluid extract (1:1 in 25%) three times daily. Commission E recommends a daily dosage of 1.5 to 3 g dried herb.

Menyanthidis folium, in *Herbal Drugs and Phytopharmaceuticals*

Mitchella repens L.
Partridgeberry
Rubiaceae

Parts Used: Aerial parts

Constituents: Largely unknown; unspecified alkaloids, saponins, glycosides, tannins, and mucilages have been reported[171]

Actions: Parturient, emmenagogue, diuretic, tonic, astringent

Indications: Partridgeberry is among the best remedies for preparing the uterus and whole body for childbirth. It should be taken for some weeks before the child is due to help ensure a safe and wonderful birth for both mother and baby. Partridgeberry may also help relieve the pain of dysmenorrhea. As an astringent, it has been used to treat colitis, especially if there is much mucus.

According to *King's*,

Partridge berry is parturient, diuretic, and astringent. Used in dropsy, suppression of urine and diarrhoea, in decoction. It seems to have an especial affinity for the uterus, exerting a powerful tonic and alterative influence upon this organ, and has hence been found highly beneficial in many uterine derangements, as in amenorrhoea, some forms of dysmenorrhoea, menorrhagia, chronic congestion of the uterus, enfeebled uterine nervous system, etc. Dose of a strong decoction, from 2 to 4 fluid ounces, 2 or 3 times a day. The berries are a popular remedy for diarrhoea and dysuria. Used as follows, partridge berry is highly recommended as a cure for sore nipples: Take 2 ounces of the herb, fresh if possible, and make a strong decoction with a pint of water, then strain, and add as much good cream as there is liquid of the decoction. Boil the whole down to the consistence of a soft salve, and when cool, anoint the nipple with it every time the child is removed from the breast.

Safety Considerations: No side effects or drug interactions have been reported.

Preparations and Dosage: Tincture dosage is 2 to 4 ml three times a day (1:5 in 40%). To make an infusion, pour 1 cup of boiling water over 1 teaspoon of herb and infuse for 10 to 15 minutes. This should be drunk three times a day.

The BHP recommends 2 to 4 g dried herb or 2 to 4 ml liquid extract (1:1 in 25%) three times a day.

Myrica cerifera L.
Bayberry
Myricaceae

Part Used: Bark

Constituents: Triterpenes (including taraxerol, taraxerone, and myricadiol); flavonoids (such as myricitrin); tannins (bark 3.9%, total aqueous extract 34.82%); miscellaneous: phenols, resins, gums[172]

Actions: Astringent, circulatory stimulant, diaphoretic

Indications: As a circulatory stimulant, bayberry may have a role in holistic approaches to many conditions. Because of its specific actions, it is a valuable astringent for diarrhea and dysentery. Bayberry is also indicated for mucous colitis. Applied as a gargle, it soothes sore throats, and when used as a douche, it helps with leukorrhea. It may also be used for the treatment of colds.

Ellingwood described bayberry as a

. . . stimulating astringent indicated where ever there is excessive mucous discharge. For atonic or persistent diarrhoea and locally for bleeding gums.

In addition, he recommended it for dysentery, stomatitis, nasal catarrh, measles and scarlet fever, convulsions, and jaundice.

Safety Considerations: No side effects or drug interactions have been reported.

Preparations and Dosage: Tincture dosage is 1 to 2 ml three times a day (1:5 in 40%). To make a decoction, put 1 teaspoon of herb into a cup of cold water and bring to a boil. Let sit for 10 to 15 minutes. This should be drunk three times a day.

Bayberry, in *Herbal Medicines: A Guide for Health-Care Professionals*

Nepeta cataria L.
Catnip
Lamiaceae

Parts Used: Leaf, flowering top

Constituents: Volatile oil (carvacrol, citronellal, nerol, geraniol, pulegone, thymol, nepetalic acid); iridoids (including epideoxyloganic acid and 7-deoxyloganic acid); tannins[173]

Actions: Carminative, antispasmodic, diaphoretic, nervine, astringent

Indications: Catnip is a traditional cold and flu remedy. It is a valuable diaphoretic helpful in any feverish condition, especially acute bronchitis. As a carminative with antispasmodic properties, catnip eases stomach upset, dyspepsia, flatulence, and colic. It is a perfect remedy for the treatment of diarrhea in children. Its nervine sedative action adds to its generally relaxing properties.

Safety Considerations: No side effects or drug interactions have been reported.

Preparations and Dosage: Tincture dosage is 2 to 6 ml three times a day (1:5 in 25%). For an infusion, pour 1 cup of boiling water over 2 teaspoons of dried herb and infuse in a covered container for 10 to 15 minutes. This should be drunk three times a day.

Dosage listed in the BHP is 2 to 4 g dried herb, 3 to 6 ml tincture (1:5 in 25%), or 2 to 4 ml liquid extract (1:1 in 25%).

Panax ginseng L.
Korean Ginseng
Araliaceae

Other Species: American ginseng is *Panax quinquefolius*, also known as Canadian ginseng.

Part Used: Root

Constituents: Triterpene glycosides, called ginsenosides or panaxosides, of which 13 have been isolated (e.g., designated ginsenosides Ra, Rb, Rgl, Rg2, and others); glycans (panaxans A-E); volatile oil[174]

Actions: Adaptogen, tonic, stimulant, hypoglycemic

Indications: Ginseng has an ancient history, and much folklore has accumulated about its actions and uses. The genus name, *Panax*, is derived from the Latin *panacea*, meaning "cure all." Unfortunately, many of the claims made for ginseng are exaggerated, but it is clear that this is an important remedy.

Ginseng is an adaptogen, a substance that acts to enhance nonspecific resistance to various external and internal stressors. Thus, it has a wide range of possible therapeutic uses. Its best therapeutic application is for weak or elderly people, for whom the adaptogenic and stimulating properties can be profoundly useful. It should not be used indiscriminately, as its stimulating properties are contraindicated in some pathologies. For example, Chinese herbalists caution against the use of ginseng in acute inflammatory diseases and bronchitis. The ginseng used by the 19th-century Eclectic physicians was *P. quinquefolius*.

Safety Considerations: No side effects or drug interactions have been reported.

Preparations and Dosage: Ginseng root is often chewed, or a decoction may be made as follows: Put ¹/₂ teaspoon of powdered root in 1 cup of water, bring to a boil, and simmer gently for 10 minutes. Drink three times a day. The tincture dose is 1 to 2 ml three times a day (1:5 in 60%).

A common daily dosage used in clinical trials is 200 mg of a 5:1 standardized extract. Commission E recommends a daily dose of 1 to 2 g of root or equivalent preparations.

Ginseng, in *Principles and Practice of Phytotherapy*

Parietaria diffusa L.
Pellitory of the Wall
Urticaceae

Parts Used: Aerial parts

Constituents: Flavonoids (glycosides of quercetin, kaempferol, and isorhamnetin); glucoproteins; bitter principle; tannins[175]

Actions: Diuretic, demulcent

Indications: Pellitory of the wall may be used to treat any inflammation of the urinary tract, especially when a soothing action is needed. It is beneficial for cystitis and pyelitis, and acts a good general diuretic when used to relieve water retention related to kidney problems. It has an especially valuable role to play in the treatment of kidney stones or gravel.

Safety Considerations: No side effects or drug interactions have been reported.

Preparations and Dosage: Tincture dosage is 1 to 2 ml three times a day (1:5 in 40%). To make an infusion, pour 1 cup of boiling water over 1 to 2 teaspoons of dried herb and infuse for 10 to 15 minutes. This should be drunk three times a day.

Passiflora incarnata L.
Passionflower
Passifloraceae

Parts Used: Leaf, whole plant

Constituents: Alkaloids (harmine, harman, harmol, harmaline, harmalol, passaflorine); flavonoids (apigenin, homoorientin, isovitexin, kaempferol, luteolin, orientin, quercetin, rutin, saponaretin, saponarin, vitexen)[176]

Actions: Nervine, hypnotic, antispasmodic, anodyne, hypotensive

Indications: *Passiflora* is used for its sedative and soothing properties and to lower blood pressure, prevent tachycardia, and relieve insomnia. It has a depressant effect on the central nervous system and acts as a hypotensive. The pharmacological actions of many of the flavonoids, such as apigenin, are well known, and include antispasmodic and anti-inflammatory effects. The alkaloids and flavonoids in passionflower have shown sedative activity in animals.

Passionflower is the herb of choice for intransigent insomnia. It eases the transition into restful sleep without causing any next-day hangover. It may be used whenever an antispasmodic is indicated (for example, for Parkinson's disease, seizures, or hysteria). It can be effective for nerve pain, such as neuralgia, and the viral infection of nerves called shingles. Passionflower may also be helpful for asthma associated with spasmodic activity and states of tension.

Safety Considerations: Passionflower will potentiate the effects of sedative drugs. Theoretically, it is contraindicated for people taking monoamine oxidase inhibitors.

Preparations and Dosage: Tincture dosage is 1 to 4 ml, taken once in the evening for sleeplessness or twice a day for other conditions (1:5 in 40%). To make an infusion, pour 1 cup of boiling water over 1 teaspoon of dried herb and infuse for 15 minutes. As with tincture, drink a cup in the evening for sleeplessness or 1 cup twice a day for other indications.

The BHP lists a dosage of 0.25 to 1 g dried herb, 0.5 to 2 ml tincture (1:8 in 45%), or 0.5 to 1 ml liquid extract (1:1 in 25%) three times a day. Dosage recommended in the BHC is 0.5 to 2 g dried herb or 0.5 to 2 ml fluid extract (1:1 in 25%) up to four times daily.

Passionflower herb, in *Herbal Medicine, Expanded Commission E Monographs*

Petroselinum crispum (Mill.) Nyman ex A. W. Hill
Parsley
Apiaceae

Parts Used: Taproot, leaf, seed

Constituents: Volatile oil (containing apiole, myristicin, β-phellandrene, and others); coumarins; flavonoids; phthalides; vitamins[177]

Actions: Diuretic, emmenagogue, carminative, antispasmodic, expectorant, hypotensive

Indications: Fresh parsley, so widely used in cooking, is a rich source of vitamin C. Medicinally, the herb has three main areas of usage. First, it is an effective diuretic that helps the body eliminate excess water, and may be used whenever such an action is desired. (Remember, however, that the cause of the problem must also be sought and treated.) It is also an emmenagogue, used to stimulate the menstrual process. Thus, medicinal use of parsley during pregnancy is not advisable, as it may cause excessive stimulation of the womb. Finally, it has value as a carminative to ease flatulence and accompanying colic pains.

Safety Considerations: Parsley can cause allergic reactions. The essential oil is a photosensitizer. Do not use the essential oil or extracts in medicinal doses during pregnancy.

Preparations and Dosage: Tincture dosage is 1 to 2 ml three times a day (1:5 in 40%). For an infusion, pour 1 cup of boiling water over 1 to 2 teaspoons of leaf or root and infuse in a covered container for 5 to 10 minutes. This should be drunk three times a day.

The BHC recommends 2 to 4 g dried herb or 2 to 4 ml fluid extract (1:1 in 25%) three times daily. Commission E suggests a daily dose of 6 g herb or equivalent preparations.

Parsley herb and root, in *Herbal Medicine, Expanded Commission E Monographs*

Peumus boldus Molina
Boldo
Monimiaceae

Part Used: Dried leaf

Constituents: Isoquinoline alkaloids (up to 0.7%): boldine, isoboldine, and isocorydine; volatile oil (2.5%): *p*-cymene, 1,8-cineole, ascaridole, linalool; flavonoid glycosides, based on isorhamnetin[178]

Actions: Cholagogue, hepatic, diuretic

Indications: Boldo is a specific for gallbladder problems, such as stones and inflammations. It is also used when there is visceral pain related to other problems in the liver or gallbladder. Boldo, in combination with cascara, rhubarb, and gentian, is effective against a variety of symptoms, including loss of appetite, digestive difficulties, constipation, flatulence, and itching.[179] Boldo also has mild urinary demulcent and antiseptic properties, and so may be useful in cystitis.

Safety Considerations: Because of the volatile oil content, excessive doses of boldo may cause renal irritation. Thus, it should be avoided by individuals with existing kidney disease. Ascaridole is toxic, and use of boldo essential oil is not recommended.

Preparations and Dosage: Tincture dosage is 1 to 2 ml three times a day (1:5 in 60%). To make an infusion, pour 1 cup of boiling water over 1 teaspoon of dried herb and infuse for 10 to 15 minutes. This should be drunk three times a day.

Average daily dose recommended by Commission E is 3 g of herb or equivalent preparations. The BHP suggests 0.6 to 2 g dried herb or 0.6 to 2 ml liquid extract (1:1 in 45%) three times a day.

Boldo leaf, in *Herbal Medicine, Expanded Commission E Monographs*

Phytolacca americana L.

Poke

Phytolaccaceae

Part Used: Root

Constituents: Triterpenoid saponins (phytolaccosides A–E, based on the aglycones phytolaccagenin and phytolaccic acid); lectins (a mixture known as "pokeweed mitogen," consisting of a series of glycoproteins)[180]

Actions: Antirheumatic, stimulant, anticatarrhal, purgative, emetic

Indications: Poke root is a strong but valuable herb. It helps eliminate catarrh and supports cleansing of the lymphatic glands, and may be seen primarily as a remedy for infections of the upper respiratory tract. It may be used to treat catarrh, tonsillitis, laryngitis, swollen glands, and mumps.

Lymphatic problems elsewhere in the body may also benefit from the use of poke, especially mastitis, for which it can be taken internally and applied as a poultice. The herb may also have value in rheumatism, particularly long-standing disorders. Used externally as a lotion or ointment, it may be used to rid the skin of scabies and other pests. Care must be taken with this herb, as it is powerfully emetic and purgative in large doses.

Priest and Priest described poke as a

> . . . stimulating and relaxing alterative: promotes the removal of catabolic wastes and the products of fatty degeneration. Specific for skeletal congestions, and for serous and glandular tissues.

They gave the following specific indications: chronic rheumatism and arthritis, neuralgia and lumbago, tonsillitis and parotitis, mastitis, ovaritis, orchitis, enlarged thyroid, and enlarged lymph nodes.

Safety Considerations: In large doses, poke is a powerful emetic and purgative.

Preparations and Dosage: Tincture dosage is 0.25 ml three times a day (1:10 in 45%). For a decoction, only a small amount of this herb should be used. Put ¼ teaspoon of root in 1 cup of water, bring to a boil, and simmer gently for 10 to 15 minutes. This should be drunk three times a day.

Poke root, in *Principles and Practice of Phytotherapy*

Pimpinella anisum L.

Anise

Apiaceae

Other Name: Aniseed

Part Used: Dried seed

Constituents: Volatile oil (1% to 4%), consisting of largely trans-anethole (70% to 90%), also dianethole and photoanethole; coumarins (such as bergapten, umbelliferone, scopoletin); flavonoids (rutin, isovitexin, quercetin, luteolin, apigenin glycosides); phenylpropanoids; miscellaneous: lipids, fatty acids, sterols, proteins, carbohydrates[181]

Actions: Expectorant, antispasmodic, carminative, antimicrobial, aromatic, galactagogue

Indications: The internal use of anise (also known as aniseed) to ease griping, intestinal colic, and flatulence is based upon its volatile oil content. The oil also has expectorant and antispasmodic actions that underlie the use of the herb in bronchitis, for tracheitis when there is persistent irritable coughing, and for whooping cough. Used externally, aniseed oil helps control lice, and the oil may be applied in an ointment base for the treatment of scabies.

Studies have demonstrated that aniseed increases mucociliary transport, which supports its use as an expectorant. The herb has mild estrogenic effects thought to be due to the presence of dianethole and photoanethole, explaining its use in folk medicine to increase milk secretion, facilitate birth, and, allegedly, increase libido.

Safety Considerations: Anise may be allergenic and photosensitizing. It may interfere with the activity of anticoagulant therapy.

Preparations and Dosage: Tincture dosage is 1 to 4 ml three times a day (1:5 in 40%). To make an infusion, the seeds should be gently crushed just before use to release the volatile oils. Pour 1 cup of boiling water over 1 to 2 teaspoons of the seeds and infuse in a covered container for 5 to 10 minutes. Take 1 cup three times daily. The tea should be drunk slowly before meals to treat flatulence. One drop of the essential oil may be taken internally by mixing it into 1 teaspoon of honey.

Commission E recommends a daily dosage of 3 g dried fruit or 0.3 g essential oil.

Anisi fructus, in *Herbal Drugs and Phytopharmaceuticals*

Piper methysticum Forst. f.
Kava Kava
Piperaceae

Part Used: Rhizome

Constituents: Kavalactones (3.5% to 15% of the root by dried weight): methysticin, dihydromethysticin, kavain, dihydrokavain; chalcones (flavokavains A–C)[182]

Actions: Relaxing nervine, hypnotic, antispasmodic, local anesthetic, antifungal

Indications: Kava is a safe treatment for anxiety, with the added benefit that it does not dampen alertness when given at normal therapeutic doses. The antianxiety effects of kava compare favorably to those of prescription medications often used to treat anxiety disorders, such as benzodiazepines, without the side effects commonly seen with these drugs.[183] Kava does not impair reaction time and appears to improve concentration.

In one double-blind, placebo-controlled study, 29 subjects were treated for 4 weeks with 100 mg kava extract (standardized to 70% kavalactones) three times daily. The kava group experienced significant decreases in symptoms of anxiety (measured on the Hamilton Anxiety Scale) compared with the placebo group.[184] Another study showed that kava was effective in relieving anxiety associated with menopause.

Kava possesses mild antidepressant properties, making it suitable for the treatment of anxiety associated with minor forms of depression. Because it is an effective muscle relaxant, it is appropriate for conditions associated with skeletal muscle spasm and tension (for example, headaches due to neck tension). It is also a relevant hypnotic in cases of mild insomnia. It has local anesthetic actions on mucous membranes, so it is helpful for control of pain related to oral conditions. The constituent kavain has demonstrated significant analgesic effects in animal studies, apparently via non-opiate pathways.[185] Subcutaneous injections provided anesthesia for several hours to several days.

Safety Considerations: A side effect of heavy kava consumption is "kava dermopathy," an ichthyosiform skin rash characterized by noninflammatory dryness and scaling of the skin. This is typically seen only in heavy, long-term consumers of a traditional kava beverage popular in Polynesia. However, the rash has also been observed in people taking doses of 300 to 800 mg daily of the isolated lactone dihydromethysticin.[186] This skin reaction is reversible upon discontinuation of kava treatment.

Kava may potentiate the effects of substances that act on the central nervous system, such as alcohol, barbiturates, and psychopharmaceutical agents. An apparently antagonistic action or incompatibility reaction may occur: In one case, 150 mg kava extract taken twice daily reduced the efficacy of levodopa used in the treatment of Parkinson's disease.[187]

A small number of reports of hepatotoxicity related to kava use have appeared. The evidence to confirm a role for kava in such liver toxicity is extremely equivocal, but has led to restrictions on availability in some countries.

Preparations and Dosage: Recommended dosage for kava depends upon the concentration of kavalactones. The important measure is the amount of kavalactones the preparation is standardized to contain. Commission E recommends preparations equivalent to 60 to 120 mg kavalactones taken three times a day.

Kava, in *Principles and Practice of Phytotherapy*

Piscidia erythrina L.
Jamaica Dogwood
Fabaceae

Part Used: Stem

Constituents: Isoflavones (lisetin, jamaicin, ichthyone); rotenoids (rotenone, milletone, isomilletone); organic acids, including piscidic acid; β-sitosterol; tannins[188]

Actions: Nervine, anodyne, antispasmodic

Indications: Jamaica dogwood is a powerful sedative, used in its West Indian homeland as a fish poison. While the herb is not poisonous to humans, it is important not to exceed the recommended dosage level. This is a powerful remedy for the treatment of painful conditions, such as neuralgia and migraine. One of its primary applications is related to nervous tension or pain. It can also be used to relieve ovarian and uterine pain.

Safety Considerations: Use Jamaica dogwood with great care. The herb may potentiate sedative effects of concomitant therapies. It should not be used during pregnancy and lactation.

Preparations and Dosage: Tincture dosage is 2 to 4 ml of the tincture as needed (1:5 in 40%). To make a decoction, put 1 teaspoon of root in 1 cup of water, bring to a boil, and simmer gently for 10 to 15 minutes. This should be drunk as needed.

The BHC recommends 2 to 4 g of dried root bark, 5 to 15 ml tincture (1:5 in 45%), or 2 to 8 ml of liquid extract (1:1 in 60%) three times daily.

Jamaica Dogwood, in *Herbal Medicines: A Guide for Health-Care Professionals*

Plantago major L.
Plantain
Plantaginaceae

Related Species: Ribwort plantain (*Plantago lanceolata*)

Parts Used: Leaf, aerial parts

Constituents: Iridoids (aucubin, catalpol); flavonoids (apigenin, luteolin, scutellarin, baicalein, nepetin, hispidulin, plantagoside); tannins; oleanolic acid; plant acids[189]

Actions: Vulnerary, expectorant, demulcent, anti-inflammatory, astringent, diuretic, antimicrobial

Indications: Both greater plantain (*Plantago major*) and its close relative ribwort plantain (*P. lanceolata*) have valuable healing properties. Plantain acts as a gentle expectorant while soothing inflamed and sore membranes, making it ideal for coughs and mild bronchitis. Its astringency is helpful in diarrhea, hemorrhoids, and cystitis accompanied by bleeding. Plantain is one of Western herbalism's primary topical healing agents, used as a lotion, ointment, compress, or poultice for cuts and bruises. It may be applied topically for hemorrhoids and skin ulcerations.

Ellingwood described plantain thus:

> The remedy is of value in the internal treatment of all diseases of the blood. Scrofula, syphilis, specific or non-specific glandular disease and mercurial poisoning. It is used in ulcerations of the mucous membrane, due to depraved conditions. It may be given in diarrhoea, dysentery, the diarrhoea of consumption, cholera infantum, and where there are longstanding hemorrhoids. It is also given in female disorders, attended with fluent discharges and in hematuria, also in dysuria and some forms of passive hemorrhage. It would thus seem to possess marked astringent properties, as well as those of an alterative character.

Safety Considerations: No side effects or drug interactions have been reported.

Preparations and Dosage: Tincture dosage is 2 to 3 ml three times a day (1:5 in 40%). To make an infusion, pour 1 cup of boiling water over 2 teaspoons of dried herb and infuse for 10 minutes. This should be drunk three times a day. An ointment may be made for treatment of hemorrhoids and cuts.

Commission E recommends 3 to 6 g of herb or equivalent preparations daily.

Plantain, in *Herbal Medicine, Expanded Commission E Monographs*

Polygala senega L.
Seneca Snakeroot
Polygalaceae

Part Used: Rhizome

Constituents: Triterpenoid saponins, based on the aglycones senegenin, polygalacic acid, and senegenic acid; phenolic acids (*p*-coumaric, ferulic, sinapic, *p*-methoxycinnamic); polygalitol, a sorbitol derivative; methyl salicylate; sterols; fats[190]

Actions: Expectorant, diaphoretic, sialagogue, emetic

Indications: Seneca snakeroot has strong expectorant effects that can be employed to treat bronchial asthma, especially in cases marked by difficulty with expectoration. It has a general ability to stimulate secretions, including saliva. It may be used as a mouthwash and gargle in the treatment of pharyngitis and laryngitis. If too much is taken, the herb may irritate the lining of the gut and cause vomiting.

A quote from *Ellingwood* is highly suggestive of the therapeutic possibilities this herb offers:

> The agent is indicated in typhoid pneumonitis, capillary bronchitis, in aged and debilitated subjects, chronic bronchitis with profuse secretion, in the declining stages of pneumonitis, bronchitis and croup, when the inflammatory condition has passed off, chronic bronchitis with pain and soreness in the chest and asthma. The agent is in use in the treatment of dropsy from obstruction and glandular enlargement, also in rheumatism, syphilis, squamous skin diseases and in amenorrhoea. In inflammation of the eyelids and iritis it is beneficial. Snake Root has been employed as a stimulating expectorant in chronic bronchitis, in aged and debilitated subjects, where a stimulating medicine is demanded and in the later stages of pneumonia and catarrhal inflammation. In these cases, given in small doses, it improves secretion, removes abnormal deposits and restores the strength. It is an energetic stimulant to the mucous membranes of the air passages; and, when given before the inflammation has subsided, aggravates the cough and does harm.

Safety Considerations: No side effects or drug interactions have been reported.

Preparations and Dosage: Tincture dosage is 1 to 2 ml three times a day (1:5 in 60%). To make a decoction, pour 1 cup of boiling water over 1/2 teaspoon of dried root and simmer for 5 to 10 minutes. Drink 1 cup three times a day.

Commission E recommends a daily dosage of 1.5 to

3 g of root, 1.5 to 3 ml of fluid extract, or 2.5 to 7.5 ml of the tincture.

Polygalae radix, in *Herbal Drugs and Phytopharmaceuticals*

Populus candicans L.
Balm of Gilead
Salicaceae

Part Used: Unopened buds

Constituents: Phenolic glycosides (salicin, populin, chrysin); volatile oil (α-caryophyllene, cineole, arcurcumene, bisabolene, farnesene, and others); alkanes; resins; phenolic acids; tannins[191]

Actions: Stimulating expectorant, antimicrobial, vulnerary

Indications: Balm of Gilead soothes, disinfects, and astringes mucous membranes, making it an excellent remedy for sore throats, coughs, and laryngitis. In fact, it is considered a specific for laryngitis accompanied by loss of voice. It may also be used to treat chronic bronchitis. Applied externally, it may help ease the inflammation of rheumatism or arthritis, and may also be of benefit in dry and scaly skin conditions, such as psoriasis and dry eczema.

Safety Considerations: No side effects or drug interactions have been reported.

Preparations and Dosage: Tincture dosage is 1 to 2 ml of the tincture three times a day (1:5 in 40%). To make an infusion, pour 1 cup of boiling water over 1 teaspoon of buds and infuse for 10 to 15 minutes. This should be drunk three times a day or more often until effective (if the patient can deal with the taste!). The herb is usually used in the form of a syrup to improve palatability.

The BHC recommends 1.5 to 3 g root, 3 to 5 ml tincture (1:5 in 45% ethanol), or 1 to 2 ml liquid extract (1:1 in 25%) three times daily.

Poplar, in *Herbal Medicines: A Guide for Health-Care Professionals*

Populus tremuloides Michx.
Quaking Aspen
Salicaceae

Part Used: Bark

Constituents: Phenolic glycosides (salicin, populin); tannins[192]

Actions: Anti-inflammatory, astringent, antiseptic, anodyne, cholagogue, bitter tonic

Indications: Quaking aspen is a relevant anti-inflammatory for arthritis and rheumatism accompanied by pain and swelling. Its use in this indication is quite similar to that of willow, and it is most effective when used as part of a broad therapeutic approach, not as the sole treatment. It is very effective for flare-ups of rheumatoid arthritis. As a cholagogue, it helps stimulate digestion, especially stomach and liver function, particularly when loss of appetite is part of the picture. It may also be appropriate for feverish colds and other infections, such as cystitis. As an astringent, it may help in the treatment of diarrhea.

Priest and Priest described quaking aspen as a

. . . bitter tonic for all general uses, especially for postfebrile debility. Stimulates appetite and aids digestion. Suitable for the elderly.

They gave the following specific indications: dyspepsia, flatulence, diarrhea, and dysentery.

Safety Considerations: No side effects or drug interactions have been reported.

Preparations and Dosage: Tincture dosage is 2 to 4 ml three times a day (1:5 in 40%). To make a decoction, put 1 to 2 teaspoons of dried herb in 1 cup of water, bring to a boil, and simmer for 10 to 15 minutes. This should be drunk three times a day. To stimulate appetite, drink 30 minutes before meals.

Prunus serotina Ehrh.
Wild Cherry
Rosaceac

Part Used: Dried bark

Constituents: Cyanogenetic glycoside (prunasin); benzaldehyde; eudesmic acid; *p*-coumaric acid; scopoletin; tannins; sugars[193]

Actions: Antitussive, expectorant, astringent, nervine, antispasmodic

Indications: Because of its powerful sedative effect on the cough reflex, wild cherry bark finds its main use in the treatment of irritating coughs. Thus, it has a role in the treatment of bronchitis and whooping cough. It is appropriate for use in combination with other herbs to control asthma. (Remember, however, that inhibiting a cough is not the same as healing the infection, which will still need treatment.) In addition to this use for coughs, wild cherry may be used as a bitter to improve sluggish digestion. A cold infusion, applied as a wash, may be helpful for eye inflammations.

Here is an excerpt from a lengthy monograph in *King's* on wild cherry:

Wild Cherry has a tonic and stimulating influence on the digestive apparatus, and a simultaneous sedative action on the nervous system and circulation. It is, therefore, valuable in all those cases where it is desirable to give tone and strength to the system, without, at the same time, causing too great an action of the heart and blood vessels, as, during convalescence from pleurisy, pneumonia, acute hepatitis, and other inflammatory and febrile diseases. Its chief property is its power of relieving irritation of the mucous surfaces, making it an admirable remedy in many gastro-intestinal, pulmonic, and urinary troubles. It is best adapted to chronic troubles. Externally, it has been found useful, in decoction, as a wash to ill conditioned ulcers and acute ophthalmia.

Safety Considerations: Theoretically, large doses of wild cherry bark are toxic.

Preparations and Dosage: Tincture dosage is 1 to 2 ml three times a day (1:5 in 40%). For a decoction, pour 1 cup of boiling water over 1 teaspoon of dried bark and simmer for 10 to 15 minutes. This should be drunk three times a day.

Pulsatilla vulgaris L.
Pasqueflower
Ranunculaceae

Other Names: Pulsatilla, wind flower

Parts Used: Aerial parts

Constituents: Sesquiterpene lactones; protoanemonin (= ranunculin), anemonin (oxidation product of protoanemonin); triterpenoid saponins (hederagenin); flavonoids (delphinidin and pelargonidin glycosides); anemone camphor; tannins; volatile oil[194]

Actions: Nervine, antispasmodic, antibacterial

Indications: Pasqueflower is a relaxing nervine especially useful for problems combining spasm in the reproductive system with overall nervous tension. It may be safely used to relieve dysmenorrhea, ovarian pain, and painful conditions of the testes. It may help alleviate tension reactions and headaches associated with such reactions, and is appropriate for insomnia and general nervous overactivity.

Pasqueflower's antibacterial actions give this herb a role in treating skin infections, especially boils. It is similarly useful in the treatment of respiratory infections and asthma. An infused oil or tincture will ease earache.

Uterine antispasmodic activity has been documented for *Pulsatilla* in laboratory studies.[195] In another study, the constituents protoanemonin and anemonin (produced when protoanemonin oxidizes) showed sedative and antipyretic properties in rodents.[196]

This remedy was far more widely used in the 19th century than it is today. The following passage comes from the extensive monograph on *Pulsatilla* in *King's*:

Pulsatilla forms an important remedy with the Eclectic physicians as well as with homeopaths, who make extensive use of it. According to Dr. Scudder, its most important use is to allay irritation of the nervous system in persons of feeble health, thus giving sleep and rest, preventing unnecessary expenditure of nerve force, and, by this means, facilitating the action of tonics and restoratives. It is a remedy of wide applicability, but more particularly for those conditions in which the mind is a prominent factor. A gloomy mentality, a state of nerve depression and unrest, a disposition to brood over real or imagined trouble, a tendency to look on the dark side of life, sadness, mild restlessness, and a state of mental unrest generally denominated in broad terms "nervousness," are factors in the condition of the patient requiring Pulsatilla. The whole condition is one of nervous depression, the nutrition of the nerve centers are at fault. Pulsatilla may be given to produce sleep, when there is great exhaustion. If the insomnia is due to nervous exhaustion it is a prompt remedy to give rest, after which sleep obtains. Where sleep is disturbed by unpleasant dreams, and the patient awakens sad and languid, Pulsatilla should be given.

In dysmenorrhoea, not due to mechanical causes, and with the above-named nervous symptoms, no remedy is more effective. Pulsatilla frequently proves a good remedy in ovaritis and ovaralgia with tensive, tearing pain. It is frequently a remedy for pain, when dependent on or associated with debility, and sometimes when due to acute inflammation. It frequently proves a useful remedy in headache of various types. It relieves the frontal headache from nasal catarrh, nervous headache.

Safety Considerations: Fresh *Pulsatilla* is poisonous and should not be ingested. External contact with the fresh plant should also be avoided. The toxic principle, protoanemonin, rapidly degrades to the nontoxic anemonin during drying. Avoid use of *Pulsatilla* during pregnancy.

Preparations and Dosage: Tincture dosage is 1 to 2 ml three times a day (1:10 in 40%). To make an infusion, pour 1 cup of boiling water over $1/2$ to 1 teaspoon of dried herb and infuse for 10 to 15 minutes. This should be drunk three times a day or as needed. Liquid extract dosage is 0.12 to 0.3 ml (1:1 in 25%).

Pulsatilla, in *Herbal Medicines: A Guide for Health-Care Professionals*

Quercus alba L.
Oak
Fagaceae

Part Used: Bark

Constituents: Tannins (15% to 20%): phlobatannin, ellagitannins, and gallic acid[197]

Actions: Astringent, anti-inflammatory, antiseptic

Indications: Oak bark may be used wherever an effective astringent is needed—for example, for diarrhea or dysentery. However, because of its high content of astringent tannins, it may be too strong in some situations. The decoction is appropriate for use as a gargle for tonsillitis, pharyngitis, and laryngitis. It may also be applied as an enema to treat hemorrhoids and as a douche for leukorrhea. However, it is primarily indicated for acute diarrhea, for which it should be taken in small, frequent doses.

Safety Considerations: No side effects or drug interactions have been reported. However, do not use for constipation.

Preparations and Dosage: Tincture dosage is 1 to 2 ml three times a day (1:5 in 60%). To make a decoction, put 1 teaspoon of bark in 1 cup of water, bring to a boil, and simmer gently for 10 to 15 minutes. This can be drunk three times a day.

Oak bark, in *Herbal Medicine, Expanded Commission E Monographs*

Rheum palmatum L.
Chinese Rhubarb
Polygonaceae

Other Names: An interchangeable species is *Rheum officinale* Baillon. Do not confuse with garden rhubarb.

Part Used: Rhizome

Constituents: Anthraquinones (chrysophanol, emodin, aloe-emodin, rhein, sennosides A–E, others); tannins; stilbene derivatives; volatile oil; rutin; fatty acids; calcium oxalate[198]

Actions: Bitter, laxative, astringent

Indications: Rhubarb root has a purgative action that makes it very effective in the treatment of constipation. However, this purgative effect is followed by an astringent effect. This means that the herb has a truly cleansing action upon the gut, as it first removes debris and then astringes the system with antiseptic properties.

According to *Priest and Priest*, rhubarb root is a

. . . mild stimulating tonic to alimentary mucous membrane, liver and gall ducts—removes viscid mucus. Small doses—tonic hepatic. Large doses—cathartic.

They gave the following specific indications: diarrhea and dysentery, and functional dyspepsia.

Safety Considerations: Rhubarb root may cause an increase in the effectiveness and toxic effects of cardiac glycosides and an effect on the action of antiarrhythmic drugs, because it enhances loss of potassium. Potassium deficiency can be increased by simultaneous use of thiazide diuretics, corticoadrenal steroids, or licorice root. Because it decreases intestinal transit time, rhubarb root may reduce the absorption time of orally administered drugs.[199] *Note:* Rhubarb root may color the urine yellow or red.

Preparations and Dosage: Tincture dosage is 1 to 2 ml morning and evening. To make a decoction, put $^{1}/_{2}$ to 1 teaspoon of the root in 1 cup of water, bring to a boil, and simmer gently for 10 minutes. This should be drunk morning and evening.

Commission E recommends a daily dosage containing 20 to 30 mg of hydroxyanthracene derivatives (calculated as rhein). Individual dosage is the smallest dosage necessary to maintain a soft stool.

Rhei radix, in *Herbal Drugs and Phytopharmaceuticals*

Rosmarinus officinalis L.
Rosemary
Lamiaceae

Parts Used: Leaf, twig

Constituents: Volatile oil (borneol, camphene, camphor, cineole, limonene, linalool); flavonoids (apigenin, diosmetin, diosmin, luteolin and derivatives); rosmarinic acid and other phenolic acids; diterpenes (carnosol, carnosolic acid, and rosmariquinone); rosmaricine; triterpenes (ursolic acid, oleanolic acid)[200]

Actions: Carminative, antispasmodic, antidepressant, rubefacient, antimicrobial, emmenagogue

Indications: Rosemary is a circulatory and nervine stimulant. It has a toning and calming effect on digestion, especially when stomach upset is accompanied by psychological tension. Thus, conditions appropriate for treatment with rosemary include flatulent dyspepsia with headache or depression associated with debility. Applied externally, it helps ease muscular pain, sciatica, and neuralgia. It also acts as a stimulant to both hair follicles and circulation in the scalp, and thus may be useful for treating premature baldness. Rosemary essential oil is most effective for this purpose.

Priest and Priest considered rosemary a

. . . diffuse stimulant and relaxing tonic with special influence upon stomach and cerebrum. It soothes the nervous system and is tonic to the vaso-motor function and peripheral circulation. It is a suitable tonic for the elderly.

They gave the following specific indications: atonic conditions of the stomach, gastric headache, adolescent hypotonia, asthenia with pallid complexion, and circulatory weakness following stress or illness.

Safety Considerations: No side effects or drug interactions have been reported.

Preparations and Dosage: Tincture dosage is 1 to 2 ml three times a day (1:5 in 40%). To make an infusion, pour 1 cup of boiling water over 1 to 2 teaspoons of dried herb and infuse in a covered container for 10 to 15 minutes. This should be drunk three times a day.

Commission E recommends a total daily dosage of 4 to 6 g herb or equivalent preparations.

Rosemary leaf, in *Herbal Medicine, Expanded Commission E Monographs*

Rubus idaeus L.
Red Raspberry
Rosaceae

Parts Used: Leaf, fruit

Constituents: Flavonoids (mainly glycosides of kaempferol and quercetin); tannins; fruit sugar; volatile oil; pectin; citric acid; malic acid[201]

Actions: Astringent, tonic, parturient

Indications: Raspberry leaf has a long tradition of use in pregnancy to strengthen and tone the tissue of the uterus. Used for this purpose, it purportedly strengthens contractions and checks hemorrhage during labor. As an astringent, it has therapeutic applications for a wide range of conditions, including diarrhea and leukorrhea. It also helps ease mouth problems, such as aphthous ulcers, bleeding gums, and inflammations, and, used as a gargle, is effective for sore throats.

Safety Considerations: No side effects or drug interactions have been reported.

Preparations and Dosage: Tincture dosage is 2 to 4 ml three times a day (1:5 in 40%). To make an infusion, pour 1 cup of boiling water over 2 teaspoons of dried herb and infuse for 10 to 15 minutes. This may be drunk freely.

The USP recommends a daily dosage of 4 to 8 g dried herb or 4 to 8 ml fluid extract.

Rubi fructicosi folium, in *Herbal Drugs and Phytopharmaceuticals*

Rubus villosus L.
Blackberry
Rosaceae

Part Used: Bark of root and rhizome

Constituents: Tannins (20%): gallic acid; saponins (including villosin)[202]

Action: Astringent

Indications: Blackberry is an excellent, safe, and gentle astringent remedy that can be used in all situations that call for this action. It is appropriate for diarrhea, dysentery, and other problems associated with "loose bowels." It was traditionally used in Britain as an external wash to treat burns and a whole range of skin eruptions. It will stanch bleeding and is helpful for leukorrhea. Ellingwood considered blackberry specific for "diarrheas of infancy."

Safety Considerations: No side effects or drug interactions have been reported.

Preparations and Dosage: Tincture dosage is 2 to 5 ml three times a day (1:5 in 40%). To make a decoction, put 1 to 2 g of dried herb in 1 cup of water, bring to a boil, and simmer for 10 minutes. Drink 1 cup three times a day.

Commission E recommends 4.5 g of dried herb daily.

Rubi idaei folium, in *Herbal Drugs and Phytopharmaceuticals*

Rumex crispus L.
Yellow Dock
Polygonaceae

Part Used: Root

Constituents: Anthraquinone glycosides (about 3% to 4%, including nepodin, physcion, and emodin); miscellaneous: tannins and oxalates[203]

Actions: Alterative, laxative, hepatic, cholagogue, tonic

Indications: Yellow dock is used extensively in the treatment of chronic skin complaints, such as psoriasis. While anthraquinones usually have a strong cathartic action on the bowel, in this herb they act mildly, possibly tempered by the tannin content. Because yellow dock works in a broader manner than herbs that simply stimulate gut action, it is a valuable remedy for constipation. Yellow dock promotes the flow of bile and has the somewhat obscure action of "blood cleansing." Its influence on the gallbladder gives it a role in the treatment of jaundice due to congestion.

Priest and Priest considered yellow dock a "general tonic alterative with special influence upon skin eruptions." They gave the following specific indications: simple deficiency anemia, eczema, psoriasis, urticaria, prurigo (a chronic skin condition characterized by persistent, intensely itchy papules), and itching hemorrhoids.

Safety Considerations: Fresh yellow dock root may cause vomiting. Yellow dock may potentiate the activity of stimulant laxatives.

Preparations and Dosage: Tincture dosage is 1 to 2 ml three times a day (1:5 in 40%). To make a decoction, put 1 to 2 teaspoons of root in 1 cup of water, bring to a boil, and simmer gently for 10 to 15 minutes. This should be drunk three times a day.

The BHP recommends 2 to 4 g dried herb, 1 to 2 ml tincture (1:5 in 45%), or 2 to 4 ml fluid extract (1:1 in 25%) three times a day.

Yellow Dock, in *Herbal Medicines: A Guide for Health-Care Professionals*

Ruta graveolens L.
Rue
Rutaceae

Parts Used: Dried aerial parts

Constituents: Volatile oil: 2-undecanone (50% to 90%) and others; flavonoids (including quercetin and rutin); coumarins (bergapten, isoimperatorin, psoralen, scopoletin, and umbelliferone); alkaloids (arborinine, graveoline); lignans (in the root): savinin and helioxanthin[204]

Actions: Antispasmodic, emmenagogue, antitussive, antimicrobial, bitter, abortifacient

Indications: Rue is an herb with an ancient history. The genus name, *Ruta*, comes from the Greek work *reuo*, meaning "to set free," an expression of its reputation for freeing people from disease. Its main modern application is to regulate the menstrual cycle and bring on suppressed menses.

Its other main area of use is related to the plant's antispasmodic action. Rue relaxes smooth muscles, especially in the digestive system, where it eases griping and bowel tension. Its ability to ease spasm gives it a role in the treatment of spasmodic coughs. It also increases peripheral circulation and lowers elevated blood pressure. Chewing the fresh leaf relieves tension headaches, eases palpitations, and alleviates other anxiety problems.

Safety Considerations: Rue essential oil is a dangerously powerful abortifacient. Therefore, the herb should be avoided during pregnancy and the essential oil avoided at all times.

Preparations and Dosage: To make an infusion, pour 1 cup of boiling water over 1 to 2 teaspoons of dried herb and infuse for 10 to 15 minutes. This should be drunk three times a day. Tincture dosage is 1 to 4 ml three times a day (1:5 in 40%).

The BHP recommends 0.5 to 1 g of dried herb or 0.5 to 1 ml fluid extract (1:1 in 25%) three times a day.

Rue, in *The Complete German Commission E Monographs*

Salix alba L.
White Willow
Salicaceae

Part Used: Bark

Constituents: Phenolic glycosides (salicin, salicylic acid); miscellaneous: tannins, catechin, *p*-coumaric acid, flavonoids[205]

Actions: Analgesic, anti-inflammatory, tonic

Indications: Willow is an ancient remedy that has been used in various forms to treat rheumatism and gout, fevers, and aches and pains of all kinds. It is generally considered to be the natural form and original source of the modern aspirin.

Safety Considerations: Willow bark has a theoretical potential to cause interactions of the type seen with salicylates, although no cases have been reported in the scientific literature. The ESCOP monograph notes no interactions with willow, and states that irreversible inhibition of platelet aggregation by aspirin cannot be induced by the structurally different salicin present in willow.

Preparations and Dosage: Tincture dosage is 3 to 6 ml three times a day (1:5 in 25%). To make a decoction, put 1 to 2 teaspoons of dried bark in 1 cup of water, bring to a boil, and simmer for 10 to 15 minutes. This should be drunk three times a day.

The BHC recommends 1 to 2 g dried bark, 5 to 8 ml tincture (1:5 in 25%), or 1 to 2 ml fluid extract (1:1 in 25% ethanol) three times a day. Commission E advises an average daily dosage corresponding to 60 to 120 mg total salicin.

Salicis cortex, in *Herbal Drugs and Phytopharmaceuticals*

Salvia officinalis var. *rubia* L.
Red Sage
Lamiaceae

Part Used: Leaf

Constituents: Volatile oil (α- and β-thujone, cineole, borneol, camphor, others); diterpene bitters: picrosalvin (carnosol), carnosolic acid, and others; flavonoids (salvigenin, genkwanin, 6-methoxygenkwanin, hispidulin, luteolin A); phenolic acids (rosmarinic, caffeic, labiatic); salviatannin (a condensed catechin)[206]

Actions: Carminative, antispasmodic, antimicrobial, astringent, anti-inflammatory

Indications: Because of the soothing action of its volatile oils upon the mucous membranes, red sage is the classic remedy for inflammations of the mouth, throat, and tonsils. It may be used internally and as a mouthwash to treat gingivitis, glossitis, and stomatitis, and is effective as a gargle for aphthous ulcers. As a gargle, it also aids in the treatment of laryngitis, pharyngitis, and tonsillitis. Used as a compress, red sage promotes wound healing.

Taken internally, red sage is a valuable carminative that may used to good effect in dyspepsia. It decreases sweating, and may also be used to lessen the production of breast milk. Red sage stimulates the muscles of the uterus and so should be avoided during pregnancy.

Safety Considerations: Adverse reactions are likely only with overdoses (more than 15 g sage leaf per dose) or prolonged use of red sage. The toxic constituent of the essential oil, thujone, causes symptoms such as tachycardia, hot flashes, convulsions, and dizziness. Avoid during pregnancy.

Preparations and Dosage: Tincture dosage is 2 to 4 ml three times a day (1:5 in 40%). To make an infusion, pour 1 cup of boiling water over 1 to 2 teaspoons of leaf and infuse in a covered container for 10 minutes. This should be drunk three times a day. To make a mouthwash, place 2 teaspoons of leaf in $^1/_2$ liter (1 pint) of water, bring to a boil, and let stand, covered, for 15 minutes. Gargle deeply with the hot infusion several times a day.

Commission E recommends a daily dose of 4 to 6 g dried herb, 2.5 to 7.5 g tincture, or 1.5 to 3 g fluid extract. For gargles or rinses, it suggests 2.5 g of dried herb or 2 to 3 drops of essential oil in 100 ml of water. The BHP recommends 1 to 4 g dried herb as an infusion or 1 to 4 ml fluid extract (1:1 in 45%) three times daily.

Salviae folium, in *Herbal Drugs and Phytopharmaceuticals*

Sambucus nigra L.
Black Elder
Caprifoliaceae

Parts Used: Flower, berry, leaf

Constituents: *Flower:* Triterpenes (ursolic acid, oleanolic acid, α- and β-amyrin, sterols); fixed oils (free fatty acids, mainly linoleic, linolenic, and palmitic acids); miscellaneous: phenolic acids (e.g., chlorogenic acid); pectin; sugars. *Leaf:* Triterpenes (similar to those found in flowers); cyanogenetic glycosides, including sambunigrin; flavonoids (kaempferol, quercetin, and many quercetin glycosides, including hyperoside, isoquercitrin, and rutin); miscellaneous: fatty acids, alkanes, tannins[207]

Actions: *Leaf:* Purgative, expectorant, diuretic, diaphoretic (internal); emollient, vulnerary (external). *Flower:* Diaphoretic, anticatarrhal, antispasmodic. *Berry:* Diaphoretic, diuretic, laxative, antirheumatic

Indications: The elder tree is a medicine chest in its own right. The leaf is used topically for bruises, sprains, wounds, and chilblains, and some reports hold that elder leaf may be effective as an ointment for tumors. Elder flower is ideal for the treatment of colds and influenza, and a standardized black elderberry extract has demonstrated antiviral properties. This extract was effective in vitro against 10 strains of influenza virus. It also reduced the duration of flu symptoms to 3 to 4 days in a double-blind, placebo-controlled, randomized study.

Elder flower is indicated for any catarrhal inflammation of the upper respiratory tract, such as hay fever or sinusitis. Catarrhal deafness responds well to elder flower. Elder berry has properties similar to those of the flower, with the addition of effectiveness in rheumatism.

Sambucus also increases cytokine production. The herb appears to strengthen cell membranes to prevent virus penetration, possibly by inhibiting the viral enzyme that weakens the membrane.[208] An infusion made from elder flower, St. John's wort herb (*Hypericum perforatum*), and soapwort root (*Saponaria officinalis*) exhibited antiviral activity against influenza types A and B both in vivo and in vitro, and against herpes simplex type I in vitro.[209]

Safety Considerations: No side effects or drug interactions have been reported.

Preparations and Dosage: Elder flower tincture dosage is 2 to 4 ml three times a day (1:5 in 40%). To make an infusion, pour 1 cup of boiling water over 2 teaspoons of dried or fresh blossoms and infuse for 10 minutes. Drink hot three times a day. To make a juice, boil fresh berries in water for 2 to 3 minutes, then express the juice. To preserve, add 1 part honey to 10 parts juice and bring to a boil. Take 1 glass diluted with hot water twice a day.

To make an ointment, heat 3 parts fresh elder leaf with 6 parts melted Vaseline until the leaves are crisp. Strain and store.

The BHP recommends 3 to 5 g dried flowers, 5 to 15 ml expressed juice, 10 to 25 ml tincture (1:5 in 25%), or 3 to 5 ml fluid extract (1:1 in 25%) three times a day.

Sambuci flos and Sambuci fructus, in *Herbal Drugs and Phytopharmaceuticals*

Sanguinaria canadensis L.
Bloodroot
Papaveraceae

Part Used: Root

Constituents: Isoquinoline alkaloids (3% to 7%), mainly sanguinarine[210]

Actions: Expectorant, antispasmodic, emetic, cathartic, nervine, cardioactive, topical irritant

Indications: Bloodroot finds its main use in the treatment of bronchitis. While its stimulating properties are apparent in its emetic and expectorant effects, the herb also demonstrates a relaxing action on the bronchial muscles. Thus, bloodroot's most important contribution by far is its effectiveness against chronic congestive conditions of the lungs, including bronchitis, emphysema, and bronchiectasis. It also has a role in the treatment of asthma, croup, and laryngitis.

Bloodroot acts as a stimulant in cases of deficient peripheral circulation. It may be used as a snuff to treat nasal polyps. Activities documented for bloodroot are usually attributable to its isoquinoline alkaloid constituents—in particular, sanguinarine. In the recent past, interest focused on the use of sanguinarine in dental hygiene products, and many studies investigated the efficacy of bloodroot extracts for oral hygiene. Oral rinses and toothpastes containing bloodroot extracts were reported to significantly reduce plaque and improve gingival and bleeding indices. No alteration of the oral microbial flora or development of resistant microbial strains has been observed with bloodroot extracts.[211]

Ellingwood considered bloodroot specific for

> . . . harsh, dry cough with relaxed tissues of the pharynx, larynx and bronchi, with a sense of constriction and constant irritation and uneasiness or tickling of the throat.

In addition, he recommended it for congestion of the lungs, bronchial coughs, strident laryngitis, membranous croup, otitis media (external), indolent ulcerative conditions, nasal catarrh, anal fissure, epithelioma, and lupus.

Safety Considerations: Although there are no published reports of human toxicity caused by bloodroot, at high doses the herb may cause nausea, vomiting, a sensation of burning in all contacted mucous membranes, bradycardia, and hypotension. Animal studies have indicated that bloodroot is nontoxic during pregnancy. However, because of the potency of its pharmacologically active constituents, use of bloodroot during pregnancy and lactation is best avoided.

Preparations and Dosage: Tincture dosage is 0.5 to 1 ml three times a day (1:5 in 60%). To make a decoction, put 1 teaspoon of rhizome in 1 cup of cold water, bring to a boil, and infuse for 10 minutes. This should be drunk three times a day.

Bloodroot, in *Herbal Medicines: A Guide for Health-Care Professionals*

Scrophularia nodosa Juss.
Figwort
Scrophulariaceae

Parts Used: Aerial parts

Constituents: Iridoids (aucubin, harpagide, acetyl harpagide, 6-α-rhamnopyranosylcatalpol); flavonoids (diosmin, iosmetin, acacetin rhamnoside, hesperidin); phenolic acids (ferulic, isoferulic, *p*-coumaric, caffeic, vanillic, chlorogenic acids)[212]

Actions: Alterative, diuretic, laxative, cardiac stimulant

Indications: Figwort is most widely used for the treatment of skin problems. As an alterative, it acts in a broad way to improve body function and bring about a state of inner cleanliness. It may be used for eczema, psoriasis, or any skin condition characterized by itching and irritation. Part of its cleansing action is related to its purgative and diuretic actions, and it may be used as a mild laxative in constipation. Because it is a heart stimulant, figwort should be avoided in people with tachycardia (abnormally rapid heartbeat).

Priest and Priest described figwort as a

> . . . gently stimulating and relaxing alterative with lower abdominal and pelvic emphasis. Deobstruent to enlarged and engorged lymph glands

They gave the following specific indications: chronic skin disease, eczema and psoriasis, mammary tumors and nodosities, hemorrhoids.

Safety Considerations: Figwort may potentiate the effects of cardiac glycosides.

Preparations and Dosage: Tincture dosage is 2 to 4 ml three times a day (1:5 in 40%). For an infusion, pour 1 cup of boiling water over 1 to 3 teaspoons of dried leaf and infuse for 10 to 15 minutes. This should be drunk three times a day.

Figwort, in *Herbal Medicines: A Guide for Health-Care Professionals*

Scutellaria lateriflora L.
Skullcap
Lamiaceae

Parts Used: Aerial parts

Constituents: Flavonoids (baicalein, baicalin, scutellarein, and wogonin); iridoids (including catalpol); volatile oil; tannins[213]

Actions: Nervine tonic, antispasmodic, hypotensive

Indications: Skullcap is perhaps the most relevant nervine available to us in the Western materia medica. It effectively soothes nervous tension while renewing and revivifying the central nervous system. It has a long history of traditional use for the control and treatment of petit mal seizures. Skullcap may be used to treat any condition associated with exhaustion or depressed states, and can be used with complete safety to ease premenstrual tension. A recent clinical trial demonstrated that the herb is an effective anxiolytic, with a proposed mechanism involving flavonoid interactions with the $GABA_A$ receptor.[214]

Priest and Priest considered skullcap a

> . . . diffusive, stimulating and relaxing nervine-cerebral vasodilator and trophorestorative. Indicated for nervous irritation of the cerebro-spinal nervous system.

They gave the following specific indications: functional nervous exhaustion, post-febrile nervous weakness, chorea, hysteria, agitation, epileptiform convulsions, insomnia, nightmares, and restless sleep.

Ellingwood considered skullcap specific for

> . . . two distinct lines of specific phenomena. Firstly irritability of the nervous system with restlessness and nervous excitability; inability to sleep without pain; general irritability with insomnia from local causes. The second is where there is nervous disorder, characterized by irregular muscular action, twitching, tremors and restlessness, with or without incoordination. Its soothing influence continues for a protracted period, after the agent is discontinued.

In addition, he recommended it for delirium tremens and nervous excitability.

Safety Considerations: Reports of hepatotoxicity attributed to skullcap were later determined to be related to adulteration with germander. Skullcap can potentiate the effects of sedative medications.

Preparations and Dosage: Tincture dosage is 2 to 4 ml three times a day (1:5 in 40%). To make an infusion, pour 1 cup of boiling water over 1 to 2 teaspoons of dried herb and infuse for 10 to 15 minutes. This should be drunk three times a day or as needed.

The BHP recommends 1 to 2 g dried herb, 1 to 2 ml tincture (1:5 in 45%), or 2 to 4 ml fluid extract (1:1 in 25%) three times a day.

Skullcap, in *Herbal Medicines: A Guide for Health-Care Professionals*

Senna alexandrina Mill.
Senna
Fabaceae

Other Names: A number of closely related species and regional sources have given rise to a range of names, including Alexandrian senna, Kartoum senna, Tinnevelly senna, and Indian senna.

Parts Used: Dried fruit pod, leaf

Constituents: Anthraquinone glycosides (leaf: sennosides A–D; fruit: sennosides A and B and a closely related glycoside, sennoside A1); naphthalene glycosides (tinnevellin glycoside and 6-hydroxymusizin glycoside); miscellaneous: mucilage, flavonoids, volatile oil, sugars, resins[215]

Action: Cathartic

Indications: Senna is a powerful cathartic used in the treatment of constipation that works via stimulation of intestinal peristalsis. However, it is vital to remember that constipation is a symptom and that the cause must always be sought and treated. Ellingwood recommended senna for the treatment of temporary constipation.

Safety Considerations: Senna may reduce absorption of oral drugs by decreasing bowel transit time. Overuse or misuse can cause potassium loss leading to increased toxicity of cardiac glycosides. Senna aggravates loss of potassium associated with diuretic use.

As an anthraquinone-containing cathartic, senna is contraindicated in chronic constipation because it can lead to dependency and other problems (see chapter 13 for more information). There are many contraindications based upon senna's power to stimulate peristalsis.

Contraindications include any intestinal obstruction, stomach inflammation due to griping, and intestinal inflammatory disease, such as appendicitis, colitis, irritable bowel syndrome, ulcerative colitis, and Crohn's disease. Senna is also contraindicated in cases of abdominal pain of unknown origin, anal prolapse, and hemorrhoids.

Ideally, senna should not be used during pregnancy or lactation or in children younger than 12 years of age. However, orthodox physicians still routinely prescribe standardized senna preparations for use during pregnancy. To avoid the development of impaired peristalsis due to intestinal smooth muscle damage, do not use for more than 10 days.

Preparations and Dosage: To make an infusion, steep dried pods or leaves in warm water for 6 to 12 hours. Drink in the morning and at night. Use 3 to 6 Alexandrian senna pods or 4 to 12 Tinnevelly senna pods per cup of water.

The BHP recommends 0.5 to 2 ml fluid extract twice daily.

Sennae folium, Sennae fructus acutifoliae, and Sennae fructus angustifoliae, in *Herbal Drugs and Phytopharmaceuticals*

Serenoa repens (Bartr.) Small
Saw Palmetto
Arecaceae

Part Used: Fruit (berry)

Constituents: Essential oil; fixed oil: 25% fatty acids (caproic, lauric, palmitic) and 75% neutral fats; sterols; polysaccharides[216]

Actions: Diuretic, urinary antiseptic, endocrine agent

Indications: Saw palmetto tones and strengthens the male reproductive system, and is specific for the treatment of benign prostatic hyperplasia (BPH). Its primary modern application is to relieve symptoms associated with this common condition, especially difficulties with urination.

BPH is thought to be caused by accumulation of testosterone in the prostate. Once in the prostate, testosterone is converted to dihydrotestosterone (DHT). Researchers believe that DHT is the compound responsible for the multiplication of prostate cells that results in prostate enlargement. Saw palmetto appears to inhibit DHT by blocking the activity of the enzyme 5-α-reductase. The herb not only inhibits the formation of DHT, but also inhibits DHT binding at cellular receptor binding sites.[217] Numerous studies show that saw palmetto extract is effective for nearly 90% of patients with BPH. The fat-soluble (lipophilic) fraction of the herb, which contains fatty acids and sterols, is considered the active component for prostate conditions.[218]

The Eclectic use of this herb went far beyond treatment of BPH. Consider the following from *Ellingwood:*

> The direct influence of this agent is exerted upon the entire reproductive apparatus, especially upon the prostate gland of the male. It is demanded in enlarged prostate, with throbbing, aching, dull pain, discharge of prostatic fluid, at times discharge of mucus, also of a yellowish, watery fluid, with weakened sexual power, orchalgia, epididymitis and orchitis, when associated with enlarged prostate. In women, ovarian enlargement, with tenderness and dull aching pains, weakened sexual activity, and small undeveloped mammary glands, are much benefited by its continued use. It increases the size and secreting power of the mammary glands where they are abnormally small and inactive. It improves the tone and overcomes irritability of the ovaries, relieving dysmenorrhoea when due to atonicity. To this agent is ascribed considerable power in reducing the size of hypertrophied prostate in older men and in quickly relieving cystic and other disorders incident to this condition. It relieves irritation of the bladder to a satisfactory extent, correcting the irritable character of the urine, increases the muscular power of the patient to expel the urine and produces a sense of relief, that is in every way gratifying and satisfactory. . . .
>
> An exceedingly important use for this remedy that I have not been able to find in the books, is its use for sterility. In simple cases where there is no organic lesion on the part of the patient, this agent has an excellent reputation for restoring the ovarian action properly and assisting in putting the patient into an excellent condition. In its influence upon the nasal and bronchial mucous membranes this agent has been given with excellent advantage in the treatment of acute catarrh, chronic bronchial coughs of all characters, including whooping cough, laryngitis and the cough of phthisis.

Safety Considerations: No side effects or drug interactions have been reported.

Preparations and Dosage: Tincture dosage is 1 to 2 ml three times a day (1:5 in 60%). To make a decoction, put 2 to 4 teaspoon of berries in 1 cup of water, bring to a boil, and simmer gently for 5 minutes. This should be drunk three times a day.

The BHP recommends 0.5 to 1 g dried herb or 0.6 to 1.5 ml fluid extract three times daily (1:1 in 60%). Commission E suggests a daily dosage of 1 to 2 g berries or 320 mg of lipophilic ingredients extracted with lipophilic solvents (this contains approximately 85% to 95% fatty acids).

Saw palmetto, in *Principles and Practice of Phytotherapy*

Silybum marianum (L.) Gaertn.
Milk Thistle
Asteraceae

Part Used: Seed

Constituents: Flavolignans (1.5% to 3.0%): The mixture known as *silymarin* is composed mainly of silybin, silydianin, and silychristin; fixed oil (30% oleic acid, 6% palmitic acid); sterols (cholesterol, campesterol, stigmasterol, and sitosterol); mucilage[219]

Actions: Hepatic, galactagogue, demulcent, cholagogue, antihepatotoxic

Indications: Milk thistle's traditional reputation as a liver tonic is now supported by research showing that its constituents protect liver cells from chemical damage. Historically, milk thistle was used in Europe as a liver tonic, and in modern phytotherapy, the herb is indicated for a whole range of liver and gallbladder conditions, including hepatitis and cirrhosis. It is effective in increasing the secretion and flow of bile from the liver and gallbladder, and may also have value in the treatment of chronic uterine problems. As the name implies, milk thistle promotes milk secretion and is perfectly safe for use by breast-feeding mothers.

Well-designed clinical research thoroughly supports the efficacy of milk thistle seed extract in protecting and treating the liver. Studies confirm that the herb can restore liver function impaired by disease, such as viral hepatitis, or by exposure to toxins, including ethanol, mushroom toxins, solvents, acetaminophen, and psychotropic medications.[220] Research has shown that a number of chemical components have a protective effect on liver cells. They are all flavones and flavolignans, the best studied of which is a complex of the flavolignans known as *silymarin*. Silymarin has been shown to reverse the effects of highly toxic alkaloids, such as phalloidine and α-amanitine from the avenging angel mushroom (*Amanita phalloides*), and to protect liver cells from their damaging impact.

Research has provided many insights into the metabolic basis of milk thistle's activity. It has also shed considerable light on the pharmacodynamics, sites of activity, and mechanisms of action of silymarin. For example, in a clinical study involving 15 patients taking hepatotoxic psychotropic medications, a twice-daily 400 mg dose of a concentrated milk thistle seed extract protected the liver from the adverse effects of simultaneously administered drugs.[221] In a case study, milk thistle extract reduced the hepatotoxic effects of phenytoin.[222] More information on the pharmacology and therapeutic indications for this important herb may be found in chapters 9, 13, and 26.

Safety Considerations: No side effects or drug interactions have been reported.

Preparations and Dosage: For daily use as a liver protectant, dosage is 175 mg a day of 30:1 seed extract standardized to 80% silymarin. For therapeutic and restorative effects, up to 600 mg/day of extract standardized to 80% silymarin may be used.

Commission E recommends an average daily dosage of 12 to 15 g seed or formulations equivalent to 200 to 400 mg of silymarin (calculated as silibinin).

St. Mary's thistle, in *Principles and Practice of Phytotherapy*

Smilax spp.
Sarsaparilla
Liliaceae

Parts Used: Root, rhizome

Constituents: Saponins, based on the aglycones sarsapogenin and smilagenin; β-sitosterol, stigmasterol, and their glucosides[223]

Actions: Alterative, antirheumatic, diaphoretic, diuretic

Indications: Sarsaparilla is a widely applicable alterative. It may be used to support proper functioning of the whole body as well as to correct diffuse systemic problems, such as skin and rheumatic conditions. It is particularly useful for scaling skin conditions, like psoriasis, especially when accompanied by irritation. Sarsaparilla should be considered as part of a wider treatment for chronic rheumatism, and is especially helpful for rheumatoid arthritis.

Ellingwood recommended it for scrofula, secondary syphilis, cutaneous disease, and rheumatic and gouty conditions.

Safety Considerations: Sarsaparilla may increase absorption of digitalis glycosides.

Preparations and Dosage: Tincture dosage is 1 to 2 ml three times a day (1:5 in 60%). To make a decoction, place 2 to 4 teaspoons of root in 1 cup of water, bring to a boil, and simmer 10 to 15 minutes. This should be drunk three times a day.

The BHP recommends 1 to 4 g dried herb or 8 to

15 ml fluid extract (1:1 in 20% alcohol and 10% glycerin) three times a day.

Sarsaparilla, in *Herbal Medicines: A Guide for Health-Care Professionals*

Solidago virgaurea L.
Goldenrod
Asteraceae

Parts Used: Dried aerial parts

Constituents: Saponins (based on polygalic acid); clerodane diterpenes (including solidagolactones I–VII and elongatolides C and E); phenolic glycosides; flavonoids (such as rutin and quercetin); miscellaneous: acetylenes, polysaccharides, tannins[224]

Actions: Anticatarrhal, anti-inflammatory, antimicrobial, astringent, diaphoretic, carminative, diuretic

Indications: Goldenrod is perhaps the first plant to consider for upper respiratory catarrh, whether acute or chronic. The plant may also be used in combination with other herbs to treat influenza. Its carminative properties point to a role in the treatment of flatulent dyspepsia. As an anti-inflammatory urinary tract antiseptic, goldenrod may be helpful in cystitis, urethritis, and similar conditions affecting this system. As a gargle, goldenrod can be effective for laryngitis and pharyngitis. It may be applied externally to promote the healing of wounds.

Safety Considerations: Goldenrod may cause allergic reactions in people sensitive to plants in the Asteraceae family.

Preparations and Dosage: Tincture dosage is 2 to 4 ml three times a day (1:5 in 40%). To make an infusion, pour 1 cup of boiling water over 2 to 3 teaspoons of dried herb and infuse for 10 to 15 minutes. This should be drunk three times a day.

Commission E recommends a daily dosage of 6 to 12 g herb or equivalent preparations.

Goldenrod, in *Herbal Medicine, Expanded Commission E Monographs*

Stachys betonica L.
Wood Betony
Lamiaceae

Parts Used: Dried aerial parts

Constituents: Alkaloids (stachydrine and betonicine); miscellaneous: betaine, choline, tannins[225]

Actions: Nervine, bitter

Indications: Betony gently tones and strengthens the nervous system while also soothing nervous tension. It is helpful for nervous debility associated with anxiety and tension. It eases headaches and neuralgia of nervous origin, especially when caused by hypertension.

Safety Considerations: No side effects or drug interactions have been reported.

Preparations and Dosage: Tincture dosage is 2 to 6 ml three times a day (1:5 in 40%). For an infusion, pour 1 cup of boiling water over 1 to 2 teaspoons of dried herb and infuse for 10 to 15 minutes. This should be drunk three times a day.

Stellaria media (L.) Villars
Chickweed
Caryophyllaceae

Parts Used: Dried aerial parts

Constituents: Saponin glycosides; coumarins and hydroxycoumarins; flavonoids; carboxylic acids; triterpenoids; vitamin C (about 150 to 350 mg per 100 g)[226]

Actions: Antirheumatic, vulnerary, emollient

Indications: Chickweed is commonly used as an external remedy for cuts, wounds, and, especially, itching and irritation. It may be used with benefit to treat eczema or psoriasis associated with this sort of irritation. Chickweed has a reputation as a remedy for rheumatism when used internally.

King's provided the following uses:

> Chickweed appears to be a cooling demulcent. I have seen the fresh leaves bruised and applied as a poultice to indolent, intractable ulcers of the leg, of many years standing, with the most decided and immediately beneficial results; to be changed 2 or 3 times a day. In acute ophthalmia, the bruised leaves will likewise be found a valuable application. An ointment, made by bruising fresh leaves in fresh lard, may be used in many forms of cutaneous disease.

Safety Considerations: No side effects or drug interactions have been reported.

Preparations and Dosage: Chickweed should be used fresh or in the form of a water extract. To make an infusion, pour 1 cup of boiling water over 2 teaspoons of dried herb and infuse for 5 minutes. This may be drunk three times a day.

To make a "green drink" of fresh chickweed, place a handful of fresh plant in the blender with some pineapple juice; blend and strain. To ease itching, a strong infusion of fresh plant is a useful addition to bathwater.

Symphytum officinale L.
Comfrey
Boraginaceae

Parts Used: Root, rhizome, leaf

Constituents: Allantoin; pyrrolizidine alkaloids, including echimidine, symphytine, lycopsamine, symlandine (found in the fresh young leaves and in the root but, according to two separate investigations, not in the dried herb); phenolic acids (rosmarinic, chlorogenic, caffeic, and lithospermic); mucilage (about 29%), composed of a polysaccharide containing glucose and fructose; miscellaneous: choline, asparagine, volatile oil, tannins, steroidal saponins, triterpenes[227]

Actions: Vulnerary, demulcent, anti-inflammatory, astringent, expectorant

Indications: The impressive wound-healing properties of comfrey are due at least in part to the presence of allantoin. This chemical stimulates cell proliferation and thus supports wound healing, both internally and externally. Because it also contains a good deal of demulcent mucilage, comfrey root is a powerful healing agent for gastric and duodenal ulcers, hiatus hernia, and ulcerative colitis. Its astringency makes it valuable in the treatment of hemorrhages, wherever they occur. The root or herb may be used to good effect in bronchitis and irritable cough to soothe and reduce irritation while promoting expectoration.

Used externally, comfrey leaf speeds wound healing and fosters proper scar formation. Care should be taken with very deep wounds, however, as external application of comfrey can cause tissue to form over the wound before it is healed deeper down, which can lead to abscess. Used as a compress or poultice, the herb may be used to treat any external ulcers, wounds, and fractures; it is an excellent treatment for chronic varicose ulcers. It has a reputed anticancer action in European folk herbalism.

Safety Considerations: Long-term studies with rats have demonstrated that the pyrrolizidine alkaloids (PAs) in comfrey are hepatotoxic, carcinogenic, and mutagenic. Two of the PAs in comfrey have proved to be mutagenic in somatic *Drosophila* cells at a concentration of 5×10^{-3}M. This herb must therefore be recognized as a potentially genotoxic carcinogen in man. However, the risk of genetic damage from these pyrrolizidine alkaloids appears to be low. An average cup of fresh comfrey leaf tea may contain up to 8.3 mg alkaloid. To minimize potential risk, lengthy internal use is to be discouraged. Only slight absorption occurs with external application. For a more detailed discussion of the toxicity of pyrrolizidine alkaloids, please refer to chapter 10.

After external application to rats of an alcoholic extract (corresponding to a dose of 194 mg/kg of alkaloid *N*-oxide mixture), 0.1% to 0.4% alkaloid was excreted in the urine, mainly as *N*-oxide. Oral administration of the same extract for the same length of time led to a 20 to 50 times greater excretion of alkaloid in the urine.

Comfrey is banned in Australia and its use restricted in New Zealand. In the United Kingdom, oral medicinal preparations containing comfrey have been withdrawn from the market.

Preparations and Dosage: Root tincture dosage is 2 to 4 ml three times a day (1:5 in 25%). To make a decoction of the root, put 1 to 3 teaspoons of dried herb in 1 cup of water, bring to a boil, and simmer for 10 to 15 minutes. This should be drunk three times a day. A cold infusion may be made by pouring 1 cup of cold water over 2 teaspoons of root; leave to stand for 6 to 8 hours. Thus, a nighttime dose may be prepared in advance in the morning and a dose for mornings set up at night.

For leaf ointments and other preparations for external application (containing 5% to 20% dried herb), Commission E recommends that the daily applied dosage not exceed 100 mcg of pyrrolizidine alkaloids with 1,2-unsaturated necine structure, including their *N*-oxides. Similarly, for root ointments and other preparations for external use (containing 5% to 20% dried herb), the daily applied dosage should not exceed 100 mcg of pyrrolizidine alkaloids with 1,2-unsaturated necine structure, including their *N*-oxides.

Symphyti radix, in *Herbal Drugs and Phytopharmaceuticals*

Symplocarpus foetidus (L.) Salisb. ex Nutt.
Skunk Cabbage
Araceae

Parts Used: Root, rhizome

Constituents: Essential oil; 5-hydroxytryptamine; resins[228]

Actions: Antispasmodic, diaphoretic, expectorant

Indications: Skunk cabbage may be used for any spasmodic condition of the lungs. It relaxes and eases irritable coughs, and may be helpful for asthma, bronchitis, and whooping cough. As a diaphoretic, it supports the body during fever.

Safety Considerations: No side effects or drug interactions have been reported.

Preparations and Dosage: Traditionally, skunk cabbage has been used as a preparation made by mixing 1 part powdered root to 8 parts honey. Dosage is ¹/₂ to 1 teaspoon of this mixture three times a day. An infusion (for leaf) or decoction (for root) may be made with ¹/₂ teaspoon of herb per cup of water. Tincture dosage is ¹/₂ to 1 ml three times a day (1:5 in 60%).

Skunk Cabbage, in *Herbal Medicines: A Guide for Health-Care Professionals*

Tanacetum parthenium (L.) Schultz-Bip.
Feverfew
Asteraceae

Other Name: Until recently, the binomial was *Chrysanthemum parthenium*.

Part Used: Leaf

Constituents: Sesquiterpene lactones (parthenolide, articanin, santamarin); onoterpenes and sesquiterpenes (thujone, sabinene, camphor, 1,8-cineole, umbellulone); flavonoids (apigenin, diosmetin, quercetin, jaceidin, jaceosidin)[229]

Actions: Anti-inflammatory, vasodilator, emmenagogue, bitter

Indications: Feverfew has regained its deserved reputation as a primary remedy for treating and preventing migraine headaches, particularly those eased by the application of warmth to the head. Feverfew may be valuable for arthritis in the painfully active inflammatory stage. The herb may also help alleviate dizziness and tinnitus, especially if used in conjunction with other remedies, and relieve painful periods and sluggish menstrual flow.

Feverfew is the only herb used in European phytotherapy that is known to be specific for the treatment of migraine. It is also the best example of a remedy well known to medical herbalists that has recently been accepted by orthodox medicine. For more information on clinical research on feverfew and migraine, please see chapter 16.

Feverfew's spectrum of pharmacological actions appears to be related to its influences on arachidonic acid metabolism and platelet functions.

- Inhibits histamine secretion
- Inhibits aggregation, granular secretion, and arachidonate-mediated responses
- Exerts cytotoxic action
- Inhibits 5-hydroxytryptamine-mediated contractile responses
- Inhibits vascular smooth muscle contractility

Safety Considerations: Feverfew may cause allergic response in people sensitive to members of the Asteraceae family. The fresh leaves may cause mouth ulcers in susceptible people. Feverfew should not be used during pregnancy because of its stimulant action on the uterus. Although no drug interactions have been documented, it is possible that feverfew may interfere with aspirin and other anticoagulant medications because of its mechanism of action.

Preparations and Dosage: The preferred dosage is the equivalent of 1 fresh leaf one to three times a day. While fresh leaf is preferable, tincture or tablets are adequate. Of these formulations, freeze-dried leaf preparations (50 to 100 mg/day) are best.

For migraine prophylaxis, recommended dosage is 25 to 125 mg a day of a standardized leaf and flower extract containing a minimum of 0.2% parthenolide. Higher doses (up to 2 g/day) may be required for acute treatment of migraine or for inflammatory conditions.

Feverfew, in *Principles and Practice of Phytotherapy*

Taraxacum officinale Weber ex Wigg.
Dandelion
Asteraceae

Parts Used: Root, leaf

Constituents: Sesquiterpene lactones (taraxacoside, others); diterpenes, including taraxacin; triterpenes (taraxasterol, arnidiol, faradiol, β-amyrin); sterols (stigmasterol, β-sitosterol); carotenoids, such as lutein and violaxanthin; xanthophylls; flavonoids (apigenin, luteolin); polysaccharides (glucans, mannans, inulin); potassium (up to 4.5% in aerial parts)[230]

Actions: Diuretic, hepatic, cholagogue, antirheumatic, laxative, tonic, bitter

Indications: Dandelion leaf is a powerful diuretic, with an action comparable to that of the drug furosemide. The usual effect of a drug that stimulates kidney function is loss of vital potassium from the body, which can aggravate any cardiovascular problem that may be present. Dandelion leaf, however, is not only an effective diuretic, but also one of the best natural sources of potassium. It is thus an ideally balanced remedy that may be used safely whenever diuretic action is needed, even for water retention related to heart problems. Overall, this herb is a most valuable general tonic and perhaps the best widely applicable diuretic and liver tonic.

In one study investigating the effects of oral administration of dandelion extracts in rats and mice, leaf extracts produced greater diuresis than root extracts, and a dose of 50 ml/kg body weight (equivalent to 2 g dried herb) produced an effect comparable to that of furosemide given at a dosage of 80 mg/kg.[231]

As a hepatic and cholagogue, dandelion root may be helpful for inflammation and congestion of the liver and gallbladder. It is specific for cases of congestive jaundice.[232] In addition, it can be very effective as part of a wider treatment for muscular rheumatism.

Ellingwood recommended dandelion root for chronic jaundice, autointoxication, rheumatism, blood disorders, chronic skin eruptions, chronic gastritis, and aphthous ulcers.

Safety Considerations: Dandelion may theoretically cause allergic reactions in people sensitive to plants in the Asteraceae family. There have been rare reports of contact dermatitis in people coming in frequent contact with the latex found in the stem.[233]

Preparations and Dosage: Root tincture dosage is 2.5 to 5 ml three times a day (1:5 in 60%). To make a root decoction, put 2 to 3 teaspoons of root into 1 cup of water, bring to a boil, and gently simmer for 10 to 15 minutes. This should be drunk three times a day.

Leaf tincture dosage is 5 to 10 ml three times a day (1:5 in 40%). To make a leaf infusion, pour 1 cup of boiling water over 1 to 2 teaspoons of dried leaf and infuse for 10 to 15 minutes. This should be drunk three times a day. The leaf may also be eaten raw in salads.

The BHP recommends 3 to 5 g dried leaf or 5 to 10 ml tincture three times a day, or 5 to 10 ml juice from fresh leaf twice daily. Its suggested dosage for root is 0.5 to 2 g dried root or 4 to 8 ml tincture three times daily. Commission E recommends 4 to 10 g of dried leaf or 4 to 10 ml fluid extract of leaf daily, or 3 to 4 g cut or powdered root per cup by decoction.

Taraxaci radix cum herba, in *Herbal Drugs and Phytopharmaceuticals*

Thuja occidentalis L.
Thuja
Cupressaceae

Other Names: Arborvitae, white cedar, Western hemlock

Part Used: Young twig

Constituents: Volatile oil (1%), including thujone; flavonoid glycosides; mucilage; tannins[234]

Actions: Expectorant, antimicrobial, diuretic, astringent, alterative

Indications: Thuja's main action is related to its content of stimulating and alterative volatile oil. In bronchial catarrh, thuja promotes expectoration and provides systemic stimulation that is especially beneficial when heart weakness is also part of the picture. However, thuja should be avoided in cases in which cough is due to overstimulation (for example, dry, irritable coughs).

Thuja has a specific reflex action on the uterus and may help with delayed menstruation. Because of this property, however, the herb is best avoided during pregnancy. Thuja may also be used for ordinary incontinence due to loss of muscle tone. It has a role to play in the treatment of psoriasis and rheumatism when used internally. Externally, it may be effective against warts, and demonstrates a marked antifungal activity against ringworm and thrush.

Ellingwood described thuja thus:

It has been used extensively by all physicians in the treatment of cancer. It is claimed to exercise an abortive influence over incipient cancer and to retard the progress of more advanced cases. In extreme cases it will remove the fetor, retard the growth and materially prolong the life of the patient. It should be given internally and the dosage increased to the extreme limit. It should be also kept in contact with the parts externally or injected into the structures. Epithelioma, condylomata and all simple cancerous growths should be treated with it.

Thuja is directly indicated in improving conditions of the blood. Again, it acts directly upon abnormal growths, such as peculiar conditions of the cell structure of the skin and other external structure. It is thus indicated in all abnormal growths of the skin or mucous membranes. It exercises a specific influence upon catarrhal discharges, correcting the glandular faults that are to blame for such a condition wherever they may be. It is specific to urinary irritation in aged people especially; also in childhood. It strengthens the sphincter of the bladder.

As an external application Thuja produces at first a sensation of smarting or tingling when applied to open sores or wounds and it is usually best to dilute it with one, two or four parts of water, or to combine the non-alcoholic extract with an ointment base in the above proportion. This constitutes an excellent mildly antiseptic and actively stimulating dressing to indolent, phagedenic or gangrenous ulcers. It is of much service in bed sores and in other open ulcers dependent upon local or general nerve exhaustion. In chronic skin diseases of either a nonspecific or specific character, it is a useful remedy. It is a useful agent in the treatment of post-nasal catarrh and nasal polypi. A small dose internally 4 or 5 times daily, with the application of fluid hydrastis in a spray, will quickly retard or remove such abnormal growths.

Safety Considerations: Due to its content of thujone, large doses of thuja may be toxic; please see chapter 10 for more information. Use in combination with other thujone-containing herbs will cause an additive effect. Avoid during pregnancy.

Preparations and Dosage: Tincture dosage is 1 to 2 ml three times a day (1:5 in 60%). To make an infusion, pour 1 cup of boiling water over 1 teaspoon of dried herb and infuse for 10 to 15 minutes. This should be drunk three times a day.

Thymus vulgaris L.
Thyme
Lamiaceae

Parts Used: Leaf, flowering top

Constituents: Volatile oil of highly variable composition, mainly thymol, with lesser amounts of carvacrol; flavonoids (apigenin, luteolin, thymonin, naringenin, others); miscellaneous: labiatic acid, caffeic acid, tannins[235]

Actions: Carminative, antimicrobial, antispasmodic, expectorant, astringent, anthelmintic

Indications: High in volatile oil, thyme makes a good carminative for use in dyspepsia and sluggish digestion. This oil is also strongly antiseptic, explaining many of thyme's other uses. It may be applied externally as a lotion for infected wounds and internally for respiratory and digestive infections. Used as a gargle for laryngitis and tonsillitis, it eases sore throats and soothes irritable coughs. It is an excellent cough remedy, producing expectoration and reducing spasm. It may be effective in the treatment of bronchitis, whooping cough, and asthma. As a gentle astringent, it may be helpful for childhood diarrhea and bed-wetting.

King's described it thus:

Thyme is tonic, carminative, emmenagogue and antispasmodic. The cold infusion is useful in dyspepsia, with weak and irritable stomach and as a stimulating tonic in convalescence from exhausting diseases. The warm infusion is beneficial in hysteria, dysmenorrhoea, flatulence, colic, headache, and to promote perspiration. Occasionally the leaves have been used externally, in fomentation. The oil is valuable as a local application to neuralgic and rheumatic pains; and, internally, to fulfil any of the indications for which the plant is used. Dose of the infusion, from 1 to 3 fluid ounces.

Safety Considerations: No side effects or drug interactions have been reported.

Preparations and Dosage: Tincture dosage is 2 to 4 ml three times a day (1:5 in 45%). To make an infusion, pour 1 cup of boiling water over 2 teaspoons of dried herb and infuse in a covered container for 10 minutes. This should be drunk three times a day.

Commission E recommends 1 to 2 g herb per 1 cup of tea as needed or 1 to 2 g fluid extract one to three times daily.

Thyme, in *Principles and Practice of Phytotherapy*

Tilia platyphyllos Scop.
Linden
Tiliaceae

Other Name: Lime blossom

Part Used: Dried flower

Constituents: Volatile oil (up to about 0.1%), containing farnesol; flavonoids (kaempferol, hesperidin, quercetin, astralagin, tiliroside, others); miscellaneous: mucilage (in the bract), phenolic acids, tannins[236]

Actions: Nervine, antispasmodic, hypotensive, diaphoretic, diuretic, anti-inflammatory, astringent

Indications: Linden is a relaxing European remedy for use in nervous tension. It is a valuable cardiotonic with a reputation for preventing the development of arteriosclerosis and hypertension. It is considered a specific for high blood pressure associated with arteriosclerosis and nervous tension. Its relaxing action, combined with a general tonic effect upon the circulatory system, gives linden a role in the treatment of some types of migraine. Its blend of diaphoretic and relaxant actions explains its value for feverish colds and flu.

Safety Considerations: No side effects or drug interactions have been reported.

Preparations and Dosage: Tincture dosage is 2.5 to 5 ml three times a day (1:5 in 40%). To make an infusion, pour 1 cup of boiling water over 1 teaspoon of blossoms and infuse in a covered container for 10 minutes. This should be drunk three times a day. For a diaphoretic effect in fever, use 2 to 3 teaspoons of blossoms per cup of water.

The BHP recommends 2 to 4 g dried inflorescence, 5 to 15 ml expressed juice, 4 to 10 ml tincture (1:5 in 25%), or 2 to 4 ml fluid extract (1:1 in 25%) three times daily. Commission E suggests 2 to 4 g of herb or equivalent preparations daily.

Linden flower, in *Herbal Medicine, Expanded Commission E Monographs*

Trifolium pratense L.
Red Clover
Fabaceae

Part Used: Flower head

Constituents: Isoflavones (biochanin A, daidzein, formononetin, genistein, pratensein, trifoside); other flavonoids, including pectolinarin and kaempferol; volatile oil (containing furfural); clovamides (L-dopa-caffeic acid conjugates); coumarins (coumestrol, medicagol, coumarin); miscellaneous: a galactomannan, resins, minerals, vitamins, phytoalexins[237]

Actions: Alterative, expectorant, antispasmodic

Indications: Red clover is a useful remedy for children with skin problems. It may be used with complete safety for any case of childhood eczema, and can be effective for other chronic skin conditions as well, such as psoriasis. While it is very appropriate for children, it may also be of value for adults.

Red clover's expectorant and antispasmodic actions give this remedy a role in the treatment of coughs and bronchitis, especially whooping cough. As an alterative, it is indicated as part of a holistic approach for a wide range of problems. There is some evidence to suggest that it has an antineoplastic action in animals.

Priest and Priest described red clover as a

> . . . mild, stimulating and relaxing alterative with a special affinity for the throat and salivary glands. Especially indicated for debilitated children with chronic bronchial or throat conditions.

They gave the following specific indications: salivary gland congestion, spasmodic or croupy coughs, pertussis; pharyngeal inflammation; and chronic skin eruptions.

Safety Considerations: Red clover may potentiate the effects of anticoagulant drugs.

Preparations and Dosage: Tincture dosage is 2 to 4 ml three times a day (1:5 in 40%). To make an infusion, pour 1 cup of boiling water over 1 to 3 teaspoons of dried herb and infuse for 10 to 15 minutes. This should be drunk three times a day.

The BHP recommends 4 g dried herb or 1 to 2 ml of tincture (1:10 in 45%) three times a day.

Red Clover, in *Herbal Medicines: A Guide for Health-Care Professionals*

Tussilago farfara L.
Coltsfoot
Asteraceae

Other Names: Coughwort, horsehoof, foal's foot

Parts Used: Dried flower, leaf

Constituents: Flavonoids (rutin, hyperoside, isoquercetin); mucilage, consisting of polysaccharides based on glucose, galactose, fructose, arabinose, xylose; inulin; pyrrolizidine alkaloids, including senkirkine and tussilagine; tannins[238]

Actions: Expectorant, antitussive, antispasmodic, demulcent, anticatarrhal, diuretic

Indications: Coltsfoot combines a soothing expectorant effect with an antispasmodic action. The leaves contain useful levels of zinc, a mineral shown to have marked anti-inflammatory actions. Coltsfoot may be helpful for chronic or acute bronchitis, irritating coughs, whooping cough, and asthma. Its soothing expectorant action gives it a role in most respiratory conditions, including emphysema. As a mild diuretic, it has been used to treat cystitis. The fresh bruised leaves can be applied externally to boils, abscesses, and suppurating ulcers.

Priest and Priest described coltsfoot as a

> . . . diffusive expectorant, sedative and demulcent: suitable for debilitated and chronic conditions, especially where there is a tubercular diathesis.

They gave the following specific indications: chronic pulmonary conditions, chronic emphysema and silicosis, pertussis, and asthma.

Safety Considerations: Several pyrrolizidine alkaloids are known to have hepatotoxic, genotoxic, or carcinogenic effects; however, there is no danger of acute poisoning when the herb is used as prescribed, particularly as the concentration of these alkaloids in a tea is very low. Nevertheless, do not use coltsfoot for a prolonged period of time. (For a more detailed discussion of the toxicity of pyrrolizidine alkaloids, please refer to chapter 10.)

Preparations and Dosage: Tincture dosage is 2 to 4 ml three times a day (1:5 in 40%). To make an infusion, pour 1 cup of boiling water over 1 to 2 teaspoons of dried flower or leaf and infuse for 10 minutes. This should be drunk three times a day, as hot as possible.

According to Commission E, the daily dosage of coltsfoot should not exceed 100 mcg pyrrolizidine alkaloids with 1,2-unsaturated necine structures. Do not use for longer than 4 to 6 weeks per year.

Farfarae folium, in *Herbal Drugs and Phytopharmaceuticals*

Ulmus rubra Muhl.
Slippery Elm
Ulmaceae

Part Used: Inner bark

Constituents: Mucilage, composed of galactose, 3-methyl galactose, rhamnose, and galacturonic acid residues[239]

Actions: Demulcent, emollient, nutrient, astringent, anti-inflammatory

Indications: Slippery elm is a soothing, nutritive demulcent that is perfectly suited for treating sensitive or inflamed mucous membrane linings in the digestive system. The herb may be used in gastritis, gastric or duodenal ulcer, enteritis, colitis, and similar conditions. Used to treat diarrhea, it simultaneously soothes and astringes the tissues of the intestinal lining.

Slippery elm makes an excellent food to be eaten during convalescence, as it is mild and easily assimilated. It makes an excellent poultice for external use in cases of boils, abscesses, and ulcers.

Priest and Priest considered slippery elm

> . . . the best demulcent for internal and external use. It lubricates and soothes alimentary mucosa, relieves intestinal irritation, and quietens the nervous system.

They gave the following specific indications: acute gastritis and duodenal ulcer, diarrhea, dysentery, enteritis, inflammation of the mouth and throat, vaginitis, burns, scalds, and abrasions, hemorrhoids and anal fissure, varicose ulcer, abscesses, boils, carbuncles, inflamed wounds, and skin ulcers.

Safety Considerations: Slippery elm may slow the absorption of orally administered drugs.

Preparations and Dosage: To make a decoction, use 1 part powdered root to 8 parts water. First add a small amount of powder to a little water and stir to facilitate mixing. Bring to a boil and simmer gently for 10 to 15 minutes. Dosage is $\frac{1}{2}$ cup three times a day. For a poultice, mix coarse powdered root with enough boiling water to make a paste.

The BHC recommends 5 to 20 ml powdered bark in hot water three times daily (1:10).

Slippery Elm, in *Herbal Medicines: A Guide for Health-Care Professionals*

Urtica dioica L.
Nettle
Urticaceae

Parts Used: Aerial parts, root

Constituents: Chlorophyll (high yields); indoles, such as histamine and serotonin; acetylcholine; flavonol glycosides (isorhamnetin, kaempferol, quercetin); miscellaneous: vitamin C and other vitamins, protein, dietary fiber[240]

Actions: Astringent, diuretic, tonic, hypotensive

Indications: Nettle is one of the most widely applicable plants in the materia medica. The herb strengthens and supports the whole body. Throughout Europe, nettle is used as a spring tonic and general detoxifying remedy. It may be very helpful internally and topically for myalgia and osteoarthritis.[241]

Topical use of nettle leaf involves actively stinging the skin around the affected joint. The inflammation, and thus the pain and stiffness, will subside for 4 to 8 days following the application. Such "self-flagellation" may seem too heroic for the 21st century, but it works!

Nettle is a specific for childhood eczema and beneficial for all varieties of this condition, especially nervous eczema. It can be helpful as a component of treatment for eczema in adults. Used internally as an astringent, nettle will relieve symptoms of hemorrhage anywhere in the body (for example, uterine hemorrhage).

Research has shown that nettle contains both hypoglycemic and hyperglycemic constituents. The hypoglycemic component, termed urticin, has been reported to lower blood sugar concentrations in hyperglycemic rabbits.[242] Nettle root has been used with success to treat the early stages of benign prostatic hyperplasia (BPH). Studies show that it improves urine flow, reduces urinary frequency and nocturia, and decreases the volume of residual urine.[243]

Safety Considerations: Fresh nettle causes urticaria if applied topically! Internal use may theoretically decrease the efficacy of anticoagulant drugs.

Preparations and Dosage: Tincture dosage is 2.5 to 5 ml three times a day (1:5 in 40%). To make an infusion, pour 1 cup of boiling water over 1 to 3 teaspoons of dried herb and infuse for 10 to 15 minutes. This should be drunk three times a day.

The BHP recommends 2 to 4 g of dried herb or 2 to 6 ml tincture three times a day (1:5 in 45%). The BHC recommends 5 to 10 ml of fresh juice three times daily. Commission E suggests a daily dosage of 8 to 12 g of herb (or equivalent preparations) and 4 to 6 g of root (or equivalent preparations).

Nettle, in *Principles and Practice of Phytotherapy*

Valeriana officinalis L.
Valerian
Valerianaceae

Parts Used: Rhizome, stolon, root

Constituents: Essential oil (mainly composed of sesquiterpenes, such as bornyl acetate, β-caryophyllene, valerone, and valerenic acid); bicyclic iridoids known as valepotriates (including valtrate, isovaltrate, acetoxy-valerenic acid, isovaleroxy-hydoxydidrovaltrate); baldrinals, found only in dried herb or extracts, are degradation products of the valepotriates[244]

Actions: Nervine, hypnotic, antispasmodic, carminative, hypotensive, emmenagogue

Indications: Valerian has a wide range of specific uses. However, its main indications are anxiety, nervous sleeplessness, and bodily symptoms of tension, such as muscle cramping and indigestion. In short, this herb may be safely used for any situation in which tension and anxiety cause problems, either psychological or physical. It is a valuable muscle relaxant, effective for muscle spasms, uterine cramps, and intestinal colic. For some people, it may serve as a mild pain reliever. A useful herbal sleep aid, valerian helps promote normal sleep, as it is not powerful enough to suppress necessary REM phases.

Valerian's sedative and antispasmodic actions can be partially attributed to its content of valepotriates, and, to a lesser extent, to the sesquiterpene constituents of the volatile oil. Various species of *Valeriana* are used worldwide as relaxing remedies for hypertension and stress-related heart conditions.

Safety Considerations: No drug interactions have been reported by Commission E or ESCOP. Valerian may potentiate the effects of sedatives. A characteristic paradoxical reaction occurs in a few people, producing an unpleasant stimulation response.

Preparations and Dosage: To be effective, valerian must be used at a sufficiently high dosage. The tincture (1:5 in 60%) is the most widely used preparation and is always useful, as long as 2.5 to 5 ml (1/2 to 1 teaspoon) is given as a single dose. Up to 10 ml may be given at one time.

To make an infusion, use 2 teaspoons of dried herb per cup of boiling water; prepare in a closed vessel to ensure no loss of volatile oils. A cold infusion may be made by pouring 1 cup of cold water over 2 teaspoons of root; leave to stand for 8 to 10 hours. In this way, a nighttime dose may be prepared in advance in the morning and a dose for morning set up at night.

The BHP recommends 4 to 8 ml of the tincture three times a day (1:8 in 60%). Commission E suggests 2 to 3 g of dried root per cup of water, taken one to several times a day.

Valerian, in *Principles and Practice of Phytotherapy*

Verbascum thapsus L.
Mullein
Scrophulariaceae

Parts Used: Dried leaf, flower

Constituents: Flavonoids (such as verbascoside and herperidin); mucilage; saponins; tannins; volatile oil[245]

Actions: Expectorant, demulcent, anti-inflammatory, antispasmodic, vulnerary

Indications: Mullein is a very beneficial respiratory remedy, useful for most conditions and ideal for toning the mucous membranes of this vital system. The herb reduces inflammation while stimulating fluid production, thus facilitating expectoration. It is considered a specific for bronchitis characterized by a hard cough with soreness. Its anti-inflammatory and demulcent properties indicate its use for inflammation of the trachea and associated conditions. For external use, an extract made by infusing mullein flowers in olive oil is excellent for soothing and healing any inflamed surface and for easing ear problems.

Safety Considerations: No side effects or drug interactions have been reported.

Preparations and Dosage: Tincture dosage is 2.5 to 5 ml three times a day (1:5 in 40%). To make an infusion, pour 1 cup of boiling water over 2 teaspoons of dried leaf or flower and infuse for 10 to 15 minutes. This should be drunk three times a day.

The BHP recommends 4 to 8 g dried herb or 4 to 8 ml fluid extract (1:1 in 25%) three times a day.

Mullein Flower, in *The Complete German Commission E Monographs*

Verbena officinalis L.
Vervain
Verbenaceae

Parts Used: Aerial parts

Constituents: Iridoids (verbenin, verbenalin, bastatoside); miscellaneous: essential oil, mucilage[246]

Actions: Nervine tonic, sedative, antispasmodic, diaphoretic, hypotensive, galactagogue, hepatic

Indications: Vervain is a gentle anxiolytic. It is helpful for easing depression and melancholia, especially after debilitating illness, such as influenza. Vervain may be beneficial in seizure and hysteria. As a diaphoretic, it can be used in the early stages of fevers. As a hepatic remedy, it is appropriate for jaundice and inflammations of the gallbladder. It may be used as a mouthwash to treat caries and gum disease.

Safety Considerations: No side effects or drug interactions have been reported.

Preparations and Dosage: Tincture dosage is 2.5 to 5 ml three times a day (1:5 in 40%). To make an infusion, pour 1 cup of boiling water over 1 to 3 teaspoons of dried herb and infuse in a covered container for 10 to 15 minutes. This should be drunk three times a day.

Dosage given in the BHP is 2 to 4 g dried herb, 2 to 4 ml liquid extract (1:1 in 25%), or 4 to 10 ml tincture (1:5 in 45%).

Verbenae herba, in *Herbal Drugs and Phytopharmaceuticals*

Viburnum opulus L.
Cramp Bark
Caprifoliaceae

Part Used: Dried bark

Constituents: Hydroquinones (arbutin, methylarbutin, traces of free hydroquinone); coumarins (such as scopoletin and scopoline); tannins (mainly catechins)[247]

Actions: Antispasmodic, anti-inflammatory, nervine, hypotensive, astringent, emmenagogue

Indications: As implied by the name, cramp bark has a richly deserved reputation for relaxing muscular tension and spasm. It has two primary areas of use: cramps of the voluntary muscles and uterine muscle problems. Cramp bark relaxes the uterus and thus relieves painful menstrual cramps (dysmenorrhea). In a similar way, it may be used to protect against threatened miscarriage. Its astringent action gives it a role in the treatment of excessive menstrual blood loss and, especially, irregular bleeding during menopause

Priest and Priest described cramp bark as a

. . . relaxing and stimulating nervine, cerebrospinal vaso-stimulant. Restores sympathetic/parasympathetic balance—has a specific action to relieve voluntary and involuntary muscular spasms.

They gave the following specific indications: colicky

pains and spasms of tubular organs, gastrointestinal and genitourinary use with *Dioscorea villosa*, and atonic conditions of pelvic organs where menses is scanty or delayed.

Safety Considerations: No side effects or drug interactions have been reported.

Preparations and Dosage: Tincture dosage is 4 to 8 ml three times a day (1:5 in 40%). To make a decoction, put 2 teaspoons of dried herb into 1 cup of water, bring to a boil, and simmer gently for 10 to 15 minutes. This should be drunk hot three times a day.

The BHP recommends 2 to 4 g dried herb or 5 to 10 ml tincture (1:5 in 45%) three times a day.

Viburnum prunifolium L.
Black Haw
Caprifoliaceae

Part Used: Dried bark of stems or trunk

Constituents: Coumarins (including scopoletin, aesculetin); phenolic acids (including chlorogenic acid, salicin); biflavones (amentoflavone); triterpenes (α- and β-amyrin, oleanolic and ursolic acids)[248]

Actions: Antispasmodic, nervine, hypotensive, astringent

Indications: Uses for black haw are similar to those for cramp bark, to which it is closely related. Black haw is a powerful uterine relaxant. It is helpful in the treatment of dysmenorrhea and false labor pains as well as for preventing threatened miscarriage. Its relaxant and sedative actions explain its ability to lower blood pressure associated with hypertension, which it accomplishes by relaxing peripheral blood vessels. Black haw's antispasmodic properties make it appropriate for the treatment of asthma.

King's described black haw in the following way:

That it has a decided affinity for the female reproductive organs is well established. Its principal use at the present day is in disorders of the female organs of reproduction. As a uterine tonic it is unquestionably of great utility. In the hyperasthetic, or irritable condition of the uterus incident to highly nervous women, or as the result of overwork, it will be found an admirable agent. In dysmenorrhoea, with deficient menses, uterine colic, and in those cases where there are severe lumbar and bearing-down pains, it will prove an efficient drug. It is specifically indicated in cramp-like menstrual pains, pains decidedly expulsive and intermittent in character and in the various painful contractions of the pelvic muscles, so common to disorders of women. Uterine congestion and chronic uterine inflammation are often greatly relieved by Black Haw. It acts promptly in spasmodic dysmenorrhoea, especially with excessive flow. It is a good remedy for uterine haemorrhage attending the menopause. In amenorrhoea in pale, bloodless subjects, the menses are restored by it. Cramps of limbs attending pregnancy yield to both black haw and cramp bark. It is considered almost specific for cramp in the legs, not dependent on pregnancy, especially when occurring at night. The condition for which black haw is most valued is that of threatened abortion. It is the most prompt drug in the materia medica to check abortion, provided the membranes have not ruptured. In all cases of habitual abortion it should be given in small doses for a considerable length of time. By its quieting effects upon the irritable womb, women who have previously been unable to go to full term have been aided by this drug to pass through the pregnancy without mishaps which would otherwise have proven disastrous to both child and mother. *Viburnum opulus* resembles this agent very closely in its effects, and may be used in the above-named conditions, for which the black haw is useful.

Specific Indications and Uses—Uterine irritability and hyperasthesia; threatened abortion; uterine colic; dysmenorrhoea with deficient menses; severe lumbar and bearing-down pains; cramp-like, expulsive menstrual pain; intermittent, painful contractions of the pelvic tissues; after-pains and false pains of pregnancy; obstinate hiccough.

Safety Considerations: No side effects or drug interactions have been reported.

Preparations and Dosage: Tincture dosage is 5 to 10 ml three times a day (1:5 in 60%). To make a decoction, put 2 teaspoons of dried herb in 1 cup of water, bring to a boil, and simmer for 10 minutes. This should be drunk three times a day.

The BHP recommends 2.5 to 5 g of dried herb or 5 to 10 ml tincture (1:5 in 70%).

Viburni prunifolii cortex, in *Herbal Drugs and Phytopharmaceuticals*

Vinca minor L.
Periwinkle
Apocynaceae

Parts Used: Aerial parts

Constituents: Indole alkaloids; tannins[249]

Action: Astringent

Indications: Periwinkle is an all-around astringent that may be used internally or externally. Its main application is excessive menstrual flow, either during the period itself (menorrhagia) or between periods (metrorrhagia). As with other remedies that affect the uterus, it may be used to address similar processes in the urinary system. Thus, it may be valuable in the treatment of hematuria (blood in the urine). In addition, periwinkle helps with digestive problems, such as colitis and diarrhea, in which it will reduce loss of fluid or blood while toning membranes. It may also be effective in cases of nosebleed, bleeding gums, mouth ulcers, and sore throat. It has a questionable reputation for aiding in the treatment of diabetes.

Safety Considerations: No side effects or drug interactions have been reported.

Preparations and Dosage: Tincture dosage is 1 to 2 ml three times a day (1:5 in 60%). For an infusion, pour 1 cup of boiling water over 1 teaspoon of dried herb and infuse for 10 to 15 minutes. This should be drunk three times a day.

Periwinkle, in *The Complete German Commission E Monographs*

Viola odorata L.
Sweet Violet
Violaceae

Parts Used: Leaf, flower

Constituents: Phenolic glycosides (including gaultherin, salicylic acid methyl ester); saponins (myrosin, violin); flavonoids (rutin, violarutin); miscellaneous: odoratine (an alkaloid), mucilage[250]

Actions: Expectorant, alterative, anti-inflammatory, diuretic

Indications: Sweet violet has a long history of use as a cough remedy, especially for bronchitis, and may be of benefit in upper respiratory catarrh. With the combination of actions this herb offers, it may also help in skin conditions (such as eczema), in urinary tract infections, and as part of a long-term approach to rheumatism. Sweet violet has a reputation as an "anticancer herb"; while the concept is inappropriate, as an alterative the herb definitely has a role to play in holistic approaches to the treatment of cancer.

Safety Considerations: No side effects or drug interactions have been reported.

Preparations and Dosage: Tincture dosage is 1 to 2 ml three times a day (1:5 in 40%). To make an infusion, pour 1 cup of boiling water over 1 teaspoon of herb and infuse in a covered container for 10 to 15 minutes. This should be drunk three times a day.

Viola tricolor L.
Heartsease
Violaceae

Parts Used: Aerial parts

Constituents: Flavonoids (including violanthin, rutin, violaquercitrin); methylsalicylate; miscellaneous: mucilage, gums, resin, saponins[251]

Actions: Expectorant, diuretic, anti-inflammatory

Indications: Traditionally used for bronchitis and rheumatism, heartsease is also an especially valued remedy for skin diseases. Used both internally and topically, it is helpful for eczema, psoriasis, acne, and, topically, in babies, for cradle cap. The herb is also employed to treat frequent and painful urination associated with conditions such as cystitis.

Both the salicylates and the rutin contained in heartsease are anti-inflammatory. This action helps explain the traditional use of the herb for arthritis. The saponins account for its expectorant action, while the mucilage it contains soothes the chest. Heartsease is used to treat a range of respiratory disorders, including bronchitis and whooping cough. Due to the high concentration of rutin in the flowers, this herb may be employed to prevent bruising and broken capillaries and to check buildup of fluid in the tissues (edema). It can be helpful in the treatment or prevention of atherosclerosis, and thus may help reduce blood pressure. Heartsease is mildly laxative.

Safety Considerations: No side effects or drug interactions have been reported.

Preparations and Dosage: Tincture dosage is 1 to 2 ml three times a day (1:5 in 40%). To make an infusion, pour 1 cup of boiling water over 1 teaspoon of dried herb and infuse for 10 to 15 minutes. This should be drunk three times a day.

Commission E recommends 1.5 g dried herb per cup of water as tea three times a day.

Violae tricoloris herba, in *Herbal Drugs and Phytopharmaceuticals*

Vitex agnus-castus L.
Vitex
Verbenaceae

Other Names: Chaste tree, chasteberry, monk's pepper

Part Used: Fruit (berry)

Constituents: Iridoid glycosides (aucubin and agnuside); labdane diterpenes (otundifuran, vitexilactone); flavonoids (casticin, vitexin, isovitexin, kaempferol); essential oil (0.4% to 0.7%), with bornyl acetate, 1,8-cineole, limonene, and α-and β-pinene[252]

Actions: Hormonal normalizer, uterine tonic, galactagogue

Indications: Vitex has the effect of stimulating and normalizing pituitary gland function, especially as it relates to relative progesterone levels. Vitex may be called an amphoteric remedy, as it can produce apparently opposite effects, although in truth it is simply normalizing.

The term *amphoteric* comes from chemistry, in which it is used to indicate the ability of a chemical to react as either an acid or an alkali. The word itself is derived from Greek roots meaning "partly one and partly the other." In the context of herbal actions, *amphoteric* implies that apparently opposite effects may be observed, but the overall result is a normalizing effect. For instance, vitex has a reputation for being both an aphrodisiac and an anaphrodisiac! In effect, the herb will generally facilitate the most appropriate action required to normalize function, no matter what aspect of function is out of balance.

The most important therapeutic application for vitex comes from its ability to normalize the activity of female sex hormones. It is thus indicated for dysmenorrhea, premenstrual syndrome (PMS), and other disorders related to hormone function. It is especially beneficial during menopause. Similarly, it may help the body regain a natural balance after discontinuation of oral contraceptives.

The precise mechanisms of action of vitex and its active constituents have not been established. Laboratory research suggests that the herb acts on the anterior pituitary gland via a dopaminergic mechanism.[253] This leads to a reduction in release of the hormone prolactin, which in turn enhances corpus luteum development and corrects any relative progesterone deficiency. It is important to note that the effect of vitex on progesterone levels is indirect, as it works through the complexities of endocrine homeostasis rather than by directly stimulating progesterone release. However, the herb is thought to act on the pituitary-hypothalamic axis, rather than directly on the ovaries.

Vitex not only eases symptoms of PMS, but also, over time, may actually cure the disorder. PMS has been linked to abnormally high levels of estrogen, and vitex has proved especially helpful for cases in which symptoms tend to disappear when menstruation begins. Positive results may be perceived as early as the second menstrual cycle, but permanent improvement may take up to one year or longer.

Vitex is also effective for irregular menstruation, especially when related to endometriosis. In addition, because progesterone production declines at menopause, vitex may reduce some of the undesirable symptoms associated with "the change." Several studies indicate that vitex can help control acne in teenagers, both young women and men. The herb is also useful for stabilizing the menstrual cycle after withdrawal from progesterone-containing birth control pills. It may help with fibroid cysts that occur in smooth muscle tissue or in subserous areas, but is less likely to help with submucous cysts.

For women who are trying to get pregnant, vitex may effectively regulate the ovulatory cycle. Clinical research shows that vitex may start correcting imbalances after about 10 days, but for full benefit, it should be taken for three cycles or longer. Studies have documented that vitex has a galactagogue action, but chemical analysis of the breast milk revealed no changes in composition.[254] This may seem surprising, as the proposed mechanism of action of vitex involves a reduction of prolactin release. However, it is simply a good example of how the actual activity of a plant is more complex than what is demonstrated in specific laboratory tests.

Safety Considerations: Commission E lists no drug interactions for vitex. However, there is a theoretical possibility that the herb may interact with dopamine antagonists and dopamine-receptor-blocking agents.

Preparations and Dosage: Tincture dosage is 2.5 ml three times a day (1:5 in 60%). To make an infusion, pour 1 cup of boiling water over 1 teaspoon of berries and infuse for 10 to 15 minutes. This should be drunk three times a day.

Commission E recommends a daily dose of aqueous-alcoholic extracts corresponding to 30 to 40 mg of the herb. Alternatively, it recommends 175 mg/day of a 20:1 standardized fruit extract containing 0.5% agnuside. According to Commission E, health benefits are seen after 3 to 6 weeks of use; most women continue treatment for 3 to 6 months.

Chaste tree, in *Principles and Practice of Phytotherapy*

Zanthoxylum americanum Mill.
Prickly Ash
Rutaceae

Parts Used: Bark, berry

Constituents: Alkaloids, coumarins, resin, tannins, volatile oil[255]

Actions: Stimulant (circulatory), tonic, alterative, carminative, diaphoretic, antirheumatic, hepatic

Indications: Prickly ash may be used in similar ways to

cayenne, although its action is slower. It is appropriate for many chronic problems, such as rheumatism and skin diseases, and its stimulating actions upon the lymphatic system, circulation, and mucous membranes give it a role in the holistic treatment of many specific conditions.

Any sign of poor circulation calls for prickly ash, including chilblains, leg cramps, varicose veins, and varicose ulcers. Externally, it may be applied as a stimulating liniment for rheumatism and fibrositis.

Priest and Priest described prickly ash as a

> . . . positive diffusive stimulant—induces free arterial/capillary circulation, restores vascular tone. It is a general stimulant for relaxed and feeble conditions and atonic digestive states. An excellent tonic and alterative for convalescence and the elderly.

They gave the following specific indications: chronic rheumatic conditions, neurasthenia and poor circulation, gastric distension, eructations and flatulence, and loss of sensitivity in injured nerves.

Safety Considerations: Theoretically, prickly ash is contraindicated for patients on anticoagulant therapy.

Preparations and Dosage: Tincture dosage is 2 to 4 ml three times a day (1:5 in 60%). For an infusion, pour 1 cup of boiling water over 1 to 2 teaspoons of herb and infuse for 10 to 15 minutes. This should be drunk three times a day.

The BHP recommends 1 to 2 g dried bark or 2 to 5 ml tincture three times a day (1:5 in 45%).

Prickly Ash, Northern, and Prickly Ash, Southern, in *Herbal Medicines: A Guide for Health-Care Professionals*

Zea mays L.
Cornsilk
Poaceae

Part Used: Stigma from female flower (fine soft threads 4 to 8 inches long)

Constituents: Saponins; allantoin; sterols (especially β-sitosterol and stigmasterol); hordenine (an alkaloid); miscellaneous: vitamins C and K, cryptoxanthin, anthocyanins, plant acids[256]

Actions: Diuretic, demulcent, anti-inflammatory, tonic

Indications: As a soothing diuretic, cornsilk is beneficial for any irritation of the urinary system. It is used for renal problems in children and, combined with other herbs, as a urinary demulcent for cystitis, urethritis, prostatitis, and similar conditions.

Ellingwood recommended cornsilk for catarrhal cystitis, lithiasis (stones), bladder irritation, gonorrhea, all catarrhal conditions of the urinary passages, and dropsy (edema) due to heart disease.

Safety Considerations: No side effects or drug interactions have been reported.

Preparations and Dosage: Tincture dosage is 5 to 10 ml three times a day (1:5 in 25%). For an infusion, pour 1 cup of boiling water over 2 to 4 teaspoons of dried herb and infuse for 10 to 15 minutes. This should be drunk three times a day.

Dosage recommended in the BHC is 2 to 8 g dried herb, 5 to 15 ml tincture (1:5 in 25%), or 4 to 8 ml fluid extract (1:1 in 25%) three times daily.

Corn Silk, in *Herbal Medicines: A Guide for Health-Care Professionals*

Zingiber officinale Roscoe
Ginger
Zingiberaceae

Part Used: Rhizome

Constituents: Volatile oil (1% to 3%, occasionally more), primarily containing the sesquiterpenes zingiberene and β-bisabolene; oleoresin (4% to 10%), containing gingerols, gingerdiols, gingerdiones, dihydrogingerdiones, shogaols; lipids (6% to 8%)[257]

Actions: Stimulant, carminative, antispasmodic, rubefacient, diaphoretic, emmenagogue

Indications: The best-known therapeutic application of this spice is as a treatment for motion sickness, a use well documented in the research literature. Ginger also effectively stimulates peripheral circulation, making it effective for bad circulation, chilblains, and cramps. In feverish conditions, ginger acts as a useful diaphoretic, promoting perspiration. As a gargle, it helps relieve sore throats. Externally, it is the base of many treatments for fibrositis and muscle sprains.

Ginger has been used around the world as an aromatic carminative and pungent appetite stimulant. In India and other countries with hot and humid climates, ginger is eaten daily and is a well-known remedy for digestive problems. It is popular not only for its flavor, but also because its antioxidant and antimicrobial properties help to preserve food, an essential action in such climates.

Research has documented a wide range of activities for ginger. Clinical studies have shown that the herb is effective as a prophylactic against seasickness.[258,259] Animal studies have suggested that it has hypoglycemic, hypotensive, hypertensive, antihypercholesterolemic, cholagogic, and stomachic properties.[260] Human pharmacological studies have shown that ginger causes a reduction in platelet aggregation.[261] Ginger demonstrates anti-inflammatory effects in rheumatoid arthritis due to a dual inhibition of cyclooxygenase and lipoxygenase.[262] It has also shown an ability to inhibit the actions of prostaglandins.[263]

Safety Considerations: Ginger may influence bleeding times and immunological parameters because it inhibits thromboxane synthase and acts as a prostacyclin agonist. However, a clinical study demonstrated no differences in bleeding times between treatment and placebo groups.[264] Large doses (12 to 14 g) may enhance the effects of anticoagulant drugs. According to Commission E, ginger should not be used to alleviate the morning sickness of pregnancy.[265] However, there is a well-established tradition of such use. Traditional Chinese medicine tells us not to use more than 2 g of dried ginger daily during pregnancy.[266]

Preparations and Dosage: Tincture dose is 1.5 to 5 ml three times a day (1:5 in 40%). To make an infusion, pour 1 cup of boiling water over 1 teaspoon of fresh root and infuse for 5 minutes. Drink whenever needed. Fluid extract dosage is 0.25 to 1 ml three times a day (1:1 in 40%).

Ginger, in *Principles and Practice of Phytotherapy*

References

1. Wren RC. *Potter's New Cyclopedia of Botanical Drugs and Preparations*, 8th edition, revised by Williamson EM and Evans FJ. Essex, UK: C. W. Daniel Co., 1988.

2. Bruneton J. *Pharmacognosy, Phytochemistry, Medicinal Plants*. Paris: Lavoisier Publishing, 1995.

3. Bisset, ed. *Herbal Drugs and Phytopharmaceuticals*. Boca Raton, FL: CRC Press, 1994.

4. Newall C, Anderson L, Phillipson J. *Herbal Medicines: A Guide for Health-Care Professionals*. London: The Pharmaceutical Press, 1996.

5. Blumenthal M, et al. *The ABC Clinical Guide to Herbs*. Austin, TX: American Botanical Council, 2003.

6. Ibid.

7. Bisler H, Pfeifer R, Kluken N, Pauschinger P. Effects of horse-chestnut seed extract on transcapillary filtration in chronic venous insufficiency. *Deutsche Medizinische Wochenschrift* 1986; 111(35):1321–9.

8. Pittler MH, Ernst E. Horse chestnut seed extract for chronic venous insufficiency. *Archives of Dermatology* 1998; 134: 1356–60.

9. Wren RC. *Potter's New Cyclopedia of Botanical Drugs and Preparations*, 8th ed.

10. Ibid.

11. Patrascu V, et al. Rezultate terapeutice favorabile in porfiria cutanata cu Agrimonia eupatoria. *Dermato-venerologia* 1984; 29:153–7.

12. Petkov V. Bulgarian traditional medicine: A source of ideas for phytopharmacological investigations. *Journal of Ethnopharmacology* 1986; 15:121–32.

13. Chakarski I, et al. Clinical study of a herb combination consisting of Agrimonia eupatoria, Hypericum perforatum, Plantago major, Mentha piperita, Matricaria chamomila for the treatment of patients with chronic gastroduodenitis. *Probl Vatr Med* 1982; 10:78–84.

14. Wren RC. *Potter's New Cyclopedia of Botanical Drugs and Preparations*, 8th ed.

15. Blumenthal M, et al. *The ABC Clinical Guide to Herbs.*

16. Bordia A, Joshi HK, Sanadhya YK, Bhy N. Effect of essential oil of garlic on serum fibrinolytic activity in patients with coronary artery disease. *Atherosclerosis* 1978; 28:155–9.

17. German K, Kumar U, Blackford HN. Garlic and the risk of TURP bleeding. *British Journal of Urology* 1995; 76:518.

18. Burnham BE. Garlic as a possible risk of postoperative bleeding. *Plastic and Reconstructive Surgery* 1995; 95(1): 213.

19. Wren RC. *Potter's New Cyclopedia of Botanical Drugs and Preparations*, 8th ed.

20. Tomodo M, et al. Hypoglycaemic activity of twenty plant mucilages and three modified products. *Planta Medica* 1987; 53:812.

21. Recio MC, et al. Antimicrobial activity of selected plants employed in the Spanish Mediterranean area, part II. *Phytotherapy Research* 1989; 3:77–80.

22. Wren RC. *Potter's New Cyclopedia of Botanical Drugs and Preparations*, 8th ed.

23. Ibid.

24. Ibid.

25. Gijbels MJM, et al. Phthalides in roots of Apium graveolens, A. graveolens var. rapaceum, Bifora testiculata, and Petroselinum crispum var. tuberosum. *Fitoterapia* 1985; 56:17–23.

26. Kar A, Jain SR. Investigations on the antibacterial activity of some Indian indigenous aromatic plants. *Flavour Industry* 1971 Feb.

27. Berkley SF, et al. Dermatitis in grocery workers associated with high natural concentrations of furanocoumarins in celery. *Annals of Internal Medicine* 1986; 105:351–5.

28. Chaudhary SK, et al. Increased furocoumarin content of celery during storage. *Journal of Agricultural and Food Chemistry* 1985; 33:1153–7.

29. Wren RC. *Potter's New Cyclopedia of Botanical Drugs and Preparations*, 8th ed.

30. Bever BO, Zahnd GR. Plants with oral hypoglycaemic action. *Quarterly Journal of Crude Drug Research* 1979; 17:139–96.

31. Schulte KE, et al. Polyacetylenes in burdock root. *Arzneimittel-Forschung* 1967; 17:829–33.

32. Morita K, et al. Chemical nature of a desmutagenic factor from burdock (A. Lappa L.). *Agricultural and Biological Chemistry* 1985; 49:925–32.

33. Morita K, et al. Desmutagenic factor isolated from burdock (*Arctium lappa* L.). *Mutation Research* 1984; 129:25–31.

34. Dombradi CA, Foldeak S. Anti-tumor activity of A. lappa ext. *Tumori* 1966; 52:173–5.

35. Tsujita J, et al. Comparison of protective activity of dietary fiber against the toxicities of various food colors in rats. *Nutrition Reports International* 1979; 20:635–42.

36. Wren RC. *Potter's New Cyclopedia of Botanical Drugs and Preparations*, 8th ed.

37. Ibid.

38. Ibid.

39. Rao VSN, Menezes Ams, Gadelha MGT. Antifertility screening of some indigenous plants of Brasil. *Fitoterapia* 1988; 59:17–20.

40. Pinto-Scognamiglio W. Connaissances actuelles sur l'activité pharmacodynamique de la thuyone, aromitisant naturel d'un emploi étendu. *Bollettino Chimico Farmaceutico* 1967; 106:292–300.

41. Wren RC. *Potter's New Cyclopedia of Botanical Drugs and Preparations*, 8th ed.

42. Ibid.

43. Costello CH, Butler CL. The estrogenic and uterine-stimulating activity of Asclepius tuberosa. *Journal of American Pharmaceutical Association Science Education* 1949; 39:233–7.

44. Mills S, Bone K. *Principles and Practice of Phytotherapy: Modern Herbal Medicine*. Edinburgh: Churchill Livingstone, 1999.

45. [No authors listed] Astragalus membranaceus. Monograph. *Alternative Medicine Review* 2003 Feb; 8(1):72–7.

46. Chang HM, But PPH. *Pharmacology and Applications of Chinese Materia Medica*, vol. 2. Hong Kong: World Scientific, 1987.

47. Chu, et al. Fractioned extract of Astragalus membranaceous, a Chinese medicinal herb, potentiates LAK cell cytotoxicity generated by a low dose of recombinant interleukin-2. *Journal of Clinical and Laboratory Immunology* 1988; 26:183–7.

48. Zhang, et al. Hepatoprotective effects of Astragalus root. *Journal of Ethnopharmacology* 1990; 30:149–54.

49. DeSmet PAGM, D'Arcy PF. Drug interactions with herbal and other non-orthodox remedies. In: D'Arcy PF, McElnay JC, Welling PG, eds. *Mechanisms of Drug Interactions.* New York: Springer-Verlag, 1996.

50. Wren RC. *Potter's New Cyclopedia of Botanical Drugs and Preparations*, 8th ed.

51. Ibid.

52. Ibid.

53. Ibid.

54. Ibid.

55. Ibid.

56. Ibid.

57. Boucard-Maitre Y, et al. Cytotoxic and antitumoral activity of Calendula officinalis extracts. *Pharmazie* 1988; 43:220.

58. Kioucek-Popova E, et al. Influence of the physiological regeneration and epithelization using fractions isolated from Calendula officinalis. *Acta Physiologica et Pharmacologica Bulgarica* 1982; 8:63–7.

59. Manolov P, Boyadzhiev Tsv, Nokolov P. Antitumorigenic effect of preparations of Calendula officinalis on Crocker sarcoma 180. *Eksperimentalna Meditsin Morfologiia* 1964; 3:41–5

60. Avramova S, Portarska F, Apostolova B, et al. Marigold (of Calendula officinalis L.) Source of new products for the cosmetic industry. *Medical Biology Information* 1988; 4:28–32.

61. Wren RC. *Potter's New Cyclopedia of Botanical Drugs and Preparations*, 8th ed.

62. Blumenthal M, et al. *The ABC Clinical Guide to Herbs.*

63. Bernstein JE, Parish LC, Rapaport M, et al. Effects of topically applied capsaicin on moderate and severe psoriasis vulgaris. *Journal of the American Academy of Dermatology* 1986; 15:504–7.

64. Scheffler NM, Sheitel PL, Lipton MN. Treatment of painful diabetic neuropathy with capsaicin 0.075 percent. *Journal of the American Podiatric Medical Association* 1991; 81(6):288–93.

65. Partsch G, Matucci-Cerinic M. Effect of capsaicin on the release of substance P from rheumatoid arthritis and osteoarthritis synoviocytes in vitro. *Annals of the Rheumatic Diseases* 1990; 49(8):65–73.

66. Wren RC. *Potter's New Cyclopedia of Botanical Drugs and Preparations*, 8th ed.

67. Ibid.

68. Ibid.

69. Ibid.

70. Ibid.

71. Ibid.

72. Blumenthal M, et al. *The ABC Clinical Guide to Herbs.*

73. Liske E. Therapeutic efficacy and safety of Cimicifuga racemosa for gynecological disorders. *Advances in Therapy* 1998; 15:45–53.

74. Wren RC. *Potter's New Cyclopedia of Botanical Drugs and Preparations*, 8th ed.

75. Ibid.

76. Ibid.

77. Tariq M, et al. Anti-inflammatory activity of Commiphora molmol. *Agents and Actions* 1986; 17:381–2.

78. Al-Awadi FM, et al. On the mechanism of the hypoglycaemic effect of a plant extract. *Diabetologia* 1985; 28:432–4.

79. Blumenthal M, et al. *The ABC Clinical Guide to Herbs.*

80. Wren RC. *Potter's New Cyclopedia of Botanical Drugs and Preparations*, 8th ed.

81. Ibid.

82. Ibid.

83. Vichkanova SA, et al. Chemotherapeutic properties of plumbagin. In: Aizenman BE, Fitontsidy Mater Soveshch, eds. Kiev: Naukova Dumka, 6th edition, 1969, 1972; 183–5.

84. Blumenthal M, et al. *The ABC Clinical Guide to Herbs.* Austin, TX: American Botanical Council, 2003.

85. Stoll A, Renz J, Brack A. *Helvetica Chimica Acta* 1950; 33:1877–93.

86. Samochowiec E, Urbanska L, Manka W, et al. *Wiadomosci Parazytologiczne* 1979; 25:77–81.

87. Facino RM, Carini M, Aldini G, et al. Echinacoside and caffeoyl conjugates protect collagen from free radical–induced degradation: potential use of Echinacea extracts in the prevention of skin photodamage. *Planta Medica* 1995; 61(6):510–4.

88. Bauer R, Wagner H. Echinacea species as potential immunostimulatory drugs. In: Farnsworth NR, et al., eds. *Economic and Medicinal Plant Research*, vol. 5. London: Academic Press, 1991.

89. Melchart D, Linde K, Worku E, et al. Immunomodulation with Echinacea—a systematic review of controlled clinical trials. *Phytomedicine* 1994; 1:245–54.

90. Mills S, Bone K. *Principles and Practice of Phytotherapy: Modern Herbal Medicine.*

91. Blumenthal M, et al. *The ABC Clinical Guide to Herbs.*

92. McCaleb R, Leigh E, Morien K. *The Encyclopedia of Popular Herbs.* Roseville, CA: Prima Health, 1999.

93. Fugh-Berman A. Herb–drug interactions. *Lancet* 2000; 335:134–8.

94. Wren RC. *Potter's New Cyclopedia of Botanical Drugs and Preparations*, 8th ed.

95. Blumenthal M, et al. *The ABC Clinical Guide to Herbs.*

96. Evans WC. *Pharmacognosy*, 13th ed. London: Baillere Tindall, 1989.

97. European Scientific Cooperative on Phytotherapy. *ESCOP Monographs on the Medicinal Uses of Plant Drugs.* Exeter, UK: ESCOP, 1997, 1999.

98. World Health Organization. *WHO Monographs on Selected Medicinal Plants*, vol. 1. Geneva: WHO, 1999.

99. Wren RC. *Potter's New Cyclopedia of Botanical Drugs and Preparations*, 8th ed.

100. Ibid.

101. Ibid.

102. Shaparenko, et al. On use of medicinal plants for treatment of patients with chronic suppurative otitis. *Zhurnal ushnykh, nosovykh i gorlovykh boleznei (Journal of Otology, Rhinology, and Laryngologie)* 1979; 39:48–51.

103. Wren RC. *Potter's New Cyclopedia of Botanical Drugs and Preparations*, 8th ed.

104. Ibid.

105. Wagner H. Immunostimulants from Medicinal Plants. In: Chang HM, et al. *Advances in Chinese Medicinal Materials Research.* Singapore: World Scientific, 1985; 159–70.

106. Wagner H, et al. Immunostimulating polysaccharides (heteroglycans) of higher plants. *Arzneimittel-Forschung* 1985; 35:1069.

107. Wren RC. *Potter's New Cyclopedia of Botanical Drugs and Preparations*, 8th ed.

108. Ibid.

109. Ibid.

110. Ibid.

111. Ibid.

112. DeSmet PAGM, et al. Kelp in herbal medicines: hyper-thyroidism. *Nedertands Tidschrift voor Geneeskunde* 1990; 134:1058–9.

113. Norman JA, et al. Human intake of arsenic and iodine from seaweed-based food supplements and health foods available in the UK. *Food Additives and Contaminants* 1987; 5:103–9.

114. Wren RC. *Potter's New Cyclopedia of Botanical Drugs and Preparations*, 8th ed.

115. Ibid.

116. Ibid.

117. Ibid.

118. Ibid.

119. Blumenthal M, et al. *The ABC Clinical Guide to Herbs.*

120. Kriegistein J. Neuroprotective properties of Ginkgo biloba constituents. *Zeit. Phytother* 1994; 15:92–6.

121. Kleijnen J, Knipschild P. Ginkgo biloba. *Lancet* 1992; 1136–9.

122. Ibid. Ginkgo biloba for cerebral insufficiency. *British Journal of Clinical Pharmacology* 1992; 34:352–8.

123. Rosenblatt M, Mindel J. Spontaneous hyphema associated with ingestion of Ginkgo biloba extract. *The New England Journal of Medicine* 1997; 336(15):1108.

124. Sikora R, Sohn M, Deutz FJ, et al. Ginkgo biloba extract in the therapy of erectile dysfunction. *The Journal of Urology* 1989; 141:188A.

125. Blumenthal M, et al. *The ABC Clinical Guide to Herbs.*

126. Paolini M, Pozzetti L, Sapone A, Cantelli-Forti G. Effect of licorice and glycyrrhizin on murine liver CYP-dependent monooxygenases. *Life Sciences* 1998; 62(6):571–82.

127. Pompei R, Flore O, Marccialis MA, et al. Glycyrrhizic acid inhibits virus growth and inactivates virus particles. *Nature* 1979 Oct 25; 281(5733):689–90.

128. World Health Organization. *WHO Monographs on Selected Medicinal Plants*, vol. 1. Geneva: WHO, 1999.

129. Wren RC. *Potter's New Cyclopedia of Botanical Drugs and Preparations*, 8th ed.

130. Ibid.

131. Ibid.

132. Ibid.

133. European Scientific Cooperative on Phytotherapy. *ESCOP Monographs on the Medicinal Uses of Plant Drugs.* Exeter, UK: ESCOP, 1997, 1999.

134. Wren RC. *Potter's New Cyclopedia of Botanical Drugs and Preparations*, 8th ed.

135. Wohlfart R, et al. The sedative-hypnotic principle of

hops. Communication: Pharmacology of 2-methyl-3-buten-2-ol. *Planta Medica* 1983; 48:120–3.

136. Chakarski I, et al. Clinical study of a herb combination consisting of Humulus lupulus, Cichorium intybus, Mentha piperita in patients with chronic calculous and non-calculous cholecystitis. *Probl Vatr Med* 1982; 10:65–9.

137. Wren RC. *Potter's New Cyclopedia of Botanical Drugs and Preparations*, 8th ed.

138. Blumenthal M, et al. *The ABC Clinical Guide to Herbs*.

139. Pizzorno JE, Murray MT. Hydrastis canadensis, Berberis vulgaris, Berberis aquifolium and other berberine-containing plants. In: *Textbook of Natural Medicine*. Seattle: John Bastyr College Publications, 1985.

140. Mills S, Bone K. *Principles and Practice of Phytotherapy: Modern Herbal Medicine*.

141. Blumenthal M, et al. *The ABC Clinical Guide to Herbs*.

142. Harrer G, Schulz V. On the clinical investigation of the antidepressant effectiveness of Hypericum. *Nervenheilkunde* 1993 Oct; 12:271–3.

143. Muller WE, Rolli M, Schafer C, Hafner U. Effects of hypericum extract (LI 160) in biochemical models of antidepressant activity. *Pharmacopsychiatry* 1997; 30(suppl):102–7.

144. Siegers CP, Biel S, Wilhem KP. Zur Frage der Phototoxiztat von Hypericum. *Nervenheilkunde* 1993; 12:320–2.

145. James JS. Hypericin. *AIDS Treatment News* 1992 Feb; 146:1–4.

146. Siegers CP, Biel S, Wilhelm KP. *Nervenheilkunde* 1993; 12:320–2.

147. Roby CA, Anderson GD, Kantor Ga, et al. St. John's wort: Effect on CYP3A4 activity. *Clinical Pharmacology and Therapeutics* 2000; 67:451–7.

148. Wren RC. *Potter's New Cyclopedia of Botanical Drugs and Preparations*, 8th ed.

149. Ibid.

150. Ibid.

151. Ibid.

152. Markkanen T, et al. Antiherpetic agent from juniper tree (Juniperus communis), its purification, identification, and testing in primary human amnion cell cultures. *Drugs under Experimental and Clinical Research* 1981; 7:691–7.

153. Wren RC. *Potter's New Cyclopedia of Botanical Drugs and Preparations*, 8th ed.

154. Ibid.

155. Ibid.

156. Kong YC, et al. Isolation of the uterotonic principle from Leonurus sibirica, the Chinese motherwort. *American Journal of Chinese Medicine* 1976; 4:373-82.

157. Wren RC. *Potter's New Cyclopedia of Botanical Drugs and Preparations*, 8th ed.

158. Ibid.

159. Ibid.

160. Ibid.

161. Ibid.

162. Ibid.

163. Blumenthal M, et al. *The ABC Clinical Guide to Herbs*.

164. Wren RC. *Potter's New Cyclopedia of Botanical Drugs and Preparations*, 8th ed.

165. Ibid.

166. Ibid.

167. Sullivan JB, et al. Pennyroyal oil poisoning and hepatotoxicity. *The Journal of the American Medical Association* 1979; 1242:2873.

168. Blumenthal M, et al. *The ABC Clinical Guide to Herbs*.

169. Wren RC. *Potter's New Cyclopedia of Botanical Drugs and Preparations*, 8th ed.

170. Todd RG, ed. *Martindale: The Extra Pharmacopoeia*, 25th ed. London: Pharmaceutical Press, 1967.

171. Wren RC. *Potter's New Cyclopedia of Botanical Drugs and Preparations*, 8th ed.

172. Ibid.

173. Ibid.

174. Ibid.

175. Ibid.

176. Ibid.

177. Ibid.

178. Ibid.

179. Borgia M, et al. Pharmacological activity of an herb extract: A controlled clinical study. *Current Therapeutic Research* 198 1; 29: 525–36.

180. Wren RC. *Potter's New Cyclopedia of Botanical Drugs and Preparations*, 8th ed.

181. Ibid.

182. Blumenthal M, et al. *The ABC Clinical Guide to Herbs*.

183. Kinzler E, Kromer J, Lehmann E. Effect of a special kava extract in patients with anxiety-, tension-, and excitation states of non-psychotic genesis. Double-blind study with placebos over 4 weeks. *Arzneimittel-Forschung* 1991; 41:584–8.

184. Volz HP, Kieser M. Kava-kava extract WS 1490 versus placebo in anxiety disorders, a randomized placebo-controlled 25-week outpatient trial. *Pharmacopsychiatry* 1997; 30:1–5.

185. Jamieson DD, Duffield PH. The antinocioceptive actions of kava components in mice. *Clinical and Experimental Pharmacology and Physiology* 1990; 17:495–507.

186. Keller F, Klohs MW. A review of the chemistry and pharmacology of the constituents of Piper methysticum. *Lloydia* 1963; 26:1–15.

187. Schelosky L, Raffauf C, Jendroska K, et al. Kava and dopamine antagonism. *Journal of Neurology, Neurosurgery, and Psychiatry* 1995; 58(5):639–40.

188. Wren RC. *Potter's New Cyclopedia of Botanical Drugs and Preparations*, 8th ed.

189. Ibid.

190. Ibid.

191. Ibid.

192. Ibid.

193. Ibid.

194. Ibid.

195. Pilcher JM, et al. The action of "female remedies" on intact uteri of animals. *Surgery, Gynecology, & Obstetrics* 1918; 18:97–9.

196. Martin ML, et al. Pharmacological effects of lactones isolated from Pulsatilla alpina subsp. apiffolia. *Journal of Ethnopharmacology* 1988; 24:185–91.

197. Wren RC. *Potter's New Cyclopedia of Botanical Drugs and Preparations*, 8th ed.

198. Ibid.

199. World Health Organization. *WHO Monographs on Selected Medicinal Plants*, vol. 1. Geneva: WHO, 1999.

200. Wren RC. *Potter's New Cyclopedia of Botanical Drugs and Preparations*, 8th ed.

201. Ibid.

202. Ibid.

203. Ibid.

204. Ibid.

205. Ibid.

206. Ibid.

207. Ibid.

208. Vivian B, Tal H, Inna K. The effect of Sambucol, a black elderberry-based, natural product, on the production of human cytokines: I. Inflammatory cytokines. *European Cytokine Network* 2001 Apr; 12(2):290.

209. Serkedjieva J, et al. Antiviral activity of the infusion (SHS174) from flowers of Sambucus nigra L., aerial parts of Hypericum perforatum L., and roots of Saponaria officinalis L. against influenza and herpes simplex viruses. *Phytotherapy Research* 1990; 4:97.

210. Wren RC. *Potter's New Cyclopedia of Botanical Drugs and Preparations*, 8th ed.

211. Godowski KC. Antimicrobial action of sanguinarine. *The Journal of Clinical Dentistry* 1989; 1:96–101.

212. Wren RC. *Potter's New Cyclopedia of Botanical Drugs and Preparations*, 8th ed.

213. Ibid.

214. Wolfson P, Hoffmann DL. An investigation into the efficacy of Scutellaria lateriflora in healthy volunteers. *Alternative Therapies in Health and Medicine* 2003 Mar–Apr; 9(2):74–8.

215. Wren RC. *Potter's New Cyclopedia of Botanical Drugs and Preparations*, 8th ed.

216. Blumenthal M, et al. *The ABC Clinical Guide to Herbs*.

217. Rhodes L, Prinika RL, Berman C, et al. Comparison of finasteride (Proscar), a 5a-reductase inhibitor, and various commercial plant extracts in vitro and in vivo 5a-reductase inhibition. *The Prostate* 1993; 22:43–51.

218. Caaroj C, Raynaud JP, Koch G, et al. Comparison of phytotherapy (Permixon) with finasteride in the treatment of benign prostate hyperplasia: a randomized international study of 1,098 patients. *The Prostate* 1996; 29:231–40.

219. Blumenthal M, et al. *The ABC Clinical Guide to Herbs*.

220. McCaleb R, Leigh E, Morien K. *The Encyclopedia of Popular Herbs*. Roseville, CA: Prima Health, 1999.

221. Palasciano G, Portincasa P, Palmieri V, et al. The effect of silymarin on plasma levels of malon-dialdehyde in patients receiving long-term treatment with psychotropic drugs. *Current Therapeutic Research* 1994; 55:537–45.

222. Fintelmann V. Toxic metabolic liver damage and its treatment. *Zeitschrift fur Phytotherapie* 1986; (3):65–73.

223. Wren RC. *Potter's New Cyclopedia of Botanical Drugs and Preparations*, 8th ed.

224. Ibid.

225. Ibid.

226. Ibid.

227. Ibid.

228. Ibid.

229. Blumenthal M, et al. *The ABC Clinical Guide to Herbs*.

230. Bisset, ed. *Herbal Drugs and Phytopharmaceuticals*.

231. Racz-Kotilla, et al. The action of Taraxacum officinale extracts on the body weight and diuresis of laboratory animals. *Planta Medica* 1974; 26:212–7.

232. Vogel G. Natural substances with effects on the liver. In: Wagner H, Wolff P, eds. *New Natural Products and Plant Drugs with Pharmacological, Biological or Therapeutic Activity*. Heidelberg: Springer-Verlag, 1977.

233. Bisset, ed. *Herbal Drugs and Phytopharmaceuticals*.

234. Wren RC. *Potter's New Cyclopedia of Botanical Drugs and Preparations*, 8th ed.

235. Ibid.

236. Ibid.

237. Ibid.

238. Ibid.

239. Ibid.

240. Ibid.

241. Chrubasik, et al. Evidence for antirheumatic effectiveness of Herba Urtica dioicae in acute arthritis: a pilot study. *Phytomedicine* 1997; 4(2):105–8.

242. Oliver-Bever B, Zahland GR. Plants with oral hypoglycaemic activity. *Quarterly Journal of Crude Drug Research* 1979; 17:139–96.

243. Sokeland J, Albrecht J. A combination of Sabal and Urtica extract vs. finasteride in BPH. *Urologie A* 1997; 36(4):327–33.

244. Blumenthal M, et al. *The ABC Clinical Guide to Herbs*.

245. Wren RC. *Potter's New Cyclopedia of Botanical Drugs and Preparations*, 8th ed.

246. Ibid.

247. Ibid.

248. Bisset, ed. *Herbal Drugs and Phytopharmaceuticals*.

249. Wren RC. *Potter's New Cyclopedia of Botanical Drugs and Preparations*, 8th ed.

250. Ibid.

251. Ibid.

252. Blumenthal M, et al. *The ABC Clinical Guide to Herbs*.

253. Mills S, Bone K. *Principles and Practice of Phytotherapy: Modern Herbal Medicine*.

254. Amann W. Amenorrhoe. Gfinstige wirkung von Agnus castus (Agnolyt®) auf amenorrhoea. *Z Allg Med* 1982; 58:228–31.

255. Wren RC. *Potter's New Cyclopedia of Botanical Drugs and Preparations*, 8th ed.

256. Ibid.

257. Blumenthal M, et al. *The ABC Clinical Guide to Herbs*.

258. Grontved A, et al. Ginger root against seasickness. A controlled trial on the open sea. *Acta Oto-laryngologica* 1988; 105:45–9.

259. Mowrey DB, Clayson DE. Motion sickness, ginger, and psychophysics. *Lancet* 1982 Mar 20; 1(8273):655–7.

260. Newall, C, Anderson L, Phillipson J. *Herbal Medicines: A Guide for Health-Care Professionals*.

261. Srivastava KC. Effect of onion and ginger consumption on platelet thromboxane production in humans. *Prostaglandins, Leukotrienes, and Essential Fatty Acids* 1989; 35:183–5.

262. Srivastava K, et al. Ginger and rheumatic disorders. *Medical Hypotheses* 1989; 29:25–8.

263. Lumb AB. Effect of ginger on human platelet function. *Thrombosis and Haemostasis* 1994; 71:110–1.

264. Ibid.

265. Blumenthal M, et al. *The ABC Clinical Guide to Herbs*.

266. Bensky D, Gamble A. *Chinese Herbal Medicine Materia Medica*. Seattle: Eastland Press, 1986.

Appendix 1

❧

GLOSSARY

abortifacient: Induces abortion or miscarriage.

abscess: A localized collection of pus and liquefied tissue in a cavity.

absolute: A highly concentrated viscous, semisolid, or solid perfume material, usually obtained by alcohol extraction from the concrete.

acetylcholine: A neurotransmitter. Its effects include cardiac inhibition and increase in blood vessel diameter.

achlorhydria: Absence of hydrochloric acid in the stomach.

acid: A compound producing hydrogen ions in aqueous solution. *Acidic* refers to a pH below 7.0.

acidosis: Abnormal state of reduced alkalinity of blood and tissues.

acrid: Leaving a burning sensation in the mouth.

ACTH: *See* adrenocorticotropic hormone.

acupressure: Manual application of pressure at points where acupuncture needles would be inserted.

acupuncture: Chinese practice that involves insertion of needles into body at specific points along meridians to treat disease and reduce pain.

acute: Designating disease with rapid onset, severe symptoms, and brief duration; opposite of *chronic*.

acute abdomen: Emergency condition caused by damage to one or more abdominal organs that results in intense pain and shock.

adaptogen: An herb that increases resistance and resilience to stress, enabling the body to avoid reaching collapse because it can adapt around the problem.

adenoma: An ordinarily benign (nonmalignant) tumor of skin tissue.

Addison's disease: Condition marked by weakness, low blood pressure, and dark pigmentation due to inadequate hormone secretion by adrenal glands.

adenitis: Regional inflammation of gland or lymph node.

adenocarcinoma: Malignant epithelial tumor in glandular pattern.

ADH: *See* antidiuretic hormone.

adhesion: Union by fibrous connective tissue of two normally separate parts.

adipose: Fat in connective tissue.

adjuvant: Any substance that enhances the immune-stimulating properties of an antigen or the pharmacological effect of a drug.

adjuvant chemotherapy: One or more anticancer drugs used in combination with surgery or radiation therapy as part of the treatment of cancer. *Adjuvant* usually means "in addition to" initial treatment.

administration: This term refers to how a drug is taken.

adrenaline: Hormone secreted by the adrenal gland, which produces the "fight-or-flight" response. Also called epinephrine.

adrenergic: Compound that acts like epinephrine or norepinephrine.

adrenocorticotropic hormone (ACTH): Polypeptide secreted by anterior pituitary that stimulates the adrenal cortex to secrete cortisol.

adverse drug reaction (ADR): Defined by the WHO as "any response to a drug which is noxious and unintended, and which occurs at doses used in man for prophylaxis, diagnosis, or therapy."

aerophagy: Swallowing of air.

aflatoxin: A toxic chemical produced by the *Aspergillus flavus* and *A. parasiticus* molds.

agar: Polysaccharide derived from seaweed, used as culture medium for microorganisms; gelatinous natural laxative.

agglutinin: Substance, especially antibody, that causes bacteria, blood cells, and antigens to clump.

agonist: A drug that both binds to receptors and has an intrinsic effect.

agranulocytosis: Acute illness caused by chemicals or drug reaction in which certain white blood cells disappear, causing rapid, massive infection.

ague: Malaria; general malaise marked by fever.

AIDS: Acquired immune deficiency syndrome; severe weakening or destruction of body's immune system by human immunodeficiency virus.

AIDS-related complex arc: Chronic enlargement of lymph nodes and persistent fever caused by AIDS virus.

albumin: Most abundant protein found in blood plasma.

albuminuria: Presence of the protein albumin in urine.

aldosterone: A hormone secreted by the zona glomerulosa of the adrenal gland, which causes the retention of sodium and the secretion of potassium.

alga: Unicellular organism distinguished from plants by having no true root stem.

alkaline phosphatase: A blood enzyme measurement that indicates the health of the liver.

alkaline: Solution having a pH above 7.0.

alkaloids: A large, varied group of nitrogen-containing compounds found in plants. Often alkaline, they react with acids to form soluble salts, many of which are physiologically active.

alkalosis: Abnormal state of increased alkalinity of blood and tissues.

allelochemicals: Chemicals involved in interspecific communication.

allelopathy: Chemical interaction between species at all levels of complexity, from microorganisms to higher plants, inextricably interwoven into ecological phenomena.

allergen: Any substance that comes into contact with body tissue (by skin absorption, ingestion, or inhalation) and causes a specific reaction within the bloodstream.

allergy: Hypersensitivity to a particular substance or antigen, such as pollen, fur, feathers, mold, dust, drugs, dyes, cosmetics, or food, causing characteristic symptoms when encountered, ingested, or inhaled.

alliaceous: Garlic- or onionlike.

allogenic transplant: Transfer of bone marrow from one person to another.

alopecia: Absence of hair from an area where it normally grows, especially progressive hair loss in men; baldness.

alterative: Herbs that gradually restore proper functioning of the body, increasing health and vitality. Some alteratives support natural waste elimination via the kidneys, liver, lungs, or skin. Others stimulate digestive function or are antimicrobial.

Alzheimer's disease: Progressive dementia and brain degeneration.

amebiasis: Infection with or disease caused by an amoeba.

amebic dysentery: Severe dysentery caused by protozoan amoebas.

amenorrhea: Absence or cessation of menstruation due to a congenital defect, hormonal deficiency, hypothalamus disorder, or emotional problem.

amino acid: Any of 25 organic acids containing an amino group that link into polypeptide chains to form proteins.

amoebicidal: A substance with the power to destroy amoebas.

amphoteric: Having the ability to act as either an acid or a base.

amylase: Enzyme that breaks down starch into disaccharides.

anabolism: Constructive metabolism in which food is changed into living tissue.

analgesic: A substance that reduces the sensation of pain.

analog (analogue): A chemical compound with a structure similar to that of another but differing from it in respect to a certain component; it may have a similar or opposite action metabolically.

anaphrodisiac: Reduces sexual desire.

anaphylaxis: Acute, allergic reaction to a substance to which a person has been previously sensitized, resulting in faintness, palpitations, loss of color, difficulty in breathing, and shock.

androgen: Any substance that produces masculinization, such as testosterone.

anemia: Reduced hemoglobin in blood, causing fatigue, breathlessness, and pallor.

anesthetic: Agent that diminishes or abolishes sensation and can produce unconsciousness.

aneurysm: Balloonlike swelling of an arterial wall.

angina: Feeling of suffocation; chest pain.

angina pectoris: A suffocating pain (angina) of the chest (pectoris). Angina is a result of the oxygen demands of the heart not being met.

angiosperm: Flowering plant.

angiotensin-converting enzyme (ACE): ACE converts angiotensin I to a biologically active form, angiotensin II. ACE inhibitors are used to combat hypertension.

annual: Plant with life cycle of one year or season.

anodyne: Substance that soothes or relieves pain.

anodynia: Absence of pain.

anorexia: Loss of appetite.

anorexia nervosa: Extreme loss of appetite, especially in adolescent females, causing severe weight loss and starvation.

anoxia: Condition in which body tissues receive inadequate oxygen.

anorexiant: A drug or substance that leads to anorexia or diminished appetite; appetite suppressant.

antacid: A substance that neutralizes acid.

antagonism: The joint effect of two or more drugs such that the combined effect is less than the sum of the effects produced by each agent separately. The *agonist* is the agent producing the effect that is diminished by the administration of the *antagonist*.

antagonist: A drug that impedes the action of another chemical substance in the body.

anthelmintic: A vermifuge, destroying or expelling intestinal worms.

anther: Part of the stamen that produces and releases pollen.

anthocyanidin: A particular class of flavonoids that gives plants, fruits, and flowers colors ranging from red to blue.

anthraquinone: Glycoside compound that produces dyes and purgatives.

antianemic: An agent that combats anemia.

antiarthritic: An agent that combats arthritis.

antibacterial: A substance that stops or checks the growth of bacteria.

antibiotic: A drug that kills microorganisms.

antibody: Protein manufactured by lymphocytes that reacts with a specific antigen to fight invasion as the principal component of immunity.

anticatarrhal: Anticatarrhals help the body remove excess mucus, whether in the sinus area or in other parts of the body.

anticoagulant: Agent that prevents blood from clotting.

anticonvulsant: Helps arrest or prevent convulsions.

antidepressant: Helps alleviate depression.

antidiarrheal: Efficacious against diarrhea.

antidiuretic hormone: ADH; peptide hormone synthesized in the hypothalamus and released from the posterior pituitary, causing retention of more water in body.

antidote: A substance that counteracts the effects of a poison.

antiemetic: An agent that reduces the incidence and severity of nausea or vomiting.

antifungal: A substance that inhibits the growth or multiplication of fungi.

antigen: Any substance or microorganism that, when introduced into the body, causes the formation of antibodies against it.

antihemorrhagic: An agent that prevents or combats hemorrhage or bleeding.

antihepatotoxic: Protects liver cells from chemical damage.

antihistamine: A chemical that blocks action of histamine.

antihypertensive: Blood pressure–lowering effect.

anti-inflammatory: Soothes inflammations or reduces the inflammation of the tissue directly.

antilithic: Prevents the formation of a calculus or stone.

antimicrobial: Antimicrobials help the body destroy or resist pathogenic microorganisms. They help the body strengthen its own resistance to infective organisms and throw off the illness.

antineuralgic: Relieves or reduces nerve pain.

antioxidant: A compound that prevents free radical or oxidative damage.

antiphlogistic: Checks or counteracts inflammation.

antipruritic: Relieves sensation of itching or prevents its occurrence.

antiputrescent: An agent that prevents and combats decay or putrefaction.

antipyretic: Reduces fever; *see also* febrifuge.

antiretroviral: A substance that stops or suppresses the activity of a retrovirus such as HIV.

antirheumatic: Helps prevent and relieve rheumatism.

antisclerotic: Helps prevent the hardening of tissue.

antiscorbutic: A remedy for scurvy.

antiseborrheic: Helps control the production of sebum, the oily secretion from sweat glands.

antiseptic: Destroys and prevents the development of microbes.

antispasmodic: Substance that relieves smooth muscle spasms.

antitoxic: An antidote or treatment that counteracts the effects of poison.

antitumor: A substance that prevents or is effective against tumors.

antitussive: Substance that reduces coughing, especially one that affects activity in the brain's cough center and depresses respiration.

antiviral: Substance that inhibits the growth of a virus.

anxiety: An unpleasant emotional state ranging from mild unease to intense fear.

aperient: A mild laxative.

aperitif: Stimulant of the appetite.

aphonia: Loss of voice.

aphrodisiac: Increases or stimulates sexual desire.

apnea: Temporary cessation of breathing.

apoplexy: Sudden loss of consciousness, a stroke, or sudden severe hemorrhage.

appendicitis: Acute inflammation of vermiform appendix.

application: Medication, remedy, or antiseptic placed externally on body part, as in a compress.

arbovirus: RNA-containing virus that can cause disease when transmitted from animals to humans by insects.

ARC: AIDS-related complex.

aril: The husk or membrane covering the seed of a plant.

aromatherapy: The therapeutic use of essential oils.

aromatic: A substance with a strong aroma or smell.

arrhythmia: Irregularity or deviation from normal rhythm or force of heartbeat.

arteriole: Microscopic blood vessel that connects the smallest arteries with the capillary beds. Arterioles together with the smaller arteries make up the resistance vessels.

arteriosclerosis: Deposit of cholesterol on artery walls; hardening of the arteries.

artery: A blood vessel that carries oxygen-rich blood away from the heart.

arthritis: Inflammation of joints.

asbestosis: A lung disease caused by inhalation of asbestos fibers, sometimes leading to lung cancer.

asepsis: Complete absence of disease-causing bacteria, viruses, fungi, and microorganisms.

aspergillosis: A disease caused by a fungus. It can cause lesions of the skin, ear, orbit, nasal sinuses, lungs, and sometimes the bones, meninges, heart, kidneys, or spleen. Symptoms include fever, chills, difficulty breathing, and coughing up blood. If the infection reaches the brain, it may cause dementia.

assay: A test.

asthenia: *See* debility.

asthma: Paroxysmal attacks of bronchial spasms that cause difficulty in breathing, often hereditary; bronchial asthma.

astigmatism: Distortion of visual images due to failure of the retina to focus light.

asymptomatic: Showing no evidence of a disease.

asystole: Absence of contraction (systole). Asystole is when the heart has stopped beating.

ataxia: Shaky movements and unsteady gait when brain fails to regulate posture or direction of limb movements.

atherogenic: Having the capacity to start or accelerate the process of atherogenesis or the formation of lipid deposits in the arteries.

atheroma: Degeneration of artery walls due to fatty plaques and scar tissue; common form of arteriosclerosis, atherosclerosis.

atherosclerosis: A process in which fatty substances (cholesterol and triglycerides) are deposited in the walls of medium to large arteries, eventually leading to blockage of the artery.

atony: Lessening or lack of muscular tone or tension.

atopy: A predisposition to various allergic conditions including eczema and asthma.

atrial fibrillation: Rapid irregular twitchings of the wall of an atrium (chamber) of the heart.

atrium: One of the upper chambers of the heart. Blood returning to the heart is stored in the atria before being ejected into the ventricles.

arthralgia: Severe joint pain.

atrophy: Wasting away of normally developed organ or tissue due to degeneration of cells.

attrition: Normal wearing away of surface of teeth.

autoimmune: Designating a disorder of the body's defense mechanism in which antibodies are produced against the body's own tissue, treating it as a foreign substance.

autoimmune disease: Disorder that permits destruction of tissue by the body's own antibodies.

autologous: Derived from the same individual or organism.

autonomic: Occurring involuntarily, controlled by the autonomic nervous system.

axil: Upper angle between a stem and leaf or bract.

axillary: In the armpit area.

axon: The long, filamentous part of a neuron (nerve cell) that carries nerve impulses away from the cell.

ayurveda: A highly developed system of therapeutics developed in the Hindu and Buddhist cultures of the Indian subcontinent.

B lymphocyte (B cell): One of the immune system cell types; B cells fight infection primarily by making antibodies.

bacteremia: Presence of bacteria in blood, indicating infection.

bactericidal: An agent that destroys bacteria (a type of microbe or organism).

bacteriostat: Substance that retards growth of bacteria.

balm: Fragrant ointment or aromatic oil with medicinal value.

balsam: A resinous semisolid mass or viscous liquid exuded from a plant. A "true" balsam is characterized by its high content of benzoic acid, benzoates, cinnamic acid, or cinnamates.

baroreceptor: Neural receptor sensitive to pressure and rate of change in pressure; stretch receptor; found in the aortic arch and carotid sinuses.

basal metabolic rate: The rate of metabolism when the body is at rest.

basal cell carcinoma: Common, usually curable, slow-growing malignant tumor on the skin.

basal rosette: Leaves radiating directly from the crown of the root.

baseline: The first or starting measurement in a study. New measurements of blood values are compared to this starting value.

basophil: A type of white blood cell that is involved in allergic reactions.

bed-wetting: *See* enuresis.

Bell's palsy: Paralysis of muscles on one side of the face and the inability to close eye, sometimes with loss of taste and excess sensitivity to noise.

benign: Consisting of a localized mass of nonmalignant specialized cells within connective tissue that do not invade and destroy tissue or spread throughout body.

berry: Small, fleshy fruit or dry seed or kernel of various plants.

beta-blocker: Drug that decreases heart activity by affecting receptors of the sympathetic nervous system.

beta cells: The cells in the pancreas, which manufacture insulin.

biennial: Plant with two-year life cycle in which the vegetative first-year growth is followed by fruiting and dying during second year.

bile: Greenish liver secretion that is stored in the gallbladder until released to emulsify fats in the small intestine.

bile salts: Steroid molecules in bile that promote solubilization and digestion of fats.

bilirubin: The breakdown product of the hemoglobin molecule of red blood cells.

bilirubinemia: Excess bile pigment in blood that causes jaundice.

binomial: Standard scientific name for an organism in Latin.

bioavailability: The amount of drug that is available to the target tissue after administration; this may not be 100% due to degradation or alteration before reaching the target tissue.

biopsy: A diagnostic test in which tissue or cells are removed from the body for examination under a microscope.

biopharmaceutics: The science and study of the ways in which the pharmaceutical formulation of administered agents can influence their pharmacodynamic and pharmacokinetic behavior.

biotransformation: Chemical alteration of an agent that occurs by virtue of the sojourn of the agent in a biological system. Pharmacodynamics involves the chemical effects of a drug on the body; biotransformation involves the chemical effect of the body on a drug. "Biotransformation" and "detoxication" are not synonyms: The product of a biotransformation may be more, not less, biologically active, or potent, than the starting material.

biotranslocation: The movement of chemicals through biological organisms.

bitters: Herbs with a bitter taste.

blade: Broad, expanded part of a leaf.

bleeding time: The time required for the cessation of bleeding from a small skin puncture as a result of platelet disintegration and blood vessel constriction. Ranges from 1 to 4 minutes.

blennorrhagia: Heavy discharge of mucus, especially from the urethra.

blepharitis: Inflammation, scaling, and crusting of eyelids.

blister: External swelling that contains watery fluid and blood or pus, caused by friction.

blocking antibody: Antibody whose production is induced by cancer cells or tissue transplants and that blocks the killing of those cells by cytotoxic T cells.

blood count: Measurement of the number of red cells, white cells, and platelets in a sample of blood.

blood pressure: The force exerted by blood as it is pumped by the heart and presses against and attempts to stretch blood vessels.

blood poisoning: Prolonged invasion of the bloodstream by pathogenic bacteria due to infectious disease or skin lesions; bacteremia; septicemia; toxemia.

blood-brain barrier: Group of anatomical barriers and transport systems that tightly control types of substances entering the extracellular space of the brain.

boil: Tender, inflamed, pustulant area of skin, usually due to staphylococcus infection; furuncle.

bolus: Single, large mass of a substance.

bone marrow: The inner core of bone that produces blood cells.

botany: Branch of biology dealing with life, structure, growth, and classification of plants.

bract: Leaflike structure growing below or encircling a flower cluster or flower.

bradycardia: Slowing of the heart rate to under 50 beats per minute.

bradykinin: Peptide vasodilator that increases capillary permeability and probably stimulates pain receptors.

bromeliad: Member of the Pineapple family of plants, usually epiphytic, with stiff, leathery leaves and spikes of bright flowers.

bronchial asthma: *See* asthma.

bronchitis: Inflammation of the walls of the bronchi in the lungs due to virus or bacteria, causing coughing and production of sputum.

bronchodilator: Substance that relaxes bronchial muscle to open air passages to the lungs.

bronchospasm: Muscular contraction that narrows the bronchi and causes difficulty especially in exhalation.

bruit: Any abnormal sound or murmur heard with a stethoscope.

bryophyte: Any member of the division of nonvascular plants, including mosses and liverworts.

bubo: Swollen and inflamed lymph node in armpit or groin.

bulb: Dormant underground bud stage of some plants.

bulimia: Psychogenic syndrome of overeating followed by vomiting.

bunion: Swelling of the joint between the big toe and the first metatarsal.

bursa: A sac or pouch that contains a special fluid that lubricates joints.

bursitis: Inflammation of a bursa.

cachexia: Weight loss, weakness, and debility associated with chronic disease.

calcinosis: Abnormal deposit of calcium salts in tissue.

calcitonin: Peptide hormone secreted by the thyroid that reduces excess of calcium in the blood by depositing it in bone.

calculus: Pebblelike mass, such as gallstone or kidney stone, formed within the body; hard tartar layer formed on teeth by plaque.

callus: Hard thickening of an area of skin undergoing rubbing, on hands or feet; mass of tissue forming around fractured bone ends.

calorie: A unit of heat. A nutritional calorie is the amount of heat necessary to raise 1 kg of water one degree C.

calyx: The sepals or outer layer of floral leaves.

cambium: Layer of formative cells beneath the bark of a tree.

cancer: General term for more than 100 diseases characterized by abnormal and uncontrolled growth of cells.

cancrum: Ulceration of the lip or mouth; canker.

candidiasis: Yeastlike fungus infection in the mouth and moist areas of the body; *see also* thrush.

canker: *See* cancrum.

capsule: A dry fruit, opening when ripe, composed of more than one carpel.

carbohydrate: Sugars and starches.

carbuncle: Staphylococcus infection of the skin that causes boils with multiple drainage channels.

carcinogen: Any agent or substance capable of causing cancer.

carcinogenesis: The development of cancer caused by the actions of certain chemicals, viruses, and unknown factors on primarily normal cells.

carcinoma: Cancer in epithelium lining skin or internal organs.

cardiac output: Volume of blood pumped by either ventricle per minute.

cardiac remedy: An herbal remedy that has a beneficial action on the heart. Some of the remedies in this group are powerful cardioactive agents such as foxglove; others are gentler, safer herbs such as hawthorn and motherwort.

cardiac arrest: Abrupt cessation of heartbeat, causing loss of pulse, consciousness, and breathing.

cardiac stenosis: Abnormal narrowing of a heart valve.

cardiomyopathy: Chronic viral, congenital, or other disorder that affects heart muscle and causes heart failure, arrhythmias, or embolisms.

cardiopulmonary: Pertaining to the heart and lungs.

cardiotonic: A compound that tones and strengthens the heart.

carditis: Inflammation of the heart.

caries: Decay of bone tissue, especially tooth; cavity.

carminative: Plants rich in aromatic volatile oils that stimulate the digestive system to work properly and with ease, soothing the gut wall, reducing any inflammation, easing griping pains, and helping the removal of gas from the digestive tract.

carotene: Fat-soluble plant pigments. Some carotenes can be converted into vitamin A by the body.

cartilage: A type of connective tissue that acts as a shock absorber at joint interfaces.

carpal tunnel syndrome: Compression of the median nerve entering the palm of the hand that causes pain and numbing in the middle and index fingers.

castor oil: Unpleasant-tasting, irritant laxative or cathartic.

catalyst: A chemical that increases the rate of a chemical reaction without itself being consumed.

cataract: Opacity of eye lens that causes blurred vision, especially in the elderly.

catarrh: Excessive secretion of thick phlegm or mucus by the mucous membrane of the nose.

catecholamines: The chemically similar neurotransmitters dopamine, epinephrine, and norepinephrine.

cathartic: A substance that stimulates the movement of the bowels, more powerful than a laxative.

catheter: A device that allows drugs to be given on an ongoing basis.

ceiling: The maximum biological effect that can be induced in a tissue by a given drug, regardless of how large a dose is administered.

cell-mediated immunity: Specific immune response mediated by cytotoxic T lymphocytes.

cephalalgia: *See* headache.

cephalic: Remedy for disorders of the head; referring or directed toward the head.

cerebral hemorrhage: Bleeding from the cerebral artery into brain tissue.

cerebral: Pertaining to the largest part of the brain, the cerebrum.

chelating agent: An organic compound capable of binding metals.

chemoreceptor: A molecular structure on the surface of a cell that is sensitive to chemical substances, such as epinephrine, released by nerve cells.

chemotaxis: Movement or response of cells to chemicals.

chemotherapy: Drug treatment of parasitic or neoplastic disease in which the drug has a selective effect on the invading cells or organisms.

chemotype: The same botanical species occurring in other forms due to different conditions of growth, such as climate, soil, and altitude.

Cheyne-Stokes respiration: Cyclical slowing of breathing to cessation, then speeding up to peak.

chilblain: Red, round, itchy swelling of skin on fingers or toes due to exposure to cold.

chiropractic: Treatment method using manipulation of the muscular and skeletal systems, especially the spine.

chlamydia: Sexually transmitted, viruslike microorganism causing conjunctivitis, urethritis, and cervicitis.

chlorophyll: Pigment in chloroplast, needed for photosynthesis.

chloroplast: Membrane-bound organelle that is the site of photosynthesis.

cholagogue: A compound that stimulates the contraction of the gallbladder.

cholecystitis: Inflammation of the gallbladder.

cholecystokinetic: Agent that stimulates the contraction of the gallbladder.

cholecystokinin (CCK): A peptide hormone secreted by the small intestine.

cholelithiasis: Presence of gallstones.

choleretic: Aids excretion of bile by the liver, so there is a greater flow of bile.

cholestasis: The stagnation of bile within the liver.

cholesterol: Steroid molecule that is a precursor of steroid hormones and bile salts, a component of plasma membranes, and present in fat and blood.

cholinergic: Pertaining to the parasympathetic portion of the autonomic nervous system and the release of acetylcholine as a transmitter substance.

chorionic: Referring to the chorion or membrane enclosing the fetus.

chromatography: Separation of chemical compounds.

chronic: Long term or frequently recurring.

chronic fatigue syndrome: Persistent, extreme exhaustion and weakness due to unknown causes.

chronotropic effect: An effect that changes the heart rate (i.e., the time between P-waves).

chyme: Solution of partially digested food in the lumen of the stomach and intestines.

cicatrisant: An agent that promotes healing by the formation of scar tissue.

cicatrix: *See* scar.

cirrhosis: Progressive liver condition from various causes.

claudication: Cramping pain from inadequate blood supply to muscle.

climacteric: Physical and emotional changes as sexual maturity gives way to cessation of reproductive function in females and testosterone decrease in males.

clot: Soft, thickened lump formed in liquid, especially blood.

clinical therapeutic index: An index of relative safety or relative effectiveness that cannot be defined explicitly and uniquely, although it is presumed that the same quantifiable and precise criteria of efficacy and safety will be used in comparing drugs of similar kinds.

clinical trial: The systematic investigation of the effects of materials or methods, according to a formal study plan and generally in a human population with a particular disease or class of diseases.

club moss: Any of various small, non-seed-bearing vascular plants with conelike, spore-bearing structures on top of stems.

clubbing: Thickening of tissue at the base of a fingernail or toenail, especially enlargement of a fingertip.

CNS: Central nervous system.

coccus: Spherical bacterium.

coenzyme: Nonprotein organic molecule that temporarily joins with an enzyme during reaction, is not consumed in reaction, and can be reused until degraded; cofactor.

cold sore: Small swelling or eruption of skin around lips that dries to leave a crusty patch; fever blister.

colic: Pain due to contraction of the involuntary muscles of the abdominal organs.

colitis: Any inflammation of the colon, causing diarrhea and lower abdominal pain.

collagen: Extremely strong fibrous protein that functions as a structural element in connective tissue, tendons, and ligaments.

collagen disease: A disease characterized by changes in the makeup of connective tissue: lupus, rheumatic fever, rheumatoid arthritis, and scleroderma.

colloid: An extremely fine particle suspended in a surrounding medium.

collyrium: Medicated solution used to bathe eyes.

coma: Prolonged state of deep unconsciousness from which patient cannot be roused.

comedo: Blackhead.

comparison trial: A trial in which experimental drugs are tested against each other or against an approved drug.

complement: Set of enzymes in the bloodstream that work with antibodies to attack foreign cells and bacteria.

complete blood count (CBC): Series of tests including cell counts, hematocrit, hemoglobin, and cell volume measurement.

compliance: The extent to which a patient agrees to and follows a prescribed treatment regimen.

compress: Moistened pad of folded cloth, often medicated, applied with heat, cold, or pressure to soothe a body part.

concrete: A concentrated, waxy, solid or semisolid perfume material prepared from previously live plant matter, usually using a hydrocarbon type of solvent.

cone: Reproductive structure of certain nonflowering plants with overlapping scales or bracts containing pollen, ovules, or spores.

congestion: Accumulation of blood within an organ; clogging of the upper respiratory system with mucus.

congestive heart failure: Inability of the heart to adequately supply blood to body tissue, often due to weakening of cardiac muscle, causing body swelling and shortness of breath.

conifer: Cone-bearing gymnosperm, usually with narrow, needlelike or small, scalelike leaves.

conjunctivitis: Inflammation of mucous membrane covering front of eye, often with discharge of pus; pinkeye.

connective tissue: The type of tissue that performs the function of providing support, structure, and cellular cement to the body.

constipation: Infrequent, difficult, often painful bowel movements with hard feces; irregularity.

contagious: A disease that can be transferred from one person to another by direct contact.

contraceptive: Medication or device to prevent conception.

continuous infusion: Uninterrupted introduction of fluid other than blood into a vein.

contractility: Refers to the strength of heart muscle contraction. This is controlled by the autonomic nervous system. The sympathetic nervous system increases and the parasympathetic nervous system decreases the strength of a contraction.

controlled trial: Trial in which one group gets the experimental drug and another group gets either a placebo or an approved drug therapy.

contusion: Surface injury in which skin is not broken; bruise.

convulsion: Involuntary muscle contraction that causes contorted movements of body and limbs.

corm: Underground stem base that acts as a reproductive structure.

corn: Area of hard or thickened skin on or between the toes.

corolla: The petals of a flower considered as a whole.

coronary: Of or pertaining to arteries of the heart.

coronary heart disease: Serious condition affecting the coronary arteries.

coronary insufficiency: The right and left coronary arteries supply blood to the heart. Flow is considered insufficient if it cannot meet the needs of the heart.

corpus luteum: The remains of the egg follicle after ovulation.

cortical: Involving external layers of brain.

corticosteroid drugs: A group of drugs similar to natural corticosteroid hormones that are used predominantly in the treatment of inflammation and to suppress the immune system.

corticosteroid hormones: A group of hormones produced by the adrenal glands that control the body's use of nutrients and the excretion of salts and water in the urine.

cortisol: A steroid hormone secreted by the adrenal cortex that regulates organic metabolism by converting fats and proteins to glucose.

corymb: Flat-topped or convex cluster of flowers in which the outer flowers open first.

cotyledon: First or second leaf of a seedling.

cough: Violent exhalation of irritant particles or congestive mucus from the respiratory system; tussis.

counterirritant: An application to the skin that relieves deep-seated pain, usually applied in the form of heat; *see also* rubefacient.

cramp: Prolonged painful contraction or spasm of muscle.

creatinine: A protein found in muscles and blood and excreted by the kidneys in the urine. The level of creatinine in the blood and urine provides a measure of kidney function.

crepitation: Soft crackling sound heard in the lungs through a stethoscope; rale.

crepitus: Crackling sound made by grating of bone on bone or on cartilage, especially in an arthritic joint.

CRH: Corticotropin-releasing hormone.

crick: Painful muscle spasm or cramp in neck or upper back.

crossover experiment: Each subject receives the test preparation at least once, and every test preparation is administered to every subject. At successive experimental sessions each preparation is "crossed over" from one subject to another.

Cushing's disease: Syndrome due to excess corticosteroid hormone, causing weight gain, excess body hair, and high blood pressure.

cutaneous: Pertaining to the skin.

cuticle: Waxy layer on the outer surface of plants.

cyanosis: Bluish discoloration of skin and mucous membranes due to inadequate oxygenation.

cycad: Any of the order of gymnosperms intermediate between ferns and palms, often with a thick, columnar trunk crowned by large, tough, pinnate leaves.

cyme: Inflorescence in which the primary axis bears a single central or terminal flower that blooms first.

cyst: An abnormal lump or swelling, filled with fluid or semi-solid material, in any body organ or tissue.

cytokine: Protein produced by white blood cells that acts as a chemical messenger between cells. CD8 (T-suppressor) cells release a cytokine that appears to block HIV replication in infected cells, at least until the advanced stage of HIV disease.

cytokinin: Plant hormone that promotes cell division.

cytomegalovirus: A virus in the herpes family that causes enlargement of epithelial cells and mononucleosis-like disease.

cytotoxic: Toxic to all cells.

cytotoxic T lymphocyte (CTL): A lymphocyte that is able to kill foreign cells that have been marked for destruction by the immune system.

cytotoxin: Substance that has a toxic effect on certain cells, used against some tumors.

debility: Weakness, lack of tone.

deciduous: Any plant that sheds all its leaves once each year.

decoction: An herbal preparation in which the plant material (usually hard or woody) is boiled in water and reduced to make a concentrated extract.

decongestant: Substance used to reduce nasal mucus production and swelling.

deficiency disease: Any disease, such as beriberi, caused by nutritional deficiency.

dehiscence: Splitting open of a wound.

dehydration: Deficiency or loss of water in body tissues marked by thirst, nausea, and exhaustion.

delirium: Acute mental disorder due to organic brain disease, causing hallucinations, disorientation, and extreme excitation.

dementia: Senility; loss of mental function.

demineralization: Loss of minerals from the bone.

demulcent: An herb rich in mucilage that soothes and protects irritated or inflamed tissue.

deodorant: Corrects, masks, or removes unpleasant odors.

dependence: A somatic state that develops after chronic administration of certain drugs; this state is characterized by the necessity to continue administration of the drug in order to avoid the appearance of uncomfortable or dangerous (withdrawal) symptoms.

depressant: Drug that lowers nervous or functional activity; sedative.

depurative: Helps combat impurity in the blood and organs.

dermal: Pertaining to the skin.

dermatitis: Skin inflammation.

detumescence: Reduction or subsidence of swelling.

diabetes: Diabetes mellitus.

dialysis: A technique using sophisticated machinery to remove waste products from the blood and excess fluid from the body in the treatment of kidney failure.

diaphoretic: Promotes perspiration, enabling the skin to eliminate waste from the body, thus helping the body ensure a clean and harmonious inner environment.

diarrhea: Frequent bowel evacuation, especially of soft or liquid feces.

diastole: Period of the cardiac cycle in which ventricles are not contracting.

diastolic pressure: Minimum blood pressure during cardiac cycle.

dicot: *See* dicotyledon.

dicotyledon: Angiosperm having two seed leaves or cotyledons; dicot.

digestion: Process of breaking down large particles and high-molecular-weight substances into small molecules.

digestive: Substance that promotes or aids the digestion of food.

diphtheria: Acute, highly contagious bacterial infection of the throat that can cause death from respiratory obstruction or carditis.

disinfectant: Cleansing agent that destroys bacteria and other microorganisms, used on surfaces and surgical tools.

disintegration time: The time required for a tablet to break up into granules of specified size (or smaller), under carefully specified test conditions.

dissolution time: The time required for a given amount (or fraction) of drug to be released into solution from a solid dosage form.

diuretic: Increases the production and elimination of urine.

diverticulum: Saclike out-pouching of the wall of the colon.

diverticulitis: Colonic diverticulosis with inflammation.

diverticulosis: Condition characterized by the existence of diverticular sacs at weak points in the walls of the alimentary tract, especially the intestine.

dizziness: Feeling off balance, unstable, confused, as though whirling in place.

dopamine: A catecholamine neurotransmitter, precursor of epinephrine and norepinephrine.

dorsal: Pertaining to the back.

dormancy: Period of time in which growth ceases.

dosage form: The physical state in which a drug is dispensed for use.

dose: The quantity of drug, or dosage form, administered to a subject at a given time.

double-blind study: A way of controlling against experimental bias by ensuring that neither the researcher nor the subject knows when an active agent or a placebo is being used.

douche: Introduction of water and/or a cleansing agent into the vagina with the aid of a bag with tubing and a nozzle attached.

dressing: Protective or healing material applied externally to a wound or a diseased body part.

dromo: Refers to speed.

dromotropic effect: A change in the amount of time it takes the heart to complete one beat.

dropsy: Excess of fluid in the tissues.

drug: Substance that affects the structure or functional processes of an organism, especially to prevent or treat diseases or relieve symptoms.

drupe: A fleshy fruit, with one or more seeds, each surrounded by a stony layer.

dysentery: Infection of the intestinal tract that causes severe diarrhea mixed with blood and mucus.

dysfunction: Abnormal function.

dysmenorrhea: Painful, difficult menstruation.

dyspepsia: Digestive disorder with abdominal pain and gas after eating, sometimes with nausea and vomiting; indigestion.

dysplasia: Any abnormality of growth.

dyspnea: Labored or difficult breathing; breathlessness.

dystrophy: Organ or muscle disorder caused by insufficient nourishment or a hereditary disorder.

ecchymosis: Bluish black mark on skin from release of blood into tissues, usually due to injury; black-and-blue mark.

eclampsia: Convulsions, especially due to toxemia during pregnancy.

ectopic pregnancy: State in which a fertilized egg implants at a site other than the uterus.

edema: Excessive accumulation of fluid in tissues; dropsy.

ED50: Median effective dose.

electrocardiogram (ECG): Machine that measures and records the activity of the heart.

electroencephalogram (EEG): Machine that measures and records brain waves.

electrolyte: Substance that ionizes in solution and conducts electric current.

electuary: Medication mixed with honey.

elimination diet: A diet that eliminates allergic foods.

elimination half-life: The time it takes for the body to eliminate or break down half of a dose of a pharmacologic agent.

elixir: Substance that contains alcohol or glycerin, used as solution for bitter or nauseating drugs.

elliptical: Shaped like an ellipse, or regular curve.

embolism: Obstruction of an artery by a lodged blood clot, fat, air, or foreign body carried by circulating blood.

embolus: Mass of matter that obstructs blood flow.

emesis: Vomiting; vomited matter.

emetic: Substance that induces vomiting.

emmenagogue: Stimulates menstrual flow and activity.

emollient: Soothes and softens external tissue.

empyema: Accumulation of pus in a body cavity, especially the pleural cavity.

emulsification: Maintenance of lipid droplets in solution.

emulsify: The dispersement of large globules into smaller, uniformly distributed particles.

endemic: Disease that is constantly present in a particular region but generally under control.

endocarditis: Inflammation and damage to the heart cavity lining due to bacterial infection or rheumatic fever.

endocrine gland: Ductless organ that synthesizes hormones and releases them directly into the bloodstream.

endocrine system: All ductless glands in the body.

endocrinology: Study of the endocrine glands and hormones.

endometrium: The mucous membrane lining the uterus.

endometriosis: A condition in which tissue similar to that normally lining the uterus is found outside of the uterus, usually the ovaries, fallopian tubes, and other pelvic structures.

endorphin: Neurotransmitter that exhibits painkilling activity.

enervation: Weakness, lack of energy.

engorgement: Congestion of a part of tissues, or fullness (as in the breasts).

enteric-coated: A way of coating a tablet or capsule to ensure that it does not dissolve in the stomach and so can reach the intestinal tract.

enuresis: Involuntary urination, especially at night, usually functional in nature; bed-wetting.

enzyme: Complex protein that is produced by living cells and catalyzes specific biochemical reactions.

eosinophil: A type of white blood cell, called a granulocyte, that can digest microorganisms.

epidemiology: Study of causes and control of epidemics.

epilepsy: One of various brain disorders that cause recurrent, sudden convulsive attacks.

epinephrine: Hormone released by the adrenal medulla that elevates blood sugar and initiates the fight-or-flight response; adrenaline.

epiphyte: Nonparasitic plant growing upon another plant for support.

epistaxis: Bleeding from the nose.

erysipelas: A skin infection from streptococcus bacteria that causes inflammation, swelling, and fever.

erythema: A superficial redness of the skin due to excess of blood.

erythrocyte: A red blood cell whose primary function is to carry oxygen to cells.

erythropoiesis: Formation of erythrocytes.

erythropoietin: Hormone secreted mainly by the kidneys that stimulates erythrocyte production.

essential fatty acid (EFA): A fatty acid that the body cannot manufacture, e.g. linoleic and linolenic acids.

essential oil: A volatile oil obtained from the leaves, stem, flower, or other part of plants, usually carrying the odor characteristic of the plant.

estrogen: Any of several steroid hormones produced chiefly by the ovaries and responsible for promoting estrus and the development and maintenance of female secondary sex characteristics.

etiology: Science of causes and origins of diseases.

evergreen: Plant that maintains functional green foliage throughout year.

excretion: The elimination of waste products from a cell, tissue, or the entire body.

exfoliant: A product or ingredient whose purpose is to remove unwanted tissue or waste products from the skin and other body surfaces.

exfoliate: To shed cells from the epithelium layer of the skin or mucosa.

exocrine gland: A gland that secretes through a duct.

exophthalmic goiter: Enlargement of the thyroid gland accompanied by protrusion of the eyeballs from their orbits.

expectorant: Soothes bronchial spasm and loosens mucous secretions, helping dry, irritating coughs.

extracellular: The space outside the cell, composed of fluid.

exudate: Escaping fluid or semifluid material that oozes from a space that may contain serum, pus, and cellular debris.

eyewash: Medicinal solution that soothes eyes.

fatty acid: Organic compound whose carbon chain ends in a carboxyl group.

febrifuge: Substance that relieves or reduces fever.

feces: Digestive waste products.

feedback inhibition: Mechanism that maintains constant secretion of a product by exerting inhibitory control.

fern: Nonflowering, vascular plant having roots, stems, and fronds and reproducing by spores instead of seeds.

fever: Rise in body temperature above normal 98.6 degrees.

fibrillation: Rapid, uncontrolled irregular twitching of heart muscle.

fibroblastic: Pertaining to fibroblasts, or connective tissue cells.

fibrocystic changes: Formation of benign cysts of various sizes in the breast.

fibrosis: Thickening and scarring of connective tissue due to injury or inflammation.

first-degree burn: Reddening of the outer layer of skin.

first pass effect: The biotransformation and/or excretion of a drug by hepatic, including biliary, mechanisms following absorption of the drug from the gastrointestinal tract, before the drug gains access to the systemic circulation.

fissure: Crack in membrane lining.

fistula: Abnormal passage that leads from an abscess or cavity to the skin or to another abscess or cavity, caused by disease or injury.

fixative: A material that slows down the rate of evaporation of the more volatile components in a perfume composition.

fixed oil: A name given to vegetable oils obtained from plants that, in contradistinction to essential oils, are fatty, dense, and nonvolatile, such as olive and sweet almond oils.

flatulence: Expulsion of intestinal gas through mouth by belching or through anus by passing flatus.

flatus: Intestinal gas.

flavonoid: Plant pigment that exerts a wide variety of physiological effects in the human body.

floret: Small flower; one of a number of individual flowers comprising the head of a composite plant.

flowering plant: Any angiosperm that produces flowers, fruit, and seeds in an enclosed ovary.

foliage: Leaves of plant or tree.

follicle: Saclike structure that forms inside an ovary when an egg is produced.

free radical: Highly reactive molecule that can bind to and destroy cellular compounds.

frond: Fern or palm foliage.

fructose: Yellowish to white, crystalline, water-soluble sugar found in many fruits.

fruit: Mature ovary of a flowering plant, sometimes edible.

functional cyst: A benign cyst that forms on an ovary and usually resolves on its own without treatment.

fungicidal: Prevents and combats fungal infection.

fungus: Unicellular or filamentous organism, formerly classified with plants.

furuncle: Boil.

galactagogue: Increases secretion of milk.

gallstone: Hard mass of bile pigments, cholesterol, and calcium salts in the gallbladder.

gamma globulin: The part of blood serum that contains antibodies, used in temporary prevention of infectious diseases.

gargle: Antiseptic, often medicated, liquid used to rinse mouth and throat; mouthwash.

gastrin: Digestive system hormone that stimulates hydrochloric acid release by stomach and secretion of digestive enzyme by pancreas.

genus: Category of closely related species ranking below family and above species.

germicidal: Destroys germs or microorganisms such as bacteria.

germinate: Sprout and start to grow from spore or seed.

gingivitis: Inflammation of gums, sometimes with bleeding.

glaucous: Covered with a fine white, often waxy film that rubs off.

glioma: Cancer of nerve tissue.

glomerular filtration rate (GFR): Milliliters of plasma per minute filtered through the kidney.

glomerulonephritis: Potentially fatal streptococcal infection of the kidney.

glucagon: Pancreatic hormone that increases blood glucose levels.

glucocorticoid: Adrenal cortex hormone that affects salt and water metabolism and stimulates conversion of noncarbohydrates to carbohydrates.

glucose: A monosaccharide that is found in the blood and is one of the body's primary energy sources.

glutamic acid: An amino acid that may be a brain neurotransmitter.

gluten: One of the proteins in wheat and certain other grains that gives dough its tough, elastic character.

glycerin: *See* glycerol.

glycerol: Syrupy liquid prepared by hydrolysis of fats and oils for use as a skin lotion.

glycogen: White polysaccharide sugar, derived from glucose, that is the principal form in which carbohydrate is stored in tissue.

glycoprotein: Carbohydrate-protein complex.

glycoside: Plant chemical that consists of molecules made up of two sections, one of which is a sugar.

glytosuria: Excretion of excess sugar in urine, as in diabetes.

goblet cell: A goblet-shaped cell that secretes mucus.

goiter: Swollen neck due to an enlarged thyroid gland.

gonadotropin: A hormone that promotes gonad (sex gland) growth and function.

granulocyte: A cell type of the immune system filled with granules of toxic chemicals that enable it to digest microorganisms. Basophils, neutrophils, and eosonophils are examples of granulocytes.

granuloma: Nodule of connective tissue and capillaries associated with tuberculosis, syphilis, or nonorganic foreign bodies.

ground substance: The thick, gel-like material in which the cells, fibers, and blood capillaries of cartilage, bone, and connective tissue are embedded.

gum: A class of carbohydrates that swell in the presence of water and increase the thickness of water-based products.

gymnosperm: Member of the division of seed plants having ovules on open scales, especially cones.

half-life: The time required for the decay of half a sample of a radioactive substance; may also apply to pharmacologic agents.

hallucinogenic: Causes visions or delusions.

hay fever: Common, usually seasonal allergy to plant pollen that causes sneezing, runny nose, and watery eyes.

HDL: High-density lipoprotein.

headache: Pain within the skull, commonly due to stress or fatigue; cephalalgia.

heart failure: Inadequate pumping of the heart ventricles due to coronary thrombosis, hypertension, or arrhythmia; congestive heart failure.

heart murmur: Blowing or swishing noise produced by blood passing through a defective heart valve.

heartburn: Pain rising from abdomen to throat, often accompanied by bitter fluid in the mouth; pyrosis.

heartwood: The central portion of a tree trunk.

helper T cell: White blood cell that helps in the immune response.

hematocrit: The percentage of packed red blood cells in a given volume of blood. Normal ranges: women 37–43%, men 43–49%.

hematuria: Blood in the urine.

hemorrhage: Outflow of blood from a ruptured blood vessel, especially internal bleeding.

hemorrhoid: An enlarged vein in the anus wall, especially due to prolonged constipation or diarrhea, characterized by fissure, painful swelling, and bleeding; piles.

hemostatic: A substance that checks bleeding.

heparin: Natural anticoagulant produced by liver cells as a polysaccharide.

hepatic: Pertaining to the liver.

hepatitis: Inflammation of the liver, due to a virus transmitted by food or drink (infectious hepatitis), blood on a needle, or transfusion (serum hepatitis), causing fever and jaundice.

hepatomegaly: Enlargement of the liver.

herbaceous: Nonwoody.

hernia: Protrusion of tissue or an organ outside the cavity it normally occupies, especially in the lower abdomen, due to physical strain or coughing.

herniated disk: Slipped disk.

Herpes: Herpes simplex; small viral blisters on the skin.

Herpes simplex: Virus in the herpes family; non-venereal blisters on mucous membranes that can cause conjunctivitis, vaginal inflammation, or cold sores; herpes.

Herpes zoster: Virus in the herpes family characterized by vesicles, often with severe pain along distribution of nerve; shingles.

hiccup: Characteristic sound made by abrupt involuntary lowering of the diaphragm and closing of the upper end of the trachea.

high-density lipoprotein (HDL): Lipid-protein aggregate with a low proportion of lipid or cholesterol that removes cholesterol from arteries.

histamine: Amine derived from the amino acid histidine that is released in allergic reaction, causing dilation of the blood vessels.

HIV: Human immunodeficiency virus.

homeostasis: Maintenance of constant internal environment.

hormone: A secretion of an endocrine gland that controls and regulates functions in other parts of the body.

humoral: Immunity defense against disease by antibodies in body fluids.

hybrid: A plant originating by fertilization of one species or subspecies by another.

hydrocarbon: Compound containing only hydrogen and carbon.

hydrocele: Accumulation of watery fluid, especially about the testis.

hydrochloric acid: Acid secreted by stomach during digestion.

hyperglycemia: High blood sugar level.

hypergonadotropic: Increased production of gonad-stimulating hormone from the anterior pituitary gland.

hyperlipidemic: Elevation of cholesterol and triglycerides in the blood.

hyperpigmentation: Abnormally increased pigmentation.

hypersecretion: Excessive secretion.

hypersensitivity: Allergic reaction.

hypertension: High blood pressure.

hypertensive: A substance that causes a rise in blood pressure.

hyperthermia: Exceptionally high body temperature of 105 degrees F or above; fever induced as treatment.

hyperthyroidism: Overactivity of the thyroid gland that causes rapid heartbeat, sweating, tremors, weight loss, and anxiety.

hypertrophy: Increase in size of tissue or organ due to enlargement of cells.

hyperventilation: Abnormally rapid breathing that lowers carbon dioxide concentration in the blood.

hypnotic: A drug that produces a state clinically identical to sleep by means of action in the central nervous system.

hypochlorhydria: Insufficient gastric acid output.

hypochondria: Obsession with real and imagined physical ailments.

hypoglycemia: Low blood sugar.

hypoglycemic: Plant remedy that lowers abnormally elevated blood sugar.

hypogonadism: Below normal gonad (sex gland) function.

hypokalemia: Low potassium levels in the blood.

hypotension: Low blood pressure.

hypotensive: Plant remedy that lowers abnormally elevated blood pressure.

hypothalamus: An area of the forebrain that regulates pituitary gland secretion, among many other functions.

hypothyroidism: Subnormal thyroid gland activity that can lead to cretinism if present at birth.

hypoxia: An inadequate supply of oxygen.

iatrogenic: Meaning literally "physician produced," the term can be applied to any medical condition, disease, or other adverse occurrence that results from medical treatment.

idiopathic: Of unknown cause.

Ig: *See* immunoglobulin.

immune response: Body's defense reaction through dual modes of antibody and cellular response.

immunity: Ability of the body to recognize and neutralize foreign matter, either natural or acquired.

immunoglobulin (Ig): Any of five classes of antibodies: Igg, Igm, Iga, and Igf.

immunodeficiency: A condition resulting from a defective immune system.

immunomodulator: Substance hoped to strengthen the immune system and help the body fight off opportunistic infections or other diseases. Not necessarily used to stimulate the immune system.

immunostimulant: A plant that stimulates some aspect of immune system functioning.

impairment: Damage to or weakening of body part or function.

in vitro: Latin for "in glass." An artificial environment created outside a living organism, used to study a disease or process.

in vivo: Latin for "in life." Study conducted within a living organism—e.g., animal or human study.

inborn immunity: Congenital resistance to a specific disease.

incidence: The number of new cases of a disease that occur during a given period (usually years) in a defined population.

inclusion/exclusion criteria: The medical or other reasons why a person may or may not be allowed to enter a clinical trial.

incontinence: Involuntary passage or leakage of urine.

incubation period: Time between entry of disease organisms into the body and onset of disease symptoms.

infarction: Death of tissue due to oxygen deprivation.

infestation: Attack on body by parasitic microorganism.

inflorescence: Flowering structure above the last stem leaves (including bracts and flowers).

infusion: An herbal remedy prepared by steeping the plant material in water.

inorganic: In chemistry, the term refers to compounds that do not contain carbon.

inotropic effect: *Ino-* is a prefix that refers to muscle. Inotropic effects are ones that change the strength of contraction of the heart muscle.

insomnia: Inability to fall asleep or to remain asleep.

insulin: Pancreatic hormone that regulates blood sugar level.

interferon: Substance produced by infected cells that inhibits specific viral growth.

interleukin: A natural blood substance that helps immune system cells to communicate.

intestinal malabsorption: A condition in which the nutrients found in food are not absorbed by the body.

intrinsic activity: The property of a drug that determines the amount of biological effect produced per unit of drug-receptor complex formed.

investigational new drug (IND): A drug allowed by the FDA to be used in clinical trials but not approved for commercial marketing.

irreversible: Impossible to halt or reverse by treatment.

irritable bowel syndrome: Recurrent chronic abdominal pain with constipation and/or diarrhea caused by abnormal contractions of colon muscles; spastic colon.

irritant: A substance that produces redness, itching, swelling, or blisters on the skin.

ischemia: Reduced blood supply to an organ or tissue.

jaundice: A condition caused by elevation of bilirubin in the body and characterized by yellowing of the skin.

keratin: An insoluble protein found in hair, skin, and nails.

kidney stone: Hard, pebblelike mass in kidney that causes pain and blood in urine; nephrolithiasis; renal calculus.

killer T cells: A class of immune system cells that function to kill cancer- and virus-infected cells; *see also* natural killer cells.

kinin: Vasodilatory polypeptide.

laceration: Tear in flesh, especially with irregular edges.

lactase: An enzyme that breaks down lactose into the monosaccharides glucose and galactose.

lactose: One of the sugars present in milk. It is a disaccharide.

lanceolate: Lance-shaped, oval, and pointed at both ends (usually a leaf shape).

laparoscopy: A surgical procedure in which a slender, light-transmitting telescope is used to view the pelvic organs.

larvicidal: An agent that prevents and kills larvae.

laryngitis: Inflammation of the larynx and vocal cords.

latency: The period when an organism is in the body but is not producing any ill effects.

laxative: Stimulating bowel movements.

LDL: *See* low-density lipoprotein.

lecithin: Phospholipid in nerve tissue and blood.

legume: A fruit consisting of one carpel, opening on one side, such as a pea.

lenticel: Spongy area of bark on a woody plant that allows exchange of gases between the stem and the atmosphere.

lesion: Any localized, abnormal change in tissue formation.

lethargy: A feeling of tiredness, drowsiness, or lack of energy.

leukocyte: White blood cell.

leucocytosis: An increase in the number of white blood cells above the normal limit.

leucoplakia: A precancerous lesion usually seen in the mouth that is characterized by a white patch.

leukemia: Overproduction of abnormal white blood cells by bone marrow and other blood-forming organs.

leukocytosis: Abnormal level in number of white blood cells, usually due to infection.

leukopenia: Reduction in number of white blood cells to below normal level.

leukotriene: Inflammatory compound produced when oxygen interacts with polyunsaturated fatty acids.

lichen: Fungus in symbiotic union with an alga.

lignin: Organic substance that serves as a binder for cellulose fibers in wood.

ligulet: A narrow projection from the top of a leaf sheath in grasses.

lipase: A fat-splitting enzyme.

lipid: A fat, phospholipid, steroid, or prostaglandin.

lipolytic: Causing lipolysis, the chemical disintegration or splitting of fats.

lipoprotein: A molecule combining protein and lipid.

lipotropic: Promoting the flow of lipids to and from the liver.

liverwort: Any of various small, flat bryophytes, usually on logs, rocks, or soil in moist areas.

lotion: An emollient emulsion, usually of the water-in-oil type.

low-density lipoprotein (LDL): Protein-lipid aggregate that is a major cholesterol carrier in plasma.

lubricant: A greasy substance applied to reduce friction on a body surface.

lumen: Cavity within a tubular structure.

lumpectomy: Surgery to remove only the abnormal breast.

lycopod: *See* club moss.

lymph: Colorless fluid derived from blood and carried in special ducts of lymphatic vessels.

lymphadenopathy: Swollen, firm, and possibly tender lymph glands.

lymphatic: Pertaining to the lymph system.

lymphocyte: A type of white blood cell found primarily in lymph nodes.

lymphoid tissue: Connective tissue containing lymphocytes.

lymphoma: A malignant tumor of lymph nodes that is not Hodgkin's disease.

macerate: Soak until soft.

macrophage: A large immune system cell that roams through the blood looking for foreign matter.

macule: Discoloration or thickening of skin in contrast to the surrounding area.

malabsorption: Impaired absorption of nutrients.

malaise: General sense of being unwell, often accompanied by physical discomfort and weakness.

malignant: A term used to describe a condition that tends to worsen and eventually causes death.

malnutrition: Insufficient food consumption to satisfy bodily needs over a prolonged period.

mammogram: An X-ray of the breast.

manipulation: As a therapy, the skillful use of the hands to move a part of the body or a specific joint or muscle.

mast cell: A cell found in many tissues of the body that contributes greatly to allergic and inflammatory processes by secreting histamine and other inflammatory chemicals.

mastectomy: Surgical removal of the breast.

mastitis: Inflammation of breasts due to bacterial infection.

measles: Highly infectious viral epidemic disease, mainly in children, that causes high fever and elevated pink rash; rubeola.

melanoma: Malignant tumor of melanin-forming cells.

memory cells: T cells that have been exposed to specific antigens and are able thereafter to proliferate upon repeat exposure to the same antigens.

menstruation: The discharge of blood and tissue from the uterus that occurs when an egg is not fertilized.

metabolic rate: Level of energy expenditure.

metabolism: A collective term for all the chemical processes that take place in the body.

metabolite: A product of a chemical reaction.

metastasis: Spread of a malignant tumor far from its site of origin, usually through the vascular system.

microflora: The microbial inhabitants of a particular region— e.g., the colon.

microorganism: Any living organism too small to be viewed by the unaided eye, including bacteria, viruses, protists, and some algae and fungi.

migraine: Recurrent, intense headache, often accompanied by blurred vision and vomiting, caused by contraction and dilation of arteries in the brain.

mineralocorticoid steroid: A salt-retaining hormone of the adrenal cortex.

miscible: The ability of a gas or liquid to mix uniformly with another gas or liquid.

mitogenic: An agent that effects cell division.

mold: Multicellular filamentous fungus.

mole: Flat or raised area of brown pigment in the skin.

monoclonal: Genetically engineered antibodies specific for one particular antigen.

monocotyledon: An angiosperm having only one seed leaf; cotyledon.

monosaccharide: A simple one-unit sugar such as fructose or glucose.

moss: Any of various small bryophytes without true stems reproducing by spores and growing in velvety clusters in moist areas on rocks, trees, and the ground.

motor: Designating muscular activity stimulated by impulses from the central nervous system.

mouthwash: Gargle.

moxa: A dried herb (usually mugwort) burnt on or above the skin to stimulate an acupuncture point or to serve as a counterirritant.

mucilage: A substance containing gelatinous constituents that are demulcent.

mucin: A protein that forms mucus when mixed with water.

mucolytic: Dissolving or breaking down mucus.

mucosa: *See* mucous membrane.

mucous membrane: Mucus-secreting membrane lining body cavities and canals connecting with external air.

mucus: Viscid watery lubricating solution secreted by mucous membranes.

muscle relaxer: Depressant or tranquilizer that acts to relieve tension in muscles.

mutagen: External agent that increases mutation rate in cells.

myalgia: Pain in one or more muscles.

mycelium: Mass of threadlike tubes forming the vegetative parts of a fungus.

mycorrhiza: Close symbiosis between the mycelia of certain fungi and the root cells of some vascular plants.

mycosis: Fungus infection.

mycotoxin: Toxin from yeasts and fungi.

myelin sheath: A white fatty substance that surrounds nerve cells and aids in nerve impulse transmission.

myeloma: Malignancy of bone marrow.

myelosuppression: The suppression of bone marrow activity, which can cause anemia.

narcotic: A substance that induces sleep; intoxicating or poisonous in large doses.

natural immunity: Inborn lack of susceptibility to a specific disease.

natural killer cells (NK cells): Large immune system cells that attack and destroy infected and cancer-causing cells.

naturopathy: Treatment of disease that employs no surgery or synthetic drugs.

nausea: Feeling that one is about to vomit.

necrosis: Death of cells in an organ or tissue.

nectary: Organ of a plant that secretes nectar.

neoplasia: Tumor formation, characterized by a progressive, abnormal replication of cells.

neoplasm: New tumor caused by uncontrolled reproduction of abnormal cells.

nephritis: Inflammation of the kidney; Bright's disease.

nephrotoxic: Poisonous to the kidneys.

nervine: Relaxants that ease anxiety and tension by soothing both body and mind.

neuralgia: A stabbing pain along a nerve pathway.

neurasthenia: Nervous exhaustion.

neuritis: Inflammation of nerves; neuropathy.

neuron: Functional unit of a nerve, including cell body, axon, and dendrites.

neuropathy: Any abnormal, degenerative or inflammatory state of the peripheral nervous system.

neurotransmitter: A substance that modifies or transmits nerve impulses.

neutropenia: A low number of neutrophils in the blood.

nitric oxide (NO): A potent vasodilator released by endothelial cells to signal smooth muscle cells to relax.

NK cells: *See* Natural killer cells.

nocturia: The disturbance of a person's sleep at night by the need to pass urine.

nonvascular: Plant bryophyte nut dry, single-seeded fruit of various trees and shrubs consisting of kernel enclosed in hard or tough shell.

obovate: Refers to leaf shape; oval, but broader toward the apex.

occlusion: Closing or obstruction of a hollow organ or body part.

oedema: *See* edema.

oestrogen: *See* estrogen.

off label: A drug prescribed for conditions other than those indicated on the label.

ointment: Substance used to soothe or heal skin; salve; unguent.

oleo gum resin: A natural exudation from trees and plants that consists mainly of essential oil, gum, and resin.

oleoresin: A natural resinous exudation from plants; an aromatic liquid preparation extracted from botanical matter using solvents.

olfaction: The sense of smell.

open trial: A drug trial is "open" when doctors and participants know which drug is being administered. *See also* double-blind study.

opiate: Derivative of opium that depresses the central nervous system, relieves pain, and induces sleep.

opportunistic: Designating disease or infection occurring only under certain conditions, as when the immune system is impaired.

organ: Collection of tissues joined in a structural unit to serve a common function.

organic disorder: Disorder associated with physiological changes in the structure of an organ or tissue.

organic: In the chemical sense, refers to all compounds containing carbon.

osteoarthritis: Joint cartilage disease that causes pain and impaired joint function and occurs in later life, due to overuse of a joint or as a complication of rheumatoid arthritis.

osteopathy: Treatment of disease by manipulation and massage of the musculoskeletal system.

osteoporosis: Loss of bony matrix that causes brittle bones due to injury, infection, or old age.

OTC (over the counter): Medication available without a doctor's prescription.

ovate: Egg-shaped.

ovulation: The release of an egg from one of the ovaries.

oxytocic: An agent that stimulates labor contractions.

pack: Folded, moistened, often medicated pad of cotton or cloth applied to the body or inserted into a cavity.

palisade cell: Chloroplast-containing cell just below the surface of a leaf.

palliative: Medicine that relieves symptoms but does not cure disease.

palmate: With three or more leaflets, nerves, or lobes radiating from a central point.

palpitation: Abnormally rapid or violent heartbeat, especially due to fear, exertion, neurosis, or arrhythmia.

panacea: A cure-all.

pandemic: Epidemic disease that spreads to different countries over a large region.

panicle: Loose, diversely branching flower clusters.

pappus: The calyx in a composite flower having feathery hairs, scales, or bristles.

papule: Small, superficial bump or spot on the skin, often part of rash.

parahormone: Chemical control agent that can be synthesized by more than one cell type.

parasite: An organism that lives in or on another living organism while contributing nothing to its host's welfare, often causing irritation or interfering with function.

parasiticide: Prevents and destroys parasites such as fleas and lice.

parathyroid hormone (PTH): Hormone that promotes vitamin D synthesis and elevates blood calcium.

paregoric: Camphorated tincture of opium used to relieve diarrhea, formerly used as a painkiller.

parenchyma: Soft tissue forming the chief substance of leaves and roots, fruit pulp, and the center of stems.

paroxysm: Sudden, violent spasm or convulsion; abrupt worsening of a symptom.

parturient: Aiding childbirth.

passive immunity: Short-term resistance to a disease from the injection of another's antibodies.

pathogen: Any agent, particularly a microorganism, that causes disease.

pathogenesis: The process by which a disease originates and develops, particularly the cellular and physiologic processes.

pathogenic: Causing or producing disease.

pectin: A white, colloidal carbohydrate, found in certain ripe fruits, that has thickening properties.

pedicel: Stalk of a single flower, fruit, or leaf.

peduncle: Stalk supporting flower or flower cluster of an angiosperm or bearing the fruiting body of a fungus.

pepsin: Stomach enzyme that degrades proteins.

peptic: Applied to gastric secretions and areas affected by them.

peptic ulcer: Breach in lining of the digestive tract due to excess acid, occurring in the esophagus, stomach, or duodenum.

peptide: Compound of two or more amino acids.

perennial: Plant that lives more than two years, especially a herbaceous plant that produces flowers from the same root structure several years in a row.

perfoliate: A leaf that appears to be perforated by the stem.

perfusion: Passage of fluid through tissue, especially blood through the lungs.

peripheral resistance: Opposition to flow of blood in vessels.

peristalsis: Successive muscular contractions of the intestines, which move food through the gastrointestinal tract.

peristaltic waves: Successive contractions of tubular wall.

pessary: Vaginal appliance or medicated suppository.

petal: One of the circle of flower parts inside the sepals.

petiole: The stalk of a leaf.

pH: A scale from 0 to 14 used in measuring the acidity or alkalinity of solutions. Pure water, at pH 7.0, is considered neutral. Acidity increases as the numbers decrease. Alkalinity increases as the numbers increase.

pharmaceutical: A drug or medication manufactured and sold by a pharmacy.

pharmacokinetic trial: A trial that studies how the drug is absorbed by the body. People in one of these trials often have blood tests every few minutes or hours.

pharmacology: Medical science of drugs, which deals with their actions, properties, and characteristics.

pharmacopoeia: An official publication of drugs, in common use in a given country.

pharmacy: Preparation and dispensing of drugs; place where this is done.

phase I study: The first step in human testing of a drug. Designed to evaluate toxicity at different dose levels and takes place with a small number of participants.

phase II study: FDA drug-testing phase for effectiveness in humans. The stage at which drug effectiveness is established. Proceeds only if Phase I studies show toxicity to be within acceptable levels. Usually involves 50 to 300 volunteers.

phase III study: FDA drug-testing phase for extensive clinical trials in humans. Expansion of phase II study to 300 to 3,000 volunteers. Designed to back up information gathered in Phase I and II testing.

phenol: Natural or synthetic aromatic compound containing a hydroxide (–OH) ring.

pheromone: Behavior- or development-mediating chemical that transmits information between individuals of the same species.

phlebitis: Inflammation of a vein wall, especially in legs as a complication of varicose veins, causing extreme tenderness.

phlegm: *See* sputum.

phospholipid: Lipid compound containing a water-soluble phosphate group.

phosphorylation: The process of adding phosphate molecular groups to a compound.

photosynthesis: Production of organic substances from carbon dioxide and water in green-plant cells, which chemically transform the energy of sunlight.

physiological: Describes the natural biological processes of a living organism.

physiology: The study of the functioning of the body, including the physical and chemical processes of its cells, tissues, organs, and systems.

phytoestrogen: A plant compound that exerts estrogen-like effects.

phytohormone: A plant substance that mimics the action of human hormones.

phytotherapy: The treatment of disease by plants; herbal medicine.

piles: *See* hemorrhoid.

pill: Small ball or tablet of medicine to be swallowed whole; oral contraceptive.

pinnate: A leaf composed of more than three leaflets arranged in two rows along a common stalk.

pituitary gland: A pea-sized structure that secretes many important hormones, located behind the hypothalamus.

placebo: (Latin: "I will satisfy.") A medicine or preparation with no inherent pharmacologic activity.

plaque: Sticky, colorless mixture of saliva, bacteria, and carbohydrates on the surface of teeth that causes tartar and caries.

plasma: Fluid portion of blood and lymph.

plaster: Pasty medicinal dressing applied to a body part on a cloth as a curative counterirritant.

pleurisy: Inflammation of the pleura that cover the lungs, usually due to pneumonia or other lung disease, causing painful breathing.

pneumoconiosis: Black lung.

pneumonia: Inflammation or infection of the lungs in which sacs fill with pus, causing coughing and chest pain.

pneumonitis: Inflammation of the lungs.

pneumothorax: Collapsed lung.

pod: Vessel enclosing one or more seeds.

poliomyelitis: Infectious viral disease of the central nervous system, formerly epidemic, causing stiffness and paralysis of muscles, especially respiratory system muscles.

pollen: Fine, dustlike grains containing male sexual cells, produced in anthers or similar structures of seed plants.

polyarthritis: Inflammation of several joints at the same time.

polymer: Natural or synthetic macromolecules formed by the repetition of an identical small molecule.

polymerase: An enzyme that forms long-chain polymers from simple molecular components; DNA polymerase, for example, forms DNA strands from nucleosides.

polyp: Benign growth on mucous membranes especially in the nose, ear, or stomach.

polypeptide: Protein, polymer of amino acid subunits.

polysaccharide: A molecule composed of many sugar molecules linked together.

pomade: A prepared perfume material obtained by the enfleurage process.

PPM: Parts per million.

poultice: The therapeutic application of a soft moist mass (such as fresh herbs) to the skin, to encourage local circulation and to relieve pain.

prednisone: Synthetic steroid, administered orally, used to treat leukemia and Hodgkin's disease.

press: Device for drying and flattening botanical specimens.

progesterone: Hormone that prepares the uterus to receive and develop a fertilized egg.

prognosis: Assessment of the future course and outcome of a patient's disease.

prophylactic: Preventive of disease or infection.

proptosis: Forward displacement of an organ, especially the eyeball.

prostaglandin: Hormonelike compound manufactured from essential fatty acids.

prostatitis: Inflammation of the prostate gland due to bacterial infection, sometimes causing urinary obstruction.

prostration: Total exhaustion.

protease: Protein-splitting enzyme.

protein: Any of a large class of organic nitrogenous substances containing amino acids.

proteinuria: Presence of protein in the urine above normal limits.

protocol: The outline or plan for use of an experimental procedure or experimental treatment.

protozoa: A group of one-celled animals, a few of which cause human disease.

pruritis: Itching.

psoriasis: Condition characterized by chronic, itchy, scaly, silvery patches of skin, especially on elbows, forearms, knees, and scalp, of unknown cause but sometimes due to anxiety.

psychomotor: Relating to disorders of muscular activity affected by cerebral disturbances.

pulmonary embolism: Obstruction by a blood clot in an artery that conveys blood from heart to lungs.

purgative: Laxative or cathartic medication.

purpura: Skin rash due to bleeding into the skin from defective capillaries or blood platelet deficiency.

pustule: Small, pus-containing blister.

putrescence: Foul smell caused by decomposition of tissue.

pyorrhea: Periodontal disease.

pyrexia: *See* fever.

pyrosis: *See* heartburn.

quinine: Alkaloid drug used to treat malaria.

quinsy: Pus-discharging inflammation of the tonsils.

raceme: Diversely branching flowers.

radiation therapy: Treatment using X-rays, cobalt-60, radium, neutrons, or other types of cell-destroying radiation.

radiosensitizer: Drug being studied to try to boost the effect of radiation therapy.

rale: *See* crepitation.

randomized clinical trial: A study in which patients with similar traits, such as extent of disease, are chosen or selected by chance to be placed in separate groups that are comparing different treatments.

Raynaud's disease: Disorder, especially in women, in which spasms of arteries to extremities cause fingertips and toes to turn pale, blue, and numb.

rays (ray flowers): The straplike, often sterile flowers, commonly called petals, surrounding the flower head of a plant in the Composite family.

receptacle: Upper part of the stem from which the floral parts arise.

receptor: A small, chemically defined area (of a cell) that initiates a biological response upon uniting with chemically complementary areas of natural or foreign molecules.

rectification: The process of redistillation applied to essential oils to rid them of certain constituents.

referred pain: Pain felt in an unexpected part of the body separate from its source.

reflex: Automatic, involuntary activity caused by simple nervous circuits.

refrigerant: Cooling; reduces fever.

regression: The state of growing smaller or disappearing; used to describe the shrinkage or disappearance of a cancer.

regurgitation: Vomiting.

rejection: Immune reaction to a transplanted organ.

REM sleep: Rapid eye movement sleep.

remission: The decrease or disappearance of evidence of a disease; also, the period during which this occurs.

renal calculus: Kidney stone.

renal colic: Severe pain in the kidney.

renin: A protease enzyme released by the kidney that cleaves angiotensinogen to angiotensin I.

resectable: Capable of being removed by surgery.

resin: A natural or prepared product, either solid or semisolid in nature. Natural resins are exudations from trees, such as mastic; prepared resins are oleoresins from which the essential oil has been removed.

resinoid: A perfumery material prepared from natural resinous matter, such as balsam and gum resin.

resolvent: An agent that disperses swelling or affects absorption of a new growth.

respiration: Exchange of gases between body tissues and the surrounding environment.

respiratory arrest: Cessation of breathing.

restorative: An agent that helps strengthen and revive the body systems.

reticulosis: Abnormal malignant overgrowth of cells of lymphatic glands or the immune system.

retrovirus: A type of virus whose genetic material consists of RNA rather than the usual DNA.

rheum: Watery discharge from mucous membranes of the mouth, eyes, or nose.

rheumatism: Any disorder causing aches and pains in muscles or joints.

rheumatoid arthritis: Common form of arthritis that affects extremities, digits, and hips.

rhinitis: Inflammation of the nasal mucosa (mucous membranes in the nasal cavities).

rhizome: Creeping horizontal stem lying at or just beneath the soil surface that bears leaves at its tip and roots from its underside.

rickettsiae: Group of parasitic organisms similar to bacteria that infest the body through ticks or mites.

ringworm: Highly contagious fungal infection of the skin, especially the scalp and feet or under a beard.

risk: The likelihood that harm will result from exposure to a hazard.

risk assessment: The process for evaluating the probability of harm resulting from a given exposure to a hazardous substance. The three steps of a risk assessment are hazard identification; dose-response assessment; and risk characterization.

risk/benefit ratio: The relation between the risks and benefits of a given treatment or procedure.

risk management: The regulatory decision-making process, which may take into account not only the risk assessment information, but also nonscience factors such as cost, competing public needs, technical feasibility, and societal values.

root: The underground part of a plant that functions in absorption, aeration, and food storage and as a support system.

rosacea: Chronic acne characterized by red, pustular lesions about the nose, cheeks, and forehead.

rosette: Leaves that are closely arranged in a spiral.

rubefacient: Generating a localized increase in blood flow when applied to the skin, helping healing, cleansing, and nourishment. Often used to ease the pain and swelling of arthritic joints.

saccharide: A sugar molecule.

saliva: Watery, slightly acidic secretion of salivary glands that moistens food and initiates its breakdown.

salt: The chemical combination of an acid and a base yielding a salt plus water.

salve: A medicinal ointment used to soothe or heal skin irritations, burns, or wounds; ointment; unguent.

saponin: A glycoside that forms a soaplike lather when shaken in water. There are two broad groups: the steroidal saponins, which seem to mimic the precursors of female sex hormones, and the tri-terpenoid saponins, which mimic the adrenal hormone ACTH.

saprophyte: A free-living organism that lives on dead or putrefying tissues.

sarcolemma: The cell membrane of a muscle cell. Like the cell membrane of nerves, the sarcolemma is able to conduct action potentials.

sarcoma: A tumor of connective tissue.

scab: A hard crust of blood, serum, or pus over a healing wound.

scabies: A skin infection from an infestation of mites that causes severe itching, especially around the groin and nipples and between fingers.

scar: Mark left on skin by a healing wound where connective tissues replace damaged tissues; cicatrix.

schistosomiasis: An intestinal disease in the tropics, due to infestation of blood flukes, that causes anemia, diarrhea, dysentery, and cirrhosis; snail fever.

sciatica: Condition marked by pain down the back of the thigh, due to disintegration of an intervertebral disk, accompanied by numbness and a stiff back.

sclerosis: Hardening of tissue due to inflammation.

scopolamine: A belladonna derivative.

scurvy: Vitamin C deficiency from absence of fresh fruit and vegetables in the diet that causes swollen, bleeding gums, subcutaneous bleeding, and death when prolonged.

seborrhea: Excessive secretion by sebaceous glands in the face, especially at puberty; *see also* seborrheic dermatitis.

seborrheic dermatitis: Skin eruption due to an excess secretion of sebum, common on the face at puberty.

secretion: Synthesis and release of a substance by a cell or an organ.

sedative: An agent that reduces functional activity; calming.

seed: Fertilized plant ovule containing the embryo, capable of germinating to produce a new plant.

seizure: Sudden attack of disease or condition.

senescence: Bodily degeneration after maturity.

sepal: Leaflike, usually green, outer circle of the calyx.

septic: Affected with putrefactive destruction by disease-carrying bacteria or their toxins.

septicemia: Tissue destruction by disease-causing bacteria or toxins absorbed from the bloodstream; blood poisoning.

serum: Liquid portion of the blood.

sessile: Lacking a stalk.

shingles: *See* Herpes zoster.

sialogogue: An agent that stimulates the secretion of saliva.

side effect: A secondary and usually adverse effect, as from a drug or other treatment.

silique: A term applied to the peculiar seedpod structure of plants in the Mustard family.

soporific: A substance that induces sleep.

spadix: A thick, fleshy flower spike usually enveloped by a spathe.

spasm: Sustained involuntary muscular contraction.

spasmolytic: *See* antispasmodic.

spastic colon: Irritable bowel syndrome.

spasticity: Resistance to passive movement of a limb; lack of motor coordination.

spathe: A modified, leaflike structure surrounding a spadix.

species: Basic unit of biological classification ranking below genus, including similar organisms capable of interbreeding.

spike: An inflorescence in which flowers bloom along the entire length of a single stalk.

splanchnic: Pertaining to the internal organs.

splenic: Relating to the spleen, the largest endocrine gland.

spondylosis: Degeneration of intervertebral disks in the backbone, causing pain and restricting movement.

sputum: Mucus coughed up from the respiratory tract; phlegm.

staging: Method used to establish the extent of a patient's disease.

stamen: The pollen-bearing anther with attached filaments.

standard treatment: A treatment or other intervention currently being used and considered to be of proven effectiveness on the basis of past studies.

stenosis: Abnormal narrowing of a blood vessel or heart valve.

steroid: Any of the large family of chemical compounds including hormones produced by the adrenal glands, ovaries, and testes; medication used for immunosuppression and hormone replacement.

STD: A sexually transmitted disease; *see also* venereal disease.

stimulant: An agent that quickens the physiological functions of the body.

stipule: An appendage resembling a small leaf at the base of leaves of certain plants.

stitch: Sudden, sharp pain, usually in muscle between ribs.

stolon: A stem that takes root at intervals along the ground, forming new plants.

stomachic: Digestive aid and tonic; improving the appetite.

stridor: Loud, harsh breathing noise due to partial obstruction of the trachea or larynx.

stroke: Sudden weakness or paralysis, often on one side of the body, due to interruption of blood flow to the brain caused by thrombosis, embolus, or hemorrhage; apoplexy; cerebrovascular accident.

sty: Acute bacterial infection of a gland at the base of an eyelash.

styptic: An astringent agent that stops or reduces external bleeding.

subclinical: Designating suspected disease or injury that is not developed enough to produce definite signs and symptoms.

subcutaneous: Giving a drug by injecting it under the skin.

submucosa: The tissue just below the mucous membrane.

succulent: Plant with thick, fleshy tissues that stores starch.

sudorific: An agent that causes sweating.

suppressor T cell: A lymphocyte controlled by the thymus gland, which suppresses the immune response.

suppuration: Formation and discharge of pus.

surfactant: A compound that reduces the surface tension in water, between water and another liquid, or between a liquid and a solid.

sympatholytic: A drug that affects the sympathetic nervous system.

symptom: Characteristic indication of disease or disorder.

synapse: Junction between two excitable cells.

syncope: Fainting.

syndrome: Set of signs and symptoms indicative of a particular disease or condition.

synergy: The summing of the simultaneous effects of two or more drugs such that the combined effect is greater than the effect of either of the drugs when they are given alone.

systemic: Affecting the entire body, not just one part.

systole: Contraction of heart muscle.

systolic: The first number in a blood pressure reading; the pressure in the arteries during the contraction phase of the heartbeat.

T cell: A white blood cell that plays an important part in the immune system. There are three types of T cells, each of which has different subsets.

T-helper cell: A subset of T cells. Physicians regularly measure T-helper cell counts in HIV-positive people. The normal range for T-helper cells is 480–1,800, but may vary.

T-killer cell (cytoxic T cell): A white blood cell that kills foreign organisms after being activated by T-helper cells.

T-suppressor cell: A type of white blood cell that helps control the body's response to an infection.

tablet: A small disk, made from compressed powders of one or more drugs, that is swallowed whole.

tachycardia: Abnormally increased heartbeat and pulse rate.

tannin: A compound that reacts with protein to produce a leatherlike coating on animal tissue (as in the process of tanning). It promotes healing and numbing (to reduce irritation), reduces inflammation, and halts infection.

taproot: Deep main root from which lateral roots develop.

taxonomy: System of classifying organisms into natural related groups based on shared features or traits.

tendril: Threadlike, often spiral part of climbing plant that clings to or coils around objects.

teratogen: Substance that can cause birth defects.

testosterone: The principal male sex hormone produced by the testes, used in replacement therapy and as an anabolic steroid.

tetany: Spasm and twitching of the muscles of the face, hands, and feet.

thallus: Nonvascular plant body without clear differentiation into stems, leaves, or roots.

therapeutic: Pertaining to treatment.

therapeutic index: A number, LD50/ED50, which is a measure of the approximate "safety factor" for a drug; a drug with a high index can presumably be administered with greater safety than one with a low index. The therapeutic index is ordinarily calculated from data obtained from experiments with animals.

thromboembolism: Condition in which a blood clot forms at one point in circulation, dislodges, and moves to another point.

thrombogenic: Causing thrombosis or coagulation of the blood.

thrombosis: Formation of a thrombus or blood clot.

thrush: Whitish spots and ulcers in the mouth due to a parasite, especially in children; candidiasis.

thyroid hormone (TH): Thyroxine.

tincture: An herbal remedy or perfumery material prepared in an alcohol base.

tinea: Athlete's foot.

tinnitus: Ringing in the ears.

tissue: Group of similar cells that perform a particular function.

tonic: Nurturing and enlivening.

tonsillitis: Inflammation of the tonsils due to bacterial or viral infection, causing sore throat and fever.

topical: Applied directly to skin surface, not taken internally.

torpor: Sluggishness; unresponsiveness to stimuli.

toxemia: Accumulation of toxins in the blood.

toxic: Poisonous.

toxin: Poisonous substance.

transaminase: An enzyme measurement that indicates the health of the liver.

transgenic: Pertaining to the insertion by biotechnical means of a foreign gene or genes into the genetic makeup of an organism.

trifoliate: A plant having three distinct leaflets.

triglyceride: Neutral fat lipid molecule composed of glycerol and three fatty acids.

troche: Small, medicinal lozenge that soothes the mouth and throat.

tuber: Fat underground stem from which some plants grow, similar to but shorter and thicker than a rhizome.

tumescence: Swelling, especially due to the accumulation of blood or other fluid in tissue.

tumor: Abnormal growth of tissue in or on a body part.

tumor necrosis factor (TNF): A protein produced by macrophages. By itself, TNF destroys cancer cells. TNF can cause fever, chills, fatigue, headache, and inflammation.

tussis: *See* cough.

ulcer: Open, inflamed, nonhealing sore in skin or a mucous membrane, especially in the lining of the alimentary canal.

ultrasound: A test in which sound waves are used to examine a fetus or view the internal organs.

umbel: Umbrella-like; a flower in which the petioles all arise from the top of the stem.

unguent: Substance used to soothe and heal skin; ointment; salve.

urea: Nitrogenous waste product of kidneys.

uremia: The retention of urine by the body and the presence of high levels of urine components in the blood.

urethritis: Inflammation of the urethra, especially among males, due to bacterial or viral infection or obstruction.

urinalysis: The analysis of urine.

uterine: Pertaining to the uterus.

vagal: Pertaining to the vagus nerve, which supplies sensory connections to the ear, tongue, and pharynx.

vaginitis: Irritation of the vagina, due to inflammation or infection, causing burning pain and discharge.

vapors: Mentholated salve applied to chest and nose to relieve congestion.

varicella: Chicken pox.

varicose vein: Distended, sometimes painful vein in the leg, rectum, or scrotum due to obstruction of blood flow.

vascular plant: Any plant, such as an angiosperm, gymnosperm, and fern, in which the xylem and phloem conduct water and organic nutrients.

vasculitis: Inflammation of a blood vessel.

vasoconstriction: The constriction of blood vessels.

vasoconstrictor: An agent that causes narrowing of blood vessels.

vasodilator: An agent that dilates the blood vessels.

vector: Any agent, such as insect or tick, that transmits parasitic microorganisms and infectious diseases from host to host.

venereal disease (VD): Any infectious disease transmitted by sexual contact, now usually called sexually transmitted disease; social disease.

ventricle: One of two lower chambers of the heart.

vermicide: A chemical agent that kills parasitic worms in the intestine.

vermifuge: A chemical agent used to expel parasites from the intestine; anthelmintic.

verruca: *See* Wart.

vertigo: Feeling that one's surroundings are in motion, especially spinning, due to disease of the inner ear or the vestibular nerve.

vesicant: Causing blistering to the skin; a counterirritant.

vesicle: A small blister or sac containing fluid.

vinca alkaloid: A pharmacologically active substance (e.g., vinblastine or vincristine) obtained from the genus *Vinca*, which includes the periwinkles.

viral load: The amount of measurable virus in the blood.

virulent: Disease-producing.

vitamin: An essential compound necessary to act as a catalyst in normal processes of the body.

volatile: Unstable, evaporates easily; *see also* essential oil and volatile oil.

volatile oil: A complex compound that is a chemical mixture of hydrocarbons and alcohols in a plant.

voucher specimen: An identifiable piece of plant lodged as a specimen at an official herbarium. This is incorporated as a permanent archival specimen for future reference and research. Archival herbaria aim for their specimens to last 400 years.

vulnerary: A remedy that promotes wound healing, especially for skin lesions and stomach ulcers.

wart: Small, hard, benign growth in skin, caused by a virus.

welt: Raised ridge on the skin caused by a slash or a blow.

wheal: Temporary, itching, red, or pale raised area of skin due to abrasion or allergy.

whorl: A circle of leaves around a node.

xanthoma: Skin condition characterized by raised patches.

xerostomia: Diminished secretion of saliva that causes an abnormally dry mouth, especially as a drug reaction.

Appendix 2

SELECTED EXAMPLES OF
BINOMIAL MEANINGS

absinthium	Gr. name of a plant in Xenophon
Achillea	Gr. Achilles, hero of Homer's *Iliad* who is said to have discovered the virtues of a certain plant
Aconitum	Gr. *akoniton*, a kind of poisonous plant, monk's hood
Acorus	Gr. the sweet flag found in Dioscorides
aculeatus	thorny, prickly
Aesculus	L. name for a kind of oak
agnus-castus	Gr. pure, innocent
Agrimonia	L. *agrestis*, pertaining to land, rural; L. *monas*, solitary
Agropyron	Gr. *agros*, a field; L. *pyr*, wheat
alba	L. white
Alchemilla	from the Arabic for alchemy
Allium	named after Charles Allioni, Italian botanist
Aloe	Gr. name for the plant
alternifolia	alternate leaves
Althaea	Gr. *althaino*, to heal
amara	bitter-tasting
Anemone	daughter of the wind, from Gr. *anemos*, the wind
Anethum	Gr. *anethon*, anise, dill
Angelica	Gr. *angelikos*, angelic, heavenly, divine
anisum	Gr. *anison*, anise, dill
Apium	Celtic *apon*, water: because of a plant's habitation
arborescens	treelike; woody
archangelica	said to have been revealed by the Archangel Gabriel
Arctium	L. *arctus*, narrow, straight
Arctostaphylos	Gr. bear and bunch of grapes
Aristolochia	Gr. *best*, birth
Artemisia	name, in Dioscorides, or a plant called after Artemis (Diana)
arvense	L. *arvensis*, of or belonging to a field
arvensis	growing on arable land
Asclepias	Gr. Asklepias, named for Asklepios, god of medicine and healing
Asparagus	from the ancient Persian name for the plant
Astragalus	Gr. *astragalos*, name of a kind of leguminous plant.
Atropa	Gr. Atropos, one of the three goddesses of fate, the unbending one
aureus	gold, bright yellow

Avena	L. *avena*, an old name for oats
Ballota	Gr. *ballote*, a name for black horehound
Baptisia	to dip under water, dye
Barosma	Gr. *baros*, weight, heaviness
basilicus	Gr. *basilikos*, royal, kingly
belladonna	beautiful lady
Bellis	L. *bellus*, neat, charming, handsome
benedictus	L. *bene*, well, agreeable
Berberis	L. *berberis*, the barberry
Betonica	Vettonica, the name in Pliny of a medicinal plant growing in the region of Spain called Vectones or Vettones
Betula	L. *betula*, the birch
Borago	L. *burra*, a shaggy garment, referring to the rough foliage
Brassica	L. *brassica*, cabbage
Brugmansia	named after Sebald Justin Brugmans (1706–1763)
bursa-pastoris	L. *bursa*, a pouch, purse made of skin; L. *pastoris*, shepherd
calamus	L. *calamus*, a reed
Camellia	named after George Josef Kamel (1661–1819)
Calendula	L. Kalendae, the first day of the month in the Roman calendar; monthly blooming
campestris	L. *campus*, a plain; relating to a plain, growing in a field
Cannabis	L. *cannabis*, hemp
Capsella	L. *capsa*, box, from the form of the fruits
Capsicum	L. *capsula*, boxed
cardamomum	L. *cardinis*, pertaining to a hinge
Carum	Gr. Karon, name for caraway in Dioscorides
Cascara	Sp. *cascara*, bark
Castanea	Gr. Kastanus, chestnut tree
cataria	L. *catarius*, of cats; old name of a plant attractive to cats
Caulophylum	Gr. *kaulos*, the stem of a plant, a cabbage stalk
Centaurea	called after Chiron the Centaur, who had wide knowledge of herbs
Centella	Gr. *kenteo*, to prick
Cephaëlis	Gr. Kephalotos, with a head
cerifera	L. *cera*, wax, or L. *cereus*, a wax candle

Cetraria	L. *cetra*, a sort of leather shield
Chelidonium	Gr. *chelidon*, a swallow
Chamaelirium	L. *chamaeleon*, ground-lion
Chamaemelum	Gr. *chamaimelon*, name, in Dioscorides, of a plant that smelled of apples
Chelone	Gr. *chelone*, a tortoise
Chionanthus	Gr. *chion*, snow, white as snow
Chondus	Gr. *chone*, funnel, tube
Chrysanthemum	Gr. *chrysos*, gold, flower
Cimicifuga	Gr. *cimicinus*, smelling like or of bugs
cinerea	L. *cinereus*, ash-colored
Cnicus	Gr. *knekos*, a thistlelike plant used for dyeing
Coleus	Gr. *koleus*, a sheath
Commiphora	Gr. *kommi*, gum
communis	L. *communis*, common, general
Conium	Gr. *koneion*, L. *conium*, names for this plant
Convallaria	L. *conulus*, a cone; L. *vallaris*, of or belonging to a wall or rampart
cordata	L. *cordis*, the heart
Coriandrum	ancient name for coriander
Crataegus	Gr. *Krataigos*, name of a tree in Theophrastus
crispus	L. *crispus*, curled, curly, with wavy margins
Curcuma	Arabic *kirkum*, turmeric
Cypripedium	Gr. *Kypridios*, belonging to Aphrodite
Datura	from Indian vernacular name
diffusa, -us, -um	loosely spreading, spread, scatter
Digitalis	translation of German name Fingerhut, thimble
dioica	Gr. *di*, two
Dioscorea	named after the Greek herbalist Dioscorides
distichon	Gr. *distoichos*, in two rows
Drosera	Gr. *droseros*, dewy, referring to the clear, dewlike drops on the leaf glands
Dryopteris	Gr. *Dryope*, daughter of Dryops and a playmate of the wood nymphs
Elattaria	L. *elatus*, elevating
Echinacea	Gr. *echinos*, a hedgehog
Ephedra	Gr. *ephedra*, sitting upon a seat
Equisetum	L. *equinus*, horse; L. *seta*, bristle, hair
erythraea	Gr. *erythros*, red, reddish
Eschscholzia	called after Johann Friedrich Eschscholtz (1793–1831)
Eucalyptus	Gr. *eu*, good, well, true, nice; Gr. *kalyptos*, covered, hidden
Eugenia	named in honor of Prince Eugene of Savoy (1663–1736)
Eupatorium	called after Eupator, a surname of Mithridates, king of Pontus
Euphorbia	called by King Juba II of Mauretania after his physician in ordinary, Euphorbus
Euphrasia	Gr. *euphrasia*, delight, mirth
felix-mas	L. *felicis*, fruitful, productive; L. *mas*, a male
ficaria	L. *ficus*, a fig tree
Filipendula	L. *filum*, a thread; L. *pendulus*, hanging
foetidus	L. *foetidus*, stinking
Fragaria	L. *fragum*, a strawberry plant
fragrans	L. *fragrans*, scented, sweet-smelling
fulvus	L. *fulvus*, reddish yellow, tawny, gold-colored
Fumaria	L. *fumus*, smoke
Galega	Gr. *galaktos*, milky
Galium	name, in Dioscorides, of *G. verum*, used to curdle milk for making cheese
Gaultheria	Gr. *gaulos*, a pail, a round-bottomed vessel
Gelsemium	It. *gelsomino*, jessamine
Gentiana	called after Gentius, an Illyrian king
Geranium	Gr. Geranos, a kind of bird called the crane, from the beaklike fruit
Ginkgo	Jap. *ginkyo*, vernacular name of the maiden-hair fern tree
glaucus	Gr. *glaukos*, silvery, gleaming, covered with a bloom like a plum
Glechoma	Gr. *glechon*, pennyroyal
globulus	L. *globulus*, a globe, ball, round as a ball
Glycyrrhiza	Gr. *glykys*, sweet, pleasant
gracilis	L. *gracilis*, slender
graveolens	L. *graveolens*, with a strong scent
Grindelia	called after David Hieronymus Grindel (1776–1836)
Guaiacum	West Indian name for *Lignum-vitae*
Hamamelis	Gr. *hama*, all together, at the same time
Harpagophytum	Gr. *hapagos*, robbing, rapacious
Hedeoma	Gr. *hedys*, sweet, scent
Hedera	L. *hedera*, ivy
hederacea	Celtic *hederaceus*, of ivy, ivy green
hipposcastanum	Gr. *hippos*, horse, and Gr. *kastanus*, chestnut, meaning chestnut unfit for food
hirtus	L. *hirtus*, hairy
Hordeum	L. *hordeum*, barley
horridus	L. *horridus*, bristly, prickly
hortensis	L. *hortensis*, cultivated in gardens
Humulus	latinized form of a Teutonic word for hops
Hydrangea	Gr. *hydro*, water; Gr. *angos*, jar
Hydrastis	Gr. *hydor*, water; Gr. *drao*, to act; an agent, performer
Hypericum	Gr. *hyperikon*, St. John's wort
Hyssopus	Gr. *hyssopos*, an aromatic plant
idaeus	Gr. *idios*, distinct
inflatus	L. *inflatus*, inflated, swollen
Inula	L. name of elecampane
Iris	Gr. *iridos*, rainbow—name of a kind of lily
Jasminum	latinized form of the Persian name Yasmin

Juglans	Jupiter's nut, L. *Jovis glans*
Lactuca	L. *lactuca*, lettuce; L. *lac*, milk, from the white juice
Lappa	L. *lappa*, a bur
Larrea	named for Juan Antonio de la Larrea
Lavandula	L. *lavo*, to wash
Leonurus	L. *leontus*, lion
Ligusticum	name of a plant growing in Liguria
Ligustrum	name, in Virgil, of a plant with white flowers
Linum	L. *linum*, flax, thread, rope
Lobelia	called after Matthias de l'Obel, Flemish botanist (1538–1616)
longus	L. *longus*, tall, long
Lophophora	Gr. *lophos*, a crest; Gr. *phoreo*, to bear
lucidus	L. *lucidus*, shining
lupulus	L. *lupus*, a wolf
luteum	L. *luteus*, golden yellow
Lycopus	Gr. *lykos*, a wolf
maculatus	L. *macula*, spotted, speckled
majalis	used in botany to signify flowering during May
major	L. *major*, greater
Malva	Gr. *malasso*, to soften
marianum	said to refer to Mary. According to legends, the white marks on the leaves of *Silybum marianum* represent drops of milk spilled when feeding the infant Jesus during the flight to Egypt
Marrubium	Gr. *maron*, a bitter herb
Matricaria	L. *matricis*, womb
media	L. *medius*, middle, intermediate
Medicago	classical name derived from the place-name Media
Melaleuca	Gr. *melas*, *melaina*, or *malania*, black, blackness, clothed in black
melano-	Gr. *melas*, black
Melissa	Gr. *melissa*, honeybee, nymph who kept bees
Mentha	Gr. *mintha*, mint
Menyanthes	Gr. *menyo*, to disclose
millefolium	L. *mille*, thousand; L. *folium*, leaf
minimum	L. *minimus*, least, smallest, very small
minor	L. *minor*, smaller
montana	L. *montanus*, growing in mountainous places
multi-, *multus*	L. *multus*, many
muralis	L. *murus*, a wall; of, growing on, walls
muscosus	L. *muscus*, moss; mosslike
Myrica	Gr. *myrike*, ancient name of the tamarisk Gr. *myro*, to flow, as it grows on banks of running streams
Myristica	Gr. *myristikos*, fit for anointing
myrtillus	Gr. Myrtilos, son of Mercury, charioteer of Oenomaus
Myroxylon	Gr. *myron*, sweet smelling oil; Gr. *xylon*, wood
napellus	L. *napus*, a kind of turnip
Nasturtium	L. *nasus*, nose; L. *tortus*, twisting away or torment
neglectus	L. *neglectus*, neglected, overlooked
Nepeta	L. *nepa*, a scorpion
niger, *-gra*, *-grum*	L. *nigra*, black
nitens	L. *nitens*, shining
nivalis	L. *nivis*, growing in or near snow
nobilis	L. *nobilis*, famous, noted, celebrated
nodosum	L. *nodus*, knotty, referring to tubers or swollen nodes
nudi-, *nudus*	L. *nudus*, naked
Nymphaea	L. Nympha, goddess of waters, meadows, and forest
occidentalis	L. *occidentalis*, Western
odorata	L. *odoratus*, sweet-smelling
officinale, *-lis*	L. *officinalis*, kept at the druggist's shop, (i.e., used medicinally).
Olea	L. *olea*, olive
Oxalis	Gr. *oxys*, sharp, acid
Paeonia	Gr. Paionia, physician of the gods
palmatum	L. *palmatus*, marked like the palm of the hand
paluster	L. *palustre*, marsh; growing in swampy places
Panax	L. *panacaea*, an herb that was supposed to heal all diseases
Papaver	L. *papa*, pap, thick milk
Parthenium	Gr. *parthenos*, virgin
Passiflora	L. *passio*, a passion, also a suffering
pellucidus	L. *pellucido*, transparent
peltatum	L. *pellatus*, armed with a shield
pendulus	L. *pendulus*, hanging down
perennis	throughout the year, through the year
perforatum	L. *perforatus*, perforated
Petroselinum	L. *petronius*, of or belonging to a mountain, rock
Peumus	latinized Chilean name
Phytolacca	Gr. *phyton*, tree, plant
Piscidia	L. *piscis*, fish; L. *caedere*, to kill
Plantago	L. *planta*, sole of the foot
Polygala	L. *polys*, many or much; L. *gala*, milk
Populus	L. *populus*, a great number; the poplar tree, so called from the number and continual motion of its leaves
Potentilla	L. *potens*, powerful
pratense	L. *pratensis*, pertaining to or growing in a meadow
Primula	L. *primus*, the first
Prunella	from the German word for croup
Psychotria	name derived from the Greek *psychotrophon* meaning to grow in a cold place
Psyllium	Gr. *psylla*, flea; Greek name of *Plantago psyllium*. The seeds of this species resemble fleas

pubescens	L. *pubescens*, hairs of puberty; covered with soft hairs
Pulmonaria	L. *pulmonarius*, beneficial to the lungs
pulsatilla	L. *pulsata*, beaten, driven about, from the beating of the flowers by the wind
purpurea	applied to various shades of purple
Quercus	L. *quercus*, an oak
racemosa	L. *racemulus*, the stalk of a cluster, a bunch of berries
Ranunculus	L. *rana*, a frog
recutita	L. *recutitus*, having a fresh or new skin
repens	L. *repo*, creeping
Rheum	Gr. *rha*, rhubarb
riparius	growing by rivers and streams
Rosemarinus	L. *rorulentus*, full of dew
rotundifolia	L. *rotundus*, round
Rubus	L. *rubeo*, to be red
Rumex	Latin name for sorrel
rupestris	L. *rupis*, rock, growing on rocks
Ruscus	L. *ruscarius*, of or for a butcher's broom
Salix	L. *salicis*, the willow
Salvia	name of a plant in Pliny, perhaps from L. *salvus*, safe, sound; L. *salus*, health
Sambucus	Latin name for the elder tree
Sanguinaria	L. *sanguis*, blood
sativa	sown, planted, cultivated
Sanguinaria	L. *sanguis*, blood
Schizandra	Gr. *schizo*, to divide; Gr. *anthos*, male
Scrophularia	from Gr. *scrophula*—i.e., tubercular glands of the neck
Scutellaria	L. *scutella*, salver, dish, referring to the pouch on the calyx
Senecio	L. *senex*, old man, because of the conspicuous white pappus
serrulata	saw-shaped, serrated
silvaticus	L. *silva*, woodland, growing in woods
Silybum	L. *silybum*, a kind of thistle with edible stem
Smilax	Gr. *smilakos*, the yew; also a bindweed
Solidago	L. *solidago*, to put together or make whole
somniferum	L. *somnus*, sleep; sleep-inducing, soporific
spicata	L. *spica*, a point
squalidus	rough, unkempt, neglected, squalid
Stachys	L. *stachys*, an ear of grain, spike
Stellaria	L. *stella*, star
sylvatica	L. *sylvaticus*, growing among trees
Symphytum	Gr. *symphyton*, name of a kind of plant with healing properties; comfrey
Symplocarpus	Gr. *symploke*, a twisting together
Syzygium	Gr. *syzygos*, joined
Tanacetum	medieval L. *tanazita* derived from the Gr. *athanasia*, immortality
Taraxacum	medieval Latin, ultimately from Persian, bitter potherb
thalictroides	Gr. *thaliktron*, meadow rue
Thuja	Gr. *thya*, an African tree with fragrant, durable wood
Thymus	Gr. *thymos*, to perfume or to sacrifice
Tilia	L. *tilia*, the linden tree
tinctoria	L. *tinctorius*, of or belonging to dyeing; bloodthirsty
tremulus	Gr. *tremo*, shivering, trembling, quake, quiver
Trichocereus	Gr. *thrix*, hair, plus Cereus; hairy cactus
Trifolium	L. *tria*, thrice; L. *folium*, leaf
Trigonella	Gr. *trigonos*, triangular, three-cornered
Trillium	L. *trillium*, an herb with leaves in whorls of three
Tropaeolum	L. *tropaeum*, trophy
tuberosa	L. *tuberosus*, full of humps
Tussilago	L. *tussis*, cough
ulmaria	medieval name for the goats-beard, a plant with elmlike leaves
Ulmus	L. *ulmus*, the elm
Urtica	the Latin name for nettles from L. *uro*, to burn
uva-ursi	L. *uva*, grape; L. *ursi*, bear
Vaccinium	classical Latin name of the plant
Valeriana	medieval name, perhaps from L. *valeo*, be well or strong
Verbascum	classical Latin name of the plant
Verbena	L. *verbenae*, sacred boughs
versicolor	changing color
veris	of the spring
Viburnum	L. *viburnum*, the wayfaring tree
villosus	L. *villosus*, hairy, shaggy, rough
Vinca	L. *vinca*, the periwinkle
Viola	L. *viola*, the violet
virgaurea	L. *virga*, rod; L. *aureus*, golden
virosa	L. *virsosus*, muddy, covered with slime, poison, fetid
Viscum	L. *viscum*, birdlime, made from the berries of mistletoe
Vitex	L. *viticis*, the chaste tree
Vitis	classical Latin name of the grapevine
vulgare	general, common, usual
xanth(o)-	Gr. *xanthos*, yellow
Zanthoxylum	Gr. *xanthos*, yellow, Gr. *xylon*, wood
Zea	classical Greek name of another cereal plant
Zingiber	Gr. *zingiber*, ginger

Appendix 3

HERBS BY LATIN AND COMMON NAMES

HERBS BY LATIN NAME

LATIN BINOMIAL	COMMON NAME
Abelmoschus moschatus	Muskseed
Abies balsamea	Balsam fir
Abrus precatorius	Jequerity
Acacia nilotica	Acacia bark
A. catechu	Black catechu
A. senega	Gum arabic
Acer rubrum	Red maple
Achillea millefolium	Yarrow
A. ptarmica	Sneezeweed
Aconitum napellus	Aconite, monkshood
Acorus calamus	Sweet flag, calamus
Adiantum capillus-veneris	Maidenhair fern
Adonis vernalis	False hellebore
Aegopodium podagraria	Ground elder, bishop's goutweed
Aesculus hippocastanum	Horse chestnut
Agathosma betulina	Buchu
Agrimonia eupatoria	Agrimony
Ailanthus altissima	Tree of heaven
Ajuga chamaepitys	Ground pine
A. reptans	Common bugle
Alchemilla vulgaris	Lady's mantle
Aletris farinosa	True unicorn root
Alkanna tinctoria	Alkanet
Allium cepa	Onion
A. sativum	Garlic
Alnus glutinosa	Black alder
Aloe spp.	Aloe
Aloysia triphylla	Lemon verbena
Alpinia officanarum	Galangal
Alstonia scholaris	Alstonia
Althaea officinalis	Marshmallow
Amaranthus hypochondriacus	Amaranth
Anacardium occidentale	Cashew
Anagallis arvensis	Scarlet pimpernel
Anemopsis californica	Yerba mansa
Anethum graveolens	Dill
Angelica archangelica	Angelica
A. sinensis	Dong quai
Antennaria dioica	Life everlasting, pussytoes
Anthemis cotula	Mayweed
Anthoxanthum odoratum	Sweet vernalgrass
Apium graveolens	Celery seed
Apocynum androsaemifolium	Bitter root, spreading dogbane
A. cannabinum	Indian hemp

LATIN BINOMIAL	COMMON NAME
Arachis hypogaea	Peanut
Aralia nudicaulis	False sarsaparilla
A. racemosa	American spikenard
A. spinosa	Angelica tree
Arctium lappa	Burdock
Arctostaphylos uva-ursi	Bearberry, kinnikinnick
Aristolochia serpentaria	Virginia snakeroot
Aristolochia spp.	Birthwort
Armoracia rusticana	Horseradish
Arnica montana	Arnica
Artemisia abrotanum	Southernwood
A. absinthium	Wormwood
A. annua	Sweet Annie
A. dracunculus	Tarragon
A. vulgaris	Mugwort
Arum maculatum	Cuckoo pint
Asarum canadense	Wild ginger
Asclepias syriaca	Milkweed
A. tuberosa	Pleurisy root
Asparagus officinalis	Asparagus
Astragalus gummifer	Tragacanth
A. membranaceus	Astragalus
Atropa belladonna	Belladonna
Avena sativa	Oats, oatstraw
Azadiracta indica	Neem
Ballota nigra	Black horehound
Baptisia tinctoria	Wild indigo
Bellis perennis	English daisy
Berberis vulgaris	Barberry
Betula lenta	Sweet birch
Betula spp.	Birch
Bidens tripartita	Burr marigold
Bixa orellana	Annatto
Borago officinalis	Borage
Boswellia carteri	Frankincense
Brassica nigra	Black mustard
Bryonia alba	White bryony
Buxus sempervirens	Boxwood
Calamintha ascendens	Calamint
Calendula officinalis	Calendula, marigold
Camellia sinensis	Tea
Cannabis sativa	Marijuana
Capsella bursa-pastoris	Shepherd's purse
Capsicum annuum	Cayenne
Carica papaya	Papaya

LATIN BINOMIAL	COMMON NAME
Carthamus tinctorius	Safflower
Carum carvi	Caraway
Castanea sativa	Chestnut
Catharanthus roseus	Madagascar periwinkle
Caulophyllum thalictroides	Blue cohosh
Ceanothus americanus	Red root
Celastrus scandens	Bittersweet, American
Centaurea cyanus	Cornflower
C. nigra	Black knapweed
Centaurium erythraea	Centaury
Centella asiatica	Gotu kola
Cephaelis ipecacuanha	Ipecacuanha
Ceratonia siliqua	Carob
Cetraria islandica	Iceland moss
Chamaelirium luteum	False unicorn root
Chamaemelum nobilis	Roman chamomile
Chelidonium majus	Celandine
Chelone glabra	Balmony
Chenopodium ambrosioides	Wormseed
Chimaphila umbellata	Pipsissewa
Chionanthus virginicus	Fringetree
Chondrus crispus	Irish moss
Chrysanthemum cinerariifolium	Pyrethrum
Cichorium intybus	Chicory
Cimicifuga racemosa	Black cohosh
Cinchona spp.	Quinine
Cinnamomum aromaticum	Cassia
C. camphora	Camphor
C. verum	Cinnamon
Citrullus colocynthis	Colocynth
Citrus aurantifolia	Lime
C. a. var. amara	Bitter orange
C. sinensis	Sweet orange
C. limon	Lemon
Cladonia pyxidata	Cupmoss
Claviceps purpurea	Ergot
Cnicus benedictus	Blessed thistle
Cochlearia officinalis	Scurvygrass
Codonopsis tangshen	Codonopsis
Coffea arabica	Coffee
Cola acuminata	Kola, cola
C. vera	Kola, cola
Colchicum autumnale	Colchicum, autumn crocus
Coleus forskohlii	Coleus
Collinsonia canadensis	Stoneroot
Commiphora molmol, C. myrrha	Myrrh
C. mukul	Guggul
Conium maculatum	Hemlock, poison hemlock
Consolida regalis	Larkspur
Convallaria majalis	Lily of the valley
Convolvulus scammonia	Scammony
Conyza canadensis	Fleabane
Copaifera officinalis	Copaiba
Copernicia prunifera	Carnauba
Coptis trifolia	Goldthread
Corallorhiza odontorhiza	Coral root
Coriandrum sativum	Coriander
Cornus florida	Dogwood
Crataegus laevigata	Hawthorn
C. monogyna	Hawthorn

LATIN BINOMIAL	COMMON NAME
Crocus sativus	Saffron
Croton eluteria	Cascarilla
C. tiglium	Croton
Cucurbita pepo	Pumpkin
Cuminum cyminum	Cumin
Curcuma longa	Turmeric
C. zedoaria	Zedoary
Cuscuta epithymum	Dodder
Cydonia oblonga	Quince
Cymbopogon citratus	Lemongrass
Cynara scolymus	Artichoke
Cynoglossum officinale	Houndstongue
Cypripedium calceolus	Lady's slipper
Cytisus scoparius	Scotch broom
Daemonorops draco	Dragon's blood
Daphne mezereum	Mezereon
Datura stramonium	Thorn apple, jimsonweed
Daucus carota	Carrot
Delphinium staphisagria	Stavesacre
Dicentra canadensis	Turkey corn
Digitalis spp.	Foxglove
Dioscorea villosa	Wild yam
Diospyros virginiana	American persimmon
Dipteryx odorata	Tonka bean
Dorema ammoniacum	Ammoniakum
Drimys winteri	Winter's bark
Drosera rotundifolia	Sundew
Dryopteris filix-mas	Male fern
Ecballium elaterium	Wild cucumber
Echinacea spp.	Echinacea, purple coneflower
Echium vulgare	Bugloss
Elettaria cardamomum	Cardamom
Eleutherococcus senticosus	Siberian ginseng
Elymus repens	Couch grass
Embelia ribes	Embelia
Ephedra sinica	Ma huang, ephedra
Epigaea repens	Arbutus
Equisetum arvense	Horsetail
Eriodictyon californicum	Yerba santa
Eryngium maritimum	Sea holly
Erythronium americanum	Adder's tongue, American
Erythroxylum coca	Coca
Eschscholzia californica	California poppy
Eucalyptus spp.	Eucalyptus
Euonymus atropurpureus	Wahoo, spindle tree
Eupatorium cannabinum	Hemp agrimony
E. perfoliatum	Boneset
E. purpureum	Gravel root, Joe pye
Euphorbia ipecacuanhae	American ipecac
E. pilulifera	Pill-bearing spurge
Euphrasia officinalis	Eyebright
Fagopyrum esculentum	Buckwheat
Fagus sylvatica	Beech
Ferula assa-foetida	Asafetida
F. gummosa	Galbanum
Ficus carica	Fig
Filipendula ulmaria	Meadowsweet

LATIN BINOMIAL	COMMON NAME	LATIN BINOMIAL	COMMON NAME
Foeniculum vulgare	Fennel	*I. germanica*	Orris
Fragaria vesca	Strawberry	*I. pseudacorus*	Yellow flag
Fraxinus excelsior	Ash	*I. versicolor*	Blue flag
F. ornus	Manna		
Fucus vesiculosus	Bladderwrack	*Jasminum grandiflorum*	Jasmine
Fumaria officinalis	Fumitory	*Jateorhiza columba*	Columbo
		Juglans cinerea	Butternut
Galega officinalis	Goat's rue	*J. nigra*	Black walnut
Galipea officinalis	Angostura	*J. regia*	English walnut
Galium aparine	Cleavers	*Juniperus communis*	Juniper
G. odoratum	Sweet woodruff	*J. oxycedrus*	Cade juniper
G. verum	Lady's bedstraw	*J. sabina*	Savin
Ganoderma lucidum	Reishi	*J. virginiana*	Eastern red cedar
Garcinia cambogia	Garcinia		
Garrya fremontii	Feverbrush	*Kalmia latifolia*	Mountain laurel
Gaultheria procumbens	Wintergreen	*Krameria triandra*	Rhatany
Gelidium amansii	Agar		
Gelsemium sempervirens	Yellow jasmine	*Lactuca virosa*	Wild lettuce
Genista tinctoria	Dyer's greenweed	*Lamium album*	Dead nettle
Gentiana lutea	Gentian	*Larix decidua*	Larch
Geranium maculatum	Cranesbill	*L. laricina*	Tamarack
Geum urbanum	Avens	*Larrea tridentata*	Chaparral
Ginkgo biloba	Ginkgo	*Laurus nobilis*	Laurel
Glechoma hederacea	Ground ivy	*Lavandula* spp.	Lavender
Glycine max	Soy	*Lawsonia inermis*	Henna
Glycyrrhiza glabra	Licorice	*Ledum groenlandicum*	Labrador tea
Gnaphalium uliginosum	Cudweed	*Lentinus edodes*	Shiitake
Gossypium hirsutum	Cotton root	*Leonurus cardiaca*	Motherwort
Grindelia camporum	Gumweed, grindelia	*Leptandra virginica*	Black root
G. squarrosa	Gumweed, grindelia	*Ligusticum porteri*	Osha
Guaiacum officinale	Guaiacum	*Ligustrum* spp.	Privet
		Lilium candidum	Madonna lily
Hamamelis virginiana	Witch hazel	*Linum catharticum*	Fairy flax
Harpagophytum procumbens	Devil's claw	*L. usitatissimum*	Flax
Hedeoma pulegioides	American pennyroyal	*Liquidambar orientalis*	Storax
Hedera helix	Ivy	*Liriodendron tulipifera*	Tuliptree
Helianthus annuus	Sunflower	*Liriosma ovata*	Muira puama
Helichrysum angustifolium	Eternal flower	*Lobelia inflata*	Lobelia
Helleborus niger	Black hellebore	*Lomatium dissectum*	Lomatium
Herniaria glabra	Rupturewort	*Lonicera* spp.	Honeysuckle
Heuchera americana	Alumroot	*Lophophora williamsii*	Peyote
Hevea spp.	Rubber	*Lycopodium clavatum*	Club moss
Hieracium pilosella	Mouse ear	*Lycopus americanus*	Bugleweed
Hordeum vulgare	Barley	*L. europaeus*	Bugleweed
Humulus lupulus	Hops	*L. virginicus*	Bugleweed
Hydnocarpus kurzi	Chaulmoogra	*Lythrum salicaria*	Purple loosestrife
Hydrangea arborescens	Hydrangea		
Hydrastis canadensis	Goldenseal	*Magnolia officinalis*	Magnolia
Hyoscyamus niger	Henbane	*Mahonia aquifolium*	Oregon grape, mountain grape
Hypericum perforatum	St. John's wort	*Malva sylvestris*	Mallow
Hyssopus officinalis	Hyssop	*Manihot esculenta*	Tapioca
		Maranta arundinacea	Arrowroot
Ilex aquifolium	Holly	*Marrubium vulgare*	Horehound
I. paraguariensis	Paraguay tea, maté	*Marsdenia condurango*	Condurango
Illicium verum	Star anise	*M. reichenbachii*	Condurango
Impatiens capensis	Jewelweed	*Matricaria recutita*	German chamomile
Inula helenium	Elecampane	*Medicago sativa*	Alfalfa, lucerne
Ipomoea orizabensis	Mexican scammony root	*Melaleuca alternifolia*	Tea tree
I. purga	Jalap	*M. quinquenervia*	Cajeput
Iris foetidissima	Stinking iris	*Melissa officinalis*	Lemon balm

LATIN BINOMIAL	COMMON NAME	LATIN BINOMIAL	COMMON NAME
Mentha aquatica	Water mint	*P. methysticum*	Kava kava
M. piperita	Peppermint	*P. nigrum*	Black pepper
M. pulegium	Pennyroyal	*Piscidia erythrina*	Jamaica dogwood
M. spicata	Spearmint	*Pistacia lentiscus*	Mastic
Menyanthes trifoliata	Bogbean	*Plantago lanceolata*	Ribwort plantain
Mitchella repens	Partridgeberry	*P. major*	Plantain
Monarda punctata	Horsemint	*P. ovata*	Psyllium
Morus alba	Mulberry	*Podophyllum peltatum*	Mayapple
Myrica cerifera	Bayberry	*Pogostemon cablin*	Patchouli
M. gale	Sweetgale	*Polemonium caeruleum*	Jacob's ladder
Myristica fragrans	Nutmeg	*P. reptans*	Abscess root
Myroxylon balsamum	Balsam of Tolu	*Polygala senega*	Seneca snakeroot
var. *balsamum*		*Polygonatum biflorum*	Solomon's seal
M. balsamum	Balsam of Peru	*P. multiflorum*	Solomon's seal
var. *pereirae*		*Polygonum bistorta*	Bistort
Myrrhis odorata	Sweet cicely	*P. hydropiper*	Smartweed
Myrtus communis	Myrtle	*P. multiflorum*	Fo-ti
		Polypodium virginianum	Polypody root
Nepeta cataria	Catnip	*Populus alba*	White poplar
Nicotiana tabacum	Tobacco	*P. balsamifera*	Balm of Gilead
Nymphaea odorata	White water lily	var. *balsamifera*	
		P. gileadensis	Balm of Gilead
Ocimum basilicum	Basil	*P. tremuloides*	Quaking aspen
Oenothera biennis	Evening primrose	*Potentilla anserina*	Silverweed
Olea europaea	Olive	*P. erecta*	Tormentil
Ononsis spinosa	Restharrow	*Primula veris*	Cowslip
Ophioglossum vulgatum	Southern adder's-tongue	*P. vulgaris*	Primrose
Origanum majorana	Marjoram	*Prunella vulgaris*	Self-heal
O. vulgare	Oregano	*Prunus armeniaca*	Apricot
Oryza sativa	Rice	*P. africana*	Pygeum
Oxalis acetosella	Wood sorrel	*P. cerasus*	Sour cherry
		P. domestica	Plum
Packera aurea	Life root	*P. dulcis* var. *amara*	Almond
Paeonia officinalis	Peony	*P. laurocerasus*	Cherry laurel
Palaquium gutta	Gutta-percha	*P. persica*	Peach
Panax ginseng	Ginseng, Korean	*P. serotina*	Wild cherry
P. quinquefolius	Ginseng, American	*Pueraria montana* var. *lobata*	Kudzu
Papaver rhoeas	Field poppy	*Pulmonaria officinalis*	Lungwort
Papaver somniferum	Opium poppy	*Pulsatilla vulgaris*	Pasqueflower
Parietaria officinalis	Pellitory of the wall	*Punica granatum*	Pomegranate
Passiflora incarnata	Passionflower		
Paullinia cupana	Guarana	*Quassia amara*	Quassia
Pausinystalia yohimbe	Yohimbe	*Quercus alba*	White oak
Petasites hybridus	Butterbur	*Q. robur*	Oak
Petroselinum crispum	Parsley	*Quillaja saponaria*	Soap bark
Peumus boldus	Boldo		
Phoenix dactylifera	Date palm	*Ranunculus ficaria*	Lesser celandine
Phyllanthus emblica	Amla	*Rauvolfia serpentina*	Rauwolfia
Physalis alkekengi	Winter cherry	*Rehmannia glutinosa*	Rehmannia
Physostigma venenosum	Calabar bean	*Rhamnus cathartica*	Purging buckthorn
Phytolacca americana	Poke	*R. frangula*	Alder buckthorn
Picrorhiza kurrooa	Kutki	*R. purshiana*	Cascara sagrada
Pilocarpus microphyllus	Jaborandi	*Rheum officinale*	Chinese rhubarb
P. jaborandi	Jaborandi	*R. palmatum*	Chinese rhubarb
Pimenta dioica	Allspice	*Rhus aromatica*	Sweet sumac
Pimpinella anisum	Anise, aniseed	*R. glabra*	Smooth sumac
P. saxifraga	Burnet saxifrage	*Ribes nigrum*	Black currant
Pinus strobus	White pine	*Ricinus communis*	Castor bean
Piper betle	Betel	*Rorippa nasturtium-aquaticum*	Watercress
P. cubeba	Cubeb	*Rosa canina*	Dog rose

LATIN BINOMIAL	COMMON NAME
R. damascena	Damask rose
Rosmarinus officinalis	Rosemary
Rubia cordifolia	Indian madder
R. tinctorum	Madder
Rubus idaeus	Raspberry
R. villosus	Blackberry
Rumex acetosa	Sorrel
R. acetosella	Sheep sorrel
R. crispus	Yellow dock
Ruscus aculeatus	Butcher's broom
Ruta graveolens	Rue
Sabatia angularis	American centaury
Saccharum officinarum	Sugarcane
Salix alba	White willow
S. cinerea	Willow
Salvia miltiorrhiza	Dan shen
S. officinalis	Sage, garden sage
S. officinalis var. *rubia*	Red sage
S. sclarea	Clary sage
Sambucus ebulus	Dwarf elder
S. nigra	European elder
Sanguinaria canadensis	Bloodroot
Sanguisorba officinalis	Burnet
Sanicula europaea	Sanicle
Santalum album	Sandalwood
Saponaria officinalis	Soapwort
Sarracenia purpurea	Pitcher plant
Sassafras albidum	Sassafras
Satureja hortensis	Summer savory
S. montana	Winter savory
Schisandra chinensis	Schizandra
Scrophularia nodosa	Figwort
Scutellaria lateriflora	Skullcap
Selenicereus grandiflorus	Night-blooming cereus
Sempervivum tectorum	Houseleek
Senecio jacobaea	Ragwort
Senna alexandrina	Senna
Serenoa repens	Saw palmetto
Sesamum orientale	Sesame
Silybum marianum	Milk thistle
Sinapsis alba	White mustard
Sisymbrium officinale	Hedge mustard
Smilax spp.	Sarsaparilla
Solanum dulcamara	Bittersweet
Solidago virgaurea	Goldenrod
Sorbus aucuparia	Mountain ash
Spigelia marilandica	Pink root
Stachys betonica	Wood betony
S. officinalis	Wood betony
S. palustris	Woundwort
Stellaria media	Chickweed
Stillingia sylvatica	Queen's delight
Strychnos nux-vomica	Nux vomica, strychnine tree
Styrax benzoin	Benzoin
Symphytum officinale	Comfrey
Symplocarpus foetidus	Skunk cabbage
Syzygium aromaticum	Clove
S. cumini	Jambul

LATIN BINOMIAL	COMMON NAME
Tabebuia avellanedae	Pau d'arco
Tamarindus indica	Tamarind
Tanacetum parthenium	Feverfew
T. vulgare	Tansy
Taraxacum officinale	Dandelion
Taxus baccata	English yew
T. brevifolia	Pacific yew
Teucrium chamaedrys	Germander
Theobroma cacao	Cocoa
Thuja occidentalis	Thuja, arborvitae
Thymus vulgaris	Thyme
Tilia cordata	Littleleaf linden
T. europaea	Linden
T. platyphyllos	Linden
Trifolium pratense	Red clover
Trigonella foenum-graecum	Fenugreek
Trillium erectum	Beth root, trillium
Triosteum perfoliatum	Feverwort
Triticum aestivum	Wheat
Tropaeolum majus	Nasturtium
Turnera diffusa	Damiana
Tussilago farfara	Coltsfoot
Ulmus glabra	Elm
U. rubra	Slippery elm
Uncaria tomentosa	Cat's claw
Urginea maritima	Squill
Urtica dioica	Nettle
Usnea spp.	Usnea
Ustilago maydis	Corn smut
Vaccinium macrocarpon	Cranberry
V. myrtillus	Bilberry
Valeriana officinalis	Valerian
Vanilla planifolia	Vanilla
Veratrum album	White hellebore
V. viride	White hellebore
Verbascum thapsus	Mullein
Verbena officinalis	Vervain
Veronica beccabunga	Brooklime
V. officinalis	Speedwell
Vetiveria zizanioides	Vetiver
Viburnum opulus	Cramp bark
V. prunifolium	Black haw
Vinca major	Periwinkle
V. minor	Periwinkle
Viola odorata	Sweet violet
V. tricolor	Heartsease
Viscum album	Mistletoe
Vitex agnus-castus	Chaste tree, vitex
Vitis vinifera	Grape
Withania somnifera	Ashwaganda
Xanthorhiza apiifolia	Yellow root
Zanthoxylum americanum	Prickly ash
Zea mays	Cornsilk
Zingiber officinale	Ginger
Ziziphus jujuba	Jujube

HERBS LISTED BY COMMON NAME

COMMON NAME	LATIN BINOMIAL
Abscess root	Polemonium reptans
Acacia bark	Acacia nilotica
Aconite	Aconitum napellus
Adder's tongue, American	Erythronium americanum
Adder's tongue, southern	Ophioglossum vulgatum
Agar	Gelidium amansii
Agrimony	Agrimonia eupatoria
Alder, black	Alnus glutinosa
Alder buckthorn	Rhamnus frangula
Alfafa	Medicago sativa
Alkanet	Alkanna tinctoria
Allspice	Pimenta dioica
Almond	Prunus dulcis var. amara
Aloe	Aloe spp.
Alstonia	Alstonia scholaris
Alumroot	Heuchera americana
Amaranth	Amaranthus hypochondriacus
Amla	Phyllanthus emblica
Ammoniakum	Dorema ammoniacum
Angelica	Angelica archangelica
Angelica tree	Aralia spinosa
Angostura	Galipea officinalis
Anise, aniseed	Pimpinella anisum
Annatto	Bixa orellana
Apricot	Prunus armeniaca
Arborvitae	Thuja occidentalis
Arbutus	Epigaea repens
Arnica	Arnica montana
Arrowroot	Maranta arundinacea
Artichoke	Cynara scolymus
Asafetida	Ferula assa-foetida
Ash	Fraxinus excelsior
Ashwaganda	Withania somnifera
Asparagus	Asparagus officinalis
Astragalus	Astragalus membranaceus
Autumn crocus	Colchicum autumnale
Avens	Geum urbanum
Balm of Gilead	Populus balsamifera var. balsamifera
Balm of Gilead	Populus gileadensis
Balmony	Chelone glabra
Balsam of Peru	Myroxylon balsamum var. pereirae
Balsam of Tolu	Myroxylon balsamum var. balsamum
Barberry	Berberis vulgaris
Barley	Hordeum vulgare
Basil	Ocimum basilicum
Bayberry	Myrica cerifera
Bearberry	Arctostaphylos uva-ursi
Beech	Fagus sylvatica
Belladonna	Atropa belladonna
Benzoin	Styrax benzoin
Betel	Piper betle
Beth root	Trillium erectum
Bilberry	Vaccinium myrtillus
Birch	Betula spp.

COMMON NAME	LATIN BINOMIAL
Birch, sweet	B. lenta
Birthwort	Aristolochia spp.
Bishop's goutweed	Aegopodium podagraria
Bistort	Polygonum bistorta
Bitter orange	Citrus aurantium var. amara
Bitter root	Apocynum androsaemifolium
Bittersweet	Solanum dulcamara
Bittersweet, American	Celastrus scandens
Blackberry	Rubus villosus
Black catechu	Acacia catechu
Black cohosh	Cimicifuga racemosa
Black currant	Ribes nigrum
Black haw	Viburnum prunifolium
Black hellebore	Helleborus niger
Black horehound	Ballota nigra
Black root	Leptandra virginica
Black walnut	Juglans nigra
Bladderwrack	Fucus vesiculosus
Blessed thistle	Cnicus benedictus
Bloodroot	Sanguinaria canadensis
Blue cohosh	Caulophyllum thalictroides
Blue flag	Iris versicolor
Bogbean	Menyanthes trifoliata
Boldo	Peumus boldus
Boneset	Eupatorium perfoliatum
Borage	Borago officinalis
Boxwood	Buxus sempervirens
Brooklime	Veronica beccabunga
Broom	Cytisus scoparius
Buchu	Agathosma betulina
Buckwheat	Fagopyrum esculentum
Bugle	Ajuga reptans
Bugleweed	Lycopus virginicus, L. americanus, L. europaeus
Bugloss	Echium vulgare
Burdock	Arctium lappa
Burnet	Sanguisorba officinalis
Burnet saxifrage	Pimpinella saxifraga
Burr marigold	Bidens tripartita
Butcher's broom	Ruscus aculeatus
Butterbur	Petasites hybridus
Butternut	Juglans cinerea
Cade juniper	Juniperus oxycedrus
Cajeput	Melaleuca quinquenervia
Calabar bean	Physostigma venenosum
Calamint	Calamintha ascendens
Calendula	Calendula officinalis
California poppy	Eschscholzia californica
Camphor	Cinnamomum camphora
Caraway	Carum carvi
Cardamon	Elettaria cardamomum
Carnauba	Copernicia prunifera
Carrot	Daucus carota
Cascara sagrada	Rhamnus purshiana
Cascarilla	Croton eluteria
Cashew	Anacardium occidentale
Cassia	Cinnamomum aromaticum
Castor bean	Ricinus communis
Cat's claw	Uncaria tomentosa

COMMON NAME	LATIN BINOMIAL	COMMON NAME	LATIN BINOMIAL
Catnip	*Nepeta cataria*	Dodder	*Cuscuta epithymum*
Cayenne	*Capsicum annuum*	Dogbane, spreading	*Apocynum androsaemifolium*
Cedar, Eastern red	*Juniperus virginiana*	Dog rose	*Rosa canina*
Celandine	*Chelidonium majus*	Dogwood	*Cornus florida*
Celery seed	*Apium graveolens*	Dong quai	*Angelica sinensis*
Centaury	*Centaurium erythraea*	Dragon's blood	*Daemonorops draco*
Chamomile, German	*Matricaria recutita*	Dyer's greenweed	*Genista tinctoria*
Chamomile, Roman	*Chamaemelum nobilis*	Echinacea	*Echinacea angustifolia, E. pallida,*
Chaparral	*Larrea tridentata*		*E. purpurea*
Chaste tree	*Vitex agnus-castus*	Eastern red cedar	*Juniperus virginiana*
Chaulmoogra	*Hydnocarpus kurzi*	Elder	*Sambucus nigra*
Cherry laurel	*Prunus laurocerasus*	Elder, dwarf	*S. ebulus*
Cherry, sour	*P. cerasus*	Elecampane	*Inula helenium*
Chestnut	*Castanea sativa*	Elm	*Ulmus glabra*
Chickweed	*Stellaria media*	Embelia	*Embelia ribes*
Chicory	*Cichorium intybus*	Ergot	*Claviceps purpurea*
Cinchona	*Cinchona* spp.	Eternal flower	*Helichrysum angustifolium*
Cinnamon	*Cinnamomum verum*	Eucalyptus	*Eucalyptus* spp.
Clary sage	*Salvia sclarea*	Evening primrose	*Oenothera biennis*
Cleavers	*Galium aparine*	Eyebright	*Euphrasia officinalis*
Clove	*Syzygium aromaticum*		
Club moss	*Lycopodium clavatum*	Fairy flax	*Linum catharticum*
Coca	*Erythroxylum coca*	False hellebore	*Adonis vernalis*
Cocoa	*Theobroma cacao*	False sarsaparilla	*Aralia nudicaulis*
Codonopsis	*Codonopsis tangshen*	False unicorn root	*Chamaelirium luteum*
Coffee	*Coffea arabica*	Fennel	*Foeniculum vulgare*
Colchicum	*Colchicum autumnale*	Fenugreek	*Trigonella foenum-graecum*
Coleus	*Coleus forskohlii*	Feverbrush	*Garrya fremontii*
Colocynth	*Citrullus colocynthis*	Feverfew	*Tanacetum parthenium*
Coltsfoot	*Tussilago farfara*	Feverwort	*Triosteum perfoliatum*
Columbo	*Jateorhiza columba*	Fig	*Ficus carica*
Comfrey	*Symphytum officinale*	Figwort	*Scrophularia nodosa*
Condurango	*Marsdenia condurango*	Flaxseed	*Linum usitatissimum*
Copaiba	*Copaifera officinalis*	Fleabane	*Conyza canadensis*
Coral root	*Corallorhiza odontorhiza*	Fo-ti	*Polygonum multiflorum*
Coriander	*Coriandrum sativum*	Foxglove	*Digitalis* spp.
Cornflower	*Centaurea cyanus*	Frankincense	*Boswellia carteri*
Cornsilk	*Zea mays*	Fringetree	*Chionanthus virginicus*
Corn smut	*Ustilago maydis*	Fumitory	*Fumaria officinalis*
Cotton root	*Gossypium hirsutum*		
Couch grass	*Elymus repens*	Galangal	*Alpinia officanarum*
Cowslip	*Primula veris*	Galbanum	*Ferula gummosa*
Cramp bark	*Viburnum opulus*	Garcinia	*Garcinia cambogia*
Cranberry	*Vaccinium macrocarpon*	Garlic	*Allium sativum*
Cranesbill	*Geranium maculatum*	Gentian	*Gentiana lutea*
Croton	*Croton tiglium*	Germander	*Teucrium chamaedrys*
Cubeb	*Piper cubeba*	Ginger	*Zingiber officinale*
Cuckoo pint	*Arum maculatum*	Ginkgo	*Ginkgo biloba*
Cudweed	*Gnaphalium uliginosum*	Ginseng, American	*Panax quinquefolius*
Cumin	*Cuminum cyminum*	Ginseng, Korean	*P. ginseng*
Cupmoss	*Cladonia pyxidata*	Goat's rue	*Galega officinalis*
		Goldenrod	*Solidago virgaurea*
Daisy, English	*Bellis perennis*	Goldenseal	*Hydrastis canadensis*
Damiana	*Turnera diffusa*	Goldthread	*Coptis trifolia*
Dan shen	*Salvia miltiorrhiza*	Gotu kola	*Centella asiatica*
Dandelion	*Taraxacum officinale*	Grape	*Vitis vinifera*
Date palm	*Phoenix dactylifera*	Gravel root	*Eupatorium purpureum*
Dead nettle	*Lamium album*	Ground elder	*Aegopodium podagraria*
Devil's claw	*Harpagophytum procumbens*	Ground ivy	*Glechoma hederacea*
Dill	*Anethum graveolens*	Ground pine	*Ajuga chamaepitys*

COMMON NAME	LATIN BINOMIAL
Guaiacum	*Guaiacum officinale*
Guarana	*Paullinia cupana*
Guggul	*Commiphora mukul*
Gum arabic	*Acacia senegal*
Gumweed	*Grindelia camporum, G. squarrosa*
Gutta-percha	*Palaquium gutta*
Hawthorn	*Crataegus laevigata, C. monogyna*
Heartsease	*Viola tricolor*
Hedge mustard	*Sisymbrium officinale*
Hemlock, poison	*Conium maculatum*
Hemp agrimony	*Eupatorium cannabinum*
Hemp, Indian	*Apocynum cannabinum*
Henbane	*Hyoscyamus niger*
Henna	*Lawsonia inermis*
Holly	*Ilex aquifolium*
Honeysuckle	*Lonicera* spp.
Hops	*Humulus lupulus*
Horehound	*Marrubium vulgare*
Horse chestnut	*Aesculus hippocastanum*
Horsemint	*Monarda punctata*
Horseradish	*Armoracia rusticana*
Horsetail	*Equisetum arvense*
Houndstongue	*Cynoglossum officinale*
Houseleek	*Sempervivum tectorum*
Hydrangea	*Hydrangea arborescens*
Hyssop	*Hyssopus officinalis*
Iceland moss	*Cetraria islandica*
Ipecac, American	*Euphorbia ipecacuanha*
Ipecacuanha	*Cephaelis ipecacuanha*
Irish moss	*Chondrus crispus*
Ivy	*Hedera helix*
Jaborandi	*Pilocarpus jaborandi*
Jacob's ladder	*Polemonium caeruleum*
Jalap	*Ipomoea purga*
Jamaica dogwood	*Piscidia erythrina*
Jambul	*Syzygium cumini*
Jasmine	*Jasminum grandiflorum*
Jequerity	*Abrus precatorius*
Jewelweed	*Impatiens capensis*
Jimsonweed	*Datura stramonium*
Joe pye	*Eupatorium purpureum*
Jujube	*Ziziphus jujuba*
Juniper	*Juniperus communis*
Kava kava	*Piper methysticum*
Kinnikinnick	*Arctostaphylos uva-ursi*
Knapweed, black	*Centaurea nigra*
Kola	*Cola vera*
Kudzu	*Pueraria montana* var. *lobata*
Labrador tea	*Ledum groenlandicum*
Lady's bedstraw	*Galium verum*
Lady's mantle	*Alchemilla vulgaris*
Lady's slipper	*Cypripedium calceolus*
Larkspur	*Consolida regalis*
Laurel	*Laurus nobilis*
Lavender	*Lavandula* spp.

COMMON NAME	LATIN BINOMIAL
Lemon	*Citrus limon*
Lemon balm	*Melissa officinalis*
Lemongrass	*Cymbopogon citratus*
Lemon verbena	*Aloysia triphylla*
Lesser celandine	*Ranunculus ficaria*
Licorice	*Glycyrrhiza glabra*
Life everlasting	*Antennaria dioica*
Life root	*Packera aurea*
Lily of the valley	*Convallaria majalis*
Lime	*Citrus aurantifolia*
Linden	*Tilia cordata, T. europaea, T. platyphyllos*
Lobelia	*Lobelia inflata*
Lomatium	*Lomatium dissectum*
Loosestrife, purple	*Lythrum salicaria*
Lucerne	*Medicago sativa*
Lungwort	*Pulmonaria officinalis*
Ma huang	*Ephedra sinica*
Madagascar periwinkle	*Catharanthus roseus*
Madonna lily	*Lilium candidum*
Magnolia	*Magnolia officinalis*
Maidenhair fern	*Adiantum capillus-veneris*
Male fern	*Dryopteris filix-mas*
Mallow	*Malva sylvestris*
Mandrake, American	*Podophyllum peltatum*
Manna	*Fraxinus ornus*
Marigold	*Calendula officinalis*
Marijuana	*Cannabis sativa*
Marjoram	*Origanum majorana*
Marshmallow	*Althaea officinalis*
Mastic	*Pistacia lentiscus*
Maté	*Ilex paraguariensis*
Mayapple	*Podophyllum peltatum*
Mayweed	*Anthemis cotula*
Meadowsweet	*Filipendula ulmaria*
Mexican scammony root	*Ipomoea orizabensis*
Mezereon	*Daphne mezereum*
Milk thistle	*Silybum marianum*
Milkweed	*Asclepias syriaca*
Mistletoe	*Viscum album*
Monkshood	*Aconitum napellus*
Motherwort	*Leonurus cardiaca*
Mountain ash	*Sorbus aucuparia*
Mountain grape	*Mahonia aquifolium*
Mouse ear	*Hieracium pilosella*
Mugwort	*Artemisia vulgaris*
Muira puama	*Liriosma ovata*
Mulberry	*Morus alba*
Mullein	*Verbascum thapsus*
Muskseed	*Abelmoschus moschatus*
Mustard, black	*Brassica nigra*
Mustard, white	*Sinapsis alba*
Myrrh	*Commiphora molmol, C. myrrha*
Myrtle	*Myrtus communis*
Nasturtium	*Tropaeolum majus*
Neem	*Azadiracta indica*
Nettle	*Urtica dioica*

COMMON NAME	LATIN BINOMIAL
Night-blooming cereus	*Selenicereus grandiflorus*
Nutmeg	*Myristica fragrans*
Nux vomica	*Strychnos nux-vomica*
Oak	*Quercus robur, Q. alba*
Oats, oatstraw	*Avena sativa*
Olive	*Olea europaea*
Onion	*Allium cepa*
Opium poppy	*Papaver somniferum*
Orange, bitter	*Citrus aurantium* var. *amara*
Orange, sweet	*Citrus sinensis*
Oregano	*Origanum vulgare*
Oregon grape	*Mahonia aquifolium*
Orris	*Iris germanica*
Osha	*Ligusticum porteri*
Pacific yew	*Taxus brevifolia*
Papaya	*Carica papaya*
Paraguay tea	*Ilex paraguariensis*
Parsley	*Petroselinum crispum*
Partridgeberry	*Mitchella repens*
Pasqueflower	*Pulsatilla vulgaris*
Passionflower	*Passiflora incarnata*
Patchouli	*Pogostemon cablin*
Pau d'arco	*Tabebuia avellanedae*
Peach	*Prunus persica*
Peanut	*Arachis hypogaea*
Pellitory of the wall	*Parietaria officinalis*
Pennyroyal	*Mentha pulegium*
Pennyroyal, American	*Hedeoma pulegioides*
Peony	*Paeonia officinalis*
Pepper, black	*Piper nigrum*
Peppermint	*Mentha x piperita*
Periwinkle	*Vinca major, V. minor*
Persimmon, American	*Diospyros virginiana*
Peru balsam	*Myroxylon balsamum* var. *pereirae*
Peyote	*Lophophora williamsii*
Pill-bearing spurge	*Euphorbia pilulifera*
Pink root	*Spigelia marilandica*
Pitcher plant	*Sarracenia purpurea*
Plantain	*Plantago major*
Pleurisy root	*Asclepias tuberosa*
Plum	*Prunus domestica*
Poison hemlock	*Conium maculatum*
Poke	*Phytolacca americana*
Polypody root	*Polypodium virginianum*
Pomegranate	*Punica granatum*
Poplar, white	*Populus alba*
Prickly ash	*Zanthoxylum americanum*
Primrose	*Primula vulgaris*
Psyllium	*Plantago ovata*
Pumpkin	*Cucurbita pepo*
Purging buckthorn	*Rhamnus cathartica*
Purple loosestrife	*Lythrum salicaria*
Pussytoes	*Antennaria dioica*
Pygeum	*Prunus africana*
Pyrethrum	*Chrysanthemum cinerariifolium*

COMMON NAME	LATIN BINOMIAL
Quaking aspen	*Populus tremuloides*
Quassia	*Quassia amara*
Queen's delight	*Stillingia sylvatica*
Quince	*Cydonia oblonga*
Quinine	*Cinchona* spp.
Ragwort	*Senecio jacobaea*
Raspberry	*Rubus idaeus*
Red clover	*Trifolium pratense*
Red maple	*Acer rubrum*
Red poppy	*Papaver rhoeas*
Red root	*Ceanothus americanus*
Rehmannia	*Rehmannia glutinosa*
Reishi	*Ganoderma lucidum*
Restharrow	*Ononsis spinosa*
Rhatany	*Krameria triandra*
Rhubarb, Chinese	*Rheum officinale, R. palmatum*
Rice	*Oryza sativa*
Rosemary	*Rosmarinus officinalis*
Rubber	*Hevea* spp.
Rue	*Ruta graveolens*
Rupturewort	*Herniaria glabra*
Safflower	*Carthamus tinctorius*
Saffron	*Crocus sativus*
Sage, garden	*Salvia officinalis*
Sage, red	*Salvia officinalis* var. *rubia*
Sandalwood	*Santalum album*
Sanicle	*Sanicula europaea*
Sarsaparilla	*Smilax* spp.
Sassafras	*Sassafras albidum*
Savin	*Juniperus sabina*
Savory, summer	*Satureja hortensis*
Savory, winter	*Satureja montana*
Saw palmetto	*Serenoa repens*
Scammony	*Convolvulus scammonia*
Scarlet pimpernel	*Anagallis arvensis*
Schizandra	*Schisandra chinensis*
Scurvygrass	*Cochlearia officinalis*
Sea holly	*Eryngium maritimum*
Self-heal	*Prunella vulgaris*
Senna	*Senna alexandrina*
Sesame	*Sesamum orientale*
Sheep sorrel	*Rumex acetosella*
Shepherd's purse	*Capsella bursa-pastoris*
Shiitake	*Lentinus edodes*
Siberian ginseng	*Eleutherococcus senticosus*
Silverweed	*Potentilla anserina*
Skullcap	*Scutellaria lateriflora*
Skunk cabbage	*Symplocarpus foetidus*
Slippery elm	*Ulmus rubra*
Smartweed	*Polygonum hydropiper*
Smooth sumac	*Rhus glabra*
Snakeroot, Seneca	*Polygala senega*
Sneezeweed	*Achillea ptarmica*
Soap bark	*Quillaja saponaria*
Soapwort	*Saponaria officinalis*
Solomon's seal	*Polygonatum biflorum, P. multiflorum*

COMMON NAME	LATIN BINOMIAL
Sorrel	*Rumex acetosa*
Southernwood	*Artemisia abrotanum*
Soy	*Glycine max*
Spearmint	*Mentha spicata*
Speedwell	*Veronica officinalis*
Spikenard, American	*Aralia racemosa*
Squill	*Urginea maritima*
St. John's wort	*Hypericum perforatum*
Star anise	*Illicium verum*
Stavesacre	*Delphinium staphisagria*
Stinking iris	*Iris foetidissima*
Stoneroot	*Collinsonia canadensis*
Storax	*Liquidambar orientalis*
Strawberry	*Fragaria vesca*
Strychnine tree	*Strychnos nux-vomica*
Sugarcane	*Saccharum officinarum*
Sundew	*Drosera rotundifolia*
Sunflower	*Helianthus annuus*
Sweet annie	*Artemisia annua*
Sweet cicely	*Myrrhis odorata*
Sweet flag	*Acorus calamus*
Sweetgale	*Myrica gale*
Sweet sumac	*Rhus aromatica*
Sweet vernalgrass	*Anthoxanthum odoratum*
Sweet violet	*Viola odorata*
Tamarack	*Larix laricina*
Tamarind	*Tamarindus indica*
Tansy	*Tanacetum vulgare*
Tapioca	*Manihot esculenta*
Tarragon	*Artemisia dracunculus*
Tea	*Camellia sinensis*
Tea tree	*Melaleuca alternifolia*
Thorn apple	*Datura stramonium*
Thuja	*Thuja occidentalis*
Thyme	*Thymus vulgaris*
Tobacco	*Nicotiana tabacum*
Tolu balsam	*Myroxylon balsamum* var. *balsamum*
Tonka bean	*Dipteryx odorata*
Tragacanth	*Astragalus gummifer*
Tree of heaven	*Ailanthus altissima*
True unicorn root	*Aletris farinosa*
Tuliptree	*Liriodendron tulipifera*
Turkey corn	*Dicentra canadensis*
Turmeric	*Curcuma longa*

COMMON NAME	LATIN BINOMIAL
Usnea	*Usnea* spp.
Valerian	*Valeriana officinalis*
Vanilla	*Vanilla planifolia*
Vervain	*Verbena officinalis*
Vetiver	*Vetiveria zizanioides*
Virginia snakeroot	*Aristolochia serpentaria*
Vitex	*Vitex agnus-castus*
Wahoo	*Euonymus atropurpureus*
Walnut, English	*Juglans regia*
Watercress	*Rorippa nasturtium-aquaticum*
Water mint	*Mentha aquatica*
Wheat	*Triticum aestivum*
White bryony	*Bryonia alba*
White hellebore	*Veratrum album*
White water lily	*Nymphaea odorata*
Wild cherry	*Prunus serotina*
Wild cucumber	*Ecballium elaterium*
Wild ginger	*Asarum canadense*
Wild indigo	*Baptisia tinctoria*
Wild lettuce	*Lactuca virosa*
Wild yam	*Dioscorea villosa*
Willow	*Salix alba, S. cinereas*
Wintergreen	*Gaultheria procumbens*
Witch hazel	*Hamamelis virginiana*
Wood betony	*Stachys betonica, S. officinalis*
Woodruff, sweet	*Galium odoratum*
Wood sorrel	*Oxalis acetosella*
Wormseed	*Chenopodium ambrosioides*
Wormwood	*Artemisia absinthium*
Woundwort	*Stachys palustris*
Yarrow	*Achillea millefolium*
Yellow dock	*Rumex crispus*
Yellow flag	*Iris pseudacorus*
Yellow jasmine	*Gelsemium sempervirens*
Yellow root	*Xanthorhiza apiifolia*
Yerba mansa	*Anemopsis californica*
Yerba santa	*Eriodictyon californicum*
Yew, English	*Taxus baccata*
Yew, Pacific	*Taxus brevifolia*
Yohimbe	*Pausinystalia yohimbe*
Zedoary	*Curcuma zedoaria*

Appendix 4

PHARMACY TERMS

LATIN TERM	COMMON ABBREVIATION	TRANSLATION
ad	ad	to, up to
ad libitum	ad lib.	at pleasure
adde	add	add (thou)
agita	agit	shake, stir
alternis horis	alt. h.	every other hour
ana	a.a. or aa	of each
ante	a.	before
ante cibum	a.c.	before food, before meals
ante meridien	a.m.	morning
aqua	aq.	water
aqua ad	aq. ad.	water up to
aqua dist.	aq. dest;	distilled water
auris	aur.; a	ear
auris dexter	a.d.	right ear
auris laevus	a.l.	left ear
auris sinister	a.s.	left ear
auris utro	a.u.	each ear
auristillae	aurist	eardrops
	a.t.c.	around the clock
bis	b.	twice
bis in die	b.i.d.	twice a day
brachium	brach.	the arm
capsula	caps	a capsule
chartulae	charts	powders
cibus	cib.; c.	food
collunarium	collun	a nose wash
collutorium	collut.	a mouthwash
collyrium	collyr.	an eyewash
compositus	comp.	compound
congius	cong.; C.	gallon
cum	c or c.	with
cum cibus	c.c.	with food; with meals
dentur	d.	give (thou); let be given
dentur tales doses	d.t.d.	give of such doses
dexter	d.	right
diebus alternis	dieb. alt.	every other day
dilutus	dil.	dilute, diluted
	disp.	dispense
	div.	divide
	DW	distilled water

LATIN TERM	COMMON ABBREVIATION	TRANSLATION
	elix.	elixir
emulsum	emuls.	emulsion
et	et	and
ex modo prescripto	e.m.p.	as directed, in the manner prescribed
fac, fiat, fiant	f.; ft.	let it be made; make
	f.; fl.	fluid
flos		flower
folium	fol.	leaf
	g; G.; gm.	gram
granum	gr.	grain
guttae	gtt.	a drop
hora	h	at the hour of
hora somni	h.s.	at bedtime
	i.m.	intramuscular
injectio	inj.	injection
	i.v.; IV	intravenous
laevus	l.	left
linimentum	lin.	liniment
liquor	liq.	a solution
	lot.	lotion
minimum	min; Mx	minum
misce	m.; M	mix
	mcg	microgram
	mEq.	milliequivalent
	mg	milligram
	ml	milliliter
nocte	n.	at night
naristillae	narist.	nasal drops
nebule	neb.	a spray
non repetatur	non.rep.	do not repeat
octarius	O.	pint
oculentum	occulent.	eye ointment
oculus	o.	eye
oculus dexter	o.d.	right eye
oculus laevus	o.l.	left eye
oculus sinister	o.s.	left eye

LATIN TERM	COMMON ABBREVIATION	TRANSLATION
oculus utro	o.u.	both eyes, each eye
omni mane	o.m.	every morning
parti affectae applicandus	p.a.a.	to be applied to affected part
per os	p.o.	by mouth
post cibum	p.c.	after meals
	p.r.	per rectum
pro re nata	p.r.n.	as needed
pulvis	pulv.	powder
quater in die	q.i.d.	four times a day
quaque	q.	each, every
quaque die	q.d.	every day
quaque hora	q.h.	every hour
quantum sufficiat	q.s.	a sufficient quantity
quantum sufficiat ad	q.s. ad	a sufficient quantity to make
radix	rad.	root

LATIN TERM	COMMON ABBREVIATION	TRANSLATION
secundum artem	s.a.	according to the art
	S.C.; subc; subq	subcutaneously
semen	semen	seed
semis	ss	one half
signa	Sig.	write, label
sine	s	without
si opus sit	s.o.s.	if necessary
	sol.	solution
statim	stat.	immediately
suppositorum	supp.	suppository
syrupus	syr.	syrup
tabella	tab.	tablet
	tbsp.	tablespoonful
ter in die	t.i.d.	three times a day
	tinc.; tr.	tincture
trochiscus	troche	lozenge
tussis	tuss.	a cough
ungentum	ung.	an ointment
ut dictum	ut dict.; u.d.	as directed

Appendix 5

WEIGHT AND MEASURE CONVERSIONS

MINIMS	MILLILITERS	FLUID DRAMS	MILLILITERS	FLUID OUNCES	MILLILITERS
1	0.06	1	3.7	1	29.57
2	0.12	2	3.39	2	59.57
5	0.31	3	11.09	5	147.87
10	0.62	4	14.79	7	207.01
15	0.92	5	18.48	10	295.73
20	1.23	6	22.18	12	354.88
30	1.85	7	25.88	14	414.02
40	2.46	8 (1 fl. oz.)	29.57	16 (1 pt.)	473.17
50	3.08			32 (1 qt.)	946.33
60 (1 fl. dr.)	3.70			128 (1 gal.)	3785.32

Apothecaries—Metric Weight Conversion

GRAINS	GRAMS	DRAMS	GRAMS	OUNCES	GRAMS
$^1/_2$	0.032	1	3.888	1	31.103
1	0.065	2	7.776	2	62.207
$1^1/_2$	0.097 (0.1)	3	11.664	3	93.310
2	0.12	4	15.552	4	124.414
5	0.30	5	19.440	5	155.517
10	0.65	6	23.328	6	186.621
15	1.00	7	27.216	7	217.724
20	1.30	8 (1 oz.)	31.103	8	248.828
30	2.00			9	279.931
				10	311.035
				12	373.242

Appendix 6

HERBAL INFORMATION SOURCES

There is a great need for herbalists to be well informed about the diversity of information and approaches within their field of interest. For the purpose of this appendix, I have grouped a wide range of activities under the category "Herbalist," even though the members of these various groups may not agree with me. There are forms of phytotherapy that embrace both the folk healers and those using a developed medical system. There are herbal approaches based within the Western biomedical model, as well as Oriental practices, such as traditional Chinese medicine and ayurveda. Pharmacognosists, phytopharmacologists, and ethnobotanists also fit within the herbal categorization, as do those involved in the various aspects of the herbal products industry.

Herbal information germane to the various subgroupings within the herbal field exists but is often unknown to those in different segments of this wide-ranging field. There is a great need to expand the usual sources of information and build bridges between these enclaves of interest. Unfortunately, there are many issues of mutual comprehension, as language often blocks communication in medicine. Nuances of vocabulary disparities can mask fundamental agreements of ideas and approach. Likewise, lack of clarity often obscures important differences in both principle and technique. Within the field, there is often a dogmatic attachment to words and specific formulations of belief, opinion, and theory. It is important that modalities that have their foundations outside the biomedical model not be ignored or discounted because they exemplify a different belief system, as they represent an enrichment of possibilities, not a challenge to the status quo.

The material that follows focuses on the information resources that relate to Western herbalism. I hope that herbalists familiar with the other cultural forms of herbalism, such as ayurveda and TCM, will create similar guides in the future.

LIBRARIES

Libraries are an astonishing resource as long as the herbalist knows how to use them and—sometimes more important—how to relate to librarians! A range of specialized libraries are described by subject area in directories such as:

Subject Collections, Lee Ash, R.R. Bowker Co., 5th. ed., 1978.
Directory of Special Libraries and Information Centers, Gale Research Co.

Of all the specialized libraries, the Lloyd Library is of paramount interest.

Lloyd Library, 917 Plum Street, Cincinnati, OH 45202, (513) 721-3707, www.lloydlibrary.org
The Lloyd Library has one of the finest collections of the literature of botany and pharmacy in the United States, specializing in plant chemistry, pharmacognosy, medicinal plants, and Eclectic medicine. It houses the accumulated libraries of all the Eclectic medical schools, as well as a vast collection of Eclectic case history files. This cornucopia of Eclectic knowledge is a unique and irreplaceable resource. To quote Michael Moore, director of the Southwest School of Botanical Medicine, the library contains "the writings of a discipline of medicine that survived for a century that was famous (or infamous) for its vast plant materia medica that treated the patient and NOT the pathology, a sophisticated model of vitalist healing every bit as usable as traditional Chinese medicine and ayurvedic medicine."

The library boasts one of the world's largest and most complete collections of pharmacopoeias, formularies, and dispensatories. The periodicals collection includes many rare journals hard to obtain elsewhere, and often in complete, unbroken sets. The library also supports the scientific research of natural products through joint publication of the *Journal of Natural Products* (Lloydia) with the American Society of Pharmacognosy. Much information from the library is distributed by mail or provided over the phone.

The Dewey Decimal and Library of Congress Classification Systems

Both the Dewey Decimal and Library of Congress classification systems facilitate access to the wealth of books published in the English language that are relevant to the multidisciplinary interests of phytotherapy.

The Dewey Decimal System

The Dewey Decimal System of Classification, used in most local and school libraries, has the advantage of a limited number of general categories and short call numbers. The system is based on ten classes of subject (000–999), which are then further subdivided. Below are examples of the listings found under the categories Herb, Botanical Science, and Medical Sciences.

Herb

Herb gardens	635.7
agriculture	635.7
commercial processing	663.96
Herb teas	641.357
cooking with	641.657
home preparation	641.877
Herbaceous flowering plants	582.13
Herbaceous plants	582.12
Herbaceous shrubs	582.14
Herbaceous vines	582.14
Herbals	
Pharmacognosy	615.321
Herbariums	580.742

580 Botanical Science

581.6	Economic botany
581.61	Beneficial plants
581.63	Edible and medicinal plants
581.64	Plants of industrial & technological value
581.65	Deleterious plants
581.67	Allergenic plants
581.69	Poisonous plants

610 Medical Sciences

615.1	Drugs (materia medica)
615.11	Pharmacopoeias
615.12	Dispensatories
615.13	Formularies
615.3	Organic drugs
615.32	Drugs of plant origin
615.321	Pharmacognosy
615.53	General therapeutic systems, including Eclectic, botanic medicine, and ayurveda
615.535	Naturopathy
615.8	Specific therapies and kinds of therapies
615.88	Empirical and historical remedies
615.882	Folk medicine
615.886	Patent medicines

The Library of Congress (LC) classification

The Library of Congress, or LC, classification consists of separate, mutually exclusive, special classifications. The arrangement roughly follows groupings of social sciences, humanities, and natural and physical sciences. It divides the references into 20 large classes and an additional class for general works. Each main class has a synopsis that also serves as a guide. Resulting order is from the general to the specific, from the theoretical to the practical. Listed below are the letters and titles of the main classes.

A—General Works
B—Philosophy. Psychology. Religion
C—Auxiliary Sciences of History
D—History: General and Old World
E—History: America
F—History: America
G—Geography. Anthropology. Recreation
H—Social Sciences
J—Political Science
K—Law
L—Education
M—Music and Books on Music
N—Fine Arts
P—Language and Literature
Q—Science
R—Medicine
S—Agriculture
T—Technology
U—Military Science
V—Naval Science
Z—Library Science

In place of standard subdivisions, each class may incorporate divisions for literary form and geography. Terminology may be explicit, exact, scientific, or popular, depending on the situation. Subdivisions in the LC system are arranged roughly on a historical basis, and the notation is mixed, combining capital letters and numerals. More combinations, and thus greater specificity, is possible, yet excessively long notations do not occur. As examples, consider some herbally relevant subcategories in Science and in Medicine:

Class Q SCIENCE

QD	1–999	Chemistry
QH	1–705.5	Biology (General)
QK	1–989	Botany
QP	1–981	Physiology

Class R MEDICINE

RM	1–950	Therapeutics. Pharmacology
RS	1–441	Pharmacy and Materia Medica
RV	1–431	Botanic, Thomsonian, and Eclectic medicine
RX	1–681	Homeopathy
RZ	201–999	Other systems of medicine

Subject headings used by the LC system under which information concerning medicinal plants and their therapeutic application in medicine may be found include:

Materia Medica	RS 153–441
Medicinal Plants	QK 99, RS 164
Herbal Teas	RM 666
Herbs—Therapeutic Use	RA 1250
Pharmacognosy	RS 160–167
Economic Botany	QH 705–705.5

National Library of Medicine (NML) Classification

The National Library of Medicine classification covers the field of medicine and related sciences. It is a system of mixed notation patterned after the Library of Congress (LC) classification where alphabetical letters that denote broad subject categories are further subdivided by numbers. The NLM classification utilizes schedules QS–QZ and W–WZ, permanently excluded from the LC classification. An outline of the National Library of Medicine classification can be found on the Web at: wwwcf.nlm.nih.gov/class/OutlineofNLMClassificationSchedule.html.

The Index to the NLM classification consists primarily of Medical Subject Headings (MeSH), a set of terms or subject headings that are arranged in both an alphabetic and a hierarchical structure to permit searching at various levels of specificity from narrower to broader. There are almost 19,000 main headings in MeSH and nearly 800 specialized descriptors, called Qualifiers.

Index entries are updated annually to reflect additions and changes to the vocabulary. A few of the significant herbal headings are as follows:

Dispensatories, formularies, etc.	QV 740
Drugs, Chinese Herbal	QV 766
Ethnobotany	GN 476.73
Ethnopharmacology	QV 752
Herbal medicine	WB 925
Materia medica	QV 760
Medicine, Chinese Traditional	WB 50
Medicine, Herbal	WB 925
Medicine, Traditional	WB 50
Pharmacognosy	QV 752
Pharmacopoeias	QV 738
Phytotherapy	WB 925
Plant Extracts	QV 766
Plant Preparations	QV 766–770
Plants, Edible	QK 98.5
Plants, Medicinal	QV 766–770

The MeSH thesaurus is used for indexing articles for the MEDLINE database. Each reference is associated with a set of MeSH terms that describe the content of the item. Similarly, a retrieval query is formed using MeSH terms to find items on a desired topic.

A number of terms directly relevant to herbal medicine are found in the MeSH thesaurus. The following are the most useful, with the number of citations found (June 2003):

Drugs, Chinese Herbal	8,554
Medicine, Herbal	3,820
Phytotherapy	7,516
Plant Extracts	39,068
Plants, Medicinal	35,774

However, there is an undefined amount of overlap. The sum of all the citations from the above list is 94,732. If a Boolean search is done using all the search terms but excluding duplicates, a total of 68,202 is found. This represents a truly impressive body of knowledge. A further search done to ascertain how many of these citations were human studies found 26,558 papers.

It is interesting to note the exponential increase in citations listed for these herbal MeSH terms over the time frame covered in the yearly database.

Year	1970	1975	1980	1985	1990	1995	2000	2003
Number of citations	6,804	12,896	17,501	23,510	31,798	42,649	58,698	68,202

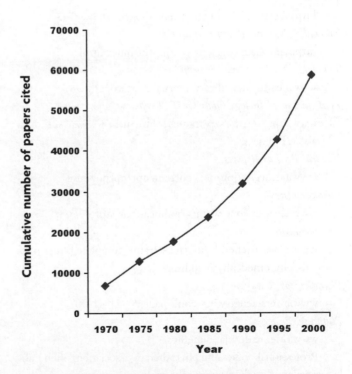

As impressive as the MeSH thesaurus is, it has some limitations when approached herbally. For the phytotherapist it is often non-MeSH words that are used for finding a particular reference. However, because only a few genus names are assigned as MeSH terms, any herb discussed in a research paper can be accessed via its genus name.

PEER-REVIEW JOURNALS AND PROFESSIONAL NEWSLETTERS

A number of peer-review journals specialize in either phytotherapy itself or studies of medicinal plants. The primary ones published in English are:

Alternative and Complementary Therapies
    www.liebertpub.com/
Alternative Medicine Review
    www.thorne.com/alternative/alter_main.html
Alternative Therapies in Health and Medicine
    www.alternative-therapies.com/at/login/index.jsp
American Journal of Botany
    www.amjbot.org/
American Journal of Clinical Nutrition
    www.ajcn.org/
Economic Botany
    www.econbot.org/
European Phytojournal
    www.ex.ac.uk/phytonet/phytojournal/index.htm
Fitoterapia
    www.elsevier.nl/locate/fitote
Journal of Alternative and Complementary Medicine
    www.liebertpub.com/ACM/default1.asp
Journal of Ethnopharmacology
    http://sciencedirect.com/science/journal/03788742
Journal of Natural Products (Lloydia)
    http://pubs.acs.org/journals/jnprdf/index.html
Journal of Naturopathic Medicine
    www.healthy.net/library/journals/naturopathic/
Pharmaceutical Biology (Journal of Pharmacognosy)
    www.szp.swets.nl/szp/frameset.htm?url=%2Fszp%2Fjournals%2Fpb.htm
Natural Product Reports
    www.rsc.org/is/journals/current/npr/nprpub.htm
Phytochemistry
    www.elsevier.com:80/inca/publications/store/2/7/3/
Phytomedicine
    www.urbanfischer.de/journals/frame_template.htm?/journals/phytomed/phytmed.htm
Phytotherapy Research
    www.interscience.wiley.com/jpages/0951-418X/
Planta Medica
    www.thieme.de/plantamedica/

Professional bodies and phytotherapy associations often publish excellent, highly relevant, although not peer-reviewed, journals and newsletters. Ones of note published in English include:

American Herb Association Quarterly
    www.ahaherb.com/
Australian Journal of Medical Herbalism
    www.nhaa.org.au/journal.html
The British Journal of Phytotherapy
    (no Web address available)

HerbalGram
    www.herbalgram.org/herbalgram/
Medical Herbalism
    www.medherb.com
Townsend Letter for Doctors & Patients
    www.tldp.com/

OUT-OF-PRINT BOOKS

As many of the primary source books are out of print, it is necessary to use the services of book-search specialists. Most bookstores can do a nationwide search but it is often more effective to go directly to the specialized search agency. The Antiquarian Booksellers Association of America publishes the *Bookman's Weekly*, the leading guide to services and books offered. There are a few antiquarian-book dealers that specialize in herbals and Eclectic material. One of these is Herbalist & Alchemist Books, run by one of America's foremost phytotherapists, David Winston. It publishes a twice-yearly catalog of books and journals relating to herbalism, Eclectic medicine, economic botany, pre-1920 pharmacy, ethnobotany, and natural products chemistry.

Herbalist & Alchemist Books, PO Box 553, Broadway, NJ 08808, (908) 689-9020.

ONLINE DATABASES

Before personal computers, creating bibliographies and finding reference material relevant to phytotherapy meant spending many hours in the library working through volumes of printed indexes and card catalogs, writing down each citation, finding the document, and then photocopying it. Online database retrieval now allows the herbal researcher access to millions of articles at the touch of a keyboard. Two databases of primary importance to herbalism are NAPRALERT and MEDLINE, although other useful sites are included as well.

AGRICOLA (Agriculture Online Access)

    www.nalusda.gov/general_info/agricola/agricola.html
A bibliographic database containing selective worldwide coverage of agriculture and related fields from 1970 to the present. AGRICOLA is the locator and bibliographic access and control system of the National Agricultural Library collections and also includes records from other cooperating institutions. Records contain bibliographic information, geographic terms, GenBank Numbers, chemical names, and CAS Registry Numbers. Abstracts are available for some records.

BIOSIS

    www.biosis.org.
A bibliographic database covering worldwide literature on all biological and biomedical topics. The database includes the printed *Biological Abstracts* (1969–present); Biological Abstracts/RRM (Reports, Review, Meetings), 1980–present; and the BioResearch Index (1969–79). Records contain bibli-

ographic data, keywords, and Biosystematic and Concept Codes. CAS Registry Numbers and chemical names are present for substances appearing in the title and keyword fields.

Chemical Abstracts

www.cas.org

The premier indexing source for chemical, biochemical, and chemical engineering literature, covering over 12,000 journals and conferences, as well as technical reports, dissertations, books, and patents. There are two parts: weekly abstracts issues arranged by topics and cumulative semiannual indexes using chemical name, formula, subject, and author.

Medicinal Plants of Native America Database (MPNADB)

herb.umd.umich.edu/

The Medicinal Plants of Native America Database, based on the book of the same name, contains data on the medicinal uses of 2,147 species by 123 different Native American peoples. The database was created by Dr. Daniel E. Moerman, and the site is a resource of the National Agricultural Library.

NAPRALERT (Natural Products Alert)

www.cas.org/ONLINE/DBSS/napralertss.html

The largest and most comprehensive computerized database covering medicinal plants is NAPRALERT, established by Professor Norman Farnsworth and colleagues at the University of Illinois at Chicago. NAPRALERT also covers the world's literature on the chemistry and pharmacology of secondary metabolites derived from natural sources. From this, a wide range of printouts can be prepared providing, for example, ethnomedical, pharmacological, and phytochemical profiles for any given plant, animal, or microbe. The database is maintained by the Program for Collaborative Research in the Pharmaceutical Sciences, College of Pharmacy, University of Illinois at Chicago. Combined, the articles contain information on more than 87,000 chemicals and more than 38,000 plant and animal species and include more than 426,000 records on biological activity associated with those species. For subscription information, call (312) 996-2246.

Phytochemical and Ethnobotanical Databases

www.ars-grin.gov/duke/

Phytochemical and Ethnobotanical Databases is a directory to various USDA plant databases. The site consists of four major areas: the Phytochemco Database, related browsable databases (listed below), documents, and additional resources. The Phytochemco Database can be searched in a variety of ways. For example, a search can list reported constituents of a specific plant, identify constituents within a specific activity, list all plants known to contain a specific chemical, and identify chemicals with a specific lethal dose value. Ethnobotany searches give ethnobotanical uses for a plant or plants with a particular ethnobotanical use. All the database references will yield reference citations. Other related databases accessible through the Phyto-

chemical and Ethnobotanical Databases are Ecosys (ecological ranges), Ethnobot DB (worldwide plant uses), Foodplant DB (Native American food plants), MPNADB (medicinal plants of Native America), and Phytochem DB (plant chemicals).

The National Library of Medicine

www.nlm.nih.gov

The National Library of Medicine (NLM) is the world's largest medical library. The library collects materials in all areas of biomedicine and health care, as well as works on biomedical aspects of technology, the humanities, and the physical, life, and social sciences. For over 100 years, the library has published the *Index Medicus*, a monthly subject/author guide to articles in 3,400 journals. This information (and much more) is now available in the database MEDLINE, the major online component of PubMed (see below), freely accessible via the World Wide Web. A number of additional databases provided by the NLM, including one covering clinical trials, are listed here below.

MEDLINE (Medical Literature, Analysis, and Retrieval System Online)

www.ncbi.nlm.nih.gov/entrez/query.fcgi

MEDLINE is the NLM's premier bibliographic database, containing citations and author abstracts from more than 4,600 biomedical journals published in the United States and 70 other countries. It lists over 12 million citations dating back to the mid-1960s. Coverage is worldwide, but most records are from English-language sources or have English abstracts. Citations prior to the mid-1960s can be found in NLM's OLDMEDLINE database. Almost 2,000 completed references are added daily. MEDLINE is available on the Internet through the PubMed URL and can be searched free of charge. No registration is required.

PubMed

www.ncbi.nlm.nih.gov/entrez/query.fcgi

Provides free access to MEDLINE and more, including selected life sciences journals not in MEDLINE. PubMed was developed by the National Center for Biotechnology Information (NCBI) at the NLM. Entrez is the text-based search and retrieval system used at NCBI for all major databases including PubMed, Nucleotide, Protein Sequences, Protein Structures, Complete Genomes, and Taxonomy. LinkOut provides access to full-text articles at journal Web sites and other related Web resources.

ClinicalTrials

www.clinicaltrials.gov/

This Web site of the NLM provides current information for patients and the general public about clinical research studies.

DIRLINE

dirline.nlm.nih.gov/

The NLM's directory of health organizations. An online database containing location and information about other resources concerned with health and biomedicine, including organizations, research resources, projects, and databases.

ADDITIONAL SITES

Herbalists

The Southwest School of Botanical Medicine/ Michael Moore

www.swsbm.com/HOMEPAGE/HomePage.html

A cornucopia of herbal wisdom and information. Michael Moore is to be commended for making his wealth of phytotherapeutic experience and insights so readily available. His site also houses online versions of many Eclectic and Thomsonian texts, which are essential reading for any medical herbalist. A brief overview of the site's sections will illustrate its importance:

> Medicinal Plant Photographs by genus
> Texts and Manuals by Michael Moore
> Eclectic Medicine, Materia Medica and Pharmacy—classic
> texts, including:
>> *American Materia Medica, Therapeutics and Pharmacognosy*
>> www.swsbm.com/Ellingwoods/Ellingwoods.html
>> *The Eclectic Materia Medica, Pharmacology and Therapeutics*
>> www.swsbm.com/FelterMM/Felters.html
> Eclectic and Pharmaceutical Journals—classic texts
> Herbology and Herb Growing—classic texts
> Thomsonian Medicine—classic texts
> Ethnobotany and Traditional Plant Uses—classic texts
> Medicinal Plants: Research, Resources, FAQs, Regional
> Plant Checklists

Henriette's Herbal Homepage

ibiblio.org/herbmed/index.html

Another treasure trove of relevant material, offered by Henriette Kress, an herbalist in Finland.

Howie Brounstein's Homepage

www.teleport.com/~howieb/howie.html

Jonathan Treasure's Herbal Bookworm

www.herbological.com

Medical Herbalism/Paul Bergner

www.medherb.com

Robyn Klein's Recommended Reading

www.rrreading.com

Rosemary Gladstar's Sagemountain

www.sagemountain.com

Christopher Hobbs Virtual Herbal

www.christopherhobbs.com

Directories/Links/Databases

Library of Congress World Wide Web

marvel.loc.gov/

WWW Virtual Library

vlib.org/

Internet Directory for Botany: economic botany, ethnobotany

www.botany.net/IDB/subject/botecon.html

Open Directory: Science, Biology, Botany, Ethnobotany

dmoz.org/Science/Biology/Botany/Ethnobotany/

Excite Directory: Science, Biology, Botany, Ethnobotany

www.excite.co.uk/directory/Science/Biology/Botany/Ethnobotany

Open Directory: Health, Alternative, Herbs

dmoz.org/Health/Alternative/Herbs/

Excite Directory: Health, Alternative, Herb

www.excite.co.uk/directory/Health/Alternative/Herbs

Omni

omni.ac.uk/browse/mesh/detail/C0025125L0025125.html

Food & Drug Administration (FDA)

www.fda.gov/fdahomepage.html

Martindale's Bio & Medical Databases

www.sci.lib.uci.edu/~martindale/RefDatabaseBio.html

NIH Office of Dietary Supplements

dietary-supplements.info.nih.gov/

NIH Web Search

search.info.nih.gov/

Phytonet

www.exeter.ac.uk/phytonet/welcome.html

Phytopharmacognosy

www.mdx.ac.uk/www/pharm/

Materia Medicas

A Modern Herbal (Mrs. Grieve)

www.botanical.com/botanical/mgmh/mgmh.html

HealthWorld Online

www.healthy.net/

HerbMed

www.herbmed.org/

King's American Dispensatory

www.ibiblio.org/herbmed/eclectic/kings/intro.html

The Raintree Tropical Plant Database
www.rain-tree.com/plants.htm

The TCM Herbal Database
www.rmhiherbal.org/ai/pharintro.html

Associations

American Association of Naturopathic Physicians
www.naturopathic.org/

American Association of Oriental Medicine
www.aaom.org/

American Botanical Council
www.herbalgram.org/

American Herb Product Association
www.ahpa.org/

American Herbal Pharmacopoeia
www.herbal-ahp.org/

American Herbalists Guild
www.americanherbalistsguild.com/

British Herbal Medical Association
www.ex.ac.uk/phytonet/bhma.html

European Scientific Co-operative on Phytotherapy (ESCOP)
www.ex.ac.uk/phytonct/cscop.html

Gesellschaft für Phytotherapie e.V.
www.phytotherapy.org/

Herb Research Foundation
www.herbs.org/

National Centre for Complementary and Alternative Medicine
altmed.od.nih.gov/

National Herbalists Association of Australia
www.nhaa.org.au/

National Institute of Medical Herbalists
www.nimh.org.uk/

New Zealand Association of Medical Herbalists
nzamh.org.nz/

The European Herbal Practitioners Association
www.users.globalnet.co.uk/~ehpa

The Ontario Herbalists Association
www.herbalists.on.ca/

United Plant Savers
www.plantsavers.org/

Phytochemicals

Phytochemistry Tutorials
www.friedli.com/herbs/phytochem/phyto_tutorial.html

The Phytochemistry of Herbs
www.herbalchem.net/

Chemfinder
chemfinder.cambridgesoft.com/

Taxomony

Integrated Taxonomic Information System
www.itis.usda.gov/index.html

Missouri Botanical Garden
www.mobot.org/

PLANTS Database (USDA)
plants.usda.gov/

GRIN Taxonomy
www.ars-grin.gov/npgs/tax/

Appendix 7

TAXONOMY HIERARCHY

Kingdom Plantae
Division Phaeophycophyta (brown algae: 1,500 species)
  Class Phaeophyceae
    Order Fucales
      Family Fucaceae
        Genus *Fucus vesiculosus*—bladderwrack
Division Rhodophycota (red algae: 4,000 species)
  Class Rhodophyceae
    Order Gigartinales
      Family Gigartinaceae
        Genus/Species *Chondrus crispus*
Division Bryophyta (mosses)
  Subdivision Musci
  Class Sphagnopsida
    Subclass Sphagnidae
      Order Sphagnales
        Family Sphagnaceae
          Genus *Sphagnum* L. (336 spp.)
Division Equisetophyta
  Class Equisetopsida
    Order Equisetales (1 family)
      Family Equisetaceae (1 genus)
        Genus *Equisetum* (32 spp.)
          Species *E. arvense* L.—horsetail
Division Lycopodiophyta
  Class Lycopsida
    Order Lycopodiales
      Family Lycopodiaceae (4–14 genera, 350–400 spp.)
        Genus *Lycopodium* (200 spp.)
          Species *L. clavatum* L.—club moss
Division Pteridophyta
  Class Filicopsida
    Order Polypodiales (28 families)
      Family Dryopteridaceae (60–78 genera, 3,000–3,500 spp.)
        Genus *Dryopteris* (150 spp.)
          Species *Dryopteris filix-mas* L.—male fern
Division Ginkgophyta
  Class Ginkgoopsida
    Order Ginkgoales (1 family)
      Family Ginkgoaceae (1 genus)
        Genus *Ginkgo* (1 sp.)
          Species *Ginkgo biloba* L.—ginkgo
Division Coniferophyta (gymnosperms)
  Class Pinopsida
    Order Taxales
      Family Taxaceae (5 genera, 17–20 spp.)
        Genus *Taxus* (8 spp.)
          Species *Taxus brevifolia* Nutt.—Pacific yew

    Order Pinales (4 families)
      Family Pinaceae (9–12 genera, 210 spp.)
        Genus *Abies* (50 spp.)
          Species *Abies balsamea*—balsam fir
      Family Cupressaceae (28 genera, 120 spp.)
        Genus *Juniperus* (60 spp.)
          Species *Juniperus communis* L.—common juniper
        Genus *Thuja* (5 spp.)
          Species *Thuja occidentalis* L.—arborvitae
Division Gnetophyta
  Class Gnetopsida (3 orders)
    Order Ephedrales (1 family)
      Family Ephedraceae (1 genus, 40 spp.)
        Genus *Ephedra* (40 spp.)
          Species *Ephedra sinica* Stapf—ma huang
Division Magnoliophyta (angiosperms, flowering plants)
  (250,000 spp.)
  Class Magnoliopsida
    Subclass Magnoliidae (8 orders)
      Order Magnoliales (10 families)
        Family Magnoliaceae (7–12 genera, 220 spp.)
          Genus *Magnolia* (180 spp.)
            Species *Magnolia* x *soulangiana* Soul.-Bod.—
            Chinese magnolia, Hou Pu
        Family Myristicaceae (18 genera, 300 spp.)
          Genus *Myristica* (120 spp.)
            Species *Myristica fragrans* Houtt.—nutmeg
      Order Laurales (8 families)
        Family Monimiaceae (30 genera)
          Genus *Peumus* (1 sp.)
            Species *Peumus boldus* Molina—boldo
        Family Lauraceae (30–50 genera, 2,000 spp.)
          Genus *Cinnamomum* (200 spp.)
            Species *Cinnamomum camphora* (L.) J. Presl.—
            camphor
          Genus *Laurus* (2 spp.)
            Species *Laurus nobilis* L.—sweet bay
          Genus *Sassafras* (3 spp.)
            Species *Sassafras albidum* (Nutt.) Nees—sassafras
      Order Piperales (3 families)
        Family Piperaceae (10 genera, 1,400–2,000 spp.)
          Genus *Piper* (1,000 spp.)
            Species *Piper betel* L.—betel pepper
            Species *Piper cubeba* L. f.—cubeb
            Species *Piper methysticum* G. Forst.—kava kava
            Species *Piper nigrum* L.—black pepper

Order Aristolochiales (3 families)
Family Aristolochiaceae (8–10 genera, 600 spp.)
Genus *Aristolochia* L. (500 spp.)
Species *Aristolochia reticulata* Jacq.—birthwort
Order Illiciales (2 families)
Family Schisandraceae (2 genera, 47 spp.)
Genus Schisandra (25 spp.)
Species *Schisandra chinensis*—schizandra
Order Papaverales (9 families)
Family Papaveraceae (26 genera, 300 spp.)
Genus *Papaver* (100 spp.)
Species *Papaver somniferum* L.—opium poppy
Genus *Chelidonium* (2 spp.)
Species *Chelidonium majus* L.—celandine
Genus *Sanguinaria* (1 sp.)
Species *Sanguinaria canadensis* L.—bloodroot
Genus *Eschscholzia* (10 spp.)
Species *Eschscholzia californica* Cham.—
California poppy
Family Fumariaceae (16 genera, 55 spp.)
Genus Fumaria (425 spp.)
Species *Fumaria officinalis* L.—fumitory
Order Ranunculales (8 families)
Family Ranunculaceae (50–52 genera, 2,000 spp.)
Genus *Aconitum* (100 spp.)
Species *Aconitum napellus* L.—aconite, monkshood
Genus *Pulsatilla* (7 spp.)
Species *Pulsatilla vulgaris* (L.) P. Mill.—pasqueflower
Genus *Cimicifuga* (15 spp.)
Species *Cimicifuga racemosa* (L.) Nutt.—black
cohosh
Genus *Coptis* (10 spp.)
Species *Coptis trifolia* (L.) Salisb.—goldthread
Genus *Ranunculus* (400 spp.)
Species *Ranunculus ficaria* L.—lesser celandine
Genus *Hydrastis* (2 spp.)
Species *Hydrastis canadensis* L.—goldenseal
Family Berberidaceae (16–18 genera, 600 spp.)
Genus *Berberis* (450 spp.)
Species *Berberis vulgaris* L.—barberry
Genus *Mahonia* (12 spp.)
Species *Mahonia aquifolium* (Pursh) Nutt.—Oregon
grape
Genus *Caulophyllum* (2 spp.)
Species *Caulophyllum thalictroides* (L.) Michx.—
blue cohosh
Genus *Podophyllum* L. (2 spp.)
Species *Podophyllum peltatum* L.—mayapple
Subclass Rosidae (18 orders)
Order Rosales (24 families)
Family Hydrangeaceae (17 genera, 170 spp.)
Genus *Hydrangea* (23 spp.)
Species *Hydrangea arborescens* L.—wild hydrangea
Family Rosaceae (100 genera, 2,000 spp.)
Genus *Agrimonia* (15 spp.)
Species *Agrimonia eupatoria* L.—agrimony
Genus *Crataegus* (200 spp.)
Species *Crataegus laevigata* (Poir.) DC.—smooth
hawthorn
Genus *Filipendula* (10 spp.)
Species *Filipendula ulmaria* (L.) Maxim.—
meadowsweet

Genus *Prunus* (430 spp.)
Species *Prunus serotina* Ehrh.—black cherry
Genus *Rubus* L. (250 spp.)
Species *Rubus idaeus* L.—common red raspberry
Order Fabales (19 families)
Family Fabaceae (590–800 genera, 14,000–20,000 spp.)
Genus *Astragalus* (1000 spp.)
Species *Astragalus membranaceus*—astragalus
Genus *Baptisia* (30–35 spp.)
Species *Baptisia tinctoria* (L.) Venten.—wild indigo
Genus *Cyamopsis* (3 spp.)
Species *Cyamopsis tetragonoloba* (L.) Taubert—guar
Genus *Galega* (6–8 spp.)
Species *Galega officinalis* L.—goat's rue
Genus *Glycine* (4 spp.)
Species *Glycine max* (L.) Merr.—soybean
Genus *Medicago* (100 spp.)
Species *Medicago sativa* L.—alfalfa
Genus *Melilotus* (25 spp.)
Species *Melilotus officinalis* (L.) Lam.—sweet
clover
Genus *Myroxylon* (2 spp.)
Species *Myroxylon balsamum* (L.) Harms—
balsam of Tolu
Genus *Trifolium* (300 spp.)
Species *Trifolium pratense* L.—red clover
Genus *Trigonella* (100 spp.)
Species *Trigonella foenum-graecum* L.—fenugreek
Genus *Acacia* (750–800 spp.)
Species *Acacia catechu* (L. f.) Willd.—black catechu
Order Myrtales (14 families)
Family Myrtaceae (140 genera, 3,000 spp.)
Genus *Eucalyptus* (600 spp.)
Species *Eucalyptus globulus* Labill.—eucalyptus
Genus *Pimenta* (4 spp.)
Species *Pimenta dioica* (L.) Merr.—allspice
Genus *Syzygium* (400–500 spp.)
Species *Syzygium aromaticum* (L.) Skeels—clove
Family Onagraceae (16–17 genera, 645 spp.)
Genus *Oenothera* (80 spp.)
Species *Oenothera biennis* L.—evening primrose
Order Santalales (10 families)
Family Viscaceae (8 genera, 350 spp.)
Genus *Viscum* (60–70 spp.)
Species *Viscum album* L.—European mistletoe
Order Celastrales (13 families)
Family Celastraceae (50–85 genera, 800 spp.)
Genus *Euonymus* (176 spp.)
Species *Euonymus atropurpurea* Jacq.—wahoo
Genus *Catha* (1 sp.)
Species *Catha edulis* (Vahl) Forssk. ex Endl.—khat
Family Aquifoliaceae (4 genera, 200–400 spp.)
Genus *Ilex* (399 spp.)
Species *Ilex aquifolium* L.—English holly
Species *Ilex paraguariensis* St.-Hil.—maté
Order Euphorbiales (4 families)
Family Euphorbiaceae (310–320 genera, 7,500 spp.)
Genus *Euphorbia* (2,000 spp.)
Species *Euphorbia pilulifera* Engelm.—pill-bearing
spurge
Genus *Ricinus* (1 sp.)
Species *Ricinus communis* L.—castor bean

Order Rhamnales (3 families)
  Family *Rhamnaceae* (50–55 genera, 900 spp.)
    Genus *Ceanothus* (55 spp.)
      Species *Ceanothus americanus* L.—red root
    Genus *Rhamnus* (110 spp.)
      Species *Rhamnus cathartica* L.—buckthorn
    Genus *Ziziphus* (100 spp.)
      Species *Ziziphus jujuba* (L.) Karst.—jujube
Order Linales (5 familes)
  Family Erythroxylaceae (4 genera, 200 spp.)
    Genus *Erythroxylum* (7 spp.)
      Species *Erythroxylum coca* Lam.—coca
  Family Linaceae (19 genera, 290 spp.)
    Genus *Linum* (230 spp.)
      Species *Linum usitatissimum* L.—flax
Order Polygalales (7 families)
  Family Polygalaceae (12–19 genera, 750 spp.)
    Genus *Polygala* (600 spp.)
      Species *Polygala senega* L.—Seneca snakeroot
  Family Krameriaceae (1 genus)
    Genus *Krameria* (17 spp.)
      Species *Krameria triandra* L.—rhatany
Order Sapindales (15 families)
  Family Sapindaceae (134–140 genera, 1,500 spp.)
    Genus *Paullinia* L. (180 spp.)
      Species *Paullinia cupana* L. Kunth—guarana
  Family Hippocastanaceae (2 genera, 16 spp.)
    Genus *Aesculus* L. (13 spp.)
      Species *Aesculus hippocastanum* L.—horse chestnut
  Family Burseraceae (16–20 genera, 600 spp.)
    Genus *Boswellia* (24 spp.)
      Species *Boswellia sacra* Flueck.—frankincense
    Genus *Commiphora* (185 spp.)
      Species *Commiphora molmol* Jacq.—myrrh
  Family Anacardiaceae (60–70 genera, 600 spp.)
    Genus *Rhus* L. (250 spp.)
      Species *Rhus aromatica* Ait.—fragrant sumac
  Family Rutaceae (150–158 genera, 900–1,500 spp.)
    Genus *Agathosma* (134 spp.)
      Species *Agathosma betulina* (Bergius) Pill.—buchu
    Genus *Citrus* (16 spp.)
      Species *Citrus limetta* Risso—bitter orange
    Genus *Pilocarpus* (22 spp.)
      Species *Pilocarpus jaborandi* Holmes—jaborandi
    Genus *Ruta* (40 spp.)
      Species *Ruta graveolens* L.—rue
    Genus *Zanthoxylum* (30 spp.)
      Species *Zanthoxylum americanum* Mill.—prickly ash
  Family Zygophyllaceae (25 genera, 240 spp.)
    Genus *Guaiacum* (6 spp.)
      Species *Guaiacum sanctum* L.—lignum-vitae
    Genus *Larrea* (3–4 spp.)
      Species *Larrea tridentata* (Sessé & Moc. ex DC.) Cov.—chaparral
Order Geraniales (6 families)
  Family Geraniaceae (11 genera, 750 spp.)
    Genus *Geranium* (400 spp.)
      Species *Geranium maculatum* L.—American cranesbill

Order Apiales (7 families)
  Family Araliaceae (47–70 genera, 700 spp.)
    Genus *Panax* (8 spp.)
      Species *Panax ginseng* C. Mey.—Korean ginseng
      Species *Panax quinquefolius* L.—American ginseng
    Genus *Eleutherococcus* (50 spp.)
      Species *Eleutherococcus senticosus* (Rupr. et Maxim.)—Siberian ginseng
    Genus *Aralia* L. (25 spp.)
      Species *Aralia racemosa* L.—American spikenard
    Genus *Hedera* (15 spp.)
      Species *Hedera helix* L.—English ivy
  Family Apiaceae (Umbelliferae) (428 genera, 3,000 spp.)
    Genus *Ammi* L. (10 spp.)
      Species *Ammi visnaga* L. Lam.—khella
    Genus *Anethum* (2 spp.)
      Species *Anethum graveolens* L.—dill
    Genus *Angelica* (80 spp.)
      Species *Angelica archangelica* L.—angelica
      Species *Angelica sinensis* (Oliv.) Diels—dong quai
    Genus *Apium* (1 sp.)
      Species *Apium graveolens* L.—celery
    Genus *Bupleurum* (100 spp.)
      Species *Bupleurum falcatum* L.—bupleurum
    Genus *Carum* (30 spp.)
      Species *Carum carvi* L.—caraway
    Genus *Centella* (100 spp.)
      Species *Centella asiatica* (L.) Urban—gotu cola
    Genus *Conium* (4 spp.)
      Species *Conium maculatum* L.—poison hemlock
    Genus *Daucus* (60 spp.)
      Species *Daucus carota* L.—wild carrot
    Genus *Ferula* (100+ spp.)
      Species *Ferula assa-foetida* L.—asafetida
      Species *Ferula gummosa* Boiss.—galbanum
    Genus *Foeniculum* (5 spp.)
      Species *Foeniculum vulgare* Mill.—fennel
    Genus *Lomatium* (70 spp.)
      Species *Lomatium dissectum* (Nutt.) Mathias & Constance—lomatium
    Genus *Petroselinum* (5 spp.)
      Species *Petroselinum crispum* (Mill.) Nyman ex A.W. Hill—parsley
    Genus *Pimpinella* (150 spp.)
      Species *Pimpinella anisum* L.—aniseed
Subclass Asteridae (11 orders)
  Order Asterales (1 family)
  Family Asteraceae (Compositae) (1,300–1,540 genera, 20,000–23,000 spp.)
    Genus *Achillea* (200 spp.)
      Species *Achillea millefolium* L.—yarrow
    Genus *Arctium* (5 spp.)
      Species *Arctium lappa* L.—burdock
    Genus *Arnica* (32 spp.)
      Species *Arnica montana* L.—arnica
    Genus Artemisia (400 spp.)
      Species *Artemisia absinthium* L.—wormwood
      Species *Artemisia annua* L.—sweet annie
      Species *Artemisia dracunculus* L.—tarragon
    Genus *Calendula* (30 spp.)
      Species *Calendula officinalis* L.—marigold

Genus *Cnicus* (1 sp.)
  Species *Cnicus benedictus* L.—blessed thistle
Genus *Cynara* (11 spp.)
  Species *Cynara scolymus* L.—globe artichoke
Genus *Echinacea* (3 spp.)
  Species *Echinacea purpurea* (L.) Moench—purple coneflower
Genus Eupatorium (1,200 spp.)
  Species *Eupatorium perfoliatum* L.—boneset
  Species *Eupatorium purpureum* L.—joe pye weed
Genus *Grindelia* (50-60 spp.)
  Species *Grindelia camporum* Greene—asthma weed
Genus *Inula* (200 spp.)
  Species *Inula helenium* L.—elecampane
Genus Lactuca (100 spp.)
  Species *Lactuca virosa* L.—wild lettuce
Genus Matricaria (40 spp.)
  Species *Matricaria recutita* L.—German chamomile
Genus *Silybum* (2 spp.)
  Species *Silybum marianum* L. Gaertn.—milk thistle
Genus *Tanacetum* (60 spp.)
  Species *Tanacetum parthenium* L. Schultz-Bip.— feverfew
  Species *Tanacetum vulgare* L.—tansy
Genus *Taraxacum* (60 spp.)
  Species *Taraxacum officinale* G.H. Weber ex Wigg.—dandelion
Genus *Tussilago* (1 sp.)
  Species *Tussilago farfara* L.—coltsfoot
Order Campanulales (7 families)
 Family Campanulaceae (70–84 genera, 2,000 spp.)
  Genus *Lobelia* L. (300 spp.)
   Species *Lobelia inflata* L.—Indian tobacco
Order Dipsacales (4 families)
 Family Caprifoliaceae (13–15 genera, 450 spp.)
  Genus *Lonicera* (200 spp.)
   Species *Lonicera caprifolium* L.—honeysuckle
  Genus *Sambucus* (40 spp.)
   Species *Sambucus nigra* L.—European elder
  Genus *Viburnum* (200 spp.)
   Species *Viburnum opulus* L.—cramp bark
   Species *Viburnum prunifolium* L.—blackhaw
 Family Valerianaceae (13 genera, 360 spp.)
  Genus *Valeriana* (200 spp.)
   Species *Valeriana officinalis* L.—valerian
Order Gentianales (7 families)
 Family Loganiaceae (20 genera, 500 spp.)
  Genus *Gelsemium* (2 spp.)
   Species *Gelsemium sempervirens* (L.) St.-Hil.— yellow jasmine
 Family Gentianaceae (75–76 genera, 1,000 spp.)
  Genus *Gentiana* (400 spp.)
   Species *Gentiana lutea* L.—yellow gentian
 Family *Apocynaceae* (168–200 genera, 2,000 spp.)
  Genus *Strophanthus* (40 spp.)
   Species *Strophanthus kombe* Oliver—strophanthus
  Genus *Rauvolfia* (100 spp.)
   Species *Rauvolfia serpentina* (L.) Benth. ex Kurz— snakeroot
  Genus *Vinca* (5 spp.)
   Species *Vinca major* L.—periwinkle

Family Asclepiadaceae (315 genera, 2,000 spp.)
  Genus *Asclepias* (120 spp.)
   Species *Asclepias tuberosa* L.—pleurisy root
Order Lamiales (4 families)
 Family Boraginaceae (110–131 genera, 2,400 spp.)
  Genus *Borago* (3 spp.)
   Species *Borago officinalis* L.—borage
  Genus *Pulmonaria* (10 spp.)
   Species *Pulmonaria officinalis* L.—lungwort
  Genus *Symphytum* (25 spp.)
   Species *Symphytum officinale* L.—common comfrey
 Family Verbenaceae (86–100 genera, 2,600 spp.)
  Genus *Verbena* (250 spp.)
   Species *Verbena officinalis* L.—vervain
  Genus *Vitex* (270 spp.)
   Species *Vitex agnus-castus* L.—chasteberry
 Family Lamiaceae (Labiatae) (200–212 genera, 3,200 spp.)
  Genus *Collinsonia* (5 spp.)
   Species *Collinsonia canadensis* L.—stoneroot
  Genus *Lavandula* (28 spp.)
   Species *Lavandula angustifolia* Mill.—English lavender
  Genus *Leonurus* (14 spp.)
   Species *Leonurus cardiaca* L.—motherwort
  Genus Lycopus (4 spp.)
   Species *Lycopus virginicus* L.—bugleweed
  Genus *Marrubium* (40 spp.)
   Species *Marrubium vulgare* L.—horehound
  Genus *Mentha* (25 spp.)
   Species *Mentha x piperita* L.—peppermint
   Species *Mentha pulegium* L.—pennyroyal
   Species *Mentha spicata* L.—spearmint
  Genus *Nepeta* (250 spp.)
   Species *Nepeta cataria* L.—catnip
  Genus *Prunella* (7 spp.)
   Species *Prunella vulgaris* L.—self-heal
  Genus *Rosmarinus* (3 spp.)
   Species *Rosmarinus officinalis* L.—rosemary
  Genus *Scutellaria* (300 spp.)
   Species *Scutellaria lateriflora* L.—blue skullcap
  Genus *Thymus* (300 spp.)
   Species *Thymus vulgaris* L.—garden thyme
Order Plantaginales (1 family)
 Family Plantaginaceae (3 genera, 250 spp.)
  Genus *Plantago* (200+ spp.)
   Species *Plantago major* L.—broadleaf plantain
   Species *Plantago ovata* L.—psyllium seed
Order Rubiales (2 families)
 Family Rubiaceae (450–606 genera, 6,500 spp.)
  Genus *Cephaelis* (100 spp.)
   Species *Cephaelis ipecacuanha* (Brot.) Tussac—ipecac
  Genus *Cinchona* (40 spp.)
   Species *Cinchona officinalis* L.—quinine
  Genus *Coffea* (40 spp.)
   Species *Coffea arabica* L.—Arabian coffee
  Genus *Galium* (400 spp.)
   Species *Galium aparine* L.—cleavers
  Genus *Mitchella* (2 spp.)
   Species *Mitchella repens* L.—partridgeberry

Order Scrophulariales (13 families)
  Family Oleaceae (24–30 genera, 600 spp.)
    Genus *Chionanthus* (3–4 spp.)
      Species *Chionanthus virginicus* L.—fringetree
    Genus *Ligustrum* (50 spp.)
      Species *Ligustrum lucidum* Ait. f.—tree privet
  Family Scrophulariaceae (190–275 genera, 4,000 spp.)
    Genus *Bacopa* (60 spp.)
      Species *Bacopa monnieri* (L.) Pennell—water hyssop
    Genus *Chelone* (5–6 spp.)
      Species *Chelone glabra* L.—balmony
    Genus *Scrophularia* (300 spp.)
      Species *Scrophularia nodosa* L.—figwort
    Genus *Verbascum* (306 spp.)
      Species *Verbascum thapsus* L.—mullein
    Genus *Digitalis* (30 spp.)
      Species *Digitalis purpurea* L.—foxglove
Order Solanales (8 families)
  Family Menyanthaceae (5 genera, 33 spp.)
    Genus *Menyanthes* (1 sp.)
      Species *Menyanthes trifoliata* L.—buckbean, bogbean
  Family Solanaceae (85–96 genera, 2,800 spp.)
    Genus *Atropa* (4 spp.)
      Species *Atropa belladonna* L.—belladonna
    Genus *Capsicum* (50 spp.)
      Species *Capsicum annuum* L.—cayenne pepper
    Genus *Datura* (10 spp.)
      Species *Datura stramonium* L.—jimsonweed
    Genus *Hyoscyamus* (20 spp.)
      Species *Hyoscyamus niger* L.—black henbane
    Genus *Nicotiana* (66 spp.)
      Species *Nicotiana tabacum* L.—tobacco
    Genus *Solanum* (1,700 spp.)
      Species *Solanum dulcamara* L.—bittersweet
    Genus *Withania* (10 spp.)
      Species *Withania somnifera* (L.) Dunal—withania
Subclass Caryophyllidae
Order Caryophyllales (13 families)
  Family Cactaceae (50–150 genera, 1,500–2,000 spp.)
    Genus *Lophophora* (30 spp.)
      Species *Lophophora williamsii* (Lem. ex Salm-Dyck) Coult.—peyote
    Genus *Selenicereus* (25 spp.)
      Species *Selenicereus grandiflorus* (L.) Britt. & Rose— night-blooming cereus
  Family Caryophyllaceae (66–75 genera, 2,000 spp.)
    Genus *Saponaria* (30 spp.)
      Species *Saponaria officinalis* L.—soapwort
    Genus *Stellaria* (120 spp.)
      Species *Stellaria media* (L.) Vill.—chickweed
  Family Chenopodiaceae (100–113 genera, 1,500 spp.)
    Genus *Chenopodium* (150 spp.)
      Species *Chenopodium ambrosioides* L.—wormseed
    Genus *Spinacia* (3–4 spp.)
      Species *Spinacia oleracea* L.—spinach
  Family Phytolaccaceae (15–19 genera, 125 spp.)
    Genus *Phytolacca* L. (35 spp.)
      Species *Phytolacca americana* L.—pokeweed
Order Polygonales (1 family)
  Family Polygonaceae (30–49 genera, 1,000 spp.)
    Genus *Polygonum* (150 spp.)
      Species *Polygonum bistorta* L.—bistort

Genus *Rheum* (50 spp.)
      Species *Rheum officinale* Baill.—rhubarb
      Species *Rheum palmatum* L.—Chinese rhubarb
    Genus *Rumex* (180 spp.)
      Species *Rumex acetosella* L.—sheep sorrel
      Species *Rumex crispus* L.—yellow dock
Subclass Dilleniidae (13 orders)
Order Capparales (5 families)
  Family Brassicaceae (Cruciferae) (350–381 genera, 3,000 spp.)
    Genus *Armoracia* (3 spp.)
      Species *Armoracia rusticana* P.G. Gaertn., B. Mey. & Scherb.—horseradish
    Genus *Capsella* (5 spp.)
      Species *Capsella bursa-pastoris* (L.) Medik.— shepherd's purse
Order Ebenales (5 families)
  Family Styracaceae (10–11genera, 150 spp.)
    Genus *Styrax* (100 spp.)
      Species *Styrax benzoin* Dryand.—styrax
Order Ericales (8 families)
  Family Ericaceae (116–125 genera, 3,500 spp.)
    Genus *Arctostaphylos* (71 spp.)
      Species *Arctostaphylos uva-ursi* (L.) Spreng.— bearberry
    Genus *Gaultheria* (210 spp.)
      Species *Gaultheria procumbens* L.—wintergreen
Order Malvales (5 families)
  Family Malvaceae (100–119 genera, 1,500 spp.)
    Genus *Althaea* (12 spp.)
      Species *Althaea officinalis* L.—marshmallow
  Family Tiliaceae (50–53 genera, 450 spp.)
    Genus *Tilia* (50 spp.)
      Species *Tilia* x *europaea* L.—European linden
  Family Sterculiaceae (65–67 genera, 10,900 spp.)
    Genus *Cola* (110–125 spp.)
      Species *Cola nitida* (Vent.) A. Chev.—kola
    Genus *Theobroma* (30 spp.)
      Species *Theobroma cacao* L.—cacao
Order Nepenthales (2 families)
  Family Droseraceae (4 genera, 103 spp.)
    Genus *Drosera* (100 spp.)
      Species *Drosera rotundifolia* L.—round-leaf sundew
Order Primulales (3 families)
  Family Primulaceae (23–30 genera, 1,000 spp.)
    Genus *Primula* (500 spp.)
      Species *Primula veris* L.—cowslip
Order Salicales (1 family)
  Family Salicaceae (2 genera, 350 spp.)
    Genus *Populus* (35 spp.)
      Species *Populus tremuloides* Michx.—quaking aspen
    Genus *Salix* (300 spp.)
      Species *Salix alba* L.—white willow
Order Theales (18 families)
  Family Clusiaceae (47–50 genera, 1,200 spp.)
    Genus *Garcinia* (200 spp.)
      Species *Garcinia indica* (Thouars) Choisy—garcinia
    Genus *Hypericum* (400 spp.)
      Species *Hypericum perforatum* L.—St. John's wort
  Family Theaceae (40 genera, 600 spp.)
    Genus *Camellia* (82 spp.)
      Species *Camellia sinensis* L.O. Kuntze—tea

Order Violales (24 families)
  Family Violaceae (16–20 genera, 800 spp.)
    Genus *Viola* (500 spp.)
      Species *Viola odorata* L.—sweet violet
      Species *Viola tricolor* L.—heartsease
  Family Turneraceae (8–10 genera, 100 spp.)
    Genus *Turnera* (60 spp.)
      Species *Turnera diffusa* Willd. ex J.A. Schultes—damiana
  Family Passifloraceae (16–17 genera, 650 spp.)
    Genus *Passiflora* (400–500 spp.)
      Species *Passiflora incarnata* L.—passionflower
Subclass Hamamelidae
  Order Hamamelidales (5 families)
    Family Hamamelidaceae (26–29 genera, 100 spp.)
      Genus *Hamamelis* (6 spp.)
        Species *Hamamelis virginiana* L.—witch hazel
  Order Fagales (3 families)
    Family Betulaceae (6 genera, 120–170 spp.)
      Genus *Betula* (60 spp)
        Species *Betula pendula* Roth—white birch
    Family Fagaceae (7 genera, 800–1,000 spp.)
      Genus *Castanea* (12 spp.)
        Species *Castanea sativa* Mill.—sweet chestnut
      Genus *Quercus* (450 spp.)
        Species *Quercus alba* L.—white oak
  Order Juglandales (1 family)
    Family Juglandaceae (8 genera, 60 spp.)
      Genus *Juglans* (20 spp.)
        Species *Juglans cinerea* L.—butternut
  Order Myricales (1 family)
    Family Myricaceae (3 genera, 60 spp.)
      Genus *Myrica* (50 spp.)
        Species *Myrica cerifera* L.—bayberry
  Order Urticales (6 families)
    Family Ulmaceae (15 genera, 150 spp.)
      Genus *Ulmus* (45 spp.)
        Species *Ulmus rubra* Muhl.—slippery elm
    Family Cannabaceae (2 genera, 5 spp.)
      Genus *Cannabis* (3 spp.)
        Species *Cannabis sativa* L.—marijuana
      Genus *Humulus* (2 spp.)
        Species *Humulus lupulus* L.—hops
    Family Urticaceae (45–48 genera, 700–1,000 spp.)
      Genus *Parietaria* (2 spp.)
        Species *Parietaria officinalis* L.—pellitory
      Genus *Urtica* (50 spp.)
        Species *Urtica dioica* L.—stinging nettle
Class Liliopsida—monocotyledons
  Subclass Arecidae (6 families)
    Order Arales (3 families)
      Family Acoraceae (105–110 genera, 1,800–2,450 spp.)
        Genus *Acorus* (2 spp.)
          Species *Acorus calamus* L.—calamus, sweet flag

Order Arecales (1 family)
  Family Arecaceae (Palmae) (200–202 genera, 2,700–3,000 spp.)
    Genus *Areca* (50 spp.)
      Species *Areca catechu* L.—betel palm
    Genus *Serenoa* (1 sp.)
      Species *Serenoa repens* (Bartr.) Small—saw palmetto
Subclass Commelinidae
  Order Cyperales (2 families)
    Family *Poaceae* (Gramineae) (651–657 genera, 10,000 spp.)
      Genus *Avena* (50 spp.)
        Species *Avena sativa* L. oats
      Genus *Zea* (1 sp.)
        Species *Zea mays* L.—cornsilk
Subclass Liliidae
  Order Liliales (15 families)
    Family Liliaceae (270 genera, 4,000 spp.)
      Genus *Aletris* (10 spp.)
        Species *Aletris farinosa* L.—false unicorn root
      Genus *Allium* (450 spp.)
        Species *Allium cepa* L.—garden onion
        Species *Allium sativum* L.—cultivated garlic
      Genus *Colchicum* (65 spp.)
        Species *Colchicum autumnale* L.—autumn crocus
      Genus *Convallaria* (1 sp.)
        Species *Convallaria majalis* L.—lily of the valley
      Genus *Trillium* (30 spp.)
        Species *Trillium erectum* L.—beth root, trillium
    Family Dioscoreaceae (5–9 genera, 620 spp.)
      Genus *Dioscorea* (600 spp.)
        Species *Dioscorea villosa* L.—wild yam
    Family Iridaceae (60–88 genera, 1,500 spp.)
      Genus *Iris* (300 spp.)
        Species *Iris versicolor* L.—blue flag
Subclass Zingiberidae
  Order Zingiberales (8 families)
    Family Zingiberaceae (45–50 genera, 1,000 spp.)
      Genus *Curcuma* (5 spp.)
        Species *Curcuma longa* L.—turmeric
      Genus *Zingiber* (90 spp.)
        Species *Zingiber officinale* Roscoe—ginger

Sources

Greuter, et al., eds. *International Code of Botanical Nomenclature* (Tokyo Code). Regnum Vegetabile No. 131. Konigstein, Germany: Koeltz Scientific Books, 1994.

Stearn, WT. *Botanical Latin*. Newton-Abbot, UK: David & Charles, 1992.

Trehane, et al. *International Code of Nomenclature for Cultivated Plants*. Wimborne, UK: Quarterjack Publishing, 1995.

BIBLIOGRAPHY

History

Griggs B. *Green Pharmacy: The History and Evolution of Western Herbal Medicine*. Rochester, VT: Healing Arts Press, 1997.

Haller JS. *Medical Protestants: The Eclectics in American Medicine*. Carbondale: Southern Illinois University Press, 1994.

Wood M. *The Magic Staff: The Vitalist Tradition in Western Medicine*. Berkeley: North Atlantic Books, 1992.

Eclectic Textbooks

Ellingwood F. *American Materia Medica, Therapeutics & Pharmacognosy*. 1898. Reprint, Sandy, OR: Eclectic Medical Publications, 1983.

Felter and Lloyd. *King's American Dispensatory*, vols. 1 and 2, 1892. Reprint, Sandy, OR: Eclectic Medical Publications, 1983.

Felter, HW. *The Eclectic Materia Medica, Pharmacology & Therapeutics*. 1922. Reprint, Sandy, OR: Eclectic Medical Publications, 1983.

Modern Herbals

Bisset, ed. *Herbal Drugs and Phytopharmaceuticals*. Boca Raton, FL: CRC Press, 1994.

Blumenthal M, et al. *The ABC Clinical Guide to Herbs*. Austin, TX: American Botanical Council, 2003.

Foster S, Hobbs C. *A Field Guide to Western Medicinal Plants and Herbs*. Boston: Houghton Mifflin Co., 2002.

Grieve M. *A Modern Herbal*, vols. I and II, New York: Dover Publications, 1971.

Hobbs C. *Medicinal Mushrooms: An Exploration of Tradition, Healing, and Culture*. Summertown, TN: Botanica Press, 2003.

Lewis WH, Elvin-Lewis M. *Medical Botany*. New York: J. Wiley, 2003.

McCaleb RS, Leigh E, Morien K. *The Encyclopedia of Popular Herbs*. Roseville, CA: Prima Publishing, 2000.

Moore M. *Medicinal Plants of the Desert and Canyon West*. Santa Fe: Museum of New Mexico Press, 1989.

———. *Medicinal Plants of the Mountain West*. Santa Fe: Museum of New Mexico Press, 2003.

———. *Medicinal Plants of the Pacific West*. Santa Fe: Red Crane Books, 1993.

Newall CA, Anderson LA, Phillipson JD. *Herbal Medicines: A Guide for Health-Care Professionals*. London: Pharmaceutical Press, 1996.

Tyler VE. *The Honest Herbal: A Sensible Guide to the Use of Herbs and Related Remedies*. New York: Haworth Herbal Press, 2002.

Wren RC. *Potter's New Cyclopedia of Botanical Drugs and Preparations*, 8th ed. Essex, UK: C. W. Daniel Co., 1988.

Modern Herbal Medicine Making

Green J. *The Herbal Medicine Maker's Handbook: A Home Manual*. Freedom, CA: Crossing Press, 2000.

Hobbs C. *Handmade Herbal Medicines: Recipes for Potions, Elixirs, and Salves*. Loveland, CO: Interweave Press, 1998.

Phytotherapy

Bove M. *An Encyclopedia of Natural Healing for Children and Infants*. Chicago: Keats, 2001.

Brown D. *Herbal Prescriptions for Better Health*. Rocklin, CA: Prima Publishing, 1996.

Gladstar R. *Family Herbal: A Guide to Living Life with Energy, Health, and Vitality*. Pownal, VT: Storey Books, 2001.

———. *Herbal Healing for Women*. New York: Simon & Schuster, 1993.

———. *Rosemary Gladstar's Herbal Remedies for Children's Health*. Pownal, VT: Storey Books, 1999.

Green J. *Male Herbal: Health Care for Men & Boys*. Freedom, CA: Crossing Press, 1991.

Hobbs C. *Natural Therapy for Your Liver: Herbs and Other Natural Remedies for a Healthy Liver*. New York: Avery, 2002.

Hoffmann D. *The Complete Illustrated Holistic Herbal: A Safe and Practical Guide to Making and Using Herbal Remedies*. London: Thorsons, 2001.

———. *An Elder's Herbal*. Rochester, VT: Healing Arts Press, 1993.

———. *Holistic Herbal*. London: Thorsons, 2002.

———. *The Information Sourcebook of Herbal Medicine*. Freedom, CA: Crossing Press, 1994.

———. *Successful Stress Control*. Rochester, VT: Healing Arts Press, 1991.

Hudson T. *Women's Encyclopedia of Natural Medicine*. Los Angeles: Lowell House; Chicago: Contemporary Books, 1999.

Keville K, Green M. *Aromatherapy: A Complete Guide to the Healing Art*. Freedom, CA: Crossing Press, 1995.

Kuhn MA, Winston D. *Herbal Therapy and Supplements: A Scientific and Traditional Approach*. Philadelphia: Lippincott, 2000.

McIntyre A. *The Complete Woman's Herbal: A Manual of Healing Herbs and Nutrition for Personal Well-Being and Family Care*. New York: H. Holt, 1995.

McKenna DJ. *Botanical Medicines: The Desk Reference for Major Herbal Supplements*. New York: Haworth Herbal Press, 2002.

McQuade Crawford A. *The Herbal Menopause Book*. Freedom, CA: The Crossing Press, 1996.

Mills S, Bone K. *Principles and Practice of Phytotherapy: Modern Herbal Medicine*. Edinburgh: Churchill Livingstone, 1999.

Moore M. *Herbs for the Urinary Tract*. New Canaan, CT: Keats Publishing, 1998.

Pizzorno JE, Murray MT. *The Textbook of Natural Medicine*. Edinburgh: Churchill Livingstone, 1999.

Weiss RF. *Herbal Medicine*. Stuttgart; New York: Thieme, 2000.

Winston D. *Saw Palmetto for Men and Women*. Pownal, VT: Storey Books, 1999.

Wood, M. *The Book of Herbal Wisdom: Using Plants as Medicine*. Berkeley: North Atlantic Books, 1997.

Yance DR. *Herbal Medicine, Healing and Cancer*. Los Angeles: Keats Publishing, 1999.

Pharmacognosy

Bruneton J. *Pharmacognosy, Phytochemistry, Medicinal Plants*. Hampshire, UK: Intercept, 1999.

Evans WC. *Trease and Evans' Pharmacognosy*, 13th ed. London: Baillere Tindall, 1989.

Phytochemistry

Cody V, Middleton E, Harborne JB: *Plant Flavonoids in Biology and Medicine*. New York: Liss, 1986.

Colegate S, Molyneux R. *Bioactive Natural Products: Detection, Isolation and Structural Determination*. Boca Raton, FL: CRC Press, 1993.

Glasby JS. *Encyclopaedia of the Terpenoids*. New York: Wiley, 1982.

———. *Encyclopedia of the Alkaloids*. New York: Plenum Publishing, 1983.

Harborne JB. *Introduction to Ecological Biochemistry*. London; San Diego: Academic Press, 1988.

Harborne JB, Baxter H. *Phytochemical Dictionary: A Handbook of Bioactive Compounds from Plants*. London; Washington, DC: Taylor & Francis, 1993.

Harborne JB, Mabry TJ, Mabry H. *The Flavonoids*. London: Chapman & Hall, 1982.

Mann J, Davidson RS, Hobbs JB, et al. *Natural Products: Their Chemistry and Biological Significance*. New York: Wiley, 1994.

Mann J. *Secondary Metabolism*. New York: Oxford University Press, 1987.

Roberts MF, Wink M. *Alkaloids: Biochemistry, Ecology, and Medicinal Applications*. New York: Plenum Press, 1998.

Schultes RE, Hofmann A. *The Botany and Chemistry of Hallucinogens*. Springfield, IL: Charles C. Thomas, 1980.

Wagner H, Bladt S. *Plant Drug Analysis: A Thin Layer Chromatography Atlas*. Berlin; New York: Springer, 1996.

Phytopharmacology

Boik J. *Cancer and Natural Medicine: A Textbook of Basic Science and Clinical Research*. Princeton, MN: Oregon Medical Press, 1996.

Der Marderosian A, Liberti L. *Natural Product Medicine: A Scientific Guide to Foods, Drugs, Cosmetics*. Philadelphia: G. F. Stickley, 1988.

Chu CK, Cutler HG. *Natural Products as Antiviral Agents*. New York: Plenum Press, 1992.

Hartwell JL. *Plants Used Against Cancer: A Survey*. Lawrence, KS: Quarterman Publications, 1984.

Hudson JB. *Antiviral Compounds from Plants*. Boca Raton, FL: CRC Press, 1990.

Mou-Tuan Huang, et al. *Food Phytochemicals for Cancer Prevention*, vols. 1 and 2. Washington, DC: American Chemical Society, 1994.

Williamson EM, Okpako DT, Evans FJ. *Selection, Preparation, and Pharmacological Evaluation of Plant Material*. Chichester; New York: J. Wiley, 1996.

Pharmacopoeias

Blumenthal M, et al. *The Complete German Commission E Monographs: Therapeutic Guide to Herbal Medicines*. Austin, TX: American Botanical Council; Boston: Integrative Medicine Communications, 1998.

Boyle, W. *Official Herbs: Botanical Substances in the United States Pharmacopoeias, 1820–1990*. East Palestine, Ohio: Buckeye Naturopathic Press, 1991.

Bradley, Peter. *British Herbal Compendium*. Bournemouth, UK: British Herbal Medicine Association, 1992.

British Herbal Pharmacopoeia. Bournemouth, UK: British Herbal Medicine Association, 1983.

British Pharmaceutical Codex. London: Pharmaceutical Press, 1911.

British Pharmacopoeia. London: Constable & Co. Ltd., 1932.

United States Pharmacopeia, 11th ed. Easton, PA: The United States Pharmacopoeial Convention, 1936.

Wood HC, Osol A. *The Dispensatory of the United States of America*, 23rd ed. Philadelphia: J. B. Lippincott, 1943.

Phytopharmacy

List PH, Schmidt PC. *Phytopharmaceutical Technology*. Boca Raton, FL: CRC Press, 1989.

Osol A, ed. *Remington's Pharmaceutical Sciences*, 15th ed. Easton, PA: Mack, 1975.

Wijesekera, ed. *The Medicinal Plant Industry*. Boca Raton, FL: CRC Press, 1991.

Toxicology

Brinker F. *Herb Contraindications and Drug Interactions*. Sandy, OR: Eclectic Medical Publications, 2001.

DeSmet P, et al. *Adverse Effects of Herbal Drug*, vols. 1–3. New York: Springer-Verlag, 1992–97.

Harborne JB, et al. *Dictionary of Plant Toxins*. Chichester; New York: J. Wiley, 1996.

McGuffin M, et al. *American Herbal Products Association's Botanical Safety Handbook*. Boca Raton, FL: CRC Press, 1997.

Ethnobotany

Akerele O, Heywood V, Synge H. *Conservation of Medicinal Plants*. New York: Cambridge University Press, 1991.

Akerele O, Kawaguchi Y, eds. *Natural Resources and Human Health—Plants of Medicinal and Nutritional Value: Proceedings of the 1st WHO Symposium on Plants and Health for All*. Amsterdam; New York: Elsevier, 1992.

Balick MJ, Cox PA. *Plants, People, and Culture: The Science of Ethnobotany*. New York: Scientific American Library, 1996.

Balick MJ, Elisabetsky E, Laird SA. *Medicinal Resources of the Tropical Forest: Biodiversity and Its Importance to Human Health*. New York: Columbia University Press, 1996.

Cotton CM. *Ethnobotany: Principles and Applications*. New York: John Wiley & Sons, 1996.

Jones T. *With Bitter Herbs They Shall Eat It: The Origins of Human Diet and Medicine*. Tucson: University of Arizona Press, 1996.

Martin GJ. *Ethnobotany: A Methods Manual*. New York: Chapman & Hall, 1995.

Schultes R, Raffauf R. *The Healing Forest: Medicinal and Toxic Plants of the Northwest Amazonia*. Portland, OR: Dioscorides Press, 1990.

Schultes RE, Hofmann A, Rätsch C. *Plants of the Gods: Their Sacred, Healing, and Hallucinogenic Powers*. Rochester, VT: Healing Arts Press, 2001.

Schultes RE, von Reis S. *Ethnobotany: Evolution of a Discipline*. Portland, OR: Dioscorides Press, 1995.

Walter KS, Gillett HJ, eds. *IUCN Red List of Threatened Plants*. Gland, Switzerland; Cambridge, UK: International Union for Conservation of Nature and Natural Resources, 1998.

INDEX